Clinical Examination

Owen Epstein MBBCh FRCP
Consultant Physician and Gastroenterologist
Clinical Tutor and Director of the Endoscopy Unit
Royal Free Hospital NHS Trust
London, UK

G David Perkin BA MB FRCP
Consultant Neurologist
Charing Cross Hospital and Hillingdon Hospital
London, UK

David P de Bono MA MD FRCP
British Heart Foundation Professor of Cardiology (University of Leicester)
Glenfield General Hospital, Leicester
Honorary Consultant Cardiologist
Groby Road General Hospital
Leicester, UK

John Cookson MD FRCP
Consultant Physician and Clinical Tutor
Department of Respiratory Medicine
Glenfield General Hospital
Leicester, UK

With a contribution by

Neil Solomons MBChB FRCS
Senior Registrar in Otolaryngology
Royal Surrey County Hospital
Guildford, UK

Foreword by

Andrew J Zweifler MD
Professor of Internal Medicine
Director, Clinical Skills Curriculum
University of Michigan, Ann Arbor
USA

Mosby
London St. Louis Baltimore Boston Chicago Philadelphia Sydney Toronto

British Library Cataloging-in-Publication Data:
Epstein, Owen
Clinical Examination
I. Title II. Perkin, David
616.07

ISBN 0-379-44723-X (Hardback)
ISBN 0-7234-1988-4 (Paperback)

Library of Congress Cataloging-in-Publication Data is available on request

First published in 1992 by Gower Medical Publishing
Reprinted in 1993 by Mosby

For full details of Mosby–Year Book titles, please write to Mosby–Year Book Inc., 11830 Westline Industrial Drive, St. Louis, MO 63146, USA.

Originated in Singpore by ChromaGraphics (Overseas) Pte Ltd
Setting & page make-up by Apple Macintosh
Output by Text Unit, London
Text set in Palatino; captions in Helvetica
Produced by Mandarin Offset
Printed and bound in Hong Kong

Project Manager: Alan Rupert Burgess

Designers: Ian Wilberforce Spick III
Jane Antonia Valerie-Brown

Illustration Designer: Marion Tasker

Illustrators: Marion Tasker
Lynda Rosemary Payne
Lee St John Smith
Jenni Ann Miller
Maurice Murphy
Dereck Bart Johnson
Sue Tyler

In-house photographic technician: Tobes Richardson

Paste-up The Hon John William Codling
Alan Wood
Olgun Genghis Hassan
Ruth Natalia Miles

Indexer: Nina Boyd

Production Manager: Susan Elizabeth Bishop

Publisher: Fiona Foley

To June, Daniel and Marc

To Louise, Michael, Emma and Matthew, not forgetting Megan Lloyd George

To Anne, John and Joe

To Anna, Alastair and Fiona

A slide atlas of Clinical Examination based on the contents of this book, is available. In the slide atlas format, the material is split into volumes, each of which is presented in a binder together with numbered 35mm slides of abbreviated slide captions for easy reference when using the slides.

Further information can be obtained from:

Mosby–Year Book Europe Ltd.
Lynton House
7–12 Tavistock Square
London WC1H 9LB
England

FOREWORD

Although physical diagnoses continues to be important in the identification of the cause of illness, dramatic advances in clinical biochemistry, microbiology, immunology and imaging technology in recent years have provided more sensitive indicators to the pretence of many pathological states. Nevertheless, the detection and quantity of physical abnormalities associated with disease continue to be of great importance in clinical medicine. In primary care, the presence or absence of physical findings in symptomatic patients is still critical to decisions related to the further workup of these individuals. In speciality practice, change in physical abnormalities during the treatment of patients with established disease is frequently of major importance in determining adjustments in the therapeutic regimen. The ability to perform an accurate physical examination remains an essential competence for health care practitioners.

Physical diagnosis is a technical skill and as such it can only be learned through practice, but written guidance is essential to mastery of this discipline. A good textbook is one which recognizes the importance of both normality and abnormality in the study of this subject. Appreciation of the normal on physical examination is rooted in comprehension of the wide range of physique and physiology among healthy individuals. The authors of *Clinical Examination* were well aware of this point and have produced a text which acknowledges it explicitly. Each chapter begins with a section on "structure and function", in all case illustrated by excellent tables and figures. Anatomy and up-to-date physiology are accurately depicted in numerous simple and colourful drawings. In each chapter this initial section is followed by one on the technique of examination, again accompanied by very helpful photographs and line-drawings. When more than one method may be useful, the different techniques available for carrying out a particular regional examination are described and illustrated.

The goal of physical diagnosis is detection of abnormalities associated with disease. Although this requires mastery of the sequence and techniques of the physical examination and an appreciation of normal bodily structure and function, it also requires knowledge of the physical abnormalities produced by diseases. In its description of common physical abnormalities and methods for eliciting pathological functioning, *Clinical Examination* excels. Choice photographic illustrations of patients with abnormal findings abound in its pages as well as useful figures and summary tables related to the clinical expression of common clinical conditions.

The entire book is very well done, but some chapters deserve special mention: Chapter 1 on the medical record is lucid and especially welcome because of its focus on the problem-oriented medical record; Chapter 4 on the skin excels because of its vivid colour photographs of dermatologic lesions; Chapter 6 on the respiratory system is distinguished by its excellent illustrative chest roentgenograms and CT scans; while chapter 12 on the nervous system, is truly remarkable with its profusely illustrated and lucid coverage of this major position of the physical examination. All in all *Clinical Examination* is a vigorous, and uniquely colourful, entrant in the field of physical diagnosis texts. Few other texts can compare to it on the basis of number and quality of illustrations and therefore it is likely to become the standard reference in its field. Both medical and nursing students will find this to be a valuable resource, and while it will be of greatest value to the novice, it would be a useful addition to the library of experienced clinicians as well.

Andrew J Zweifler MD
Professor of Internal Medicine
Director, Clinical Skills Curriculum
University of Michigan
October 1991

PREFACE

The techniques and skills required for a competent clinical examination can only be mastered by practice at the bedside. However, a thorough and intelligent clinical examination relies heavily on an understanding of normal and abnormal anatomy and physiology as well as "pattern recognition" of disease. *Clinical Examination* has been written as a companion for medical students and postgraduates acquiring or revising clinical skills. The book guides the user through the anatomy and physiology of each system and builds on this information to describe the normal and abnormal examination.

Examining patients draws on the senses of sight (inspection), touch (palpation) and hearing (percussion and auscultation). The text is complemented by almost 1,000 coloured figures, clinical photographs, tables and question boxes. A slide atlas of the figures is available and this unique collection should be of great value to clinical teachers.

The first chapter in the book illustrates the problem orientated approach to case notes and record-keeping and emphasises the centrality of good note taking and record keeping in patient management. This chapter is followed by a general introduction to history-taking with more detailed elements of the history incorporated into the chapters dealing with individual systems. Chapter 3 deals with the general physical examination, focusing information (appearance, nutritional, status, hydration and temperature), syndrome recognition, and deals with those systems which do not fall neatly into the regional examination (endocrine and lymphatic systems). The clinical characteristics of most of the common skin, hair and nail disorders, an area of medicine which is notoriously badly assessed by students and doctors, are described in Chapter 4, followed by chapters on regional examination including the ears, nose and throat, cardiovascular system, chest and lungs, abdomen, male and female genitalia, the musculo-skeletal system and the nervous system. These chapters are introduced by a description of anatomy and physiology (structure and function), the history and the normal and abnormal examination. Aspects of the clinical history are highlighted in question boxes which summarize a series of questions asked in response to a patient's symptoms. Wherever possible, the description of the physical examination is accompanied by artwork and clinical photographs to illustrate the examination technique.

The book deals only with the clinical examination of the adult. Neonatal and paediatric examination is a specialized skill with considerable variation from the adult in anatomy, physiology and pathology. However, many of the principles outlined in this book are applicable across all age groups and the book may be used as a companion to be read alongside specialists texts.

It is well to remember that most medical problems can be solved by a careful history and examination. This book is a rich "multimedia" resource to help learn and teach these clinical skills.

ACKNOWLEDGEMENTS

We wish to thank the following individuals and organizations for generously providing illustrative material: Dr Philip Bardsley, Dr Russell Lane, Dr Mike Morgan, Dr P H McKee, and Dr John Wales; Joan Slack, Dept of Clinical Genetics, Royal Free NHS Trust (Figs 3.5, 3.7, 3.9, 3.11, 3.12, 3.16–3,18, 3.20, 3.22, 3.24–3.26); Dr Les Berger, Dept of Radiology, Royal Free NHS Trust (Figs 3.51, 3.52, 8.17a); Dr Malcolm Rustin (Figs 4.13, 4.16, 4.26–4.29, 4.33, 4.34, 4.73–4.75); King's College Hospital (Figs 4.14, 4.15, 4.18, 4.39, 4.40, 4.42–4.46, 4.48–4.50, 4.57, 4.68, 4.76, 4.77) for slides reproduced from Anthony du Vivier: *Atlas of Clinical Dermatology* (Gower Medical Publishing UK,, 1986); Dame Margaret Turner-Warwick *et al* (Figs 6.2, 6.9–6.12, 6.16, 6.36, 6.49) for slides reproduced from *Clinical Atlas Respiratory Diseases* (Gower Medical Publishing UK, 1989); Professor Robert H Anderson and Dr Sally P Allwork (Figs 7.4, 7.6, 7.7) for slides reproduced from *Cardiac Anatomy* (Gower Medical Publishing UK, 1980); Dr James S Bingham (Figs 9.37, 9.45–9.48, 10.19, 10.20, 10.34) for slides reproduced from *Sexually Transmitted Diseases* (Gower Medical Publishing UK, 1984); Dr Paul A Dieppe *et al* (Figs 11.25–11.27, 11.43, 11.44, 11.52, 11.53, 11.56, 11.57, 11.62–11.64, 11.74, 11.76, 11.80, 11.83, 11.86–11.89, 11.96, 11.97) for slides reproduced from *Atlas of Clinical Rheumatology* (Gower Medical Publishing UK, 1986); Mr David Spalton *et al* (Figs 12.23, 12.31–12.33, 12.35, 12.36, 12.38–12.47, 12.62, 12.75, 12.79, 12.80) *Atlas of Clinical Ophthalmology* (Gower Medical Publishing UK, 1984).

The figures listed below were derived with permission from the following sources: Figs 12.7 and 12.14 from R B Strub and F William Black: *The Mental Status Examination in Neurology* (F A Davis Co); Figs 12.19–12.21, 12.23–12.25, 12.31–12.33, 12.36–12.53, 12.58, 12.59, 12.62, 12.71, 12.75, 12.77–12.80, 12.86) from David Spalton: *Atlas of Clinical Ophthalmology* (Gower Medical Publishing UK, 1984); Figs. 12.49 (right), 12.87, 12.99 from Haymaker, Webb: *Bing's Local Diagnosis in Neurological Diseases*, 15th ed, (St Louis, The C V Mosby Co, 1989); Figs 12.54 and 12.55 from J S Glaser: *Neuro-ophthalmology* (Harper & Row); Figs 12.56 and 12.57 from R John Leigh and David S Zee: *The Neurology of Eye Movement* (F A Davis Co); Figs 12.113, 12.133, 12.169 from Drs J W Lance and J G McLeod: *A Physiological Approach to Clinical Neurology* (Butterworths); Figs 12.117, 12.129, 12.170, 12.174 from Lord Walton of Detchant: *Introduction to Clinical Neuroscience* 2nd ed, (Balliere Tindall Ltd); Fig. 12.122 from Professor R S Snell: *Clinical Neuroanatomy for Medical Students* 2nd ed, (Little Brown & Co); Figs 12.131 and 12.132 from Dr V B Brooks: *Neural Basis of Motor Control* (Oxford University Press); Figs 12.152, 12.158, 12.159 from A K Ashbury *et al*: *Diseases of the Nervous System* (W B Saunders); Fig.12.160 from Drs L R Caplan and R W Stein: *Stroke a Clinical Approach* (Butterworths); Fig. 12.171 from "Somaesthetic Pathways" Br Med Bull, **33**, 113–120, 1977; Fig. 12.172 from Dr A G Brown: "Subcortical Mechanisms Concerned in Somatic Sensation" Br Med Bull, **33**, 121–128, 1977; Fig. 12.182 from Sir G Holmes: *An Introduction to Clinical Neurology* 3rd ed, (Edinburgh: E & S Livingstone, 1968); Fig. 12.185 from Professor Ian A D Bouchier, CBE, and J S Morris: *Clinical Skills* 2nd ed, (W B Saunders); Fig. 12.197, 12.199, 12.200 from Dr F Plum: *Diagnosis of Stupor and Coma* 3rd ed, (F A Davis Co).

We are indeed grateful to the following for their secretarial help, often at short notice: Fiona Legate and Rachel Hayto, Beryl Laatz, June Hegarty, and Jennifer Kerry

Finally, we are especially indebted to Fiona Foley, UK Managing Director of Gower Medical Publishing, to whom the original idea for a highly illustrated text on clinical examination rightly belongs, to Alan Burgess for his persistence and unflagging enthusiasm, to Marion Tasker for her excellent illustrations which were created from 'stick men' and our best artistic efforts, and to Ian Spick and Jane Brown for the imaginative and concise design.

OE, GDP, DPdB, JC
London and Leicester
May 1992

CONTENTS

THE MEDICAL RECORD

1

Before setting out to learn about clinical examination, it is important to know how to write up a full medical record. Almost every encounter between doctor (or student) and patient involves recording information. The initial record will include a detailed history and examination as well as plans for investigation and treatment. Whenever the results of investigations become available, this new information is added to the record and at each follow-up visit, progress and change in management is recorded.

The medical record chronicles the patient's medical history from the first illness through to death. Over a lifetime, patients present with distinct episodes of acute disease or chronic, intractable, or progressive conditions. At each presentation, the emphasis of diagnosis and treatment is focused on the isolated episode and little consideration is given to less pressing problems unless they have an obvious bearing on the main complaint. A number of different doctors and health-care professionals may contribute to the medical record over a period of hours, days, months, years, and even decades. In addition, this multi-author document may follow the patient whenever they move home.

There is a heavy responsibility on the author of each medical entry to recognize the historical importance of each record and to ensure that the entry conveys a clear and accurate account which can be easily accessed by others.

The medical record has other uses: it is the prime resource used in medical audit, a practice widely adopted in the quest for quality control in the medical practice. In addition, the record provides much of the evidence used in medico-legal practice. At some time or other, you will probably have to either appear in court or provide an affadavit in connection with a patient whom you have treated. It is imperative the medical record fully documents the assessment and treatment of the patient, for it is somewhat unlikely that you will remember the details of the patient's complaint or injuries months or even years later. If much of your time is spent working in a busy casualty/emergency room, you may not even recollect treating the patient. When under judicial examination your professional credibility, if your memory fails, relies solely on the medical record you wrote.

As medical care becomes more specialized and complex and increasingly dependent on teamwork, it has become necessary to standardize the approach to clinical note-keeping. Problem orientated medical records (POMR) has emerged as a widely accepted framework designed to standardize the structure and enhance the quality of medical records. The system encourages a logical approach to diagnosis and management, and addresses the problem of maintaining order in the multi-disciplinary, highly specialized practice of modern medical care. This chapter describes the problem orientated approach to medical records first advocated in 1969 by Lawrence Weed. There are critics of POMR and you may be taught around different frameworks. However, most systems overlap with POMR and a basic understanding of this approach will provide you with a useful benchmark to compare with other systems.

THE PROBLEM ORIENTATED MEDICAL RECORD

The accuracy of information gathered from a patient during the course of an illness influences the precision of diagnosis and treatment. POMR stresses the need to gather all the information (demographic, personal, symptoms and signs and special tests) and to use this 'database' to constuct a list of problems. This problem list provides a summary of the 'whole' patient and offers a resource for planning management. The problem list encourages you to look for relationships between problems and develop an integrated overview of the patient; moreover, it distinguishes problems needing active management from those which may only be of historical significance. The list does not provide a perspective of the relative importance of each problem; this draws on the skill of clinical judgment. The database and problem list evolve through the course of an illness and change with subsequent presentations.

In addition to the problem list, POMR provides a framework for standardizing the structure of follow-up notes (Fig. 1.1). This element stresses changes in the patient's symptoms and signs and the evolution of the clinical assessment and management plans. The final element of the POMR structure is the flow sheet which is designed to record sequential changes in clinical and biochemical measurements.

Extracting information from notes for research purposes is notoriously difficult and unreliable. The rigorous structure of POMR and the discipline it imposes can make a considerable contribution to research which relies on retrospective data collection.

THE HISTORY

For generations, there has been little change in the method of recording information from the history. The interview is the focal point of the 'doctor-patient' relationship and establishes the bonding necessary for the patient's care (see Chapter 2). The history guides the patient through a series of questions designed to build a profile of the individual and their problems. The order of the history should be clearly indicated with appropriate headings. By the end of the first interview you should have a good grasp of the patient's personality, social habits, and clinical problems. Additionally, you will have considered a differential diagnosis which might explain the patient's symptoms.

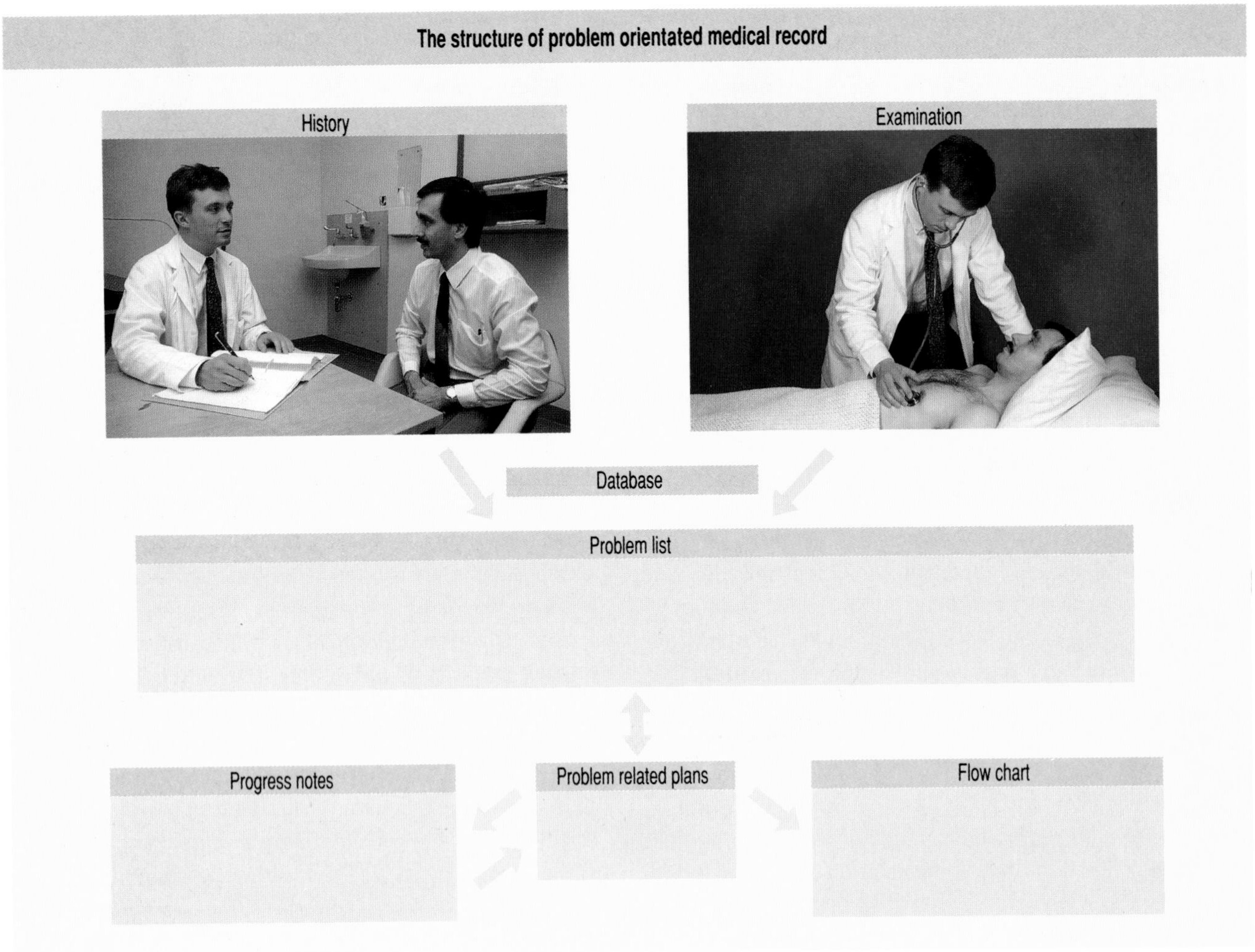

Fig. 1.1 Diagramatic representation of the structure of POMR.

The medical history ranges over a spectrum of questions ranging from the presenting complaint to the social history, education, employment history, personal habits, travel, home circumstances, family history and review of the major systems. It is easy to churn through this series of questions, neglecting the reason for asking each question. The POMR model encourages ordered, logical history-taking and emphasizes that this information should be easily accessible from the notes.

When trying to analyze a patient's symptoms, order the questions to answer four key questions: From where does the symptom arise? What is the likely cause? Are there any predisposing or risk factors? Are there any complications? These focused questions will help you to maintain an economical flow of questions and to write an intelligible transcript in the notes. This series of structured questions can also be applied to any symptoms complained of by the patient.

A new history and examination is recorded in the notes whenever a patient presents with a fresh problem. Some information remains unchanged over long periods (past history, psycho-social and family history, education, and occupation). If this has been accurately recorded at the time of the first presentation there is no need to re-enter unless there has been change.

Doctors often blame their illegible handwriting on all the writing entailed in the systems review. You might well question the purpose of asking a lengthy series of routine questions when all you expect (and usually get) from the patient is a series of negative monosyllabic responses. Remember that at some time in the future, the systems review might provide an important source of information not only for you but also for your colleagues. A patient admitted to hospital with intense pain, altered consciousness, or severe breathlessness may be unable to provide a history. In these circumstances, a detailed systematic history recorded sometime in the past might provide crucial information. A routine systems enquiry also prompt your patient to remember events or illnesses which might othewise have been forgotten.

THE EXAMINATION

Like the history, the format of the clinical examination has remained unchanged for generations. The examination may confirm or refute a diagnosis suspected from the history and by adding this information to the database you will be able to construct a more accurate problem list. Like the history, the examination is structured to record both positive and negative findings in

Initial problem list

Patient's name : **Hospital No :**

No	active problems	date	inactive problems	date
1	jaundice (Jan'91)	9/1/91		
2	anorexia (Dec '91)	9/1/91		
3	weight loss	9/1/91		
4	recurrent rectal bleeding	9/1/91		
5	smoking (since 1964)	9/1/91		
6	unemployed (Nov '90)	9/1/91		
7	stutter	9/1/91		
8			duodenal ulcer (1960)	9/1/91

Fig. 1.2 Problem list entered on 9th January 1991.

detail. Remember that the record of negative findings might be an important reference point at some stage in the future. For example, if on examination of the abdomen you detect an enlarged liver, it is helpful to read from the notes that a year previously 'a liver edge was not palpable'.

THE PROBLEM LIST

The problem list lies at the heart of POMR. The entries provide a summary and historical record of all the patient's important health-related problems. The master problem list is placed in the front of the medical record and each entry is dated (Fig. 1.2). This date refers to the date of the entry, not the date when the patient first noted the problem (this can be indicated in brackets alongside the problem). The dates entered into the problem list provides not only a chronology of the patient's health-related problems but also a 'table of contents' which serves the medical record. Using the entry date as a reference and assuming that each entry in the clinical record is dated, there should be no difficulty finding the original entry in the notes. In addition to providing a summary and index, the problem list also assists the development of management plans.

Setting up the problem list

Once the history and examination is complete, glance through your notes and decide which problems should be entered into the problem list. Divide the problems into those which are active (or require action) and those which are inactive (problems which have resolved or require no action, but may be important at some stage in the patient's present or future management). An entry of 'Peptic ulcer (1971)' in the 'inactive' column will provide a reminder to someone considering the use of a non-steroidal anti-inflammatory drug in a patient presenting 20 years later with arthritis. The problem list is dynamic and the page is designed to allow you to shift problems from the active to inactive columns and vice versa (Fig. 1.3).

Your entries into the problem list may include established diagnoses (e.g. ulcerative colitis), symptoms (e.g. dyspnoea), physical signs (e.g. ejection systolic murmur), laboratory tests (e.g. anaemia), psychological and social history (e.g. depression, unemployment, parental/marital problems) or special risk factors (e.g. smoking, alcohol/narcotic abuse). The diagnostic level at which you make the entry depends on the information available at a particular moment in time. Express the problem at the highest level possible but update the list if new findings alter or refine your understanding of the problem. The problem list is designed to accommodate change; consequently, it is not necessary to delete an entry once a higher level of diagnosis (or understanding) is reached. For example, a patient may present with the problems of jaundice, anorexia, and weight loss. This information will be entered into the problem list (see Fig. 1.2). If, a few days later, serological investigation confirms that the patient was suffering from type A viral hepatitis, this new level of diagnosis can be entered on a new line in the block reserved for active problem 1 (see Fig. 1.3). Other problems explained by the diagnosis (anorexia and weight loss) should be amended with an arrow and asterisk to indicate the connection with the solved problem. At this point, viral hepatitis represents the highest level of diagnosis, so the date of this entry should allow anyone reviewing the notes to turn to the page in the medical record where the evidence for the final diagnosis was first recorded. Once the disease has resolved, an arrow to the opposite 'inactive' column will indicate the point during follow up that the doctor noted return of the liver tests to normal (see Fig. 1.3). Unexpected problems may become evident in the course of investigation (e.g. hypercholesterolaemia) and these are added to the problem list.

Some diseases have many symptoms and signs, so judgment is required when deciding which problems should be added to the list. In general, it is reasonable to omit problems which have little importance in investigations or treatment. If you feel that extra information obtained over 24–48 hours might help consolidate a more accurate entry into the master problem list, you might then consider delaying that entry for a day or two. The problem list should be under constant review to ensure that the entries are accurate and up to date. This review can be undertaken once a week during the major ward round.

Updated problem list

Patient's name :   Hospital No :

No	active problems	date	inactive problems	date
1	jaundice (Jan'91)	9/1/91		
	→ type A hepatitis	13/1/91	→ resolved	14/2/91
2	anorexia (Dec '91)	9/1/91		
	→ *1			
3	weight loss	9/1/91		
	→ *1			
4	recurrent rectal bleeding	9/1/91		
	→ haemorrhoids	13/1/91	haemorrhoid banding	1/2 /91
5	smoking (since 1964)	9/1/91		
6	unemployed (Nov '90)	9/1/91		
7	stutter	9/1/91		
8			duodenal ulcer (1960)	9/1/91
9	hypercholesterolaemia			
		13/1/91		

Fig. 1.3 Problem list updated to 14th February indicating the diagnosis of hepatitis A on the 13th January and return of liver tests to normal by the 14th February. The anorexia and weight loss are readily explained by the hepatitis and these problems are arrowed to indicated the relationship to problem 1 (hepatitis). Note, the haemorrhoids were diagnosed on 13th January and this problem became 'inactive' when banding was performed on 1st February. When the biochemical tests were returned on 13th January, hypercholesterolaemia was diagnosed for the first time and this was entered into the problem list on the same day. On 14th February three unresolved problems remained.

INITIAL PROBLEM-RELATED PLANS

POMR offers a structured approach to the management of patients' problems. By constructing the problem list you will have clearly defined those problems requiring active management (i.e. investigation and treatment), so it should be reasonably easy to develop a plan (Fig. 1.4) for each problem by considering four headings (see below). All or only some of these headings may be applicable to a particular problem.

Problem related plans

	Problem	Differential Diagnosis	Investigation
Dx	jaundice		liver tests, prothrombin time
		acute hepatitis	hepatitis screen (A,B, & C)
			auto-antibodies (SMA,ANA,AMA)
		alcohol	mean cell volume gamma GT
		drugs	check with family doctor
		obstructive jaundice	ultrasound liver
	anorexia	see jaundice	urea & electrolytes
	weight loss	see jaundice	basal weight
	recurrent rectal bleeding	haemorrhoids	full blood count
		polyp/colon cancer	proctoscopy
			colonoscopy/barium enema
	smoking		chest X-ray

	Problem	Monitor
Mx	jaundice	twice weekly liver tests
	anorexia	monitor diet and caloric intake (ask dietician)
	weight loss	twice weekly weight
	recurrent rectal bleeding	check haemoglobin weekly

	Problem	Treatment
Rx	jaundice	bed-rest
	anorexia	encourage caloric intake (favourite foods)
	weight loss	special high caloric drink supplements
	recurrent rectal bleeding	treat cause
		(haemorrhoids/tumor) seek surgical opinion
	smoking	encourage relaxation/stress management
	unemployed	arrange meeting with social worker

	Problem	Education
Ed	jaundice	discuss differential diagnosis
	anorexia	explain association with jaundice
	smoking	discuss dangers, techniques for coping
	rectal bleeding	explain need for colonic investigation

Fig. 1.4 An example of a problem related plan following the creation of the problem list.

Dx – diagnostic tests
Mx – monitoring tests
Rx – treatments
Ed – education

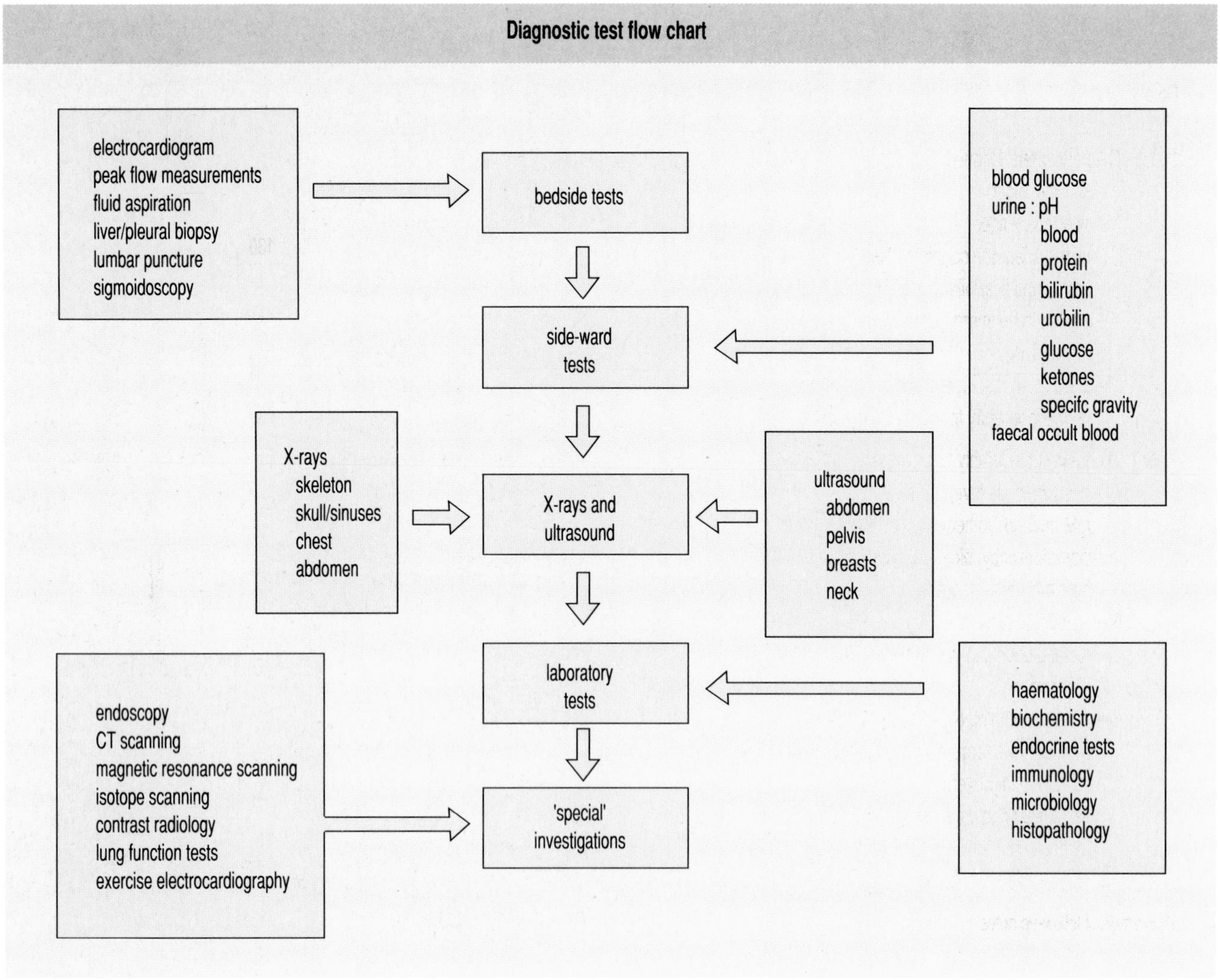

Fig. 1.5 A flow diagram to help plan diagnostic tests.

Diagnostic tests (Dx)

The choice of diagnostic tests will be guided by the differential diagnosis of the problem. Write differential next to each problem. Adjacent to each of the possible diagnoses, enter the investigation which might aid diagnosis. There are a large number of special tests which might be applicable to a particular problem; therefore, it is useful to evolve a general framework for investigation and to adapt this to each problem. You can construct a logical flow of investigations by considering bed-side tests, side-ward tests, plain X-rays, ultrasound, blood tests, and specialized imaging examinations (Fig. 1.5).

Monitoring tests (Mx)

Monitoring information may be necessary to provide evidence of the patient's progress. Consider whether a particular problem can be monitored; if so, document the appropriate tests and the frequency with which they should be performed so as to provide meaningful information.

Treatments (Rx)

Consider each problem in turn with a view to deciding whether active treatment is necessary. 'Treatment' includes drugs, radiotherapy, surgery, physiotherapy, occupational therapy, and psychotherapy. If drug treatment is indicated, note the drug and dosage. Include a plan for monitoring both side-effects and the effectiveness of treatment if you anticipate drug-related side effects.

Education (Ed)

An important component of your patient's treatment is education. Patient's are better able to cope with their illness if they understand its nature, its likely course, and the effect of treatment. By including this heading in your plans, you will be reminded of the need to talk to your patient about their illness and encouraged to develop an educational plan for your overall management strategy.

Progress notes

Date

11/1/91 S – nauseated, fatigued
O – less jaundiced
liver less tender
taking adequate calories & fluid
ultrasound liver/biliary tract: normal
A – seems to be improving
no obstruction
P – check liver tests tomorrow
phone laboratory for hepatitis markers

13/1/91 S – feels considerably better, appetite improving
O – transaminase levels & bilirubin falling
IgM antibody to hepatitis A positive
sigmoidoscopy: bleeding haemorrhoids
hypercholesterolaemia
A – resolving hepatitis A
rectal bleeding in young patient likely to be due to haemorrhoids
P – reassess patient, explain 'hepatitis A'
consider discharge if next set of liver tests show sustained improvement
ask surgeon to consider treating haemorrhoids
recheck cholesterol in 3 months

Fig. 1.6 Example of follow-up notes.

Flow sheet

Tests \ Date	9.1.91	11.1.91	13.1.91	14.1.91	7.2.91	14.12.91
Bilirubin (<17)	233	190	130		28	10
AST (<40)	1140	830	500		52	23
ALT (<45)	1600	650	491		61	31
Albumin (35 – 45)	41	40	41	discharged	42	43
Pro-time (seconds)	14/12	14/12	13/12		13/12	12/12
Haemoglobin (11.5 – 16.2)	12.1	12.3	12.1		12.2	12.6
Blood urea (3.5 – 6.5)	3.1	4.2	4.8		6.0	6.2
Blood glucose (3.5 – 6.5)	5.5	6.8	5.0		5.6	6.0
Hepatis screen			IgM Hep A +ve			
Cholesterol (3.5-6.8)			8.1			8.4

Fig. 1.7 Example of a flow sheet.

Progress notes

Progress is often poorly documented in the medical record; conversely, POMR provides a disciplined and standardized structure to the follow-up note. Follow-up notes should be succinct and brief, focusing mainly on change. There are four headings to guide you through the progress note (Fig. 1.6):

Subjective (S)

Record any change in the patient's symptoms and when necessary, comment on compliance with a particular regimen (e.g. stopping smoking) or tolerance of drug treatment.

Objective (O)

Record any change in physical signs and investigations which might influence diagnosis, monitoring, or treatment.

Assessment (A)

Comment on whether the subjective and objective information have confirmed or altered your assessment and plans.

Plan (P)

After making the assessment, consider whether any modification of the original plan is needed. Structure this section according to the headings listed earlier (Dx, Mx, Rx, Ed).

If there is no subjective or objective change from one visit to the next, simply record 'No change in assessment or plans'.

Flow charts

Clinical investigations and measurements are often repeated to monitor the course of acute or chronic illness. For example, patients presenting with diabetic ketoacidosis require frequent checks of blood suger, urea, electrolytes, blood pH, urine output, and central venous pressure. In chronic renal failure, the course of the disease and its treatment is monitored by repeating measurements of blood urea and electrolytes, creatinine, creatinine clearance, haemoglobin, and body weight. A flow sheet is convenient for recording this data in a format which, at a glance, provides a summary of trends and progress (Fig. 1.7). Graphs may be equally revealing (Fig. 1.8) although a single graph showing the flow of two or more different tests may be confusing. Case-notes become bulky when numerous

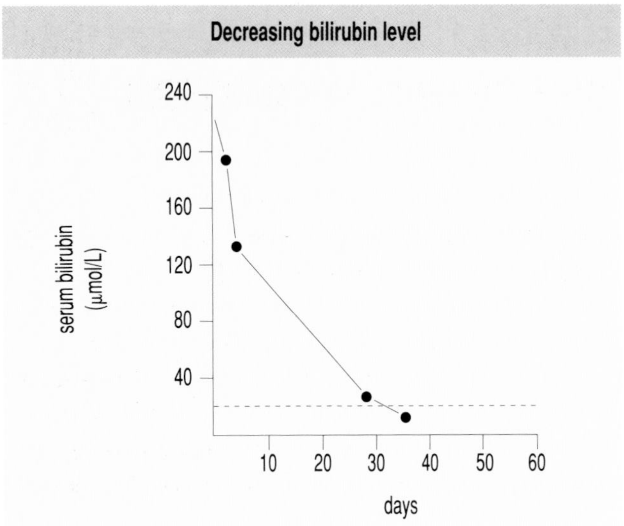

Fig. 1.8 Example of the use of a graph to illustrate change in bilirubin following acute type A hepatitis.

laboratory reports are filed. This is avoided if a flow sheet is maintained in the main medical record and the individual reports sent from the laboratory are stored in a subsidiary file.

Advantages of POMR

POMR encourages all the members of the healthcare team to standardize their approach to record-keeping. This, in turn, enhances communication and guarantees that all those involved in the patient's care can contribute to the medical biography. Furthermore, careful structuring of the problem list, care plans, and follow-up notes encourages logical, disciplined thinking and ensures that the record is not only comprehensive but accurate. The POMR approach to record keeping counteracts the tendency for the 'weight' of a single problem to overwhelm and to distract from other subsidiary but potentially important problems.

Peer review and medical audit have become an integral part of quality assurance and continuing medical education. The structure of POMR exposes the clinician's thoughts and decision-making processes. This, in itself, is educational both for the clinician and anyone else reading the notes and makes the system particularly suited to the process of medical audit. The pressure to record meticulous and detailed information is also of intrinsic value to research workers embarking on retrospective or prospective clinical studies. Perhaps most important, POMR helps us maintain a perspective of the 'whole' patient, thereby providing an overview of physical, psychological, and social problems and their interaction in health and disease.

CONFIDENTIALITY

Clinical notes contain confidential information and it is of vital importance that you protect this confidentiality. Ensure that there is control over access to the medical record and only those directly involved in the patient's care should read, or write in the notes. In certain circumstances special security may be necessary. Patients with HIV infection and AIDS and those attending venereology or psychiatric clinics may have a separate set of clinical notes which are maintained as distinct from the general medical records. Access to these classified records is usually restricted to those doctors working in that department and the notes never leave the area of the specialist unit.

Armed with these guidelines on keeping well-constructed notes you should be ready to set off on the adventure of clinical examination described in detail in the following chapters.

2 INTERVIEWING TECHNIQUES AND HISTORY-TAKING

It would be unwise for the student to assume that, with the advent of increasingly sophisticated investigative techniques, history-taking becomes of lesser value. Surveys suggest that over 80 per cent of diagnoses in a general medical clinic are based on the interview. It is clear that the way in which the interview is conducted, and what questions are asked, determine the amount of diagnostically useful information which the patient is prepared to reveal.

For many patients, particularly those seen in the out-patient clinic, the process of history-taking is liable to take longer than the physical examination.Your first step should be to read the referral letter. Sometimes the information provided is inadequate and barely legible (Fig. 2.1). Often, however you will find a wealth of clinical detail (Fig. 2.2) relating to the past history which the patient has either forgotten or chosen not to reveal. During the interview, you will be using a combination of open-and close-ended questions. The former deal in generalizations: how are you? how are you feeling? The latter require a more specific response: do you experience chest pain when you exercise? A history confined to close-ended

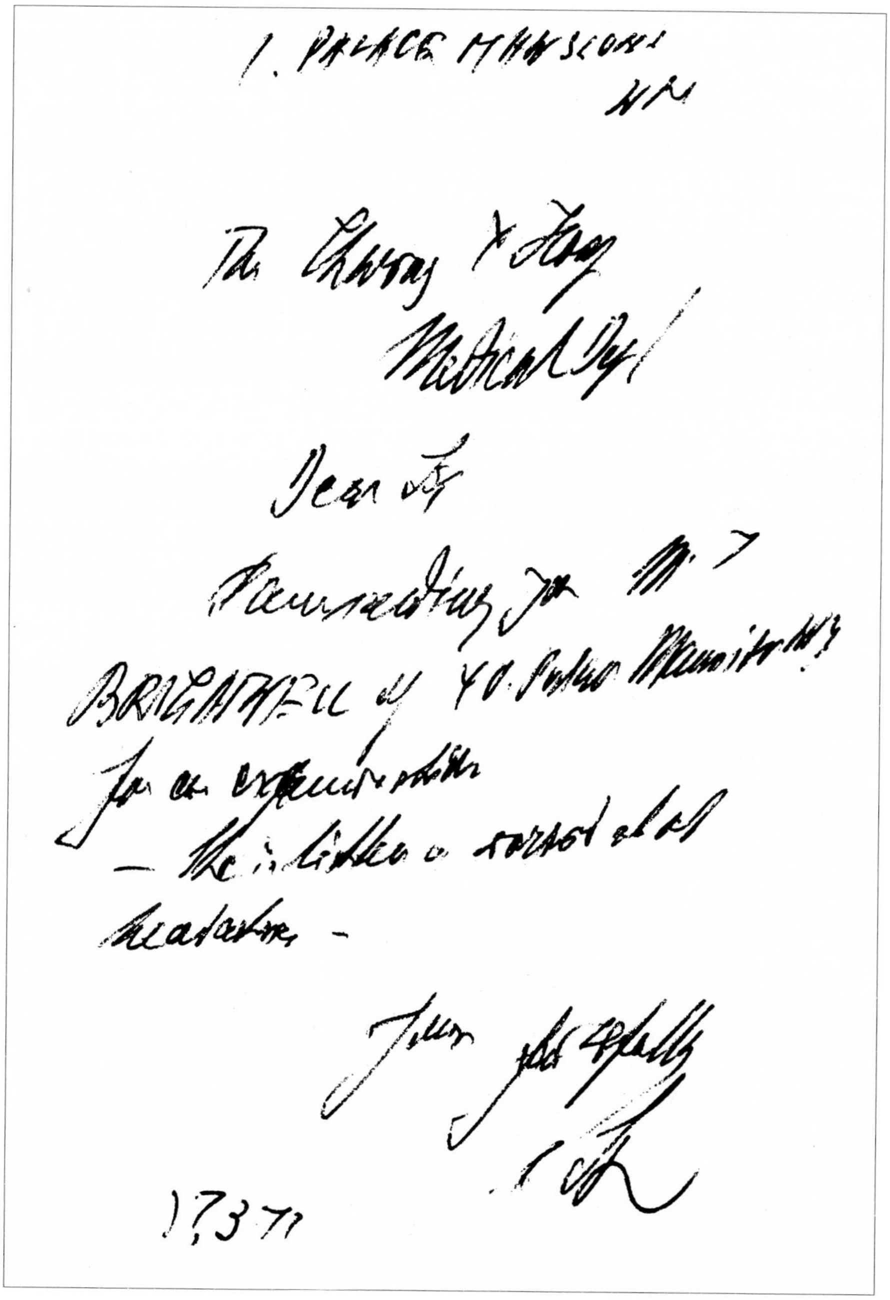

Fig. 2.1 A less than satisfactory referral letter. The writing is virtually illegible and the clinical information is inadequate.

questions will be quickly completed but will be denuded of any personal element. Taken to its extreme, the patient would simply need to answer yes or no to a succession of questions. Open-ended questions allow the patient far more freedom to respond, but therein lies the danger of their use. A history confined to such questions would occupy hours for some patients as they meander through a great deal of irrelevant material. As you learn to structure history-taking, a balance between these two types of question will emerge. Generally you will start with open-ended questions, then gradually introduce close-ended questions if certain aspects of the history remain unclear.

Both students and doctors tend to overlook the psychiatric component of a physical illness, or fail to recognize that bodily complaints can reflect a primary psychiatric disorder. The way in which the patient conducts himself during the interview, whether submissively or aggressively, can tell a great deal about the underlying problem.

Before considering the formal stages of history-taking, how can the interview be planned so that as much information as possible is forthcoming?

THE INTERVIEW

Setting

Most of the patients you interview will be on the ward rather than in the out-patient department. The noise and interruption of a busy

17 April 1992

[Consultant neurologist's name
Address
Address]
London

Dear Sir,

Re: [Patient's name, date of birth: 1 September 1951, and address]

I would be grateful if you could see this obsessive epileptic gentleman. His main problems at present are increasing, what he describes as, petit mal attacks which may be associated with incontinence. These are of such frequency that he is having trouble at work. He works in the civil service.

He was born by forceps delivery and there was the possibility of neonatal convulsions. In 1953, he was found to have a spastic right hemiplegia. In 1963, he had a grand mal fit and an EEG at that time showed left temporal lobe dysfunction and, he was placed on phenobarbitone and phenytoin. Over the years he has seen a variety of neurologists, including [names of two neurologists]. He last saw [...] in 1982 when the diagnosis of temporal lobe epilepsey was confirmed. His regular medication was phenytoin 100 mgs four times a day and 25 mgs at night, mysoline 250 mgs three times a day and ethosuximide 500 mgs four times a day.

I sent him in April for some anti-convulsant levels which showed phenobarbitone 19, phenytoin 12.1 and ethosuximide 81. All these results are in the therapeutic range. As his phenytoin was slightly low, I increased his phenytoin by an extra 25 mgs at night. He then developed what he described as 'abdominal tightening' over the epigastrium. He saw my partner who prescribed cimetidine. This further aggravated what appeared to be a dystonic reaction. When I subsequently saw him, I stopped his cimetidine and restored his phenytoin dose to the original level. His abdominal symptoms have disappeared but his petit mal attacks are as frequent as before.

Again, I tried a cautious increase in his phenytoin; he is now taking 100 mgs four times a day plus an extra 50 mgs at night.

I would be grateful if you could see him to offer some suggestions as to how we might improve his treatment. I rather fear if we keep on like this he will lose his job. He lives at home with his elderly mother. He unfortunately continues to drink alcohol, despite having been advised to stop.

Yours sincerely,

[General Practitioner's name]

Fig. 2.2 A comprehensive and complete letter of referral. The presenting complaint and its effects on the patient's life-style are clearly stated . In the context of this complaint, very full details are provided of the patient's past history, including the results of previous investigations. Both his previous and present medication is detailed. Finally, the major reasons for the referral are summarized.

ward can prove a hindrance particularly when discussing sensitive issues. If a quiet room is available, use that to obtain the history. If you are seeing the patient in the out-patient department, arrange the patient's seat close to yours (Fig. 2.3), rather than confront the patient across a desk (Fig. 2.4).

Time

You need to ascertain that the time you have chosen to see the patient is an appropriate one. Rest periods are generally regarded as sacrosanct by the nursing staff though ironically they often offer the best, because the quietest, time to see the patient. With the increasing flexibility of visiting times, the likelihood of finding the ward quiet for your visit diminishes. Again, use of a separate interview room is valuable.

Yourself

The patient's first judgment of any doctor or student who sees them is based on their appearance. Fashions in dress have altered, and the range of accepted apparel is correspondingly broader, but certain fundamentals remain. You will be wearing a freshly laundered white coat (except, probably, for your visits to the paediatric and psychiatric wards). Your hands and nails must be meticulously clean. Nothing is more offensive to a patient than being palpated by grubby fingers. Your hair should be so constrained that it does not fall over the patient as you perform fundoscopy. Your shoes should betray some sign of contact with polish in the recent past. Some of these points may seem trivial, but they will not seem so to the patient. If you have no regard for your own appearance, might the patient wonder whether you are able to consider his welfare?

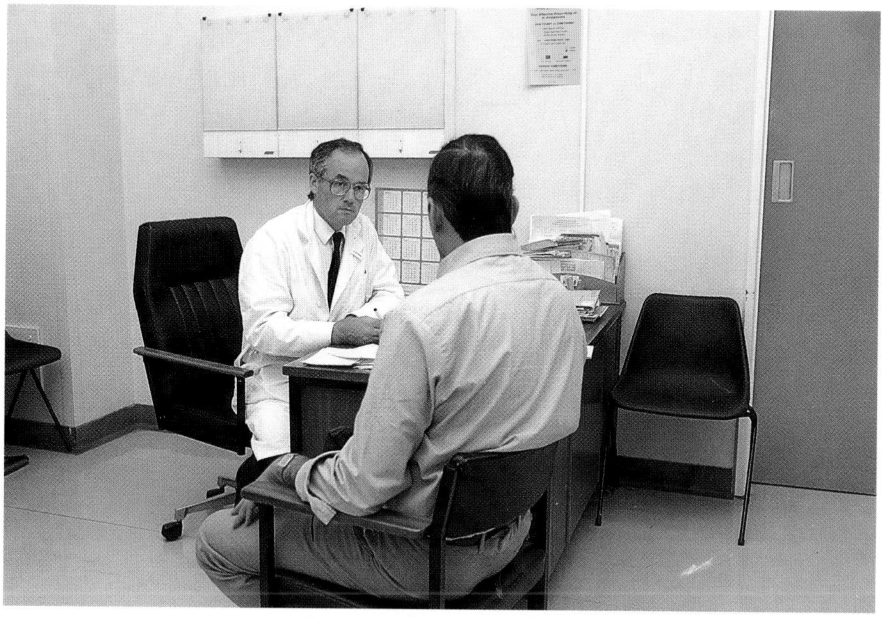

Fig. 2.3 The preferred arrangement of chairs when interviewing the patient. You are physically closer to the patient, without any intervening barrier.

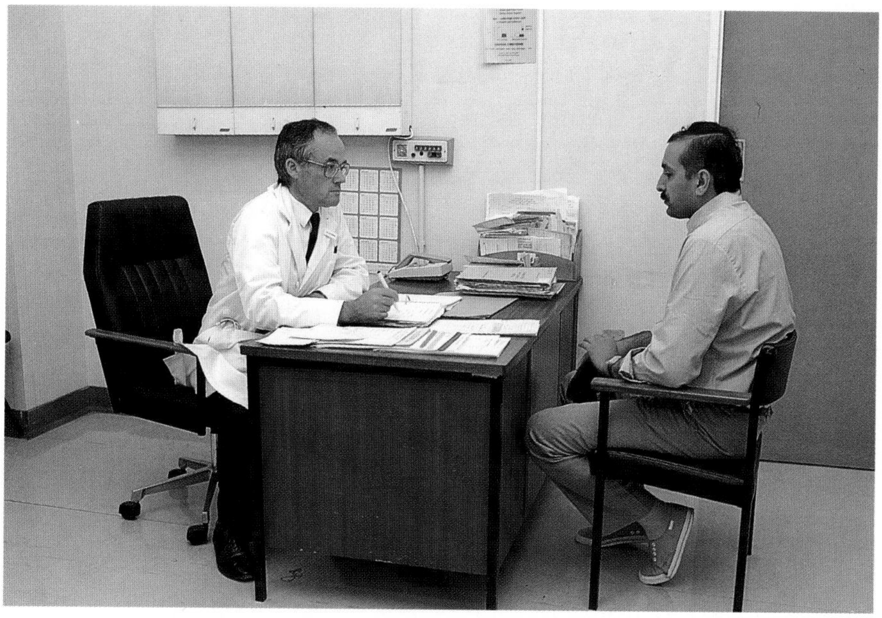

Fig. 2.4 This arrangement is less satisfactory. For the more sensitive or nervous patient, it will seem as if an additional physical barrier has been placed between him and the doctor, thereby hindering the exchange of information.

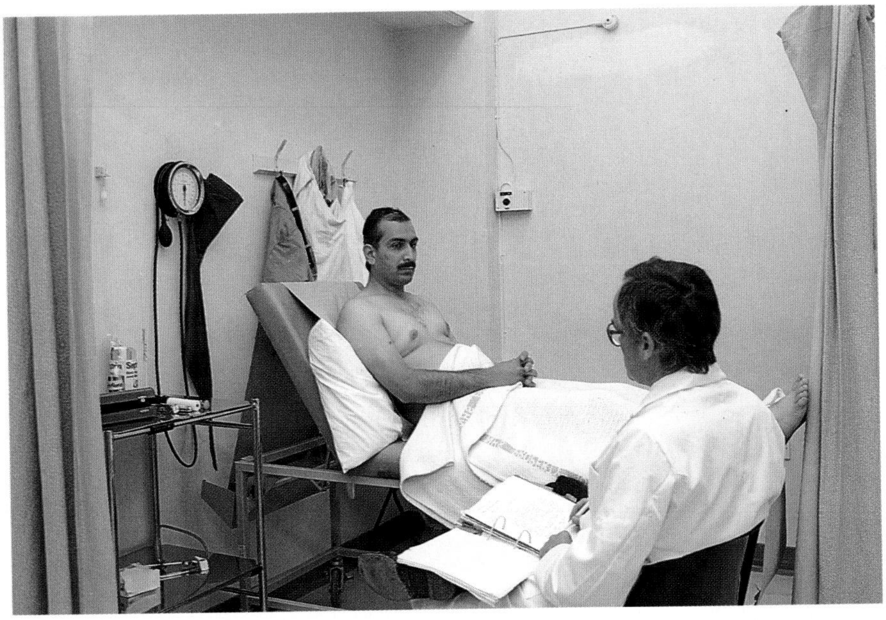

Fig. 2.5 For the bedside interview sit in a chair alongside the bed. Ensure that the patient is comfortable and is able to look at you without straining.

H.M. aged 57 Housewife
1. Increasing shortness of breath for 3 months 2. Bouts of night time shortness of breath for 3 weeks 3. A dry cough for the last 6 days

Fig. 2.6 Summarize the presenting complaints.

Symptoms
1. Mode of onset 2. Static, decreasing, or increasing in severity 3. Exacerbating and relieving factors

Fig. 2.7 For any symptom, cover all three points.

INITIAL APPROACH

Though most hospitals now provide their staff and students with badges bearing their name and position, many personnel fail to use them. Introduce yourself, indicating that you are a student and that you would like the opportunity to take a history and to carry out a physical examination. Some patients will refuse. Don't take this as a personal insult unless, of course, your appearance is such that any sensible individual would have reacted in the same way. The vast majority of patients are endlessly obliging, but they expect, and should receive, the courtesies due to them. Having obtained the patient's consent, pull up a chair rather than sit on the patient's bed or, even worse, on part of their anatomy (Fig. 2.5). Although you may feel it more intimate to carry out the interview on a first-name basis, many patients will find that offensive. Address the patient by their surname unless they have indicated that they would prefer their Christian name to be used. At this point, give the patient an outline of what you intend to do and also some idea of how long it might take. Although both history-taking and examination are ideally completed at one sitting, you may have to complete the examination at a later time if the patient has another commitment.

First questions

There is little point in attempting to take an elaborate history from someone who is dementing. Though you may obtain definite answers to your questions, particularly if they are not open-ended, the patient's relatives will soon disabuse you of their accuracy. Better, therefore, to begin the interview with a few questions which will help you to decide whether the patient is capable of providing a detailed history. Do not confine yourself to asking the patient's name and address, details which are often preserved in quite severely demented individuals; it is preferable to ask the patient how long they have been in hospital, who is their doctor (they will often name the houseman rather than the consultant!) and what has been happening to them in the previous twenty-four hours. If the answers appear coherent and accurate, proceed with reasonable confidence.

Begin by asking the patient to outline the problem. You can ask either 'what is the problem' or 'what has brought you to hospital'. If the patient has multiple complaints, list them chronologically rather than in the sometimes haphazard order in which the patient offers them. At this stage you will be writing down a precis of the

Pain
1. Type
2. Site
3. Spread
4. Periodicity or constancy
5. Relieving factors
6. Exacerbating factors
7. Associated symptoms

Fig. 2.8 Assessment of pain.

patient's comments, but avoid becoming so immersed in your writing that you seldom again look at the patient until you come to the physical examination. An example of what you may have written by this stage is shown in Figure 2.6.

THE HISTORY

HISTORY OF THE PRESENTING COMPLAINT(S)

You now need to explore each of the patient's symptoms in greater detail. If they give you a diagnosis as their complaint, (e.g. 'I've got angina') explore that diagnosis in detail so that you are confident of its accuracy. First, establish when the symptoms began. Some patients will have forgotten, others approximate, a few furnish a specific date. The ability to provide such detail is influenced by the patient's personality and determined by whether or not the problem began abruptly. At this point, some patients will provide a written account of their history. Though the appearance of such a list can be the forerunner of a protracted interview, it can provide a helpful precis and will certainly suggest how the patient views the illness.

For each symptom, explore the items listed in Figure 2.7. Patients often relate their symptom to a recent physical or emotional event. A facial paralysis is often attributed to a draughty window, or a headache to a recent bereavement. Avoid being too ready to accept a physical complaint as the reflection of a psychological problem, even if the patient presses that interpretation upon you. It is important, nonetheless, to take account of these beliefs and also to discover if the patient fears a particular disease.

For the assessment of pain, cover the topics shown in Figure 2.8. Sometimes the patient finds it difficult to describe a pain's quality. Help them by providing a list to choose from: dull, throbbing, tight, knife-like, and so on. Moreover, it is particularly difficult to assess pain severity. You can ask whether medication has been used to alleviate the pain and whether the pain interferes with work or social activities. The answers, however, tell you as much about an individual's stoicism as it does about the severity of their pain.

For each presenting complaint, assessment of severity is best achieved by determining its effect on lifestyle. For example, if the patient has vascular claudication, how far can they walk before pain forces them to rest.

Social history

Here you will cover the patient's schooling, their employment, both previous and present, their drug history, and the use of tobacco and alcohol.

Education

Enquire at what age the patient left school, whether they attended university and what qualifications were obtained. You will gain some measure of their premorbid intelligence and an appreciation as to whether their present occupation may be beyond their intellectual capacity.

Employment history

The employment history may be of critical importance if it suggests that exposure to a particular environment (e.g. an asbestos factory) could have triggered the patient's illness. Here again patients can enthusiastically provide an explanation for their illness. Some patients with headache, for instance, will attribute it to watching a VDU screen, while a proportion with chronic fatigue and malaise will suggest that they suffer from the sick building syndrome. Though many such attributions owe more to prejudice than reality, avoid dismissing them too readily. Frequent job changes may reflect the patient's personality or instability as, in some cases, can chronic unemployment. Patients sometimes describe their employment with imagination rather than accuracy. Hence a clerk becomes a secretarial assistant, and a labourer describes himself as a building operative. It is sensible to enquire whether there is specific stress in the patient's employment, particularly if that employment began at about the same time as the presenting complaints. Stress is an over-used concept, so remember that a patient's description of a situation as stressful is personal and may not be shared by others.

Drug history

Many patients bring their medication to the clinic, whereas for in-patients, information is readily available from the drug chart. Determine, for over-the-counter drugs, whether the patient is self-prescribing or on instructions from a doctor. Find out for how long the patient has been taking a particular drug and for what reason it was first prescribed. It will surprise you how often the patient has forgotten the indication for the drug they are taking. Sometimes the side effects of the medication explain the source of some of the patient's symptoms. Ask women of reproductive age whether they are on an oral contraceptive and document its oestrogen content. For postmenopausal women, enquire about hormone replacement therapy (HRT). List any drug allergies.

Now ask the patient about the use of illicit drugs. Your enquiry needs to be sensitively phrased and will be influenced by the patient's age and background. Few 80 year-olds are smoking pot or eating magic mushrooms! Ask first about marijuana, LSD, and amphetamine derivatives. If the response suggests exposure, enquire about the use of the harder drugs (e.g. cocaine and heroin).

Tobacco consumption

Patients usually give a fairly accurate account of their smoking. Ask what form of tobacco they consume and for how long they have been smoking. Do they inhale cigarette smoke? If they previously smoked, when did they stop?

Alcohol consumption

Some patients tell you they drink 'the usual' or 'socially'. The terms are meaningless. First, establish the type of alcohol the patient consumes: many will admit to predominantly one type, making an estimate of consumption more straightforward. Calculate the amount in units (Fig. 2.9). If the patient is vague, ask them how long a bottle of sherry or spirits lasts. Many patients who are alcohol-dependent will lie to you about their consumption. Certain questions may reveal dependency without asking the patient to specify consumption. You can ask if the patient vomits in the morning, if they drink alone, or if they drink during the course of the day. Do they have days without alcohol?

Foreign travel

Ask the patient if they have been abroad recently. If so, determine the countries visited and the levels of hygiene maintained. If the patient has returned from an area where malaria is endemic, ask if the patient has taken adequate prophylaxis for the appropriate period.

Units of alcohol

1 unit equals
- 1/2 pint beer
- 1 glass sherry
- 1 glass wine
- 1 standard measure of spirits

Fig. 2.9 Alcohol equivalents.

Home circumstances

It is necessary at this stage to ascertain how the patient was managing in the community prior to their present illness. The issue is particularly relevant for elderly patients. Do they live on their own, have they any support systems, provided by either the community or their family? If the patient's condition has been present for some time, determine how the patient is managing. For example, in a patient with motor neurone disease, is work still possible? Can the patient climb stairs? If not, what provisions will have to be made if the patient is to remain at home? Can the patient get in and out of a bath? What assistance might be on hand during the day or at night? What effects will the patient's illness have on the financial status of the family?

PAST HISTORY

Patients recall their past medical history with varying degrees of detail and accuracy. Some will provide a meticulously-typed sheet, others will need reminding of quite major events. You can jog their memory by asking the patient if they have ever been admitted to hospital. If the patient has had an operation, check whether there were postoperative complications. Include caesarian sections in your enquiry. If the patient mentions specific illnesses or diagnoses, explore them in detail rather than accepting them verbatim. For example, a patient might say that she had a heart attack four years previously. Further enquiry might reveal that this referred to an episode of chest discomfort which a doctor, visiting in the middle of the night, suggested might be a 'small heart attack'. Alternatively, it might relate to an episode of severe central chest pain which led to the patient's admission to hospital for a period of two weeks. Similarly, if the patient mentions migraine, ask them to describe an attack so that you can decide whether or not the diagnosis is correct.

Medical students are often encouraged to go through a list of specific illnesses when enquiring about the past medical history. The list tends to be derived from old textbooks and contains diseases less relevant to the present generation. It is unlikely, for instance, that a patient under the age of thirty will have had rheumatic fever. The enquiry about past illnesses should be guided by the presenting complaints. If a patient has cardiac failure, ask if there is a history of myocardial infarction. It is preferable to list substantial illnesses in chronological order, even if this means 'tidying-up' the history after the patient has given it.

FAMILY HISTORY

Though enquiry into the family history will primarily seek evidence of an inherited disorder, information about the immediate family may have considerable bearing on the patient's symptoms. Start by asking if the patient is married, or has a regular partner. If so, determine if that individual is well, or whether they have had a recent or more chronic illness. If the patient has children, determine their ages and state of health. Find out if any offspring died in childhood and from what cause? Now move on to the patient's siblings and parents. Did any family members die at a relatively young age and if so, from what cause. Where there is suspicion of a familial disorder, (e.g. Huntington's disease) it is helpful to construct a family tree (Fig. 2.10). Ages can be added to the tree, or listed separately. If the pattern of inheritance suggests a recessive trait, ask whether the parents were related, in particular whether they were first cousins.

SYSTEMS REVIEW

Before concentrating on individual systems ask some general questions about the patient's health. Is the patient sleeping well? If not, is there a problem getting to sleep or a tendency to wake in the middle of the night or in the early hours of the morning? Does the patient feel tired, though when you ask this question beware of the fact that a large proportion of individuals will respond positively. Has the appetite diminished and has it been accompanied by weight loss? Does the patient feel reasonably well outside the presenting complaint, or chronically ill?

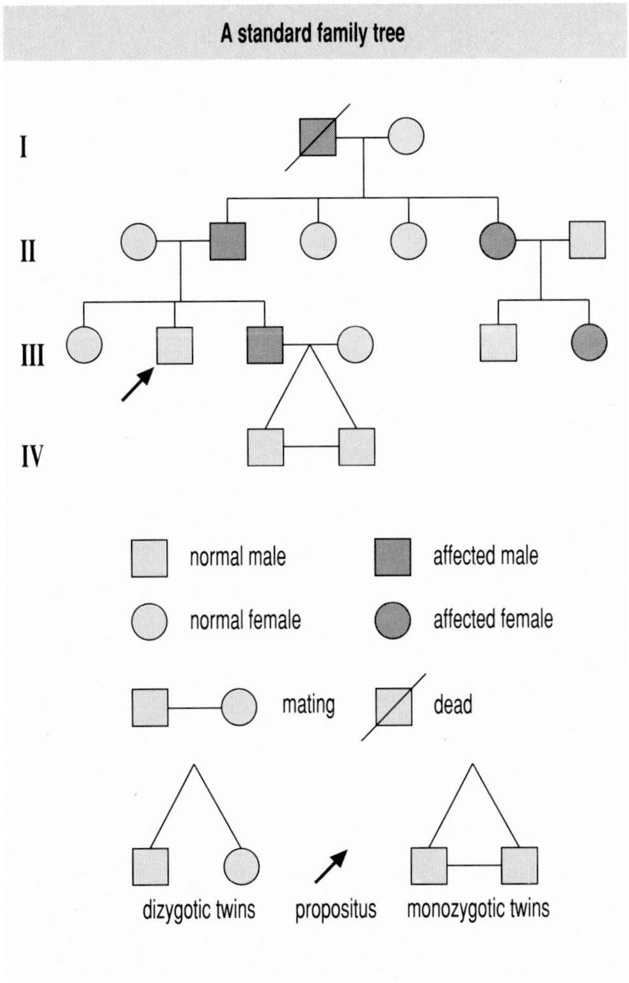

Fig. 2.10 A standard family tree.

Now enquire about symptoms referable to a particular system. It is probably logical to start with the system to which the patient's presenting complaints belong. Thereafter continue in the following order. Having such a routine helps to avoid missing out a particular system.

CARDIOVASCULAR SYSTEM

Chest pain

Determine the position of any chest pain, its quality, and its periodicity. Find out if there are specific triggering factors. Does the pain radiate? If the patient describes an exercise-induced pain, remember that angina can be confined to the throat or jaw, rather than centering on the chest.

Dyspnoea

Ask the patient if they are readily short of breath. Quantify the problem: does it occur after climbing one flight of stairs, after walking on the flat for 100 metres, and so on? Does the patient become short of breath on lying flat (orthopnoea) or do they wake up breathless in the middle of the night (paroxysmal nocturnal dyspnoea)?

Ankle swelling

Has the patient noticed any ankle swelling? Is it confined to one leg, or does it affect both? Is the swelling persistent, or only noticeable towards the end of the day

Palpitations

Few patients record their pulse, but most will register an abnormal heart rhythm, particularly one that is rapid. Try to establish whether the abnormal rhythm is regular or irregular, and for how long it lasts. Can the patient give you an idea of the frequency by beating out the rhythm with the hand? Do any other symptoms appear while the heart is beating abnormally?

RESPIRATORY SYSTEM

Cough

Many patients, particularly smokers, assume that coughing is a normal life experience. It may be difficult to quantify the problem, particularly if the cough is dry. If productive, work out the amount – an eggcupful a day perhaps? Is the sputum mucoid or purulent, i.e. is the sputum white or grey in colour, or more yellow/green in appearance?

Haemoptysis

If the patient has coughed up blood, find out whether this represents fine blood-streaking of the sputum or a more conspicuous amount. Is it a recent event, or has it happened periodically over several years? Did it follow a particularly violent bout of coughing?

Wheezing

Is the wheezing constant or intermittent, does it appear in particular environments, and can it be triggered by exercise? If the patient is using bronchodilators, determine the dosage and the frequency of use, particularly if an aerosol preparation has been prescribed.

GASTROINTESTINAL SYSTEM

Change in weight

Ask the patient if there has been any weight loss or gain. Those whose weight gain is due to excessive food intake seldom recognize the fact. If there is uncertainty about weight change, ask the patient if they have noticed any alteration in the fit of their clothes.

Abdominal pain

Avoid asking the patient about indigestion. Many use the term to describe flatulence. Ask specifically about abdominal pain. Determine its site, its quality, and its relationship to eating. Does it appear soon after a meal, or 3–4 hours later? Is it then relieved by the use of alkalis, or the ingestion of more food? Is the pain relieved by adopting a certain posture? Can the pain disappear for weeks or months, or is it more persistent?

Vomiting

Ask about both nausea and vomiting. If vomiting occurs, does it affect any accompanying pain? Is the vomiting violent (projectile) or does it represent little more than regurgitation of the stomach contents? Is the vomiting lightly blood-stained, or does it look like coffee-grounds suggesting partly altered blood? Are items of food eaten some hours before still recognizable?

Flatulence and regurgitation

Does the patient complain of flatulence, leading to burping or the passage of flatus? Is there retrosternal burning, particularly in certain postures? Does the mouth suddenly fill with regurgitated fluid (waterbrash)?

Dysphagia

Has there been a problem in swallowing? Does this affect solids more than liquids, or the reverse? The degree of weight loss is a good measure of the severity of the problem. Can the patient identify a site where they believe the obstruction occurs, though you must realize that this correlates poorly with the site of the relevant pathological process.

Bowel habit

Enquire about the patient's bowel habits. Many patients believe they are constipated simply because they do not have a daily bowel action. If the patient has always emptied his bowels three times a week and the motions are normally formed, then he is not constipated. Of significance is a change in bowel habit whether in terms of frequency or consistency of stool. Has the appearance of the stool altered? Are they unusually dark or pale, or are they difficult to flush away? If there has been a change in bowel habit, ask the patient what drugs they are taking. A common cause of constipation is the use of analgesics containing a codeine derivative. Has the patient noticed bleeding with defaecation, or the presence of a mucous discharge? Finally, ask about perianal pain and whether there is discomfort during defaecation.

GENITOURINARY SYSTEM

Frequency

Determine the daytime and night time frequency of micturition. Summarize the findings as a ratio; for example

$$\frac{D}{N} = \frac{6\text{-}8}{0\text{-}1}$$

Has there been an increase in the actual volume of urine passed (polyuria)? This is usually then associated with increased thirst and fluid intake.

Pain

Ask the patient if there is any pain either during or immediately after micturition. Has the patient noticed a urethral discharge? Is the urine offensive, cloudy, or blood-stained?

Altered bladder control

Determine if there has been urgency of micturition, with or without incontinence. Does the patient have urinary incontinence without warning? Has the urinary stream become slower, perhaps associated with difficulty in starting or stopping (terminal dribbling)? Does the patient have the desire to empty the bladder soon after micturition?

Menstruation

Ask about the menstrual history. Use a ratio to summarize the duration of menstruation and the number of days between each period (e.g. 7/28). Are the periods heavy (menorrhagia) or painful (dysmenorrhoea)? Have they changed in quality or quantity?

Sexual activity

Finally, ask about the patient's sexual activity, though many will be reluctant to discuss this with you in detail. Is the patient willing to tell you how many different partners they have had in the past, and whether they have had any homosexual encounters? Does the patient practice safe sex? Have they ever had a sexually transmitted disease? In addition, ask whether intercourse is painful, or whether the patient is concerned about a lack of sexual activity, whether due to loss of libido or to actual impotence.

THE NERVOUS SYSTEM

Headache

Ask about headache, though few individuals have never experienced the problem. Follow the enquiry you use for other forms of pain (Fig. 2.8); but, in addition, ask if the pain is affected by head movement, coughing, or sneezing. If the patient mentions migraine, find out what the individual means by that term. One of the most important questions to ask about headache is whether it has been a recent problem, or whether it has occurred over months or years.

Loss of consciousness

Has the patient lost consciousness? Avoid terms like blackouts even if the patient tries to use them. Find out if there are any warning symptoms before attacks, whether they have been witnessed; and whether they have led to incontinence, injury, or a bitten tongue. Do the episodes occur only in certain environments, or can they be triggered by certain activities (e.g. standing suddenly)? How does the patient feel after the attack? Most patients recover quickly from a simple faint, but after an epileptic seizure, patients often complain of headache then sleep deeply for several hours. If the patient mentions epilepsy, get him to specify the exact nature of the attacks. There may be specific symptoms accompanying the attack which assist in making a diagnosis. Is there first pallor followed by facial flushing, or is there a clear cut warning with faintness, sweating, and nausea?

Dizziness and vertigo

Dizziness (or giddiness) is a common complaint, describing an ill-defined sense of dysequilibrium usually without any objective evidence of imbalance. Some patients describe a continuous feeling of dizziness but most refer to attacks. If the symptom is paroxysmal, does it occur in particular environments or with particular actions? For instance, hyperventilation attacks, in which dizziness is often prominent, tend to occur in crowded places (e.g. supermarkets), while patients with postural hypotension will notice dizziness triggered by standing suddenly. Only use the term vertigo if the patient describes a sense of rotation, either of the body or of the environment. Again, detail any triggering factors. In one particular type, benign positional vertigo, the symptom is induced by lying down in bed at night, but only when on one particular side.

Speech and related functions

Ask about the patient's speech. Is there simply a problem of articulation, or does the patient use wrong words, with or without a reduction in total speech output? Carefully note the patient's handedness which should include questions about the limb used for a variety of skilled tasks, rather than just writing. Does the patient have difficulty understanding speech? Has there been any change in reading or writing ability? For the latter, ask not just about the quality of the script, but also the content.

Memory

The patient may not complain of a disturbance of memory, but if he does determine whether this simply applies to recent events, to events further back in the patient's youth, or to both. Is the memory problem persistent, or does the patient have 'good and bad days'? Many individuals mention difficulties with memory, though further enquiry often indicates that the problem is largely determined by the patient's psychological state.

CRANIAL NERVE SYMPTOMS

Vision

Ask about any visual disturbances. Do these take the form of negative symptoms (i.e. visual loss) or positive symptoms in the form of scintillations or shimmerings? Most patients assume that the right eye is concerned with vision to the right, and the left eye with vision to the left. Consequently, few will cover test during attacks of visual disturbance to determine whether the problem is monocular or binocular. Ensure you ask whether the patient has cover tested before accepting their account of the distribution of the symptoms. Is the visual disturbance intermittent or continuous? Is it accompanied or followed by headache?

Diplopia

If the patient has or has had diplopia, determine whether the images were separated horizontally or in an oblique fashion. Can the patient tell you in which direction of gaze the diplopia is most evident? Is it relieved by covering one eye or the other?

Facial numbness

Can the patient outline the distribution of any facial sensory loss? Does the involvement include the tongue, the gums, and the buccal mucosae?

Deafness

Has the patient become aware of deafness? Is it bilateral or unilateral? Has the patient a history of chronic exposure to noise, or is there a family history of deafness? Is the hearing particularly troublesome when there is an increased level of background noise? Is the hearing problem accompanied by tinnitus?

Dysphagia

Has the patient problems with swallowing? Does this principally affect fluids or solids? Is the problem mainly concerned with transferring the food from the mouth to the pharynx or at a slightly later stage?

Limb motor or sensory symptoms

Is the problem confined to one limb, or to the limbs on one side of the body, to the lower limbs alone, or to all four limbs? Does the patient describe loss of sensation or some distortion of sensation (e.g. a feeling of tightness round the limb)? If the patient complains of weakness, find out whether it is intermittent or continuous, and, if the latter, whether it is progressing. Does the weakness mainly affect the proximal or the distal part of the limb? Has the patient noticed muscle wasting or any twitching of limb muscles?

Loss of coordination

Few patients with a cerebellar syndrome will describe their problem in terms of loss of coordination. Some will complain of clumsiness, many will simply refer to the problem as weakness. When assessing the loss of limb coordination, it is useful to ask the patient about everyday activities, (e.g. writing and eating). Ask the patient about their sense of balance. Do they tend to deviate to a particular side, or in either direction? Have they had falls as a consequence?

MUSCULOSKELETAL SYSTEM

Has the patient had bone or joint pain? If the latter, has it been accompanied by swelling, tenderness, or redness? Is the problem confined to a single joint, or is it more diffuse? Does the pain predominate on waking, or does it appear as the relevant joint is used (for example in walking) Is there a history of trauma to the joint now painful, or is there a family history of joint disease?

SKIN

Has the patient had rashes? What was their distribution? Were or are they accompanied by itching? Is the patient's occupation a possible guide to the cause of the rash? Find out what chemicals or cosmetics could have been in contact with the skin. Have metal bracelets or bra fasteners been worn; this is particularly relevant if the rash has a very focal distribution.

PARTICULAR PROBLEMS

The patient with depression or dementia

There is some logic in coupling these clinical problems. In both cases the patient can appear withdrawn and uncommunicative. Patients with depression may well dwell on their vegetative symptoms (e.g. insomnia and loss of appetite) and be reluctant to discuss their mood change.

A critical part of that questioning is the determination of whether or not there has been any suicidal intent. Patients with dementia initially retain some insight; nevertheless, even then they are likely to be bewildered by the effects of their illness. It is important to gain additional information from friends or relatives, though this needs to be pursued with tact if the patient is present.

The hostile patient

If a patient is hostile to the idea of being interviewed by a student then respect those feelings and abandon the discussion. For some patients, the hostility arises out of a sense of frustration over perceived delays or inefficiences in the system. Patients whose conditions elude diagnosis can become embittered. As a representative of the medical profession, albeit unqualified, you may encounter their criticism. Commonly, anger or hostility hides an underlying fear that the patient harbours over their illness. It is disastrous to respond aggressively in such situations. Start by asking the patient why he or she feels angry. Having gained the patient's confidence you can then begin to explore the history more formally. If the hostility persists, then terminate the interview and discuss the problem with one of the medical staff.

Sometimes, patients who are anxious or depressed can appear irritable or angry. Similarly, certain physical illnesses can affect mood, particularly those in which pain is a prominent feature. Patients with damage to the frontal lobes of the brain tend to lose both insight and self-control.

History-taking in the presence of students

Usually, when eliciting the history, you will be seeing the patient on a one-to-one basis. At other times, you will observe the process in the outpatient department. Patients can find your presence overwhelming and sometimes will ask you to leave before revealing intimate details (Fig. 2.11).

OTHER PROBLEM PATIENTS

Sometimes you may feel that the patient is being sexually provocative during either the interview or the examination. It will seldom be possible for a nurse to accompany you so, instead, find a fellow student to join you. If one is not available, it is wise to postpone or terminate your examination.

You will seldom be asked to examine 'VIPs', simply because the patient is usually spared the possible hazard of seeing you! That is a pity, since you need to learn to see such people in exactly the same way that you would any other patient. Eminent people (including doctors) are often disadvantaged in their contacts with the medical profession. Corners tend to be cut; painful or embarrassing procedures are avoided.

THE USE OF NEBULOUS TERMS

Many terms used by patients suggest a descriptive certainty which does not withstand close scrutiny. Sometimes a broad term can be of value (e.g. stroke) when a more accurate diagnosis, such as cerebral infarction, cannot be assumed on the evidence available. Patients with a restricted vocabulary can have difficulty describing their problem, but you will also encounter patients whose history reveals more of their intelligence than of their illness. Many nebulous terms are used in medicine (e.g. sciatica, dizziness, and numbness). Make sure that you ask the patient to define what is meant by a particular complaint. Use the patient's own words in your history, rather than attempting what may well be an inaccurate simplification.

THE USE OF SPECIFIC DIAGNOSES

As you take the past history, inevitably you will ask about specific illnesses the patient may have suffered. A string of surgical procedures can sometimes reflect aspects of the patient's personality rather than ill-fortune. If the patient mentions a particular illness (e.g. pneumonia), determine the symptoms, the duration of the illness, and its treatment. A longstanding history of multiple bodily complaints, including pain, is often helpful when trying to understand the current problem. Though this may not concern you as a student, remember that data can be obtained from other hospitals and from the general practitioner. Finally, remember that memory is fickle, and it is unreasonable to expect complete recall of events occurring many years previously.

PRESENTING YOUR FINDINGS

Most hospitals provide continuation sheets reserved for the use of students. It is imperative that you write your history and examination findings on them, signing each entry. It is a good idea to take copies of these notes which you can then keep in a personal file for future reference (Fig. 2.12).

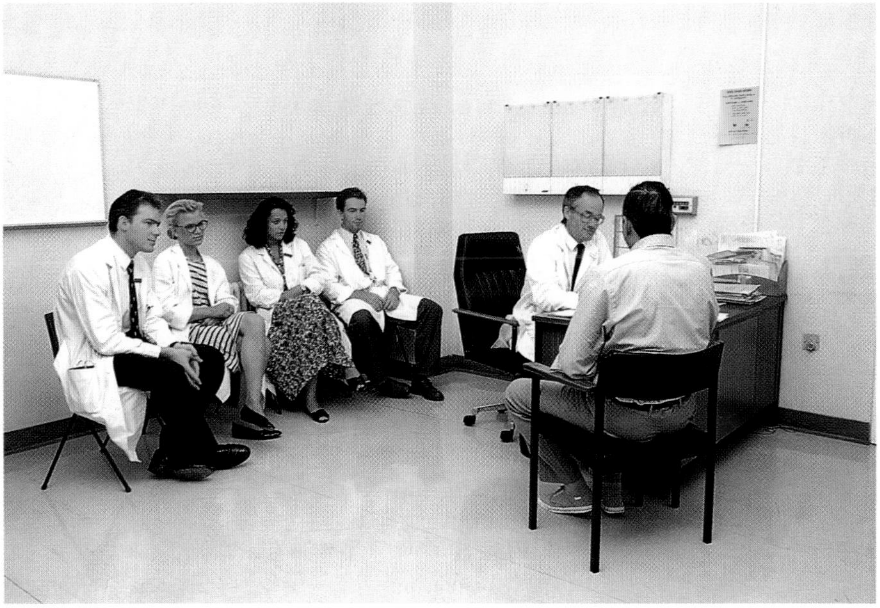

Fig. 2.11 The patient has to face not only the doctor but a number of students. Some patients will have difficulty coping with a 'mass' audience.

Patient history

Mrs G. W. — 70 years old Female
Date of Birth: 11/1/21 — Retired Shop Assistant

Date: 1/8/91

Presenting Complaint(s): (1) Constipation
(2) Stomach Pain

HISTORY OF PRESENTING COMPLAINT:
(1) Constipation: Started on 7/6/91. Normally bowels open once a day, but didn't go for six days. Subsequently has been going once every 2–4 days.
(2) Stomach Pain: Pain started at the same time. Site of pain is the left iliac fossa. Patient thought it was due to 'straining'. Episodes of pain are of sudden onset and are a 'sagging dull ache'. They last one hour and occur anything between 2–3 times a day to once every three days. There are no alleviating or exacerbating factors. Pain unrelated to eating or defaecation and there are no preceeding events. Pain appears to be staying the same.

Patient went to visit GP after 6 days constipation. GP felt a mass on abdominal palpation which on bimanual examination was though to be of ovarian origin. Patient referred to the gynaecological outpatient department.

SOCIAL HISTORY:
Retired at age of 60 as shop assistant. Married. Husband is a retired bus driver. Alive and well. Live together in own terraced house. Self-sufficient. No pets.

SMOKING:
Ex-smoker, 4–5 a day for five years as a teenager.

ALCOHOL:
Only on Christmas day and Birthdays.

PAST OBSTETRIC HISTORY:
Menarche – 12   Menopause – 50   Gravidity 3   Parity 3

(1) Female 41   Spontaneous vaginal delivery full term (7lb)

(2) Female 38   Spontaneous vaginal delivery full term (8lb 4oz)

(3) Female 35   Spontaneous vaginal delivery 39 weeks (6lb 8oz)

PAST MEDICAL HISTORY:
Hypertension for last 6 years treated by GP with Atenolol.
No previous operations.

DRUG HISTORY: Atenolol

ALLERGIES: None known

TRAVEL ABROAD: Never

FAMILY HISTORY:

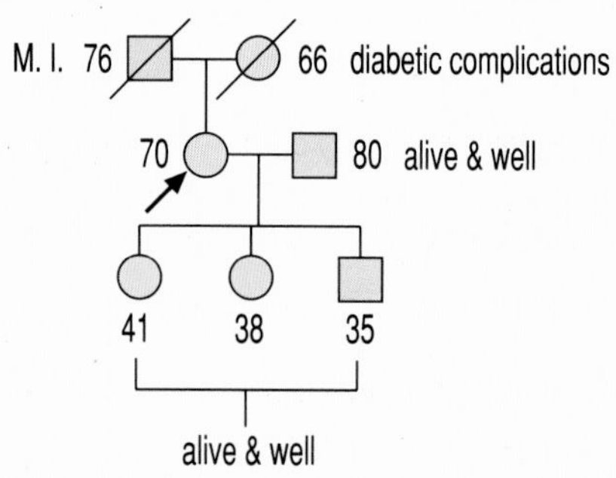

No family history of TB,

SYSTEMS REVIEW

GENERAL:
No weight change, appetite normal, no fevers, night sweats, fatigue or itch.

CARDIOVASCULAR SYSTEM:
No chest pain, palpitations, exertional dyspnoea, paroxysmal nocturnal dyspnoea, orthopnoea or ankle oedema.

RESPIRATORY SYSTEM:
No cough, wheeze, sputum or haemoptysis.

GASTROINTESTINAL SYSTEM:
No abdominal swelling noticed by patient, no nausea or vomiting, no haematemesis. Bowels open once every 2–3 days. Stool normally formed. No blood or slime. No melaena.

GENITOURINARY SYSTEM:
No dysuria, haematuria. Frequency $\frac{D}{N} = \frac{2\text{–}3}{1}$
No vaginal discharge. Not sexually active.

NERVOUS SYSTEM:
No fits, faints or funny turns. No headache, paraesthesiae, weakness or poor balance.

MUSCULOSKELETAL SYSTEM:
No pain or swelling of joints. Slight stiffness in morning.

SUMMARY:
This is a 70 year old hypertensive woman, referred to gynaecological outpatients with a short history of constipation and stomach pain. She has no other previous medical history.

Fig. 2.12 A specimen case-history taken from a student's notes. Note the brief summary at the end, the writing of which gives useful practice in the art of condensing a substantial volume of information.

The dividing line between the history and examination is artificial. The examination really begins from the moment you set eyes on the patient. During the course of the history you will examine the patient's intellect, personality, family and genetic background, as well as gather information on the presenting complaint and previous medical history. In addition, you will have the opportunity to assess speech, orientation for person, place, and time, and mood (affect). Throughout the history and examination you should sense information from the patient's 'unspoken' body language. These physical signs are rarely taught in the medical curriculum, although the examination of body language may provide many useful signs. The patient's facial expression and tone of voice often impart more information than verbal communication. Hunched shoulders, a slow gait, and poor eye contact might convey a reluctant patient, unable or unwilling to confront or expose anxieties or fears. The facial expression, tone of voice, and body attitude might signal depression even if the patient does not complain of feeling depressed. Regretably, many doctors write the history without looking at the patient or acknowledging their physical presence. Try to look, listen, and then write; this will give you the opportunity to see as well as listen to the patient's complaints.

The formal physical examination follows on the history and calls on your major senses of sight, touch, and hearing. Inspection, palpation, percussion, and auscultation form the foundation of the physical examination and this formula is repeated each time you examine an organ system. The otoscope and ophthalmoscope extend your vision into the ear and eye, respectively, whilst the stethoscope provides a handy, portable amplification system to help you listen to the heart, lung, and bowel sounds. With the help of technology we are now able to extend our vision deep into the body; X-rays (including CAT scanning), ultrasound, magnetic resonance, and fibre-optics greatly broaden our powers of observation.

The examination begins with a general examination and is followed by examination of the skin, head and neck, heart and lungs, abdominal organs, musculoskeletal, and neurological systems (Fig. 3.1). With practice it is possible to perform the entire 'routine' examination in 10–15 minutes, although if you discover an abnormality, considerably more time will be spent refining the findings. In time you will develop a set examination routine and from the outset you should aim to choreograph an economical, aesthetic, and complete examination.

THE GENERAL EXAMINATION

The general examination permits you to obtain an overview of the general state of health and provides an opportunity to examine those systems which do not fall neatly into a regional examination. For the patient, the general examination is also a gentle introduction to the more intense systems examination to follow.

First impressions

The examination commences as the patient walks into the consulting room or as you sit down at the bedside to take a history. At this first encounter, even before you initiate the history, decide whether the patient looks well or not and whether there is any striking physical abnormality. You will also gain an immediate impression of dress, grooming, and personal hygiene.

As the patient approaches you in the consulting/examination room, observe the gait and character of their stride. Diseases of nerves, muscles, bones, and joints are associated with abnormal gaits and postures. You should quickly recognize the slow shuffling gait and 'pill rolling' tremor of Parkinson's disease, or the unsteady broad-based gait of the ataxic patient. Patients with proximal muscle weakness may have difficulty rising from the waiting room chair and the gait may have a waddling appearance. Patients with osteoporosis lose height as the vertebrae progressively collapse. You might be struck by the typically stooped (kyphotic) appearance and 'round shoulders' of these patients. Take note if the patient walks with a stick or some form of additional physical support. A white stick indicates partial or complete blindness. The gait also conveys body language: the patient may have a spring in his step, make rapid eye contact, and immediately offers a firm handshake. This contrasts with the patient with drooping shoulders, a slow (but otherwise normal) step who avoids eye contact.

When making your initial acquaintance with the patient, a warm handshake serves a number of functions (Fig. 3.2). The touching of hands may reassure the patient and serve as a gentle and symbolic introduction to the more intimate physical contact of the examination which follows the history. Before shaking hands, glance momentarily at the hand to ensure that you will not be grabbing a prosthesis or deformed hand. A well-made prosthesis may cause considerable embarrassment as you suddenly realize that the hand you are shaking is hard and lifeless. You might also note other abnormalities such as a potentially painful rheumatoid hand or missing fingers. The grip of the handshake usually provides some useful information. A normal grip conveys quite different information from a weak, lethargic handshake which might imply distal muscle weakness, general ill-health, or depression. The handshake is a useful physical sign in patients with myotonia dystrophica, a rare autosomal dominant inherited disease of muscle. A feature of this disease is the abnormally slow relaxation of the grip on completion of the handshake. The syndrome is also characterized by premature frontal balding, testicular atrophy, and cataracts.

On first contact with the patient, you might be struck by an unusual physical stature. Unusually short stature might reflect constitutional shortness, a distinct genetic syndrome, or the

The examination

General examination

First impressions
Clinical syndromes (including endocrinopathies)
Nutritional status
Hydration
'Colour'
Oedema
Temperature
Lymphoreticular examination

Skin examination

Skin inspection
Palpation
Description of lesions
Hair
Nails

Ears, nose, and throat examination

Inspection outer ear, drum, test hearing and balance
Inspection of nose and palpation/percussion of sinuses
Inspection of lips, teeth, tongue, oral cavity, and pharynx inspection and palpation of salivary glands
Palpation of regional lymph nodes

Cardiovascular examination

Hands (splinters, clubbing)
Pulses
Blood pressure
Jugular venous pressure
Heart (inspect, palpate, auscultate)
Lungs (basal crackles, effusions)
Abdomen (liver pulsation)
Extremities (peripheral circulation, oedema)

Respiratory examination

Hands (clubbing, cyanosis, CO_2 retention)
Blood pressure (pulsus paradoxus)
Neck (JVP, trachea)
Lungs (inspect, palpate, percuss, auscultate)
Heart (evidence of cor pulmonale)

Abdominal examination

Hands (flapping tremor, nails, palms)
Jaundice and signs of liver failure
Parotids
Mouth and tongue
Chest (gynaecomastia, spiders, upper border of liver)
Abdomen (inspect, palpate, percuss, auscultate)
Groins
Rectal examination

Male genitalia

Sexual development
Penis
Scrotum
Testes and spermatic cord
Inguinal region

Female breasts and genitalia

Sexual development
Breast (inspection, palpation)
Vulva (inspection, palpation)
Vagina (speculum inspection)
Uterus and adnexae (palpation)

Musculoskeletal examination

Proximal and distal muscles (inspection, palpation)
Large joints
Small joints
Spine

Neurological examination

Psychological profile
Mental status
Cranial nerves
Motor and sensory examination (central and peripheral) cerebellar examination
Autonomic nervous system

Fig. 3.1 A format for the general and regional examinations.

consequence of intrauterine, childhood, or adolescent growth retardation (Fig. 3.3). Unusually tall stature is most often constitutional, although hypothalamic tumors in childhood or adolescence may cause excessive growth hormone release resulting in abnormally rapid linear growth and gigantism. If excess growth hormone release occurs after the bony epiphyses have fused, the body shape changes (acromegaly).

Both severe malnutrition and obesity are readily recognized on the first encounter with the patient.

THE FORMAL EXAMINATION

On completion of the history, prepare the patient for the formal examination. Always remain sensitive to the apprehension most patients feel when laid out in a near naked state on the examination couch or bed. Imagine yourself in that position, confronted by a near stranger who is about to inspect, palpate, percuss, and auscultate your body – a daunting thought. The history should have provided you with the opportunity to build a confident professional relationship with the patient. This is superimposed on a cultural and established fact that it is quite acceptable for a doctor to examine a patient. This acceptance usually extends to medical students who can be reassured that most patients welcome students and recognize their need to learn the examination technique. Explain the necessity of undertaking a full physical examination. The examination adds information to the clinical database and a thorough examination provides considerable reassurance to the patient.

The examination requires full exposure; both men and women should be asked to remove superficial clothing and vests/undershirts. For a chest examination, women should be asked to remove their brassiere. Ensure a clean and presentable examination gown is available in the examination room for the patient to don before you enter the room. When the opposite sex is to be examined, always ask the chaperone to check whether the patient is ready.

Setting

A separate examination room or adequate screening should be provided to ensure privacy whilst the patient is undressing and being examined. The room should be comfortably warm. Ensure that there are fresh sheets (either linen or disposable) and a clean blanket for cover. The examination couch should be positioned to allow you to examine from the patient's right side and there must be good general illumination. You should be fully equipped to undertake the examination without disruption. Ensure you have a working penlight torch and stethoscope. Close at hand there must be a sphygmomanometer, ophthalmoscope, otoscope, tongue depressors, and disposable gloves (for the genital and rectal examination). Basic equipment for the neurological examination should be available. This includes a patellar hammer, tuning fork, cotton wool buds, sterile disposable needles for testing pin-prick, test tubes to fill with hot and cold water for temperature testing, and hat pins with red and white tops to assess visual fields. A cupful of drinking water should also be available as you might ask the patient to swallow a mouthful to check for a thyroid goitre or other neck swelling.

As you approach the patient, re-establish both verbal and eye-contact. You might ask the patient whether they feel comfortable and are prepared for the examination. Start the examination with the patient supine and the head and shoulders raised to about 45° above the horizontal. Most modern examination couches and hospital beds are designed to allow easy adjustment of the upper body. Most of the examination takes place with the patient

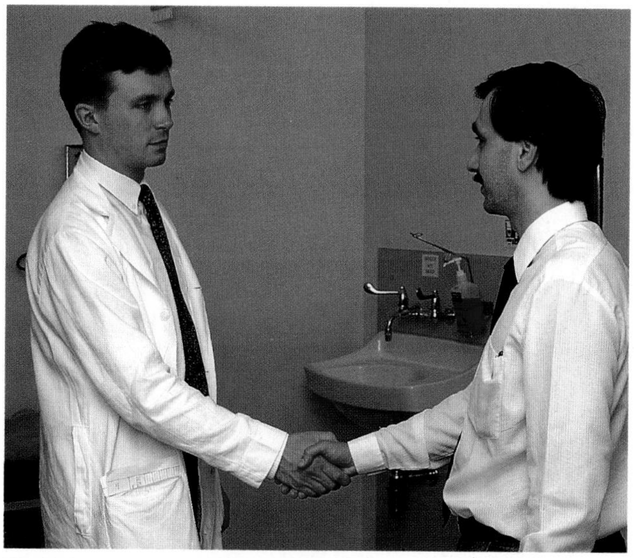

Fig. 3.2 The handshake serves as a gentle introduction to the physical contact which will occur during the formal physical examination.

Causes of growth failure

Cause	Example
Genetic	Genetic achondroplasia, Turner's syndrome, Down's syndrome
Constitutional	Family members who have short stature
Endocrine	Hypopituitarism, hypothyroidism
Systemic disease	Crohn's disease, ulcerative colitis, renal failure
Malnutrition	Intrauterine growth retardation, marasmus, kwashiorkor, starvation

Fig. 3.3 Causes of growth failure

comfortably resting in this position (Fig. 3.4). Three further adjustments will be made in the course of the examination. When auscultating the mitral area of the heart it is helpful to roll the patient towards the left lateral position as this brings the apex closer to the stethosope. To examine the neck, posterior chest, back, and spine you will ask the patient to sit forward. For assessing the abdomen, reposition the patient to lie flat, as this provides optimal access for the abdominal examination. Plan the examination to ensure the most economical movements for both you and the patient.

Based on the history you should already have reflected on the physical signs which might help you to confirm or refine your initial assessment. Anticipation of physical signs will help you to direct and focus the examination. For example, if a patient complains of breathlessness, you might anticipate anaemia, respiratory, or cardiac disease; therefore, you should gear the examination towards determining which of these possibilities is responsible for the symptoms.

Begin with a global inspection of overall appearance. Does the patient look comfortable or distressed? Is there a recognizable syndrome or external manifestation of disease? Is the patient normally nourished and hydrated?

RECOGNIZABLE SYNDROMES AND FACIES

Certain diseases are readily identified by a distinctive combination of physical characteristics. There are a large number of recognizable congenital syndromes which were likely diagnosed during childhood and should not present as an undiagnosed problem to physicians caring for teenagers or adults. In addition, only a proportion survive into adulthood. There are several recognizable genetic or chromosomal syndromes which may present to clinicians caring for adults; examples include Down's syndrome (Figs 3.5 and 3.6), Turner's syndrome (Figs 3.7 and 3.8), Marfan's syndrome (Figs 3.9 and 3.10), tuberous sclerosis (Figs 3.11–3.13), albinism (Figs 3.14 and 3.15), the fragile X chromosome

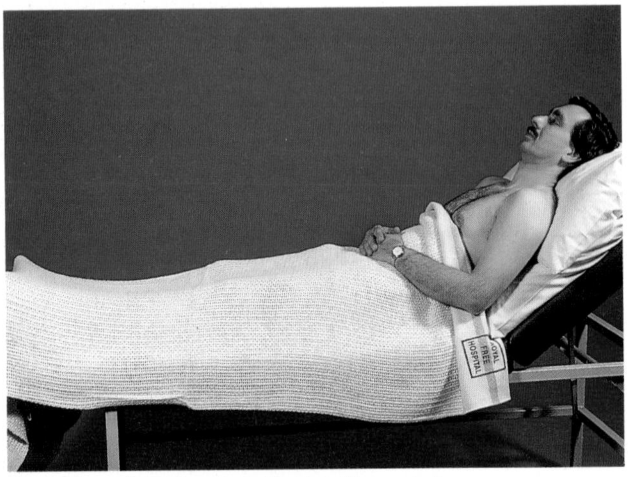

Fig. 3.4 The position of the patient at the start of the examination.

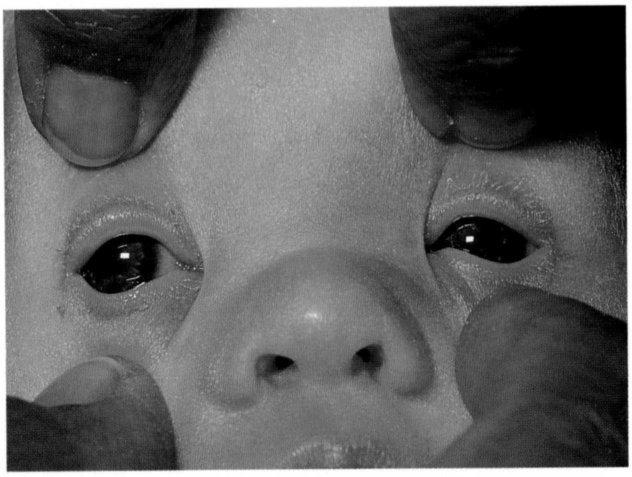

Fig. 3.5 Down's syndrome showing prominent epicanthic folds, Brushfield's spots, and hypertelorism.

Down's syndrome (Trisomy 21)

Facies – oblique orbital fissures, epicanthic folds, small ears, flat nasal bridge, protruding tongue, Brushfield's spots on iris.

Short stature

Hands – single palmar crease, curved little finger, short hands

Heart disease (endocardial cushion defects)

Gap between first and second toes

Educationally subnormal

Fig. 3.6 Down's syndrome

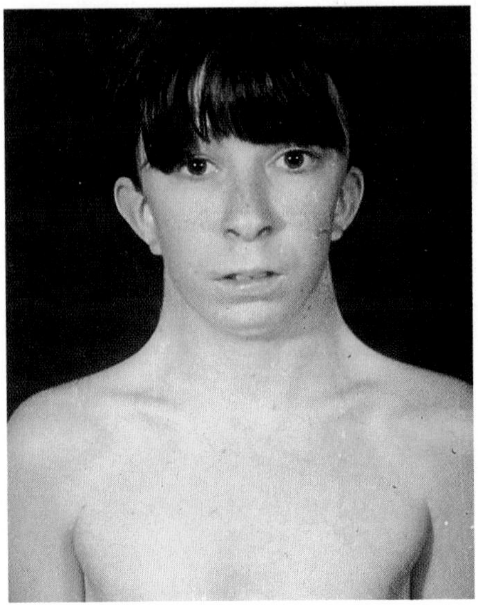

Fig. 3.7 Turner's syndrome; typical facial appearance, webbed neck, widely-spaced nipples.

Turner's syndrome (XO karyotype)

Failure of sexual development

Short stature

Facies – micrognathia (small chin), low set ears, fish-like mouth, epicanthic folds.

Short webbed neck with low hairline
widely-spaced nipples (shield-shaped chest)

Heart disease (coarctation)

Short 4th metacarpal/metatarsal

Abnormally wide carrying angle of the elbow

Fig. 3.8 Turner's syndrome.

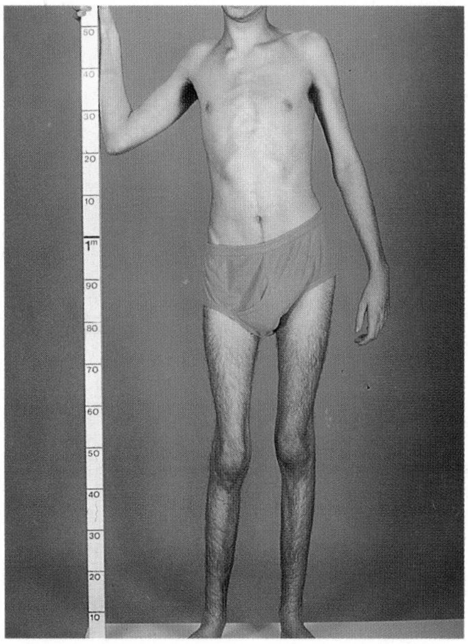

Fig. 3.9 Marfan's syndrome.

Marfan's syndrome

Armspan greater than height

Above average crown to heel height

Long slender fingers

Hyperextensible joints

Kyphoscoliosis and anterior chest wall deformity

High-arched palate

Aortic incompetence and dissecting aortic aneurysms

Subluxation or dislocation of the lens

Fig. 3.10 Marfan's syndrome.

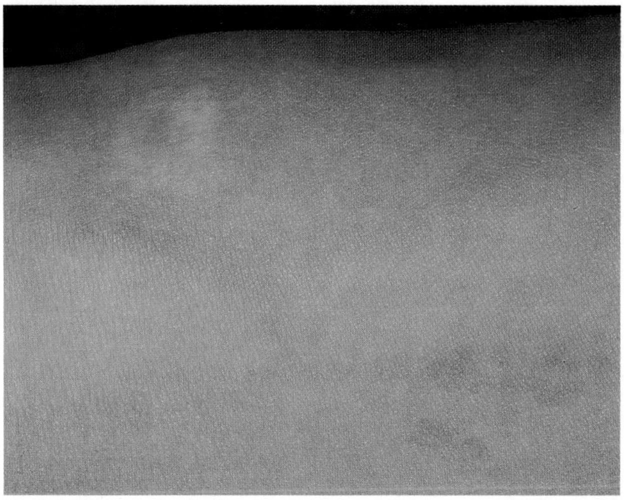

Fig. 3.11 Tuberous sclerosis. Shagreen patch.

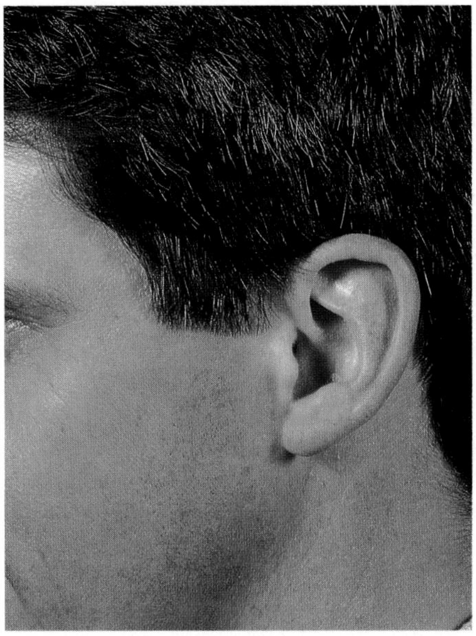

Fig. 3.12 Tuberous sclerosis. Flecks of white hair.

Tuberous sclerosis (Bourneville's disease) (autosomal dominant chromosome 9)

Epilepsy

Mental deficiency (in 2/3rds)

Skin lesions (facial adenoma sebaceum, Shagreen patch, fibromas near toenails and eyebrows)

Flecks of white hair

Retinal haemorrhages

Fig. 3.13 Tuberous sclerosis.

(a common genetic cause of mental subnormality where affected males have unusually large testes), Peutz Jeghers syndrome (Figs 3.16–3.19), Waardenburg's syndrome (Figs 3.20 and 3.21), familial hypercholesterolaemia (Figs 3.22–3.27), and neurofibromatosis. Other readily recognizable syndromes include the endocrine disorders and major organ failure (liver, heart, lungs, and kidneys).

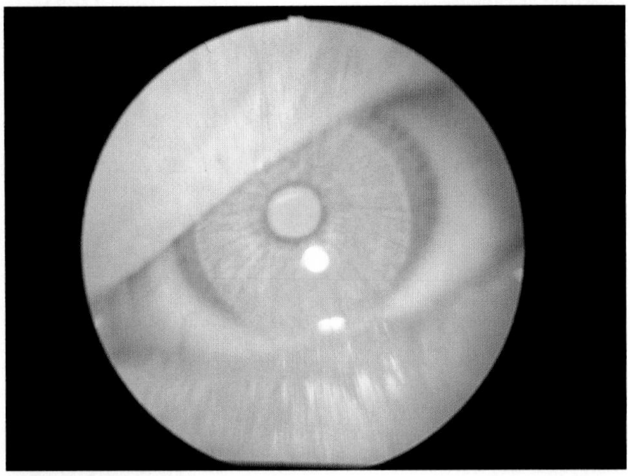

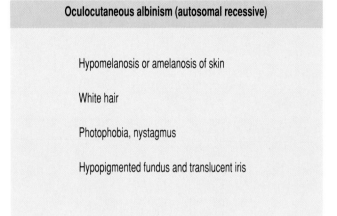

Fig. 3.14 The typical translucent iris of albinism.

Oculocutaneous albinism (autosomal recessive)

- Hypomelanosis or amelanosis of skin
- White hair
- Photophobia, nystagmus
- Hypopigmented fundus and translucent iris

Fig. 3.15 Oculocutaneous albinism.

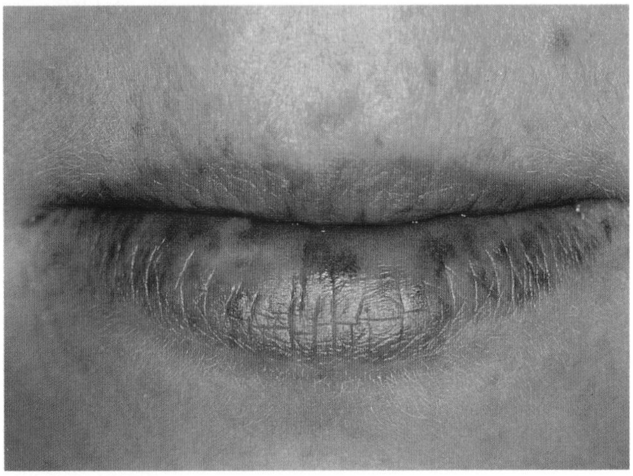

Fig. 3.16 Peutz Jeghers syndrome. Freckles on lips.

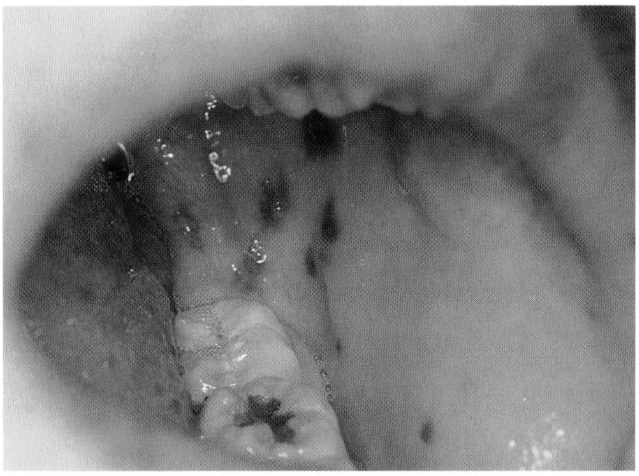

Fig. 3.17 Peutz Jeghers syndrome. Pigmented buccal mucosa.

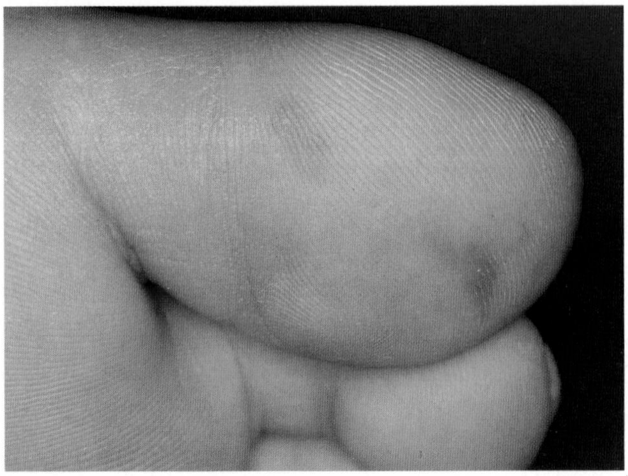

Fig. 3.18 Peutz Jeghers syndrome. Pigmentation of the big toe.

Peutz Jeghers syndrome (autosomal dominant)

- Pigmented macules (1–5mm in diameter)
- Occurs in profusion on lips, buccal mucosa, and fingers
- Gastric, small intestinal and colonic hamartomatous polyps
- Sometimes gives rise to abdominal pain, bleeding, and intussusception

Fig. 3.19 Peutz Jeghers syndrome.

ENDOCRINE SYNDROMES

The endocrine glands are scattered throughout the body (Fig. 3.28) and, unlike the other major organ systems, cannot be assessed in a regional examination; therefore, it is practical to consider the examination of the endocrine glands in the context of the overall general examination. Both over and underactivity of the endocrine glands can be suspected from the patient's facies, body build, and

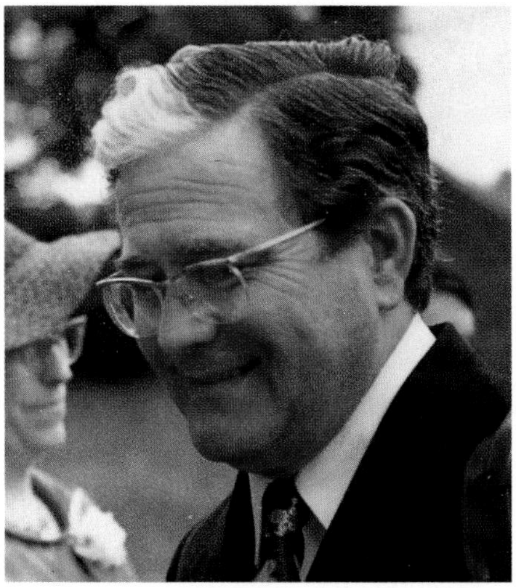

Fig. 3.20 The typical white forelock of Waardenberg's syndrome.

Waardenberg's syndrome (autosomal dominant)

- Cochlear deafness
- Frontal white lock of hair
- Wide set eyes
- Differing colour irises
- White eyelashes
- Piebaldism

Fig. 3.21 Waardenberg's syndrome.

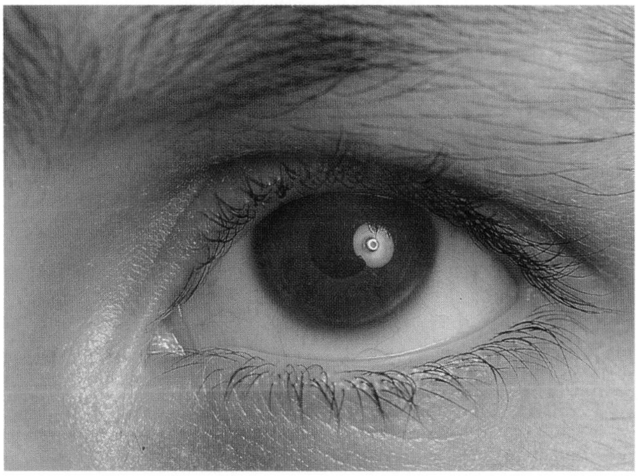

Fig. 3.22 Familial hypercholesterolaemia. Arcus senilis.

Familial hypercholesterolaemia (autosomal dominant)

- Xanthelasmas, skin xanthomas
- Tendon xanthomas
- Arcus senilis
- Marked atherosclerosis
  - Ischaemic heart disease
  - Peripheral vascular disease

Fig. 3.23 Familial hypercholesterolaemia.

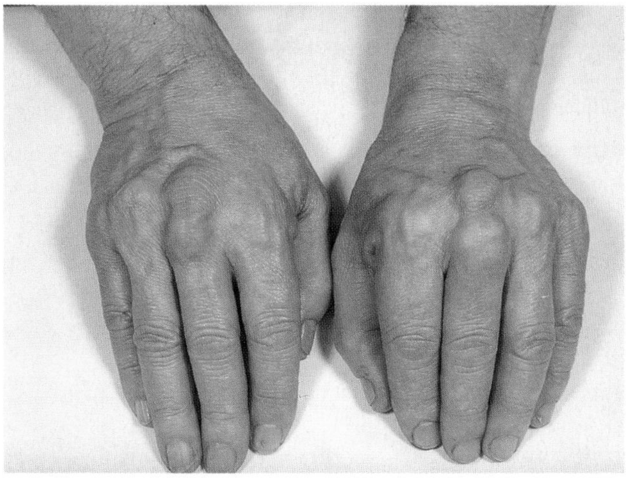

Fig. 3.24 Familial hypercholesterolaemia. Tendon xanthomas.

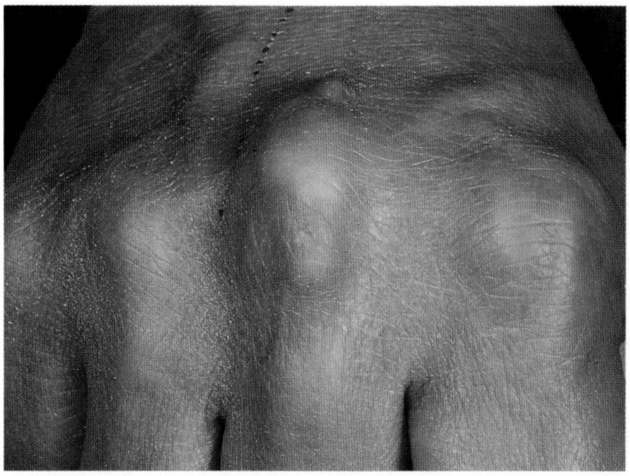

Fig. 3.25 Familial hypercholesterolaemia. Tendon xanthomas.

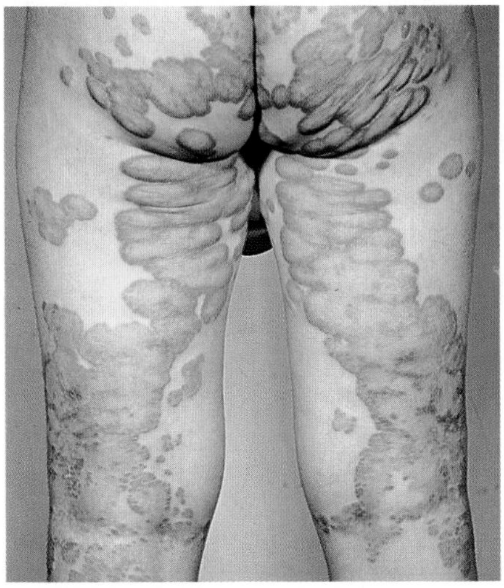

Fig. 3.26 Familial hypercholesterolaemia. Skin xanthomas.

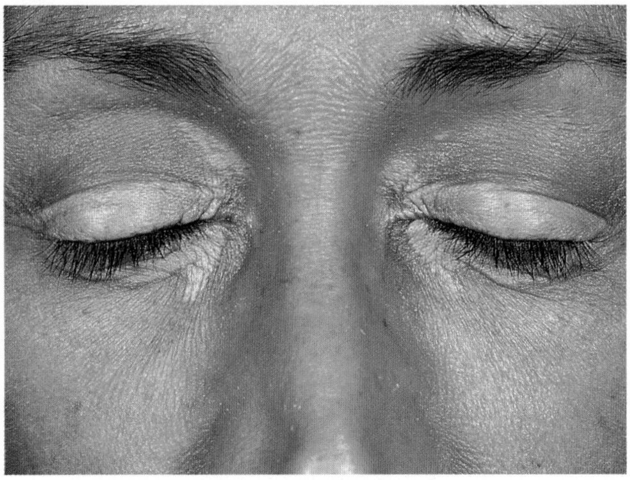

Fig. 3.27 Familial hypercholesterolaemia. Xanthelasmata around eyelids.

The endocrine organs

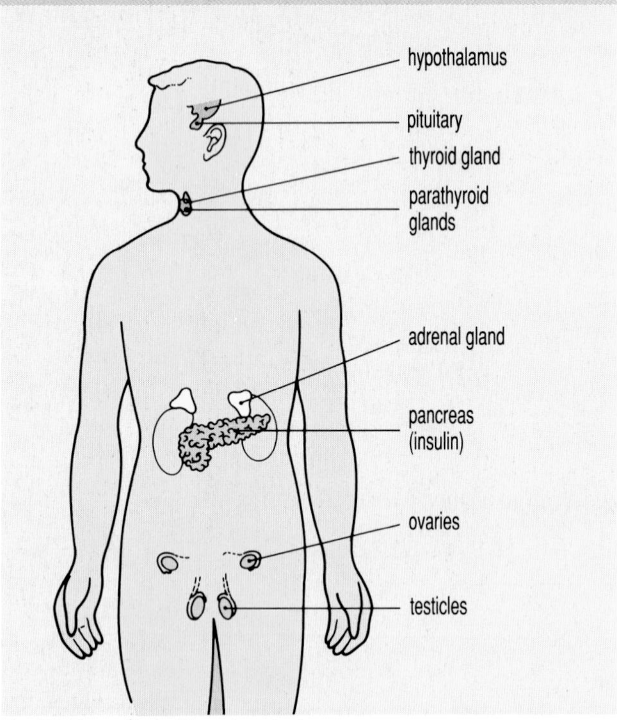

Fig. 3.28 The positions of the main endocrine organs.

Thyroid anatomy

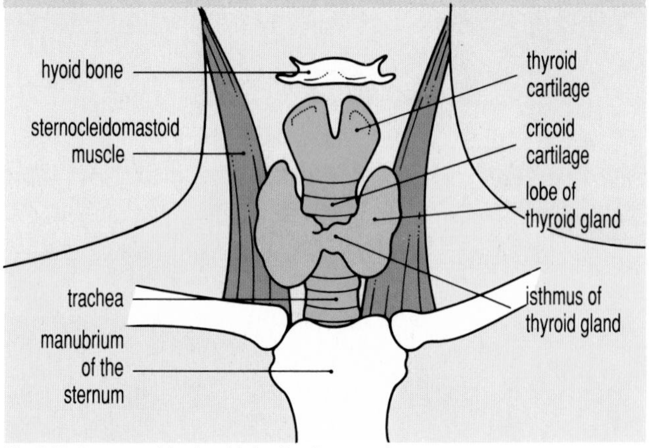

Fig. 3.29 Anatomy of the thyroid gland and surrounding structures.

skin colour; the endocrinopathies are often readily recognized in the course of the general examination.

Distinct clinical syndromes occur in diseases of the thyroid, parathyroid, adrenal, and pituitary glands. An overview of structure and function of each of these organs will help your clinical assessment and syndrome recognition.

STRUCTURE AND FUNCTION OF THE THYROID GLAND

The thyroid gland develops from a ventral pouch of the foetal pharynx. This pouch evolves into the thyroid gland by migrating caudally to a resting place in front of the trachea. The migration may leave thyroid remnants along the embryonic tract which extends from the back of the tongue (where a residual lingual thyroid 'rest' may occur). A midline thyroglossal cyst may develop if the migration tract fails to obliterate.

The thyroid gland consists of two lateral lobes joined by an isthmus. The gland lies in front of the larynx and trachea with the isthmus overlying the 2nd to 4th tracheal rings (Fig. 3.29). The lateral lobes extend from the side of the thyroid cartilage to the 6th tracheal ring. Two nerves lie in close proximity to the thyroid gland: the recurrent laryngeal nerve runs in the groove between the trachea and the thyroid, and the external branch of the superior laryngeal nerve lies deep to the upper poles. In thyroid cancer, these nerves may be invaded and damage may occur in the course of thyroid surgery.

Thyroxine synthesis and secretion

The anterior pituitary hormone, thyroid stimulating hormone (TSH), stimulates the synthesis of thyroxine (Fig. 3.30). The

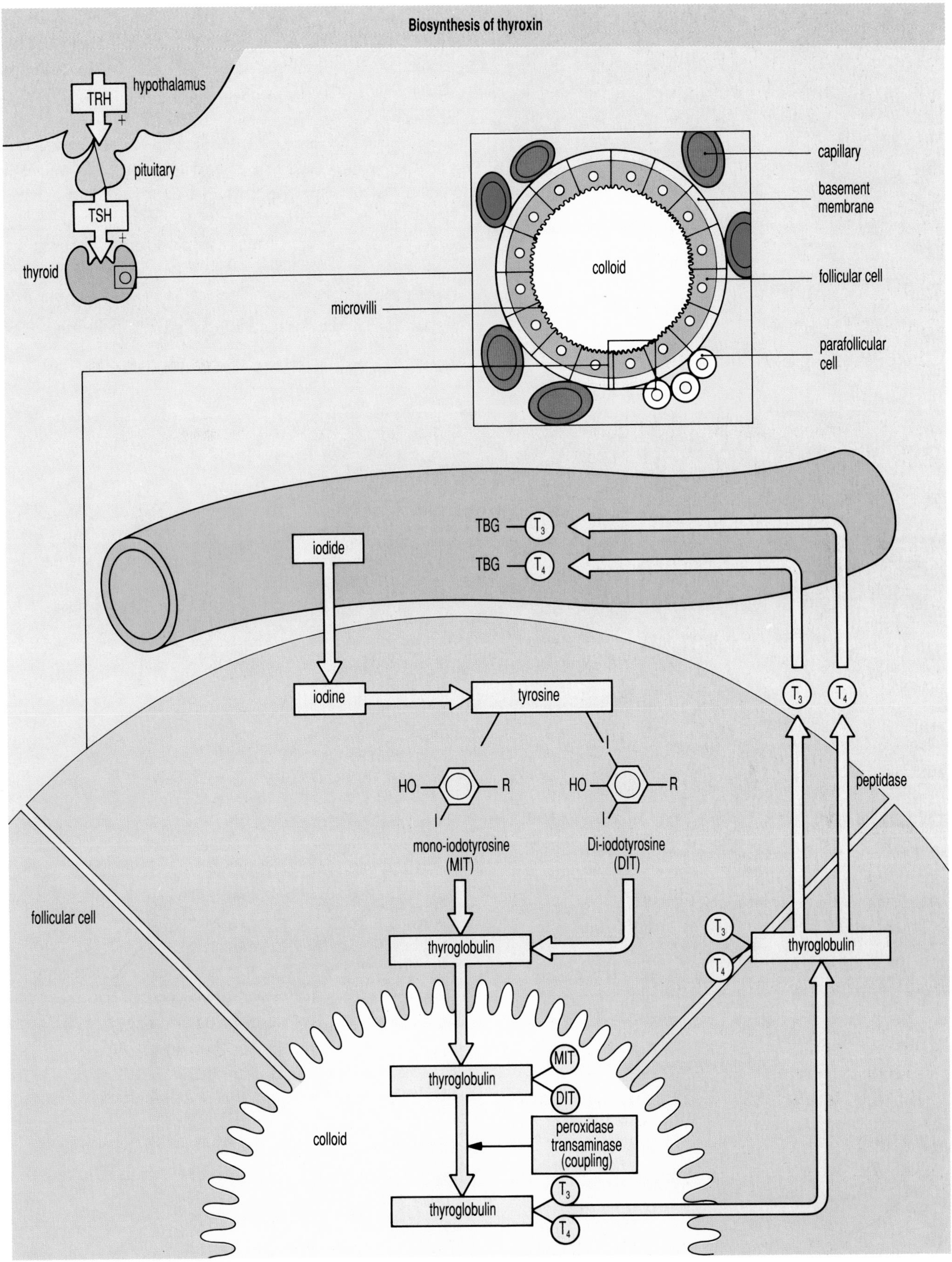

Fig. 3.30 The hypothalamus secretes TRH which stimulates the anterior pituitary to produce TSH. This simulates the synthesis of thyroxine in the follicles. Iodide taken up into the follicular cell is oxidised to iodine and then incorporated into tyrosine to form MIT and DIT which binds with thyroglobulin and is secreted into the colloid where T3 and T4 is synthesized. This is taken back into the follicular cells where the T3 and T4 is split from thyroglobulin and released into the circulation where it is bound to TBG.

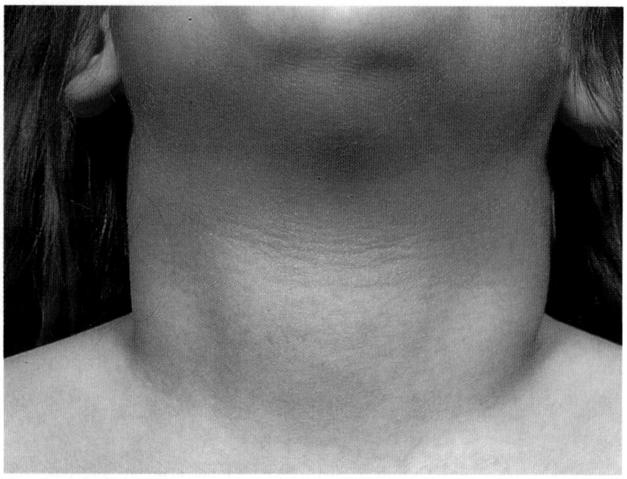

Fig. 3.31 Smooth goitre appearing as fullness in the anterior neck.

functioning unit of the thyroid is the follicle which consists of epithelial cells lining a central colloid space. The epithelial cells concentrate iodide which is oxidized to iodine and incorporated with tyrosine to form mono-iodotyrosine and di-iodotyrosine. These two iodinated tyrosines are combined in the colloid to form either tri-iodothyronine (T3) or tetra-iodothyronine (T4). The two active hormones, T3 and T4, are stored in the colloid and bound to a specific binding protein (thyroglobulin). The protein-bound hormones are taken back up into the follicle epithelium by endocytosis. In the cells, the colloid droplets are disrupted by proteolytic enzymes, allowing the release of T3 and T4 into the circulation where most circulate bound to thyroid binding globulin (TBG). Free hormone levels dictate the metabolic effects of

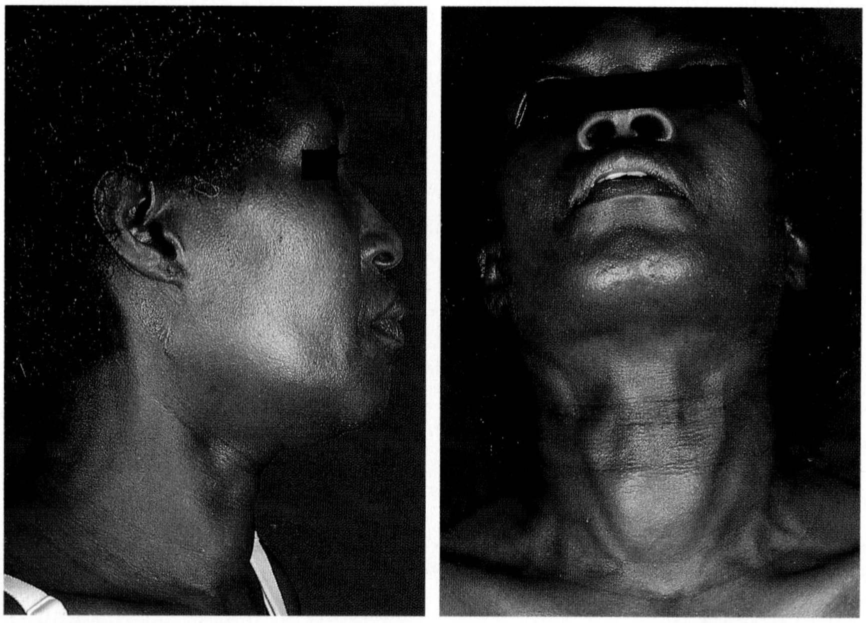

Fig. 3.32 Readily visible multinodular thyroid goitre.

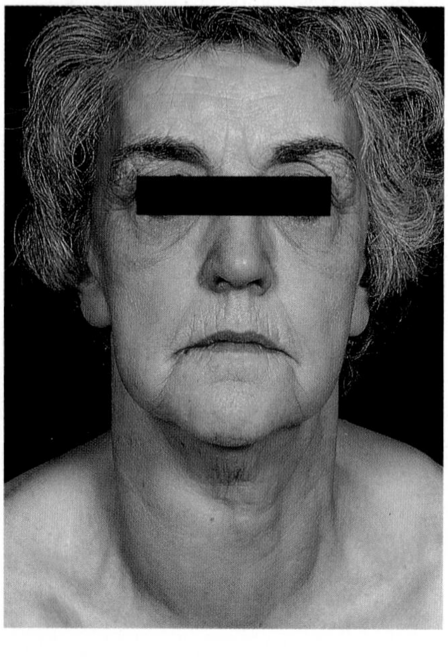

Fig. 3.33 Asymmetrical multinodular goitre.

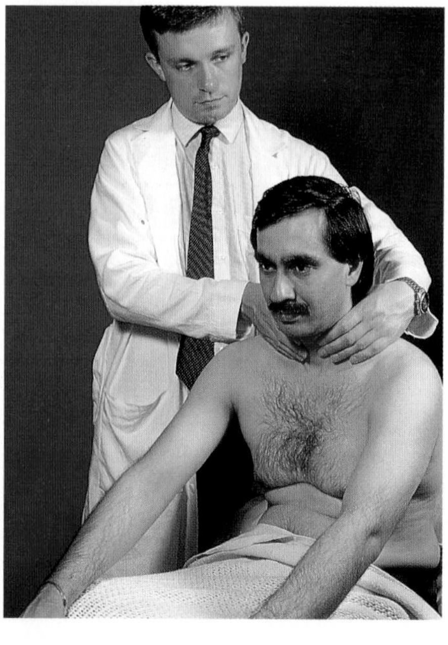

Fig. 3.34 Position for palpation of the lateral lobes and isthmus of the thyroid.

thyroxine. T4 is only synthesized in the thyroid, but T3 can also be produced from conversion of circulating T4 in the liver, the kidney, and other tissues. The heptic conversion of T4 results in two species of T3: an active T3 and an inactive reverse T3.

CLINICAL EXAMINATION OF THE THYROID GLAND AND FUNCTION

Like any other organ, the thyroid examination relies on inspection, palpation, percussion, and auscultation. Examine the thyroid gland with the patient sitting forward in bed or seated in a chair.

Ensure complete exposure of the neck and upper chest. Inspect the thyroid from the front of the neck. The normal thyroid gland is neither visible nor palpable. An enlarged thyroid (known as a goitre) is seen as a fullness on either side of the trachea below the cricoid cartilage, or as a distict, enlarged, nodular organ with one or both lobes easily visible (Figs 3.31–3.33). If the lobes are visible, determine whether they look symmetrical or irregular. Ask the patient to sip a little water and hold it in the mouth. When you give the instruction to swallow, watch for the characteristic upward movement of the goitre as the pharyngeal muscles contract. This test is helpful in distinguishing a thyroid mass from other neck masses (e.g. enlarged lymph nodes which hardlly move with swallowing). The midline remnant of the thyroid (thyroglossal cysts or thyroid remnants) also moves with swallowing.

Next, explain to the patient that you wish to feel the front of the neck for the thyroid gland. Position yourself to the right and slightly behind the patient. Feel for the left and right lobes with the finger pulps of both hands (Fig. 3.34). Ensure a gentle examination as your hands are postitioned in a throttling posture; reassure the patient by standing to the side rather than at the rear so that you remain in the patient's peripheral field of vision. Assess the texture (hard or soft, single or multiple nodules), symmetry, and extent of the goitre. A soft, smooth goitre may be more easily seen than felt. It is unusual for the goitre to be tender unless the enlargement is caused by acute inflammatory thyroiditis. In the course of thyroid palpation, again ask the patient to take a sip of water and to swallow when you indicate. As the patient gulps you should feel the goitre move beneath your fingers. Complete the palpation by feeling for the carotids which may be encased by a malignant thyroid gland. Thyroid carcinoma may spread to local neck lymph nodes, so it is important to conclude the palpation by checking for palpable regional lymph nodes.

The thyroid gland may also enlarge in a downward direction behind the manubrium sterni. This retrosternal goitre may extend quite deeply into the superior mediastinum and may even cause compression symptoms (i.e. breathlesness and dysphagia). Retrosternal extension can be assessed by percussing over the manubrium and upper sternum (Fig. 3.35). Normally, this area resonates, yet when there is retrosternal enlargement the percussion note is dull. Auscultate the gland for bruits by applying the diaphragm of the stethoscope to each lobe in turn (Fig. 3.36). Ask the patient to stop breathing for a moment whilst you listen on either side for a bruit. A soft bruit is characteristic of the smooth symmetrical hyperthyroid goitre of Graves' disease.

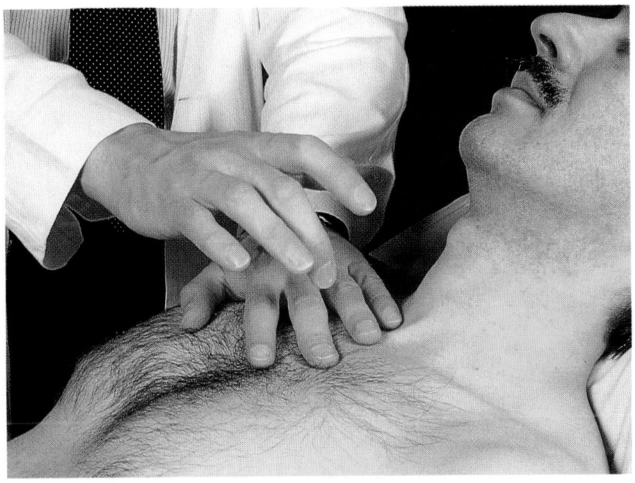

Fig. 3.35 A retrosternal goitre is suggested by dullness to percussion over the manubrium sterni.

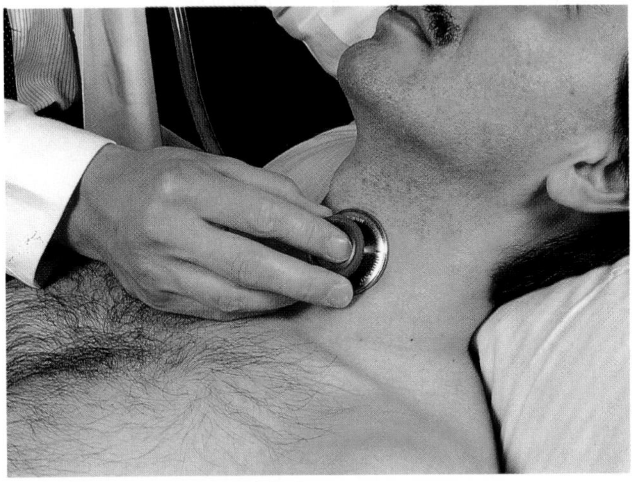

Fig. 3.36 Auscultation of the thyroid gland.

CLINICAL ASSESSMENT OF THYROID FUNCTION

Thyroxine has a number of crucial metabolic effects and over or under activity results in characteristic clinical syndromes which may readily be recognized. Diagnosis of hyperthyroidism is confirmed by measuring serum level of T4 and T3, whilst in hypothyroidism the serum TSH level is increased.

Hyperthyroidism

Hyperthyroidism occurs most commonly in young women with smooth diffuse goitres (Graves' disease). Although in the elderly, hyperthyroidism may be caused by an autonomous 'toxic'

Hyperthryroidism

Have you lost weight recently?

Has your appetite changed (e.g. increased)?

Have you noticed a change in bowel habit (e.g. increased)?

Have you noticed a recent change in heat tolerance?

Do you suffer from excessive sweating?

Does your heart race or palpitate?

Have you noticed a change in mood?

adenoma and, rarely, a functioning carcinoma (Fig. 3.37). In both young and old thyrotoxic patients, you might be alerted to the diagnosis by a history of weight loss, recent intolerance to hot weather, sweating, palpitations, abnormal irritability and nervousness, and increased bowel frequency. Most hyperthyroid patients feel warm and sweaty, have a tachycardia, staring eyes (due to lid retraction), and abnormally brisk tendon reflexes. A fine peripheral tremor is common in thyrotoxicosis. This can be demonstrated by placing a sheet of paper on the back of the outstretched hand and watching the tremor which is amplified through the sheet of paper which trembles (Fig. 3.38). Although similar signs of hyperthyroidism may occur in the young and old, Graves' disease is more readily recognizable from the characteristic facial appearance and associated physical signs (Fig. 3.39).

Graves' disease

The facies in Graves' disease is dominated by a staring appearance caused by retraction of the upper eye-lid (Fig. 3.40). Normally, in relaxed forward gaze, the upper lid protects the eye by lying in a

Clinical feature of hyperthyroidism.
Weight loss, increased appetite
Recent onset heat intolerance
Agitation, nervousness
Hot, sweaty palms
Fine peripheral tremor
Bounding peripheral pulses
Tachycardia, atrial fibrillation
Lid retraction and lid lag
Goitre, with/out overlying bruit
Brisk tendon reflexes

Fig. 3.37 Clinical feature of hyperthyroidism.

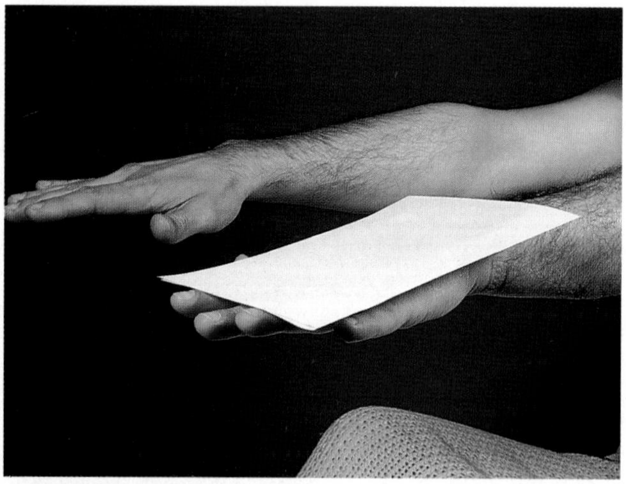

Fig. 3.38 Place a sheet of paper on the outstretched fingers to demonstrate the fine tremor of hyperthyroidism.

Hyperthyroidim in Graves' disease and toxic nodular goitre.

	Graves' disease	Toxic nodular goitre
Sex	Female>>Men	Female = Men
Eye signs	Very common, exopthalmos	Less severe
Goitre	Diffuse, overlying bruit	May be multinodular
Heart	Tachycardia, atrial fibrillation	Also angina, CCF
Weight	May lose weight	Often profound

Fig. 3.39 Hyperthyroidim in Graves' disease and toxic nodular goitre.

horizontal position which crosses the eye in a plane just above the upper pole of the pupil. In Graves' disease, autonomic overactivity causes increased tone and spasm of levator palpebrae superioris. This causes retraction of the upper lid which exposes most, if not all of the iris, exposing sclera above the iris and creating the typical staring appearance (Fig. 3.41). Spasm of the muscles supplying the upper lid also results in an abnormal following reflex. Normally, if you ask a patient to follow the movement of an object (e.g. your fingertip) (Fig. 3.42) from a point above eye level to a vertical point below eye level, you will note that as the eye moves, the upper lid follows the upper margin of the pupil in a fully synchronized downward movement. In hyperthyroidism, this coordination is lost and the movement of the upper lid lags well behind the pupil (this is termed 'lid lag') (Fig. 3.43).

In progressive Graves' disease, abnormal connective tissue deposits in the orbit and external ocular muscles. The globes are pushed forward resulting first in proptosis and in the more severe form exophthalmos (>18mm protrusion). To examine for exophthalmos seat the patient in a chair and inspect the globes from above by looking over the forehead or from the side of the profile (Fig. 3.44). A Hertel exophthalmometer can be used to make an accurate baseline measurement of the degree of exophthalmos and this measurement is used to monitor progression and regression. Other eye signs of Graves' disease include ophthalmoplegia caused by weakness and infiltration of the external ophthalmic muscles. These patients complain of double vision (diplopia) and on examination there is loss of gaze symmetry. Conjunctival oedema (chemosis) may also occur. The

Signs of Graves' disease (autoimmune hyperthyroidism).

Diffuse goitre with audible bruit

Pretibial myxoedema, finger clubbing

Onycholysis (Plummer's nails)

Eye signs: lid retraction, lid lag

Proptosis, exophthalmos

Ophthalmoplegia

Conjunctival oedema (chemosis)

Fig. 3.40 Signs of Graves' disease (autoimmune hyperthyroidism).

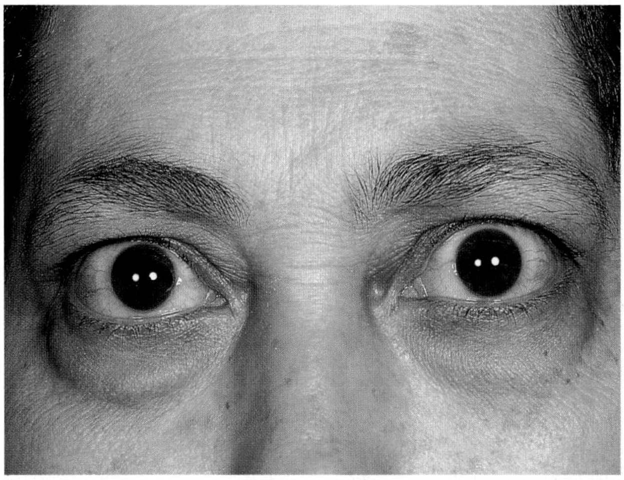

Fig. 3.41 Bilateral lid retraction in a patient with Grave's disease. Note that the upper lid is positioned well above the pupil and the palpebral fissure is widened.

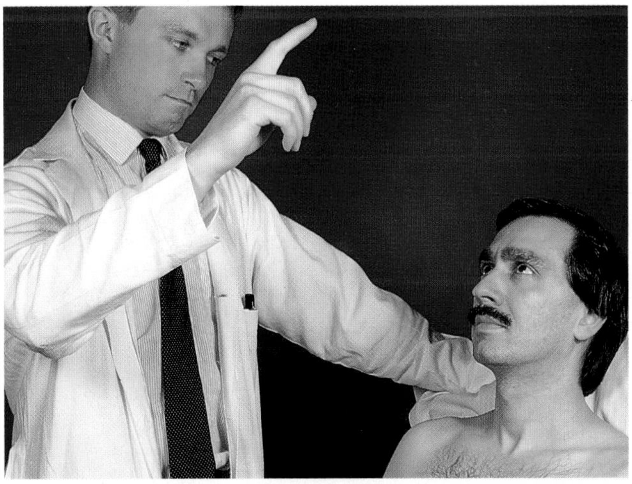

Fig. 3.42 Lid lag. With the patient sitting, position yourself on the patient's right side. Watch how the lid moves with the downward movement of the eye as the patient follows your finger moving from a point approximately 45° above the horizontal to a point below this plane. Normally, there is perfect coordination as the lid follows the downward movement of the eye.

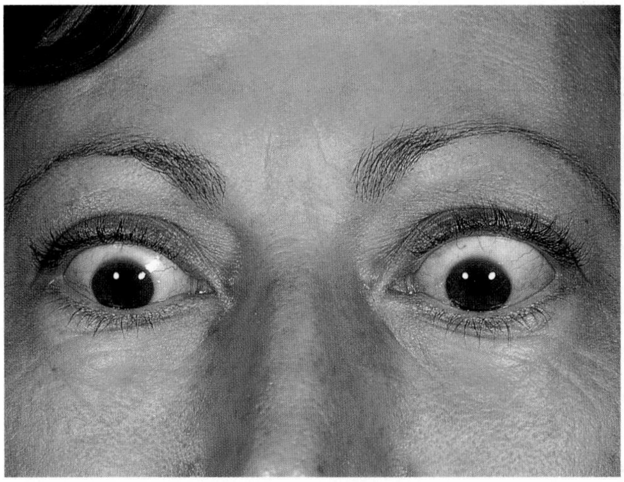

Fig. 3.43 In hyperthyroidism, the downward movement of the lid lags behind the movement of the bulb as it follows your finger through an arc.

eye signs can be either bilateral or unilateral (Fig. 3.45), although in the latter, always consider a space occupying lesion of the orbit. Other features of Graves' disease include finger clubbing, onycholysis, pretibial myxoedema (swelling of lower legs), and periostitis.

Hypothyroidism

Hypothyroidism presents insidiously; the diagnosis may be readily apparent on general examination. Suspect in patients complaining of unexplained lethargy, weight gain, newly-noted cold intolerance, constipation, generalized hair loss, and pain in the hand suggestive of a carpal tunnel syndrome (Fig. 3.46). Poor memory and general intellectual deterioration may also be presenting features. You might notice the unusually hoarse voice whilst taking the history. The disorder may occur at any age although it is most common in the elderly. There are a number of possible causes to consider (Fig. 3.47). On first sight you might notice the characteristic puffy facial appearance, the pale 'waxy' skin, and diffuse hair loss from the scalp and eyebrows. Look for other signs to confirm your clinical suspicion of myxoedema (Fig. 3.48). The delayed relaxation phase of the Achilles tendon jerk is especially helpful (Fig. 3.49).

Hypothyroidism

Has your weight changed?

Has your bowel habit changed (e.g. constipation)?

Is your hair falling out?

Have you noticed a change in weather preference (e.g. cold intolerance)?

Has there been a change in your voice (e.g. hoarse)?

Do you suffer from pain in your hands (e.g. carpal tunnel syndrome)?

STRUCTURE AND FUNCTION OF THE PARATHYROID GLANDS

There are usually four parathyroid glands (two superior and two inferior). Ninety per cent of parathyroid glands lie in intimate

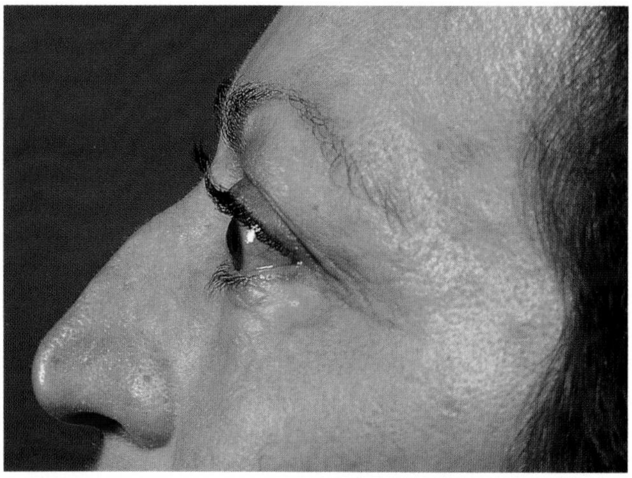

Fig. 3.44 Proptosis of the eye in Graves' disease.

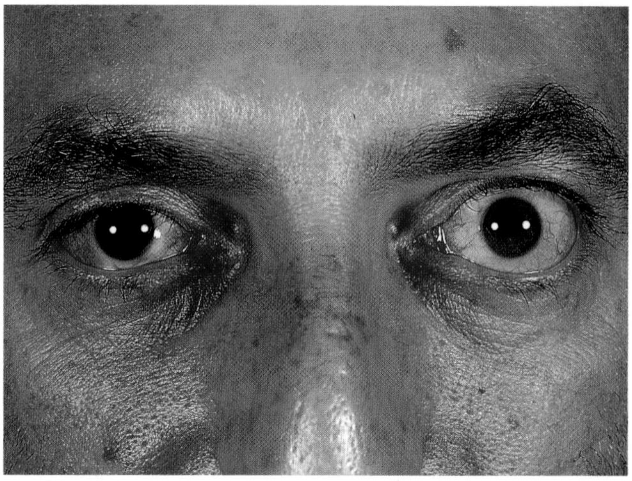

Fig. 3.45 Unilateral eye disease in Grave's disease

Clinical features of hypothyroidism
Constipation, weight gain
Hair loss
Angina pectoris
Hoarse, croaky voice
Dry flaky skin
Balding and loss of eyebrow (beginning laterally)
Bradycardia
Xanthelasmas (hyperlipidaemia)
Goitre (especially with iodine deficiency)
Effusions (pericardial/pleural)
Delayed relaxation phase of tendon reflexes
Carpal tunnel syndrome

Fig. 3.46 Clinical features of hypothyroidism,

Causes of hypothyroidism.
Congenital
Congenital absence
Inborn errors of thyroxine metabolism
Acquired
Iodine deficiency (endemic goitre)
Autoimmune thyroiditis (Hashimoto's disease)
Post-radiotherapy for hyperthyroidism
Post-surgical thyroidectomy
Antithyroid drugs (e.g. carbimazole)
Pituitary tumors and granulomas

Fig. 3.47 Causes of hypothyroidism.

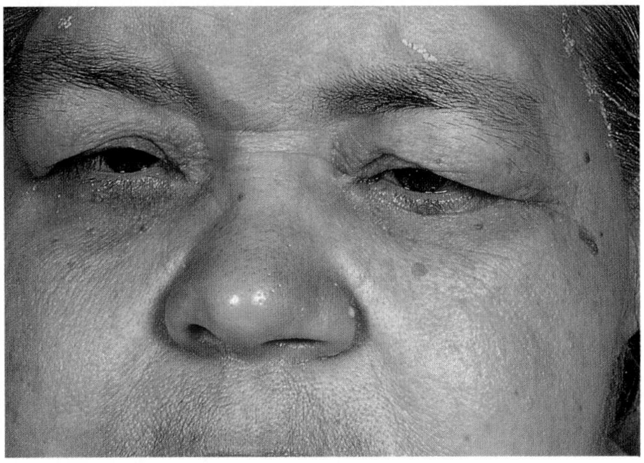

Fig. 3.48 Myxoedema.

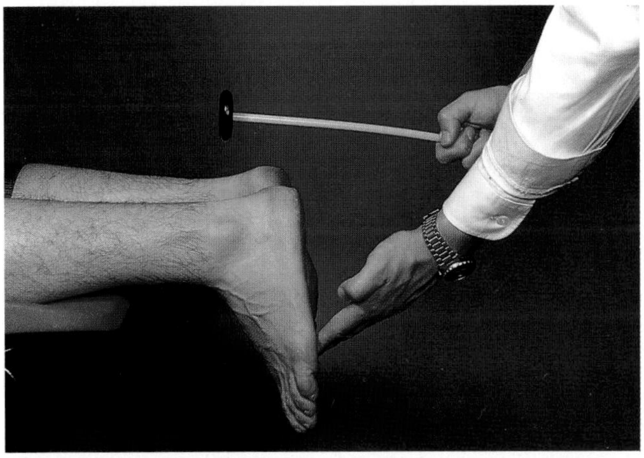

Fig. 3.49 The ankle jerk in hypothyroidism. Although all the reflexes demonstrate a distinct slowing of the relaxation phase of the tendon reflex, this sign is best observed and felt with the Achilles tendon jerk. Ask the patient to kneel on a chair or examination couch with the feet hanging over the edge. Expose the Achilles tendon and percuss with a patellar hammer whilst gently resting one hand on the sole of the foot. Watch and feel for the unusually delayed return of the foot to its resting position after the reflex

contact with the thyroid gland, although in 10 percent the inferior glands lie in an aberrant position. The pea-sized glands usually lie embedded in the posterior aspect of the upper and lower poles of the thyroid, or superficially on the surface of the thyroid.

Parathyroid hormone

This hormone is synthesized in a precursor form known as pre-pro-PTH which is first cleaved to pro-PTH and then cleaved again to the 84 amino-acid polypeptide, PTH (Fig. 3.50). PTH secretion is regulated by the level of calcium in the blood; hypocalcaemia stimulates release. In the circulation, the 84 amino acid PTH is cleaved to smaller fragments, most of which are inactive. The only active fragments are those containing the first 32 amino acids. The hormone's prime effect is on the renal tubule where it stimulates calcium resorption from the tubular fluid and phosphate excretion in the urine. PTH also stimulates calcium resorption from bone.

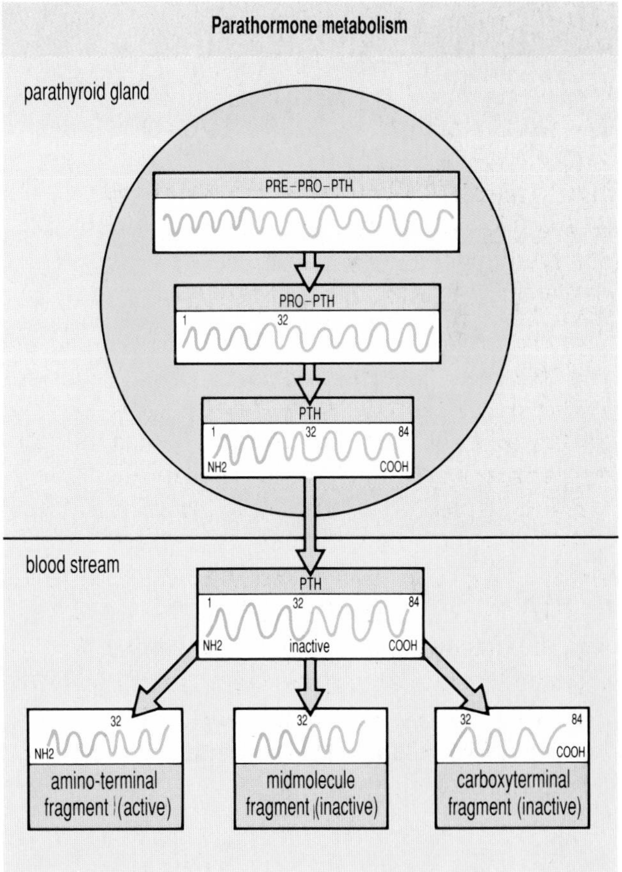

Fig. 3.50 Parathormone metabolism: a large precursor molecule is cleaved to form an 84 amino acid molecule PTH which is secreted into the blood stream. The molecute has an amino and a carboxy terminal which is cleaved to smaller fragments. Only fragments with the first 32 amino terminal amino acids are metabolically active.

Hyperparathyroidism

Hyperparathyroidism is usually detected by finding an abnormally high serum calcium level on routine blood testing or in patients presenting with renal colic due to stones. Hyperparathyroidism may be caused by hyperplasia or one or more autonomous adenomas (often associated with the multiple endocrine neoplasia syndromes). In chronic renal failure, longstanding stimulation may result in loss of feedback and an autonomous secretion of PTH leading to hypercalcaemia (this is known as tertiary hyperparathyroidism). The clinical syndrome may be difficult to recognize, as the symptoms ('moans') dominate the signs ('stones and bones'). The patient complains of tiredness and lethargy, excessive thirst (polydipsia), and symptoms of increased urine output (nocturia and frequency). There may be quite profound changes in the mental state and in severe cases, drowsiness and even coma may occur. The patient may complain of gastrointestinal symptoms including nausea and constipation. Renal stones are common and the patient might present with severe acute unilateral abdominal pain radiating towards the groin. On examination, there may be proximal muscle weakness (due to a myopathy), a thin opaque ring around the limbus of the cornea, and bone pain or radiological evidence of hyperparathyroidism (Figs 3.51 and 3.52).

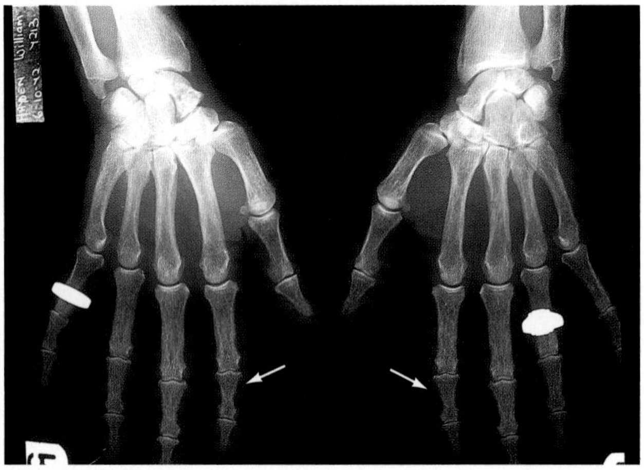

Fig. 3.51 In hyperparathyroidism, an X-ray of the phalanges may show subperiosteal erosions and bone cysts.

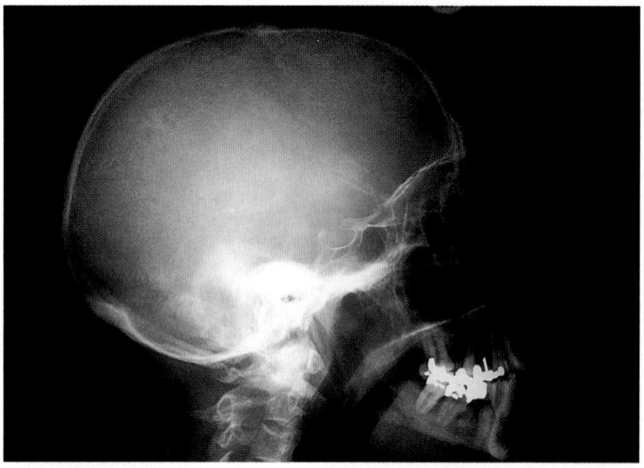

Fig. 3.52 Skull X-ray shows thinning of the cortex and small osteolytic areas – known as 'pepper pot' skull.

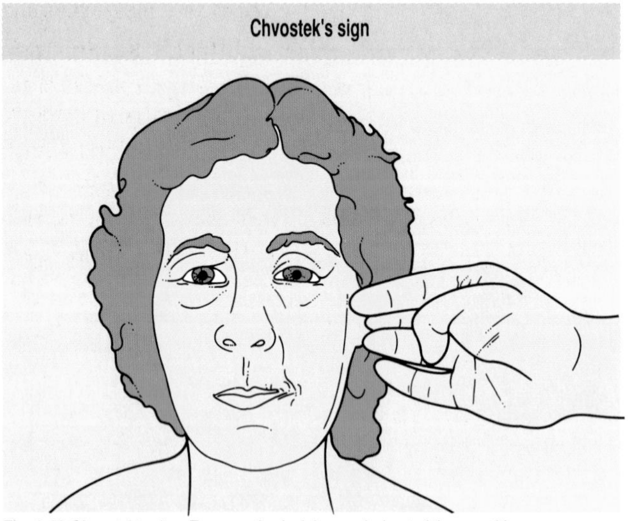

Fig. 3.53 Chvostek's sign. Tap over the facial nerve in front of the ear; this causes a momentary twitch of the corner of the mouth on the same side as the irritable facial muscles contract.

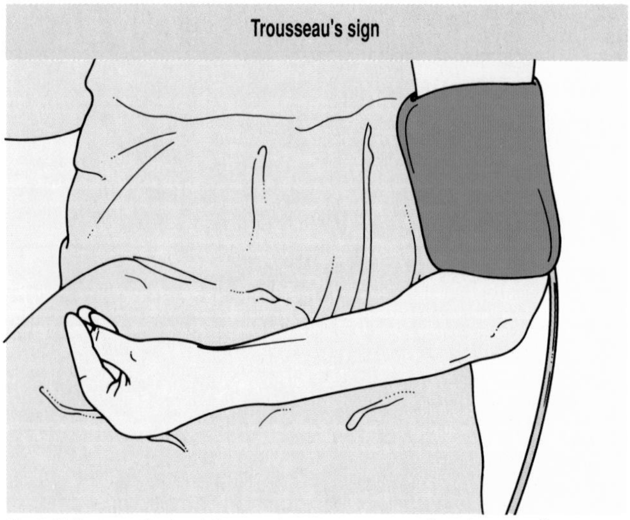

Fig. 3.54 Trousseau's sign. Inflate a sphygmomanometer cuff to above systolic pressure. Within about 4 minutes, there is characteristic 'carpopedal' spasm of the hand. There is opposition of the thumb, extension of the interphalangeal joints and flexion of the metacarpophalangeal joints. This posture reverses spontaneously when the cuff is deflated.

Hypoparathyroidism

Surgical damage or removal of three or four parathyroid glands during neck surgery (usually thyroid) is the commonest cause of hypoparathyroidism. Rarely, autoimmune destruction may cause hypoparathyroidism. The serum calcium level is low (in the presence of a normal serum albumin). The major symptoms of acute hypoparathyroidism are paraesthesiae around the mouth, fingers, and toes. Abnormal irritability of the nerves and muscles can be elicited with Chvostek's (Fig. 3.53) and Trousseau's signs (Fig. 3.54). In chronic hypoparathyroidism, the physical effects develop slowly. The symptoms include tiredness, fatigue, muscle cramp and epilepsy. Premature cataracts should also alert you to the possibility of underlying chronic hypoparathyroidism.

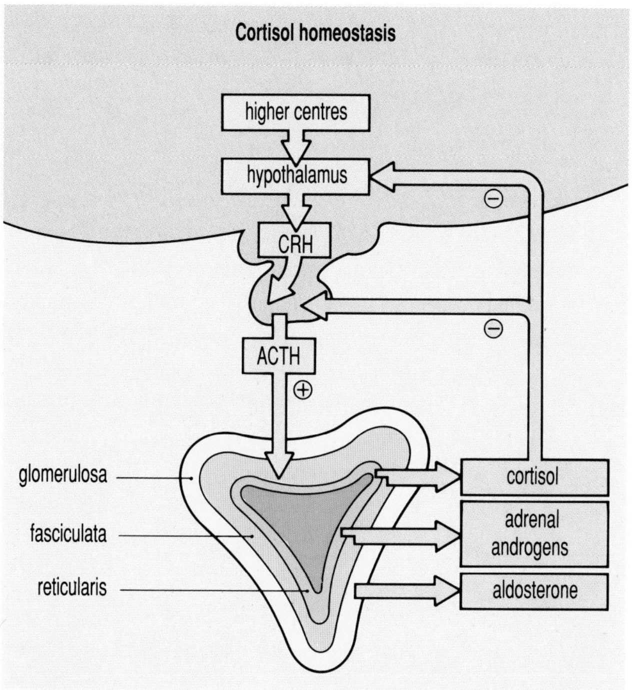

Fig. 3.55 The secretion of cortisol is stimulated by ACTH secretion and this, in turn, is under negative feedback control by circulating cortisol. Aldosterone is secreted from the zona glomerulosa by the stimulatory effect of angiotensin II.

STRUCTURE AND FUNCTION OF THE ADRENAL GLAND

The high fat content of the adrenal glands (suprarenal) gives the organ a distinctive yellow colour. The adrenals lie on the upper poles of the kidneys abutting on the diaphragm. Each gland weighs about four grams and has a rich arterial blood supply from vessels derived from the aorta, renal, and phrenic arteries. A single adrenal vein drains from the hila of the glands to the inferior vena cava on the right and to the renal vein on the left. The gland has an outer cortex derived from mesoderm and central medulla, which is derived from neuro-ectoderm.

The cortex comprises 90 per cent of the gland and consists of three distinct layers: the subcapsular zona glomerulosa, the middle zona fasciculata, and the zona reticularis which lies adjacent to the medulla (Fig. 3.55).

Hormone regulation

The adrenal cortex synthesizes three steroid hormones: the mineralocorticoids, glucocorticoids, and androgens. Aldosterone is produced in the cells of the zona glomerulosa. Aldosterone secretion is primarily regulated by the renin angiotensin system, which in turn is influenced by the intravascular volume (Fig. 3.56).

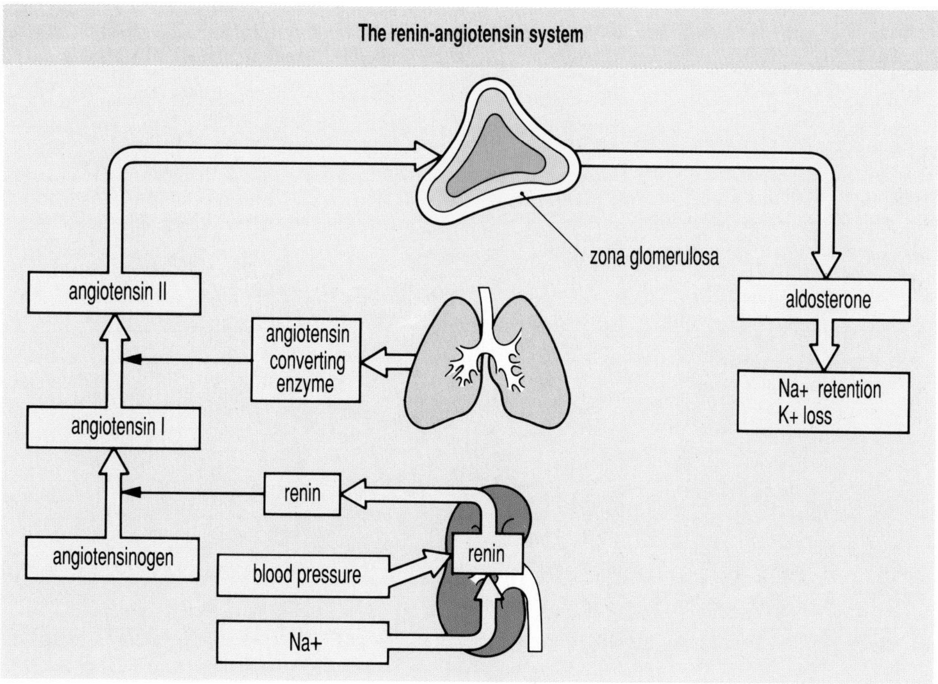

Fig. 3.56 The renin-angiotensin system. Renin is secreted from the juxta glomerular apparatus of the kidney in response to reduced serum sodium or reduced renal blood pressure. Renin converts angiotensinogen to angiotensin I which in turn is converted to angiotensin II by ACE from the lung. The angiotensin II stimulates aldosterone release from the cells of the zona glomerulosa.

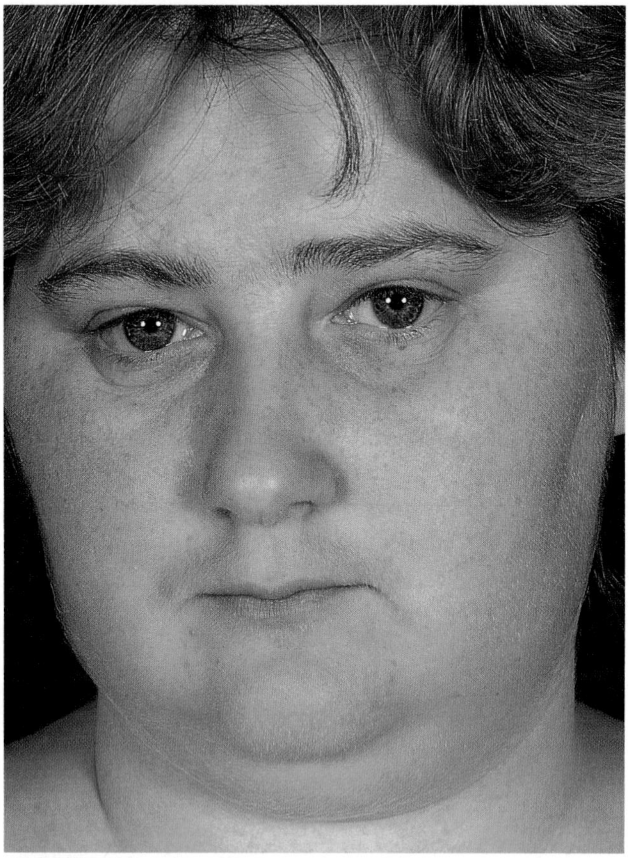

Fig. 3.57 Cushing's syndrome. Plethoric 'moon shaped' facies.

In contrast to the glucocorticoids, mineralocorticoid metabolism is not influenced by corticotrophin (ACTH). When adrenal failure is secondary to pituitary failure, mineralocorticoid function is preserved, whereas glucocorticoid function may be seriously impaired. Aldosterone promotes the entry of sodium into cells and the secretion of potassium from cells; consequently, the overall effect of aldosterone is to cause sodium retention and potassium loss. This effect on renal tubular cells plays a central role in the regulation of sodium, potassium, and water balance. Aldosterone-producing tumors of the adrenal cortex cause Conn's syndrome which is characterized by hypertension, oedema (due to sodium and water retention), and hypokalaemia.

The cells of the zona fasciculata and reticularis synthesize cortisol and adrenal androgens. Glucocorticoid synthesis and secretion is under direct control of ACTH secreted by the anterior pituitary. The secretion of ACTH is itself regulated by the release of hypothalamic corticotrophin releasing hormone (CRH). There is a feedback loop between the hypothalamus and pituitary on one side of the axis and the adrenal on the other. Whilst ACTH stimulates glucocorticoid and adrenal androgen synthesis and secretion, cortisol (and exogenous corticosteroids as well) inhibit ACTH secretion by impairing the release of CRH and directly inhibiting ACTH release from the anterior pituitary.

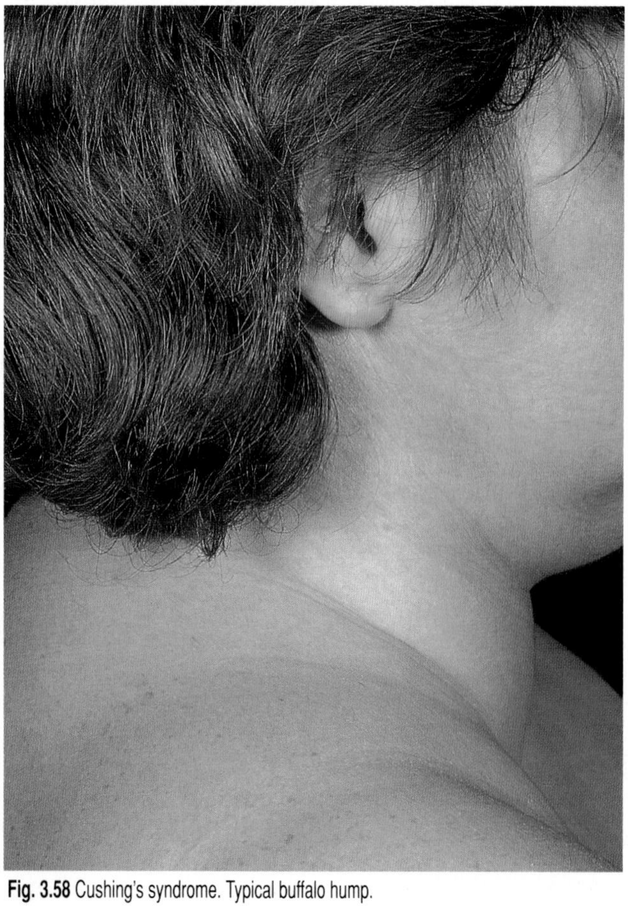

Fig. 3.58 Cushing's syndrome. Typical buffalo hump.

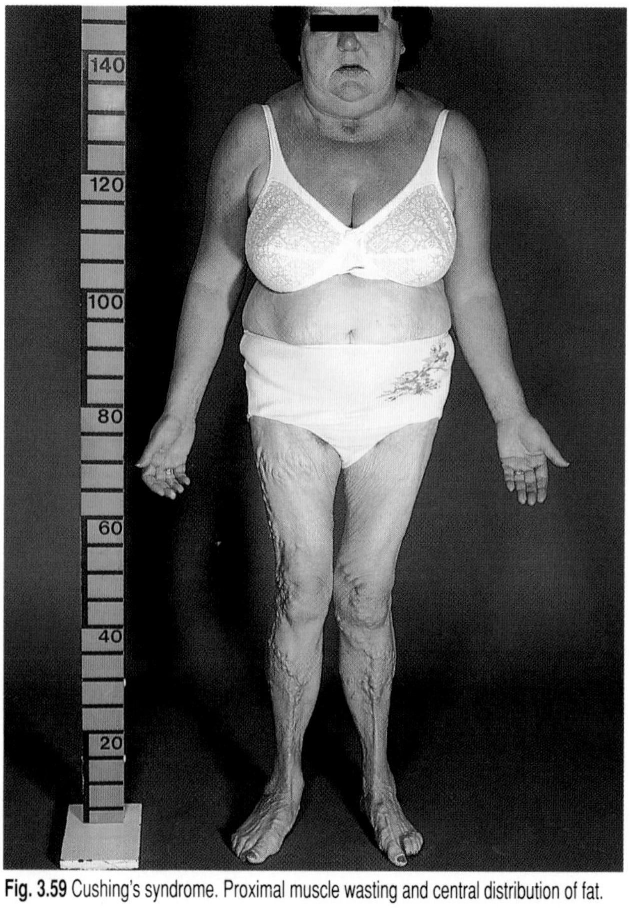

Fig. 3.59 Cushing's syndrome. Proximal muscle wasting and central distribution of fat.

The hormones of the adrenal cortex have a circadian rhythm: blood levels of cortisol and aldosterone are highest on waking and lowest at and around midnight. Glucocorticoids promote the conversion of protein to glucose (gluconeogenesis) and inhibit the peripheral utilisation of glucose. The corticosteroids increase blood pressure, support kidney function by increasing the glomerular filtration rate. Diagnosis of adrenal disease is based on measurement of ACTH, blood cortisol, and the adrenal response to ACTH stimulation.

Hyperadrenalism (Cushing's syndrome)

Excessive glucocorticoids (either endogenous or exogenous) cause significant change in body appearance which can be readily recognized as Cushing's syndrome. A Cushingoid appearance is most commonly caused by treatment with exogenous steroids. The syndrome is also typical of bilateral adrenal hyperplasia, adrenal adenomas, and occasionally carcinoma of the adrenal. In addition, certain tumors (e.g. lung) can secret ACTH-like peptides which stimulate the adrenals to hypersecrete. The most characteristic feature is the rounded, 'moon-shaped' face (Fig. 3.57), the obese body (Fig. 3.58), and, thin limbs (Fig. 3.59). Look for the other features to try and confirm a clinical diagnosis (Fig. 3.60). A typical Cushingoid appearance may also occur in chronic alcoholism and in this setting, it is called pseudo-Cushing's syndrome. The diagnosis is suspected if the physical appearance of Cushing's syndrome occurs against a background of excessive alcohol consumption. The physical and biochemical abnormalities of pseudo-Cushing's syndrome regresses when alcohol is discontinued.

Hypoadrenalism and Addison's disease

Acute adrenal failure may occur in septicaemic illnesses (especially meningococcal septicaemia), in patients chronically treated with exogenous steroids whose treatment is accidently discontinued, and in steroid-dependent patients whose drug dosage is not increased at times of physical stress (e.g. when undergoing surgery).

In acute adrenal failure the clinical features may be non-specific and puzzling. The patient usually presents with malaise, weakness, nausea and vomiting, and abdominal pain with an acute change in bowel habit (constipation or diarrhoea). The most helpful physical sign is the profound drop in blood pressure when the patient quickly changes position from lying to standing (postural hypotension). Collapse and prostration may occur. Because of a mineralocorticoid deficiency, serum potassium levels are actually elevated.

Chronic, progressive adrenal failure may be caused by tuberculous involvement of the adrenals, metastatic secondaries or Addison's disease, an auto-immune destructive disease of the adrenals. On examination, there are usually clinical clues to the diagnosis. Increased pigmentation develops in the skin (especially sun-exposed areas, pressure points, areolae and skin creases) (Fig. 3.61) and mucous membranes (seen best in the buccal mucous membrane). In Addison's disease, patients may also develop characteristic symmetrical patches of depigmented skin (vitligo). Vague abdominal pain, altered bowel habit, weight loss, and weakness also occur. Like the acute disease, postural hypotension is a helpful clinical sign which, later in the course of the disease, may dominate the patient's symptoms.

Clinical features of Cushing's syndrome
Round, moon-shaped, plethoric facies
Hirsutes
Acne
Hypertension
Buffalo hump on neck (fatty deposit)
Central distribution of fat
Proximal muscle weakness and wasting
Purple skin striae

Fig. 3.60 Clinical features of Cushing's syndrome.

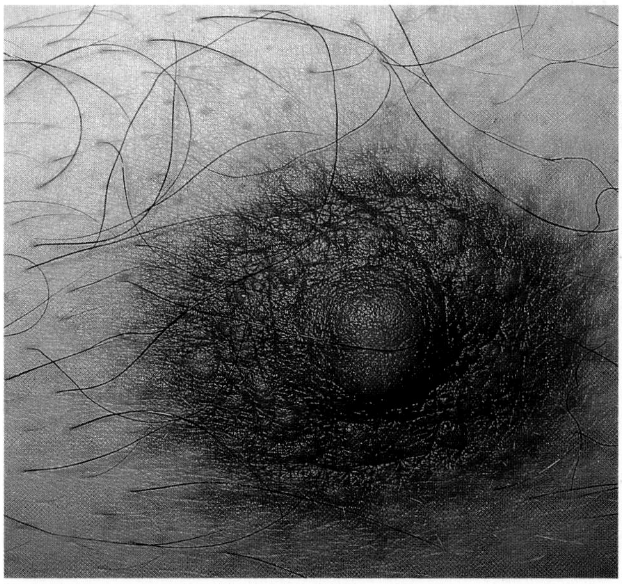

Fig. 3.61 Hyperpigmentation of the areola in Addison's disease.

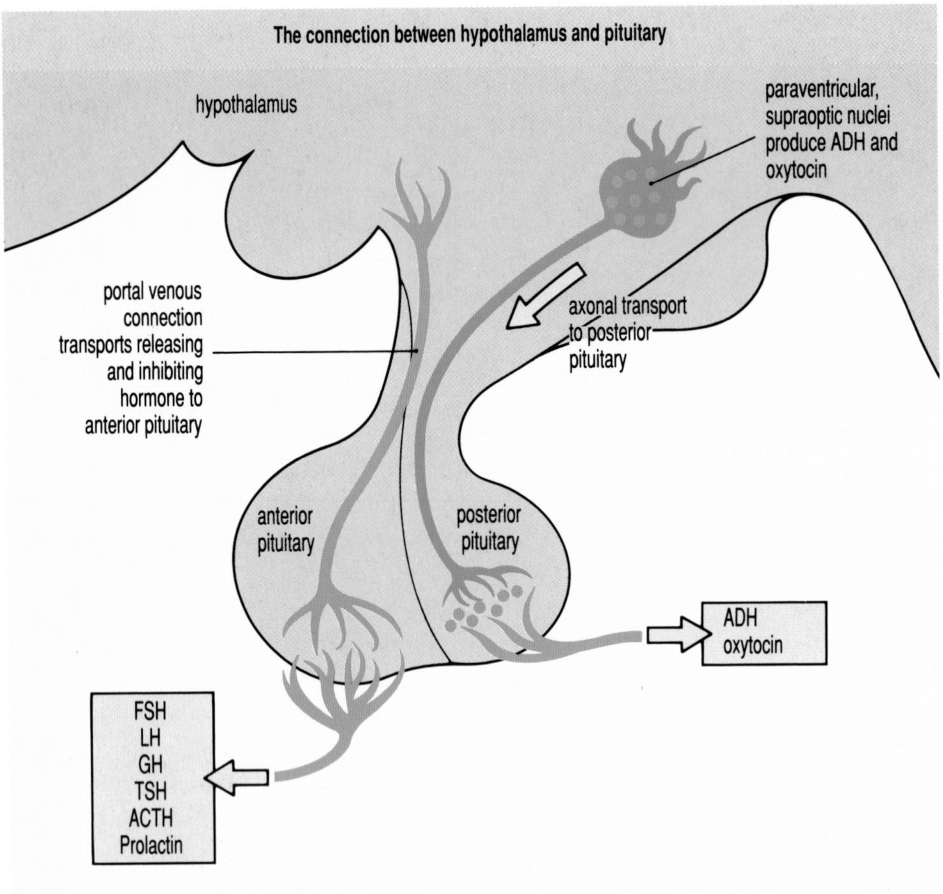

Fig. 3.62 The hypothalamus connects to the anterior pituitary by a portal venous network which carries releasing and inhibiting hormones to stimulate the release of hormones into the circulation. By contrast, the posterior pituitary hormones are synthesized in the supraoptic and paraventricular nuclei of the hypothalamus and transported to the posterior pituitary along axons which discharge directly into the systemic circulation.

STRUCTURE AND FUNCTION OF THE PITUITARY GLAND

The pituitary gland lies suspended from the hypothalamus by the infundibulum and lies in the pituitary fossa at the base of the skull (Fig. 3.62). The hypothalamus communicates with the anterior pituitary (or adenohypophysis) via a unique portal blood system which transports chemical stimuli to the anterior pituitary. A different form of communication occurs with the posterior pituitary (or neurohypophysis). The supraoptic and paraventricular nuclei of the hypothalamus synthesize ADH (vasopressin) and oxytocin and these hormones flow along the axons to nerve endings in the posterior pituitary where they released into the circulation so that they can assert their distant effects.

Hormones synthesized and secreted by the anterior pituitary include follicle stimulating hormone (FSH), luteinizing hormone (LH), growth hormone (GH), prolactin, thyroid stimulating hormone (TSH) and adrenocorticophic hormone (ACTH). These hormones are regulated by the secretion of specific releasing factors produced in the hypothalamus and transported to the pituitary by the hypothalamopituitary portal circulation (Fig. 3.63). The regulation of the anterior pituitary hormones is controlled by the balance between the stimulating effects of the release factors and the inhibitory feedback from the target circulating hormone. There are also inhibitory hypothalamic hormones (somatostatin and dopamine). Prolactin release is inhibited by hypothalamic dopamine. This neurotransmitter is secreted into the portal circulation causing tonic inhibition of prolactin release (Fig. 3.64).

Hypothalamic osmoreceptors and volume receptors sense blood osmolality and effective circulating volume, and regulate the secretion of ADH from the posterior pituitary. ADH reduces free water clearance by the distal tubules of the nephron resulting in concentration of the urine and water conservation. Oxytocin from the posterior pituitary causes uterine contraction during childbirth. In addition, the hormone promotes milk ejection during lactation by stimulating contraction of the smooth muscles surrounding the gland's ducts.

Pituitary tumors may cause overstimulation syndromes or destruction of the gland and deficiency syndromes. Both over and understimulation cause recognizable clinical syndromes which can be identified on general examination. Remember that pituitary tumors may be associated with other endocrine adenomas, especially parathyroid adenomas which cause hypercalcaemia. Diagnosis of pituitary disease depends on the responsiveness of stimulatory influences (e.g. effect of administration of hypothalamic releasing hormones or insulin induced hypoglycaemic stress).

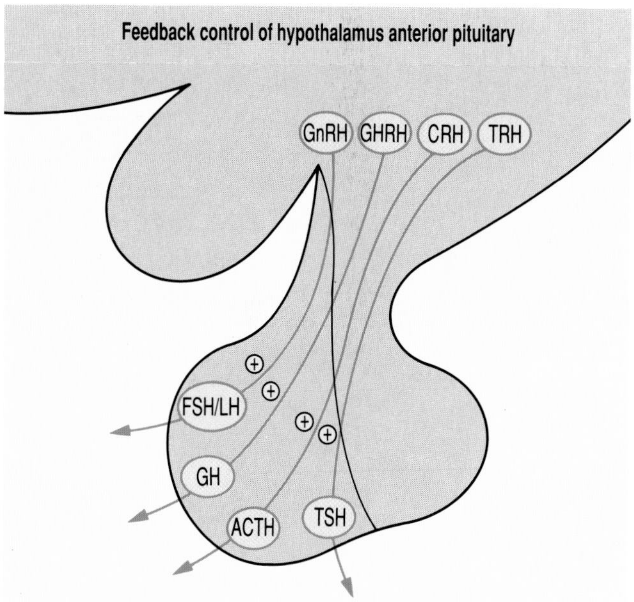

Fig. 3.63 The regulation of the hypothalamic-anterior pituitary endocrine axis.

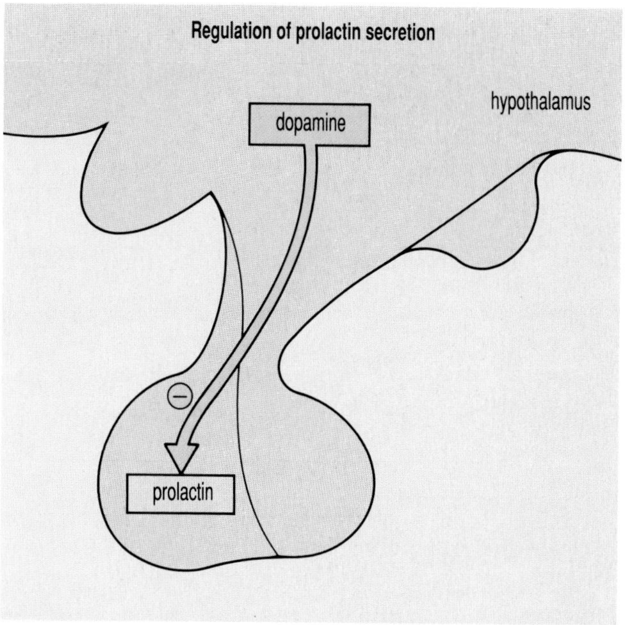

Fig. 3.64 Prolactin secretion from the anterior pituitary in inhibited by the tonic secretion of dopamine from the hypothalamus.

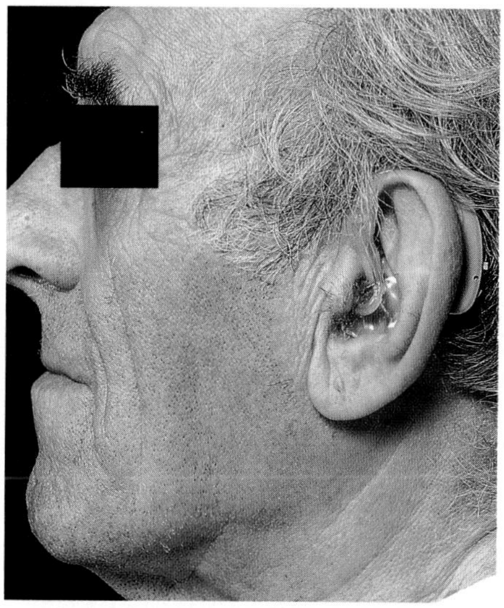

Fig. 3.65 Acromegaly. Typical appearance of the face.

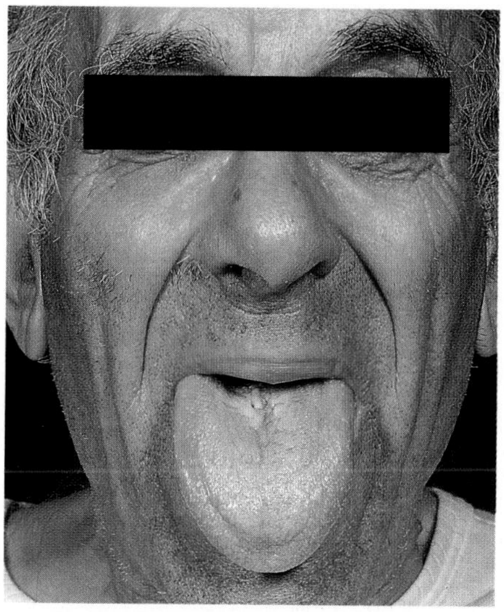

Fig. 3.66 Large tongue of acromegaly.

SYNDROMES ASSOCIATED WITH OVERPRODUCTION OF PITUITARY HORMONES.

Acromegaly

Acidophil (or more rarely chromophobe) tumors of the anterior pituitary may cause inappropriate release of GH resulting in gigantism if the epiphyses have not fused and acromegaly in adults where fusion has occurred. Acromegalic patient may present complaining that their shoes, gloves, or rings no longer fit, or they might recognize a change in facial appearance. There may also be symptoms suggestive of visual field defects. Ask for a previous photograph to compare physical features. On physical examination, a typical syndrome reflects the overgrowth of bone and other tissues resulting from GH hypersecretion (Figs 3.65–3.68).

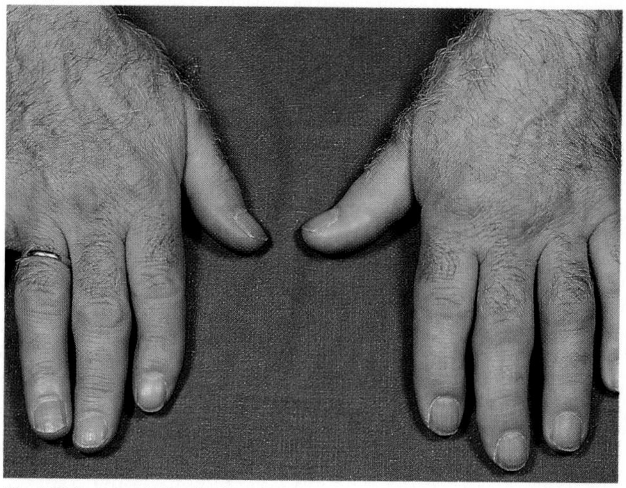

Fig. 3.67 Acromegaly. Spade-shaped hands.

Clinical features of acromegaly
Coarse, prominent facial features
Prognathoid jaw
Prominent nose and forehead
Thickened lips and large tongue
'Spade-shaped' hands
Excessive sweating/greasy skin
Kyphosis
Hypertension
Bitemporal hemianopia develops
Carpal tunnel syndrome
Impaired glucose tolerance

Fig. 3.68 Clinical features of acromegaly.

Clinical features of hyperprolactinaemia	
Women	**Men**
Present earlier	Present later
Galactorrhoea (30–80%)	Galactorrhoea (<30%)
Infertility	Impotence
Menstrual disorders	Signs of pituitary tumor
	Visual field defects
	Anterior pituitary failure

Fig. 3.69 Usual clinical features of hyperprolactinaemia in women and men.

Hyperprolactinaemia

Disruption of the tonic inhibition of prolactin release by dopamine results in the syndrome of hyperprolactinaemia (Fig. 3.69). The syndromes associated with the overproduction may be dominated by either the effect of the prolactin or the destructive effect of the pituitary tumor. Breast secretion (galactorrhoea) may develop in both women and men. The usual presenting symptom in women is alteration in the menstrual pattern (usually oligomenorrhoea or amenorrhoea). Men may present with impotence or with symptoms of pituitary expansion and malfunction (headaches, visual defects, hypothyroidism, hypoadrenalism).

SYNDROMES ASSOCIATED WITH PITUITARY HYPOFUNCTION

Hypopituitarism

The syndrome of hypopituitarism (Fig. 3.70) may become recognizable if the pituitary is destroyed by a tumor, granulomatous disease (e.g. sarcoidosis, tuberculosois, histiocytosis X), trauma or following a post-partum haemorrhage (Sheehan's syndrome). Secondary pituitary failure may also occur with disease of the hypothalamus. The clinical features progress in a characteristic sequence. GH and LH failure occurs first, followed by FSH and TSH, and finally ACTH (Fig. 3.71).

Impaired ADH secretion causes a typical syndrome known as cranial diabetes insipidus. Patients have inappropriate polyuria and produce a dilute urine even when deprived of water for prolonged periods. Often there is no obvious cause for the isolated defect. Head injury or cranial surgery may be complicated by posterior pituitary damage and diabetes insipidus. Other rare causes include pituitary tumors (e.g. destructive adenomas, craniopharyngiomas, metastases), granulomatous diseases (e.g. sarcoidosis, eosinopholic granulomas), infections (e.g. bacterial meningitis, tuberculosis) and familial disease. The symptoms of cranial diabetes insipidus can be confused with compulsive water drinking (i.e. where water deprivation causes appropriate urine concentration) and nephrogenic diabetes insipidus (i.e. where water deprivation is associated with dilute urine and high serum levels of ADH).

Clinical features of hypopituitarism	
gonadotrophin deficiency	
Men	**Women**
Loss of libido	Amenorrhoea, infertility
Impotence, infertility	Vaginal atrophy, dyspareunia
Soft atrophic testes	Atrophic breasts
Loss of secondary sexual characteristics	Loss of axillary/pubic hair
TSH deficiency – mild to moderate hypothyroidism	
ACTH deficiency – weakness postural hypotension pallor hypoglycaemia	

Fig. 3.70 Clinical features of hypopituitarism

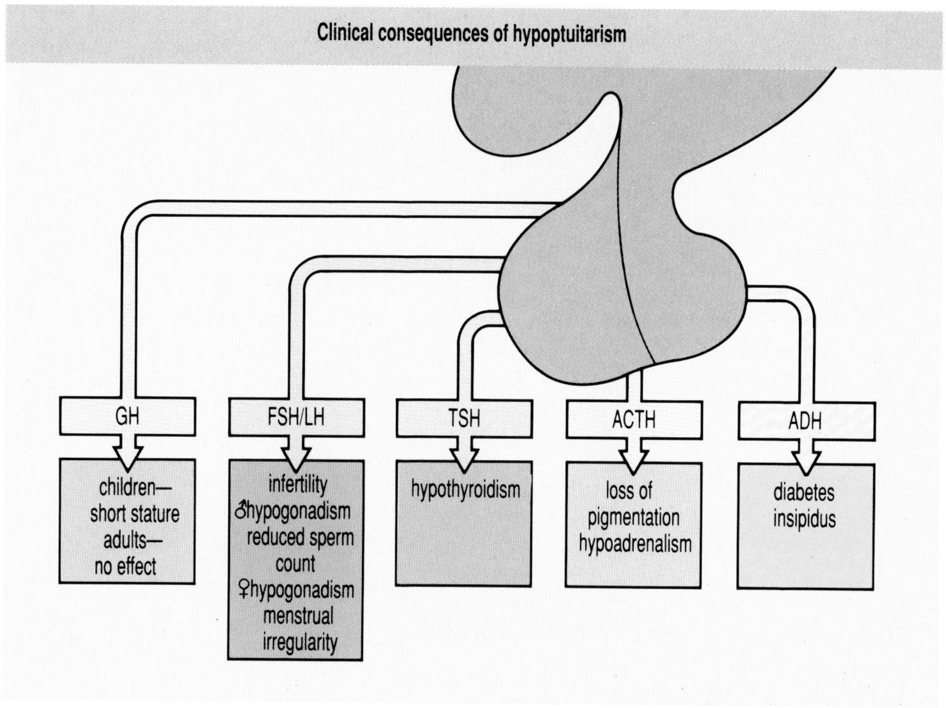

Fig. 3.71 Clinical consequences of pituitary failure. Posterior pituitary failure with diabetes insipidus is a rare manifestation of the hypopituitary syndrome.

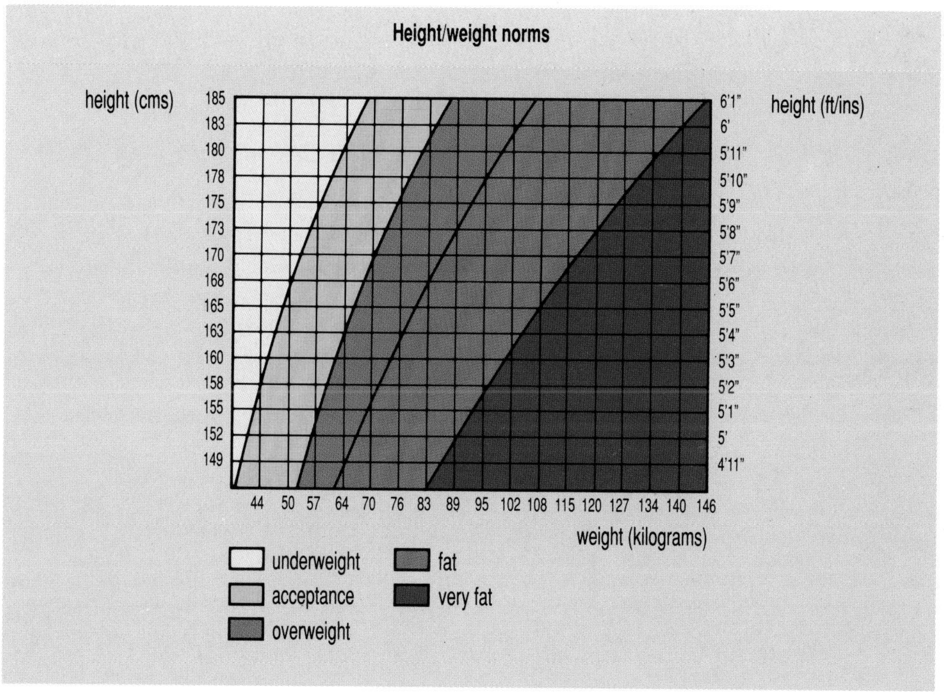

Fig. 3.72 Chart indicating height and weight norms in adults.

NUTRITION

Nutritional status may be an important marker of disease and the progression or regression of a disorder. Poor nutrition is readily treatable and nutritional support can hasten recovery and protect against complications. Malnutrition may seriously impair immunological and healing responses and attention to nutritional status may positively influence the course of disease. By contrast, obesity is also associated with morbidity, so weight loss in these individuals can be advantageous.

Assessment of nutrition

The clinical assessment of nutritional status includes overall appearance, weight, height, assessment of muscle and fat bulk, and assessment of vitamin, mineral, and haematinic status.

Either at the beginning or conclusion of the first examination, you should weigh the patient and measure their height. This provides, for useful baseline information, for standard growth charts are available to help you judge whether the patient falls within the normal range of weight for height (Fig. 3.72). Always

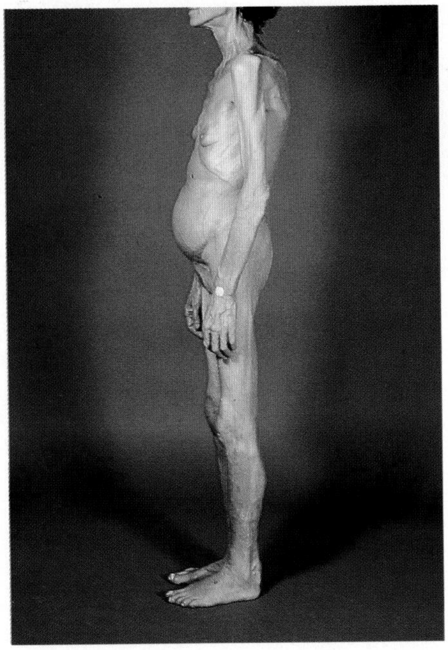

Fig. 3.73 Malnutrition in liver disease. Muscle wasting is readily recognized by the prominence of the skeleton due to loss of muscle bulk and fatty tissue.

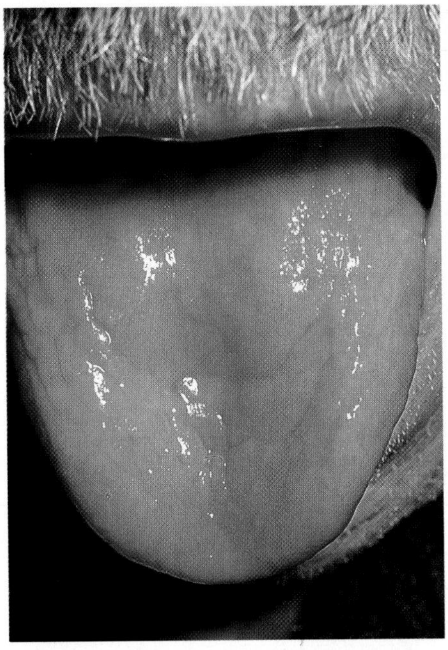

Fig. 3.74 Malnutrition. Smooth shiny tongue of atrophic glossitis.

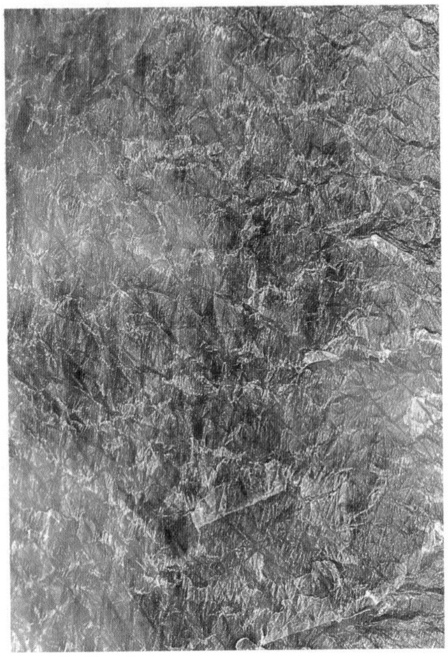

Fig. 3.75 Photosensitive 'crazy-paving'. Skin rash in pellagra.

Biochemical and immunological markers of malnutrition
Haemoglobin (iron, B_{12}, folate deficiency)
Low serum albumin
Low serum transferrin
Reduced creatinine (reflects reduced muscle bulk)
Creatinine: height ratio
Reduced white cell count
Impaired delayed cell mediated immunity (skin tests)

Fig. 3.76 Biochemical and immunological markers of malnutrition.

adopt a standard procedure for weighing the patient. In the outpatient department, it is customary to weigh the patient in socks and basic clothing. Patients in hospital can be weighed either naked or with a light linen gown. Ensure that all subsequent weighings are performed in a standard manner. Standard weight charts indicating expected percentiles and norms for height assume that the patient has been weighed naked.

Standardize the method for measuring height. The height measurement is usually made on the vertical height ruler attached to the scale. Ensure that the patient stands bolt upright with heals firmly on the surface and back flush against the rule. Measure the height by sliding the height marker to touch the crown. The sitting height is also useful; from the teens to adulthood, this height should be near 50 per cent of the total height. In osteoporosis, the collapse of vertebrae causes shortening which is reflected in a reduction of the sitting height. Armspan may occasionally be helpful. Ask the patient to fully extend the arms and hands and measure the distance between the tips of the middle fingers. This distance should equal the linear height. In Marfan's syndrome, the armspan exceeds the height.

When the patient is exposed during the course of the physical examination, take the opportunity to evaluate whether the patient

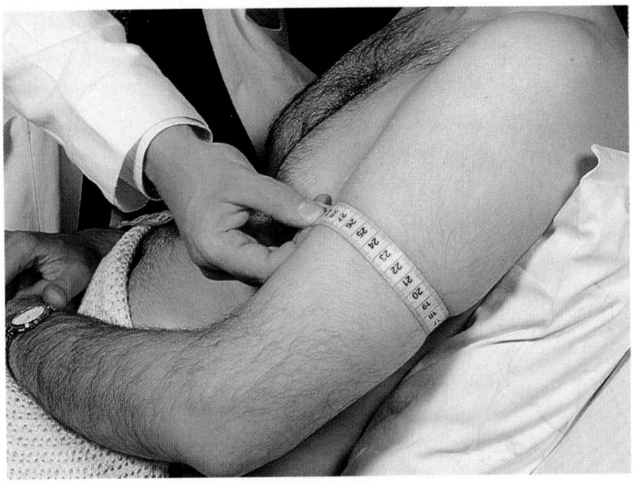

Fig. 3.77 Measurement of the midarm muscle circumference.

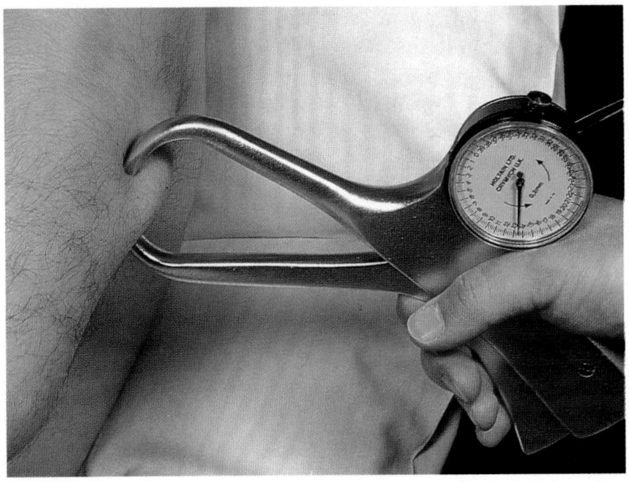

Fig. 3.78 Measurement of the triceps skinfold thickness.

Table of vitamin deficiency syndromes	
Fat soluble vitamin	**Clinical features of deficiency**
A	Dry eyes and skin, night blindness corneal thinning (keratomalacia)
D	Proximal muscle weakness, bone pain, osteomalacia
K	Easy bleeding, bruising

Fig. 3.79 Table of fat-soluble vitamin deficiency syndromes.

is of usual body build, unusually thin, or overweight. Weight loss and 'wasting' are suggested by drawing of the cheeks and unusual prominence of the cheekbones, head of humerus and major joints, the rib cage, and bony landmarks of the pelvis (Fig. 3.73). Muscle wasting may exaggerate the skeletal prominence. Atrophy of the deltoid muscles may be particulary striking. Hypoalbuminaemia may cause white nails (leukonychia, see page 4.24) and loss of capillary osmotic pressure results in pedal oedema. Iron deficiency may cause spooning of the nails (koilonychia, see page 4.26). Other features of nutritional deficiency include inflammation and cracks at the angle of the mouth (angular stomatitis); the tongue may become smooth and lacking in papillae (atrophic glossitis) (Fig. 3.74); and skin rashes may occur (e.g. pellagra) (Fig. 3.75). Although an 'eyeball' assessment provides quite an accurate assessment of general nutritional status, more objective measures, clinical and biochemical (Fig. 3.76), are necessary, especially when it is important to establish a baseline for nutritional support and where progress needs monitoring.

Midarm muscle circumference

This measurement provides an estimate of muscle and fat status. The standard position for measurement is the midpoint between the tip of the olecranon and acromial process. The patient's arm should be relaxed and flexed to a right angle. Take the measurement by wrapping the tape-measure around the upper arm midpoint (Fig. 3.77), taking care not to pull too tight or to leave excessively slack. Take three measurements at the same point and calculate the average. The measurement is itself a useful baseline measure for follow-up purposes; in addition, the single measurement can be compared with percentiles in standard age and sex charts.

Triceps skinfold thickness

In adults, the skin overlying the triceps muscle can be lifted and the subcutaneous tissue can be distinguished from the underlying muscle bulk. This fold of skin and subcutaneous tissue (the fatfold) provides an indirect assessment of fat stores. Measure the fatfold thickness from the patient's rear and make the measurement at the same midarm landmark used for measuring the midarm muscle circumference. It is useful to mark this point so that you can lift the skinfold between your thumb and index finger and position the jaws of the calipers on either side of the midarm mark on the raised skinfold (Fig. 3.78). Like the tape measurement of midarm muscle circumference, ensure that the caliper jaws are neither too tight nor too loose. Repeat the measurement three times and take the average to compare with standard tables.

CLINICAL ASSESSMENT OF VITAMIN STATUS

Vitamins are essential cofactors obtained from the diet. Reduced dietary intake may result in recognizable deficiency syndromes. Specific deficiencies of the fat soluble vitamins (A, D, K) occur in patients with chronic steatorrhoea due to chronic cholestasis, and malabsorption syndromes complicated by steatorrhoea (Fig. 3.79).

Deficiencies of water soluble vitamins occur in all forms of malnutrition. The syndromes are especially prevalent in malnutrition due to famine, malnourished alcoholics, patients on chronic renal dialysis, and in underdeveloped countries where processing of staple foods reduces vitamin content and deprives the population of necessary vitamins (Fig. 3.80).

Clinical manifestations of water soluble vitamin deficiency	
B_1 (thiamine)	Wet beriberi Peripheral vasodilatation High output cardiac failure Oedema Dry beriberi Sensory and motor peripheral neuropathy Wernicke's encephalopathy Ataxia, nystagmus, lateral rectus palsy Altered mental state Korsakoff's psychosis Retrograde amnesia, impaired learning Confabulation
B_2 (riboflavin)	Inflamed oral mucous membrane Angular stomatitis Glossitis, normocytic anaemia
B_3 (niacin)	Pellagra Dermatitis (photosensitive) Diarrhoea Dementia
B_6 (pyridoxine)	Peripheral neuropathy Sideroblastic anaemia
B_{12}	Megaloblastic, macrocytic anaemia Glossitis Subacute combined degeneration of the cord
Folic acid	Megaloblastic, macrocytic anaemia Glossitis
C	Scurvy Perifollicular haemorrhage Bleeding gums, skin purpura Bleeding into muscles and joints Anaemia Osteoporosis

Fig. 3.80 Clinical manifestations of water soluble vitamin deficiency

CLINICAL ASSESSMENT OF HYDRATION

Fluid and electrolyte balance is carefully regulated. The intake of fluid and electrolytes is closely matched by loss in urine, stool, and sweat. Dehydration can occur if there is a mismatch between fluid intake and loss. Ill patients may be anorexic and fail to take in the minimal fluid intake necessary to maintain fluid balance; the kidney may lose its ability to regulate the quality and quantity of urine; and there may be excessive gastrointestinal fluid loss (diarrhoea and vomiting) or abnormal sweating (pyrexia).

The history may be helpful when assessing hydration. Dehydration rapidly provokes thirst, the first clinical symptom of dehydration. Ask the patient whether they feel abnormally thirsty and whether they have noticed a dry, parched mouth. Physical signs of dehydration are usually only apparent with moderate to severe dehydration. Inspect the tongue and note whether the mucosa is wet and glistening. Touching the tongue may help you assess its moistness. Look at the eyes which should have a glistening, shiny appearance; however, this sparkle is lost as dehydration develops. With moderate dehydration, the eyes may appear sunken into the orbits; the pulse rate may increase to compensate for intravascular volume loss; blood pressure may drop; and the patient may experience symptoms of postural hypotension.

With marked dehydration skin turgor is lost. This can be demonstrated by gently pinching-up a fold of skin on the neck or anterior chest wall, holding the fold for a few moments (Fig. 3.81) and letting it go. Well-hydrated skin immediately springs back to its original position, whereas in dehydration, the skinfold only slowly melts back to normal. This sign is unreliable in the elderly whose skin may have lost its normal elasticity. Urine output falls and the urine is concentrated. In severe dehydration, the patient may be profoundly hypotensive, anuric, and renal failure due to tubular necrosis may occur.

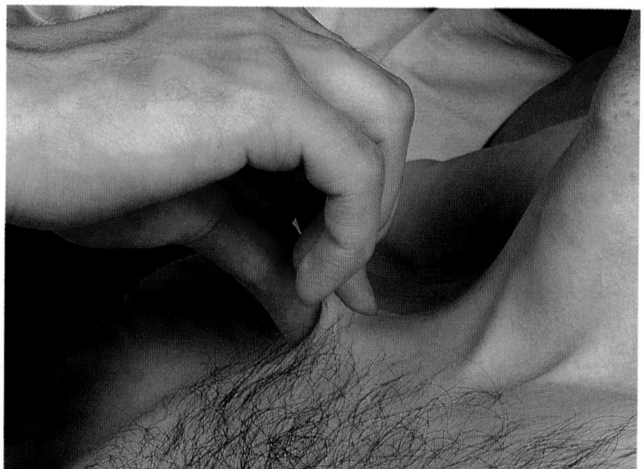

Fig. 3.81 To assess for moderate to severe dehydration, assess skin turgor by lifting the skin, pinching it and observing the rate at which it springs back to its normal position.

COLOUR

Once you have assessed nutrition and hydration, look at the patient's 'colour'. Look for pallor or plethora, central and peripheral cyanosis, jaundice and skin pigmentation.

Pallor

The cardinal sign of anaemia is pallor. Severe anaemia may be readily recognized by a pale facial appearance and shortness of breath on exertion. The red colour of arterial blood is easiest to assess where the horny layer of the epidermis is thinnest; this includes the palpebral conjunctiva, nail bed, lips, and tongue. Inspect the palpebral conjunctiva by gently everting the lower eyelid to expose the palpebral conjunctiva (Fig. 3.82),. normally a healthy red colour. In anaemia, the palpebral conjunctiva appears a pale pinker colour than is expected.

Experience will teach you to assess normal from abnormal. Conjunctival pallor should be accompanied by pallor of the nail bed and palmar skin creases (only assess this if the hands are warm). Pallor is an unreliable sign in cold or shocked patients because peripheral vasoconstriction causes skin and conjunctival pallor even when not associated with blood loss.

Plethora

This refers to a ruddy 'weather beaten' facial appearance where the skin has an unusually red or bluish (cyanosed) appearance. Facial plethora is usually caused by an abnormally high haemoglobin concentration (polycythaemia). This is usually caused by chronic cyanotic lung disease where hypoxia stimulates erythropoietin release from the macula densa of the proximal renal tubular cells. This hormone stimulates the marrow to increase red cell production with consequent increase in haemoglobin concentration. The plethora causes a bloated facial appearance and together with the cyanosis, these patients have a typical 'blue bloater' appearance.

Polycythaemia rubra vera is a myeloproliferative disorder which causes very high haemoglobin levels and plethora occurs in the absence of hypoxic cyanosis. The conjunctiva have a characteristic 'plum' colour and on fundoscopy the increased blood viscosity causes the venules to assume a thickened 'sausage-shaped' appearance.

Cyanosis

Cyanosis refers to a bluish or purplish discoloration of the skin or mucous membranes caused by excessive amounts of reduced haemoglobin in blood. At least 5g/dl of reduced haemoglobin is necessary for cyanosis to appear. In peripheral cyanosis, the extremities are cyanosed (Fig. 3.83), but the tongue retains a healthy pink colour. This is caused by any condition resulting in slowing of the peripheral circulation. In cold weather, there is reflex peripheral vasoconstriction with slowing of the circulation, allowing more time for the extraction of oxygen from haemoglobin. A similar mechanism accounts for peripheral cyanosis in heart failure, peripheral vascular disease, Raynaud's phenomenon, and shock. A reduction in arterial oxygen saturation results in central cyanosis. The extremities are cyanosed; moreover, the tongue and mucous membranes also have a bluish or purple discoloration. Central cyanosis may develop in any lung disease where there is a mismatch between ventilation and perfusion. In right-to-left shunts caused by congenital heart disease the admixture of venous blood to the systemic circulation causes cyanosis.

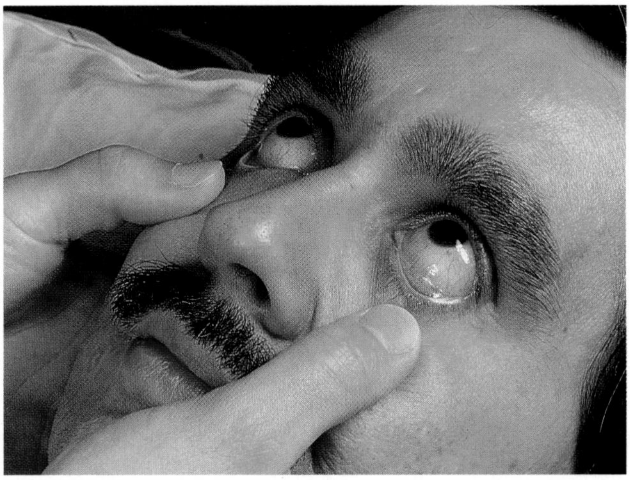

Fig. 3.82 Evert the lower lid to inspect the palpebral conjunctiva for pallor.

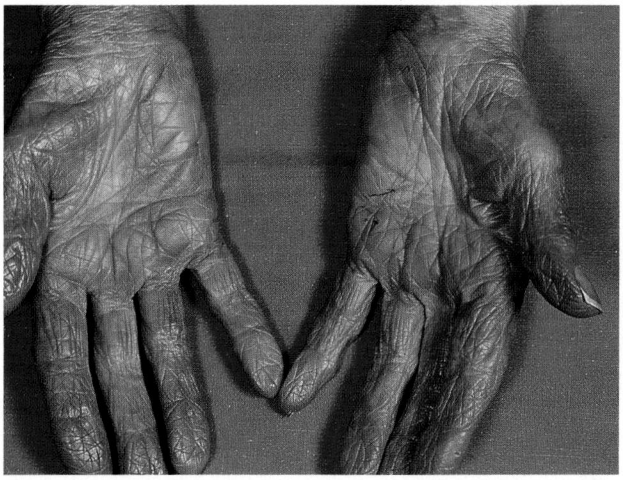

Fig. 3.83 Peripheral cyanosis; note the blue discoloration of the fingers.

Jaundice

Skin pigmentation influences the ease with which jaundice can detected. The yellow discoloration is most easily recognized in fair-skinned individuals and is more difficult to detect in darkly pigmented patients. Bilirubin has a high affinity for elastic tissue. This, together with the sclera's white colour, makes the sclera the most sensitive area for looking for the yellow discoloration of jaundice.

Mild jaundice is best seen in natural daylight. Expose the sclera by gently holding down the lower lid and asking the patient to look upwards. With progression, the yellow discoloration becomes obvious on the truncal skin. In chronic, severe obstructive jaundice, the skin develops a yellow-green appearance. Eating large amounts of carrots or other carotene-containing vegetables or substances causes carotenaemia which can be confused with jaundice. The yellow discoloration is prominent in the face, palms, and soles, in contrast to jaundice, the sclera remains white.

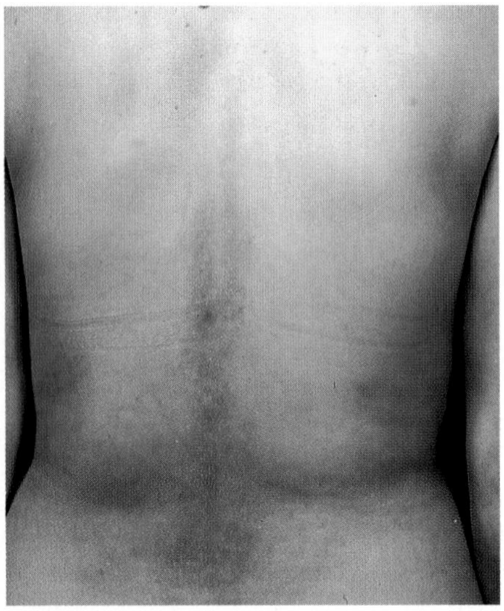

Fig. 3.84 Typical skin pigmentation in chronic cholestasis (primary biliary cirrhosis).

Pigmentation

Sunburn is the commonest cause of increased pigmentation and this should be readily distinguished from the history. In iron overload (haemochromatosis) the skin colour may appear slate-grey. A silver-grey colour develops in silver poisoning (argyria). In chronic cholestasis (e.g. primary biliary cirrhosis), skin hyperpigmentation may develop (Fig. 3.84). Marked increase in pigmentation occurs following bilateral adrenalectomy for adrenal hyperplasia. This condition (Nelson's syndrome) is caused by unopposed pituitary stimulation. Addison's disease may also be associated with deepening pigmentation.

OEDEMA

Fluid movement between the intravascular and extravascular space occurs through the walls of capillaries. The efflux of fluid across the capillary wall is governed mainly by the hydrostatic pressure transmitted by the arterial blood pressure through the pre-capillary arteriole, and also by the capillary permeability and the opposing osmotic (oncotic) pressure exerted by the serum proteins (especially albumin). In addition, the oncotic pressure of the interstitial fluid may contribute to the efflux of intravascular fluid. The reabsorption of interstitial fluid is driven primarily by the plasma oncotic pressure, the hydrostatic pressure in the interstitial

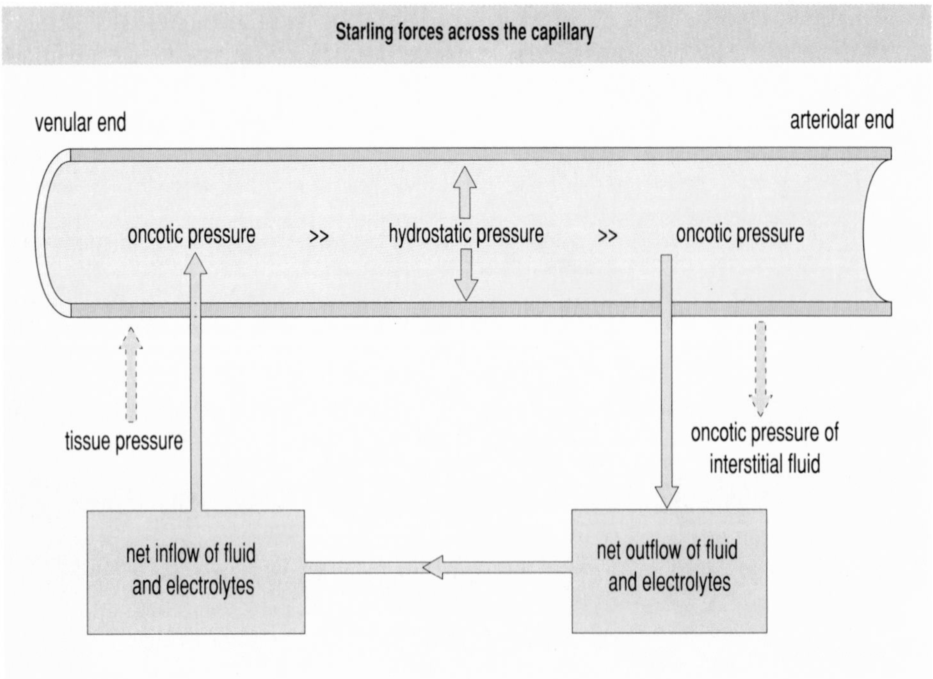

Fig. 3.85 The Starling forces across the capillary bed. At the arteriolar end, the hydrostatic and interstitial oncotic pressures exceed the plasma oncotic pressure resulting in efflux of fluid and electrolytes. At the venular end, plasma oncotic pressure exceeds hydrostatic pressure, resulting in net influx.

space (known as the tissue pressure) and the fall in hydrostatic pressure at the venular end of the capillary. These forces (known as the Starling forces) determine the movement of fluid and electrolytes between the intravascular and interstitial compartments (Fig. 3.85).

Any imbalance of the Starling forces will cause expansion of the interstitial space. In heart failure, the increased central venous pressure causes increased capillary pressure, reduced resorption, and oedema; moreover, renal hypoperfusion also stimulates the renin-angiotensin system which, in turn, causes inappropriate sodium and water retention, and further contributes to oedema. When serum albumin levels fall there is a loss of plasma oncotic pressure. This favors the the movement of fluid into the interstitial space. The consequent fall in intravascular volume causes activation of the renin-angiotensin system which adds further to fluid retention and oedema. Hypoalbuminaemia occurs in nephrotic syndrome (albuminuria, hypoalbuminaemia, hyperlipidaemia, and oedema), liver failure, malabsorption syndromes, protein losing enteropathy, severe burns, and malnutrition.

In liver disease complicated by portal hypertension, there is pooling of blood in the splanchnic bed with increased splanchnic capillary pressure. The pooling results in a fall in the effective intravascular volume which, in turn, activates the renin-angiotensin system. These factors all contribute to fluid retention which complicates portal hypertension. Ascites complicating portal hypertension usually only develops when there is hypoalbuminaemia and a fall in oncotic pressure (Fig. 3.86).

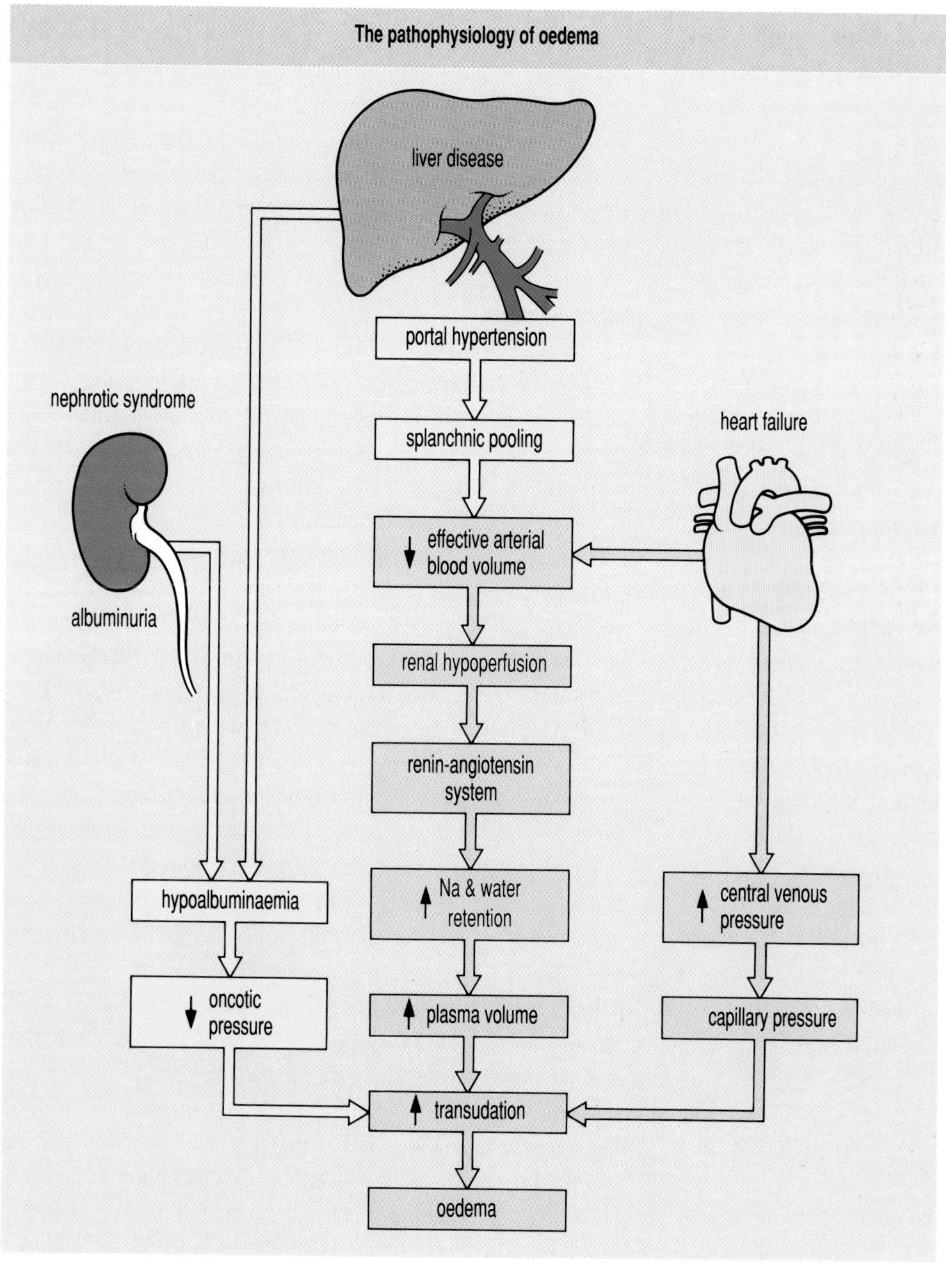

Fig. 3.86 The formation of oedema in liver disease with portal hypertension, cardiac failure and nephrotic syndrome.

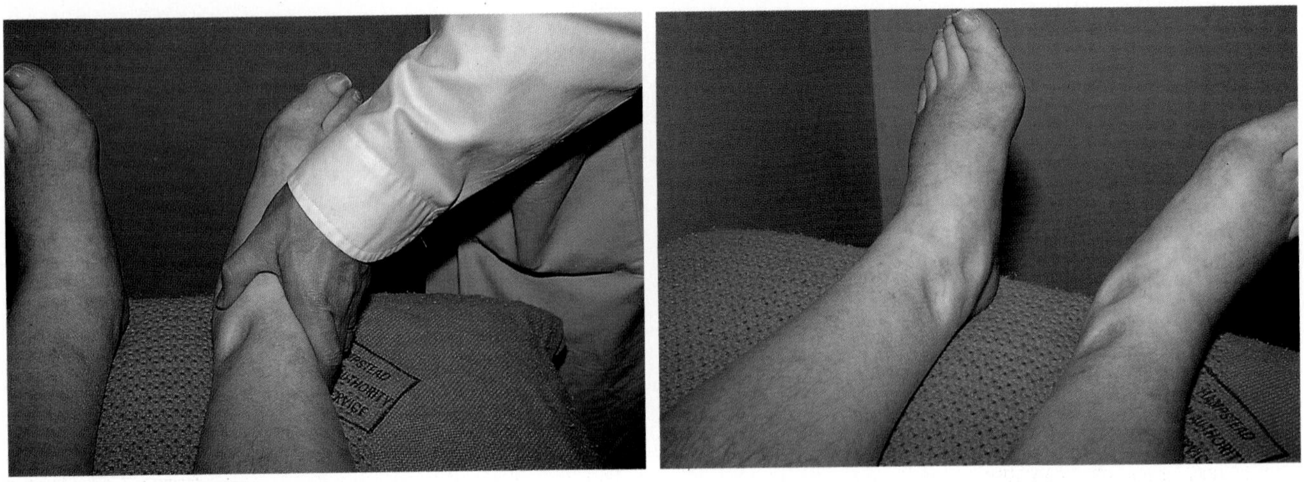

Fig. 3.87 Finger indentation to demonstrate ankle oedema.

Inflammation increases capillary permeability, allowing movement of albumin and other colloidal proteins as well as fluid into the interstitial space. The increase in interstitial oncotic pressure encourages the shift of fluid and electrolytes out of the capillaries into the interstitium. This causes the swelling which invariably accompanies the inflammatory response. Lymph is particularly rich in protein and when lymphatic flow is obstructed, the abnormal accumulation of lymph in the interstitial space increases the interstitial oncotic pressure with consequent retention of interstitial fluid.

The distribution of excess fluid depends on its underlying cause, the shifting effect of gravity, and the capacity of the tissue in which it accumulates. In congestive heart failure, patients often notice marked ankle swelling (dependent oedema) which becomes more noticeable as the day wears on and appears to resolve through the night. In the upright posture, increased capillary pressure is transmitted to the lower limbs: this favors the regional accumulation of excess fluid around the loose connective tissue around the ankles. At night, the recumbent position causes redistribution of the transcapillary and gravitational forces so that by early morning the oedema is most prominent in the sacral region, and appears to have resolved from around the ankles. When the left ventricle fails, interstitial oedema accumulates in the lungs causing pulmonary oedema. The fluid settles in the most dependent (basal) areas of the lung causing the basal alveoli to collapse during expiration. The opening of these collapsed alveoli during inspiration can be heard with a stethoscope as 'crackles'. Facial and periorbital tissue is particularly compliant. In superior vena caval obstruction and chronic renal failure, facial 'puffiness' is prominent, especially on waking. Anasarca refers to gross, generalized oedema which accompanies profound hypoproteinaemic states.

Symptoms of oedema

If the oedema is generalized, patients may notice tight fitting shoes, frank swelling of the legs, or an unexplained increase in weight. There may be associated symptoms linked to underlying diseases such as heart failure, liver, kidney, bowel, or nutritional disease. Localized oedema may be quite obvious if there is venous thrombosis, regional lymphatic obstruction, or a painful, inflamed area of swelling. Fluid accumulation in the pleural space (hydrothorax or pleural effusion) may cause breathlessness. Ascites may be noticed as an increase in girth, weight gain, or the eversion of the umbilicus.

Signs of oedema

In ambulant patients, generalized oedema is readily demonstrated in the tissue space behind the medial malleolus. Fluid accumulates in the loose connective tissue of this dependent area; the skin between the medial maleolus and Achilles tendon is normally concave but with fluid accumulation becomes flattened and then convex. You might notice a skin impression made by tight-fitting socks. In long-standing oedema, the skin may become shiny, thin, and even ulcerated due to poor local tissue circulation. Mild pedal oedema may not be obvious on inspection. Palpation is, however, a sensitive test for oedema. Press the ball of your thumb or the tips of your index and middle fingers into the posterior malleolar space and maintain moderate pressure for a few seconds. The skin has a 'boggy' feel. The extrinsic pressure will squeeze oedema fluid away from the pressure point. On removing your thumb or fingers, the finger impression remains imprinted in the skin for a short while before fading as the oedema redistributes. Repeat the compression test more proximally to assess the upper margin of oedema (Fig. 3.87).

In the recumbant posture, oedema is less obvious around the ankles and most prominent over the sacrum and lower back. This is often forgotten when examining ill patients confined to bed. Ask the patient to sit well forward in bed and expose the lower back and sacral region. Press the thumb or fingers into the skin over the mid-sacrum. Like pedal oedema, abnormal fluid retention is indicated by the residual impression left at the pressure point. In anasarca, the signs of oedema extends to the thighs, scrotum, and anterior abdominal wall. Anasarca occurs in hypoproteinaemic states (especially nephrotic syndrome, malnutrition, and malabsorption), severe cardiac or renal failure and where there is generalized increase in capillary permeability (septic shock and severe allergic reactions).

The veins of the lower legs have valves which protect the vessels from the pressure effect of the column of blood from the right ventricle. Damaged and incompetent valves in the deep and perforating veins of the lower limb cause a marked increase in hydrostatic pressure to the lower limb veins, causing varicose veins and pedal oedema. Localized oedema may occur in deep venous thrombosis of the leg veins. The affected limb becomes swollen and if there is thrombophlebitis and rapid muscle swelling, the calf muscle may be tender to palpation (Homan's sign).

Lymphatic oedema has a high protein content and the oedema is localized to the area drained by the lymphatics. The swelling is pronounced and on palpation the skin has an indurated, thickened feel. This 'brawny' oedema is the clinical hallmark of lymphoedema (filariasis is a common cause of brawny oedema in certain tropical countries). Surgical removal of axillary lymph nodes in the treatment of breast cancer commonly results in troublesome lymphoedema of the arm.

Ascites is characterized by abdominal distention (especially in the flanks) and on examination, there is shifting dullness (see page 8.33). Look for signs of localized abdominal disease such as peritoneal infection, peritoneal carcinomatosis, or liver disease with portal hypertension (e.g. splenomegaly or liver flap). Removing a small volume of ascitic fluid is often helpful in reaching a diagnosis. A blood-stained sample suggests malignancy; cytology, pH, protein content, gram and direct stains for tuberculosis can facilitate a rapid diagnosis. Pleural effusions are readily detected on clinical examination and chest X-ray (see Chapter 6). Like ascites, an aspiration sample can provide valuable diagnostic information.

TEMPERATURE AND FEVER

In all warm blooded animals, core body temperature is set within closely regulated limits and is stabilized by a combination of convection, conduction, and evaporation. The major regulatory organ for heat loss and retention is the extensive vascular plexus in the subcutaneous tissue. Though metabolism produces most of the body heat, ventilation and ingestion of hot or cold substances also make a small contribution to heat exchange in the body. Vasodilatation of skin vessels allows dissipation of heat transferred from the deep organs. Sweating facilitates heat loss through evaporation: the eccrine sweat glands are innervated by cholinergic sympathetic nerve fibres. Conservation of heat by adreneric autonomic stimuli reduces blood flow through the subcutaneous vascular plexus. The integrated response to temperature regulation is under the control of the hypothalamus.

Measuring temperature

Temperature may be measured by placing a thermometer under the tongue, into the rectum, or under the axilla. If you use a mercury thermometer, shake the instrument to ensure that the mercury is well below 37°C and leave for at least 90 seconds. Electronic temperature sensors are available which provide more rapid stabilization.

Normal temperature

Temperature depends on the site of measurement. The mouth, rectum and axilla are common sites. 'Normal' oral temperature is usually considered to be 37°C. Rectal temperature is 0.5°C higher than the mouth and the axilla is 0.5°C lower than oral readings. Remember that 'normal' temperature is not set at a precise level and there are small variations between individuals (which may range from 35.8–37.1°C). There is also a distinct diurnal variation: oral temperature is usually about 37°C on waking in the morning rising to a daytime peak between 6.00pm and 10.00pm and falling to a low point between 2.00 and 4.00am. In menstruating women, ovulation is accompanied by a 0.5°C increase in body temperature. Daily temperature measurement can be used as an accurate marker of ovulation.

Fever

Abnormally high body temperature is an important physical sign. Pathological temperatures often show an exaggerated diurnal pattern with evening high points and the lowest temperatures in the early morning. Fever may be caused by microbes, immunological reactions, hormones (e.g. thyroxine and progesterone), inability to lose heat (e.g. absence of sweat glands and icthyosis), drugs (e.g. penicillin and quinidine), and malignancy (e.g. Hodgkin's disease, hypernephroma).

Seqential recording of the temperature may show a variety of patterns (Fig. 3.88). These patterns are neither specific nor sensitive signs of individual diseases. Typhoid fever may show a 'step-wise' increase in temperature associated with a relative bradycardia. Occasionally, patients with Hodgkin's disease have a Pel–Ebstein fever, characterized by 4–5 days of persistent fever, followed by a similar period when the temperature hovers around the normal baseline. Abcess and collections of pus often present with a high spiking fever.

Chills and rigors

High fever may be accompanied by a subjective sensation of chill which may be accompanied by goose-pimples, shivering, and chattering of the teeth. As the fever subsides, the defervescence is accompanied by hot sensations and intense sweating. When shivering is extreme, the presentation is dominated by the rigors.

Sequential temperature variation

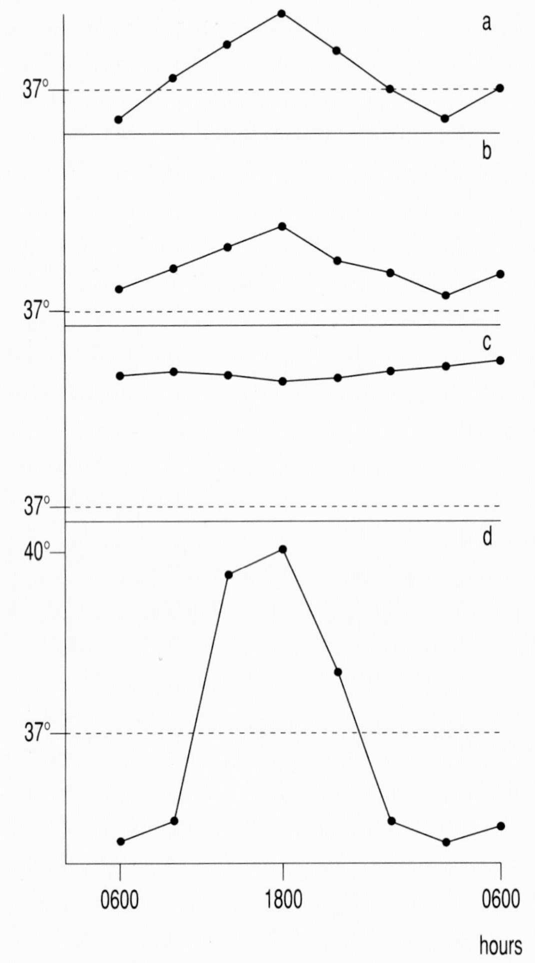

Fig. 3.88 Temperature may be described as (a) intermittent, (b) remittent, (c) persistent, or (d) spiking.

Charcot's triad

Jaundice

Right hypochondrial pain

Fever and rigors

Fig. 3.89 Biliary sepsis causes Charcot's triad.

Severe rigors and spikng fevers are characteristic of biliary sepsis (Fig. 3.89), pyelonephritis, abscess formation, and malaria.

Hypothermia

This usually occurs with prolonged exposure to winter cold. Predisposing factors include old age, myxoedema, pituitary dysfunction, Addison's disease, and abuse of drugs or alcohol. Patients are pale, the skin feels cold and waxy, and the muscles are stiff. Consciousness is depressed and when the temperature drops to below 27°C, consciousness is lost. A special low-reading thermometer is required to establish the baseline temperature. The most convenient measuring device is a rectal probe (thermocouple) which provides real-time temperature measurement.

EXAMINATION OF THE LYMPHATIC SYSTEM

As the lymphoreticular system is so widespread, it is convenient to consider its examination in the general examination. You may choose to examine for lymphadenopathy as part of the preliminary general examination, though most clinicians integrate the examination into the regional examination of the head and neck, chest and abdomen.

Primary and secondary lymphoid tissue

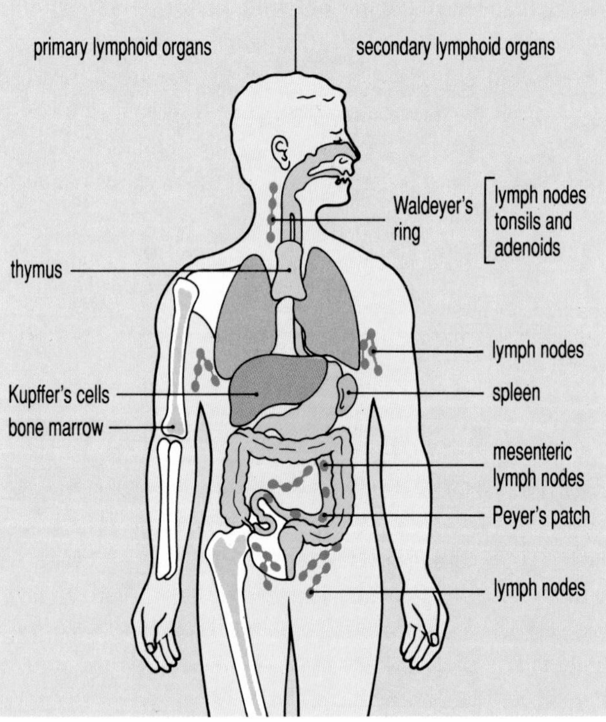

Fig. 3.90 The primary lymphoid organs include the bone marrow (which produces B lymphocytes) and thymus (which produces T lymphocytes). The secondary lymphoid organs provide a 'base camp' for interaction between lymphocytic subtypes and antigens (i.e. macrophages, antigen presenting cells, T and B lymphocytes). The immune response is generated in the secondary lymphoid tissues.

STRUCTURE AND FUNCTION OF THE LYMPHATIC SYSTEM

The lymphatic system comprises the lymphatic ducts, lymph nodes, spleen, tonsils, adenoids and the thymus gland (Figs 3.90 and 3.91). Lymphoid tissue is also present in the Peyer's patches of the terminal ileum. The lung also contain significant islands of lymphoid tissue and the hepatic reticulo-endothelial cells are an integral component of the lymphoreticular system.

A network of lymphatic ducts accompany the blood vessels; these lymphatics transport lymph from the interstitial tissues to the lymph nodes. Lymph is an opalescent fluid derived from the protein-rich fluid, enriched with lymphocytes which bathes the interstitial space. The lymphatic vessels drain distinct regions of the body into groups of regional lymph nodes. Efferent lymph vessels leave the regional nodes, converging to form larger vessels. Ultimately, the larger lymphatic vessels converge into two main lymph vessels; the lymphatic trunk drains the right upper body into the right subclavian vein, with the remainder of the body ultimately draining to the thoracic duct which drains into the left subclavian vein (Fig. 3.92). Fat from the small intestine is not absorbed into the portal circulation. Triglyceride in the enterocyte is coated with protein to form chylomicrons and these are absorbed into mesenteric lymphatics which drain through the thoracic duct into the systemic circulation.

The lymph nodes are comprised of lymphocyte-rich lymphoid follicles and sinuses which are lined with reticulo-endothelial cells (histiocytes and macrophages). The follicles in the cortex of the node have a germinal centre populated by rapidly dividing B lymphocytes and macrophages. The germinal centre is surrounded by a cuff of T lymphocytes. Antigens from a distant region drain through the lymphatic vessels into the regional nodes where they are presented to the lymphocytes which respond by proliferating into antibody-producing B lymphocytes or antigen specific T lymphocytes (Fig. 3.93).

Enlargement of the lymph nodes (lymphadenopathy) may be caused by proliferation of cells in response to antigen challenge. Abnormal cells may populate the nodes. Malignant transformation of the lymphoid cells in lymphomas may cause lymphadenopathy. The glands may become populated by leukaemic cells or metastatic carcinoma. In the lipid storage diseases, lipid-laden macrophages may infiltrate and enlarge the nodes.

Before setting out to examine the lymphatic system, it is important to know the regional arrangement of the major groups of superficial nodes (see Fig. 3.92).

The lymph nodes of the head and neck are grouped in an encircling and vertical arrangement (Fig. 3.94). The circle of nodes drain the superficial structures of the head and neck. This ring of nodes includes the submental, submandibular, pre-auricular (superficial parotid), posterior auricular (mastoid), and occipital nodes. The vertical nodes also drain the deep structures of the head and neck. The deep cervical chain extends along the internal jugular vein from the base of the skull to the root of the neck (deep

Functions of the lymphatic system

Drains the interstitial space

Antigen presentation and lymphocyte activation

Antibody production and phagocytosis

Pathway for absorption of chylomicrons from enterocytes

Fig. 3.91 Functions of the lymphatic system.

The lymphatic drainage system

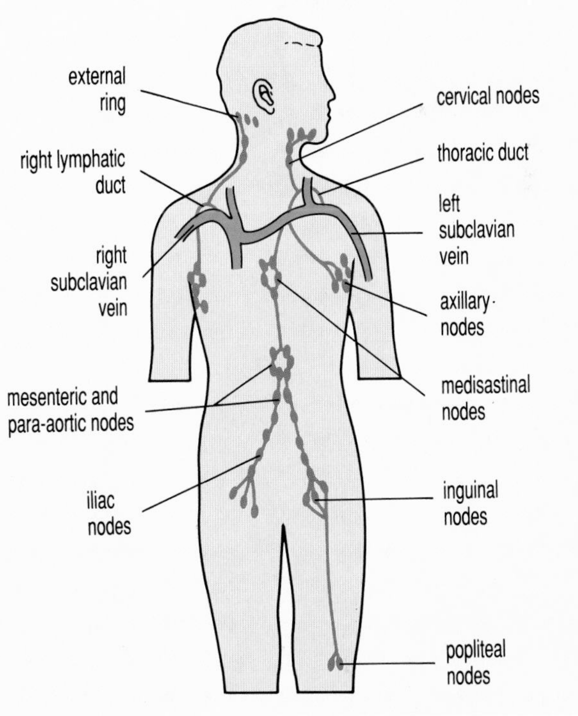

Fig. 3.92 The regional drainage of the lymphatic system. The right upper quadrant drains via the right thoracic duct into the right subclavian vein. The remainder of the lymphatic network drains into the left subclavian vein via the thoracic duct.

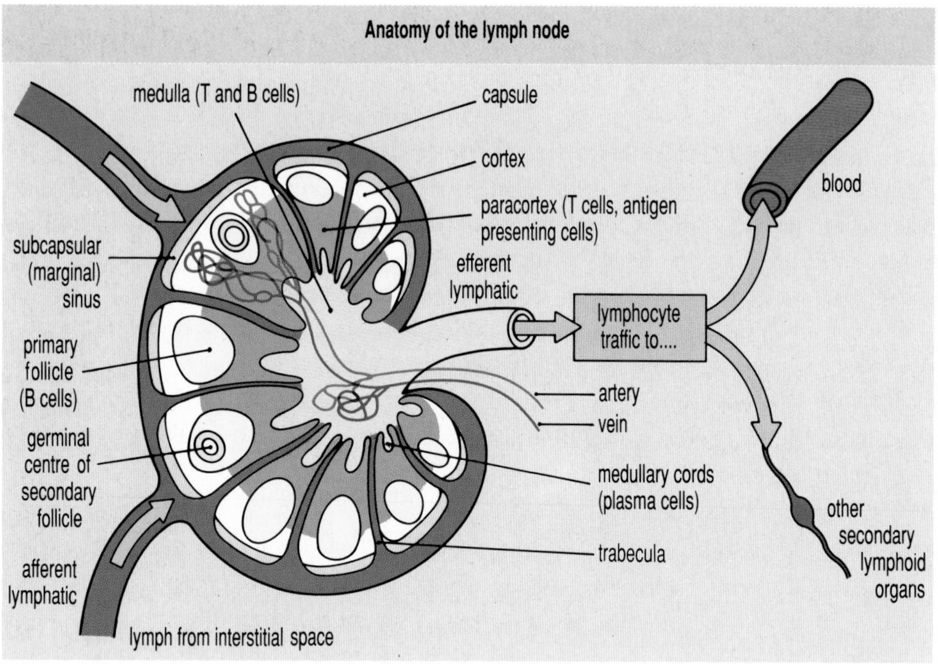

Fig. 3.93 Structure of the lymph node.

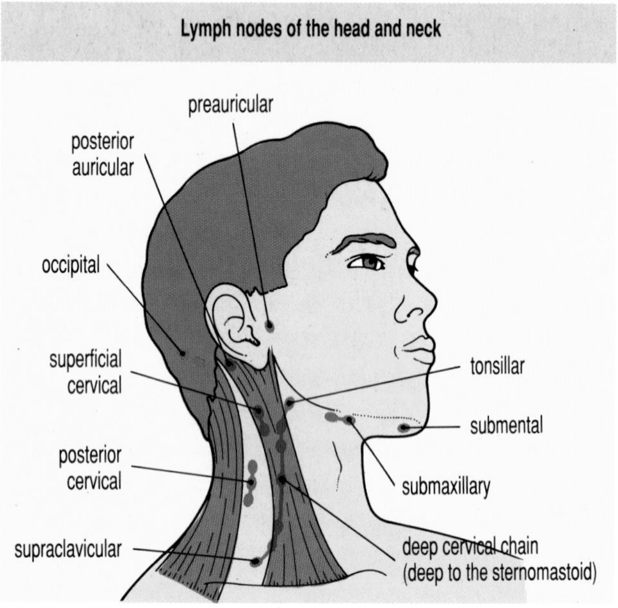

Fig. 3.94 The horizontal ring of facial node's and the vertical chain or cervical neck nodes.

to sternocleidomastoid) and then to the thoracic and right lymphatic ducts. A chain of superficial cervical nodes lie along the external jugular vein, draining the parotid glands and the inferior portion of the ear. This chain drains into the deep cervical nodes. The tip of the tongue drains to the submental nodes, the anterior two thirds to the submental and submandibular nodes, and then to the lower deep cervical nodes; the posterior tongue drains to the tonsillar nodes at the upper limit of the deep cervical chain.

The lymphatics of the hand and arm drain to the axillary and infraclavicular group of nodes (Fig. 3.95). The epitrochlear node is the most distal node in the arm. The anterior chest wall (and breast)

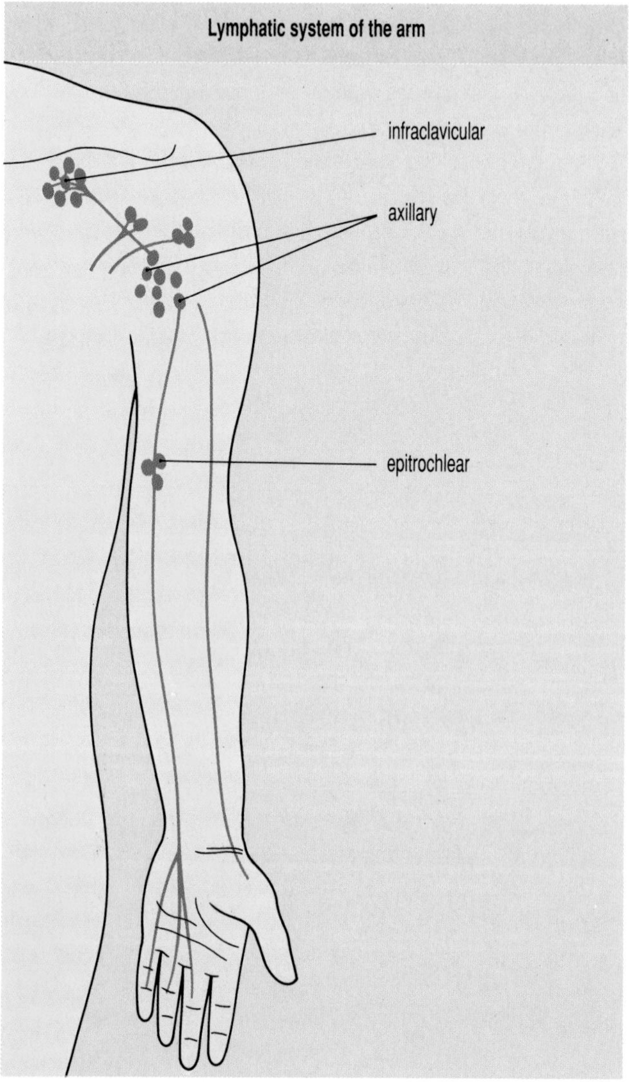

Fig. 3.95 The lymphatic drainage of the arm.

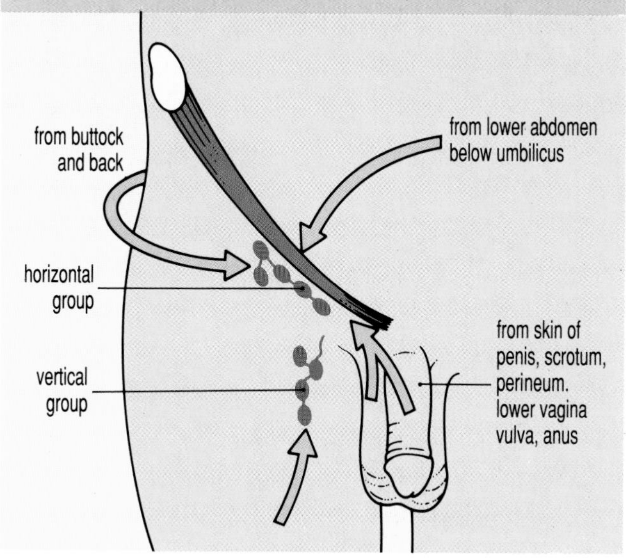

Fig. 3.96 The inguinal nodes drain the lower limbs, lower trunk, penis, scrotum, perineum, lower vagina, and anus.

Causes of generalized lymphadenopathy
Lymphoma
Acute and chronic lymphatic leukaemia
Viral infections (HIV/AIDS, infectious mononucleosis, CMV)
Bacterial infections (tuberculosis, brucellosis, syphilis)
Toxoplasmosis
Sarcoidosis
Phenytoin pseudolymphoma, serum sickness
Autoimmune diseases (SLE, rheumatoid arthritis)
Lipid storage disease (Gaucher's and Niemann-Pick)

Fig. 3.97 Causes of generalized lymphadenopathy.

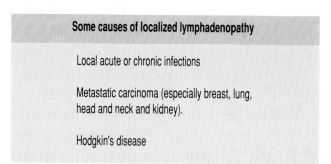

Some causes of localized lymphadenopathy
Local acute or chronic infections
Metastatic carcinoma (especially breast, lung, head and neck and kidney).
Hodgkin's disease

Fig. 3.98 Causes of localized lymphadenopathy.

drains medially to the internal mammary chain and laterally to the axillary and brachial nodes (see page 9.6). The lung parenchyma and visceral pleura drains to the hilar nodes, whereas the parietal pleura drain to the axillary nodes (this is why the axilla is palpated in the course of the lung examination). The lymphatics of the lower limb drain to the popliteal nodes and then up to the vertical group of superficial inguinal nodes lying close to the upper portion of the great saphenous vein (Fig. 3.96). The perineum, scrotal skin, penis, lower vagina and vulva, and lower trunk and the back below the umbilicus drain into the horizontal group lying below the inguinal ligament. The testes drain to the para-aortic nodes, whilst the female genitalia drain to pelvic, intra-abdominal, and para-aortic nodes.

EXAMINATION OF THE LYMPHATIC SYSTEM

Examination of the lymph nodes involves inspection and palpation. Large nodes may be clearly visible on inspection. If nodes are infected they are enlarged and tender (lymphadenitis) and the overlying skin may be red and inflamed. When superficial lymphatic vessels leading to a group of nodes are inflamed (lymphangitis), the channels can be seen as thin red streaks leading from a more distal site of inflammation.

Use your fingertips to palpate the regional nodes. Feel for the node by applying moderate pressure over the region and moving your fingers in an attempt to feel a node or nodes slipping under your fingers. Normal nodes are not palpable. If you feel nodes, assess size (length and width), consistency (soft, firm, rubbery, hard, craggy), tenderness, mobility or fixity to surrounding nodes and tissues. Whenever you discover an enlarged node, inspect the draining area in an attempt to find a source. Painful, tender nodes usually indicate an infected source which may be hidden from obvious view (e.g. infected cracks between toes). Malignant lymph nodes (either primary or secondary) are not usually tender. Malignant nodes vary in size from tiny barely palpable structures to large glands 3–4cm in size. Malignant lymph nodes may feel unusually firm (often described as 'rubbery') or hard and irregular. Fixation to surrounding tissue is highly suspicious of malignancy. Matted glands may occur in tuberculous lymphadenitis.

Often, in the course of routine examination, you will discover one or more small, mobile, non-tender 'pea-sized' lymph nodes. The 'significance' of these 'shotty' nodes may be difficult to assess. Prior to embarking on a major exercise to diagnose the cause of the lymphadenopathy, it is reasonable to re-examine the node a few weeks later. If there is no change in symptoms and signs or gland size over this period, it is reasonable to consider the node a relic of a previous illness.

On completion of of the lymphoreticular examination, it should be clear whether the lymphadenopathy is localized or generalized. This, in turn, helps with the differential diagnosis (Figs 3.97 and 3.98). If there is widespread adenopathy, consider HIV infection and AIDS, lymphomas, and leukaemia.

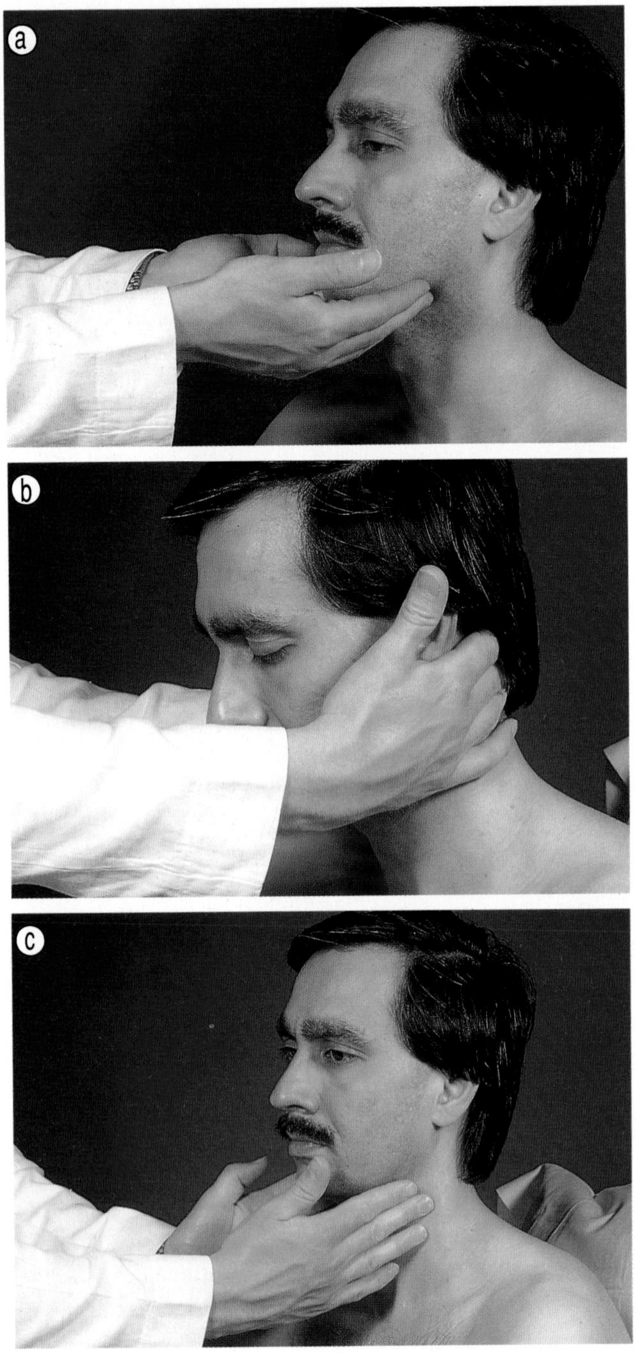

Fig. 3.99 Examination of the lymph nodes of the head and neck from the patient's front (a) submandibular nodes, (b) occipital node, and (c) deep cervical nodes.

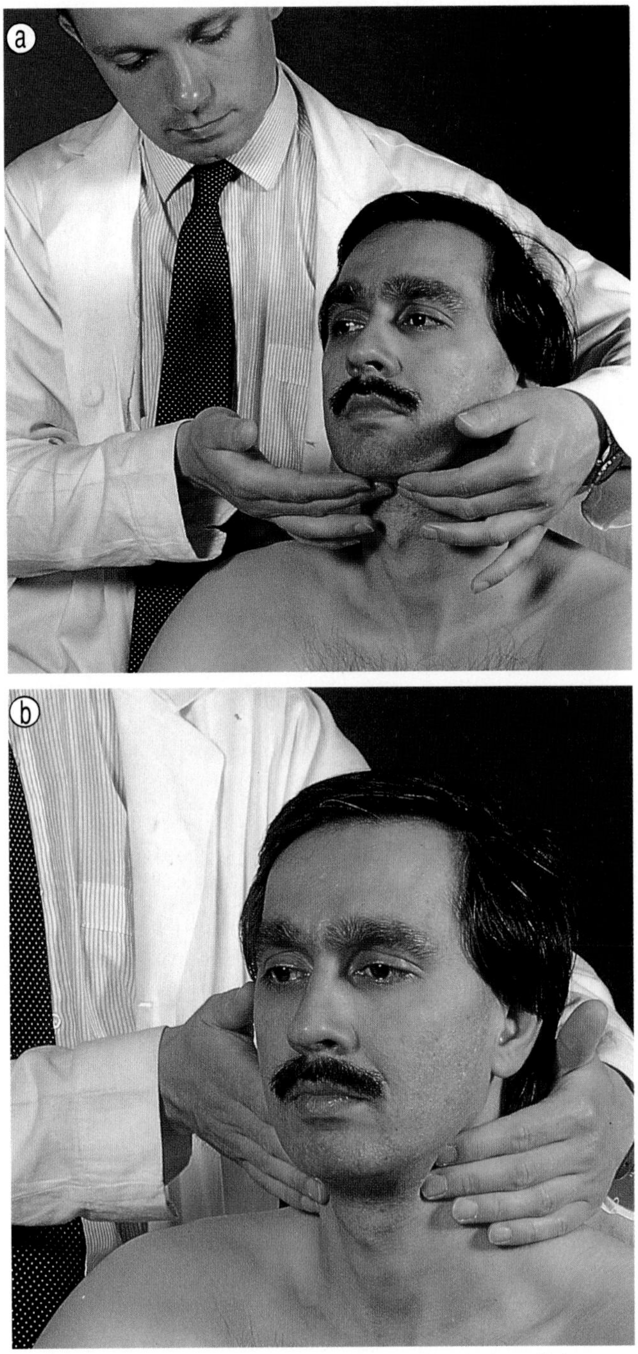

Fig. 3.100 Examination of the lymph nodes from the posterior; (a) submandibular nodes, and (b) cervical nodes.

The head and neck nodes

First, examine the nodes encircling the lower face and neck. Sit the patient forward. You may choose to examine these nodes from the front (Fig. 3.99a) or back (Fig. 3.100). Both left and right sides can be examined simultaneously using the fingers of your left and right hands. Palpate the nodes in sequence starting with the submental group in the midline behind the tip of the mandible. Next, feel for the submandibular nodes midway and along the inner surface of the inferior margin of the mandible. Feel for the tonsillar node at the angle of the jaw, the pre-auricular nodes immediately in front of the ear, the post-auricular nodes over the mastoid process, and finally, the occipital nodes at the base of the skull posteriorly. Follow this examination with palpation of the vertical groups of neck nodes. It may be helpful to flex the patient's neck slightly to relax the strap muscles. Feel for the superficial cervical nodes along the body of sternocleidomastoid (see Fig. 3.94). The posterior cervical nodes run along the anterior border of trapezius. The deep cervical chain is difficult to feel as they are deep to the long axis of sternocleidomastoid; explore for these nodes by palpating more firmly through the body of this muscle. Conclude the examination by probing for the supraclavicular nodes which lie in the area

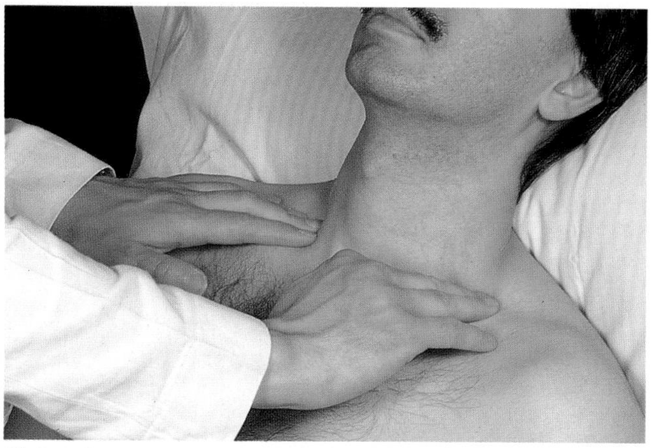

Fig. 3.101 Palpate the supraclavicular nodes in the supraclavicular fossa.

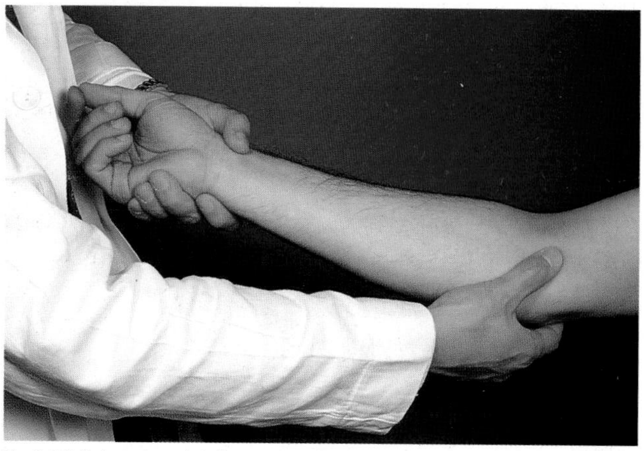

Fig. 3.102 Palpate the epitrochlear nodes which lie in a groove above and posterior to the medial condyle of the humerus.

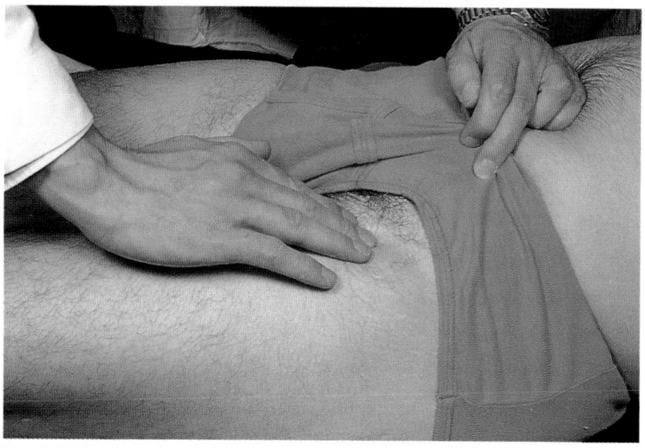

Fig. 3.103 Palpating the inguinal nodes.

bound by the clavicle inferiorly and the lateral border of sternocleidomastoid medially (Fig. 3.101). A palpable left supraclavicular node (Virchow's node) should always alert you to the possibility of stomach cancer.

The epitrochlear and axillary nodes

To palpate the epitrochlear node, passively flex the patient's relaxed elbow to a right angle. Support this position with one hand whilst feeling with your fingers for the epitrochlear nodes which lie in a groove above and posterior to the medial condyle of the humerus (Fig. 3.102). The axillary group includes anterior, posterior, central, lateral, and brachial nodes. Examine the axillary nodes from the patient's front. The technique for examining this region is described in Chapter 9.

The nodes in the inguinal region and leg

Examine these nodes with the patient lying (Fig. 3.103). The superficial inguinal nodes run in two chains. Palpate the horizontal chain which runs just below the line of the inguinal ligament and the vertical chain which runs along the saphenous vein. Relax the

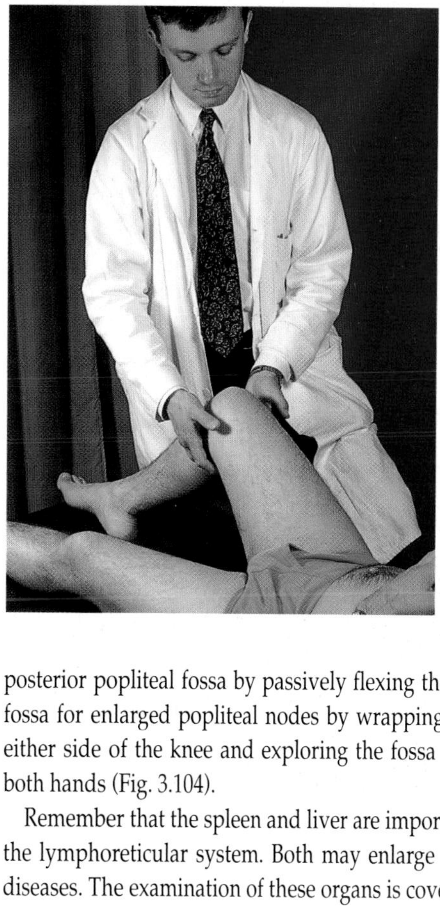

Fig. 3.104 Palpating the popliteal nodes.

posterior popliteal fossa by passively flexing the knee. Explore the fossa for enlarged popliteal nodes by wrapping the hands around either side of the knee and exploring the fossa with the fingers of both hands (Fig. 3.104).

Remember that the spleen and liver are important components of the lymphoreticular system. Both may enlarge in lymphoreticular diseases. The examination of these organs is covered in Chapter 7.

PRESENTING YOUR FINDINGS

The general examination if the stepping stone to the specific regional examinations outlined in the following chapters. The context of the general examination is illustrated in the specimen report (Fig. 3.105). Once you have read through the chapters on regional examination, return to Figure 3.105, as it may serve as a useful model to develop a 'template' for your own examination case-notes.

Recording of an examination

General Examination

Recognizable syndromes — Cushingoid facial appearance
liver decompensation
flapping tremor
jaundice
bruising (forearms)
spider naevi (face, chest)

Hydration	dry tongue but normal tissue turgor
Nutrition	wasted proximal muscles
	angular stomatitis
Colour	pallor, no cyanosis, jaundice
Temperature	37.7°C
Lymphatics	no lymphadenopathy
Oedema	obvious pedal oedema with pitting to mid-shin
Endocrine	clinically euthyroid

Head and Neck Examination

Bilateral parotid enlargement
Ears – normal drums, normal Rinne and Weber's tests
Nose – sebaceous skin nodules (rhinophyma)
Mouth and throat – severe dental caries, gum pyorrhoea
Thyroid not enlarged
JVP not raised, both carotids palpable and equal, no bruit
Trachea central

Chest Examination

Chest wall - prominent ribs suggestive or marked weight loss
Heart - pulse rate 76/minutes, regular rate, normal character
Blood pressure 110/80, 100/60

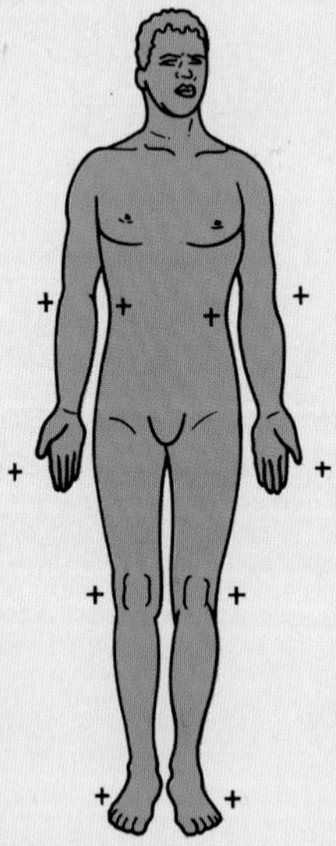

Apex beat not displaced and normal character
No parasternal heave, no thrills
1st and 2nd heart sounds normal, no 3rd/4th sounds

Lungs — respiratory rate 16/minute
normal chest wall movement
normal tactile fremitus
normal percussion anteriorly and posteriorly
breath sounds vesicular

Abdominal Examination

Distended flanks
Distended veins draining away from umbilicus
No tenderness to light or deep palpation
Smooth firm liver edge 4cm below right costal margin
Spleen palpable (2cm)
Abdomen too distended to feel for kidneys
No bladder enlargement
Dull to percussion in flanks, shifts – moderate ascites
Normal bowel sounds
No arterial or liver bruits

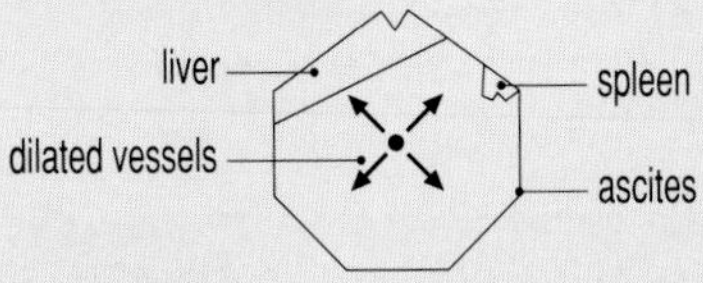

Normal hernial orifices
Rectal examination — firm, regular prostate
longitudinal sulcus prominent
normal stool on glove

Neurological Examination

Mental state	orientated for person, place but not time
Cranial nerves	no abnormality (I–XII)
	fundi – normal discs, some silver wiring

Motor
gait – mild cerebellar ataxia
cerebellum – finger-nose and heel to shin – mild ataxia

Muscle power – normal upper and lower limbs and trunk
tone – normal
reflexes:

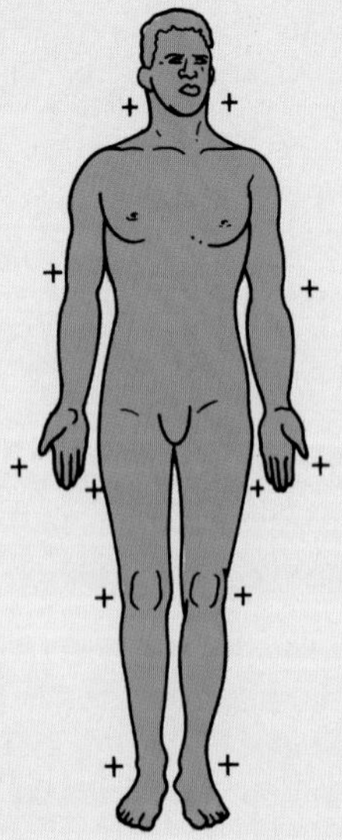

Sensation

Normal light touch, pin prick and temperature
Normal proprioception
Normal vibration sense

Summary

Signs of malnutrition and chronic liver disease with portal hypertension complicated by fluid retention and portasystemic encephalopathy. Cushingoid appearance, parotid enlargement and cerebellar signs consistent with chronic alcoholism.

Fig. 3.105 Example of an examination recorded by a medical student. The patient was admitted with a history of long-term alcohol abuse and recent onset of abdominal swelling.

THE SKIN, NAILS, AND HAIR

Skin disorders are extremely common complaints and most doctors feel uneasy with diagnosis. This section aims to familiarize you with the clinical features of skin disease and illustrates some of the more common skin disorders.

The relatively sparse distribution of hair in the human species contrasts starkly with most other mammals and reflects an evolutionary event which must, in some way, have been advantageous. Perhaps human nakedness provided a strong stimulus for developing alternative 'coats' and from this emerged the creative attributes which characterize the species.

The environment in which we live is harsh, variable, and unpredictable. In contrast, the efficiency with which the body operates is set within narrow limits of temperature and hydration. Skin has evolved to encapsulate, insulate, and thermoregulate. Recently, other functions have been recognized: the skin is an important link in the immune system; the Langerhans cells of the dermis are closely related to monocytes and macrophages and are probably important in delayed hypersensitivity reactions and allograft rejection. Skin also has an important endocrine function, being responsible for the modification of sex hormones produced by the gonads and adrenals. In addition, skin is the site of vitamin D synthesis.

STRUCTURE AND FUNCTION

SKIN

There are two layers: the epidermis, derived from embryonic ectoderm; and the dermis and hypodermis, derived from mesoderm.

The epidermis

This layer consists of a modified stratified squamous epithelium and arises from basal, germinal columnar keratinocytes which evolve as they migrate towards the surface through a prickly cell layer (where the cells acquire a polyhedral shape), a granular cell layer (where the nucleated cells acquire keratohyalin granules), and eventually form the superficial keratinized layer (horny layer of stratum corneum) where the cells lose their nuclei and form a tough superficial barrier (Fig. 4.1). The migratory cycle from the basal to horny layer takes about 30 days, with the cornified cells shedding from the surface some 14 days later. Abnormalities of this transit time may lead to certain skin diseases such as psoriasis, where the migration rate is greatly accelerated. Epidermal cells are linked by structures known as desmosomes. The epidermis rests on a thin basement membrane and is anchored to the dermis by hemidesmosomes and other anchor proteins such as laminin, basement membrane proteoglycan, and type IV collagen. These and other proteins are of importance in the pathogenesis of diseases occurring at the epidermal-dermal junction (e.g. bullous pemphigoid and epidermolysis bullosa).

Melanocytes develop amongst the basal cells. These cells are derived from neural crest cells and synthesize melanin pigment which is transferred to keratinocytes through dendritic processes. Melanin is responsible for skin and hair pigmentation. The pigment protects the skin from the potentially harmful effects of ultraviolet irradiation. Skin colour is determined by the total number, size, and distribution of melanin granules, not the number of melanocytes. Hereditary failure to synthesize melanin results in albinism.

The dermis

This layer provides the supporting framework on which the epidermis rests and consists of a fibrous matrix of collagen and elastin set in a ground substance of glycosaminoglycans, hyaluronic acid, and chondroitin sulphate (see Fig. 4.1). The skin appendages are set in the dermis. Nerves, blood vessels, fibroblasts, and various inflammatory cells also populate this layer. The dermis is divided into two layers: the papillary dermis apposes the undulating dermal-epidermal junction, whilst the reticular dermis lies beneath, forming the bulk of collagen, elastic fibres, and ground substance. Dermal fibroblasts synthesize and secrete the dermal collagen subtypes (I and III) and elastin. If there is disruption of dermal elastin, disorders such as wrinkles and a loose skin syndrome (cutis laxa) occur.

The hypodermis

The dermis rest on the hypodermis which is the subcutaneous layer of fat and loose connective tissue. This layer serves both as a fat store and an insulating layer.

SKIN APPENDAGES

Sebaceous glands

Skin sebaceous glands can function throughout life, although activity is latent between birth and puberty. There glands are partly responsible for the production of vernix caseosa which covers and waterproofs the foetus during the latter stages of gestation. The glands become particularly active during puberty. The secretion is holocrine (i.e. the secretion is caused by complete degeneration of the acinar cells) and is stimulated by androgens and opposed by oestrogens. Sebaceous glands are absent from the

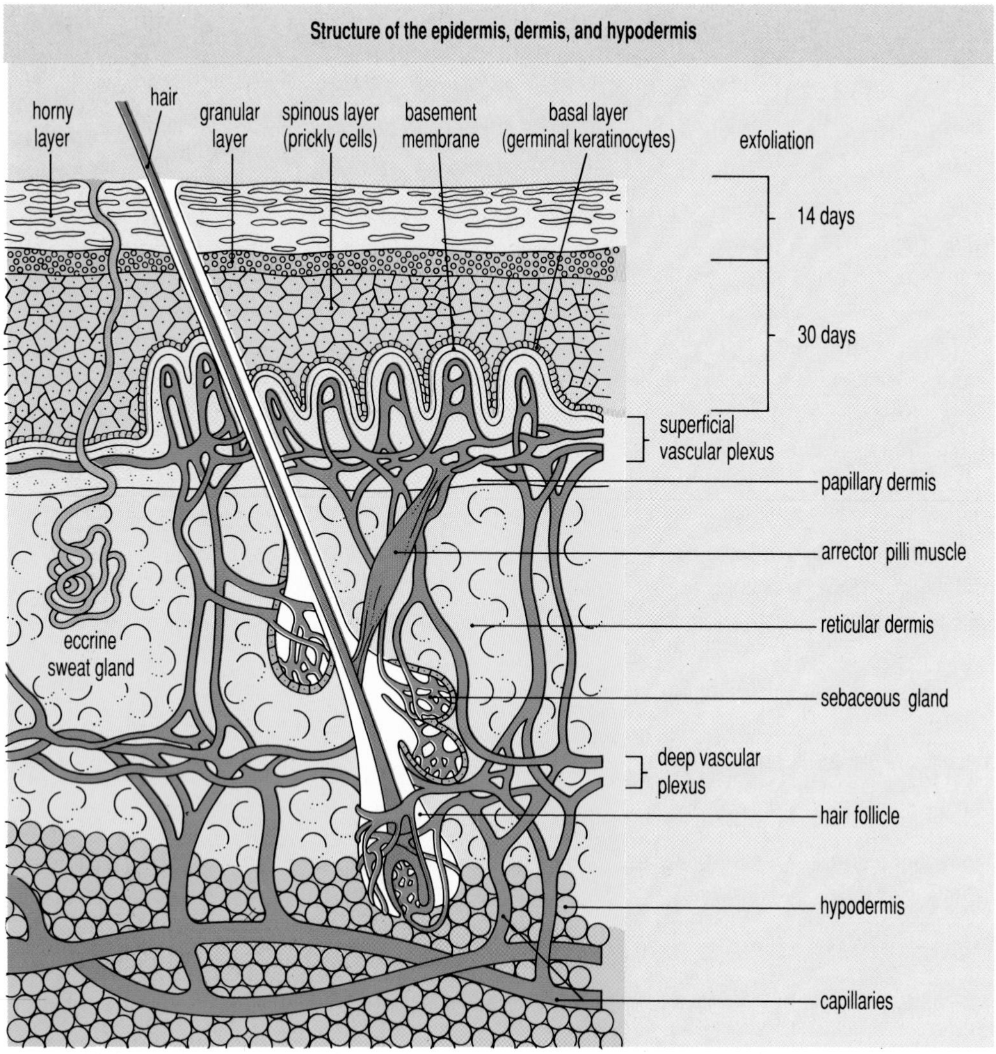

Fig. 4.1. Section through full thickness of skin demonstrating the structure of the epidermis, dermis and hypodermis.

palms and soles and concentrated on the face, scalp, midline of the back, and the perineum. Sebum contains triglyceride, scalene, and wax esters and functions to waterproof and lubricate the skin, as well as inhibiting the growth of skin flora and fungi. Skin disorders such as acne vulgaris and rosacea occur in areas where sebaceous glands concentrate.

Apocrine and eccrine glands

The apocrine glands are concentrated in the axillae, areolae, nipples, anogenital regions, eyelids, and external ears. These glands become functionally active at puberty and are responsible for an odourless secretion which is acted on by skin flora causing the characteristic body odour to develop. The eccrine sweat glands are widely distributed and are extremely important in heat regulation and fluid balance. Whilst the eccrine cells secrete an isotonic fluid, the duct cells modify the fluid to render it hypotonic. Secretion and its modification is under cholinergic and hormonal control. Sweating in response to temperature change is under hypothalamic control.

HAIR

In most mammals, hair is important in the control of temperature. In man, however, hair is mainly important as a tactile organ which also has a sensual function, important in both sexual attraction and stimulation. Hair covers all of the body except the palms, soles, prepuce and glands, and inner surface of the labia minora. During gestation the foetus is covered by a fine coat of lanugo hair which is lost shortly before birth, except for the scalp, eyebrows, and lashes. Hair may be vellus, which is short, fine, and not pigmented, or terminal, which is thicker and pigmented. Puberty is characterized by the development of coarse pigmented hair in a pubic, axillary, and facial distribution.

Hair is formed by specialized epidermal cells which invaginate deeply into the dermal layer. Hair develops from the base of the hair follicle where the papilla, a network of capillaries, supports the nutrition and growth of the hair. Hair growth is cyclical; the active growth phase is termed anagen, whilst involution of the hair is termed catagen, followed by a resting stage known as telogen.

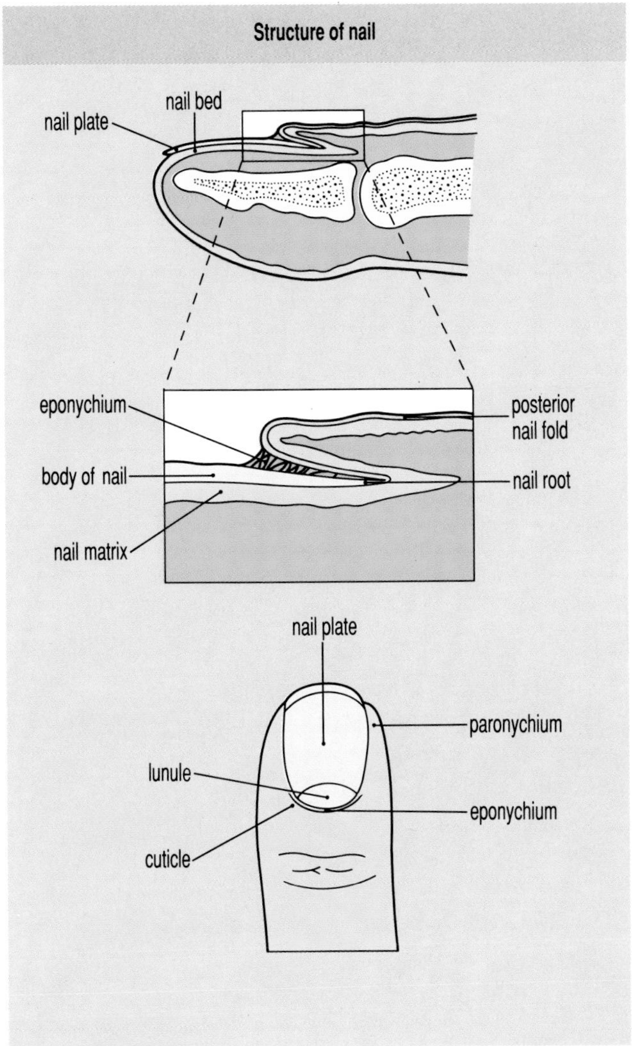

Fig. 4.2. Structure of nail.

The shaft of hair consists of a cuticle, cortex, and medulla. The arrectores pilorum muscles anchor in the papillary dermis and insert into the perifollicular tissue (see Fig. 4.1). Contraction of these muscles cause, goose pimples (cutis anserina) to occur. Hair colour is determined by the density of melanosomes within the cortex of the hair shaft. No pigment is present in white hair, whilst grey hair is caused by a reduction in number. Red hair has different melanosomes, chemically and structurally to black hair.

THE NAIL

Nail is a specialized skin appendage derived from an epidermal tuck which invaginates into the dermis. The highly kerastinized epithelium is strong but flexible and provides a sharpened surface for fine manipulation, clawing, scraping, or scratching.

The nail has three major components: the root, the nail plate, and the free edge (Fig. 4.2). The proximal and lateral nail folds overlap the edges of the nail and a thin cuticular fold, the eponychium, overlies the proximal nail plate. The lunula is the crescent-shaped portion of the proximal nail formed by the distal end of the nail matrix. The free margin of the distal nail is continuous along its under-surface with the hyponychium, a specialized area of thickened epidermis. The nail plate lies on the highly vascularized nail bed which gives the nail its pink appearance. The paroncyhium is the soft, loose tissue surrounding the nail border; it is particularly susceptible to bacterial or fungal infection infiltrating from a breach in the eponychium (a paronychia). Fingernails grow about 0.1mm per day, with more rapid growth in summer compared to winter.

SYMPTOMS OF SKIN DISEASE

The history should attempt to extract the patient's version of the disorder, evaluate possible precipitating factors, and determine whether the skin problem is localized or a manifestation of systemic illness.

The skin is readily examined and for this reason the history often assumes less importance than with other systems. However, a

Skin history

Was the onset sudden or gradual?

Is the skin itchy or painful?

Is there any associated discharge (blood or pus)?

Where is the problem located?

Have you recently taken any antibiotics or other drugs?

Have you used any topical medications?

Were there any preceding systemic symptoms (fever, sore throat, anorexia, vaginal discharge)?

Have you travelled abroad recently?

Were you bitten by insects?

Any possible exposure to industrial or domestic 'toxins'?

Any possible contact with venereal disease?

Was there close physical contact with others with skin disorders?

Any possible exposure to AIDS?

thorough history might unearth crucial information to aid diagnosis. Attempt to gain some insight into the patient's social conditions as overcrowding and close physical contact are important when considering infectious disorders such as scabies and impetigo. Enquire in some depth as to possible precipitating factors, especially contact with occupational or domestic toxins or chemicals. Ask whether waterproof gloves are worn when washing up dishes or dusting and cleaning the home. Question the patient about recent exposure to medicines, especially antibiotics which often cause skin rashes. Cosmetics are an important cause of skin sensitization so enquire about the use of new soaps, deodorants, and toileteries Ask about hobbies (e.g. gardening, model building, and dark-room developing), foreign travel, and insect bites. Ascertain whether or not the skin complaint is seasonal.

Systemic disorders may also present with skin symptoms. Infectious diseases often present with skin rashes or lesions. Ask about a recent sore throat, as streptococcal infection may be accompanied by typical rash (scarlet fever), painful red nodules on the extensor surface (erythema nodosum), or guttate psoriasis. In a cutaneous candidal infection, the patient often complains of an itchy rash, sore tongue, or in women, a vaginal discharge. Candida albicans infection often follows a course of broad spectrum antibiotics. Skin rashes developing in sun-exposed areas (in the absence of strong sunburn; these are known as photosensistive rashes) should raise the possibility of systemic lupus erythematosis, drugs, or porphyria. If the patient complains of skin lesions around the genitalia, enquire about possible contact with venereal disease. AIDS may present with the nodular lesions characteristic of Kaposi's sarcoma or thrush affecting the mucosa or skin. Therefore, it is important to take a history of risk factors (e.g. male homosexuality, high risk heterosexual contact, blood transfusion, and intravenous drug abuse). Skin itching (pruritus) in the absence of an obvious rash should alert you to an underlying systemic disorder (Fig. 4.3).

Topical steroids and other topical substances are commonly prescribed to treat a variety of skin lesions. Always ask about topical treatment as this may alter the appearance of a skin lesion, thus making the diagnosis more difficult.

Systemic diseases causing pruritus
Intrahepatic and extrahepatic biliary obstruction (cholestasis)
Diabetes mellitus
Polycythaemia rubra vera
Chronic renal failure
Lymphoma (especially Hodgkin's disease)

Fig. 4.3. Systemic diseases causing pruritus.

SYMPTOMS OF HAIR DISEASE

Hair thinning

Balding (alopecia) worries patients and you will often be asked to assess scalp hair loss. Male pattern baldness is common; the patient will note the slow onset of hair loss with the hairline receding from the frontal and temporal scalp and crown. Ask about a family history of baldness as male alopecia is an expression of autosomal dominance and may begin early in life. After the menopause, many women note thinning of the hair (Fig. 4.4); this is often associated with growth of facial hair.

Hair history

Was the hair loss sudden or gradual?

Does the loss only occur on the scalp or is the body hair involved as well?

Is the baldness localized or general, symmetrical or asymmetrical?

Is there a family history of baldness (especially men)?

What drugs have you taken recently?

Any recent illnesses, stress, or trauma?

Are there other systemic symptoms (e.g. symptoms of hypothyroidism).

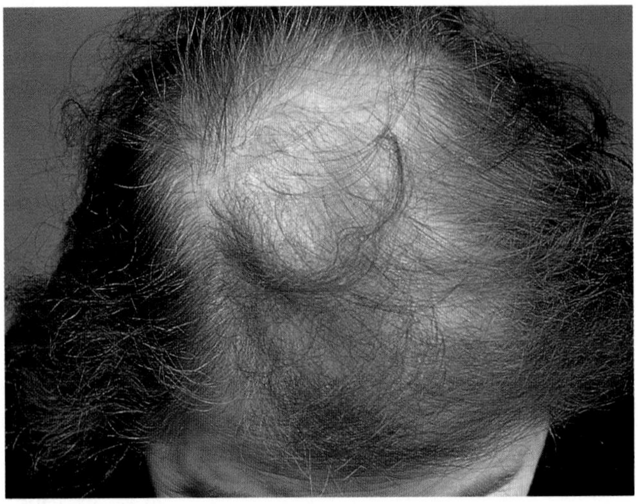

Fig. 4.4 Alopecia.

Hair loss may also be a feature of disease and the alopecia characteristics may be helpful. Patients complaining of localized alopecia (alopecia areata) (Fig. 4.5) may have an autoimmune disease (e.g. Hashimoto's thyroiditis with myxoedema). Patients with stress or anxiety neurosis may nervously pluck hair from the scalp, causing a local area of thinning or baldness. Severe illness and malnutrition, as well as sudden psychological shock may be associated with hair loss which usually recovers once the stress has been resolved.

Abnormal hair growth

Remember to warn patients undergoing cytotoxic treatment for cancer that they can expect generalized hair loss. Failure to develop axillary and pubic hair at the expected time of puberty should alert you to the possibility of pituitary or gonadal dysfunction.

Abnormal facial hair growth (hirsutes) is a distressing symptoms in women. It is important to recognize that a certain degree of facial hair growth occurs naturally in postpubertal women. There are racial differences: physiological hirsutes is least apparent in Japanese and Chinese women and most apparent in women of Mediterranean, Middle Eastern, Indian, and Negroid extraction. The unexpected occurrence of hirsutes, especially if accompanied by other symptoms and signs of virilism should alert you to the possibility of an hormonal imbalance (e.g. polycystic ovary, ovarian failure, adrenal tumor). Ask about drugs, as phenytoin, progestogens, and anabolic steroids may cause hirsutes.

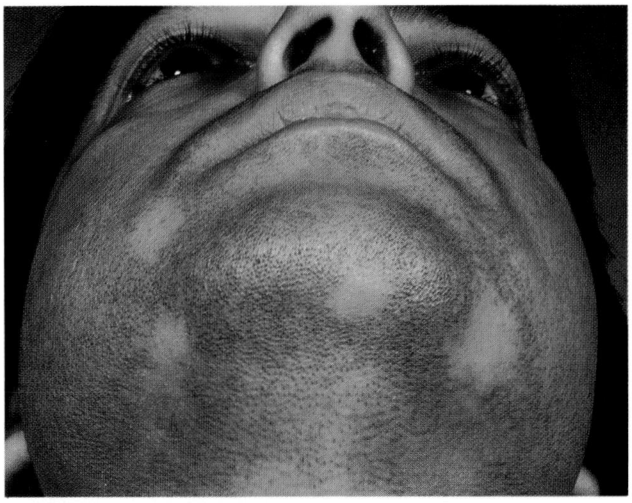

Fig. 4.5 Alopoecia areata characterized by localized patches of hair loss.

> **Hirsutes**
>
> Is there a family history of hirsutes?
>
> Are your menstrual periods normal or absent (or scanty)?
>
> Is there a history of primary or secondary infertility?
>
> Do you experience visual disturbances or headaches (pituitary disease)?
>
> What medications do you take (e.g. phenytoin, anabolic steroids, progestogens)?

SYMPTOMS OF NAIL DISEASE

Whereas examination of the nails may be very revealing, nail-related symptoms are usually non-specific. Patients may relate symptoms suggestive of bacterial infection along the nail edge; these include intense pain, swelling, and often a purulent discharge. Complaints of brittleness, splitting, or cracking provide little diagnostic information. Ask specifically about skin disease which may affect the nail such as psoriasis, sever eczema, lichen planus, or a susceptibility to fungal skin infection.

EXAMINATION OF THE SKIN NAILS AND HAIR

Examining the skin

When examining the skin, there is a tendency to focus on the local area noticed by the patient. Nonetheless, you should consider the skin as an organ in its own right and like other any examination, the whole organ should be examined to gain maximum information. The patient should be stripped to the underwear, covered with a gown or blanket, and the examination area should be well-lit (preferably natural daylight or fluorescent light).

Inspection and palpation

Scan the skin, looking for skin lesions and noting their position and symmetry. Remember to expose hidden areas like the axillae, inner thighs, and buttock with its natal cleft. Many skin lesions can be diagnosed by their appearance and localization. Unlike any other organ system, the examination relies almost entirely on careful inspection and meticulous use of descriptive terminology.

Measurement of the length and breadth of skin lesions is useful, especially when monitoring progression or regression. A small ruler or tape is handy for this purpose. A broad beam torch or electric light helps to define the outline of the border of a skin lesion; a thin beam is helpful if you wish to check whether or not a lesion transilluminates. A fluid-filled but not solid lesion emits a red glow when the torch light shines through. A Wood's lamp helps to distinguish a fluorescing lesion. By shining the lamp at a suspect lesion, it may be possible to show the characteristic blue-green fluorescence of fungal infections.

Skin colour

Skin colour varies between individuals and races, and is usually even and symmetrical in distribution. Normal variations occur in freckling and sun-exposed areas. During pregnancy, there may be darkening of the skin overlying the cheek bones and the areolae surrounding the nipple (melasma and chloasma).

Abnormal skin colour

Generalized changes in skin colour occur in jaundice, iron overload, endocrine disorders, and albinism. The yellow tinge of jaundice is best observed in good daylight, appearing initially as yellowing of the sclerae and then as a yellow discolouration on the trunk, arms, and legs. Jaundice is less apparent in unconjugated as opposed to conjugated hyperbilirubinaemia. In long-standing, deep obstructive jaundice, the skin might turn a deep yellow-green. Remember that people eating large quantities of carrots or other forms of vitamin A may develop yellow skin pigmentation (carotenaemia) and that the absence of scleral discolouration distinguishes this syndrome clinically from jaundice.

Iron overload (haemosiderosis and haemochromatosis) causes the skin to turn a slate-grey colour. The astute observer might recognize this metabolic disease by the characteristic skin pigmentation. Addison's disease (autoimmune adrenal destruction) is characterized by darkening of the skin, occuring first in the skin creases of the palms and soles, scars, and other skin creases. The mucosa of the mouth and gums also becomes pigmented. Striking pigmentation also arises after bilateral adrenalectomy for adrenal hyperplasia: this syndrome (Nelson's syndrome) is due to unopposed pituitary overstimulation. In hypopituitarism, the skin is soft, pale, and wrinkled.

Albinism is an autosomal recessive disorder caused by failure of melanocytes to produce melanin. The skin and hair are white and the eyes are pink due to a lack of pigmentation of the iris (there may also be nystagmus).

Common localized abnormalities of skin pigmentation include vitiligo (Fig. 4.6), café au lait spots (Figs 4.7 and 4.8), pityriasis versicolor, and idiopathic guttate hypomelanosis. Erythema of the skin is caused by capillary dilatation; when pressure is applied the red lesion blanches and reforms. When examining a patient, you may notice an erythematous flush in the necklace area which is caused by anxiety. Purpura is the term used for red-purplish lesions of the skin caused by seepage of blood of skin blood vessels. Unlike erythema, these lesions do not blanche with pressure. If the lesions are small (<5mm) they are called petechiae (Fig. 4.9), whereas larger

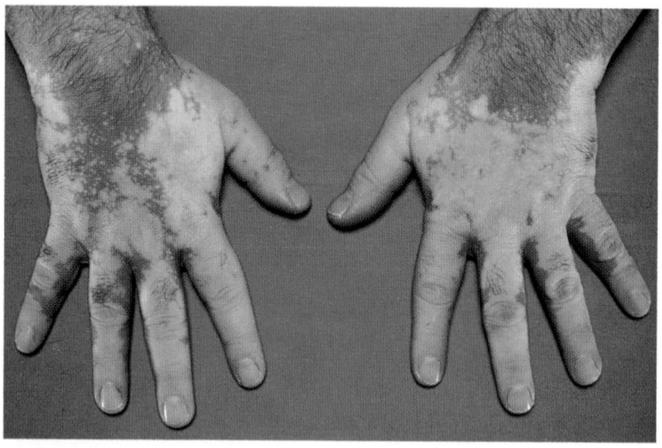

Fig. 4.6. Depigmented skin (vitiligo). White discoloration of brown hand.

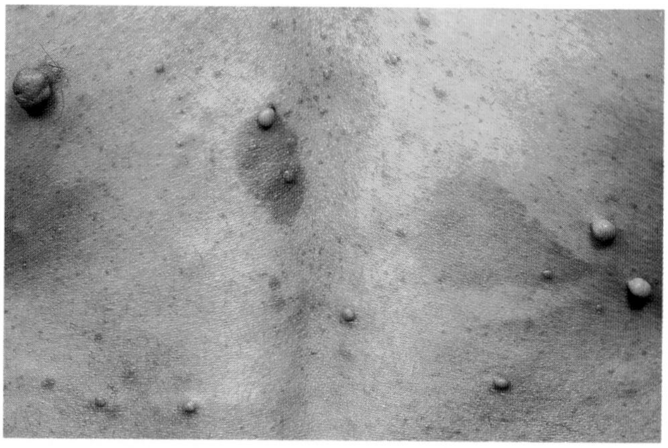

Fig. 4.7 Café au lait patches with neurofibromas.

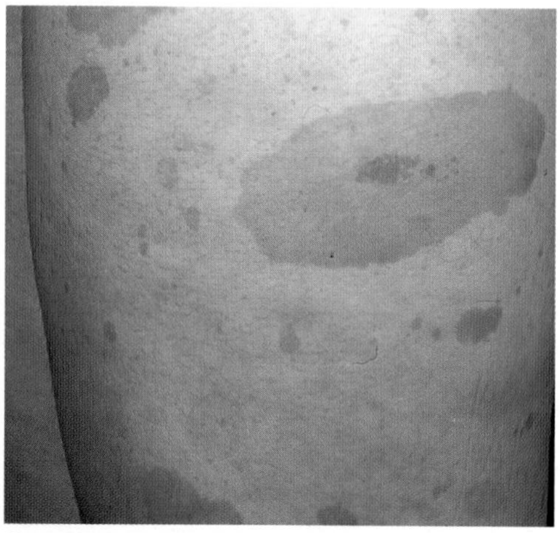

Fig. 4.8 Café au lait patches in neurofibromatosis.

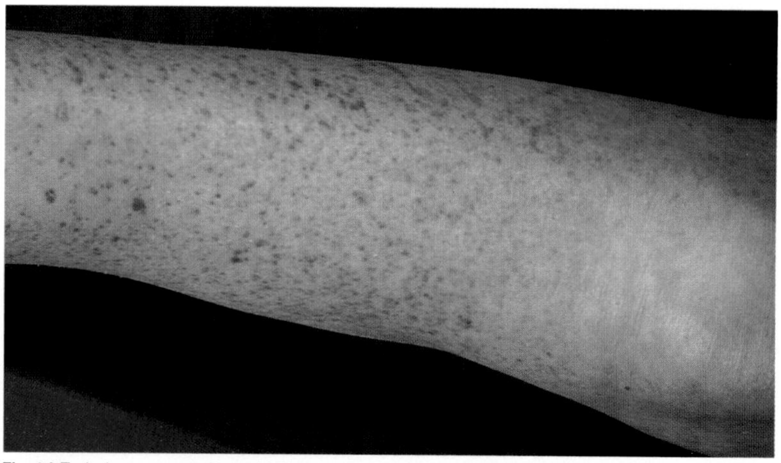

Fig. 4.9 Typical appearance of petechial haemorrhage in a patient with thrombocytopoenia.

lesions are called purpura. Traumatic bruises are called ecchymoses. Telangiectasia refers to fine blanching vascular lesions caused by superficial capillary dilatation (Fig. 4.10).

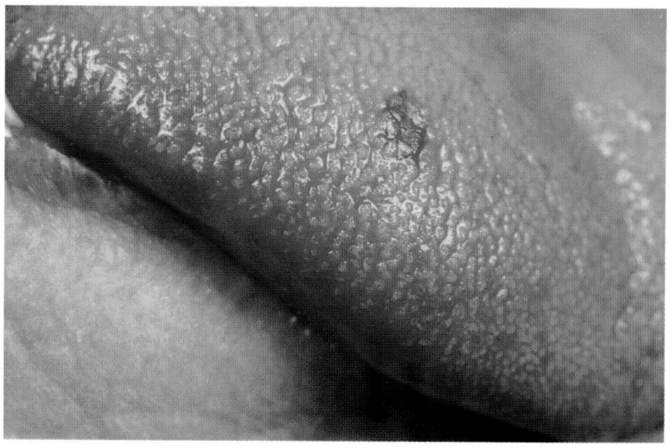

Fig. 4.10 Telangiectasia on the tongue.

Localized skin lesion

Careful descriptions of size, shape, colour, texture, and position of skin lesions is helpful in skin diagnosis. Try to ascertain a primary and secondary description of the skin lesion. To establish the primary nature of the skin lesion decide whether the lesion is flat, nodular, or fluid-filled. Flat circumscribed changes in colour are termed macules (if <1cm) or patches (if >1cm). If the lesion is raised and can be palpated, assess whether the mass is a papule, plaque, nodule, tumor, or wheal. If a circumscribed elevated lesion is fluctuant and fluid-filled, describe whether it is a vesicle, bulla, or pustule (Fig. 4.11). If possible, describe the arrangement of the lesions, i.e. whether linear, annular (ring-shaped), or clustered. In shingles (herpes zoster), the rash occurs in the distribution of one or more skin dermatomes.

Add to the primary description any secondary characteristics such as superficial erosions, ulceration, crusting, scaling, fissuring, lichenification, atrophy, excoriation, scarring, necrosis, or keloid formation.

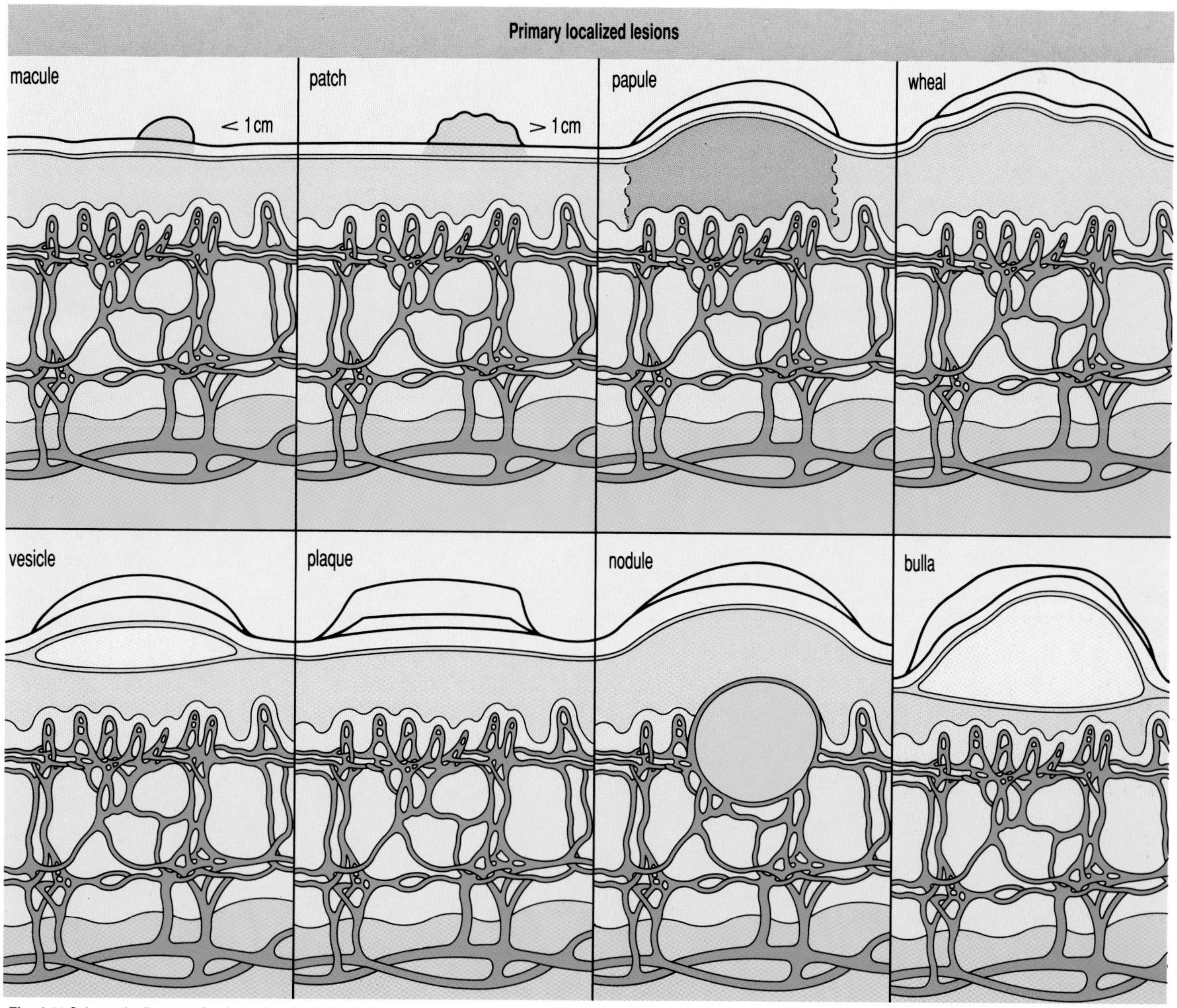

Fig. 4.11 Schematic diagram of primary localized skin lesions.

Palpation is used to decide whether a lesion is flat, raised, or tender. Compression may be helpful (e.g. demonstration of the characteristic arteriolar dilatation of spider naevi occuring in decompensated liver disease) (Fig. 4.12). Use the back of your hand to assess temperature. Inflamed lesions (e.g. cellulitis) are hotter than surrounding tissue, whilst skin overlying a lipoma (subcutaneous fat tumors) is cooler than adjacent tissue. Skin turgor may be used as a measure of moderate to severe hydration. Pinch a small area of skin between index finger and thumb. Hold firmly for 2–3 seconds and then release. Healthy, well-hydrated skin immediately springs back into its resting position. In significant dehydration and when skin elastic tissue is lost (e.g. ageing), the skin behaves like putty and only slowly reshapes to its resting position. Skin oedema can be demonstrated by pressing your thumb or fingers into the skin, maintaining the pressure for a short while and then releasing. Your thumb or finger impression will remain indented in the skin if there is excessive fluid ('pitting' oedema).

Although most disorders can be diagnosed from their appearance, special techniques such as microscopy of skin biopsies or skin scrapings, immunofluorescent staining, and culture of specimens may be required to confirm diagnosis.

Common skin lesions

Common skin lesions are often readily recognizable and you should be able to distinguish some common conditions.

Acne vulgaris

This common disorder of the pilosebaceous apparatus occurs at puberty. Plugging of the duct, increased sebum production, bacterial growth, and hormonal changes all predispose to the condition. Acne presents with greasy skin, blackheads (comedones), papules, pustules, and scars (Fig. 4.13). The lesions are common, vary in severity, and most teenagers recognize the problem before visiting the doctor. The disorder affects the face, chest, and back. Acne usually subsides in the third decade.

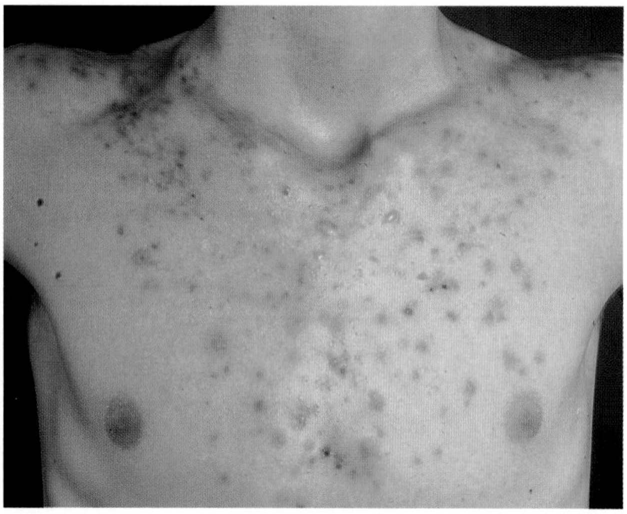

Fig. 4.13 Papules, pustules, and scarring in acne vulgaris.

Rosacea

This facial rash usually presents in the fourth decade, although in women, it may present after the menopause. Papules and pustules erupt on the forehead, cheeks, bridge of the nose, and the chin. The erythematous background highlights the rash (Figs 4.14 and 4.15). Comedones do not occur, distinguishing the condition clinically from facial acne. Occasionally, the rash may be localized to the nose. Eye involvement is characterized by grittiness, conjunctivitis, even corneal ulceration. There appears to be vasomotor instability and patients flush readily in response to stimuli such as hot drinks, alcohol, and spicy foods. If this disorder is treated with potent topical corticosteroids there may be a temporary response, but a marked relapse occurs on cessation of treatment. It is important to check carefully whether or not steroids have been applied and to disuade your patient from using this treatment (like acne vulgaris, antibiotics are the treatment of choice).

Fig. 4.12 Spider naevi in hepatocellular disease.

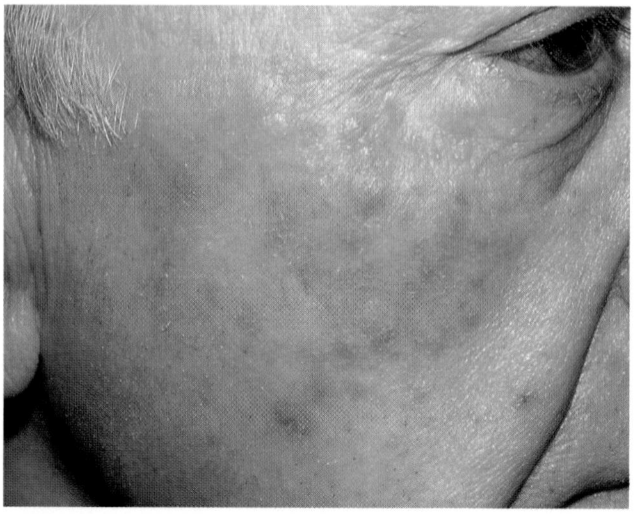

Fig. 4.14 Rosacea. Papules and pustules occur on the face.

Drug reaction

Drugs are probably the most common cause of acute skin disease and your history must include a complete history of all drugs the patient may have been exposed to over the preceding month. Antibiotics such as ampicillin, penicillin, and sulphonamides commonly cause drug rashes (Fig. 4.16). It may be difficult to distinguish between a drug reaction and the manifestations of the disease under treatment. In addition, drug reaction may closely mimic skin diseases. Diagnosis may be further confused in patients taking more than one drug, for it may be difficult to decide which is the offending agent. Also remember that drugs may cause secondary skin eruptions; broad spectrum antibiotics may encourage the growth of candida which in turn can present as a 'drug related' skin rash. Drug reactions may occur within minutes or hours of taking the medication, but there may also be delays of up to two weeks for the reaction to manifest. This may even follow the discontinuation of the drug (best recognized with ampicillin). It is important to recognize different expressions of drug sensitivity.

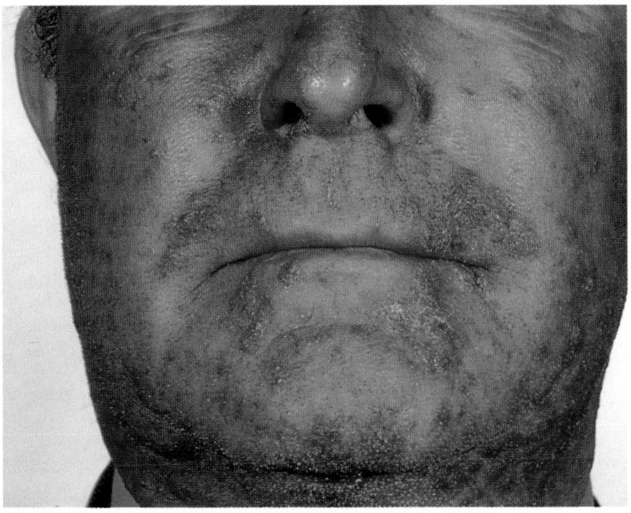

Fig. 4.15 Rosacea. The lesions occur on the nose, cheeks, and chin.

Skin lesions associated with drug sensitivity
Toxic erythema
Exfoliative dermatitis
Urticaria
Angioneurotic oedema
Erythema nodosum
Erythema multiforme
Fixed drug reaction
Photosensitive drug reactions
Pemphigus

Fig. 4.16. Skin lesions associated with drug sensitivity.

Toxic erythema

Profuse eruptions affect most of the body. Red macules appear which overlap and coalesce to give the appearance of diffuse erythema (Fig. 4.17). The erythematous skin desquamates as it heals. This condition is most often caused by ampicillin, but also by sulphonamides (including cotrimoxazole), phenobarbitone and infections.

Exfoliative dermatitis

Also known as erythroderma, this form of dermatitis is characterized by diffuse erythema and desquamation of the epithelium. If

Exfoliative dermatitis

Is there any loss of hair or nails?

Have you ever had psoriasis or or eczema?

What drugs have you taken recently (barbituates, sulphonamides, phenylbutazone, streptomycin)?

Do you have a fever?

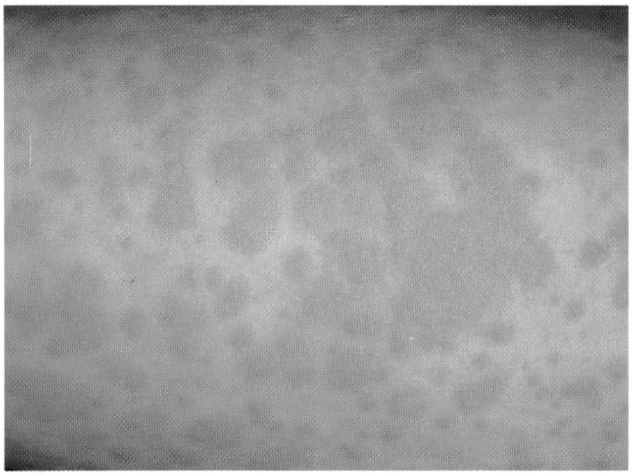

Fig. 4.17 Toxic erythema.

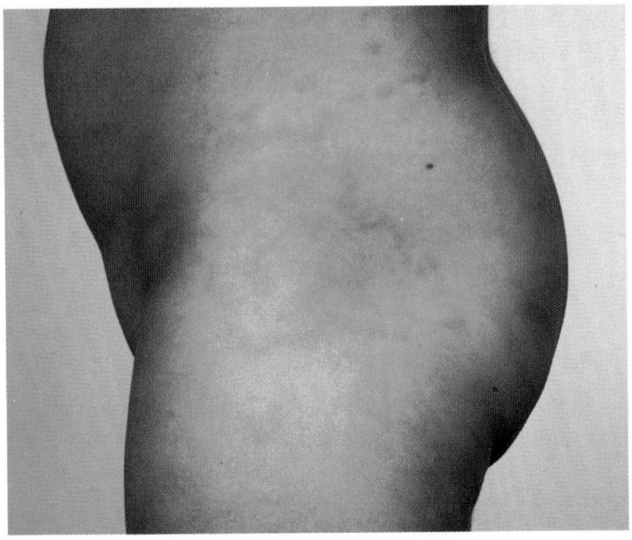

Fig. 4.18 Urticaria. The lesions vary in size and shape.

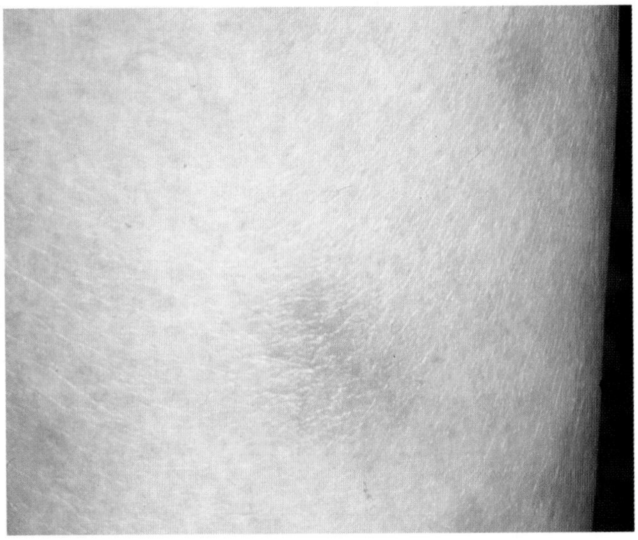

Fig. 4.19 Erythema nodosum. Painful, smooth red nodules on the lower leg.

severe, the patient may lose both heat and fluids. Many drugs are implicated, though barbiturates, sulphonamides, streptomycin, and gold are especially predominant.

Urticaria

Urticaria presents with intense itching and localized swellings of the skin which may occur anywhere on the body. Typically, wheals occur which are red at the margins with paler centres (Fig. 4.18). The characteristic feature of the rash is its tendency to disappear within a few hours. Angio-oedema usually occurs in association with urticaria and is characterized by swelling of the face and hands.

Erythema nodosum

Symmetrical in distribution, the acute crops of painful, tender, raised red nodules usually affect the extensor surfaces, especially the shins, but also the thighs and upper arms (Figs 4.19 and 4.20). Over 7–10 days, the lesions change colour from bright red through shades of purple to a yellowish area of discoloration. Erythema nodosum is caused by vasculitis, may be recurrent, and is most commonly associated with sulphonamides, oral contraceptives and barbiturates (Fig. 4.21).

Erythema multiforme

Erythema multiforme is characterized by symmetrical, round (annular) lesions occurring especially on the hands and feet but may extend more proximally (Figs 4.22 and 4.23). Central blistering may occur giving the appearance of 'Target' lesions. In severe forms, bullae may appear. This skin disease occurs with drugs, vaccination, and frequently with a herpes simplex infection.

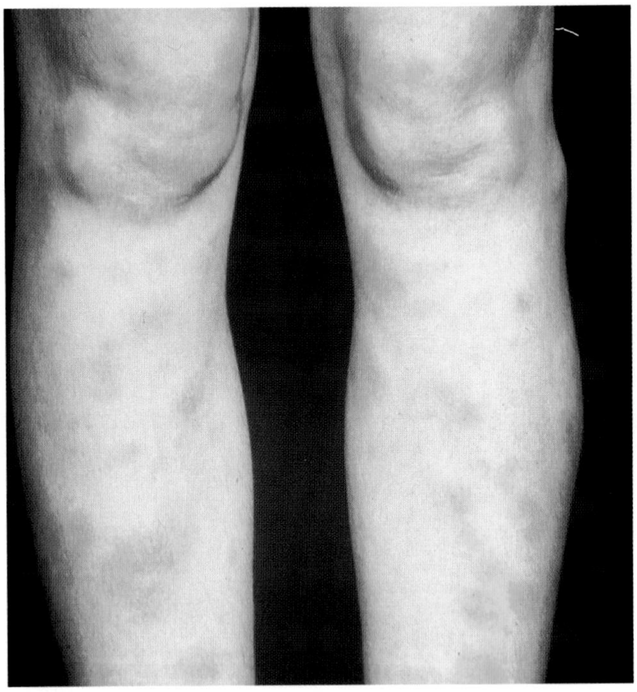

Fig. 4.20 Erythema nodosum. The nodules are raised and tender.

Stevens–Johnson syndrome

A severe blistering form of erythema multiforme with blistering and ulceration affecting mucous membranes of the mouth and often affecting the eyes, nasal and genital mucosa (Fig. 4.24).

Fixed drug eruption

One or more red blotches which may become swollen and even bullous. The rash always recurs in the same anatomical site, usually mouth, limb or genital area. The rash fades, leaving area of skin

Causes of erythema nodosum

Infections
- Streptococcal infections
- Tuberculosis
- Leprosy
- Syphilis
- Deep fungal diseases

Drugs
- Sulphonamides
- Barbiturates
- Oral contraceptives

Systemic diseases
- Sarcoidosis
- Inflammatory bowel disease

Fig. 4.21 The causes of erythema nodosum.

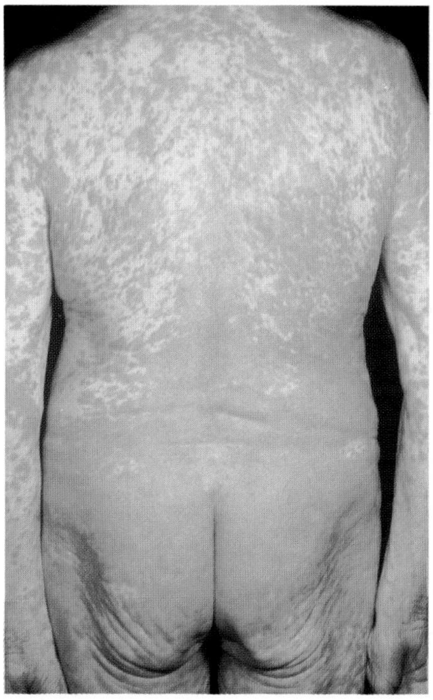

Fig. 4.22 Erythema multiforme. The lesions are widespread on this patient.

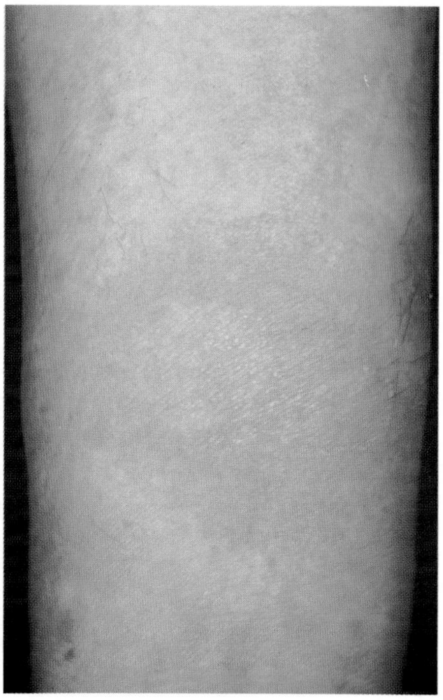

Fig. 4.23 Erythema multiforme.

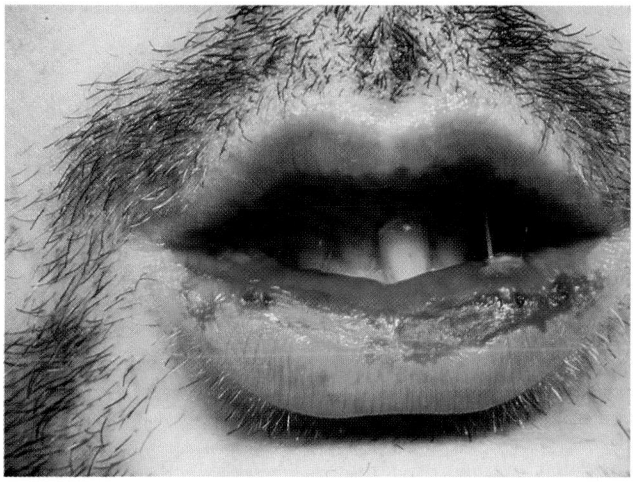

Fig. 4.24 Stevens–Johnson syndrome. Ulceration is present on the lips and in the mouth.

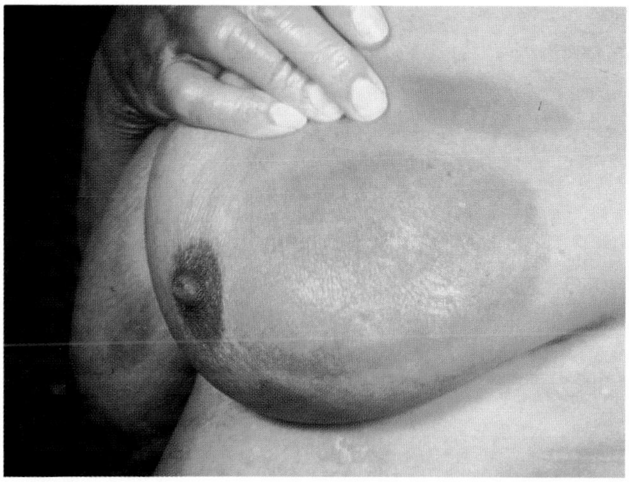

Fig. 4.25 Fixed drug eruption, with hyperpigmentation of the breasts.

discoloration (Fig. 4.25). Associated with many drugs but especially phenolphthalein (common in laxatives), sulphonamides, tetracycline, and barbiturates.

Photosensitive drug rashes

The rash occurs in sun exposed areas (face, necklace region and extensor surfaces of limbs). May appear as erythema, oedema, blistering, or an eczematous rash. Commonly implicated drugs include tetracyclines, sulphonamides, and phenothiazines. Remember that photosensitve rashes occur in systemic diseases such as lupus erythematosus and porphyria (cutanea tarda).

Eczema

This common skin abnormality is caused by a number of different mechanisms and the disease may be acute, subacute, or chronic, all of which may coexist. Itching is a major symptom. Acute eczema is characterized by oedema, vesicle formation (Fig. 4.26), exudation (weeping) (Fig. 4.27), and finally, crusting. In chronic eczema there are dry, scaly, hyperkeratotic patches thickening and fissuring of the skin (Fig. 4.28). The appearance of eczema is often modified because the patient scratches causing secondary changes such as excoriation, and secondary infection. The boundaries of an area of chronic eczema is less well-defined than psoriasis and this may be a helpful sign in the differential diagnosis (Fig. 4.29).

Discoid (nummular) eczema

Unlike other forms of eczema this subtype has a well-defined (coin-shaped [L. nummularius = of money]) outline and may be confused with psoriasis. However, nummular eczema tends to occur on the back of the fingers and hands, weeps, and does not have the characteristic scales typical of psoriasis.

Atopic eczema

Atopic eczema usually presents in infancy, yet the disorder occasionally presents for the first time in adulthood. There is usually a family history of eczema or some other atopic disorder (e.g. asthma, hay fever, urticaria). The rash is symmetrical, usually starting on the face and migrating to the trunk and limbs (where it tends to affect the flexures of the elbows, knees, wrists, and ankle).

Contact dermatitis

This variant of eczema is caused by an exogenous irritant (Fig. 4.30). The lesion may be a primary irritant phenomenon occuring almost predictably when skin contact is made with a concentrated toxic agent, or an allergic contact dermatitis, which only occurs in patients who generate a delayed (type IV) immune response to a substance in contact with the skin. The distribution of the eczema may provide an important clue to the nature of the topical irritant. Individuals who regularly immerse their hands in water containing detergents or other sensitizing substances will present with the rash restricted to the hands. Jewellery may cause an allergic contact dermatitis; nickel is an important sensitizing agent. Rubber, dyes, cosmetics, and industrial chemicals are common allergens implicated in this immune-mediated form of eczema. Plants such as primula and chrysanthemums have also been implicated.

Fig. 4.26 Eczema. Note the vesicle formation.

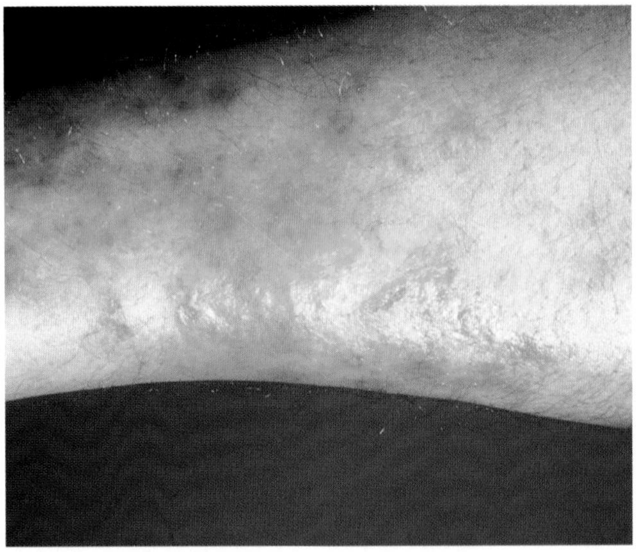

Fig. 4.27 Acute eczema. The red exudative eruption is quite painful.

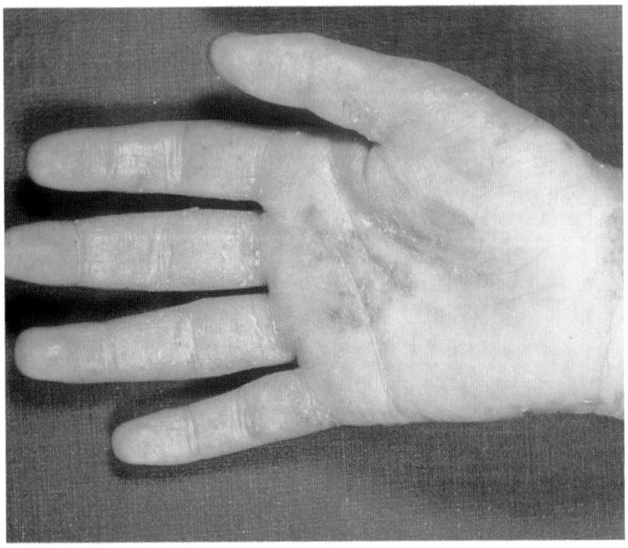

Fig. 4.28 Chronic eczema. The skin is dry and scaly.

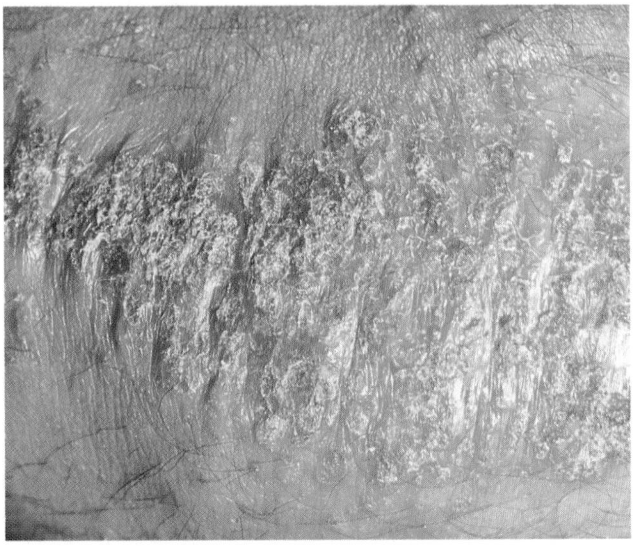

Fig. 4.29 Typical appearance of eczematous lesion. Note that the boundary is less distinct than plaques of psoriasis.

Seborrhoeic dermatitis

Seborrhoeic dermatitis is an eczematous condition occuring in infants (Fig. 4.31), adolescents, and young adults. There is erythema and scaling, with a symmetrical rash (Fig. 4.32). Secondary infection may occur, altering the appearance of the primary lesion. The scalp is most commonly involved and is distinguished from dandruff by the associated erythema of the skin due to inflammation. Other areas involved include the central areas of the face, eyelid margins, nasolabial folds, cheeks, eyebrows, and forehead. Involvement of the outer ear occurs (otitis externa). The vulva may be affected.

Pompholyx

Pompholyx is another variant of eczema affecting the hands and feet (Figs 4.33 and 4.34). This variant is characterized by the eruption of itchy vesicles, especially on the lateral margins of the fingers and toes, as well as the palms and soles.

Varicose eczema

This subtype occurs in patients with longstanding varicose veins. The eczematous patches affect the lower leg and may or may not be associated with other skin disorders caused by varicose veins (e.g. venous ulcers which occur in the region of the medial maleolus, pigmentation, and oedema).

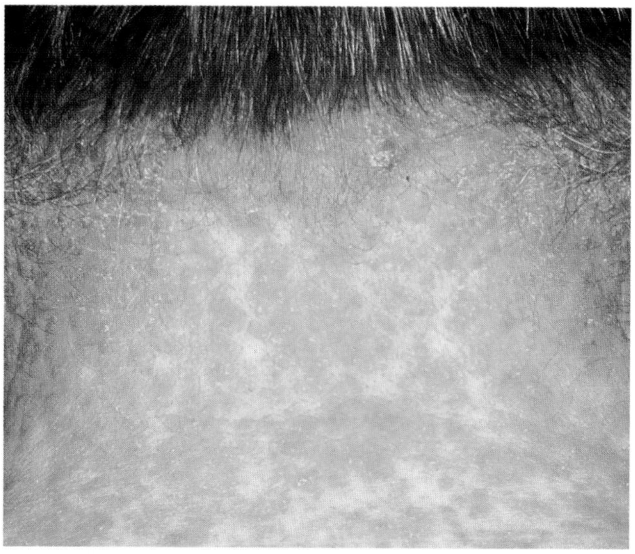

Fig. 4.30 Contact dermatitis caused by shampoo.

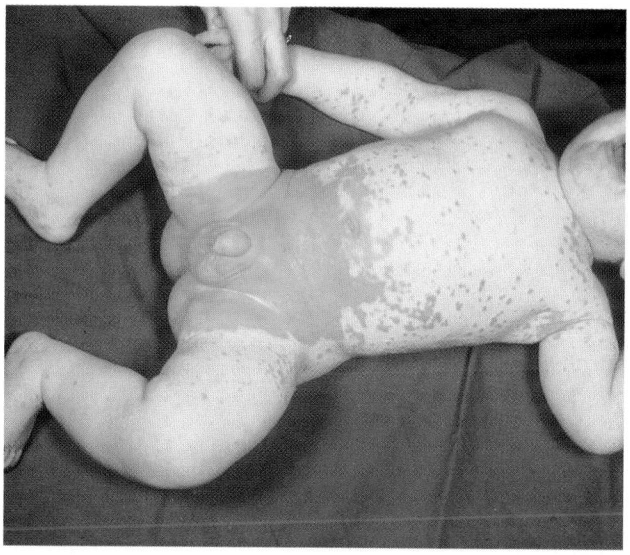

Fig. 4.31 Seborrhoeic dermatitis in an infant.

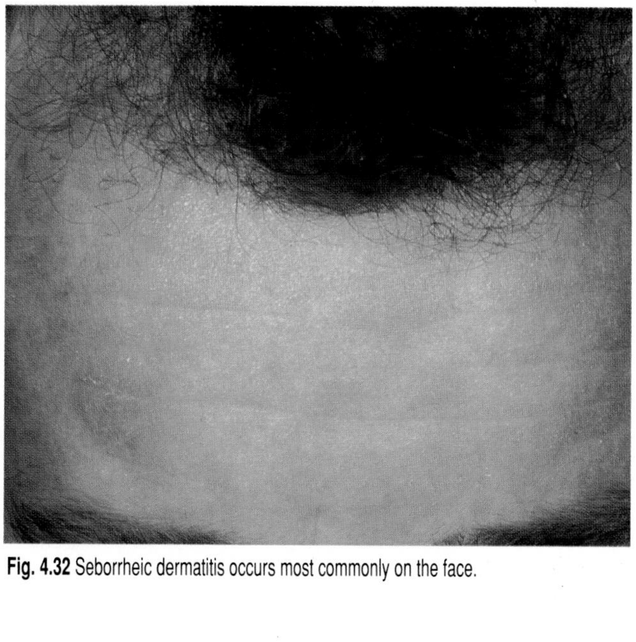

Fig. 4.32 Seborrheic dermatitis occurs most commonly on the face.

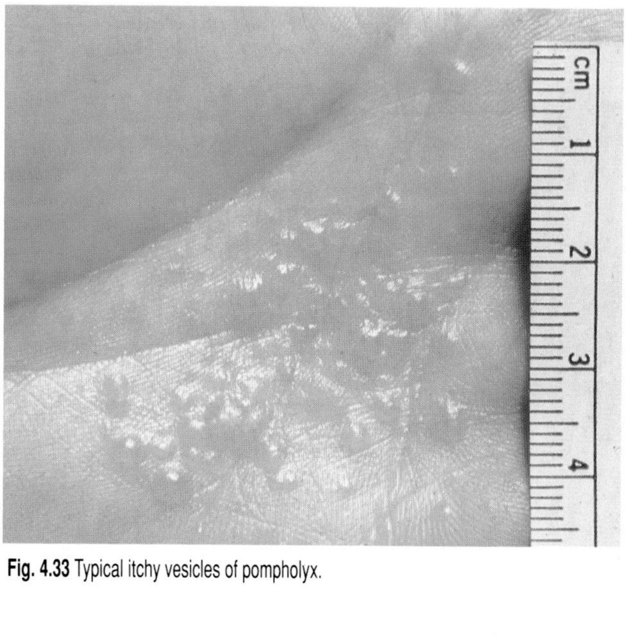

Fig. 4.33 Typical itchy vesicles of pompholyx.

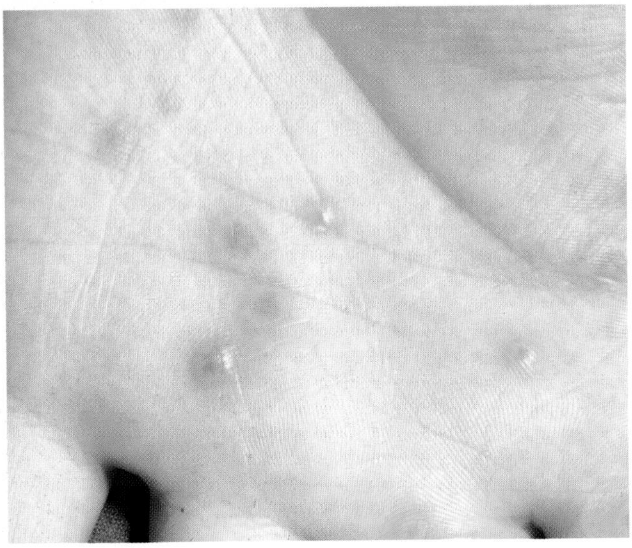

Fig. 4.34 Pompholyx. Pruritic vesicles on the hand.

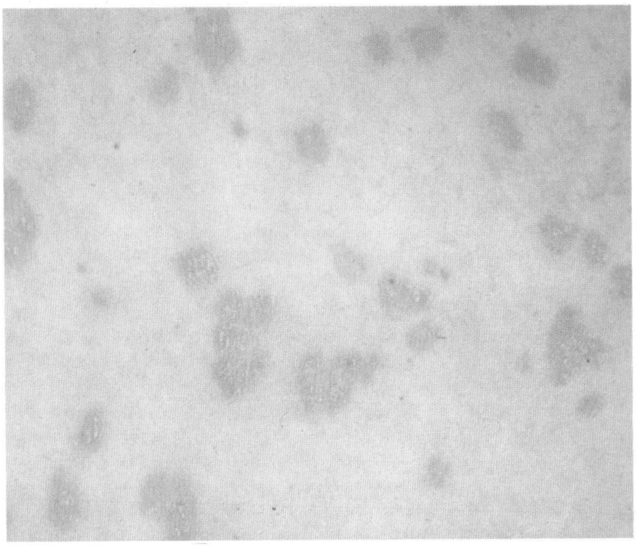

Fig. 4.35 Guttate (teardrop) psoriasis.

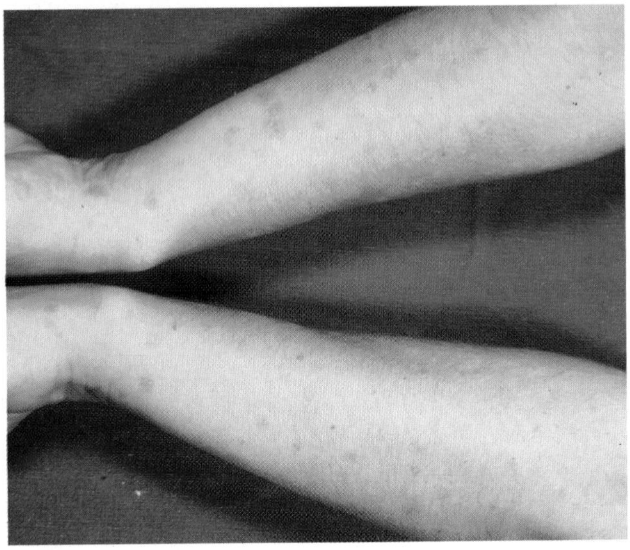

Fig. 4.36 Acute guttate psoriasis.

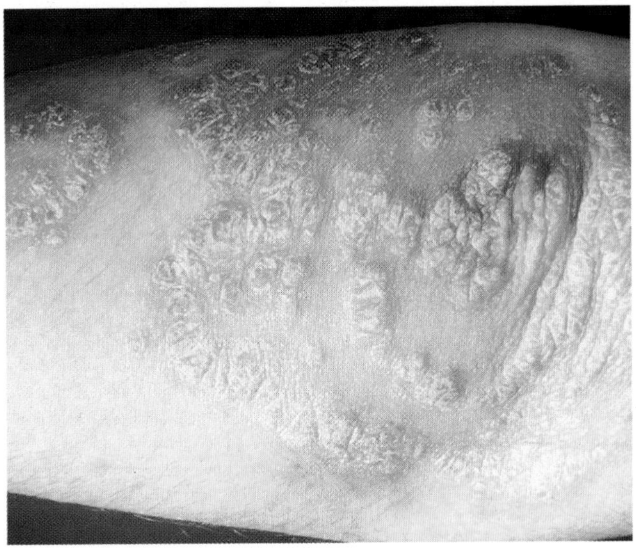

Fig. 4.37 Psoriatic plaque covered with a silvery scale.

Psoriasis

The lesion is well-defined, slightly raised, and erythematous. In the chronic phase, silvery scales cover the surface. The lesions vary in size from small (guttate) (Figs 4.35 and 4.36) to large plaques (Figs 4.37 and 4.38). These 1–3cm guttate lesions are widely distributed over the body and may either resolve or persist as chronic psoriasis. Guttate psoriasis may follow streptococcal pharyngitis.

Chronic psoriasis

The plaques of chronic psoriasis have a predeliction for the scalp, elbows, knees, perineum, umbilicus, and submammary skin. The lesions are usually symmetrical. A characteristic feature of psoriasis is the development of new psoriatic lesions where the skin is traumatized (the Koebner phenomenon). If you gently scratch the surface of a psoriatic plaque, tiny bleeding points appear.

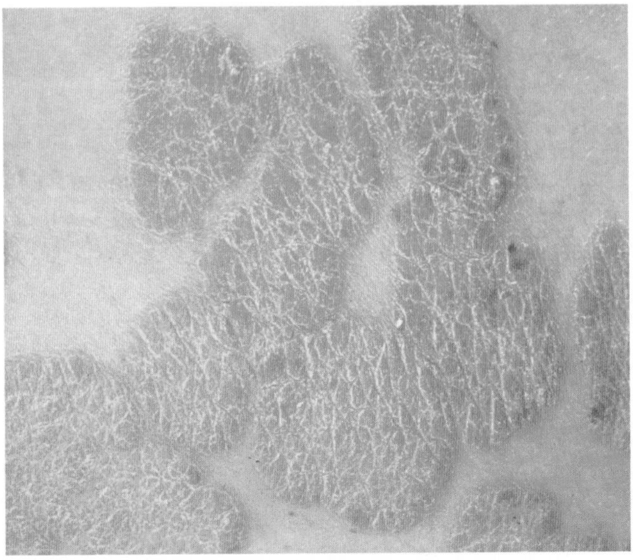

Fig. 4.38 Psoriatic plaque. Note the scaly, shiny surface and the sharp border.

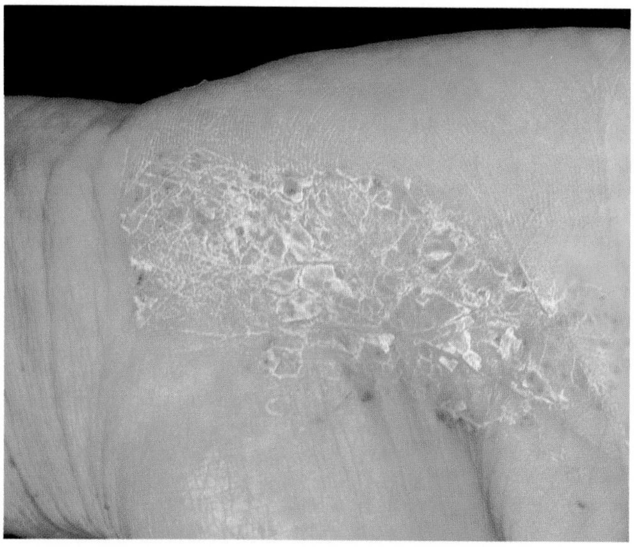
Fig. 4.39 Pustular psoriasis of the palm with well-defined scaling and erythema.

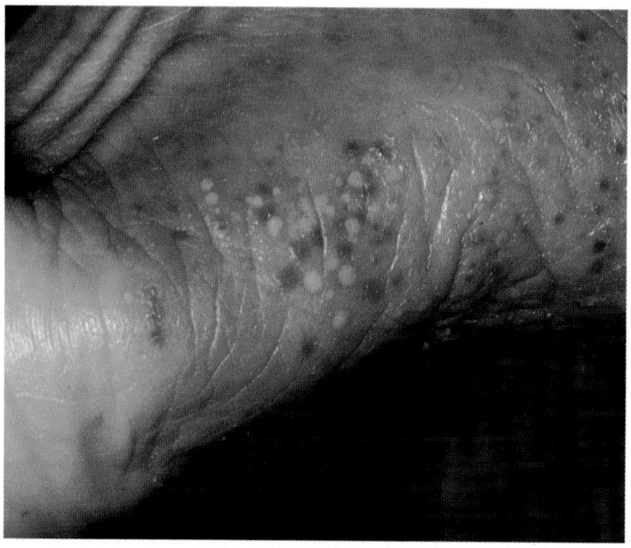
Fig. 4.40 Pustular psoriasis of the foot. The yellow pustules turn brown.

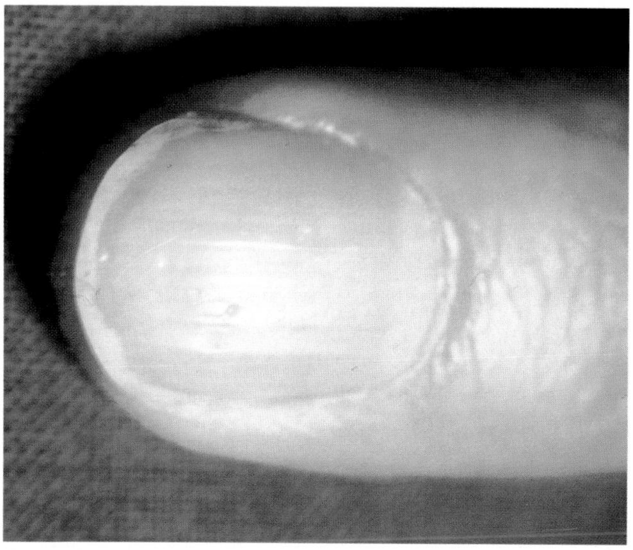
Fig. 4.41 Pitting of the nails in psoriasis.

Fig. 4.42 Pityriasis rosea. The pink papules become oval macules.

Pustular psoriasis

Pustular psoriasis is a variant, usually confined to the palms (Fig. 4.39) and soles but are occasionally more diffuse. The pustules, 2–5mm in diameter, are a yellow colour (Fig. 4.40). On the palms and soles they become pigmented and hyperkeratotic. Rarely, psoriasis may be so extensive that most of the skin is involved and exfoliation occurs.

Psoriatic arthropathy

In psoriatic arthropathy, the distal interphalangeal joints are affected. Large joints may also be affected either singly or symmetrically. Rarely, patients may have sacroileitis or even spinal ankylosis. The nails may be involved even in the absence of skin disease. The typical features include pin-point pitting of the nail (Fig. 4.41) and onycholysis (lifting of the distal nail from the nail bed). Unlike fungal nail lesions, nail psoriasis is symmetrical. Severe nail dystrophy may occur.

Pityriasis rosea

This is a common skin disorder in the younger patient. A single patch rash occurs days or even weeks before the more general eruption. This 'herald patch' may be confused with ringworm. The full blown rash affects the upper arms, trunk, and upper thighs ('shirt and shorts' distribution). Pink papules evolve into 1–3cm itchy oval macules (Fig. 4.42) which scale near the edge giving a characteristic appearance (Figs 4.43 and 4.44). The rash resolves spontaneously within approximately six weeks.

Lichen planus

This is another itchy rash which can usually be diagnosed at the bedside by its typical appearance (Fig. 4.45). Occasionally, a lichenoid rash may be associated with systemic disorders (e.g. primary biliary cirrhosis, chronic graft versus host disease) or drugs (e.g penicillamine and gold), but most commonly there is no associated disease.

The rash affects both the skin and mucous membranes. It has a predeliction for the volar (front) aspect of the forearm and wrists, the dorsal (back) surface of the hands, the shins, ankles, and lower back region. The rash is symmetrical and characterized by small, shiny, purple or violaceous papules which have a polygonal rather than rounded outline. A network of white lines on the surface of the papules are termed Wickham's striae (best seen after coating the lesion with mineral oil). As the papules resolve, the affected skin becomes pigmented. Eruptions occur after trauma (Koebner phenomenon) (Fig. 4.46) and linear lesions are tell tale signs occurring in scratched areas. The buccal mucous membrane is commonly involved (Fig. 4.47). Use a spatula and light to inspect the mouth, looking for the lace-like network of white lines or spots. The scalp is usually, although not always, spared. The disease may affect the nails and penis.

SKIN INFECTIONS

BACTERIAL

Impetigo

This is a highly contageous skin lesion caused by β-haemolytic streptococci. The face is most commonly infected (Fig. 4.48). The lesions start as a papular eruption around the mouth and nose, then evolves into a vesicular eruption, and spreads locally. The lesion breaks down to leave a typical honey-coloured crust. Secondary infection with Staphylococcus aureus is common.

Furuncle (boil)

A furuncle is an infection by S. aureus of a hair follicle which spreads locally into the surrounding tissue. A head of pus may be obvious at its apex. Furuncles usually affect adolescents. A local collection of furuncles is called a carbuncle. A stye (or Hordeoli) is a small furuncle affecting an eyelash.

Erysipelas and cellulitis

Infection of the superficial skin layers by *S. pyogenes* is termed erysipelas, whilst an infection of the deeper skin layers is called cellulitis. The lower limbs are most commonly affected. Erysipelas is characterized by the abrupt onset of a well-demarcated slightly raised and tender erythematous rash (Fig. 4.49). Left untreated, the margins of the lesion advance rapidly. The patient is usually pyrexial and toxic. The infection responds quickly to antibiotics. The margin of an area of cellulitis is less well-defined than erysipelas; in addition, superficial bullae may develop in the centre of an affected area of skin (Fig. 4.50).

Syphilis

There are numerous skin manifestations of syphilis and you should always suspect this disease when confronted with an unexplained, non-itchy rash, especially when the patient is generally unwell or where there is a high risk of venereal disease. In primary syphilis, a painless ulcer with an indurated edge (primary chancre) (Figs 4.51 and 4.52)) appears at the site of infection (usually on the genitalia but occasionally on the lips or even fingers). About two months after the appearance of the chancre, the secondary rash appears. A pink macular rash appears on the trunk (Fig. 4.53) and then becomes papular, affecting the genital skin, palms, and soles.

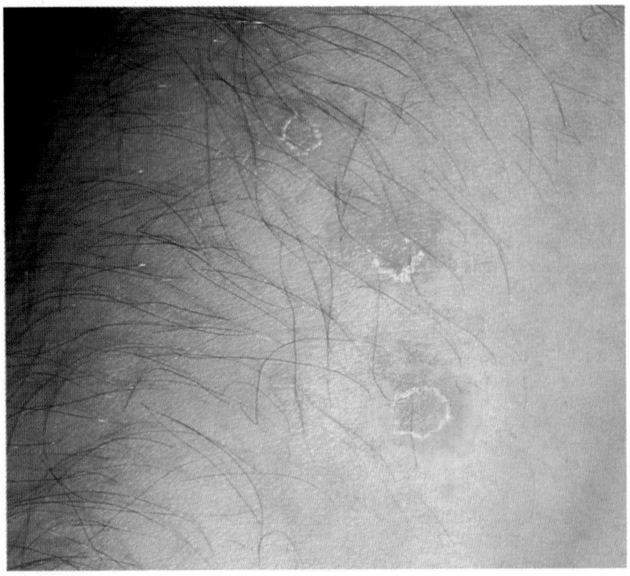

Fig. 4.43 In pityriasis rosea, the typical lesions are ovoid macules with scaling.

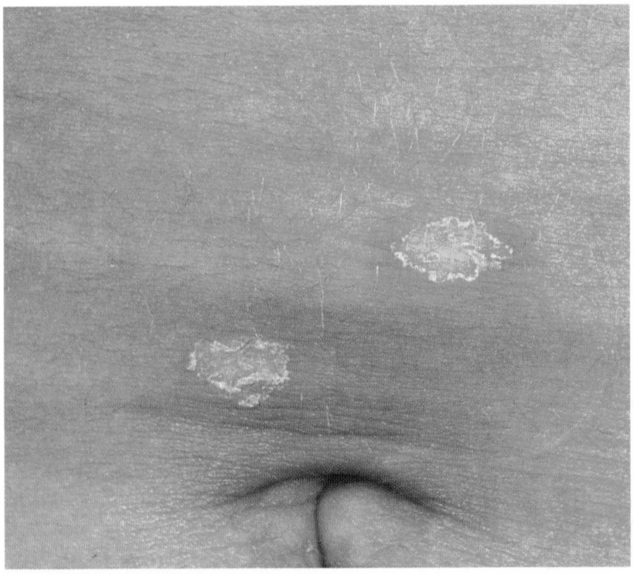

Fig. 4.44 Pityriasis rosea with obvious scaling.

In the anal and groin regions, the moistness may cause erosions (condylomata accuminata) (Fig. 4.54). Raised oval patches occur in the mucous membrane of the mouth (snail track ulcers). In the tertiary stage, granulomas form (gummas); these can be felt as skin nodules which are prone to degenerate and ulcerate.

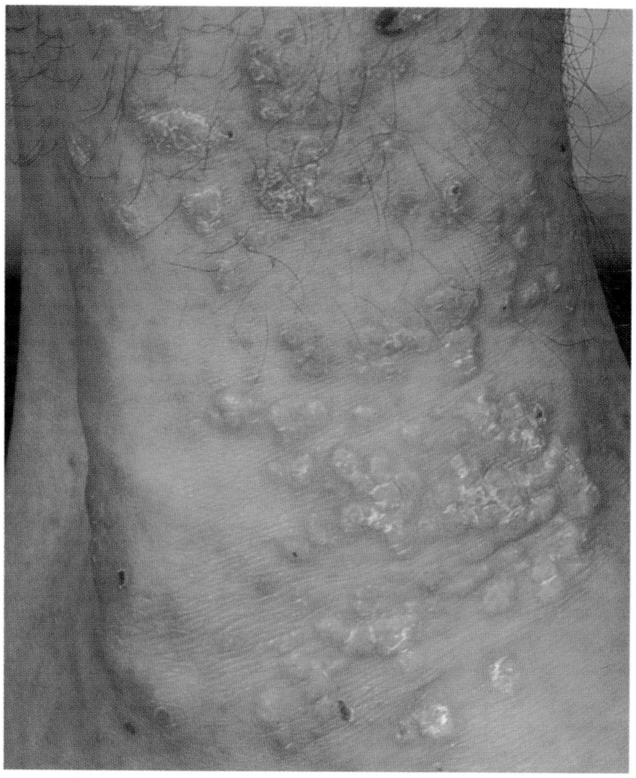

Fig. 4.45 Polygonal papules in lichen planus.

VIRAL

Warts

Common warts caused by papilloma viruses are self-limiting and usually occur at younger ages. Warts usually occur on the fingers and hands as discrete papules with a typical irregular surface (Fig. 4.55). Plantar warts occur on the pressure bearing areas of the feet and are consequently flattened rather than raised.

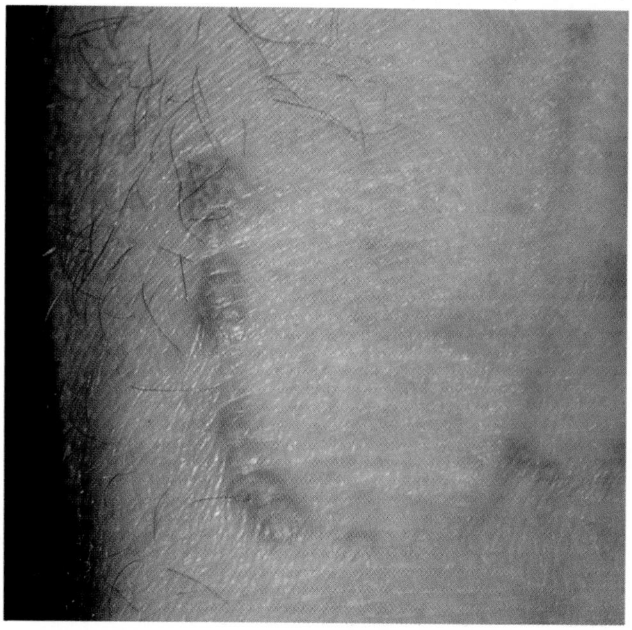

Fig. 4.46 Lichen planus. The linear lesion of the Koebner syndrome.

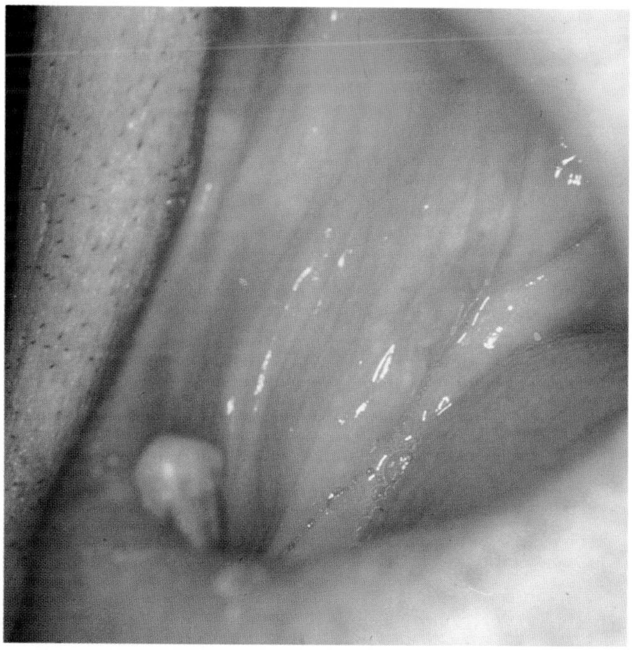

Fig. 4.47 Buccal involvement in lichen planus.

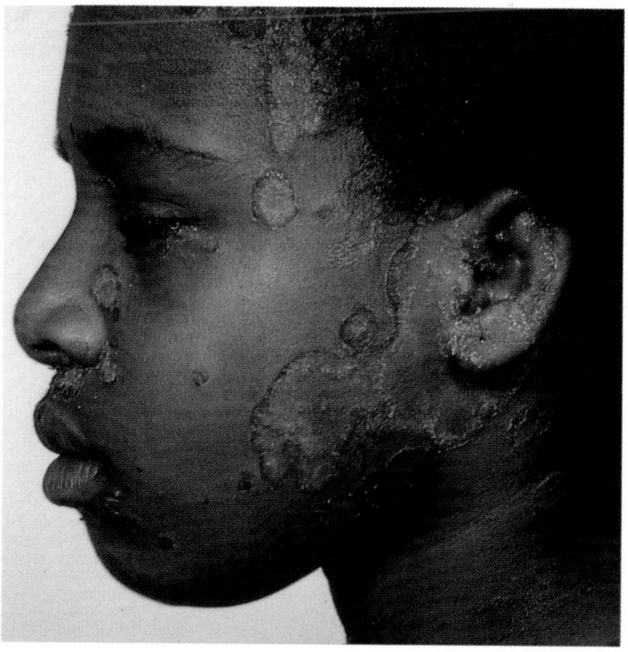

Fig. 4.48 Facial impetigo with crusting of the lesion.

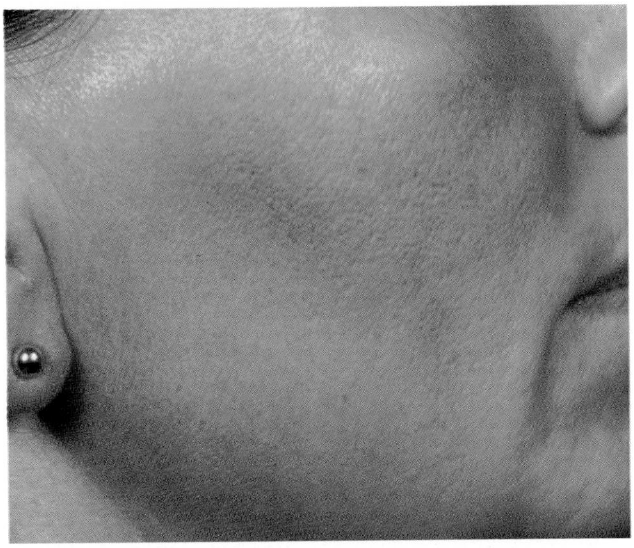

Fig. 4.49 Erysipelas. Note the erythema and oedema.

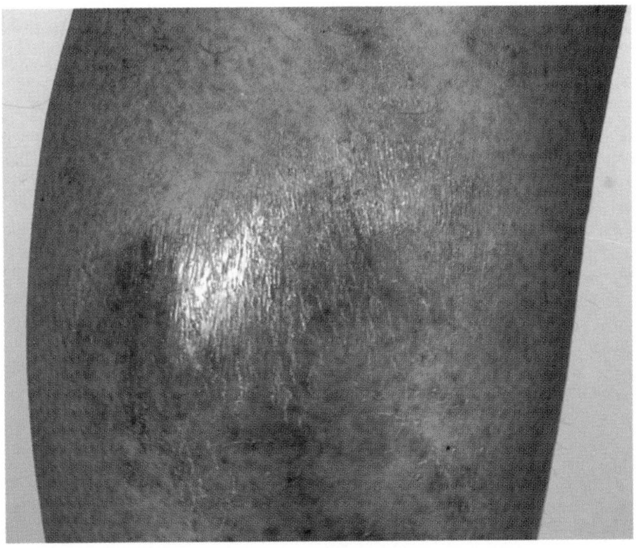

Fig. 4.50 Erythema and oedema associated with cellulitis.

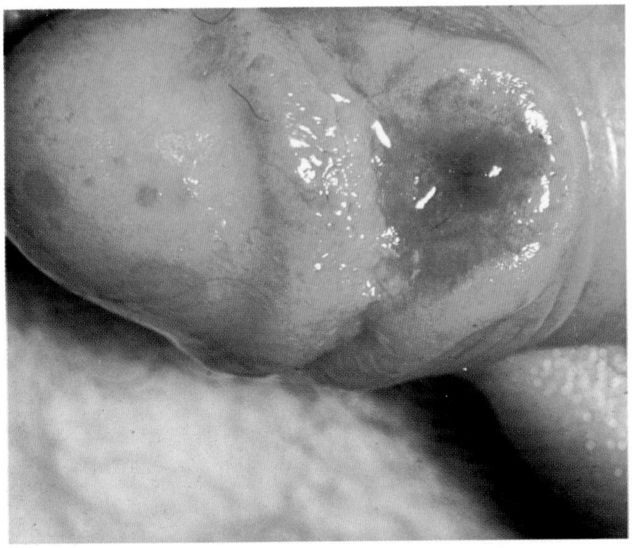

Fig. 4.51 Primary chancre in syphilis.

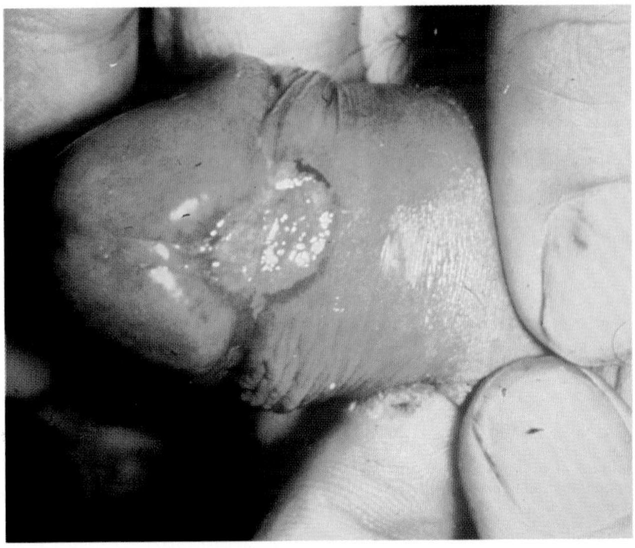

Fig. 4.52 Primary syphilitic chancre on the frenulum.

Molluscum contagiosum

This is a common infection caused by a member of the pox virus group. The lesions appear as flesh-coloured, dome-shaped papules varying in size from a pinpoint to 1cm in diameter. The most characteristic feature of the lesion is umbilication (a central depression of the surface). In children, the lesions are especially common on the face and trunk, whilst in adults, the genitalia may be affected. As the lesions resolve, an area of often develops in the surrounding skin.

Herpes simplex

There are two types of herpes simplex virus (HSV). Type 1 virus normally affects the mouth and lips (Fig. 4.56), whilst type 2 usually causes genital herpes. Crossover infections do sometimes occur. The primary HSV infection presents with crops of painful superficial vesicles surrounded by an area of erythema. The vesicles erode superficially, then crust, and finally heal without scarring. After the primary infection, the virus lies dormant in the dorsal root nerve ganglion, with recurrences occuring predictably in the same area as the initial infection. Reactivation is heralded by a tingling sensation in the skin which is followed within 1–2 days by the eruption of a crop of vesicles. Exacerbations may be precipitated by infection, stress, fever (hence the term fever blisters), abnormal exposure to sunlight, menstruation, and trauma. Often, no obvious precipitating cause is discovered.

Herpes zoster (shingles)

After an attack of chicken pox, the varicella-zoster virus lies dormant in a dorsal root or cranial nerve ganglion. Reactivation of the virus causes a localized eruption called shingles. The cause of

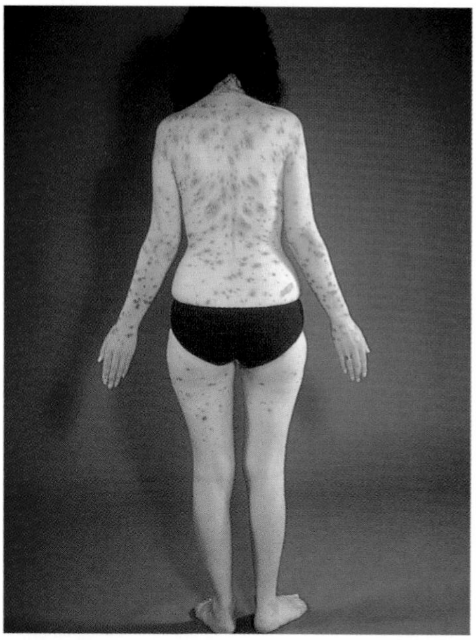

Fig. 4.53 The maculo-papular rash of secondary syphilis.

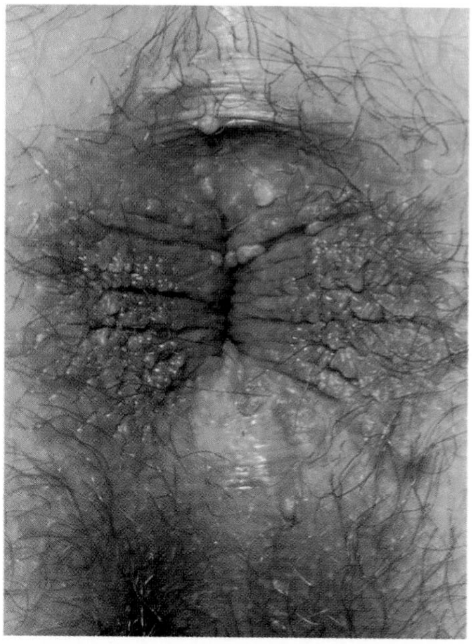

Fig. 4.54 Condylomata accuminata.

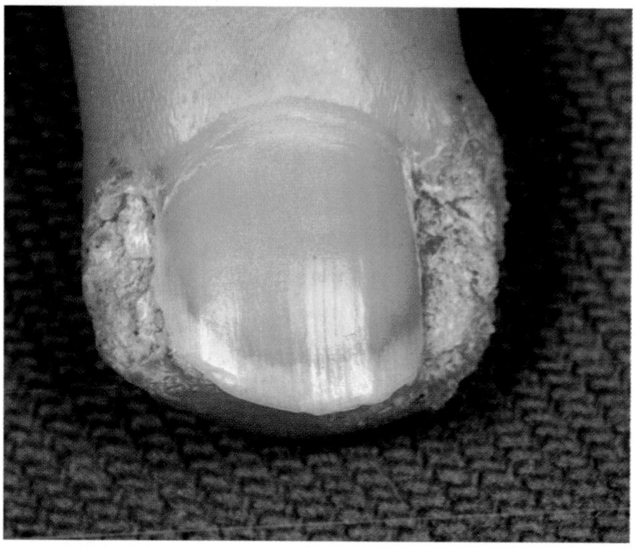

Fig. 4.55 Finger warts.

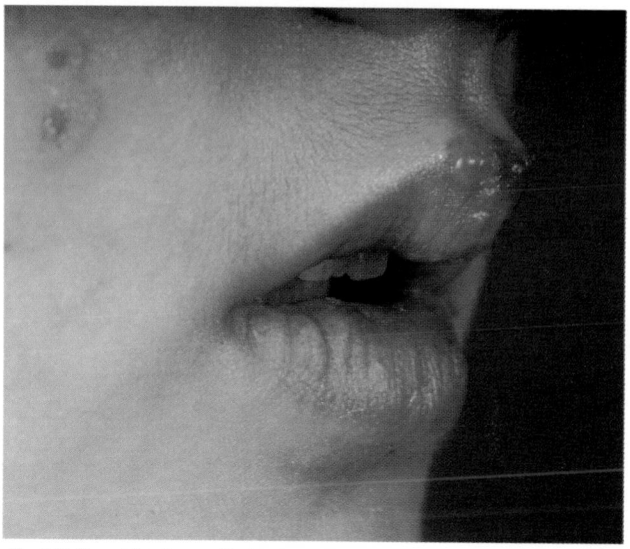

Fig. 4.56 'Fever blister' caused by herpes simplex.

reactivation is often not apparent although immunosuppression, lymphomas, and ageing may be implicated.

The patient complains of pain or discomfort in a localized area of skin and within a few days, a crop of vesicles appear in a characteristic dermatomal distribution (Fig. 4.57). Over 2–3 weeks, the vesicles evolve into pustules, then scab; finally healing occurs. Often there is some residual scarring. The thoracic, cervical, lumbar, and sacral dermatomes are affected in order of frequency. If the ophthalmic branch of the trigeminal nerve is involved, there may be serious damage to the cornea. This is associated with a typical distribution of the vesicles on the tip and side of the nose. Involvement of the geniculate ganglion of the facial nerve causes a facial palsy with involvement of the outer ear (Ramsay Hunt syndrome). The most debilitating long-term effect of shingles, even when healing has occured, is chronic pain and hyperasthesia in the affected dermatome.

FUNGAL

Candida albicans

This is a common infection of the skin and mucous membranes. Oral candidosis tends to occur in immunosuppressed patients, diabetics, and after treatment with antibiotics. Candidosis is a major manifestation of AIDS. Look for candidosis in the mouth; the oral infection is characterized by white or off-white plaques which can be scraped off leaving a raw red base. Other manifestations include angular stomatitis, vulval and vaginal infections, and involvement of contact surfaces (e.g. the natal cleft, inner thighs, scrotum, and infra-mammary fold [intertrigo]).

Pityriasis versicolor (Tinea versicolor)

This common condition of young adults is caused by Malassezia furfur and presents as small pigmented or hypopigmented macules on the upper trunk and arms. The macules tend to coalesce, resulting in lesions which vary in size and shape. Scales can be demonstrated by scraping or teasing the lesions with a scalpel blade. In sunburnt areas, the lesions appear to be hypopigmented in comparison to the surrounding skin.

Dermatophytes (Tinea)

The dermatophytes inhabit stratum corneum and the dead keratin of the nails and hair. Hair infection (tinea capitis) presents with localized patches of hair loss and skin inflammation. Skin infection (tinea corporis) affects the non-hairy parts of the body. This presentation is often referred to as 'ringworm', as the lesion has an inflamed annular edge with a paler central area of healing (Fig. 4.58). Athlete's foot (tinea pedis) appears as a scaling erythematous rash between the toes. A nail infections (tinea unguium) is often asymmetrical and affects the toenails more often than the fingernails. The nail becomes yellow and thick; there is onycholysis and, at a later stage, the nail crumbles and breaks. If suspected, take nail clippings for mycology.

INFESTATIONS

Pediculosis

Infestation with lice causes skin irritation. Headlice (pediculosis capitis) is common in children. The diagnosis is made by careful inspection of the hair for eggs (nits) which unlike dandruff, cannot be shaken off the hair. Scratching may give rise to secondary inflammation and itching. Body lice (pediculosis corporis) is rare and almost always occurs in malnutrition and where hygiene is poor. Infection of the pubic hair (pediculosis pubis) is caused by the crab louse and is usually sexually transmitted. Like other lice infections, the infestation causes intense pruritus and the nits (and lice) are seen with the naked eye.

Scabies

Consider scabies in any patient presenting with widespread pruritus. The mite (Sarcoptes scabei) burrows into the skin where the female lays her eggs. The burrows can be seen on inspection; look for these along the sides of the fingers, the webs (Fig. 4.59) and the wrist. The burrows are linear, just palpable, and the white dot of the mite can often be seen. The lesions may develop into inflamed papules and may affect the elbows, axilla, and genitalia. Scratching causes secondary excoriation and infection,

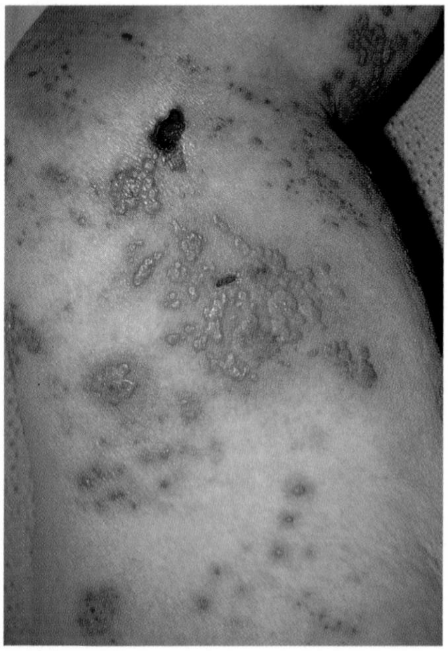

Fig. 4.57 Herpes zoster. Note the haemorrhagic lesions (distribution of L2).

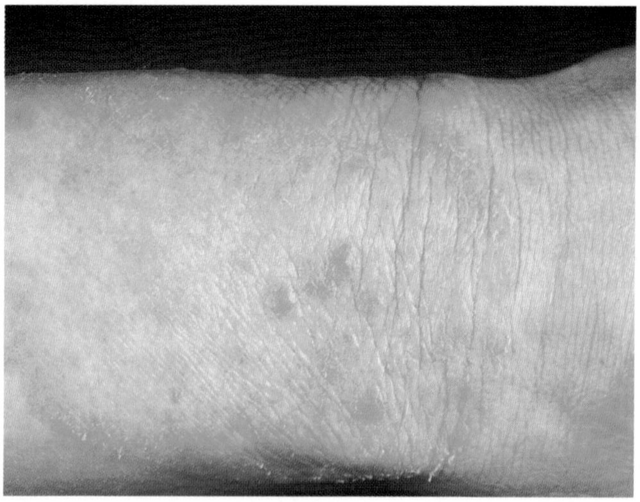

Fig. 4.58 Ringworm rash with inflamed periphery.

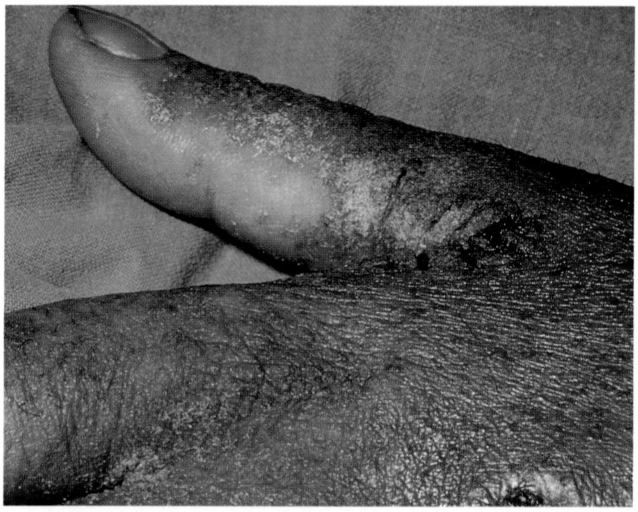

Fig. 4.59 Chronic scabies in the webs between fingers.

BLISTERING LESIONS

Bullous pemphigoid

This disorder occurs most commonly in the elderly. The lesions are itchy and appear as tense, mainly symmetrical blisters overlying and surrounded by an area of erythema (Fig. 4.60). The blisters are initially small but enlarge to a considerable size over a few days (Fig. 4.61). Although truncal involvement also happens, the blisters occur mainly on the limbs, especially along the inner aspects of the thighs and arms. The blisters become haemorrhagic and then degenerate, causing erosions which are susceptible to secondary infection (Fig. 4.62). Healing occurs without scarring.

Pemphigus

This auto-immune disorder occurs most commonly in middle-aged Ashkenazi Jews. The onset is usually insidious and the earliest lesions often start in the mouth or genital mucous membrane. However, patients usually present to the doctor once the skin is involved. Pemphigus is characterized by painful, flaccid blisters which rupture to reveal a raw base which heals slowly (Figs 4.63 and 4.64). The skin adjacent to the bullous lesion slides over the underlying dermis (Nikolsky's sign). The umbilicus, trunk, intertrigenous areas, and scalp are most commonly affected. The clinical diagnosis is confirmed by typical immunofluorescent staining which shows IgG and complement deposition in the epidermis.

Dermatitis herpetiformis

This disorder usually occurs in the third and fourth decades and is characterized by strikingly symmetrical groups of intensely itchy vesicles which most commonly erupt on the elbows, below the knees, buttocks, back, and scalp (Fig. 4.65). Scratching causes local excoriation. Healing leaves telltale areas of hyperpigmentation. The disorder is almost always associated with gluten-sensitive enteropathy (coeliac disease). Although almost all patients have villous atrophy, it is unusual for patients to present with features of malabsorption.

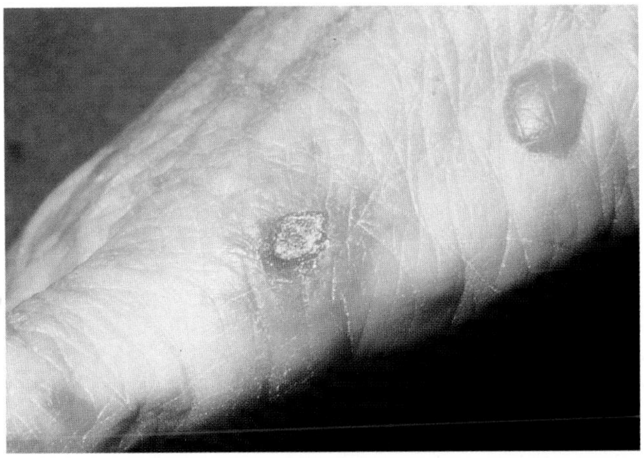

Fig. 4.60 Bullous pemphigoid with surrounding erythema.

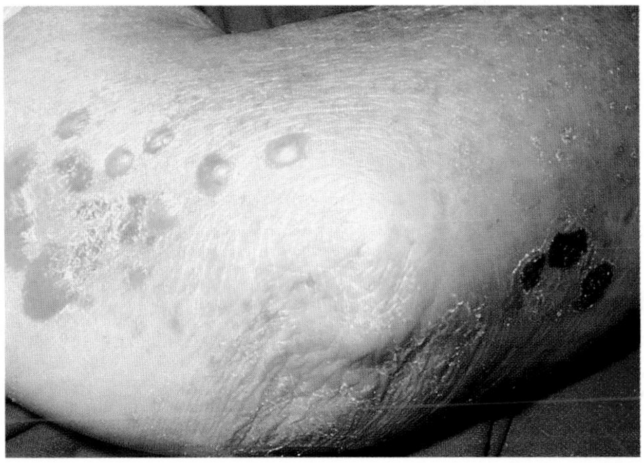

Fig. 4.61 Tense blisters of bullous pemphigoid.

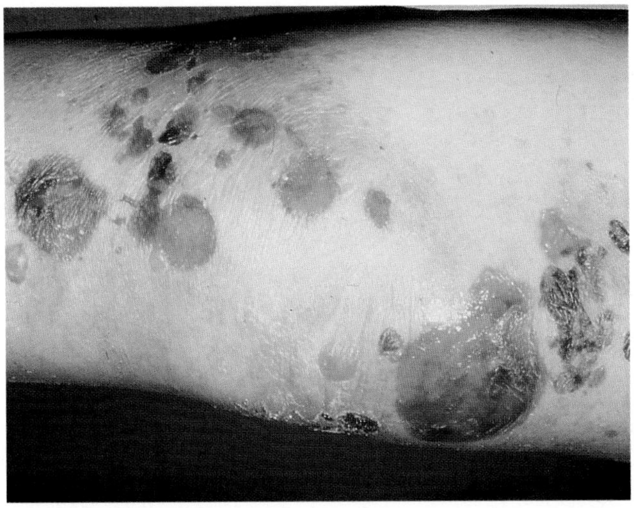

Fig. 4.62 Haemorrhagic blisters of bullous pemphigoid.

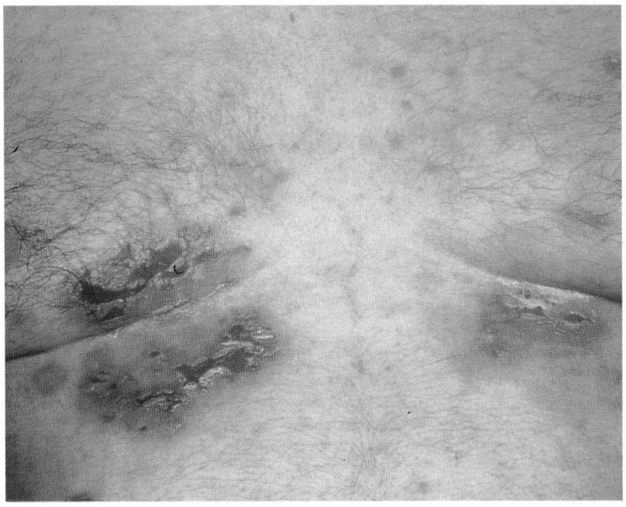

Fig. 4.63 Skin pemphigus.

Naevi

There are numerous skin blemishes collectively called naevi. Pigmented naevi cause the greatest concern because of the seriousness of malignant change. The junctional naevus is distinguished as a flat or slightly raised smooth lesion which has a uniform colour and varies in size up to about 1cm (Fig. 4.66). A compound naevus is a raised, rounded, pigmented papular lesion from which hairs may project (Fig. 4.67). Dermal naevi are raised, flesh-coloured, dome-shaped lesions with a wrinkled surface, occuring most commonly on the face (Fig. 4.68).

Café au lait patches

These are flat coffee-coloured patches, usually centimetres in size, which may occur as a benign blemish or a marker of neurofibromatosis (Von Recklinghausen's disease) (see Fig. 4.8). The presence of five or more of these patches is a sure sign of the disorder. Neurofibromas appear as soft, sessile, pedunculated lesions or discrete subcutaneous nodules.

TUMORS

Squamous cell carcinoma

There is usually a risk factor predisposing to this cancer. Consider excessive sun exposure, carcinomatous change in a chronic leg ulcer, and areas of leukoplakia. The tumor presents as an ulcer or nodule with a firm indurated margin; the ulcer margin is often everted (Fig. 4.69). The cancer usually occurs in sun-exposed areas (face, back of hands, and forearm), or for women, in an area of vulval leukoplakia (Fig. 4.70).

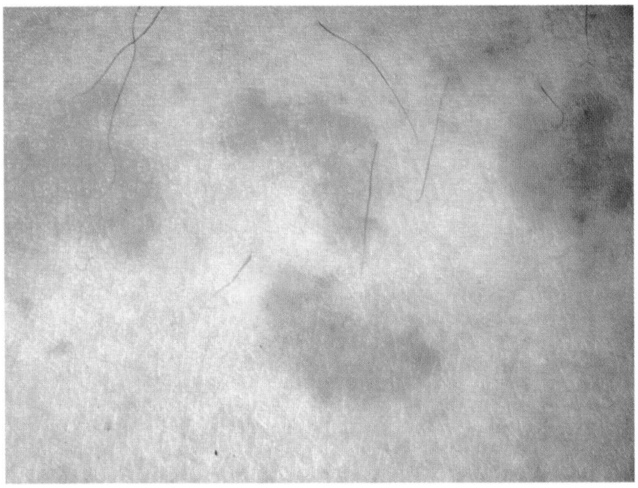

Fig. 4.65 The skin lesions of dermatitis herpetiformis.

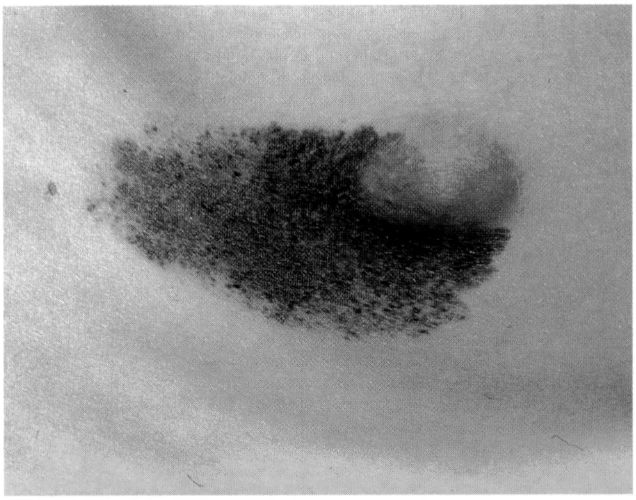

Fig. 4.66 Junctional naevus.

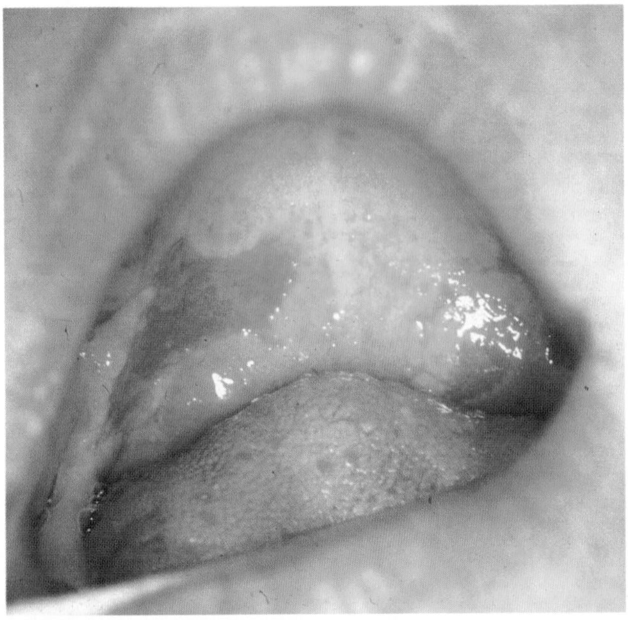

Fig. 4.64 Oral mucous membrane involvement in pemphigus.

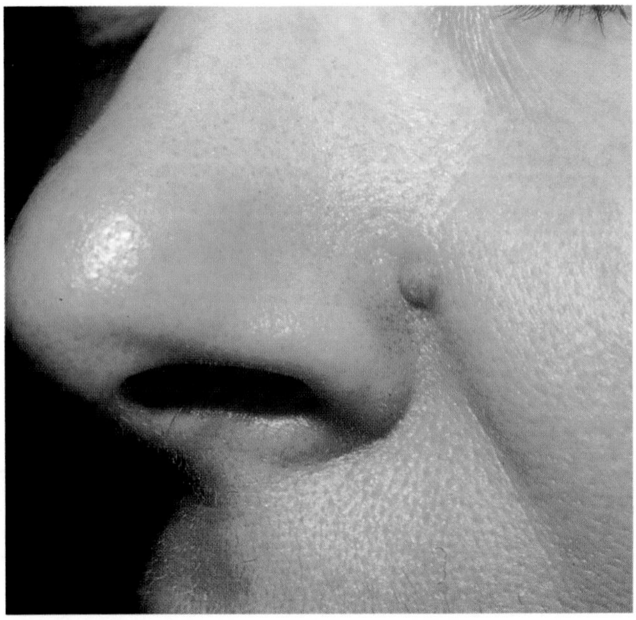

Fig. 4.67 Cellular naevus.

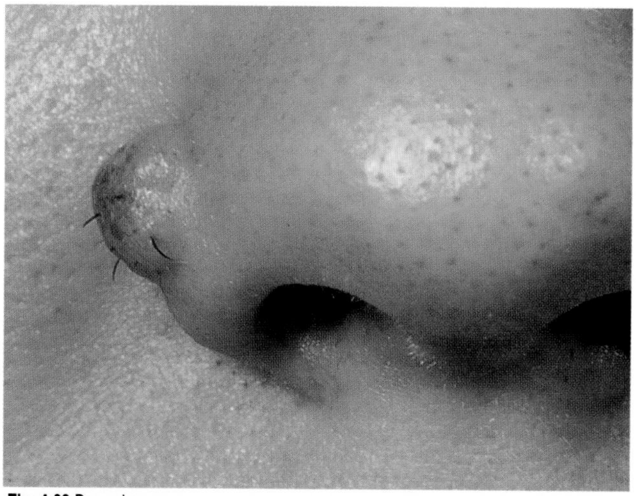

Fig. 4.68 Dermal naevus.

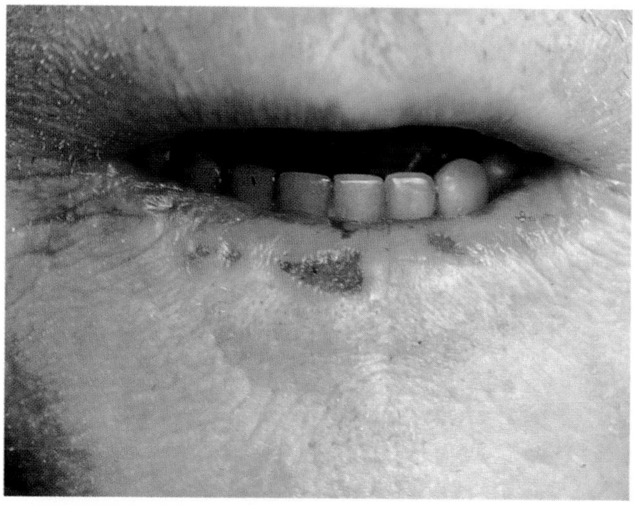

Fig. 4.69 Squamous cancer of the lip.

Basal cell carcinoma

This tumor most commonly affects the face and like squamous carcinoma, sun-exposure is an important predisposing factor. The rodent ulcer starts as a small painless papule (Fig. 4.71) which ulcerates. The ulcer margin is well-defined and rolled at the edges. The tumor bleeds and scabs. Your index of suspicion must be aroused if any skin ulcer fails to heal.

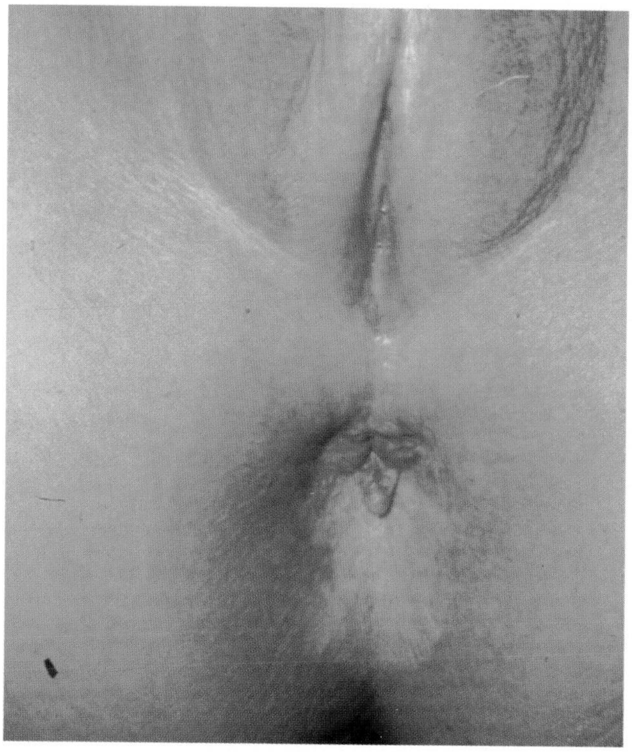

Fig. 4.70 Leukoplakia of the vulva. (The pubic area has been shaved.)

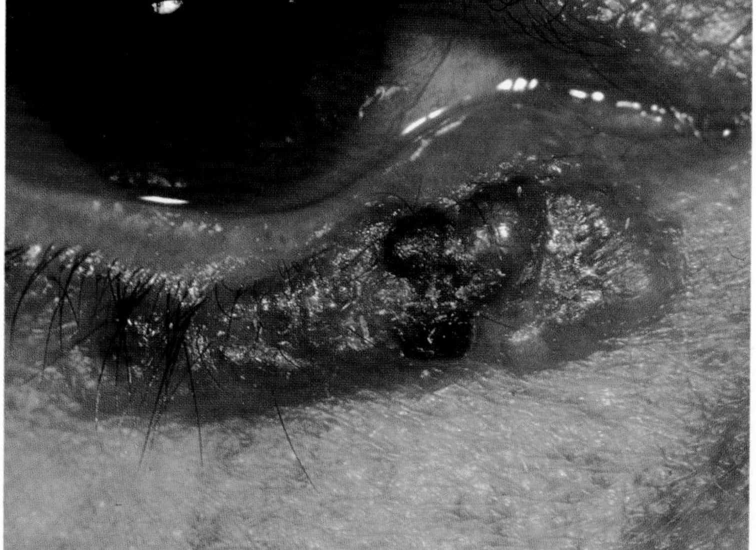

Fig.4.71 Papular form of basal cell carcinoma.

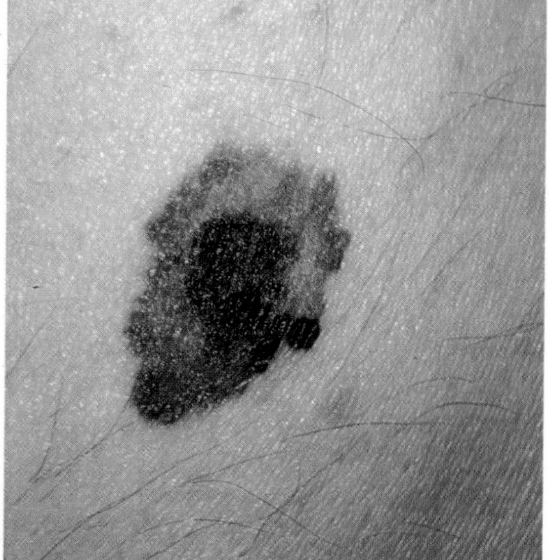

Fig. 4.72 Spreading malignant melanoma.

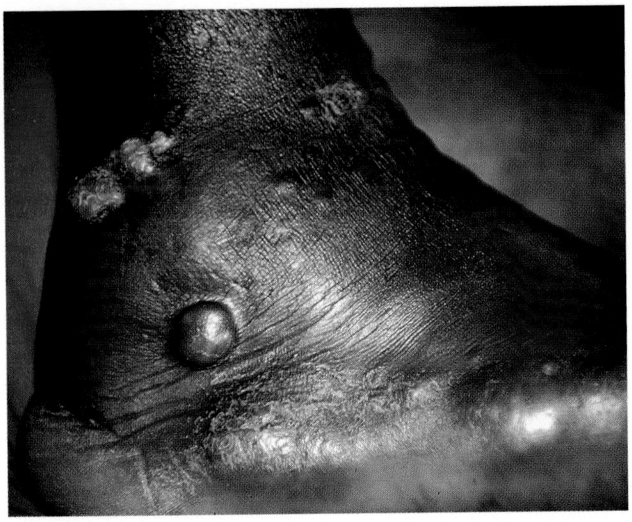

Fig. 4.73 Kaposi's sarcoma in a Black African. The nodules are mutiple and dark blue in colour.

Malignant melanoma

This is less common than squamous or basal cell carcinoma but is the most serious, as it spreads by the lymphatics and blood. Most lesions are not associated with a pre-existing pigmented lesion, but about one third are associated with a junctional pigmented naevus. The tumor is usually pigmented and presents either as a nodule or a spreading area of pigmentation (Fig. 4.72). Consider the diagnosis if a pigmented lesion is nodular, grows, darkens in colour, changes shape, or bleeds. The back is a common site in men, whereas in women, the legs are most often involved.

Kaposi's sarcoma

This tumor was once restricted to equatorial black Africans (Fig. 4.73) and elderly Ashkenazi Jews (Fig. 4.74). Immunosuppression is an important predisposing factor and the sarcoma occurs in transplant recipients on immunosuppressive drugs and is particularly association with AIDS (Fig. 4.75). The Kaposi lesion is characterized by red-blue nodules, especially affecting the lower legs but also involving the hands.

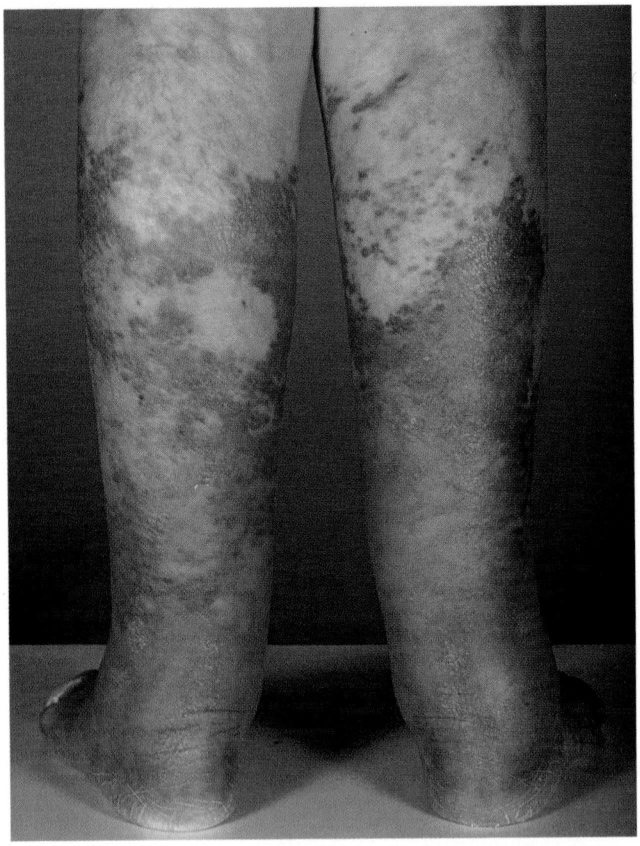

Fig. 4.74 Kaposi's sarcoma in an Ashkenazi Jew. The purple plaques particularly occur on the lower legs and feet.

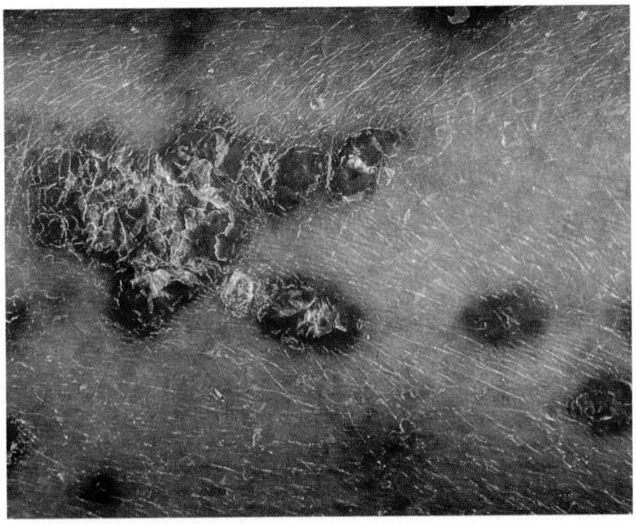

Fig. 4.75 Kaposi's sarcoma in an immunosuppressed AIDS patient.

NAIL DISORDERS

Examination of the nails can provide useful and often diagnostic physical signs. Patients often complain of cracking, ridging, and brittleness of the nail. This may be caused by nail-biting, picking, and poor nail care rather than disease. In addition, nails may have white spots which have no significance. First examine the nail face-on. Asymmetrical splinter-like lesions (splinter haemorrhages) may indicate micro-emboli from infected heart valves (sub-acute bacterial endocarditis) or vasculitis. Remember that manual laborers may have traumatic nail lesions which resemble splinter haemorrhages. Pitting of the nail occurs in psoriasis (Fig. 4.76) and may even occur in the absence of the typical skin rash. Premature lifting of the distal nail is called onycholysis (Fig. 4.77). This occurs in many chronic nail disorders and is also associated with hyperthyroidism ('Plummer's' nails). White nails with loss of the lunule (leukonychia) is typical of hypoalbuminaemia and severe chronic ill-health (Fig. 4.78).

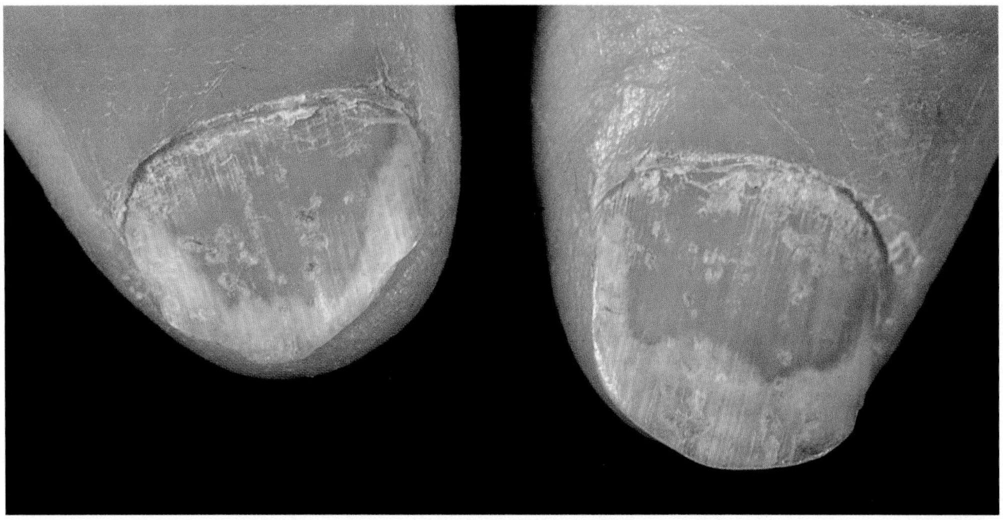

Fig. 4.76 Pitting and onycholysis of the nail caused by psoriasis.

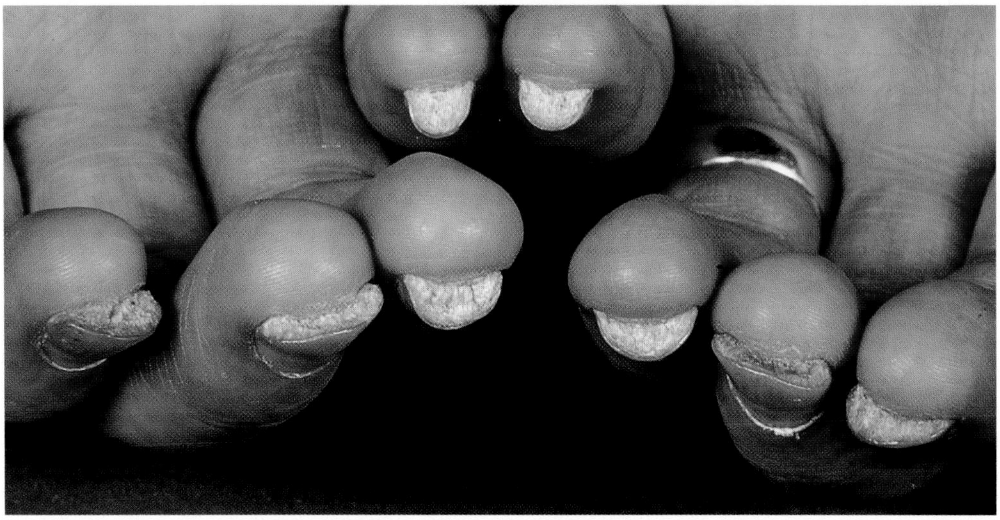

Fig. 4.77 Onycholysis caused by hyperkeratotic psoriasis beneath the nail.

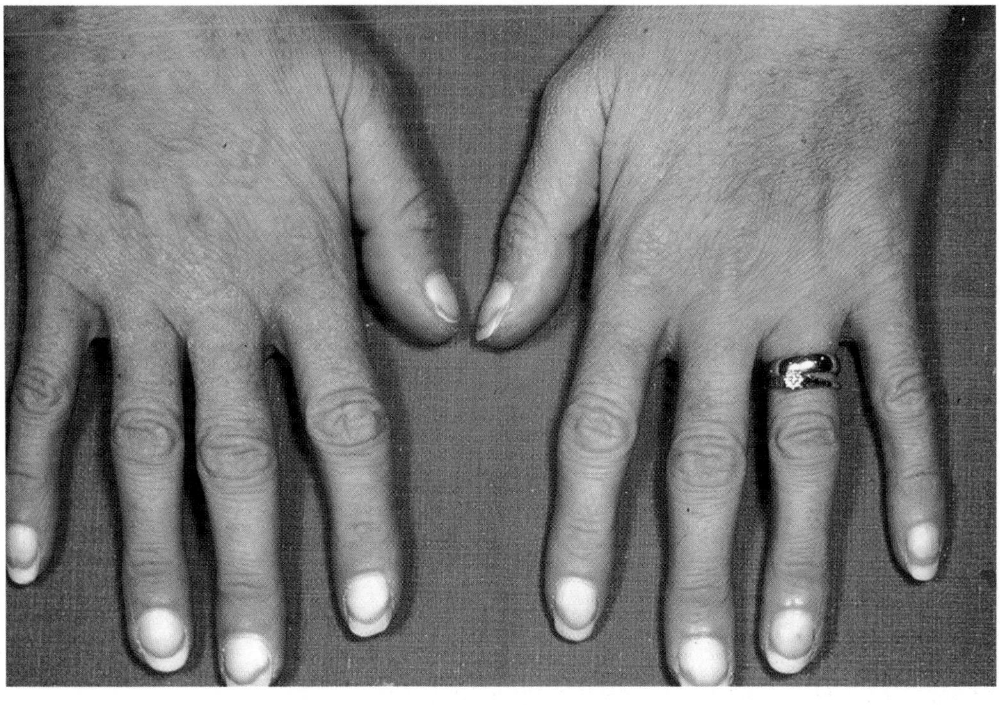

Fig. 4.78 Leukonychia in a patient with liver disease and hypoalbuminaemia.

Acute severe illness may be associated with the later appearance of transverse depressions in the nail (Beau's lines) (Fig. 4.79) which grow out with normal nail growth on recovery. Infection of the skin adjacent to the nail is called paronychia and is characterized by pain, swelling, redness, and tenderness of the skin at its interface with the nail (Fig. 4.80). Fungal infection of the nail causes opacification and distortion of the nail. Spooning of the nail (koilonychia) occurs in iron deficiency (Figs 4.81 and 4.82).

Always examine the lateral outline of the nails and fingertip to check for clubbing (Fig. 4.83). The normal angle between the finger nail and nail base is 160° (Fig. 4.84) and the base is firm to palpation. Clubbing occurs when abnormal connective tissue and capillaries fill up this angle. In early clubbing, the angle increases and if you press the nail base, the nail appears to 'float'. In severe clubbing, such as occurs with lung cancer, the fingers may have a drumstick appearance and may be associated with wrist pain and tenderness due to periostitis (hypertrophic pulmonary osteoarthropathy).

SKIN MANIFESTATIONS OF SYSTEMIC DISEASES

Many systemic disorders involve the skin and careful examination of the skin often helps in diagnosis. A summary of associated signs is represented in Fig. 4.85.

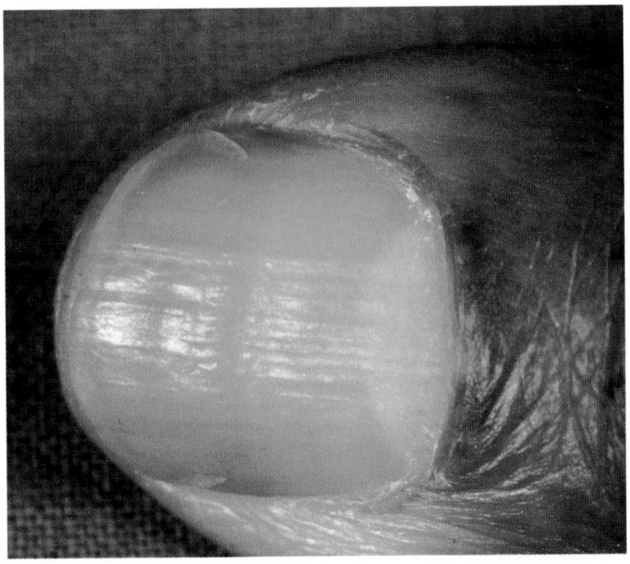

Fig. 4.79 Beau's lines.

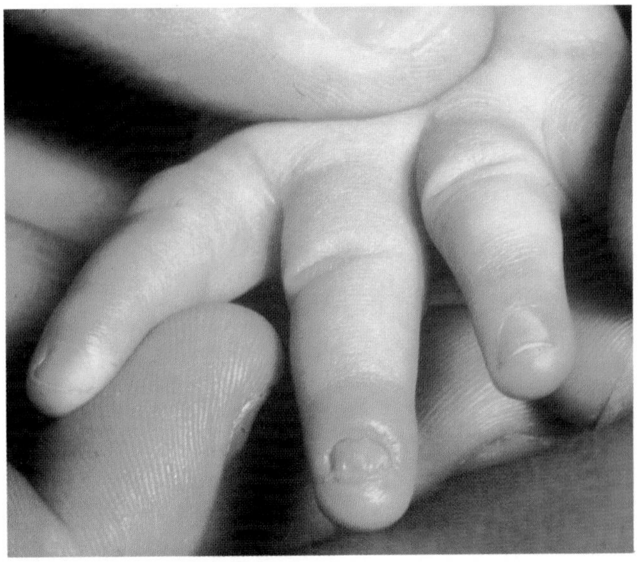

Fig. 4.80 Bacterial paronychia.

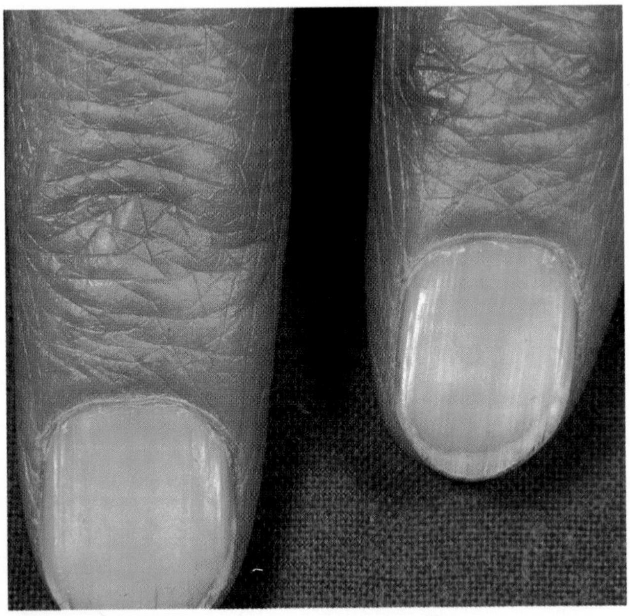

Fig. 4.81 Koilonychia with spooning of the nail in a patient with chronic iron deficiency anaemia.

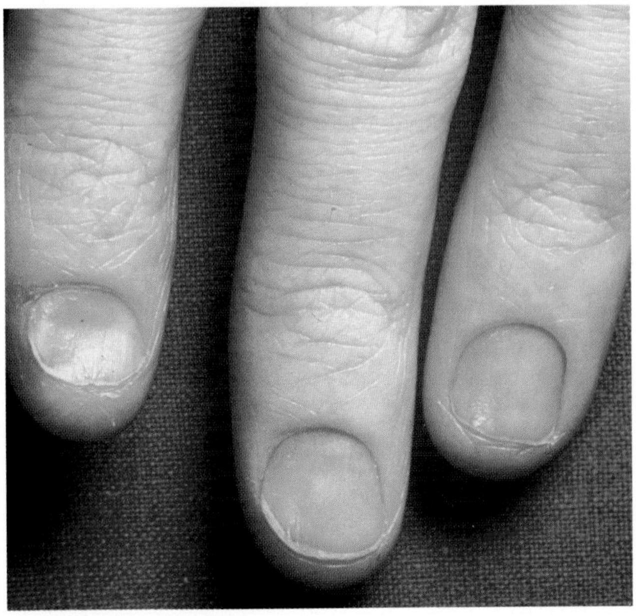

Fig. 4.82 Spooning of the nails.

Causes of clubbing

Lung disease	Pyogenic (abscess, bronchiectasis, empyema) Bronchogenic carcinoma Fibrosing alveolitis
Heart disease	Cyanotic congenital heart disease Subacute bacterial endocarditis
Gastrointestinal	Cirrhosis Ulcerative colitis Crohn's disease
idiopathic/congenital	

Fig. 4.83 Causes of clubbing.

Clubbing

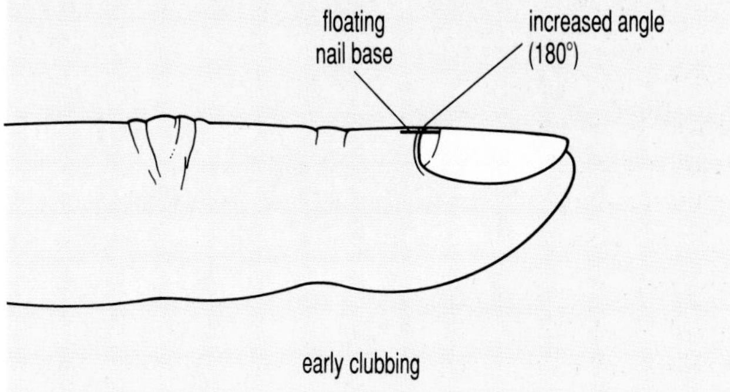

Fig. 4.84 Clubbing. The angle is increased and filled in, and the nail base has a spongy consistency.

Skin manifestations of systemic disease

Disease	Skin findings
Sarcoidosis	Erythema nodosum, lupus pernio, nodules in scars
Scleroderma	Thickened tight skin (especially fingers), skin telangiecasia, calcified skin nodules.
Hyperlipidaemia	Xanthelasmata of eyelids, xanthomas of elbows, knuckles, buttock, soles and palms, and Achilles tendon
Diabetes mellitus	Necrobiosis lipoidica – symmetrical plaques on shins with atrophic, yellow appearance and waxy feel; cutaneous candida, ulcers on feet
Hyperthyroidism	Pretibial myxoedema – thickened skin on front of shin, clubbing
Cushing's syndrome	Purple striae, thin skin, easy bruising
Ulcerative colitis/Crohn's disease	Pyoderma gangrenosum – large ulcer
Dermatomyositis	Oedema and mauve discoloration of eyelid, erythema of the knuckles and other bony points such as elbow and shoulder tip; photosensitive 'butterfly rash' on face
Cancer	Acanthosis nigricans – brown, velvet-like thickening of skin in axilla and groin; teilosis – thickening of palms/soles; icthyosis – fish-skin appearance

Fig. 4.85 Skin manifestations of systemic disease.

EAR, NOSE, AND THROAT

5

Disorders of the ears, nose, and throat are extremely common. The examination of these organs in particular and the head and neck in general should be performed in a systematic manner, as with other organ systems. An adequate and appropriate history is an essential prerequisite of the examination, and more often than not will lead you to the diagnosis.

STRUCTURE AND FUNCTION

The symptoms and signs of diseases of the ears, nose, and throat reflect disorder in the anatomy and physiology of these organs. Diseases of this organ system involve their relationship with the head and neck in terms of both referred symptoms and lymphatic drainage.

The mouth and throat

Although the mouth may be thought of merely as a receptacle for food and a vehicle for speech, several anatomical structures within the oral cavity may be the foci of disease.

The lips act as a seal to close the oral cavity and play a role in the articulation of speech. They have skin on the outer surface, and a mucous membrane lines the inner surface. The mucous glands of the lips open into the cavity. The oral cavity is lined by the buccal mucosa which is rich in mucous glands. The parotid ducts also open into the buccal mucosa on each side opposite the second upper molar tooth. The mouth cavity itself is limited anteriorly and laterally by the alveolus, gums, and teeth and communicates posteriorly with the pharynx. The floor of the mouth contains the tongue and the openings of submandibular and sublingual salivary glands. The roof of the mouth is formed by the upper alveolus, gums, teeth, and the hard and soft palates.

The gums are firmly adherent to the alveolus and are closely related to the teeth whose roots are embedded in the alveolus. The deciduous or 'milk' teeth are 20 in number, 10 in each jaw (Fig. 5.1), while the permanent or adult teeth are 32 in number, 16 in each jaw (Fig. 5.2).

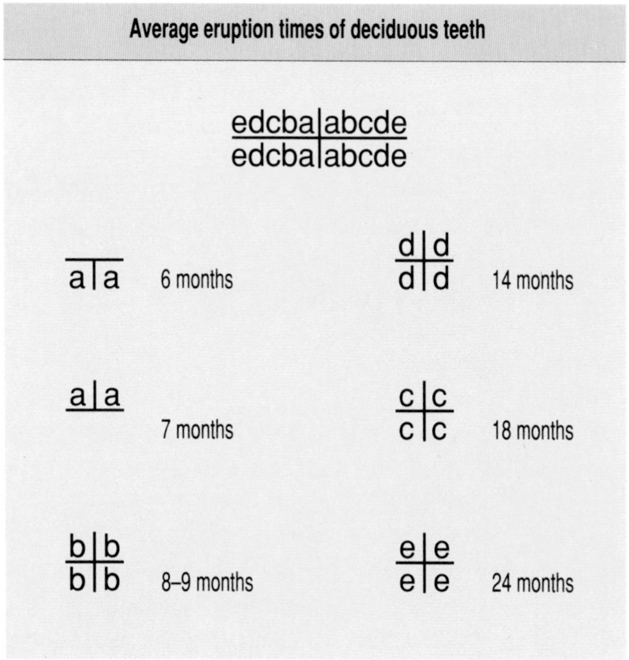

Fig. 5.1 Average eruption times of the deciduous teeth.

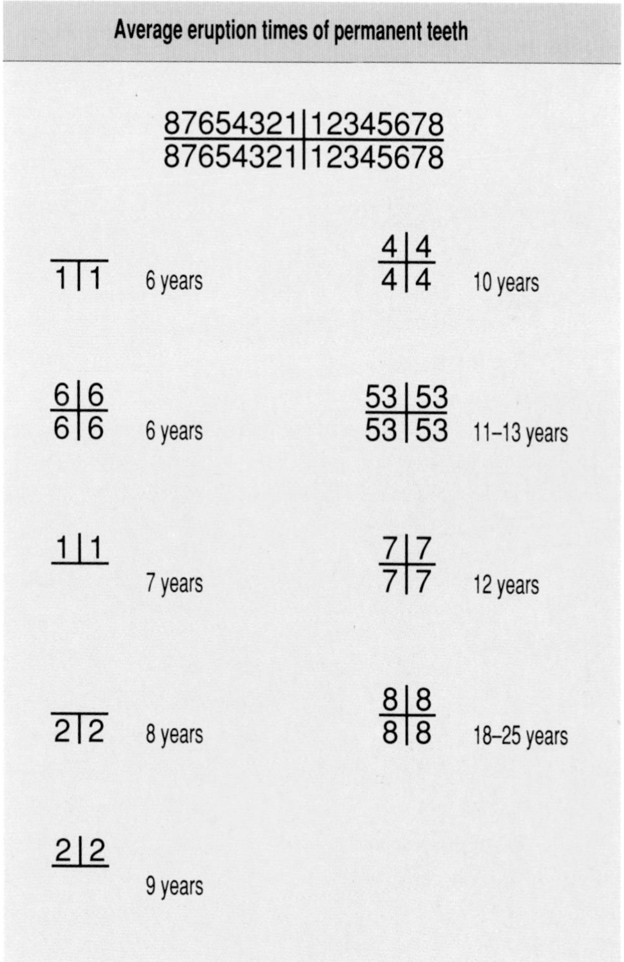

Fig. 5.2 Average eruption times of the permanent teeth.

Examination of the mouth and throat

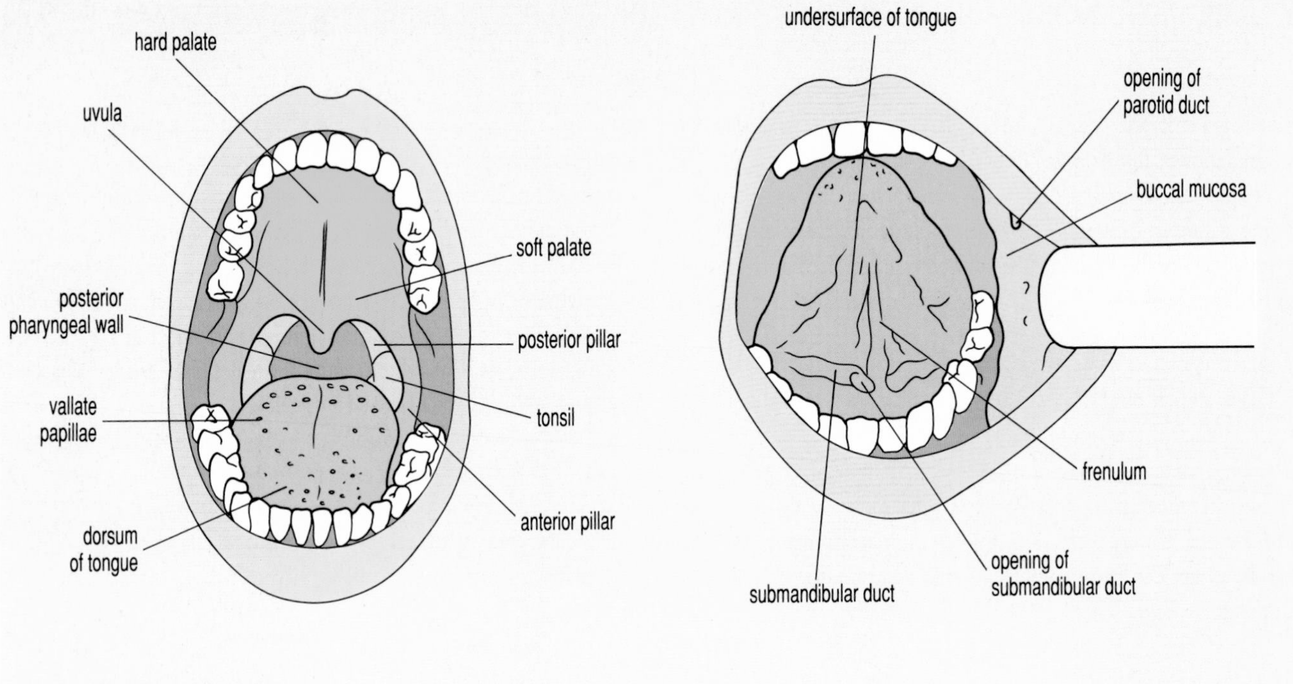

Fig. 5.3 Examination of the mouth and throat.

The tongue

This large, mobile organ consists of several muscles and is covered by a mucous membrane. The base of the tongue is bounded laterally by the anterior and posterior tonsillar pillars between which and on either side lie the tonsils (Fig. 5.3).

The parotid, submandibular, and sublingual salivary glands secrete saliva into the oral cavity, keeping it moist and aiding the first stage of swallowing. Food entering the mouth is chewed and mixed with saliva to facilitate swallowing. Taste buds on the tongue and within the buccal mucosa, together with olfactory stimuli delivered anteriorly through the nose and posteriorly via the nasopharynx, give food its characteristic tastes and smells. As well as an important organ of speech, the tongue has a role both in the mixing of the food bolus and in propelling the food towards the pharynx.

The pharynx

The pharynx consists of the combined upper parts of the respiratory and digestive tracts. It can be divided into three parts: the nasopharynx (above the soft palate and behind the choanae of the nose) the oropharynx (the posterior extension of the oral cavity), and the laryngopharynx (below the upper border of the epiglottis, including the larynx and piriform fossae).

The tonsils

The tonsils lie on either side of the oropharynx between the anterior and posterior pillars of the fauces. Ten to fifteen crypts open onto the surface of the tonsil. Mucous glands open into these crypts and they may also be the site of food debris accumulation. The tonsil parenchyma is largely composed of lymphoid tissue. Tonsillar tissue also occurs on the posterior wall of the nasopharynx (the adenoid) and on the posterior third of the tongue (the 'lingual' tonsil). The sensory nerve supply of the mouth and pharynx derives from the Vth, IXth, and Xth cranial nerves. This is very important when one considers referred pain (see 'otalgia' on page 5.10)

The larynx

The larynx is made up of several muscles and cartilages. It has three main functions: respiration, preventing food and saliva from entering the respiratory tract, and the production of voice. The sensory supply of the larynx is from the IXth and Xth cranial nerves and its motor supply is from the Xth cranial nerve.

The nose and paranasal sinuses

The external shape of the nose is determined by the shape of the nasal bones and cartilages. The anterior nares are separated by a membranous columella (Fig. 5.4). The dorsum of the nose is bony in its upper third to a half and cartilaginous (septum) in its lower half to two thirds. The nasal skin continues into the anterior nares (the vestibule) where it contains hairs and sebaceous glands. The two nasal cavities or nostrils are separated by the nasal septum which is both cartilaginous and bony. The paranasal sinuses (see Fig. 5.4) – maxillary, frontal, ethmoid, and sphenoid – of each side,

The nose and paranasal sinuses

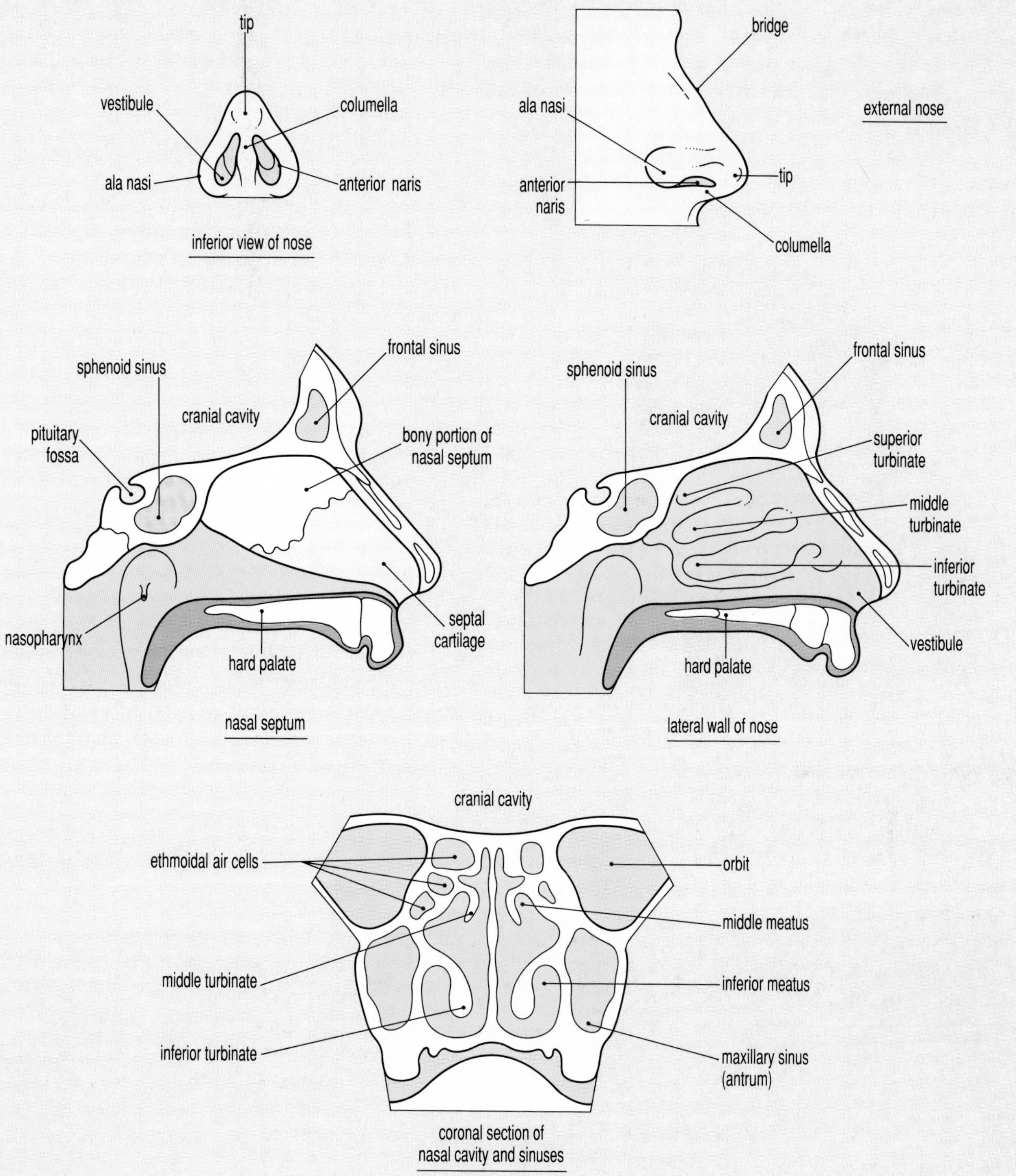

Fig. 5.4 The nose and paranasal sinuses.

drain into the respective nasal cavities. All the paranasal sinuses are present from birth except for the frontal sinuses which develop only after birth and reach their maximum size around puberty. Any of the sinuses may also be congenitally absent, with one or both frontal sinuses being most commonly absent.

The lateral wall of each nasal cavity contains the inferior, middle and, sometimes, superior turbinates. These divide the cavity into superior, middle, and inferior meati. Some ethmoidal air cells and the sphenoid sinuses drain into the superior meatus; however, the maxillary, anterior ethmoidal, and frontal sinuses open into the middle meatus. The nasolacrimal duct opens into the inferior meatus. The mucous membrane of the nose consists of respiratory and olfactory epithelium. This reflects the dual function of the nose. The olfactory epithelium lies in the roof of the nose with a variable extension to the superior turbinate, upper part of the middle turbinate and upper part of the nasal septum. Ciliated columar epithelium which is rich in mucous glands lines the rest of the nose and paranasal sinuses.

Paranasal sinuses

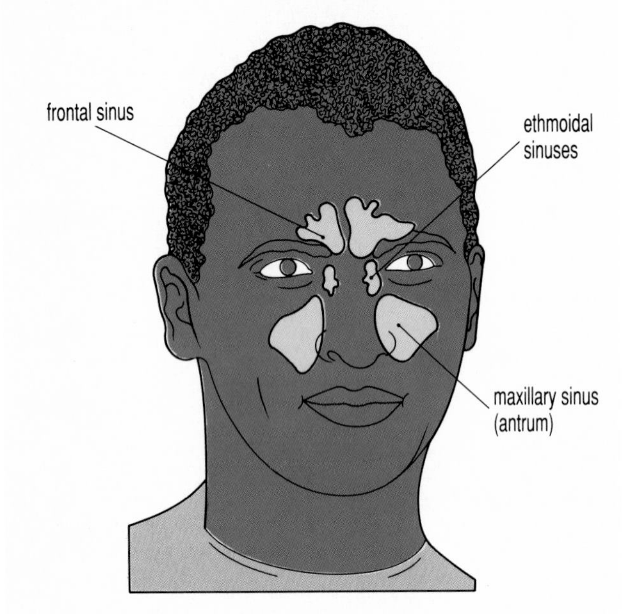

Fig. 5.5 Topographical representation of the paranasal sinuses.

EARS

The ear can be conveniently divided into the outer ear, the middle ear and the inner ear. The outer or external ear (Figs 5.6 and 5.7) consists of the pinna, the external auditory meatus, and the lateral surface of the tympanic membrane (eardrum). The pinna has a cartilage framework which is covered tightly with skin, whereas the ear lobe consists of fat with no cartilage. The outer ear canal is cartilaginous in its outer third and bony in its inner or medial two-thirds. The skin is tightly adherent to the external auditory meatus and contains hairs, sebaceous glands, and ceruminous glands in the cartilaginous meatus. These structures are absent in the bony meatus.

The sensory nerve supply of the ear is illustrated in Fig. 5.8.
The middle ear consists of the medial surface of the tympanic membrane, the tympanic cavity, the Eustachian tube, and the mastoid air cells. Within the tympanic cavity are the three auditory ossicles (Fig. 5.9). Their function is to transmit and to amplify sound from the external ear and tympanic membrane to the inner ear. The Eustachian tube serves to equalize the air pressure between the middle ear and the atmosphere. The exact function of the mastoid air cell system is uncertain and its degree of aeration is extremely variable (Fig. 5.10).

The inner ear or labyrinth communicates with the middle ear via the oval and round windows. The inner ear can be divided into two parts: the cochlea and the vestibule. The cochlear part is concerned with hearing; the hair cells of the cochlea transmit their energy to the cochlear division of the VIIIth cranial nerve. The vestibular part of the inner ear is concerned with balance and consists of the lateral, superior, and posterior semicircular canals, together with the utricle and saccule.

Pinna

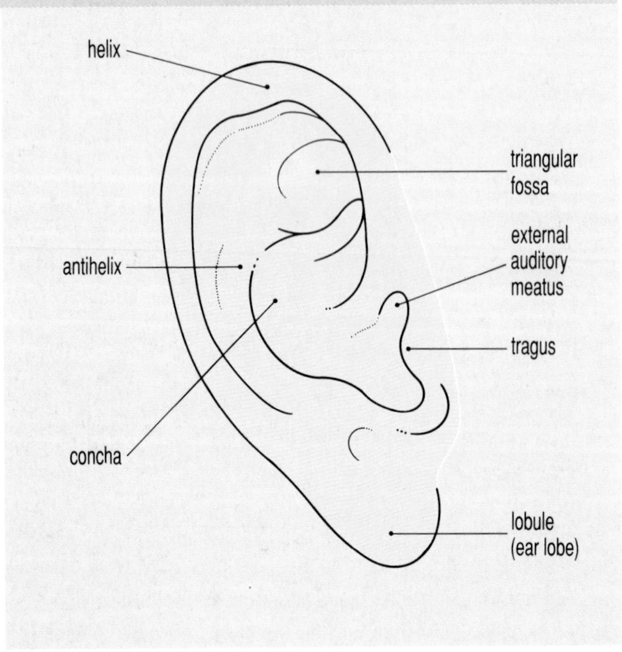

Fig. 5.6 The pinna.

Cross-section of the ear

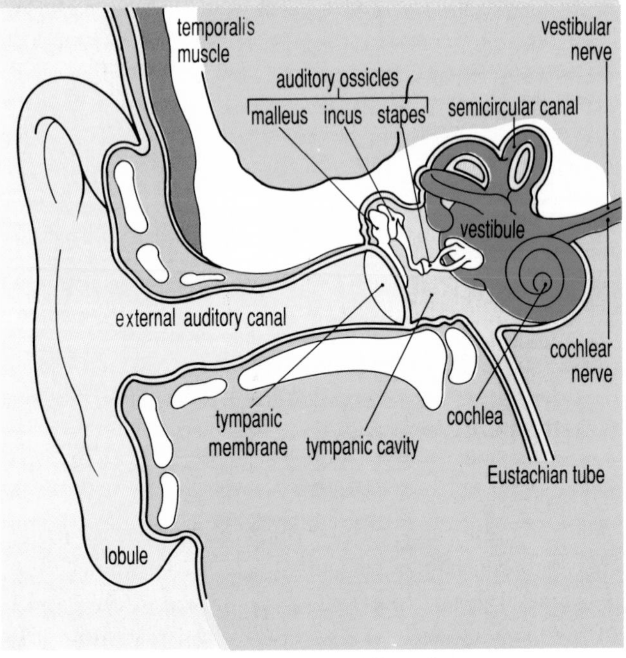

Fig. 5.7 Diagrammatic cross-section of the outer, middle, and inner ears.

The bony framework of the inner ear is called the bony or osseous labyrinth, whilst the communicating sacs and ducts within it comprise the membranous labyrinth. There are two fluid compartments within this system: one consists of perilymph whose composition resembles the extracellular fluid; the other consists of endolymph whose higher potassium concentration is closer in composition to the intracellular fluid of the body. The structure and function of the cochleo-vestibular apparatus is outlined on pages 12.51–12.53.

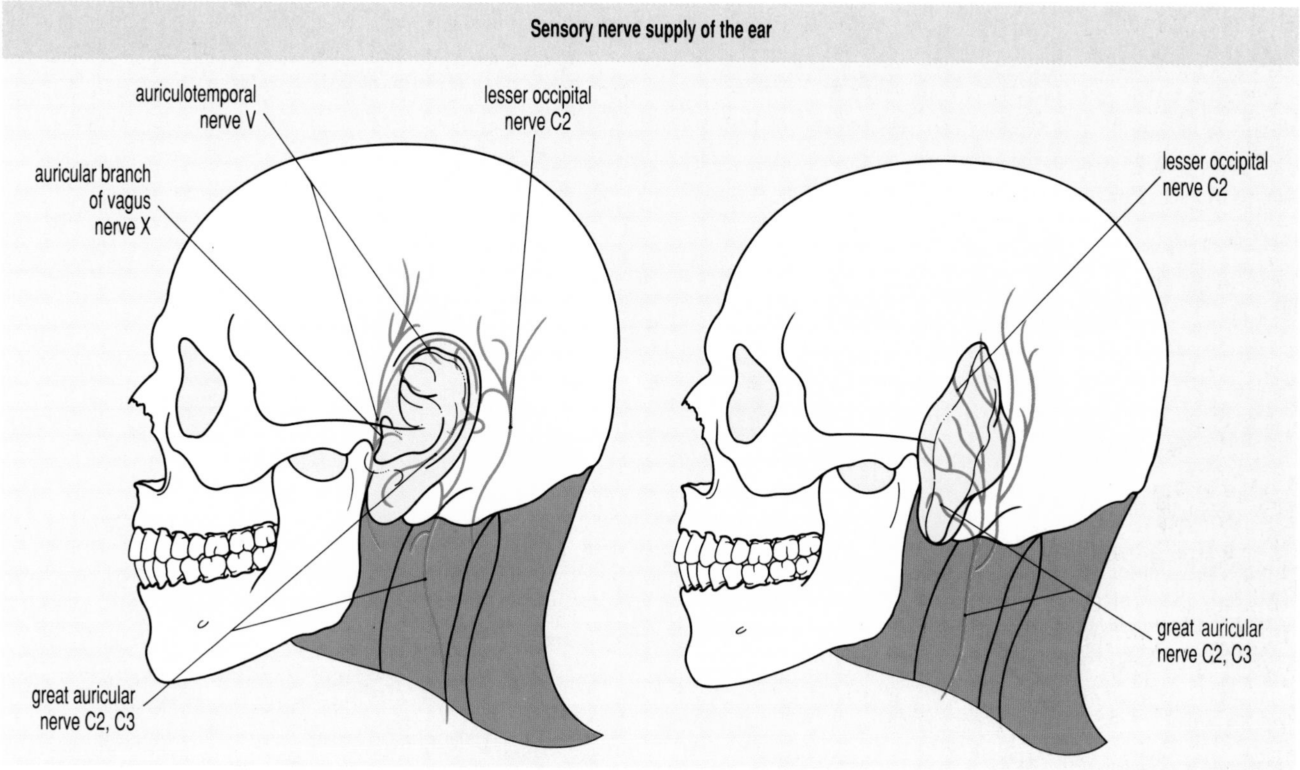

Fig. 5.8 Sensory innervation of the external ear: (a) lateral aspect and (b) medial aspect.

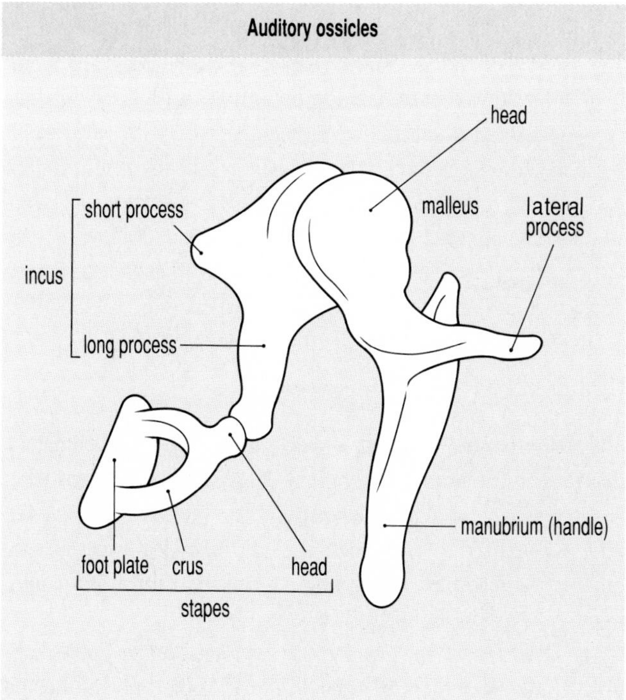

Fig. 5.9 Auditory ossicles.

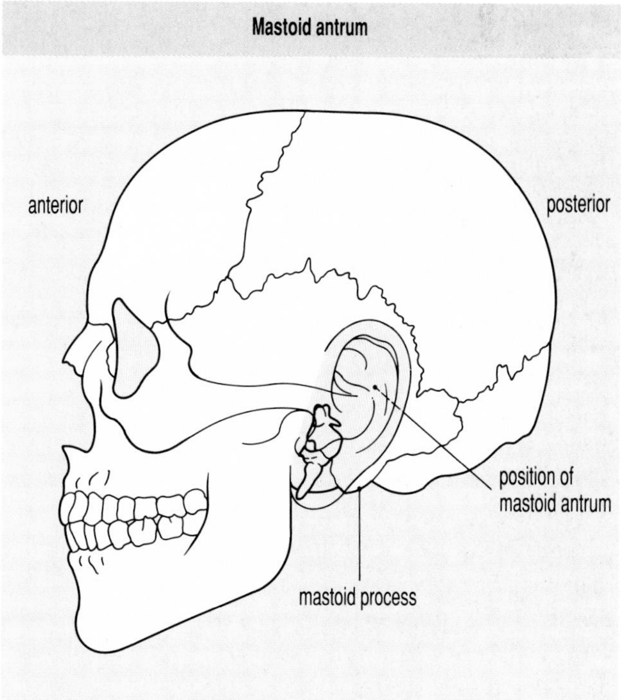

Fig. 5.10 Surface marking of the mastoid antrum.

SYMPTOMS OF MOUTH AND THROAT DISORDERS

Patients with disorders arising in the mouth or throat usually complain of pain, a sensation of a lump in the throat, a hoarse voice, difficulty in breathing (upper airway obstruction), difficulty in swallowing (dysphagia), pain on swallowing (odynophagia), a lump in the neck, and halitosis.

The sore mouth/throat

Localized pain in the mouth usually arises from lesions that can easily be seen or palpated. Pain may arise from the teeth or from the buccal and lingual surfaces. The oral mucosa may be diffusely inflamed in vitamin deficiency states, in fungal infections of the oral cavity ('thrush' or candidiasis), or following radiotherapy for malignant disease. The presence of diffuse fungal infection should alert you to the possibility of AIDS, although it may also occur following broad-spectrum antibiotic therapy or in any state of immune deficiency (eg. leukaemia, lymphoma). Pain arising more posteriorly may be due to tonsillitis or pharyngitis which can be seen but may also be due to disease of the hypo- and laryngopharynx.

Specific lesions of the oral and buccal mucosa are inflammatory (most commonly aphthous ulcers), traumatic, or due to a localized malignancy. Painful inflammatory lesions may occur in isolation or they may be associated with a generalized disorder of other mucous membranes and/or the skin.

Sore mouth/throat

How long have you had the pain?

Does the pain change in severity?

What aggravates, relieves the pain?

Is the pain local or diffuse?

What other illnesses do you have?

Are you taking any medication; if so, then what type?

How much do you smoke a day?

How much alcohol do you consume in a week?

Lump in the throat

Previously known as globus hystericus this is now more appropriately called globus pharyngeus or the globus syndrome. This is described as a sensation of something or a lump in the throat.

Lump in the throat

How long have you noticed this sensation?

Is it getting better or worse?

Do you have trouble swallowing (dysphagia)?

Is the act of swallowing painful (odynophagia)?

Have you experienced any weight loss?

What factors aggravate, relieve the pain?

Do you suffer from heartburn, indigestion, taste of acid in the mouth, i.e. symptoms of gastro-oesophageal reflux?

The majority of patients have no serious disease process and merely need assurance. A small percentage will have gastro-oesophageal reflux or excessive postnasal mucus, with a very small percentage (less than one per cent) having a malignancy. Factors pointing to a malignancy include progression of symptoms of dysphagia, odynophagia, and weight loss. A barium swallow may be indicated and may exclude local pathology; nevertheless, any doubt requires specialist assessment.

Hoarse voice

The majority of patients with a hoarse voice have an inflammatory disorder of the larynx (laryngitis). However, any patient with hoarseness that has not resolved after three weeks should have the larynx visualized. If hoarseness is associated with upper airway obstruction (stridor), emergency referral to an ENT surgeon is required.

The history will often give the examiner a good idea of the diagnosis. Any alteration in the smooth lining of the true vocal cords (vocal folds) will give rise to hoarseness. If one of the vocal folds is

Hoarse voice

How long has the hoarseness been present?

Has there been any previous upper respiratory tract infection?

Have you abused your voice, i.e. shouting at sports events or singing at a party or concert?

Do you smoke; if so, how many a day?

How much alcohol do you drink?

What type of work do you do?

paralyzed or if there is inadequate apposition of the vocal folds, a more 'breathy' quality of the voice is noted, and is more accurately called dysphonia; it requires considerable experience to make the distinction between hoarseness and dysphonia on merely listening to the patient speak. A preceding upper respiratory tract infection will usually point to a diagnosis of laryngitis, as may excessive voice abuse (traumatic laryngitis). A history of excessive smoking, alcohol (especially spirits), and poor periodontal and dental hygiene should alert you to the possibility of a malignancy. The causes of hoarseness also vary in different age groups (Fig. 5.11)

Obstructed airway

Patients with any difficulty in breathing may not be able to indicate the exact anatomical level of the obstruction. With upper airway obstruction they may point to the throat or neck or describe a feeling of 'tightness' in the throat. The causes of an obstructed upper airway differ according to the age of the patient (Fig. 5.12).

Snoring is also caused by an obstructed airway. The obstruction may be nasal, postnasal (e.g. enlarged adenoid), oropharyngeal (e.g. tonsils, lax palate and fauceal pillars), or laryngeal (e.g. con-

Likely causes of hoarseness/dysphonia

Neonate (abnormal cry)	Infant	Toddler	Children	Adults
Congenital abnormality Neurological disorder	Congenital abnormality Neurological disorder Inflammation (croup or upper respiratory tract infection [URTI])	Inflammation (croup or URTI)	Inflammatory (laryngitis) Vocal nodules (voice abuse)	Inflammatory and traumatic laryngitis Vocal nodules (voice abuse) Dysphonia (voice abuse or misuse) Carcinoma

Fig. 5.11 Likely causes of hoarseness/dysphonia.

Likely causes of obstructed upper airway

Neonate	Infant	Toddler	Children	Adults
Congenital abnormality	Congenital abnormality Inflammation (croup)	Inflammation (croup/epiglottis) Foreign body Congenital abnormality	Inflammation (croup/epiglottis) Foreign body	Inflammatory (croup/epiglottis) Carcinoma (usually over 50)

Fig. 5.12 Likely causes of an obstructed upper airway.

genital abnormalities in children). If snoring is severe this may be associated with apnoeic episodes during sleep. This in turn may lead to daytime irritability and somnolence. The hypoxic episodes during sleep may lead to cardiorespiratory abnormalities.

Difficulty in swallowing (dysphagia)

For a discussion of dysphagia see page 8.9.

Pain on swallowing:

Painful swallowing is called odynophagia. Swallowing is usually painful in the presence of inflammation in the hypopharynx or oesophagus (e.g. candidiasis), but is rarely the presenting complaint in oesophageal carcinoma. These patients usually present initially with dysphagia before the act of swallowing becomes painful. However, carcinoma of the piriform fossa or posterior third of the tongue may present with odynophagia (also see page 8.10)

Lymph nodes in the head and neck

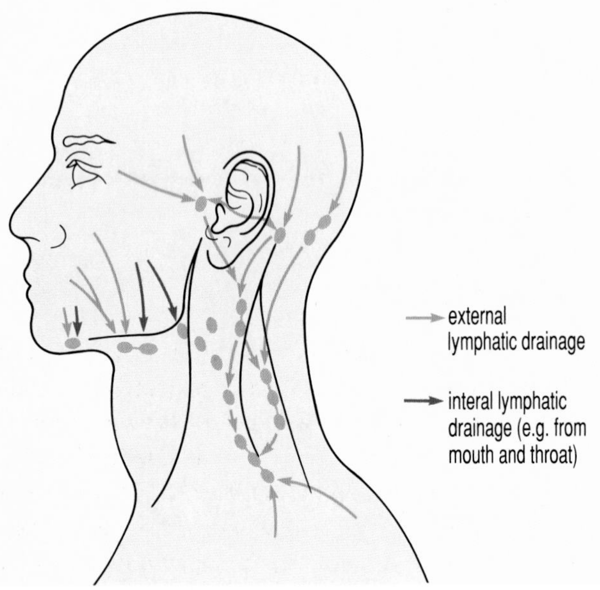

Fig. 5.13 Lymphatic drainage of the head and neck.

Lump in the neck

Patients with a lump in the neck have either felt the lump themselves or it has been noticed by someone else. Most neck lumps are due to enlarged lymph nodes, in which case questioning is directed

Lump in the neck

How long has it been present?

Has the lump changed in size?

Is the lump painful?

Do you sweat at night?

Have you lost weight recently?

Do you have thyroid problems?

Do you have a cough?

Is there anything abnormal about your mouth or throat?

Are you generally well?

Hearing loss

Infants	Toddlers & young children	Teenagers & adolescents	20–40	40–60	60+
Congenital	'Glue ear'	Congenital	Otosclerosis	Otosclerosis	Presbycusis
Secretory otitis media ('glue ear')	Congenital	Malingering	Post-infective	Noise-induced	Noise-induced
	Post-infective (measles, mumps, meningitis)	Post-infective	Noise-induced	Early presbycusis	Acoustic neuroma
		Noise-induced (often temporary in this age group)	Acoustic neuroma	Acoustic neuroma	
			Menière's disease	Menière's disease	

Fig. 5.14 Likely causes of hearing loss.

to a potential source of origin (Fig 5.13). Lymph nodes in the neck may arise from sources in the head and neck or they may arise from disease in the chest and abdomen (carcinoma). Enlarged neck nodes may also be part of generalized disease of the lymphatic system such as lymphoma. Thyroid swellings would require a history of symptoms of hyper- or hypothyroidism. Most neck lumps are painless unless there is associated inflammation or abscess formation.

Halitosis

Bad breath may arise from a variety of sources. The commonest cause of halitosis is probably poor dental and oral hygiene. Paranasal sinus infection with a purulent postnasal discharge may lead to halitosis, as may tonsillar infection and the accumulation of excessive debris in the tonsillar crypts. Infection of the oral cavity, the gums in particular (gingivitis), may give rise to a foul-smelling breath.

SYMPTOMS OF NASAL DISORDERS

Nasal disorders may present with local symptoms or symptoms some distance from the nose.

Blocked Nose

The examiner must establish whether the patient is describing true nasal obstruction or the physiological nasal cycle with alternating vasoconstriction and vasodilatation of the nasal vasculature. Mechanical abnormalities (e.g. a deviated septum or enlarged turbinates or nasal polyps) will usually cause constant obstruction whereas the nasal cycle and seasonal allergic rhinitis are usually intermittent, the former alternating between left and right sides.

Blocked nose

Is the nose blocked constantly or only some of the time (day or night)?

Does it vary with the seasons?

Is there an associated nasal discharge?

Are both nostrils affected, or only one?

What aggravates, relieves the condition?

Do you use nose drops?

Do you sniff glue or illicit substances (e.g. cocaine)?

Have you had previous nose surgery?

Do you suffer from asthma?

Runny nose (rhinorrhoea)

It is important to ascertain whether there is associated nasal obstruction and whether the discharge is constant (as in parasympathetic-dominant vasomotor rhinitis seen in the elderly) or intermittent (as in seasonal rhinitis associated with sneezing and nasal obstruction). The discharge may be watery or mucoid, purulent in the presence of infection or a foreign body (children or mentally handicapped adults), and blood–stained in the presence of a tumor or foreign body. In addition, if rhinorrhoea is associated with an itchy nose, sneezing, and itchy eyes, a diagnosis of allergic rhinitis can easily be made.

The injured nose

The importance of the history in the acute injury of the nose relates to the timing of any fracture reduction if necessary and to medicolegal implications if a report is required.

The bleeding nose (epistaxis)

Patients either give a history of intermittent nose bleeds, possibly with a precipitating cause, or they actually present with a bleeding nose. If the patient is actively bleeding, resuscitative measures may precede the history-taking or this can be done whilst staunching the flow! A history of a bleeding disorder is relevant as is a history of previous nasal surgery: septal perforations often crust and bleed. Nose bleeds may be caused by excessive nasal picking or an injury to the nose may result in epistaxis. Hypertension *per se* is not a cause of epistaxis, but an elevated venous or arterial pressure will prolong any established epistaxis.

Nasal deformity

Patients complaining about the shape of their nose may or may not have associated nasal obstruction. Nasal 'deformity' may be traumatic or congenital in origin.

The 'non-smelling' nose

Patients may complain of a diminished sense of smell (hyposmia) or no sense of smell (anosmia). There may be a history of head injury, though this needs to have been severe to tear the olfactory fibres emerging through the cribriform plate. Some patients may report a loss of the sense of smell after an upper respiratory tract infection (so-called 'post-influenza neuritis'). Patients with mechanical obstruction of the upper part of the nose, (e.g. due to nasal polyps or mucosal oedema in allergic rhinitis) will also complain of anosmia. However, in many patients the cause is unknown.

Nasal and paranasal disorders may also present with 'regional' symptoms such as headache, facial pain, epiphora (excessive tear production) if the nasolacrimal duct is obstructed, diplopia (double vision), proptosis, and orbital pain (if a tumor invades the orbit.)

SYMPTOMS OF EAR DISORDERS

Painful ear (otalgia)

Pain in the ear arises from the ear itself or is referred from several other anatomical sites. The sensory nerve supply of the ear is, therefore, very important as the same sensory derivations apply to other areas of the head and neck. (see Fig. 5.8). Thus, disorders of the nose and sinuses, nasopharynx, teeth, jaws, temporomandibular joints, salivary glands and ducts, oropharynx, laryngo- and hypopharynx, tongue, and cervical spine, may all give rise to earache. The history must establish the nature of the pain, its radiation and aggravating factors.

Otalgia

Where does it hurt?

Does the pain spread?

What exacerbates the pain?

Is there a discharge?

Have you ever had an ear operation or your ears syringed?

Do you use cotton buds?

Have you hurt your ear recently?

Have you been swimming or on an airplane recently?

Is your hearing ability affected?

The discharging ear (otorrhoea)

Discharge from the ear may contain mucus or pus, and it may be bloodstained. The questions to ask the patient are similar to those asked if the complaint is of earache. The two symptoms, earache and discharge, often co-exist.

Hearing loss or deafness

It is more appropriate to talk of hearing loss than deafness, as the latter often implies a total lack of hearing and also has a certain stigma attached to it. Hearing loss can be qualified as being mild, moderate, severe, and profound, according to the degree measured in decibels.

Hearing loss

How long have you noticed a hearing loss?

Is it partial or complete?

Are both ears affected or just one?

Is there a family history of hearing problems?

Have you had an injury or surgery to your ears?

Have you had any serious illnesses such as tuberculosis or septicaemia (ototoxic drugs)?

Have you been exposed to loud noise for any length of time?

Is there associated vertigo?

The age of onset of the hearing loss is important, as is the suddenness of its onset. The more likely causes of hearing loss in the different age groups is indicated in Figure 5.14. In patients whose hearing loss is severe and occurs prior to their acquisition of language, their speech will be unusual (pre-lingual speech). The family history is relevant, for syndromal disorders may have some hereditary basis. In otosclerosis where the stapes footplate is fixed, there may also be a family history of the same disorder. If the hearing loss follows trauma, this may be due to blood in the external auditory meatus, a perforation of the tympanic membrane, or disruption of the ossicular chain. In addition, the inner ear may have been damaged, especially in fractures of the temporal bone.

Discharge from the ear may cause a hearing loss from the accumulation of debris in the external ear. In chronic inflammation, the hearing loss may be associated with a tympanic membrane perforation or disruption of the ossicular chain. Certain drugs (e.g. the aminoglycoside antibiotics, some diuretics, and cytotoxics) may damage the inner ear and a history of the use of such drugs or the illnesses requiring them is important (eg. tuberculosis, Streptomycin; severe septicaemic illness, other aminoglycosides; cancer, cytotoxics) Previous ear surgery may have resulted in a reduction in hearing.

Eighth nerve involvement by syphilis was seen more commonly in the past, but this is now rare. Patients should be asked about prolonged exposure to loud noise either in their employment or in the armed services in case they have suffered some noise-induced hearing loss. Finally, children with a hearing loss due to secretory otitis media (glue ear) may present with problems related to a hearing loss but where the hearing loss itself is not the presenting complaint. They may present with delay in language development, inattention at school, or poor scholastic performance.

The noisy ear (tinnitus)

Tinnitus is the preception of abnormal noise in the ear or head. Tinnitus may be subjective, i.e. only the patient can hear it: this is the commonest form of tinnitus. Alternatively, tinnitus may be objective, i.e. the patient and the examiner can hear it: this is much less common and usually arises from arteriovenous malformations or clicking muscles in the middle ear or palate.

Accessory auricles

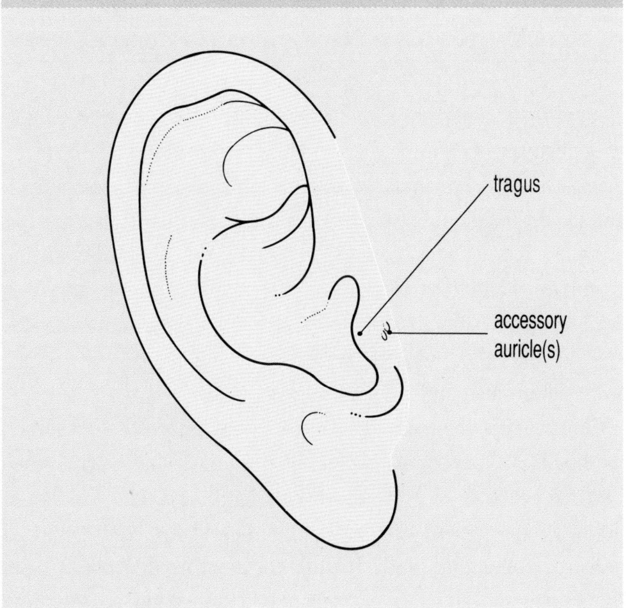

Fig. 5.15 Site of accessory auricles.

Tinnitus is usually buzzing, whistling, hissing, ringing, or pulsating, and must be distinguished from complex noises (e.g. voices, orchestras), as these constitute auditory hallucinations, an indication of a psychiatric disorder. Tinnitus is usually associated with a degree of hearing loss, yet it may occur without any hearing loss. The cause and site of origin of the noise in subjective tinnitus is usually unknown.

Ask questions similar to those asked in patients with a hearing loss. In addition aspirin overdosage can cause reversible tinnitus. It is important to ask how much the tinnitus bothers the patient, i.e. if it keeps the patient awake at night or interferes with daily living. Any history of ear disease is relevant as these are the few patients in whom, if the disease is treated, the tinnitus may disappear.

The deformed ear

Patients may complain of deformity of the ear arising from congenital causes and trauma. Congenital ear deformities include complete or partial absence of the pinna (anotia or microtia). This may be associated with middle and inner ear abnormalities. There may be accesory auricles, often seen just anterior to the tragus (Fig. 5.15) or there may be a preauricular sinus (see Fig. 5.30). The latter may become infected and require excision if it is troublesome.

Patients may also complain about the size or shape of their ears, particularly if the ear or ears protrude; 'bat ears'. This may result in children being teased at school and may cause social embarrassment. This condition can be corrected surgically.

Injury to the ear

Injury to the ear may be blunt or sharp. Patients who have had an ear injury may have sustained trauma to the pinna resulting in a haematoma auris. Trauma may have occurred in the external meatus, usually self-inflicted (e.g. with cotton-buds, hair-grips, or pencils). These objects may also injure the tympanic membrane and ossicles but rarely the inner ear. Blunt trauma in the form of a blow to the side of the head or in diffuse head injury may rupture the tympanic membrane, dislocate the ossicles, and cause damage to the inner ear. Any of these injuries may result in hearing loss, dizziness, and damage to the facial nerve as it passes through the temporal bone. The damage can be either temporary or permanent.

Vertigo

Dizziness is a common complaint and means different things to different people. The key to making a diagnosis in the dizzy patient involves taking a good history. It is important to establish exactly what the patient means by feeling dizzy. The aim is to find out whether the dizziness is in fact true vertigo (also see pages 12.55–12.56). Vertigo is an hallucination of movement. Feelings of 'light headedness', 'about to black out or faint', do not constitute true vertigo. Whilst the hallucination of movement is not always rotatory, this is often the complaint mentioned by the patient. Once the

Vertigo

Can you describe the dizziness? N.B. Don't ask leading questions.

How long does it last?

Does anything precipitate the attack?

Is there associated nausea or vomiting?

Does rapid head movement cause dizziness?

Is there associated hearing loss or tinnitus?

Are you on any medication, (e.g. hypertensive)?

Have you ever had ear problems or ear surgery?

symptom of vertigo is verified, establish whether it is of central origin or arising from peripheral receptors (e.g. the vestibule of the inner ear).

Encourage the patient to describe in detail a typical attack of dizziness in his own words. This is better than suggesting sensations like 'feeling faint' or asking if the room spins around.

In general terms, central causes of vertigo are more constant and are progressive, whereas vestibular causes tend to be intermittent and paroxysmal and are not usually progressive. However, the symptoms of peripheral causes of vertigo (e.g. the vomiting and the vertigo itself) may be as severe as in central causes.

Facial pain

Facial pain is a common complaint and arises from many different sources. The source may be relatively obvious (e.g. the patient may say 'I have toothache') or the pain may be referred from a distant site, (e.g. the patient with tonsillitis who complains of earache). It is important to remember that not all facial pain is due to sinusitis and not all earache is due to ear disease.

Facial nerve palsy

Patients may present with an isolated facial nerve palsy or the palsy may be part of a more generalized neurological disorder (e.g. a cerebrovascular accident). The suddenness of onset and any association with other neurological complaints should be elicited. A history of ear disease is particularly relevant as the facial nerve makes a considerable journey through the temporal bone, crossing the medial wall of the middle ear, the mastoid, before making its exit at the stylomastoid foramen. Questions relating to the function of branches of the facial nerve, such as dry eyes (if the greater superficial petrosal nerve is involved) or altered taste (if the chorda tympani is involved) can give you an idea of the level of nerve disruption.

Facial pain

Where does it hurt?

How long has your face been painful?

What is the pain like (e.g. throbbing, piercing)?

What aggravates, relieves the pain?

Do you have any dental problems?

Do you ever have trouble with your jaw, with eating?

Any ENT disease in the past?

Do you suffer from migraine headaches?

EXAMINATION OF THE MOUTH AND THROAT

To perform an adequate examination of this system requires certain basic instruments (Fig. 5.16), a good light source, and a systematic approach to the system as in any other organ system. The patient and the doctor should be sitting opposite each other. The ideal situation involves using a headlight or head-mirror, as this leaves the examiner with both hands free.

Observe the patient's face and facial expression for any immediately obvious abnormalities: these may include lumps and bumps, scars, deformities, and facial asymmetry.

Conveniently, the mouth and throat are examined first. Examine the lips for telangiectasia, ulcers, pigmentation, and cracks. Also look for evidence of previous surgery (e.g. the repair of a 'harelip'). Ask the patient to open the mouth and inspect the buccal mucosa, gums, and teeth. If the patient wears dentures, these should be removed. Note the state of periodontal hygiene and any evidence of gingivitis (inflammation of the gums). Look for ulcera-

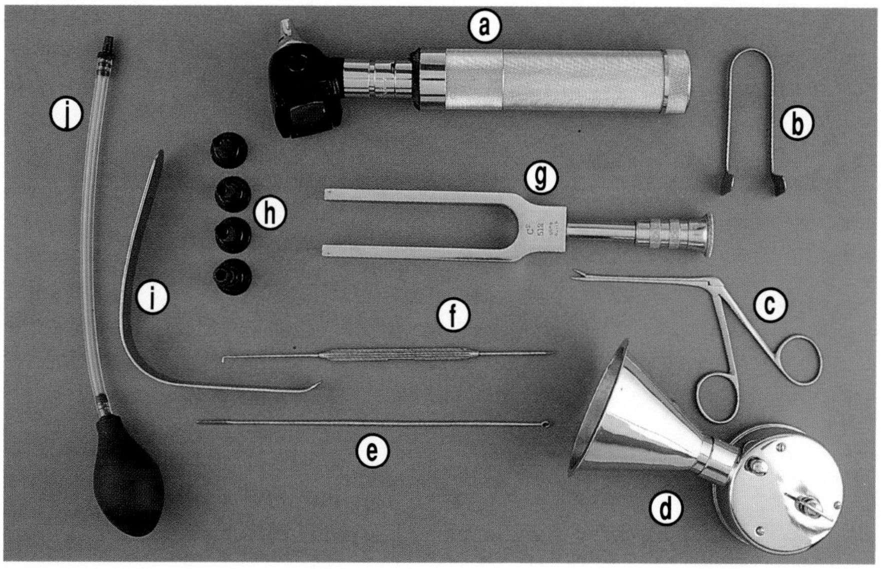

Fig. 5.16 Basic instruments necessary for the ENT examination: (a) auroscope; (b) Thudicum speculum; (c) crocodile forceps; (d) Barany noise-box; (e) Jobson–Horne or ring probe; (f) wax hook; (g) 512Hz tuning fork; (h) aural specula; (i) tongue depressor; and, (j) auroscope puffer.

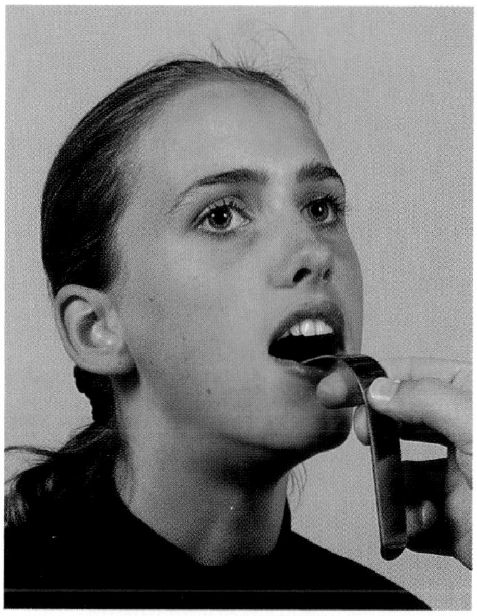

Fig. 5.17 Examining the mouth using a tongue depressor.

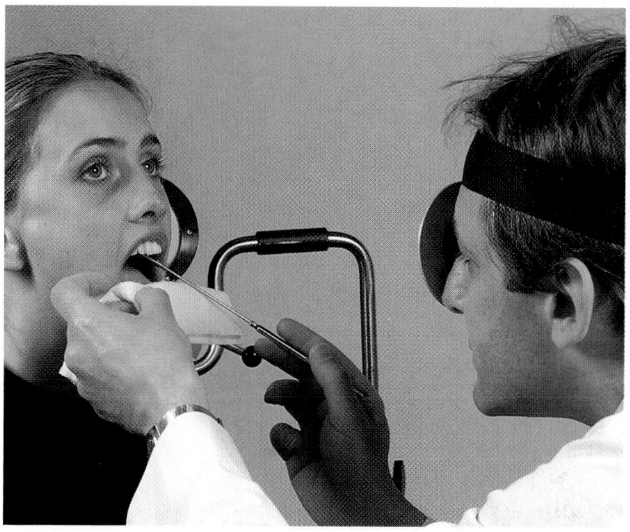

Fig. 5.18 Technique of indirect laryngoscopy.

tion, nodules, and pigmentation. Inspect the hard palate for evidence of a cleft-palate or a repaired cleft, and for telangiectasia.

Next, examine the tongue and floor of the mouth. Ask the patient to protrude the tongue. This not only allows more of the tongue to be seen but also gives an indication of XIIth nerve function. Ask the patient to touch the palate with his tongue to allow you to see the floor of the mouth with the submandibular ducts opening on either side of the frenulum. Look for ulcers, nodules, furring, and leukoplakia (white patches) on the tongue. Then, ask the patient to say 'aaah'. This will allow you to see the tonsils, the posterior pharyngeal wall, and the movement of the soft palate (the Xth cranial nerve is the motor supply). You may require a tongue depressor to obtain an adequate view of the posterior aspects of the oral cavity and oropharynx (Fig. 5.17).

Finally, put on a glove and feel any suspicious areas within the mouth. This often gives a better idea of a lesion than inspection alone. At this stage of the examination, the ENT surgeon would perform an indirect laryngoscopy (Figs 5.18 and 5.19) and

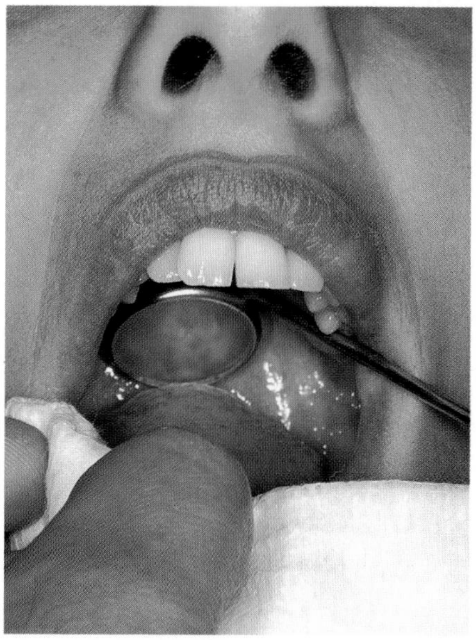

Fig. 5.19 Technique of indirect laryngoscopy.

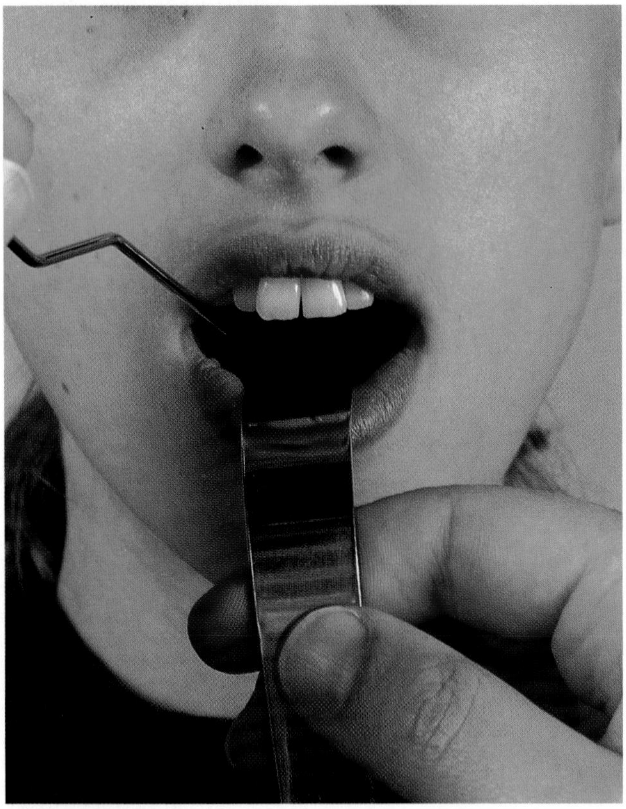

Fig. 5.20 Technique of mirror examination of postnasal space (posterior rhinoscopy).

examination of the postnasal space (posterior rhinoscopy) using the appropriate mirrors (Figs 5.20, 5.21, and 5.22). These techniques would not be expected to be part of the clinical expertise of non-ENT surgeons.

EXAMINATION OF THE NOSE

First, observe the external appearance of the nose, as this may give an indication of a more generalized skin disorder or deformity of the nasal skeleton, and may point to previous injury as the cause of nasal obstruction. Secondly, examine the nasal vestibule. In children, the cartilages of the nasal tip are soft and a good view of the nasal vestibule, anterior end of the septum, and anterior ends of the inferior turbinates can be obtained by simply elevating the tip of the nose (Fig. 5.23). In adults the cartilages are firmer, and the use of a Thudicum speculum is usually necessary to obtain a similar view (Fig. 5.24).

Posterior rhinoscopy

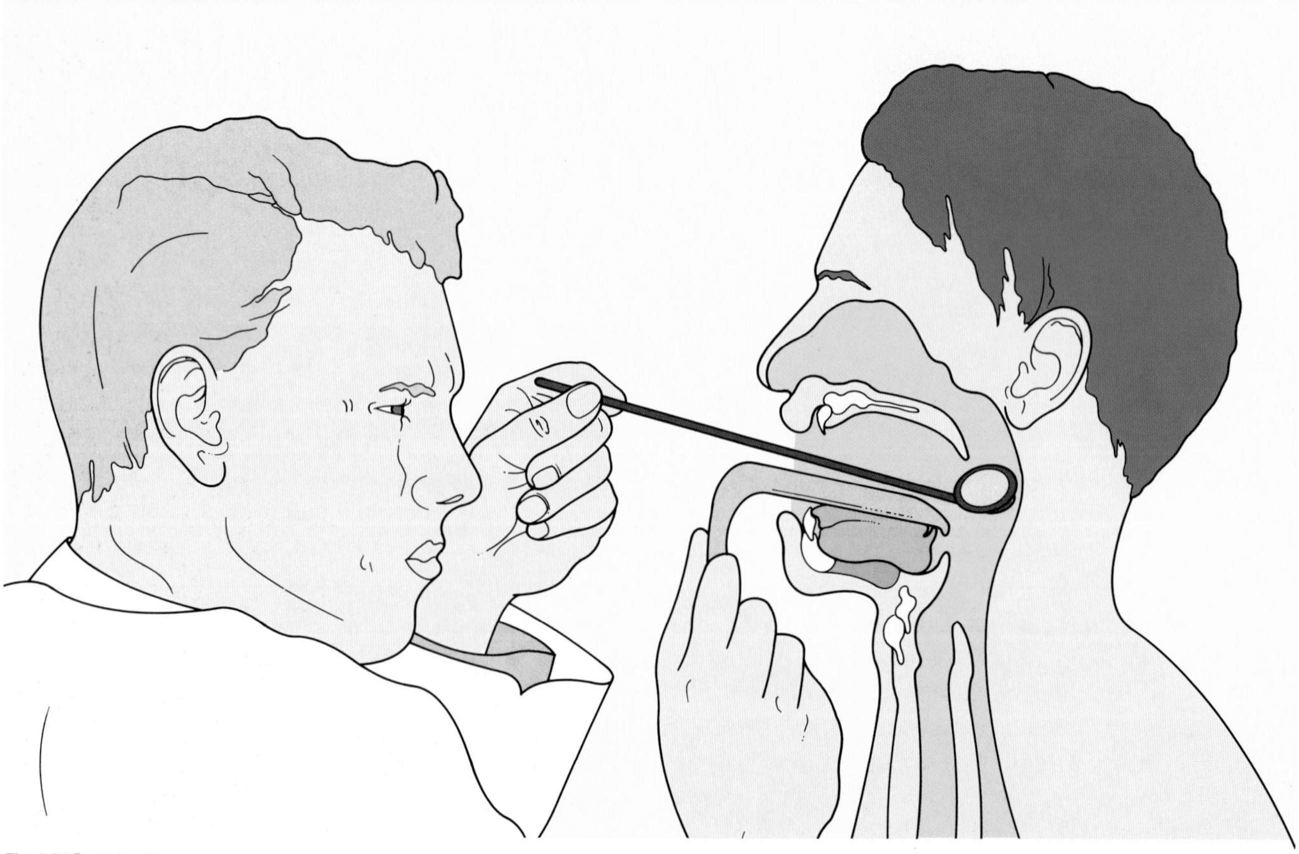

Fig. 5.21 Posterior rhinoscopy.

Indirect laryngoscopy

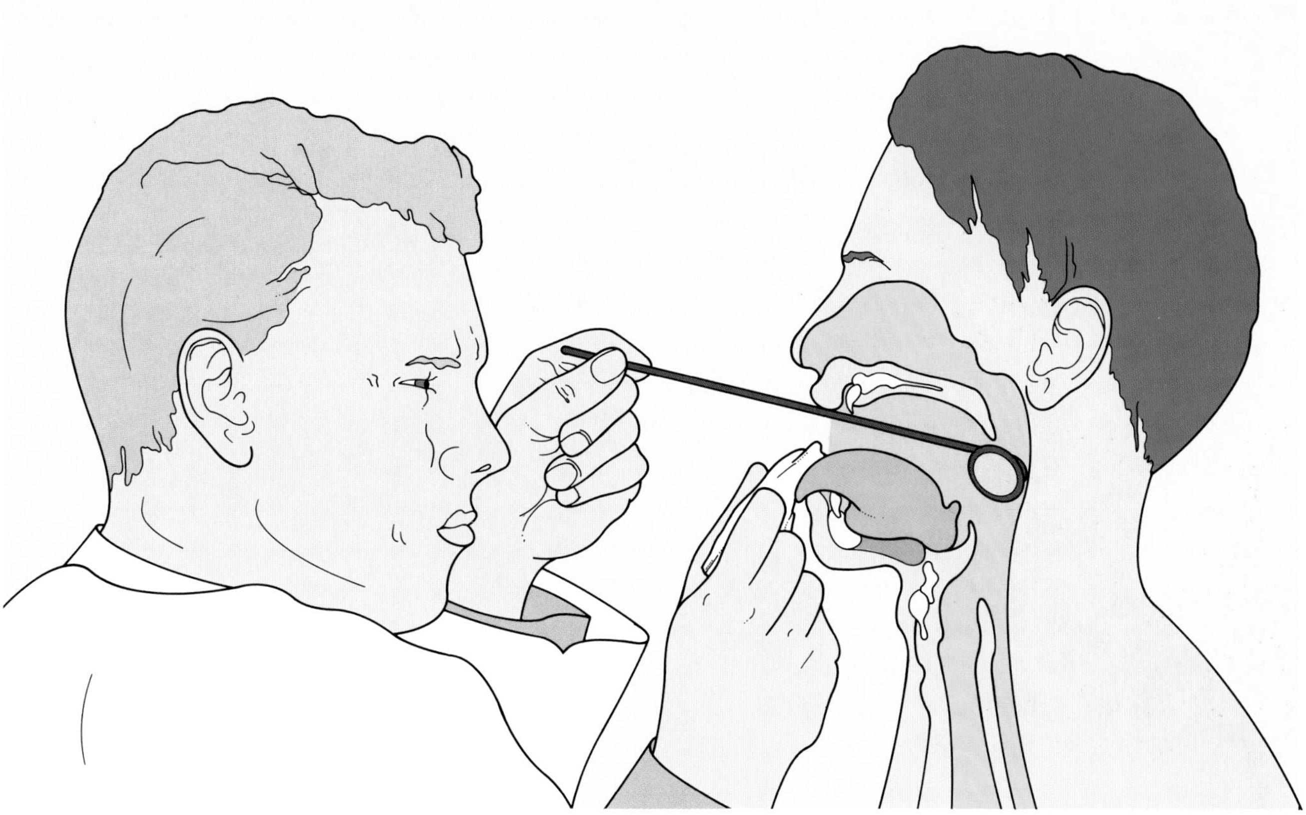

Fig. 5.22 Indirect laryngoscopy.

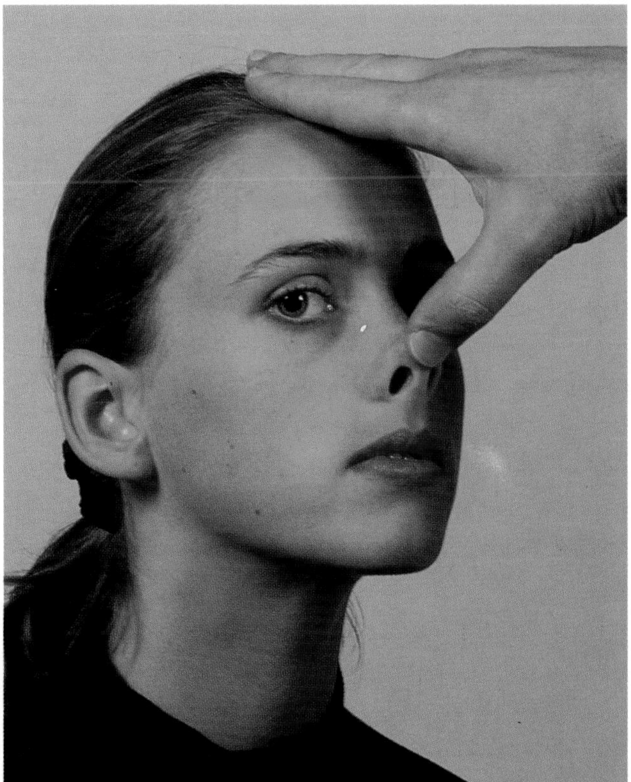

Fig. 5.23 Anterior rhinoscopy by elevating the tip of the nose.

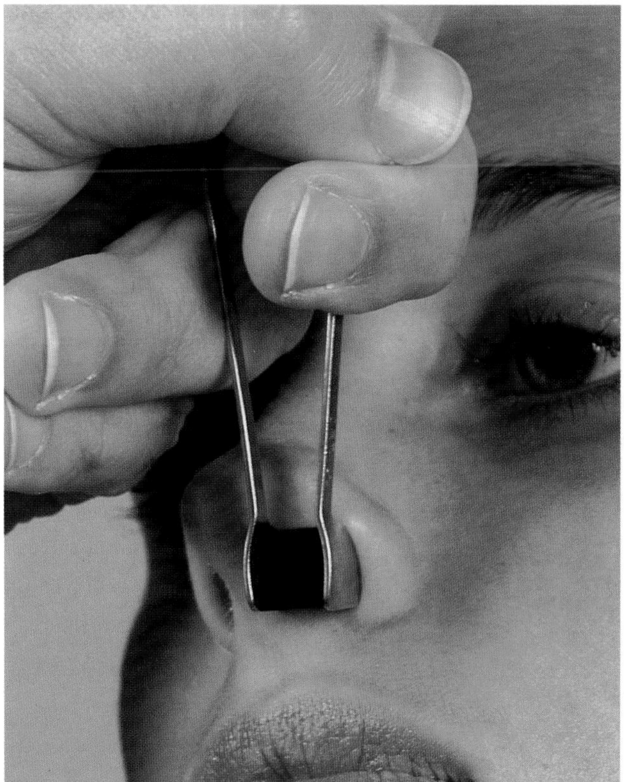

Fig. 5.24 Anterior rhinoscopy using a Thudicum speculum.

A more detailed view of the nasal cavities can be obtained using rigid Hopkins Rod telescopes or a flexible nasendoscope (Fig. 5.25) which can then be advanced through the nasal cavity to view the postnasal space (Fig. 5.26) and larynx (Fig. 5.27). There are significant advantages in viewing the larynx by this method. If the patient gags on indirect laryngscopy this is minimized by flexible nasendoscopy. When performing indirect laryngoscopy using a laryngeal mirror, the examiner must hold the tongue (see Fig. 5.18); consequently, this permits only limited phonation by the patient. This method is suitable for seeing laryngeal tumors and other obvious laryngeal pathology; nevertheless, the more subtle changes of dysphonia can be better diagnosed by using the flexible nasendoscope.

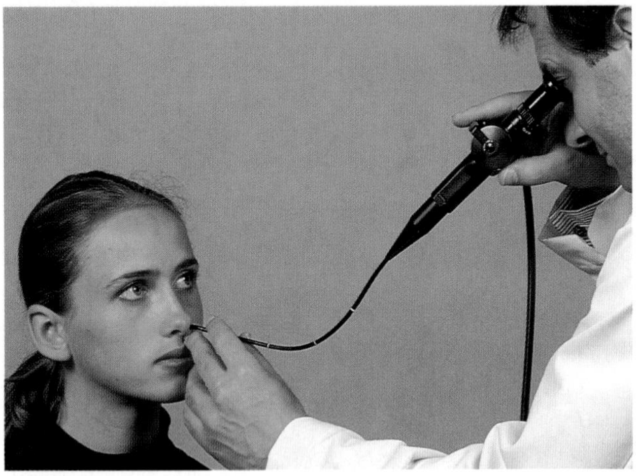

Fig. 5.25 Examination of the nose, postnasal space, and larynx using a flexible nasendoscope.

On anterior rhinoscopy, the non-specialist should be able to comment on deflection of the nasal septum, the state of inferior turbinates (both size and colour), and identify abnormal lesions (e.g. papillomata and polyps). Then assessment of the nasal airflow follows. Ask the patient to breath out nasally and observe the resultant moisture on a silver tongue depressor or mirror positioned at the anterior nares (Fig. 5.28). The inspiratory flow can crudely be assessed by occluding the undersurface of one nasal cavity at a time and asking the patient to sniff inwards (Fig. 5.29). To assess the sense of smell ask the patient to identify the smells from simple smell bottles, though this is not particularly reliable. Objective and quantitative tests of smell are as yet not available for clinical practice.

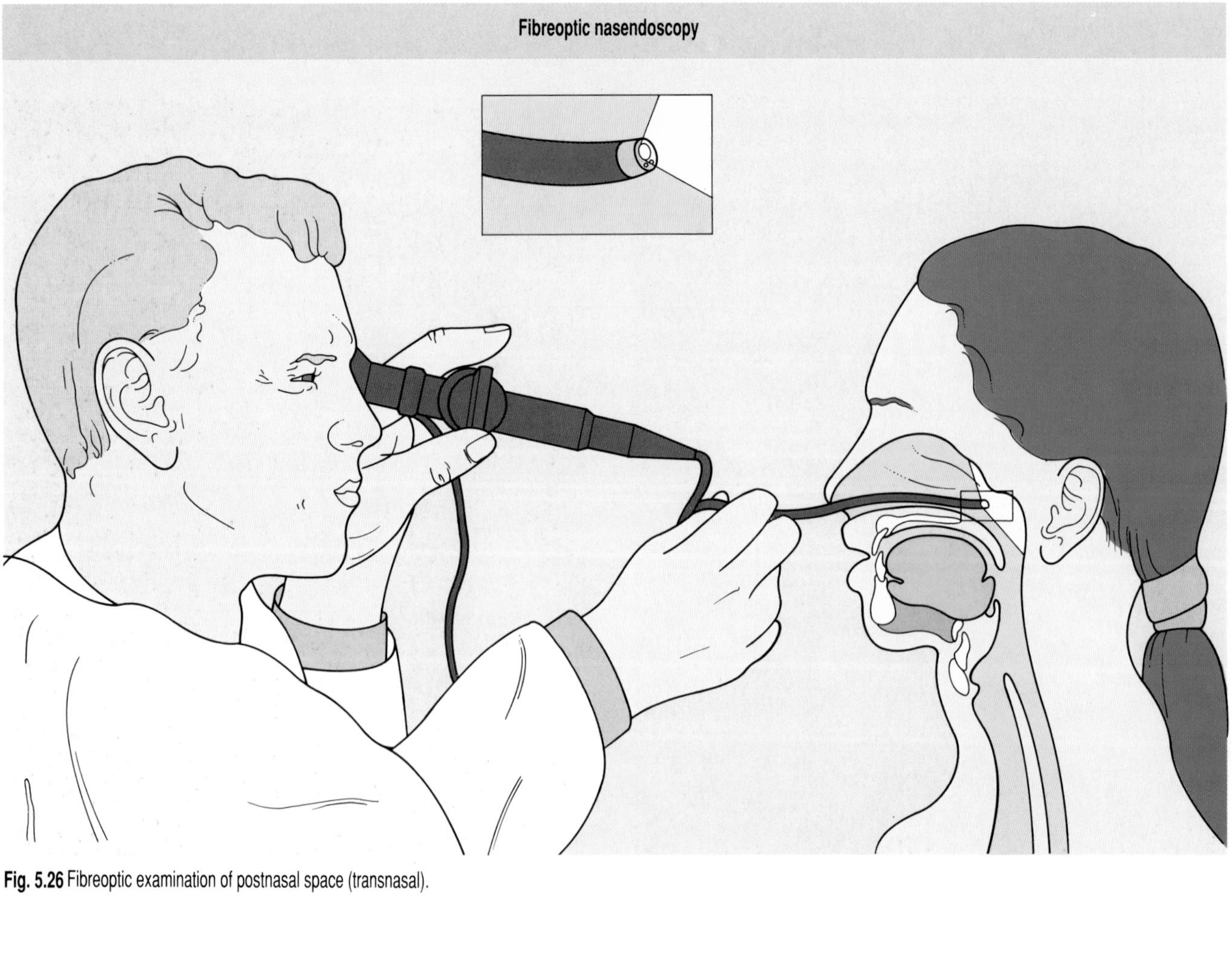

Fig. 5.26 Fibreoptic examination of postnasal space (transnasal).

Fibreoptic nasendoscopy

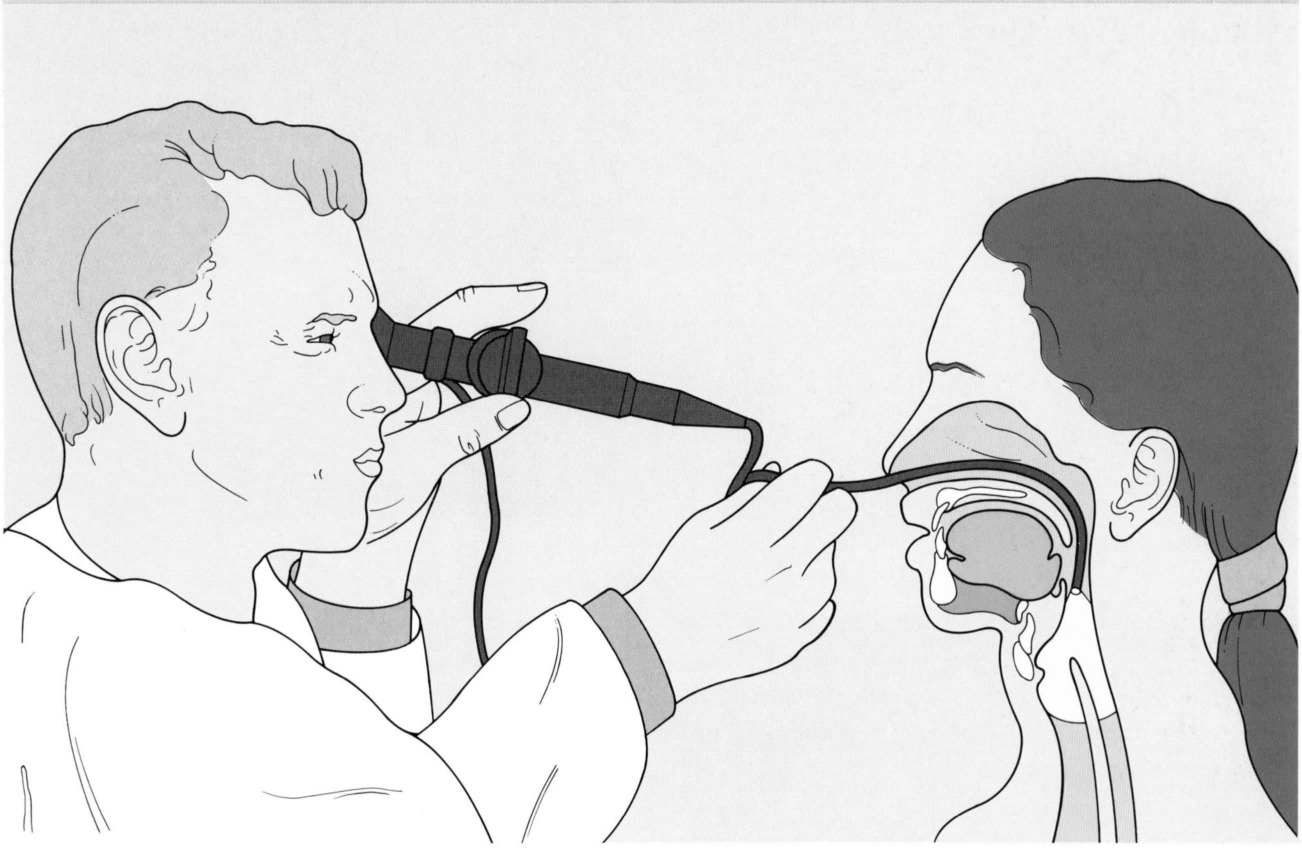

Fig. 5.27 Fibreoptic examination of the larynx (transnasal).

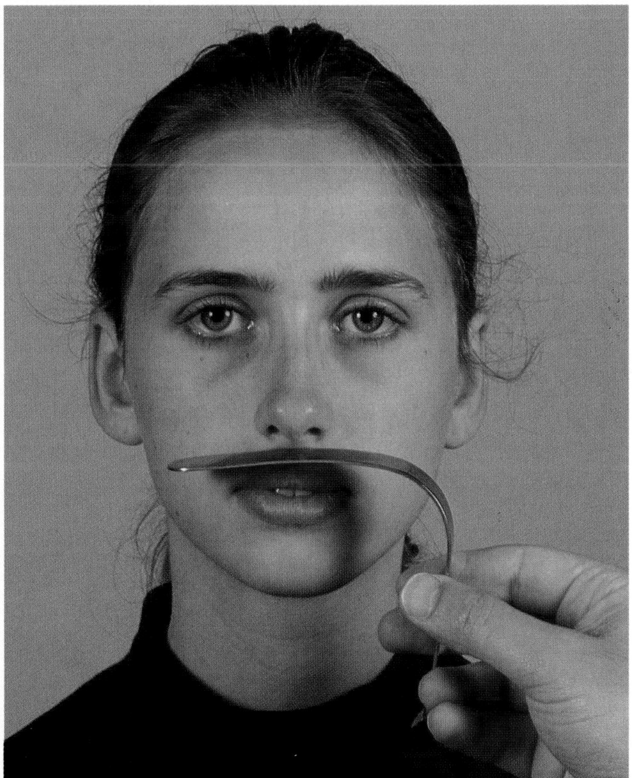

Fig. 5.28 Assessment of nasal airflow on breathing out.

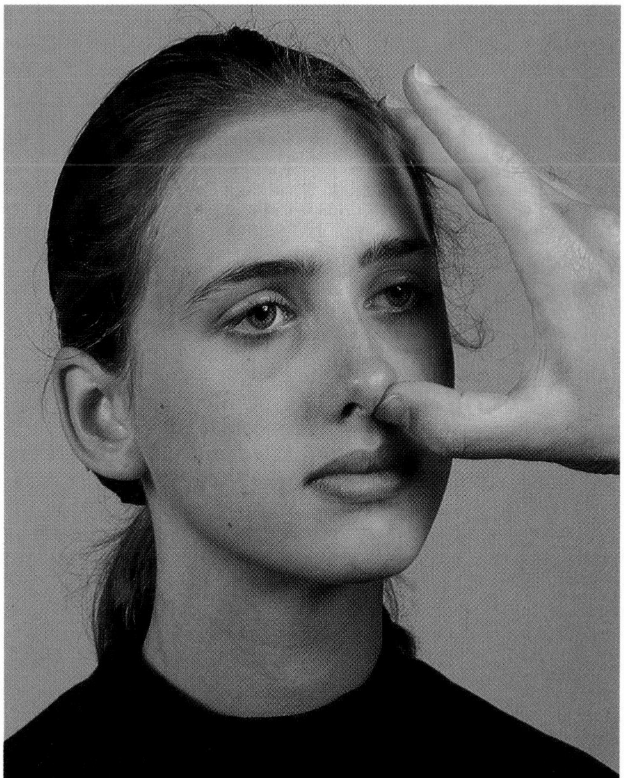

Fig. 5.29 Assessing nasal inspiratory airflow by occluding one nostril at a time.

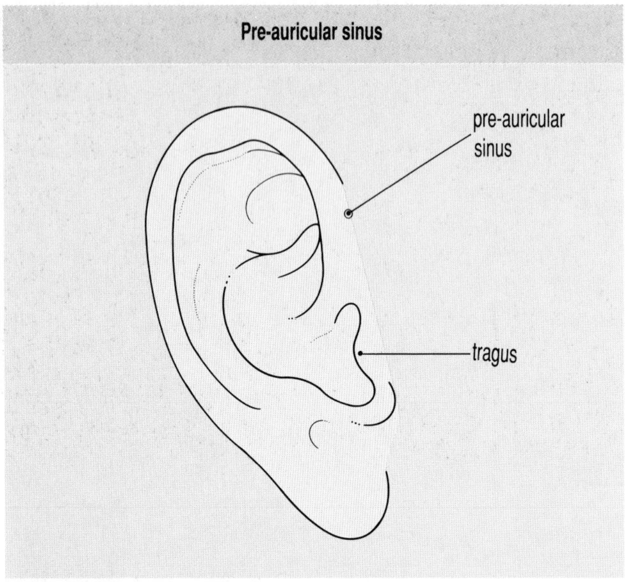

Fig. 5.30 Site of pre-auricular sinus.

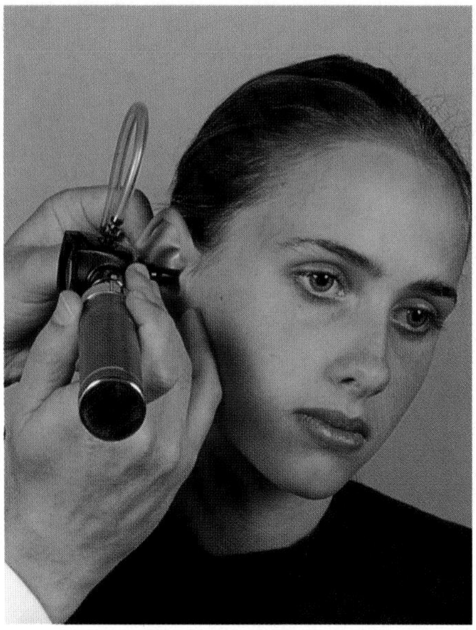

Fig. 5.31 Examination of the ear using an auroscope. Note the position of the right hand against the patient's face.

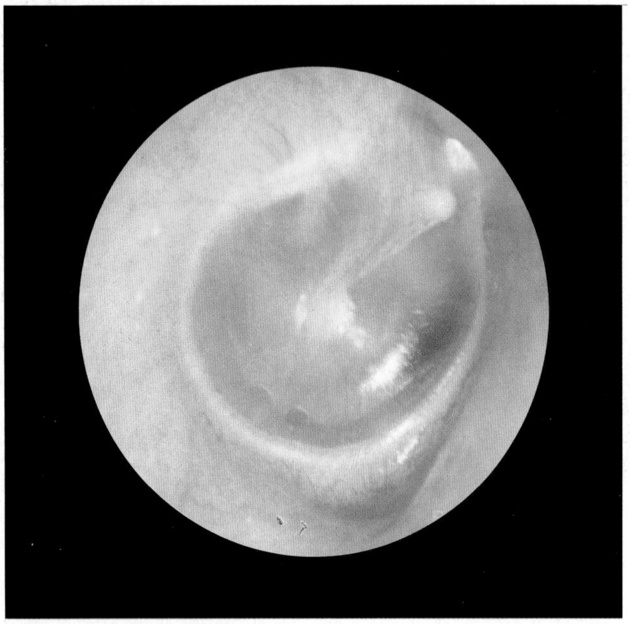

Fig. 5.32 Normal tympanic membrane.

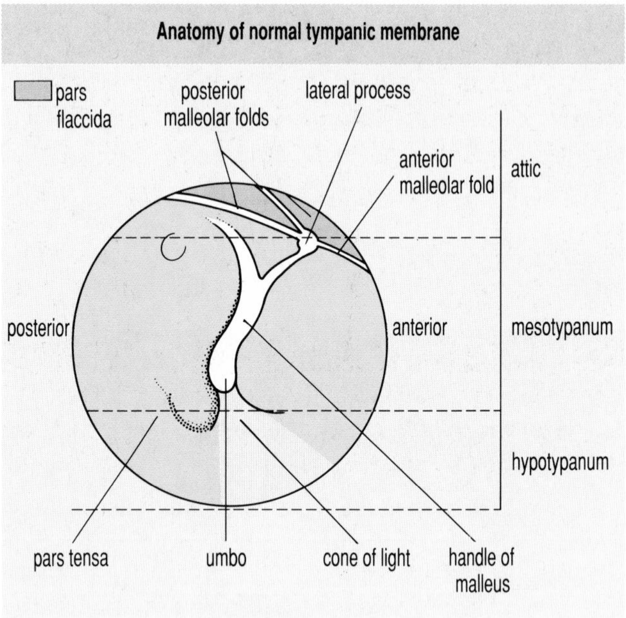

Fig. 5.33 Anatomy of normal tympanic membrane.

EXAMINATION OF THE EARS

Examine the pinna, note its shape, size, and any deformity. Look for pits (preauricular sinuses) just inferior and anterior to the origin of the helix (Fig. 5.30). Look behind the ear for any scars from previous surgery and note whether or not the patient wears a hearing aid. This will obviously need removal prior to examination. Tug gently on the pinna: tenderness here will be the result of external ear disease or of temporomandibular joint pain. Feel for pre-, post, and infra-auricular lymph nodes, again the result of external ear disease, *not* middle or inner ear disease.

Observe the meatus. If this is particularly wide it may be the result of previous mastoid surgery in which a meatoplasty was fashioned. An auroscope with a puffer attached is then used to examine the deep meatus and tympanic membrane. Ensure the light works properly and the batteries are not too old! Apply gentle traction on the ear to straighten the external ear canal (exert the traction in whichever direction serves to straighten the canal) and gently insert the auroscope. Use a black speculum (grey specula lose too much light) and use the biggest speculum that will fit the ear canal, as this permits you to see in your visual field as much of the topographical anatomy as possible. Always use the longer variety of aural speculum to allow adequate vision of the deep canal and tympanic membrane. A larger diameter speculum facilitates an airtight seal when using the puffer. It is important to hold the auroscope correctly (Fig. 5.31). This guards against injury, particularly in children, if the patient suddenly moves.

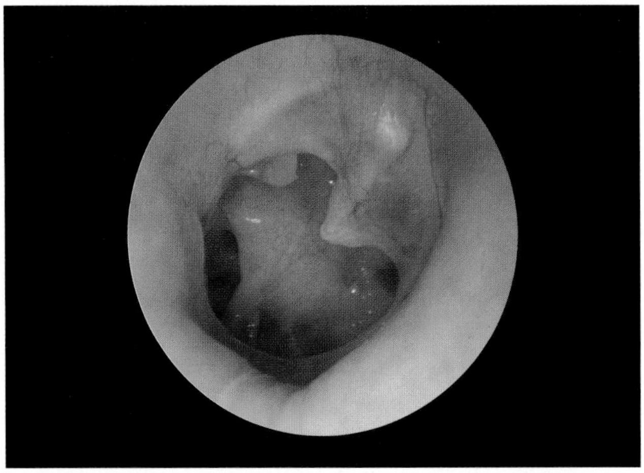

Fig. 5.34 Large tympanic membrane perforation. Incudostapedial joint just visible posterosuperiorly; round window visible posteriorly.

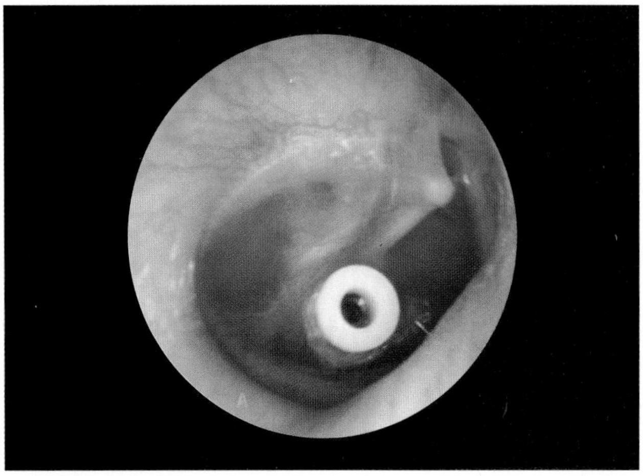

Fig. 5.35 Ventilation tube (grommet) *in situ*.

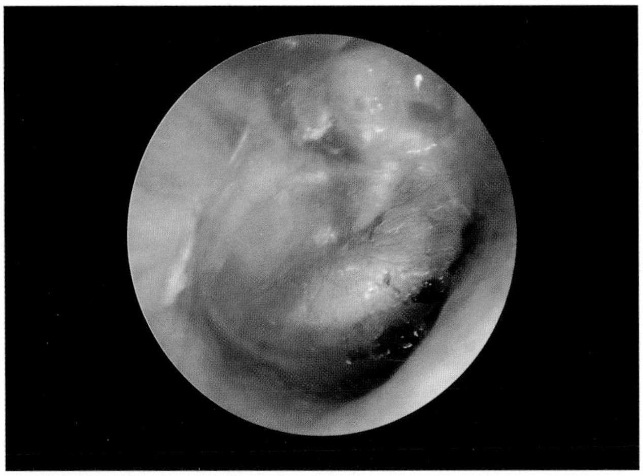

Fig. 5.36 Cholesteatoma in attic region. Note perforation of tympanic membrane in this area as well as erosion of bony outer attic wall.

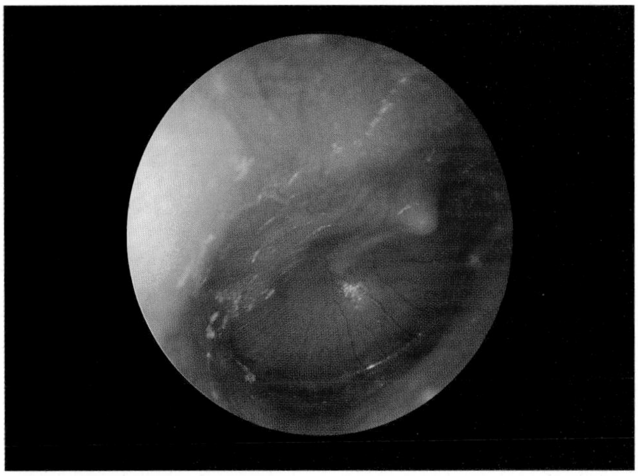

Fig. 5.37 Middle ear effusion ('glue ear').

Introduce the auroscope and look at the canal wall skin for otitis externa and exostoses (bony outgrowths from the deep canal wall). Severe otitis externa or a boil (furuncle) of the external meatus may totally occude the meatus, making visualisation impossible. At this stage the canal and tympanic membrane may be obscured by wax. Wax is a normal phenomenon and is not 'dirt' as believed by many patients. Gently remove the wax by using a ring-probe, a wax hook (see Fig. 5.16), syringing of the ear, or using a suction apparatus under the operating microscope.

If removing wax causes pain or bleeding – STOP! If the wax is very hard, it may be possible to use a wax softener (e.g. olive oil or sodium bicarbonate ear drops) for a few days before attempting its removal. If wax cannot be removed without the risk of damage to the ear, a specialist referral is necessary. Do not syringe an ear if there is a history of a perforated tympanic membrane as this may introduce infection into the middle ear.

The tympanic membrane is inspected next (Fig. 5.32). All the anatomical features of the drum should be actively sought and noted (Fig. 5.33). There are great variations of normality and accurate assessment comes from the experience of adequately assessing many ears. Note the presence or absence of any perforations (Fig. 5.34). White chalk-like deposits are commonly seen in the substance of the drum and result from infection or a previous history of grommets (ventilation tubes) (Fig. 5.35). Fluid bubbles are occasionally seen if an effusion is present in the middle ear. An accumulation of white epithelial debris within a retracted pocket of the tympanic membrane indicates the presence of cholesteatoma, a serious disease of the middle ear (Fig. 5.36).

The puffer is used next, and the patient must be warned of the impending puff of air. This is extremely valuable in assessing mobility of the tympanic membrane. As the puffer is gently squeezed, the drum should be seen to move medially then laterally. An immobile tympanic membrane indicates (a) there is an inadequate seal with escape of air, (b) a tympanic membrane perforation is present, or (c) an effusion (collection of fluid) is present in the middle ear (Fig. 5.37). If this simple test is performed accurately, a lot of useful information is obtained.

The patient's hearing should then be assessed using tuning forks.

It is also possible to perform a crude assessment of the hearing by whispering at various distances; however, this is difficult to quantify. Tuning forks will give you an idea of whether any hearing loss is conductive or sensorineural, and whether one or both ears are affected. A 512Hz tuning fork is best used, as the 256Hz tuning fork imparts too much tactile sensation.

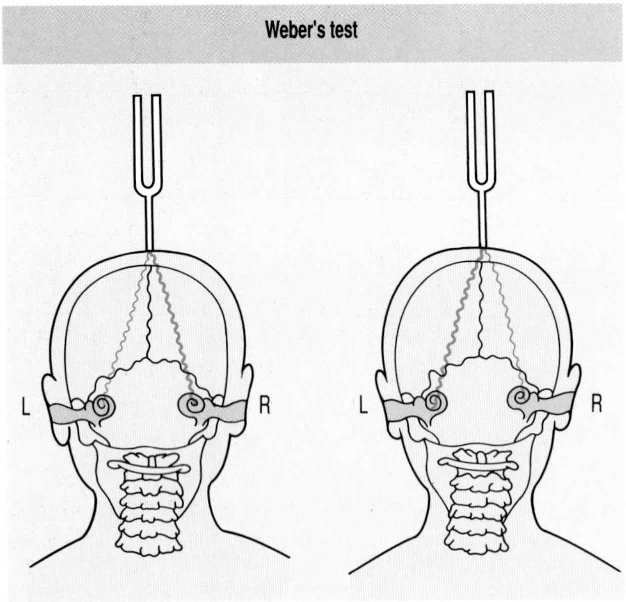

Fig. 5.38 Weber's test. Left-sided perceptive deafness (left), and left-sided conductive deafness (right).

The Weber test

The Weber test is first performed by putting the vibrating tuning fork (Fig. 5.38) on the midline of the patient's skull. This may be over the vertex, on the forehead, nasal bridge, or on the teeth. Ask the patient where the vibration is heard. If the hearing is normal in both ears or the hearing loss is symmetrical, the vibration will be heard in the midline or equally in both ears. The vibration is heard in only one ear if that particular ear has a conductive hearing loss or if the other ear has no hearing at all, i.e. a 'dead ear'.

You can simulate the test by putting a finger in your ear (creating a conductive hearing loss) and then hum (to create a noise): the sound of your hum will be heard in the occluded ear as long as this ear isn't 'dead'.

The Rinne test

The Rinne test (Fig. 5.39) should always be performed in conjunction with the Weber test, as it will help verify the findings of the latter. The base of the vibrating tuning fork is placed against the patient's mastoid process. When the patient can no longer hear the vibration, the tuning fork is placed next to his ear on that side. If the sound is now heard, the Rinne test is positive. This implies that air conduction is better than bone conduction and that there is no significant conductive hearing loss. The test is then repeated for the opposite ear.

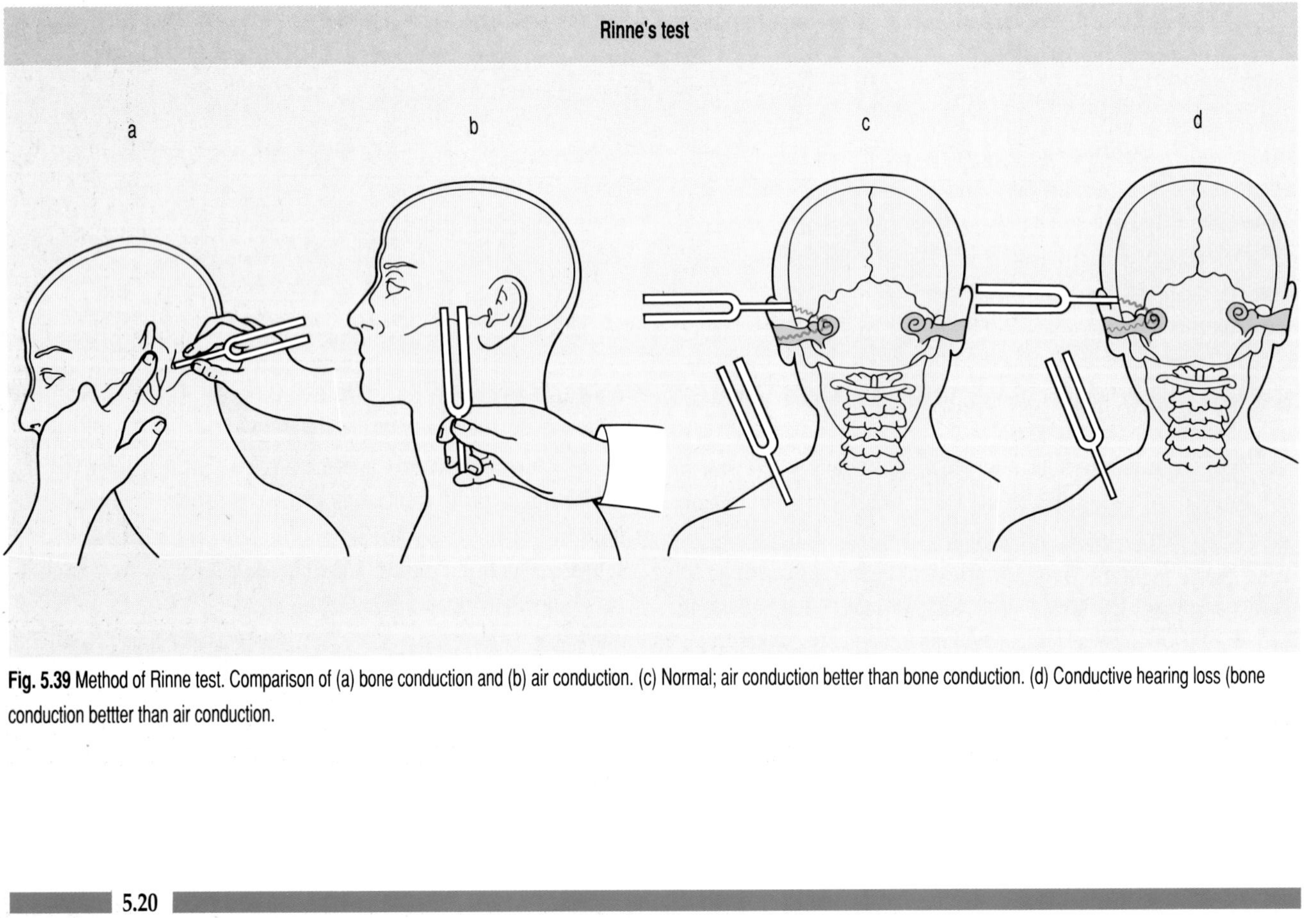

Fig. 5.39 Method of Rinne test. Comparison of (a) bone conduction and (b) air conduction. (c) Normal; air conduction better than bone conduction. (d) Conductive hearing loss (bone conduction bettter than air conduction.

If the tuning fork is heard better over the mastoid process, then the Rinne test is negative, i.e. bone conduction is better than air conduction. There is one exception to the rule. If the Rinne test is performed on the side of a non-hearing or 'dead' ear, the test may appear to be negative, i.e. bone conduction appears to be intact, indicating a functioning cochlea on that side. But if the ear is in fact a non-hearing ear, the sound waves are being transmitted through the skull bones to the opposite cochlea, thus the vibration is heard. This is then known as a false negative Rinne test and can be confirmed by masking the 'good' ear with a Barany noise box (see Fig. 5.16) or other sounds. Here the good ear will be 'flooded' with noise from the noise box and will not be able to perceive the sound of the tuning fork from the opposite ear.

Formal audiometric testing

Tuning fork tests may be difficult to interpret in young children and malingerers, so the help of an audiologist should be sought if there is an element of doubt. Formal audiometric testing is usually performed in the hospital's audiology department and takes a variety of different forms depending on the age of the patient and the hearing deficit being tested. Audiometric testing is broadly divided into subjective tests such as pure-tone and speech audiometry and objective tests such as stapedial reflexes, tympanometry, and evoked response audiometry.

In pure tone and speech audiometry, the patient is asked to respond to different pure tones and speech, and the response is recorded. Objective testing aims to eliminate subjectivity and malingering. Testing of the vestibular part of the inner ear is also performed in the audiology department (see page 12.34) and may consist of caloric tests and electronystagmography.

EXAMINATION OF THE NECK AND TEMPOROMANDIBULAR JOINTS

The neck and temporomandibular joints should be examined next. Both these examinations are best performed standing behind the seated patient (Fig. 5.40). The temporomandibular (TM) joints are palpated just anterior to the tragus of the ear (Fig. 5.41). The patient is asked to open his mouth as the joint is palpated. Excessive pressure on palpation will cause pain in normal joints, so this must not be interpreted as diagnostic of TM joint dysfunction. Feel for clicking or crepitus over the joint and ask the patient if palpation is painful. More often than not the tenderness is unilateral.

The neck should be palpated after looking at its shape and contours. If the patient is wearing a tie this should be loosened and the top buttons of his shirt undone. Similarly if a patient has a shirt or dress with buttons up to the neck or collar, these should be undone to expose the supraclavicular fossae and suprasternal notch. It is

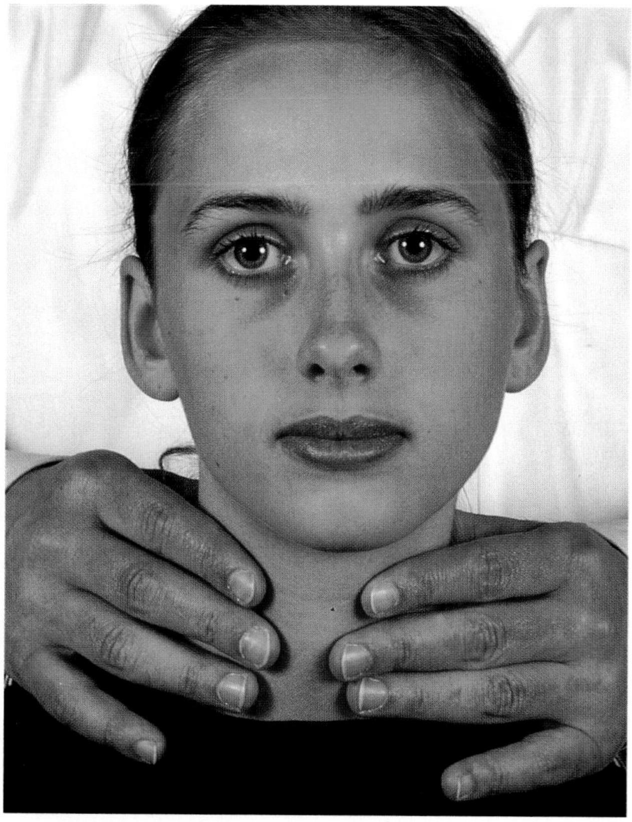

Fig. 5.40 Palpation of the neck.

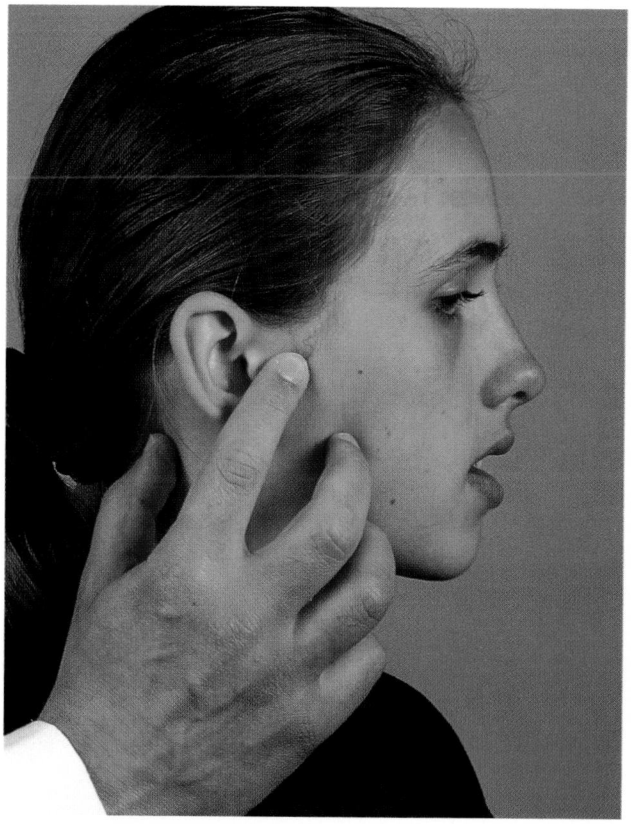

Fig. 5.41 Palpation of the temporomandibular joint.

useful to palpate the neck in a systematic pattern (e.g. submental triangle, submandibular regions, posterior, and anterior triangles). With the patient swallowing, locate and assess the thyroid gland and any thyroid or midline neck swellings. The thyroid gland and thyroglossal duct remnants move upwards on swallowing. Feel and auscultate the carotid arteries for any bruits. Cystic swellings of the neck may be transilluminated with a torch. Finally, assess the cervical spine as problems here can present with earache due to the similarity in nerve supply. Active and passive movements of flexion, extension, rotation, and lateral flexion should be performed to assess limitation of movement, induction of pain, or paraesthesiae in the upper limbs.

THE RESPIRATORY SYSTEM

6

Disease of the respiratory tract accounts for more consultations with general practitioners than any other of the body systems. It is also responsible for more new spells of incapacity for work and more days lost from work.

For example, asthma now affects about ten per cent of the population of the UK; lung cancer is the commonest male cancer and in some places has already exceeded breast as the commonest female cancer. Tuberculosis, for so long in the past the staple of the respiratory physician, may be declining in the West, but the respiratory complications of HIV infections have taken its place. Increases in pollution, new industrial processes, and the growing worldwide consumption of tobacco all have implications for the lungs. The average general practitioner, therefore, is likely to spend more of his working day examining the respiratory system than any other.

Respiratory disease is common in hospital practice. It accounts for about four per cent of all hospital admissions and about thirty-five per cent of all acute medical admissions. Surgeons and anaesthetists are very interested in ensuring an adequate respiratory system in any patient who needs a general anaesthetic.
Radiologists, pathologists, and microbiologists are intimately involved in the diagnosis of lung conditions. Consequently, doctors in many branches of medicine spend a very substantial portion of their professional working life in the diagnosis and treatment of lung disease.

A good history is the basis for a diagnosis of lung disease, as of any other disease, particularly as an examination may be normal even in quite advanced disease. Both are aided by a knowledge of structure and function. Fortunately, two fairly straightforward techniques, radiography and spirometry (the analysis of the volume of expired air over time) illustrate normality and help to understand the abnormal.

STRUCTURE AND FUNCTION

The respiratory tract extends from the nose to the alveoli and includes not only the air conducting passages but the blood supply as well. The arrangement of the major airways is shown in Figure 6.1. An appreciation of this arrangement helps in the interpretation of radiographs (Fig. 6.2) and is essential for the bronchoscopist.

The bronchial tree

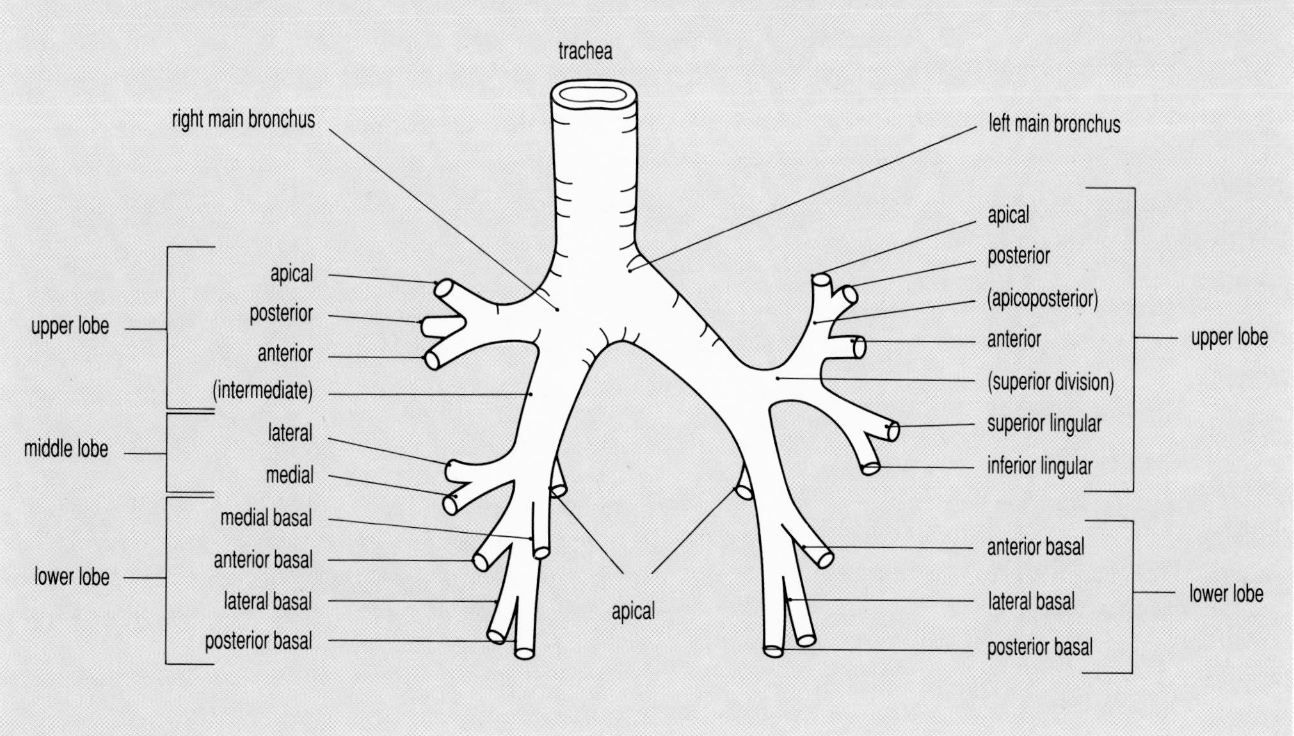

Fig. 6.1 The arrangement of the major airways.

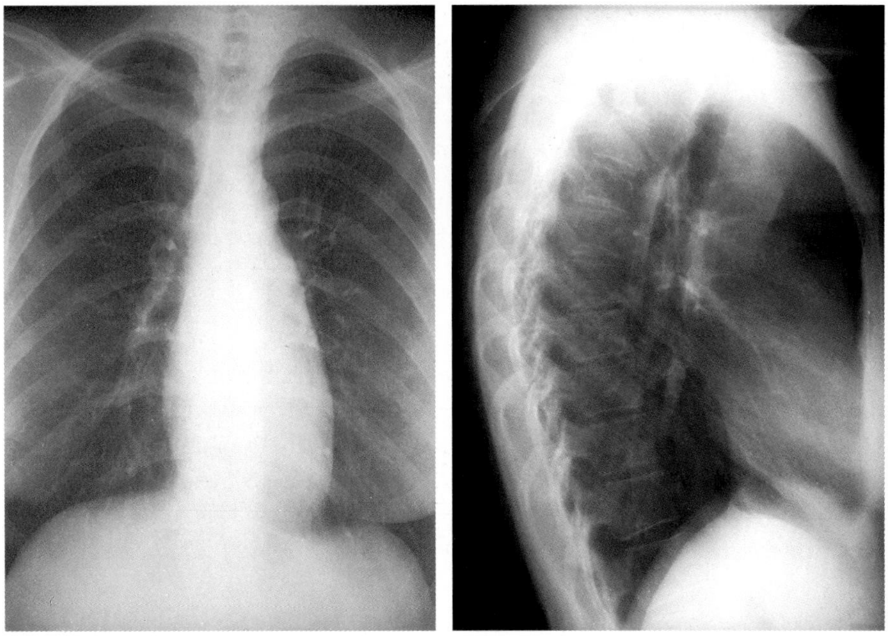

Fig. 6.2 Normal radiograph: postero-anterior view (left) and lateral view (right).

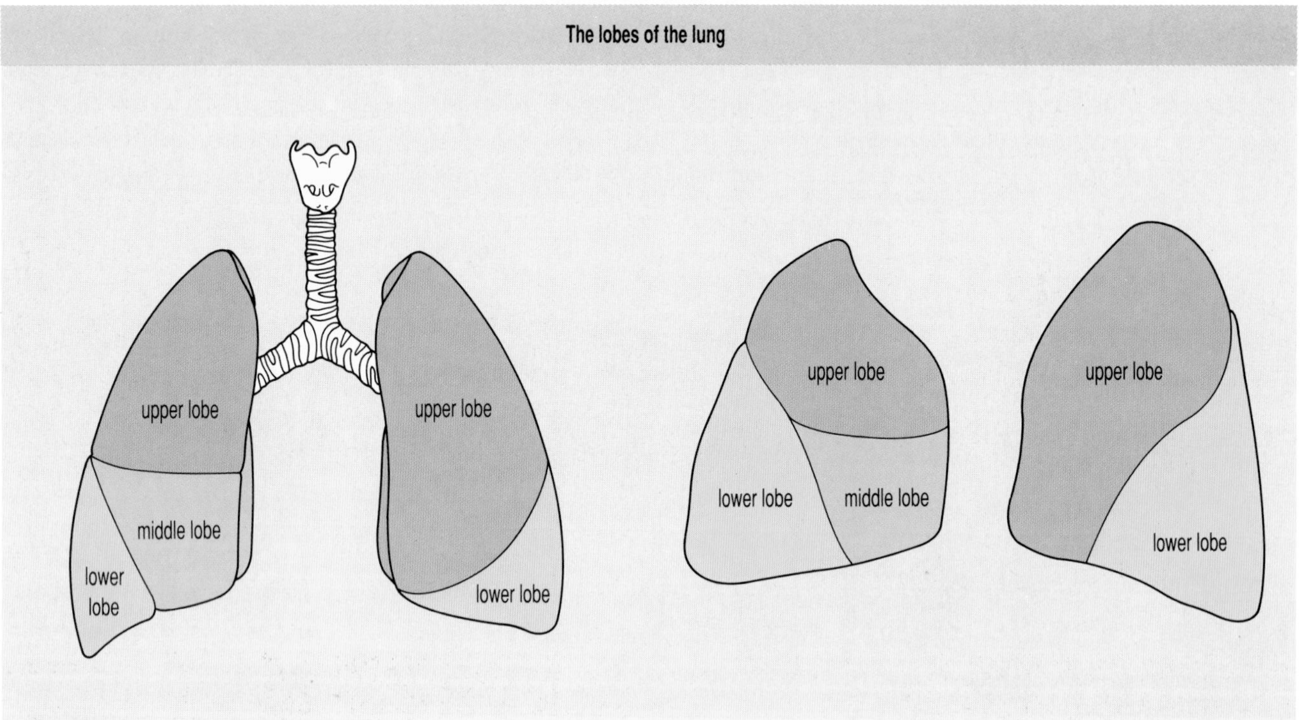

Fig. 6.3 The lobes of the lung: anterior view (left) and lateral view (right).

More important for the examiner is the arrangement of the lobes of the lung (Fig. 6.3). It will be seen that both lungs are divided into two, and the right lung is divided again to form the middle lobe. The corresponding area on the left is the lingula, a division of the upper lobe. Figure 6.4 transposes this pattern on to a subject, outlining the surface markings of the lungs. Examination of the front of the chest is largely that of the upper lobes, examination of the back the lower lobes. It will be seen how much more lung there is posteriorly than anteriorly, so it comes as no surprise that lung disease primarily affecting the bases is best detected posteriorly. Note how much lung is against the lateral chest wall. Students often examine a narrow strip of chest down the front and the back. Many signs are found laterally and in the axilla.

Computerised tomography (CT) adds an extra dimension to vizualization of the chest (Figs 6.5–6.8).

The fine detail of the airways is beautifully illustrated by wax injec-

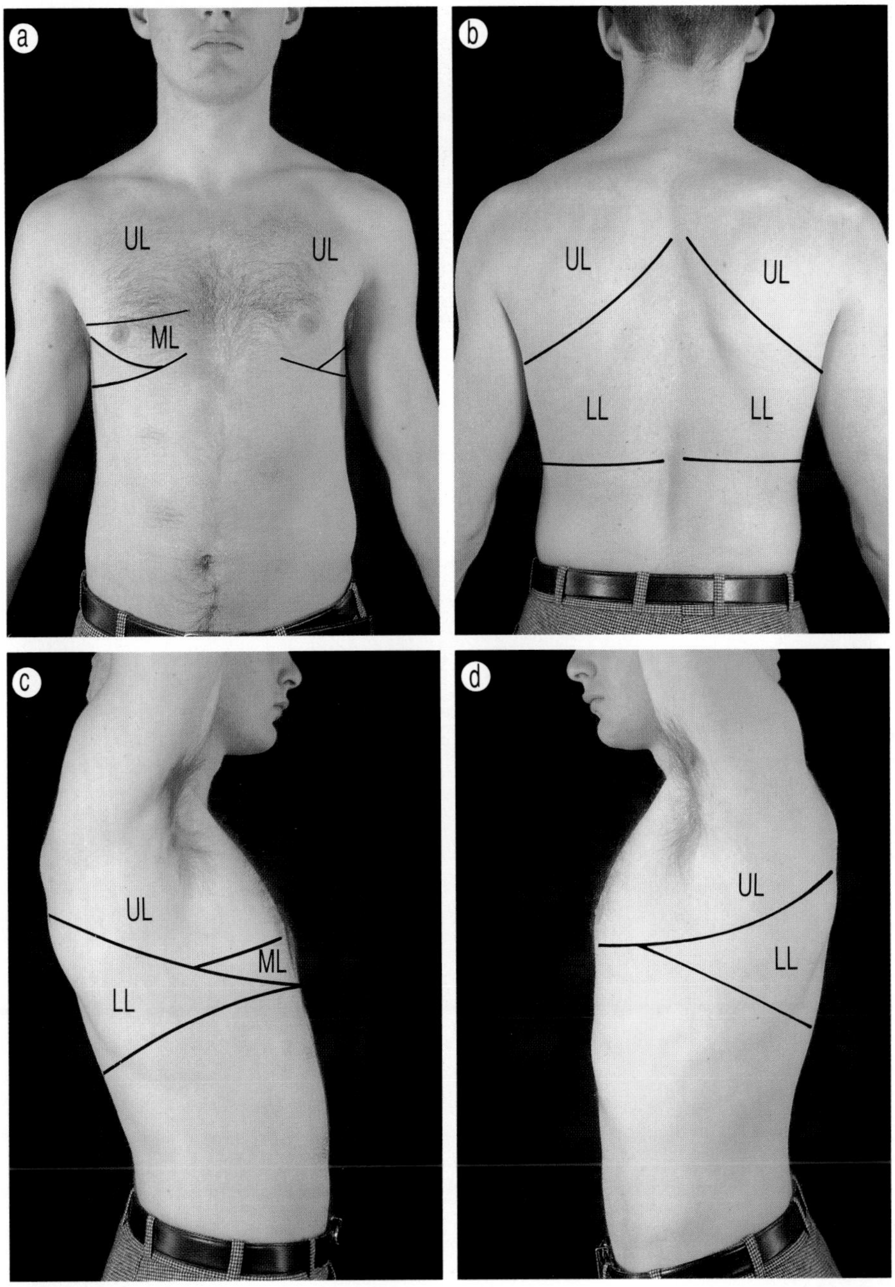

Fig. 6.4 Surface markings of the lobes of the lung: (a) anterior, (b) posterior, (c) right lateral, and (d) left lateral. UL, upper lobe; ML, middle lobe; LL, lower lobe.

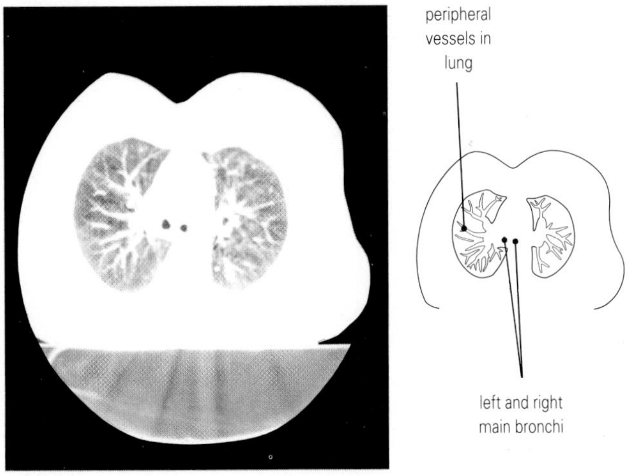

Fig. 6.5 CT scan just below carina: lung window setting.

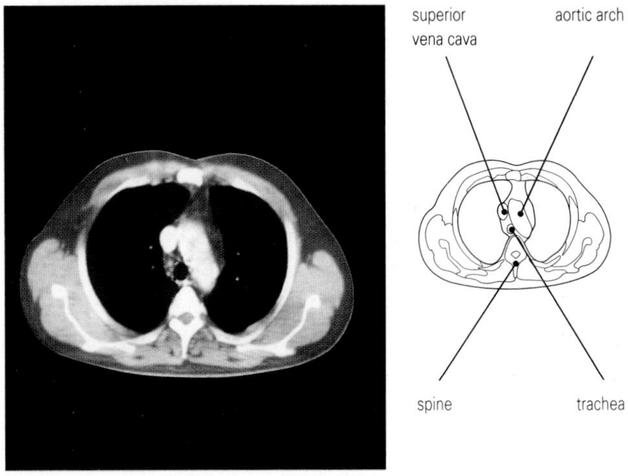

Fig. 6.6 CT scan at the level of the aortic arch.

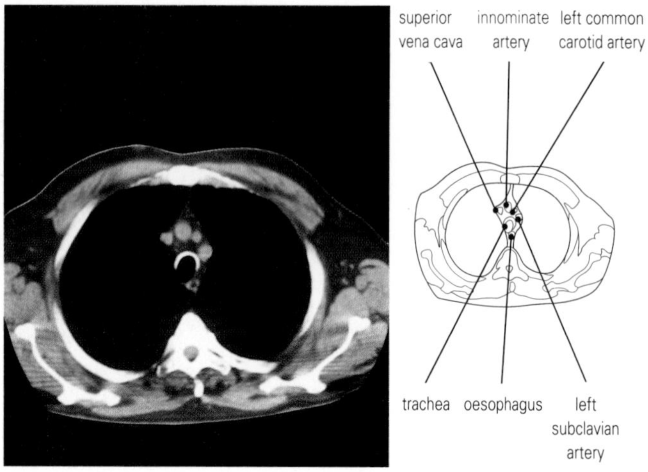

Fig. 6.7 CT scan of the superior mediastinum above the aortic arch.

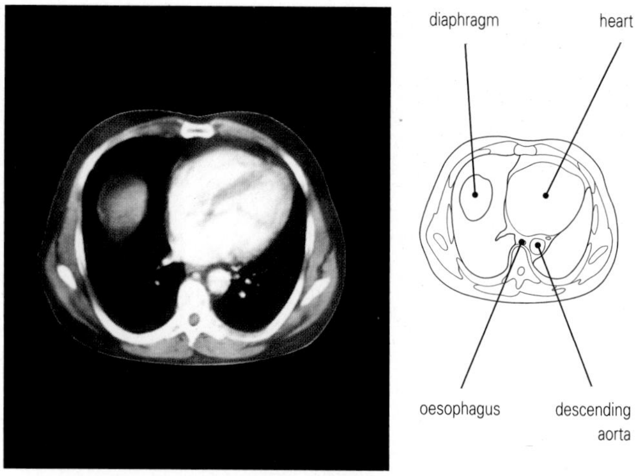

Fig. 6.8 CT scan at the level of the right diaphragm.

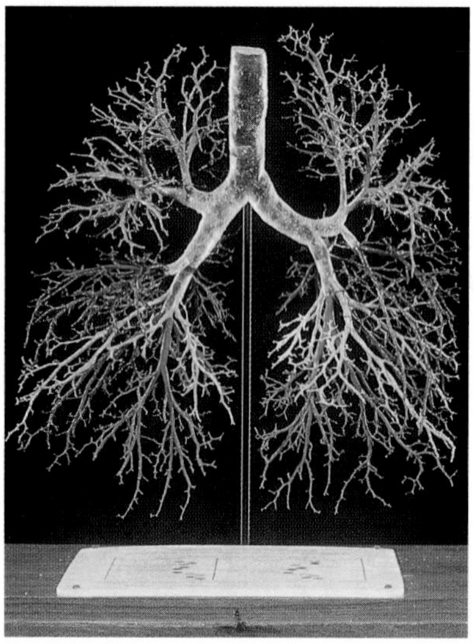

Fig. 6.9 A cast of the bronchial tree with the segments outlined in different colours.

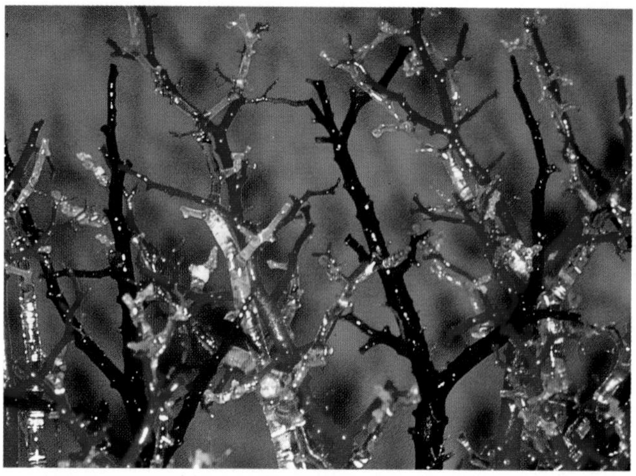

Fig. 6.10 Injection model showing bronchi (white), arteries (red – but carrying deoxygenated blood), and veins (blue – but carrying oxygenated blood).

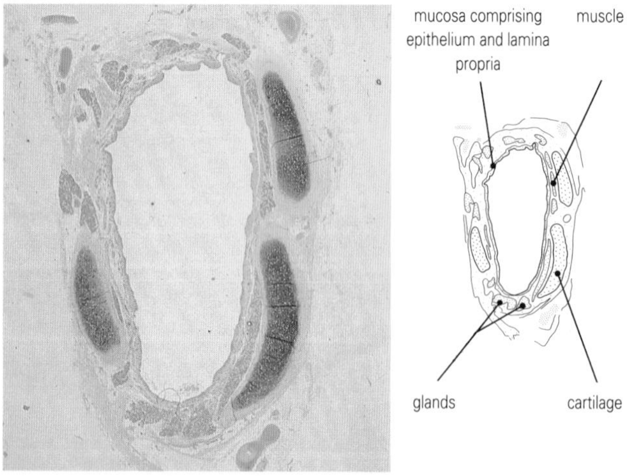

Fig. 6.11 The structure of an intrapulmonary bronchus.

tion models (Fig. 6.9). The same technique can be used to illustrate the intimate relationships between the supply of blood and air to the lungs. (Fig. 6.10)

LUNG DEFENCE AND HISTOLOGY

The lung is exposed to six litres of potentially infected and irritant-laden air every minute. There are, therefore, numerous defence mechanisms to ensure survival. The nose humidifies, warms, and filters the air, and contains lymphocytes of the B series which secrete immunoglobulin A. The epiglottis protects the larynx from inhalation of material from the gastrointestinal tract.

The cough reflex is both a protective and a clearing mechanism. Cough receptors are found in the pharynx, larynx, and larger airways. A cough starts with a deep inspiration followed by expiration against a closed glottis. Glottal opening then allows a forceful jet of air to be expelled.

The main clearance mechanism is the remarkable mucociliary escalator. Bronchial secretions from bronchial glands and goblet cells together with secretions from deeper in the lungs form a sheet of fluid which is propelled upwards continuously by the beat of the cilia lining the bronchial epithelium (Figs 6.11 and 6.12). This cilial action can fail either from the rare immotile cilia syndromes or

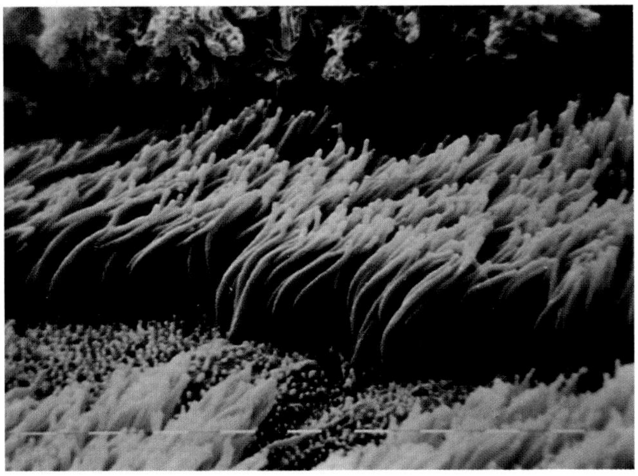

Fig. 6.12 Electronmicrograph of bronchial cilia and the mucus sheath.

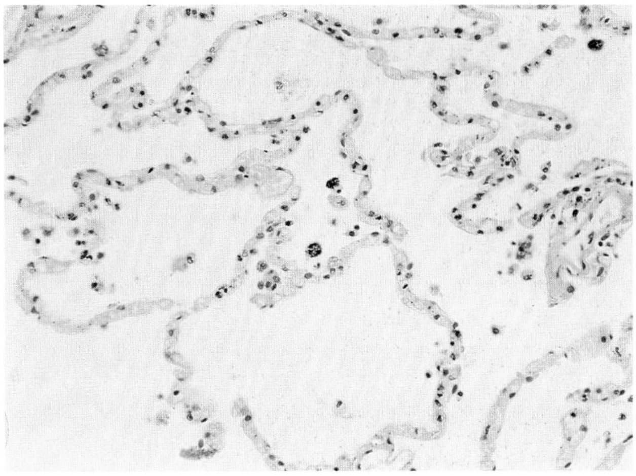

Fig. 6.13 Normal lung. Occasional pigment-containing macrophages are present within the alveolar spaces. H & E stain. (x25).

commonly from cigarette smoke.

The chief defence of the alveoli is the alveolar macrophage (Fig. 6.13) which in conjunction with complement and immunoglobulin ingests foreign material which is then transported either up the airways or into the pulmonary lymphatics. T and B lymphocytes are present throughout the lung substance and most of the immunoglobulin in the lung is made locally. The blood supplies neutrophils which pass into the lung structure in inflammation.

LUNG FUNCTION

The function of the lung is to oxygenate the blood and to remove carbon dioxide. To achieve this, ventilation of the lungs is performed by the respiratory muscles under the control of the respiratory centre in the brain. The rhythm of breathing depends upon various inhibitory and excitatory mechanisms within the brain stem. These can be influenced voluntarily from higher centres and from the effect of chemoreceptors. The medullary or central chemoreceptors in the brain stem respond to changes in partial pressure of carbon-dioxide in the blood (pCO_2). Chemoreceptors in the aortic and carotid body respond to low partial pressure of oxygen (pO_2) but only when this falls below 8kPa; thus alteration in pCO_2 is the most important factor in respiratory control in health.

The sensitivity of the medullary chemoreceptor to pCO_2 can be reset either upwards in prolonged ventilatory failure or downwards as when a patient is placed on a mechanical ventilator. The first situation is most commonly seen in chronic airflow limitation (chronic obstructive lung disease) when patients may become dependent on hypoxic drive to maintain respiration. The injudicious administration of oxygen can then lead to ventilatory failure and death. In the second situation, 'weaning' a patient away from a ventilator is difficult because the medullary centre demands a low pCO_2 which cannot be maintained by the patient unaided.

Ventilation is largely performed by nerve impulses in the phrenic nerve acting to contract the diaphragm and expand the volume of the chest. Scalene and intercostal muscles act mainly by stabilizing the chest wall. The result is to decrease the pressure in the pleura (already less than atmospheric). Since the air inside the airways is at atmospheric pressure, the lungs must follow the chest wall through pleural apposition and expand, sucking in air. Expiration is largely a passive process; when the muscles relax the lung recoils under the influence of its own elasticity. Ventilation is, therefore, much more than just forcing air through tubes. Higher brain centres, the brain stem, spinal cord, peripheral nerves, intercostal muscles, spine, ribs, and diaphragm are all involved. Moreover, the lung tissue itself must overcome its own inertia and stiffness. Malfunction of any of these can lead to respiratory failure.

Diaphragm function is in two parts. Contraction leads to descent of the diaphragm, though the costal parts also elevate the lower ribs. A common consequence of chronic airflow limitation and hyperinflation is a low flat diaphragm which may pull the ribs inwards rather than out.

ASSESSING RESPIRATORY FUNCTION

Since the function of the lungs is to add oxygen to the blood and to remove carbon dioxide, it might be thought that measurement of the pO_2 and pCO_2 in the blood would be an adequate assessment of its efficiency. However, the lung has such an enormous reserve capacity that it can sustain considerable damage before blood gases are affected. There are, nonetheless, a number of other tests of lung function which can be briefly described. These are tests of static lung volumes, ventilation or dynamic lung volumes, and gas exchange across the alveolar-capillary membrane.

Static lung volumes

When attempting to take as deep an inspiration as possible we are eventually stopped partly by the resistance of the chest wall to further deformation and partly by the inability to stretch the lung

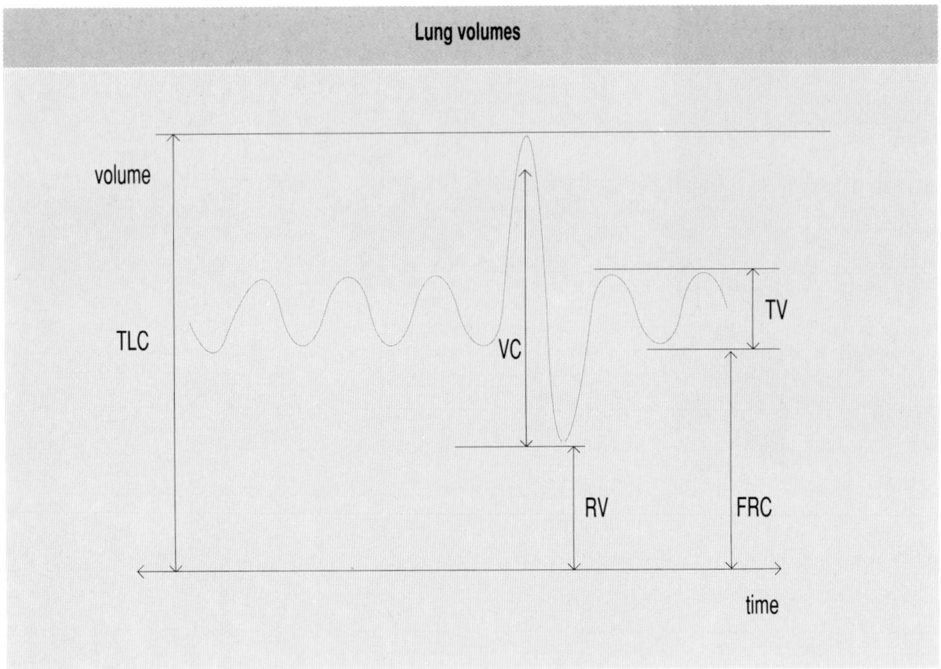

Fig. 6.14 Subdivisions of lung volume.
TLC = total lung capacity
VC = vital capacity
TV = tidal volume
FRC = functional residual capacity
RV = residual volume

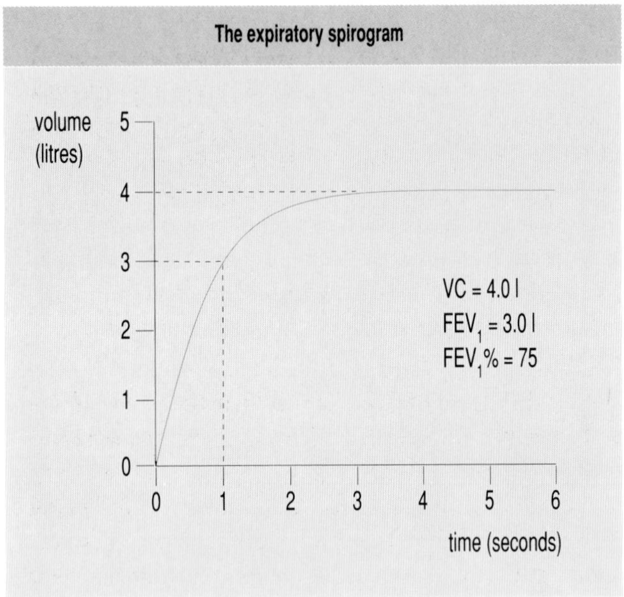

Fig. 6.15 The normal expiratory spirogram.

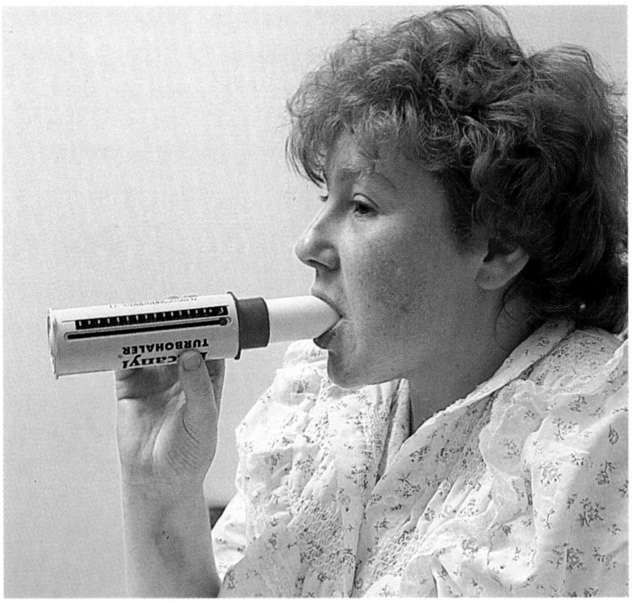

Fig. 6.16 The Mini-Wright Flow Meter in use.

tissues any further (Fig. 6.14). Total lung capacity (TLC) at one end is, therefore, largely influenced by this 'stretchability' or elasticity of the lung. The stiffer the lung, as in fibrosis or scarring, the less distensible it will be. Conversely, damage to the elastic tissue of the lung (e.g. emphysema) with destruction of the alveolar walls will make it more distensible and there will be an increase in TLC. TLC is also high is some patients with asthma and chronic obstructive bronchitis probably because the lungs are overexpanded in an attempt to widen the airways.

As indicated above, breathing out from TLC is largely passive by progressive retraction of the lung; this process will end at functional residual capacity (FRC) when the tendency of the lung to contract is balanced by the thorax resisting further deformation. This point is also the end of normal expiration. Further expiration is an active process involving expiratory muscles. By using these muscles more air can be forced out until, at least in older subjects, the limiting factor is closure of the small airways which have been getting smaller along with the alveoli. Beyond this the lungs can only become smaller by direct compression of the gas (Boyle's law) by the expiratory muscles. At this point, the amount of air left in the lung is designated residual volume (RV).

In chronic bronchitis the small airways are narrowed and inflamed; in emphysema the elastic tissue supporting the small airways is lost and they collapse in expiration. Both mechanisms lead

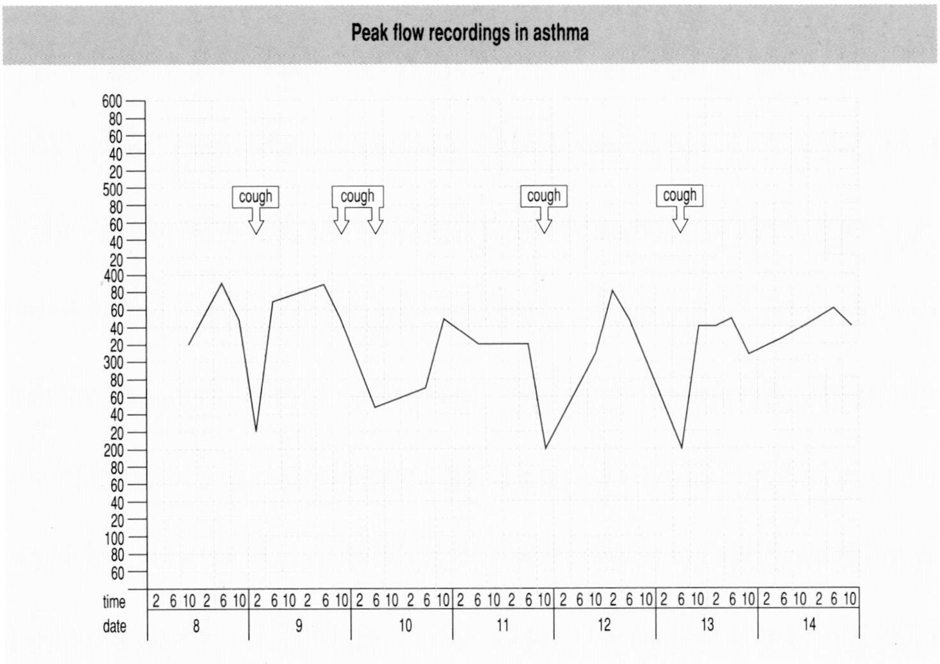

Fig. 6.17 Peak flow chart in a child with asthma whose main symptom was cough. The dips coincide with the symptoms.

to an increase in RV. Conversely, if the lungs are stiffer (fibrosis) the increased tension in the lung tissue holds the airways open with closure occuring later in expiration thus reducing the RV.

In summary, stiff lungs from fibrosis cause a low TLC and low RV; emphysema causes a high TLC and a high RV; and chronic bronchitis causes a high RV. VC depends on the relative changes in RV and TLC, but usually the overall effect in lung disease is a reduction.

Dynamic lung volumes

Assessment of airflow involves measuring volume exhaled in unit time by use of a spirometric trace (Fig 6.15). This is produced by a forced exhalation from TLC to RV. The conventional parameters derived from this trace are the forced vital capacity (FVC) and the forced expiratory volume in one second (FEV_1). FVC is the amount exhaled forcefully from a single deep inspiration, FEV_1 the fraction of that volume exhaled in the first second. These are then expressed as a ratio of the FEV_1 over the FVC ($FEV_1\%$). This is normally around seventy-five per cent which indicates that a normal person can exhale forcibly three quarters of their vital capacity in one second. VC and FVC, one in slow and the other in fast expiration, give similar results in normal subjects; though FVC is reduced due to premature airway closure in many disease states.

In diseases causing airway obstruction, the proportion of the vital capacity that can be exhaled in one second is reduced and the $FEV_1\%$ falls. Conversely, in restrictive lung disease the airways are held open by the stiff lungs and the $FEV_1\%$ is normal, even increased. Nevertheless, the FVC will be reduced because the TLC is reduced. In restrictive lung disease, FEV_1 is reduced in proportion to FVC; in airways obstruction, it is reduced disproportionately.

Peak flow

The Peak Expiratory Flow Rate is the flow generated in the first 0.10 second of a forced expiration, the resulting figure is extrapolated over one minute. It can be measured easily by a variety of portable devices (Fig. 6.16) and serial recordings can be very useful in the diagnosis and monitoring of asthma (Fig. 6.17).

Gas exchange

Measurements of diffusion (D_L)

The transfer factor is a measurement of gas transference across the alveolar-capillary membrane. For technical reasons carbon monoxide is used as the test gas, but oxygen is affected in a similar way. The transfer factor is reduced when there is destruction of the alveolar-capillary bed as in emphysema and also when there is a barrier to diffusion. This may occur when the alveolar-capillary membrane is thickened or where there is lack of homogeneity in the distribution of blood and air at alveolar level. Both mechanisms are important in lung fibrosis.

Transfer factor will naturally be reduced if the lungs are small or if one has been removed (pneumonectomy). The transfer co-efficient (KCO or D_LCO divided by alveolar volume – calculated separately) is a more useful measurement, as it reflects the true situation in ventilated lung.

Lung volumes in disease

In summary, it is possible to distinguish two main patterns of abnormal lung function. An 'obstructive pattern' is seen in asthma, chronic obstructive bronchitis, and emphysema. FVC, FEV_1, and $FEV_1\%$ are all reduced, RV increased, TLC often reduced but high

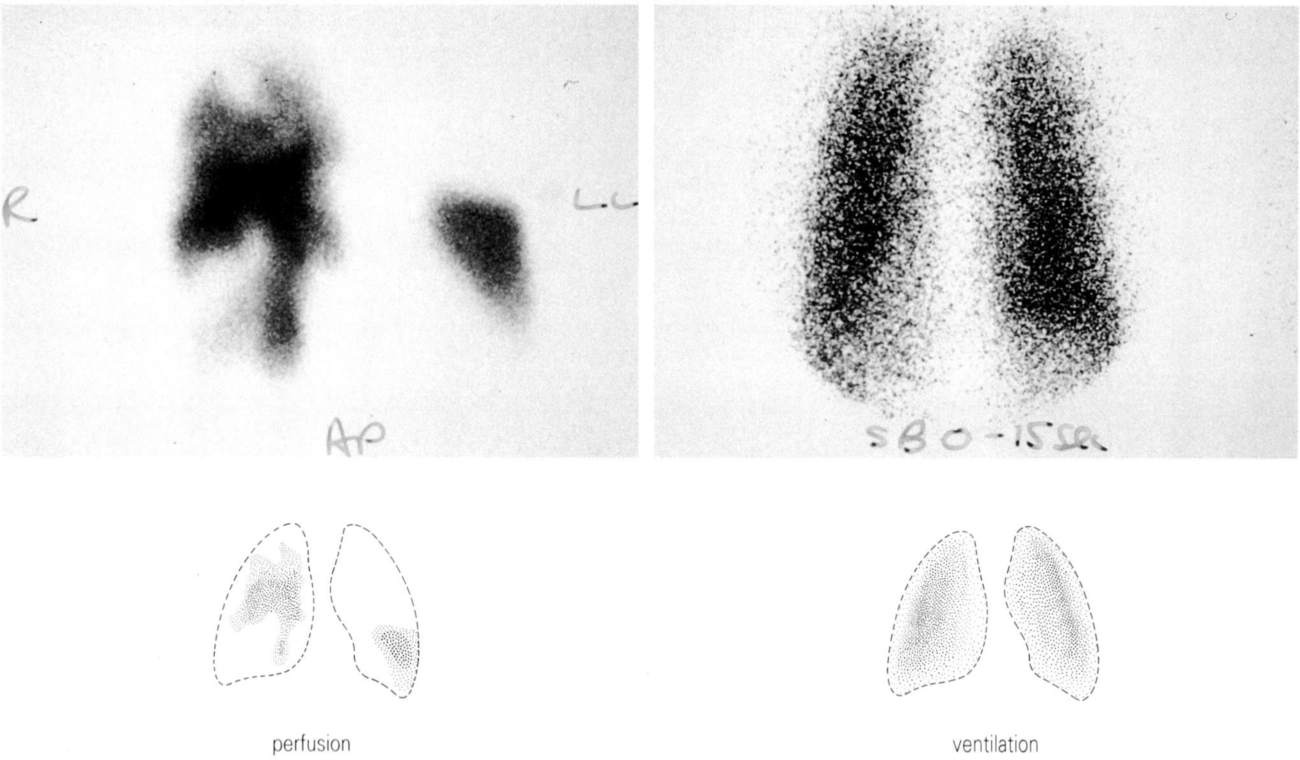

Fig. 6.18 Perfusion (left) and ventilation (right) scans in pulmonary emboli. Note the multiple perfusion defects but the normal ventilation pattern.

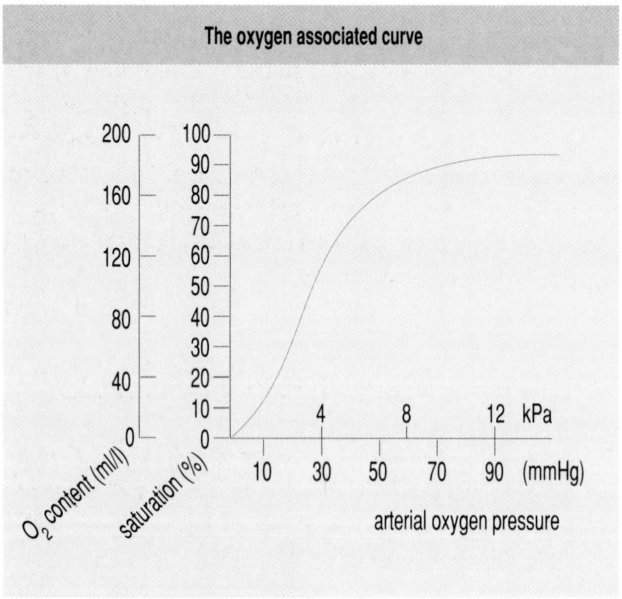

Fig. 6.19 The oxygen dissociation curve relating the partial pressure of oxgen in the blood to saturation of haemoglobin and amount of oxygen carried (assuming Hb normal).

in emphysema. Transfer factor is low in emphysema but otherwise normal. A 'restrictive pattern' is seen in lung fibrosis, such as occurs in cryptogenic fibrosing alveolitis. TLC, VC, FEV_1, RV, and transfer factor are all reduced, but FEV_1% is normal or high.

Where other results do not give a clear pattern, RV can be very helpful being high in airways obstruction and low in fibrosis.

Distribution of ventilation and perfusion

Distribution of air within the lung is best assessed for clinical purposes by radioactive isotopes. The usual tracer gas is radioactive xenon. The measurement of radioactivity over the lung gives a measure of the distribution and also the rate at which gas enters and leaves various parts of the lung. Thus, it can be used to detect 'air trapping' or absence of ventilation. Perfusion of blood can be measured in a similar way usually by micro-aggregates of albumin labelled with technetium 99m and injected into a peripheral vein. These micro-aggregates form small emboli within the lung and the radioactivity they give off is a measure of blood distribution. These tests are most useful in the diagnosis of pulmonary embolism when perfusion to an area of lung is reduced but ventilation is maintained (Fig. 6.18). If both ventilation and perfusion are reduced, then the defect probably lies within the airways and is a failure of ventilation with secondary changes in the blood supply.

Blood gases

Blood gases can be measured directly by electrodes in blood obtained by arterial puncture. The results are expressed as partial pressure of gas in the plasma (pO_2 and pCO_2). It is important to realise that this is not the same as the amount of gas carried by the blood. If all the red cells were removed, the pO_2 would be unchanged, yet the patient would be in a parlous state! The

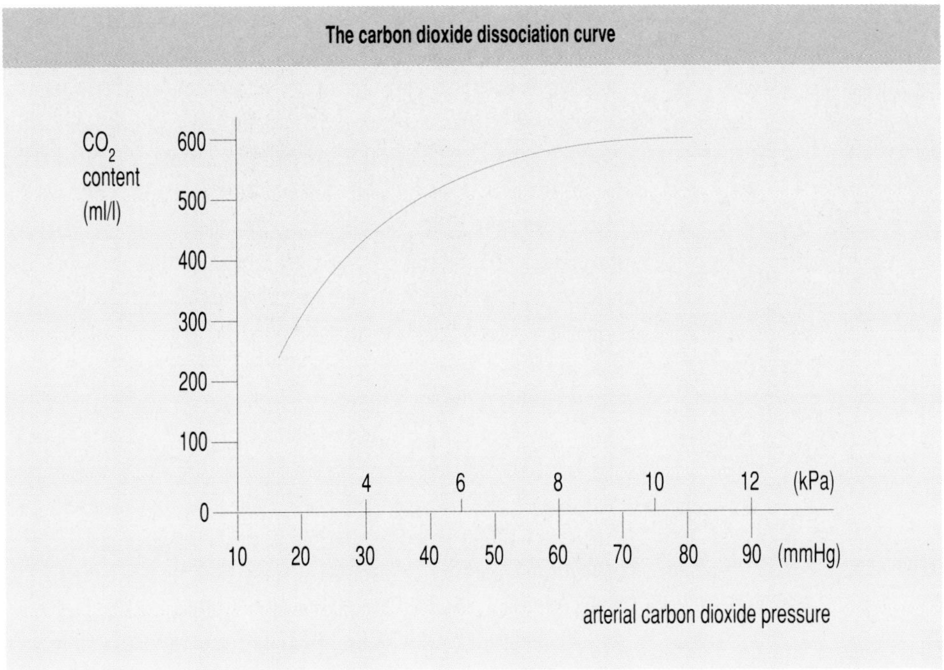

Fig. 6.20 The carbon dioxide dissociation curve relating partial pressure of gas in the blood to amount carried.

haemoglobin in the red cell packages and transports oxygen and carbon dioxide just as a tubetrain packages and transports passengers.

The relationship between pO_2 and saturation of the haemoglobin by oxygen (and hence the volume of oxygen carried) is given by the oxygen dissociation curve (Fig. 6.19). It will be seen that the pO_2 can drop significantly before there is a drop in the saturation, clearly a good thing in the early stages of lung disease. Nevertheless, it means that overventilation of the lung's good parts cannot fully compensate for under-ventilation of bad parts, as the good parts on the flat part of the curve cannot increase the carriage of oxygen in the blood supplied to them beyond a certain maximum. Thus, when there is a shunt of blood from the right to the left heart, either directly through the heart or through unventilated lung, then the total amount of oxygen carried is bound to be reduced and cannot be restored to normal either by increasing ventilation or administering oxygen.

The steep part of the curve indicates that a small increase in inspired oxygen gives a large increase in the amount of oxygen carried: clearly useful for oxygen therapy in sick patients. It also indicates how readily hypoxic tissues can remove large amounts of oxygen from the blood.

The dissociation curve for carbon dioxide is quite different to that of oxygen; lowering the partial pressure of carbon dioxide continuously lowers the saturation and hence the volume of gas carried (Fig. 6.20). This means that over-ventilation in one part of the lung can compensate for under-ventilation elsewhere. Arterial pCO_2 is a good measure of overall alveolar ventilation, being increased in alveolar hypoventilation (e.g. severe chronic airflow limitation) and decreased in alveolar hyperventilation (e.g. anxiety states and heart failure, pulmonary embolus and asthma, where hypoxia and other factors stimulate an increase in ventilation).

The lungs help to regulate acid-base balance by their ability to excrete or to retain carbon dioxide. In cases of metabolic acidosis (e.g. diabetic ketoacidosis and renal failure), the lungs can 'blow off' carbon dioxide to restore the pH towards normal. In cases of metabolic alkalosis (e.g. prolonged vomiting with loss of acid from the stomach), the retention of carbon dioxide again restores the pH towards normal. Retention or secretion of carbon dioxide as a result of lung disease (respiratory acidosis and alkalosis) alters pH which is then secondarily restored by excretion or retention of bicarbonate by the kidney. Thus, changes in arterial pCO_2 (whether primary or secondary) can be regarded as functions of the lung, changes in bicarbonate (again either primary or secondary) can be regarded as functions of the kidney.

SYMPTOMS OF RESPIRATORY DISEASE

History taking must follow the principles outlined earlier. Here we will be concerned with the analysis of the main symptoms of respiratory disease in turn. These are dyspnoea, cough, sputum, haemoptysis, pain, and wheeze.

DYSPNOEA

Most lung diseases will cause dyspnoea or difficulty in breathing. Patients will express this in different ways as 'shortness of breath', 'shortwindedness', 'can't get my breath' or in terms of functional disability ('can't do the housework').

Some patients will talk about 'tightness'. It may not be immediately clear whether they are describing breathlessness or pain. If the complaint is really a pain then this may well be angina which is in itself associated with breathlessness. If asked directly, patients

Some causes of breathlessness
Control and movement of the chest wall and pleura
Hyperventilation syndrome
Hypothalamic lesions
Neuromuscular disease
Kyphoscoliosis
Ankylosing spondylitis
Pleural effusion and thickening
Bilateral diaphragm paralysis
Diseases of the lungs
Airways disease
Chronic bronchitis and emphysema
Asthma
Bronchiectasis
Cystic fibrosis
Parenchymal disease
Pneumonia
Cryptogenic fibrosing alveolitis
Extrinsic allergic alveolitis
Primary and secondary tumor
Sarcoidosis
Pneumothorax
Pulmonary oedema
Reduced blood supply
Pulmonary embolism
Anaemia

Fig. 6.21 Some causes of breathlessness.

Duration of breathlessness		
Immediate (minutes)	**Short (hours to days)**	**Long (weeks to years)**
Pulmonary embolism	Pulmonary oedema	Chronic airflow limitation
Pneumothorax	Pneumonia	Cryptogenic fibrosing alveolitis
	Asthma	
Pulmonary oedema	Pleural effusion	Extrinsic allergic alveolitis
Asthma	Anaemia	Anaemia

Fig. 6.22 Duration of breathlessness.

can usually tell you whether their tightness means pain or breathlessness. Some patients with pleuritic pain complain of breathlessness, yet what they really mean is that they are unable to take a deep breath because of pain. It is of interest to consider why patients complain of breathlessness. Most normal people do not regard themselves as ill when they are short of breath running for a bus. It seems probable that the sensations reported by patients are the same as the rest of us, but they recognize that the work the lungs are being asked to do is disproportionate to the task the body is performing, i.e. it feels inappropriate.

Causes of breathlessness

The causes of breathlessness may be listed as those to do with the control and movement of the chest wall, lung disease itself, and problems with the blood and its supply to the lungs (Fig. 6.21). The control of breathing can start with psychological factors in the brain (see the hyperventilation syndrome on page 6.12), problems with the control centre in the medulla (rare), and the increased effort needed to overcome the effects of spinal cord disease (trauma or degeneration), neuropathies (e.g. Guillain-Barré syndrome), myopathies, and chest wall problems (e.g. kyphoscoliosis and ankylosing spondylitis).

Lung diseases may require more work to be done so as to overcome obstruction to airflow (e.g. chronic obstructive bronchitis, emphysema, asthma) or to stretch stiff lungs (e.g. pulmonary oedema and lung fibrosis).

Allergic and non–allergic factors in asthma	
Allergic	**Non–allergic**
House dust	Exercise
Animals (especially cats)	Emotion
Pollens (especially grass)	Sleep
	Smoke
	Aerosol sprays
	Cold air
	Upper respiratory tract infections

Fig. 6.23 Allergic and non-allergic factors in asthma.

Hypoxia needs to be severe to stimulate respiration but may be the mechanism in pneumonia, severe heart failure and other causes of pulmonary oedema. Pulmonary embolism leads to wasted ventilation in the affected area. Severe anaemia reduces the oxygen-carrying capacity of the blood.

J-receptors are adjacent to pulmonary capillaries. Stimulation of them by pulmonary oedema, fibrosis and lung irritants is an additional mechanism causing breathlessness.

Duration of dyspnoea

The duration of dyspnoea may give a clue to the cause, and can conveniently be divided into immediate (over minutes), short (hours to days), and long (weeks to years) (Fig. 6.22). There is some overlap but contrast for example the patient with a large pulmonary embolism who collapses in minutes in acute distress with the progressive relentless disability extending over a decade in the patient with smoking-related airflow limitation. Some patients find it difficult to remember duration accurately. Many report symptoms as lasting for only 'a few weeks' when they mean i.e. 'worse for a few weeks'. A question like 'when could you last run for a bus' may indicate problems stretching back for years. A spouse is often more accurate in this respect than the patient.

Variability of dyspnoea

Questions about variability can be couched as 'does it come and go, or is it much the same' or 'do you have good days and bad days or is it much the same one day to another' A reply suggesting variability is highly characteristic of variable airflow limitation, i.e. asthma. If asthma is suspected, this can be followed up by questions on aggravating factors. Follow this up with some more directed questions about particular factors (Fig. 6.23). These are important not only as potentially preventable causes but positive replies strengthen the diagnosis. House dust mite is the commonest allergen; patients will report worsening on sweeping, dusting, or making the beds. Exercise, at least in children, is a potent trigger of asthma but exercise will also make other forms of breathlessness worse. The difference is that in asthma the attack is caused by the exercise, may indeed follow it, and may last for 30 minutes or more. In other causes of breathlessness, recovery starts as soon as exercise stops.

Dyspnoea

Is the breathlessness recent or has it been present for sometime?

Is it constant or does it come and go?

What can't you do because of the breathlessness?

What makes the breathing worse?

Does anything make it better?

Asthma

Asthma due solely to emotional causes probably does not exist; nonetheless, most patients who have asthma are worse if emotionally upset. Patients may feel that admitting to stress is respectable when they would deny other emotions. Nocturnal asthma is very common. Few asthmatics smoke because they know it makes them worse. Ask what happens if they go into a pub. Many will say they are unable to do so because of smoke. The response to household aerosol sprays can be helpful. Many breathless patients with a variety of illnesses will think it logical – rightly or wrongly – that 'dust' or 'fumes' will make them worse, but only true asthmatics seem to notice a deterioration with the ubiquitous domestic spray can.

Asthma

Does anything make any difference to the asthma?

What happens if you are worried or upset?

Does your chest wake you at night?

Does cigarette smoke may any difference?

Do household sprays affect you?

Have you lost time from work/school?

What happens when sweeping or dusting the house?

Does exposure to cats or dogs make any difference?

Severity of dyspnoea

Severity can be assessed by rating scales, though it is much better to use some functional measure. Ask the patient in what way their breathlessness restricts their activities; can they go upstairs, go shopping, wash the car, or do the garden? If they are troubled with stairs, how many flights can they manage? Do they stop half way up or at the top? Questions about gardening are useful, at least in the summer, as it is possible to grade activity from pulling out a few weeds to digging the potato patch. It is important to as certain that any restriction is due to breathlessness and not some other disability (e.g. an arthritic hip or angina).

Orthopnoea and paroxysmal noctural dyspnoea

Orthopnoea and paroxysmal nocturnal dyspnoea (PND) need special consideration. Both are usually thought of as manifestations of left ventricular failure, yet this is an over-simplification. Orthopnoea is defined as breathlessness lying flat but relieved by sitting up. It is quite common in patients with severe fixed airways obstruction, as in chronic bronchitics who will sometimes admit to not having slept flat for years. Normal subjects when they lie flat, breathe more with the diaphragm and less with the chest wall. In patients with airways obstruction, the diaphragm is often flat and inefficient and may even draw the ribs inwards rather than out. Thus, when they lie down the diaphragm cannot provide the ventilation required.

Features suggestive of the hyperventilation syndrome
Breathlessness at rest
Breathlessness as severe with mild exertion as with greater exertion
Marked variability in breathlessness
More difficulty breathing in than out
Paraesthesiae of the fingers
Numbness around the mouth
'Lightheadedness'
Feelings of impending collapse or remoteness from surroundings
Chest wall pain

Fig. 6.24 Features suggestive of the hyperventilation syndrome.

The term paroxysmal nocturnal dyspnoea is self-explanatory and a feature of pulmonary oedema from left ventricular failure. However, many asthmatics develop bronchoconstriction in the night and wake with wheeze and breathlessness very similar to the symptoms of left ventricular failure. By contrast, patients with severe fixed flow limitation usually sleep well even if they do have to be propped up.

The hyperventilation syndrome

The hyperventilation syndrome is commoner than is generally realized but produces a distinct pattern of symptoms (Fig. 6.24). It is usually associated with anxiety patients over breathe inappropriately. The initial complaint is often, though not always, of breathlessness. The hyperventilation is the response to this sensation. It may be described by the patient as a 'difficulty in breathing in' or an inability to 'fill the bottom of the lungs'. The hyperventilation induces a reduction in the pCO_2, creating a variety of other symptoms; parasthesiae in the fingers, tingling around the lips, 'dizziness', 'lightheadedness', and sometimes frank tetany. Chest pain is the probable consequence of increased chest wall movement. The onset is often triggered by some life event especially work-related (e.g. redundancy or dismissal). The diagnosis can be confirmed by the '20 deep breaths test'.

Dyspnoea and hypoxia

Dyspnoea should be distinguished from tachypnoea (increased rate of breathing) and from hypoxia. It is a symptom, not a sign. Nor is it necessarily an indication of lung disease; psychological factors as in the hyperventilation syndrome and acidosis from diabetic ketosis or renal failure may produce tachypnoea which may be felt as dyspnoea. Many patients think that if they are short of breath, they must be short of oxygen. This is sometimes the case, but as mentioned earlier hypoxia only stimulates respiration when relatively

Pointers to the significance of an episode of haemoptysis

Probably serious	Probably not serious
Middle aged or elderly	Young
Spontaneous	Recent infection
Previous or current smoker	Never smoked
Recurrent	Single episode
Large amount	Small amount – if single episode

Fig. 6.25 Pointers to the significance of an episode of haemoptysis.

severe. To illustrate the distinction between hypoxia and dyspnoea many patients with airflow limitation from chronic bronchitis have hypoxia severe enough to cause right-sided heart failure, yet they have relatively little dyspnoea (blue bloaters). In contrast, some patients with emphysema seem to need to keep their blood gases normal by a heroic effort of breathing (pink puffers): they are very dyspnoeic.

COUGH

Cough arises from the cough receptors in the pharynx, larynx, and bronchi; cough, therefore, results from irritation of these receptors either from infection, inflammation, tumor, or foreign body. Cough may be the only symptom in asthma, particularly childhood asthma. Cough in children occurring regularly after exercise or at night is virtually diagnostic of asthma. Many smokers regard cough as normal: 'only a smokers cough' or may deny it completely despite having just coughed in front of the examiner! In these patients, a change in the character of the cough can be highly significant.

Patients can often localize cough to above the larynx ('a tickle in the throat') or below. Postnasal drip from rhinitis can cause the former and may be accompanied by sneezing and nasal blockage.

Laryngitis will cause both cough and a hoarse voice. Recurrent laryngeal nerve palsy causes a hoarse voice and an ineffective cough because the cord is immobile. The usual cause is involvement of the left recurrent laryngeal nerve by tumor in its course in the chest. Cough from tracheitis is usually dry and painful. Cough from further down the airways is often associated with sputum production (bronchitis, bronchiectasis, or pneumonia). In the latter, associated pleurisy makes coughing very distressing and reduces its effectiveness. Other possibilities are carcinoma, lung fibrosis, and increased bronchial responsiveness (this is an inflammatory condition of the airways, thought to be part of the mechanism underlying asthma and often made worse by the factors in Figure 6.23). An uncommon cause of cough, and often overlooked, is aspiration into the lungs from gastro-oesophageal reflux or a pharyngeal pouch. Cough will then follow meals or lying down. Prolonged coughing bouts can cause both unconsciousness from reduction of venous return from the brain (cough syncope) and also vomiting. Sometimes the story of cough is omitted making diagnosis difficult!

SPUTUM

Patients will understand the term 'phlegm' better than sputum. It is the result of excessive bronchial secretion; itself a manifestation of inflammation and infection. Like cough, smokers may not acknowledge its existence. Children usually swallow their sputum. It is essential to be certain that the complaint relates to the chest, as some patients have difficulty in distinguishing sputum production from gastrointestinal reflux, post-nasal drip, or saliva. Sometimes asking the patient to 'show me what you have to do to get it up' can be helpful. If the patient denies sputum, a cough producing a rattle (a 'loose cough') suggests that it is present.

> **Sputum**
>
> What colour is the phlegm?
>
> How often do you bring it up?
>
> How much do you bring up?
>
> Do you have trouble getting it up?

Sputum due to chronic irritation is usually white or grey, particularly in smokers; if infected it becomes yellow from the presence of leukocytes and this may turn to green by the action of the enzyme verdoperoxidase. Yellow or green sputum in asthma can be due to the presence of eosinophils, not necessarily infection. Questions on frequency are most useful in the diagnosis of chronic bronchitis, an epidemiological definition of this is sputum production on most days for three consecutive months for two successive years. Sputum production is common in asthmatics and is occasionally the main complaint. The diagnosis of bronchiectasis is made on a story of daily sputum production stretching back to childhood.

Patients can often given an estimate of the amount of sputum they bring up each day usually in terms of an eggcup or teaspoon and so on. Large amounts occur in bronchiectasis, lung abscess and in the rare bronchiolo-alveolar cell carcinoma.

Sticky 'rusty' sputum is characteristic of lobar pneumonia and frothy sputum with streaks of blood is seen in pulmonary oedema.

Highly viscous sputum sometimes with plugs is characteristic of asthma and in some patients with chronic bronchitis. Small bronchial casts, like twigs, may be described by a patient with the condition of bronchopulmonary aspergillosis associated with asthma.

HAEMOPTYSIS

The coughing up of blood is often a sign of serious lung disease. Nevertheless, it is common in trivial respiratory infections. Like sputum production, it is essential to establish that it is coming from the lungs and not the nose, mouth, or being vomited. Bleeding from the nose may run into the pharynx and be coughed out, but usually the patient will also describe bleeding from the anterior nares. Bleeding in the mouth causes confusion, it is usually related to brushing the teeth (gingivitis).

The blood in haemoptysis is usually bright red at first, then followed by progressively smaller and darker amounts. This would be unusual in haematemesis.

All haemoptysis is potentially serious, though the most important

Some causes of haemoptysis	
Common	**Uncommon**
Infection including bronchiectasis	Mitral stenosis and left ventricular failure
Bronchial carcinoma	Bronchial adenoma
Tuberculosis	Idiopathic pulmonary haemosiderosis
Pulmonary embolism and infarction	Anticoagulation and blood dyscrasias
No cause found	

Fig. 6.26 Causes of haemoptysis.

Features suggesting the sleep apnoea syndrome
Excessive daytime somnolence
Intellectual deterioration and irritability
Early morning headaches
Snoring
Restless nights
Social deterioration (e.g. job, marriage, driving difficulties)

Fig. 6.27 Features of the sleep apnoea syndrome.

is carcinoma of the bronchus (Fig. 6.25). Repeated small haemoptyses every few days over a period of some weeks in a middle-aged smoker is virtually diagnostic of bronchial carcinoma.

Other serious causes are pulmonary embolism (sudden onset of pleuritic chest pain, and dyspnoea followed by haemoptysis), tuberculosis (weight loss, fever, cough, and sputum), and bronchiectasis (long history of sputum production and the haemoptysis associated with an exacerbation and increased sputum purulence) (Fig. 6.26). Blood-tinged sputum in pneumonia and pulmonary oedema has been mentioned above.

PAIN

The lungs and the visceral pleura are devoid of pain fibres, whereas the parietal pleura, chest wall, and mediastinal structures are not. The characteristic 'pleuritic pain' is sharp, stabbing, and worse on deep breathing and coughing, and arises from either pleural inflammation or chest wall lesions. Pain from the pleura is due to the two pleural surfaces rubbing together. The pain may interfere with breathing: 'I have to catch my breath'. Inflammation of the pleura occurs chiefly in pneumonia and pulmonary infarction from pulmonary emboli. Pneumothorax can produce acute transient pleuritic pain.

Most pains from the chest wall are due to localized muscle strain or rib fractures (persistent cough can cause the latter). These pains are often worse on twisting or turning or rolling over in bed; an uncommon feature of other disease. Bornholm disease is thought to be a viral infection of the intercostal muscles and produces very severe pain. True pleuritic pain is often accompanied by a pleural rub; this is absent in chest wall pain, but there may be striking local rib tenderness reproducing the symptoms. Unfortunately, this is not entirely reliable, for pleurisy can be associated with local tenderness. A particular type of chest wall pain is due to swelling of one or more of the upper costal cartilages (Tietze's syndrome); however, this is quite rare and it is much more common to find tenderness without swelling. Severe constant pain not related to breathing but interfering with sleep usually indicates malignant disease involving the chest wall. Moreover, spinal disease and herpes zoster may cause pain in a root distribution round the chest.

Pleural pain is usually localized accurately by the patient, yet if the pleura overlying the diaphragm is involved pain may be referred either to the abdomen from the costal part of the diaphragm or to the tip of the shoulder from the central part because the pain fibres run in the phrenic nerve (C345). Pain may subside when an effusion develops.

Although the lungs are insensitive to pain, the mediastinal structures are not. Cancer of the lung and other central lesions produces a dull, poorly localized pain presumably from pressure on mediastinal structures.

A third type of pain is a central soreness over the trachea in acute tracheitis.

WHEEZE AND STRIDOR

Wheeze

Most patients will understand wheeze as a high-pitched whistling sound although some require a demonstration by the doctor before they recognize it. It occurs in both inspiration and expiration but is always louder in the latter. Spouses sometimes pick this up better than patients particularly if the wheeze is mainly at night. It implies airway narrowing and is, therefore, common in asthma and chronic obstructive bronchitis. In asthma, the wheeze is episodic and clearly associated with shortness of breath, fulfilling the definition of 'variable wheezy breathlessness'. Nevertheless, some asthmatics may have little wheeze and acute severe attacks can be associated with a 'silent chest'. In chronic obstructive bronchitis and emphysema, the associations are less clear cut, with wheeze, shortness of breath, cough, and sputum occuring in various proportions.

Stridor

Stridor is a harsh inspiratory and expiratory noise which is imitated by abducting the vocal cords and breathing in and out. It is often more evident to the observer than the patient.

OTHER IMPORTANT POINTS IN THE HISTORY

Other body systems

The lungs do not exist in isolation from the rest of the body. Lung disease can affect other structures and disease elsewhere can affect the lungs. The closest relationships are naturally with the heart. Lung disease can affect the right side of the heart (cor pulmonale). An early manifestation is peripheral oedema (ankle swelling). Disease of the left heart causes pulmonary oedema (orthopnoea, paroxysmal nocturnal dyspnoea, cough, and frothy sputum). Diseases of other systems which affect the lungs include rheumatoid arthritis, other connective tissue disease (scleroderma, dermatomyositis), immune deficiency syndromes (including AIDS), and renal failure. A variety of neuromuscular diseases and skeletal problems affect the mechanics of breathing.

Weight loss is an important manifestation of lung carcinoma, though by the time it occurs there are usually metastatic deposits in the liver. Less well-known is chronic airflow limitation, presumably because the increased respiratory effort impairs appetite and diverts calories to the respiratory muscles. Chronic infection, particularly tuberculosis, causes weight loss. Gain in weight may be a cause of increased dyspnoea. One cause is steroid therapy for lung disease (iatrogenic Cushing's syndrome).

Fever must be distinguished from feeling hot or sweating and generally implies infection, particularly pneumonia or tuberculosis. Less commonly, it is caused by malignancy or connective tissue disease affecting the lungs. If pulmonary embolism is suspected, pain or swelling in the legs suggest a deep venous thrombosis.

Sleep

Sleep disturbance may be due to pain, breathlessness and cough from airways obstruction, or from depression. In the sleep apnoea syndrome, patients are aroused repeatedly in the night from obstruction of the upper airways. The cause is not always clear, but obesity and hypertrophied tonsils often contribute. Sudden obstruction leads to greater and greater inspiratory efforts by the patient who, in a half-awake state, will thrash around and eventually overcome the obstruction to the accompaniment of loud snoring noises. This may be repeated many times during the night. Wives (the patients are usually men) will describe this in graphic detail! The poor quality of sleep leads to daytime somnolence and the carbon dioxide retention to morning headaches. (Fig. 6.27)

Many diseases of the respiratory system produce lasting disability and some are fatal. Therefore, depression and anxiety are to be expected and may influence the history.

PAST HISTORY

A previous history of tuberculosis may explain abnormal shadowing on a chest radiograph. Current symptoms may be due to relapse, especially if the patient was treated before the start of the antibiotic era (1950). Some operations for tuberculosis from those days (thoracoplasty, phrenic crush) produce life-long chest or radiographic deformity. Bronchial damage from tuberculosis can lead to bronchiectasis.

BCG vaccination reduces the risk of tuberculosis. In most areas in the UK it is performed at school at the age of 12 or 13. Babies born to immigrant mothers often receive it at birth. In children Heaf testing to assess sensitivity to tuberculin is performed first. A history of these procedures help in the assessment of a possible case of tuberculosis.

A history of wheeze in childhood suggests asthma. This may have gone into remission and been forgotten only to occur in later life. Whooping cough or pneumonia in childhood may lead to bronchiectasis, and the patient may have been told by his parents that his problems started with such an episode.

Chest injuries, operations, or pneumonia can all lead to permanent radiographic changes which otherwise would be very difficult to explain. Previous radiographs can be invaluable in these circumstances and may be available. At one time 'Mass Miniature Radiography' was performed on large sections of the population to screen for tuberculosis. In some areas these films are still retained. Many patients will have had chest radiography prior to an operation.

SOCIAL HISTORY

Smoking

The importance of enquiry about smoking in lung disease can hardly be overemphasized (Figs 6.28 and 6.29). Smoking is, for practical purposes, the cause of chronic bronchitis and carcinoma of the bronchus, with neither diagnosis likely to be correct in a life-long non-smoker. Patients seem to be generally accurate about their tobacco consumption contrasting sometimes with alcohol.

It is important not to appear censorious when enquiring about smoking. Tobacco is highly addictive, most patients would give up if only they could and are not being perverse when they continue despite evidence of lung damage. You should be aware that some patients claim to be non-smokers when they only stopped last month, last week, or even on the way to hospital! Ask non-smokers 'have you smoked in the past?'. The risk of disease increases with the amount smoked. Cigarettes are the most dangerous; pipes and cigars are not free of risk. Risk declines steadily when smoking stops; it takes 10–20 years for the risk of lung cancer to equal that of life-long non-smokers.

Inhalation of an other person's smoke at home or at work is increasingly recognized as a factor in lung disease. This is particularly true for asthma. Children in households with smokers have more respiratory infections.

Pets and hobbies

For many asthmatics, cats and dogs are common sources of allergen. The cause is skin dander (scurf) rather than hair and this may remain in the house long after the offending animal has been banished. Exposure to racing pigeons, budgerigars, parrots, and other caged birds can cause extrinsic allergic alveolitis characterized by cough and breathlessness. The cause is protein material derived from feathers and droppings.

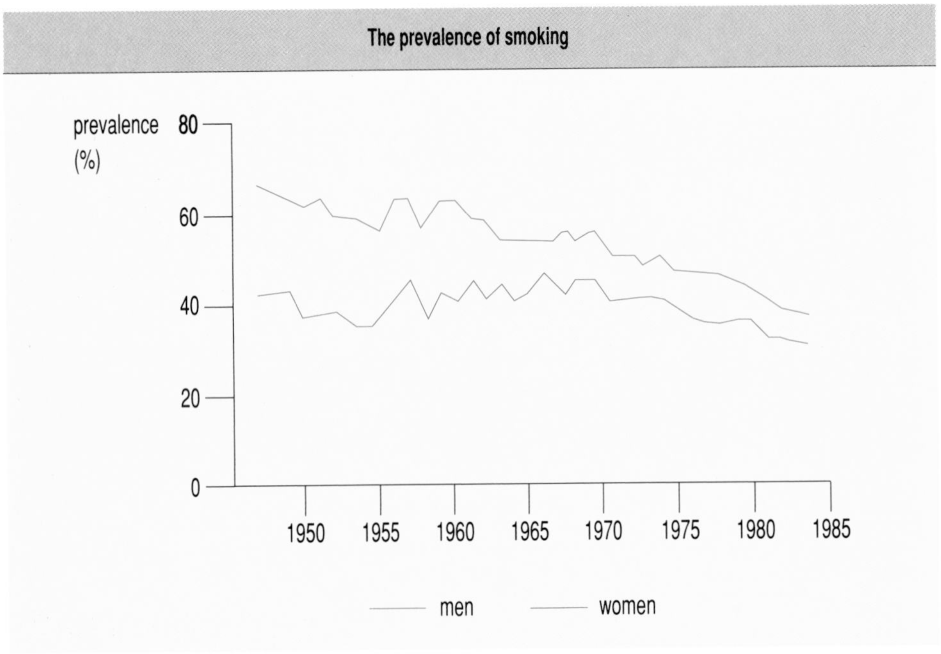

Fig. 6.28 The prevalence of smoking in the UK.

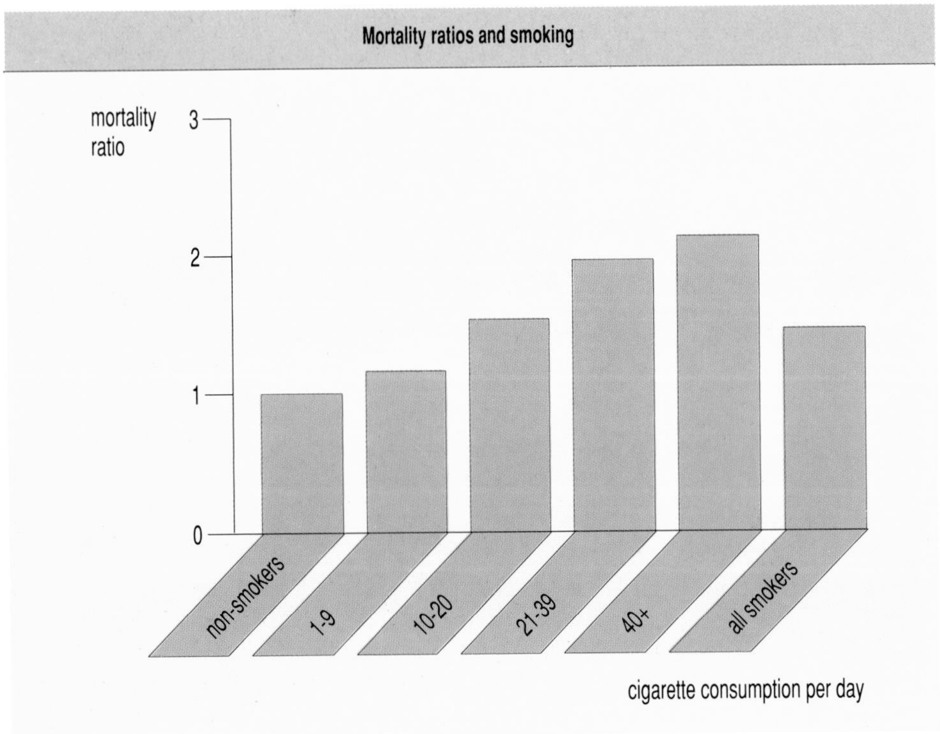

Fig. 6.29 Standardized mortality ratios in men related to smoking habit.

Acute symptoms are usually seen in pigeon fanciers who a few hours after cleaning out their birds develop cough, breathlessness, and 'flu-like symptoms. Recovery takes place over the next day or two unless there is re-exposure. Chronic symptoms are seen in budgerigar owners presumably because they are exposed continuously to low doses of antigen. Their complaint is of progressive breathlessness. Parrots and related species transmit the infectious agent of psittacosis, a cause of pneumonia. You may need to extend your enquires beyond the home, as patients may be exposed to birds belonging to friends and relations.

Occupation

The question 'what do you do?' is more important in respiratory disease than in any other (Fig. 6.30). The nature of the job and not just the title is important, as the latter may convey no meaning at all. The question is important in two ways. Respiratory disease may affect a patient's ability to perform a job but may also be the result of the occupation. Any job involving exposure to noxious agents of a respirable size is potentially damaging, the most obvious example is pneumoconiosis in coal miners.

Enquiry may need to be searching and if occupational lung disease is suspected then a full list of all jobs performed will need to be constructed. For example, in the case of asbestos there can be an interval of 30 years between exposure, say in shipyard work, and the development of asbestosis or mesothelioma. Some will deny working with asbestos but nevertheless were exposed when others were performing lagging (putting asbestos on pipes) or stripping (taking it off). Other occupations where exposure may not be obvious though real nonetheless are building and demolition work, electrical repair work, railway engineering, and gas mask and cement manufacture. Environmental exposure, including that of wives of asbestos workers, seems important occasionally.

The easiest way to diagnose pneumoconiosis is to ask the patient. Miners in the UK undergo regular chest radiography whilst working. If significant pneumoconiosis is diagnosed the patient will be told.

Some occupational causes of lung disease

Occupation	Agent	Disease
Mining	Coal dust	Pneumoconiosis
Quarrying	Silica dust	Silicosis
Foundry work	Silica dust	Silicosis
Asbestos (Mining, heating, building, demolition)	Asbestos fibres	Asbestosis Mesothelioma Lung cancer
Farming	*Actinomycetes*	Alveolitis
Paint spraying	Isocyanates	Asthma
Plastics manufacture	Isocyanates	Asthma
Soldering	Colophony	Asthma

Fig. 6.30 Occupational causes of lung disease.

Occupational asthma

The list of causes of occupational asthma grows longer yearly. A good screening question to any asthmatic is 'does your work make any difference to your symptoms' and follow this up with questions about improvement at weekends or on holiday. The latter is important because symptoms caused at work may not be manifest until the evening or night and the patient may not make the association.

Common causes are isocyanates, (paint hardeners and plastic manufacture) and colophony (soldering, electronics). The lack of an obvious culprit should not put you off the scent if the evidence is otherwise suggestive. Much detective work is necessary in individual cases.

Extrinsic allergic alveolitis

Extrinsic allergic alveolitis can be due to occupation as well as birds. The best example is farmer's lung: the agent is the microorganism *thermophilic actinomycetes* contaminating stored damp hay. The story is of shortness of breath, cough, and chills a few hours after forking out fodder for cattle in the winter. Other occupations with similar risks are mushroom workers, sugar workers (bagassosis: mouldy sugar cane), maltworkers, and woodworkers, although the antigens vary in each case.

FAMILY HISTORY

The commonest lung disease with a genetic basis is asthma, though the development of the disease in an individual is much more complicated. A family history of asthma and the related conditions of hay fever or eczema is often found, but these diseases are so prevalent that enquiry beyond the immediate family is of little value. Other diseases which run in the family include cystic fibrosis and α-1-antitrypsin deficiency, a rare cause of emphysema.

Tuberculosis is usually passed on within families. In the UK, TB is common in Asian migrants, particularly in their first ten years in the country and in those who have revisited the subcontinent.

Enquiry into sexual habits will be necessary if the illness could be a manifestation of AIDS, remembering that this is now becoming more common in the heterosexual population and in those who have travelled abroad, particularly to Africa.

DRUG HISTORY

The most useful questions are those concerning past treatment.

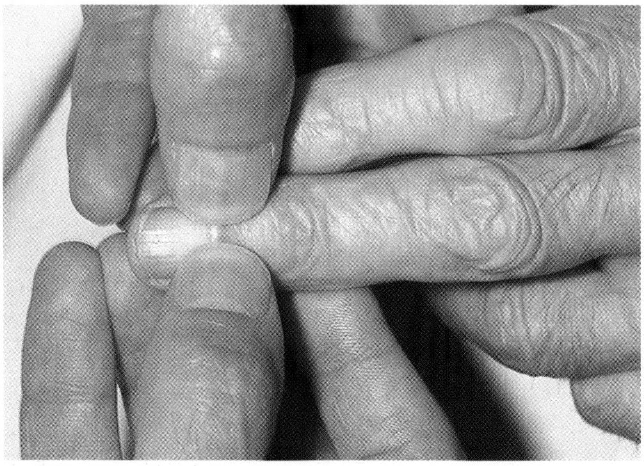

Fig. 6.31 Rocking the nail on the nail bed in clubbing.

Successful use of bronchodilators and corticosteroids in airways obstruction will indicate asthma. Aspirin and sometimes other non-steroidal anti-inflammatory drugs and β-adrenergic receptor blockers can make asthma worse and angiotensin-converting enzyme inhibitors cause chronic dry cough. Steroid therapy predisposes to infections including tuberculosis.

GENERAL EXAMINATION

Examination starts on first encounter. You should be able to continually pick up and store clues whilst talking and listening to the patient. As with all body systems, a good look at the patient as a whole will provide important evidence that will be missed in a rush to lay a stethoscope on the chest. Your findings should be divided into first impressions, then a more directed search for signs outside the chest likely to be helpful in lung disease, and finally examination of the chest itself.

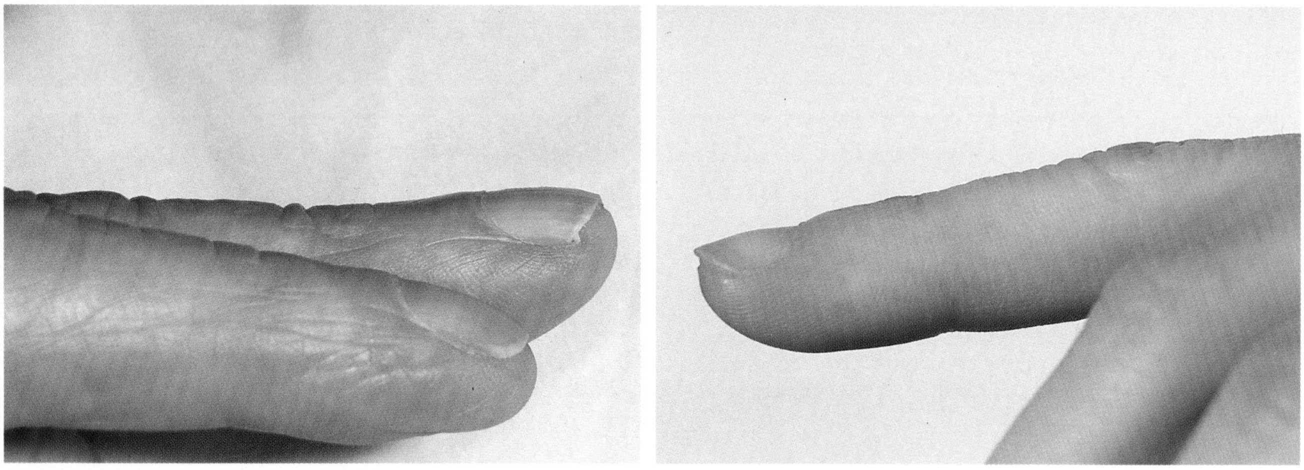

Fig. 6.32 Mild clubbing. The nail on the left shows obliteration of the angle at the nailfold compared with a normal nail on the right.

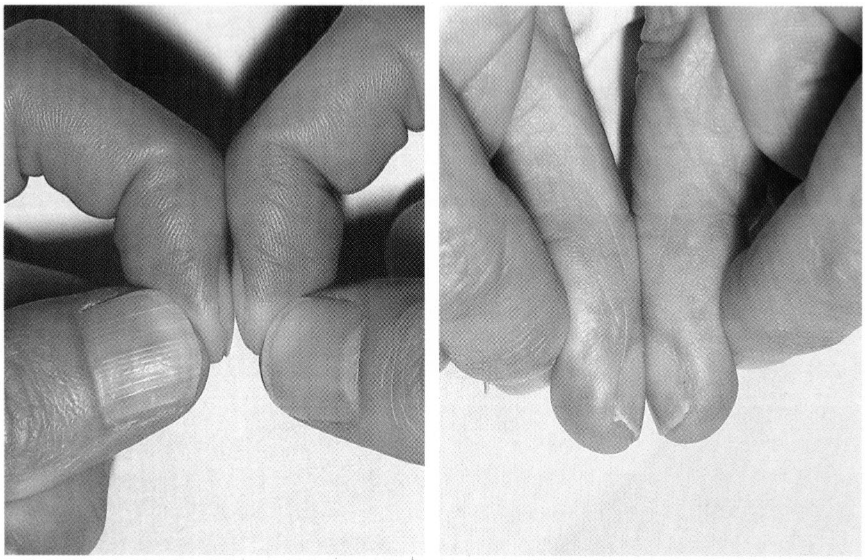

Fig. 6.33 Clubbing, showing how the diamond-shaped area formed between two normal nails (left) is obliterated (right).

First impressions

How breathless does the patient appear? Is it consistent with the story? If seen in the clinic can he walk in comfortably and sit down or does he struggle to get in? Perhaps he is in a wheelchair; if so is it because of breathing troubles or something else? Can he carry on a conversation with you or does he break up his sentences? How breathless is he getting undressed? Details of breathing patterns are considered later but is the patient obviously distressed or quite comfortable? Is there stridor or wheeze? Is there cough? confirming or perhaps at variance with the history. Is there evidence of weight loss suggesting carcinoma or weight gain from steroid therapy?

Do not ignore clues around the patient. An air compressor by the bed will be used to deliver bronchodilator drugs. A packet of cigarettes in the pyjama jacket will have the opposite effect! In hospital you will be deprived of some of these features but not how the patient is positioned – does he have to sit up to breath? – confirming a history of orthopnoea. Is he receiving oxygen?

After extracting as much information as you can, position the patient comfortably on the bed or couch with enough pillows to support his chest at an angle of about 45°, and begin the formal examination. This can conveniently start with the hands and a search for clubbing.

Clubbing

This refers to an increase in the soft tissues of the nail bed and the finger tip. The earliest stage is some softening of the nail bed which can be detected by rocking the nail from side to side on the nail bed (Fig. 6.31). This sign can be present to some extent in normal subjects but is exaggerated in the early stages of clubbing. Next, the soft tissue of the nail bed fills in the normal acute angle between the nail and the nail bed. This is usually about 160° but the area becomes flat, even convex in clubbing (Fig. 6.32). This is seen best by viewing the nail from the side against a white background, say the bedsheets. Not surprisingly, there can be considerable disagreement about the presence or absence of clubbing in the early stages. When normal nails are placed 'back to back' there is usually a diamond-shaped area between them. This is obliterated early in clubbing (Fig. 6.33).

In the next stage, the normal longtitudinal curvature of the nail increases. Some normal nails have quite a pronounced curve, but in clubbing the increase in soft tissue in the nail beds needs to be present as well. In the final stage the whole tip of the finger becomes rounded (a club) (Fig. 6.34). Clubbing less commonly affects the toes. Some causes are given in Figure 6.35.

The pathogenesis of clubbing is unknown. There is increased vascularity and tissue fluid and this seems to be under neurogenic control since it can be abolished by vagotomy.

Clubbing is sometimes associated with hypertrophic pulmonary osteoarthropathy; this presents with pain in the joints particularly the wrists, ankles, and knees. The pain is not in the joint itself but over the shafts of the long bones adjacent to the joint. It is due to

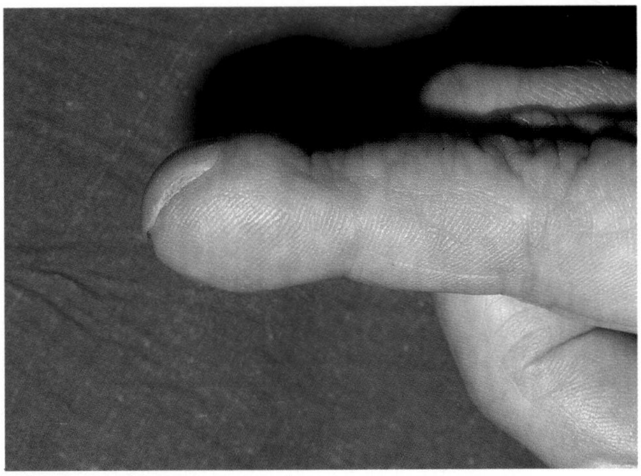

Fig. 6.34 Gross clubbing.

Some common causes of clubbing
Pulmonary
Bronchial carcinoma
Chronic pulmonary sepsis
Empyema
Lung abscess
Bronchiectasis
Cystic fibrosis
Cryptogenic fibrosing alveolitis
Asbestosis
Cardiac
Congenital cyanotic heart disease
Bacterial endocarditis
Other
Idiopathic/familial
Cirrhosis
Ulcerative colitis
Coeliac disease
Crohn's disease

Fig. 6.35 Some causes of clubbing (see also Fig. 4.84).

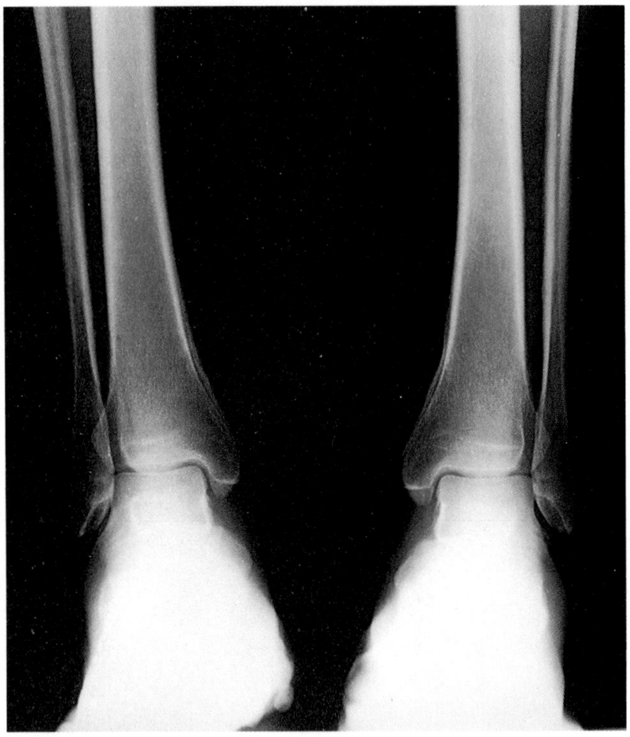

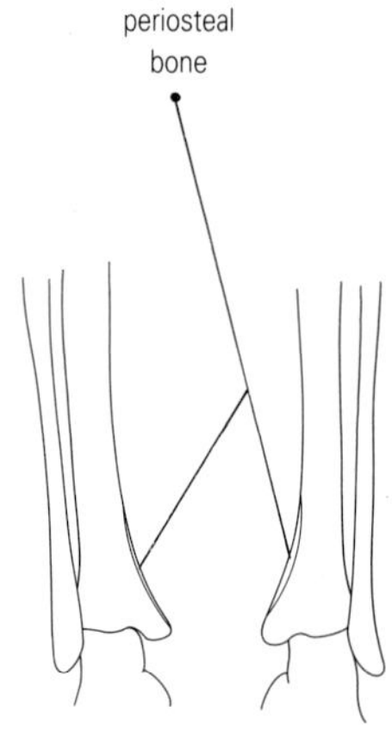

Fig. 6.36 Hypertrophic pulmonary osteoarthropathy.

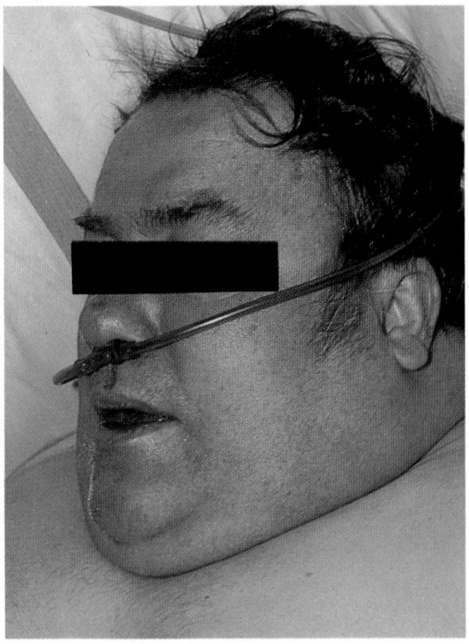

Fig. 6.37 Cyanosis in a patient with chronic airflow limitation.

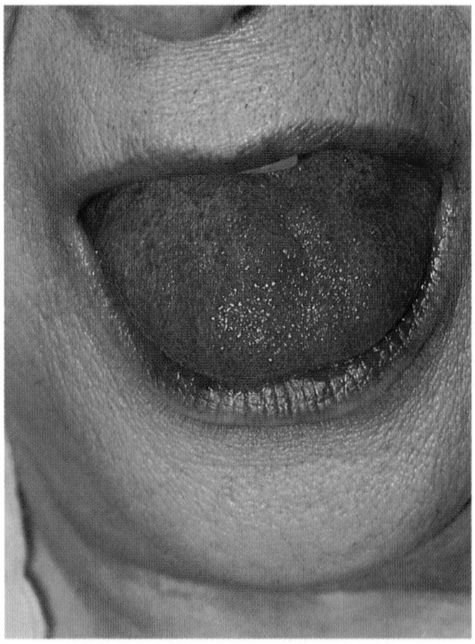

Fig. 6.38 Central cyanosis of the tongue.

subperiosteal new bone formation which can be seen on a radiograph. (Fig. 6.36). The condition is almost invariably associated with clubbing although it can occur alone. Any cause of clubbing can also cause hypertrophic pulmonary osteoarthropathy; however, it is usually associated with a squamous carcinoma of the bronchus. The condition is often mistaken for arthritis with consequent delay in diagnosis. Successful treatment of the cause will relieve clubbing and the pain of hypertrophic pulmonary osteoarthropathy. While searching for clubbing note any nicotine staining of the fingers.

Cyanosis

Cyanosis, a bluish tinge to the skin and mucous membranes, is seen when there is an increased amount of reduced haemoglobin in the blood. (Fig. 6.37). Traditionally, it is thought to become visible when there is about 5g/dl or more of reduced haemoglobin corresponding to a saturation of about eighty-five per cent. However there is a good deal of inter-observer variation. Severe anaemia and cyanosis cannot co-exist otherwise most of the haemoglobin would be reduced. Conversely, in polycythaemia where there is an

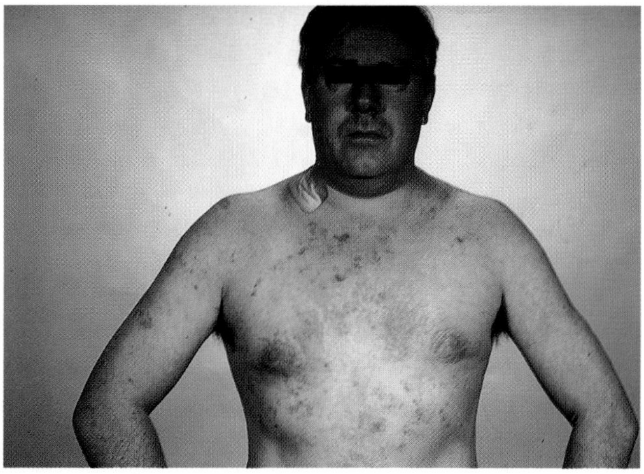

Fig. 6.39 Superior vena caval obstruction showing a swollen face and neck, dilated veins over the trunk and the site of a lymph node biopsy.

increase in red cell mass there may be enough reduced haemoglobin to produce cyanosis even though there is enough oxygenated haemoglobin to maintain a normal oxygen carrying capacity.

Cyanosis can be divided into central and peripheral varieties. Central cyanosis is due to disease of the heart or lungs and the blood leaving the left heart is blue. Peripheral cyanosis is due to decreased circulation and increased extraction of oxygen in the peripheral tissues. Blood leaving the left heart is normal.

Central cyanosis

Although the whole patient may appear cyanosed, the best place to look is the mucous membranes of the lips and tongue (Fig. 6.38). Good natural light is best. Any severe disease of the heart and lungs will cause central cyanosis, but the commonest causes are severe airflow limitation, left ventricular failure, and pulmonary fibrosis.

Peripheral cyanosis

Here the peripheries, the fingers, and the toes are blue, with normal mucous membranes. The usual cause is reduced circulation to the limbs, as seen in cold weather, Raynaud's phenomena or peripheral vascular disease. The peripheries are usually also cold. There may be an element of peripheral cyanosis in heart failure when the perfusion of the extremities is reduced.

Cyanosis can rarely be caused by the abnormal pigments methaemoglobin and sulphaemoglobin. Arterial oxygen tension is normal.

Tremors and carbon dioxide retention

The commonest tremor in patients with respiratory disease is a fine finger tremor from stimulation of β-receptors in skeletal muscle by bronchodilator drugs. Carbon dioxide retention is seen in severe chronic airflow limitation. Clinically, it can be suspected by a flapping tremor (indistinguishable from that associated with hepatic failure), vasodilation manifested by warm peripheries, bounding pulse, papilloedema, and headache.

Pulse and blood pressure

Pulsus paradoxus is a drop in blood pressure on inspiration. A minor degree occurs normally. Major degrees occur in pericardial effusion and constrictive pericarditis but also in severe asthma. A pulse above 120 per/min and pulsus paradoxus of greater then l0mm Hg correlate well with hypoxia and indicate a severe attack. For further discussion see Chapter 7.

The jugular venous pulse and cor pulmonale

The jugular venous pulse may be raised in cor pulmonale (right heart failure due to lung disease). The common cause in the UK is chronic airflow limitation leading to hypoxia. The main mechanism is pulmonary vasoconstriction. Other signs are peripheral oedema (probably due as much to renal hypoxia as back pressure from the right heart), hepatomegaly, and a left parasternal heave indicating right ventricular hypertrophy. In severe cases, functional tricuspid regurgitation will lead to a pulsatile liver, large V waves in the jugular venous pulse and a systolic murmur in the tricuspid area (see Chapter 7). Sometimes overinflation of the lungs will displace the liver downwards and also obscure the cardiac signs leaving the jugular venous pulse as the only sign.

Superior vena cava (SVC) obstruction is a common presentation of carcinoma of the bronchus but can rarely be caused by lymphoma, benign tumors, and mediastinal fibrosis. The tumor compresses the SVC near the point where it enters the right atrium. The resulting high pressure in the SVC causes distension of the neck, fullness and oedema of the face, dilated collateral veins over the upper chest (Fig. 6.39), and chemosis or oedema of the conjunctiva. The internal jugular vein is, of course, distended but may be difficult to see because it does not pulsate (The dog-in-the-night-time syndrome). The external jugular vein should be visible. The patient may have noticed that his collar has become tighter.

Lymphadenopathy

Lymph nodes may enlarge either because of generalized disease (e.g. lymphoma) or from local disease spreading through the lymphatics to the nodes. Both may be important in respiratory disease. Palpation of lymph nodes is considered in Chapter 3, so here we will consider the examination only of those lymph nodes draining the chest.

Lymphatics from the lungs drain centrally to the hilum then up the paratracheal chain to the supraclavicular (scalene) or cervical nodes. Chest wall lymphatics, especially from the breasts drain to the axillae. Lung disease, therefore, rarely involves the axillary

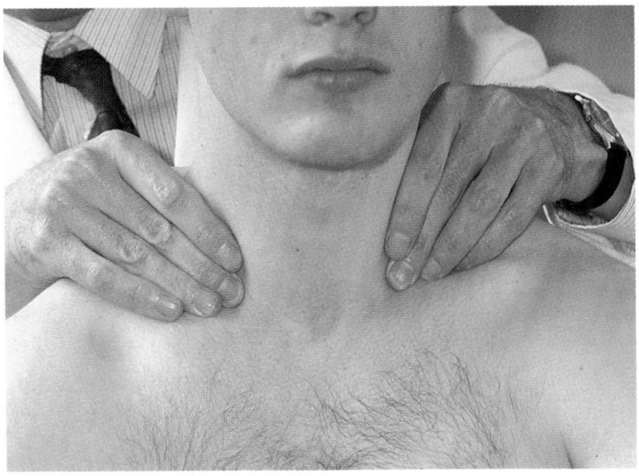

Fig. 6.40 Palpation of the supraclavicular lymph nodes from behind.

nodes. Examination of the cervical chain can be carried out by palpation from the front of the patient. Supraclavicular lymphadenopathy is best detected from behind the patient by placing your fingers either side of the neck behind the tendon of the sternomastoid muscle. It helps if the neck is bent slightly forward. (Fig. 6.40). Cervical nodes can be palpated this way too.

It is sometimes quite difficult to examine in the supraclavicular area, as lymph nodes may be only slightly enlarged. If palpable, the nodes are usually the site of disease. Careful comparisons should be made on the two sides. If lymph nodes are enlarged then biopsy or aspiration may be a simple way to confirm a diagnosis. Beware of performing a cervical node biopsy too readily. Throat cancer can involve these nodes and painstaking block dissection is the correct treatment.

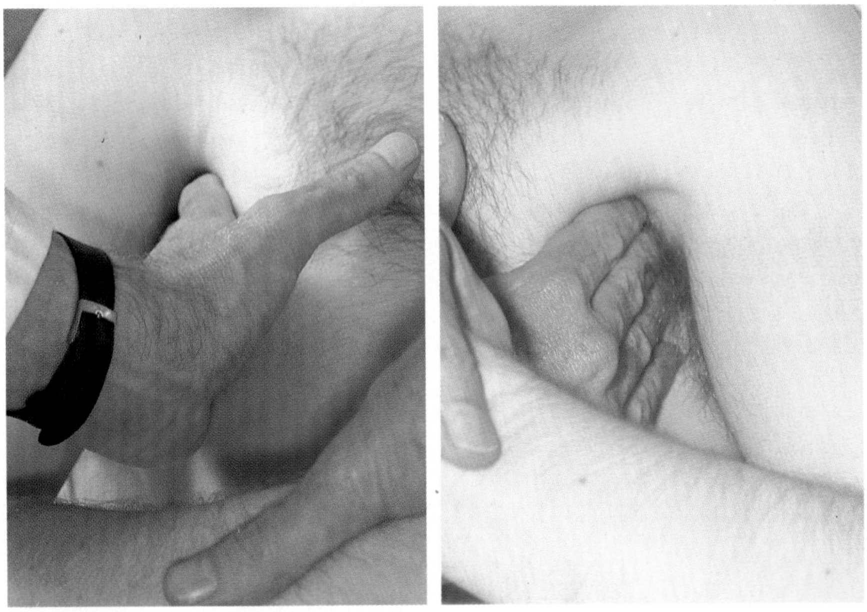

Fig. 6.41 Palpation of the axillary lymph nodes.

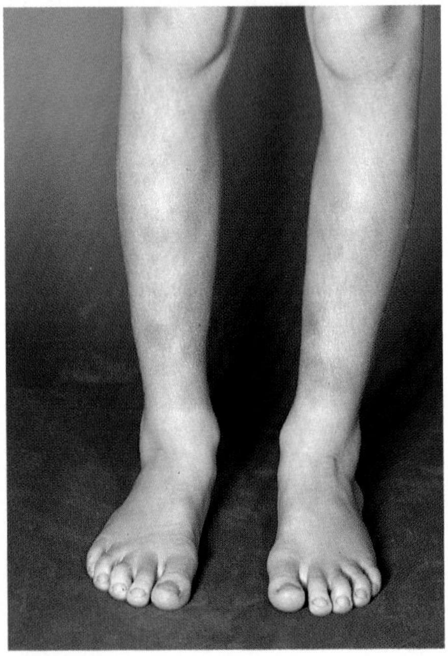

Fig. 6.42 Erythema nodosum, showing raised red lumps on the shins.

Some causes of erythema nodosum
Infections
Streptococci Tuberculosis Systemic fungal infections Leprosy
Others
Sarcoidosis Ulcerative colitis Crohn's disease Sulphonamides Oral contraceptive pill and pregnancy

Fig. 6.43 Causes of erythema nodosum.

Respiratory diseases that involve these nodes are carcinoma, tuberculosis, and sarcoidosis. Nodes containing metastatic carcinoma are hard and fixed. Tuberculous nodes are common in Asian patients in the UK and are soft and matted, and may have discharging sinuses. Healing and calcification leaves small hard nodes.

Examination of the axillary nodes is shown in Figure 6.41. Abduct the patient's arm, place the fingers of your hand high up in the axilla, press the tips of the fingers against the chest wall, relax the patient's arm and draw your fingers downwards over the ribs to roll the nodes between your fingers and ribs.

The skin

The early stages of sarcoidosis and primary tuberculosis are often accompanied by erythema nodosum (Fig. 6.42), painful red indurated areas usually on the shins, though occasionally more extensive; they fade through bruising. Severe cases may also have arthralgia. The commonest cause of erythema nodosum in the UK is sarcoidosis (Fig. 6.43). Sarcoidosis can also involve the skin – particularly old scars and tattoos – with nodules and plaques. Lupus pernio is a violaceous swelling of the nose from involvement by sarcoidosis.

The eyes

Horner's syndrome (miosis, enophthalmos, lack of sweating on the affected side of the face, and ptosis) (see also page 12.36) is usually due to involvement of the sympathetic chain on the posterior chest wall by a bronchial carcinoma

Sarcoidosis and tuberculosis can cause iridocyclitis. Miliary tuberculosis can produce tubercles visible on the retina by ophthalmoscopy. Papilloedema can be caused by carbon dioxide retention and cerebral metastases.

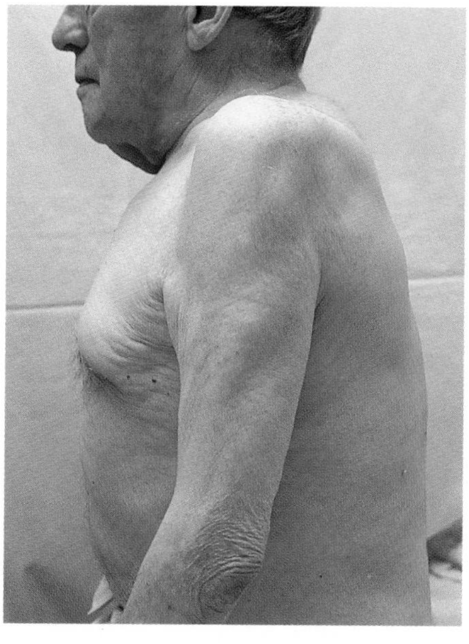

Fig. 6.44 'Barrel chest'. Note the increased AP diameter of the chest.

EXAMINATION OF THE CHEST

You should follow the classical sequence of inspection, palpation, percussion, and auscultation, not forgetting contemplation (Osler).

Inspection of the chest wall

First look for any deformities of the chest wall. In 'barrel chest' the chest wall is held in hyperinflation (Fig. 6.44). In normal people the anteroposterior (AP) diameter of the chest is less than the lateral diameter, but in hyperinflation the AP diameter may be greater than the lateral. The amount of trachea palpable above the suprasternal notch is reduced. The normal 'bucket handle' movement of the ribs upwards, and outwards pivoting at the spinous processes and the costal cartilages is converted into a 'pump handle' up and down motion. Barrel chest is seen in states of chronic airflow limitation, with the degree of deformity correlating with its severity.

In pectus excavatum (funnel chest) (Fig. 6.45), the sternum is depressed, the condition is benign and needs no treatment but can

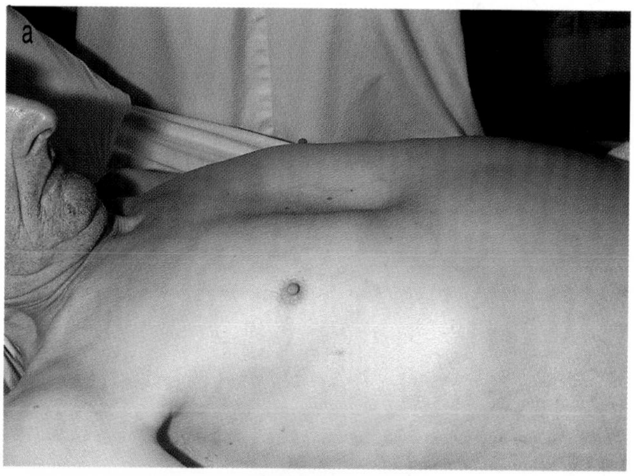

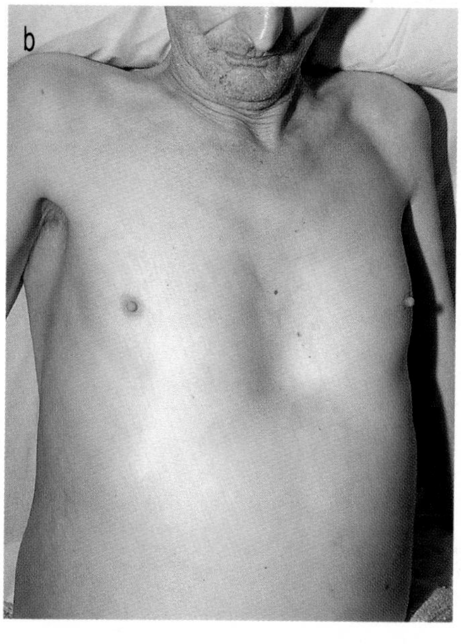

Fig. 6.45 Pectus excavatum, showing the depressed sternum.

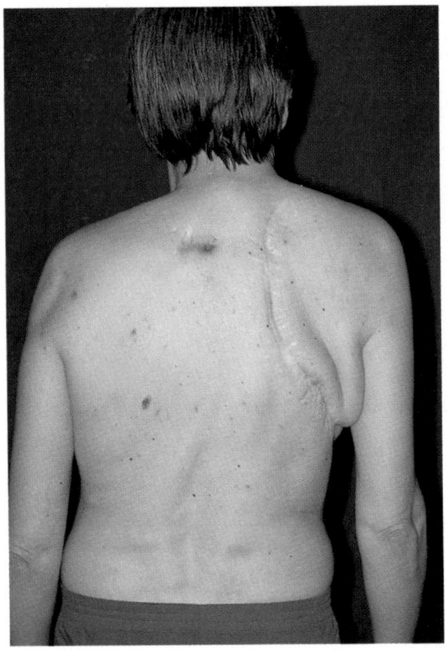

Fig. 6.46 Thoracoplasty with secondary changes in the spine.

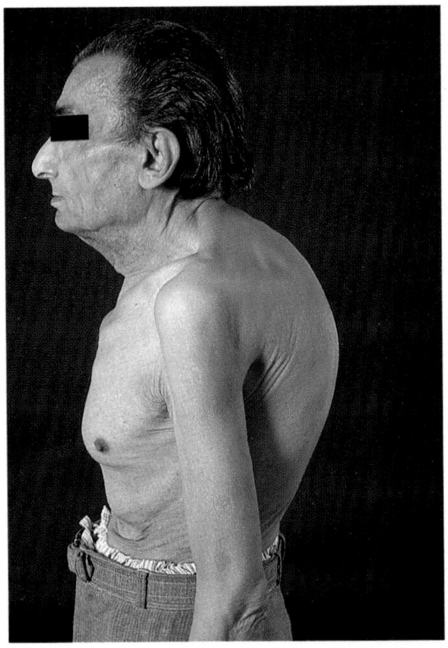

Fig. 6.47 Kyphosis.

produce unusual chest radiographic appearances, with the heart apparently enlarged and displaced to the left. In pectus carinatum (pigeon chest), the sternum and costal cartilages project outwards. It may be secondary to severe childhood asthma.

Examine the chest wall for any operative scars or the changes of thoracoplasty. This was an operation performed in the 1940's and 1950's for tuberculosis and designed to reduce the volume of the chest. It can produce marked distortion of the chest wall, more clearly seen from the back (Fig. 6.46).

Flattening of part of the chest can be due either to underlying lung disease (which usually has to be long standing) or to scoliosis. Kyphosis is forward curvature of the spine (Fig. 6.47) and scoliosis lateral curvature. Both, but scoliosis in particular, can lead to respiratory failure.

Air in the subcutaneous tissue is termed surgical emphysema, although it is as commonly associated with a spontaneous pneumothorax as trauma to the chest. The tissues of the upper chest and neck are swollen, sometimes grossly so (Michelin man), although the condition is not dangerous in itself. They have a characteristic crackling sensation on palpation. In pneumothorax the air probably tracks from ruptured alveoli, through the root of the lungs to the mediastinum, thence up into the neck. On auscultation of the precordium, you may hear a curious extra sound in time with the heart (mediastinal crunch), but this can occur in pneumothorax without pneumomediastinum. Mediastinal air may be visible on a radiograph.

Breathing patterns

A good deal can be learnt from simple observation of the chest wall movements. Note rate, depth, and regularity. Does the chest move equally on the two sides? Does breathing appear distressing? Is it noisy?

Counting the respiratory rate is a traditional nursing observation, yet the precise rate is rarely of practical importance. You should note an increase in rate or depth. An increase in rate may occur in any severe lung disease and in fever. Patients with hyperventilation may breath both faster and more deeply, though the increase can be quite subtle and easily missed. Patients with acidosis from renal failure, diabetic ketoacidosis, and aspirin overdose will have deep sighing (Kussmaul) respirations as they try to excrete carbon dioxide. Acute massive pulmonary embolism gives a similar pattern.

Is the breathing regular? Cheyne–Stokes respiration is a waxing and waning of the respiratory depth over a minute or so from quite deep respirations to virtually no breathing at all. It is thought to be due to failure of the central respiratory control to respond adequately to changes in carbon dioxide and is often seen in those with terminal disease. Patients may seem unaware of the condition.

Is there any prolongation of expiration? The typical patient with airflow limitation has trouble breathing out. Inspiration may be quite brief, even hurried, but expiration is a prolonged laboured manoeuvre. Many of these patients breath out through pursed lips as if they were whistling, this mechanism maintains a higher airway pressure and keeps open the distal airways to allow fuller though longer expiration.

Note if the chest expands unequally. If so and there is no structural abnormality of the chest or spine to account for this then air is probably not entering the lung so well on the affected side. The difference has to be quite marked to be appreciated. The causes will be considered under palpation (see page 6.27). It is possible to measure overall expansion with a tape measure (the result is of little value and certainly no substitute for measures of lung volume). Breathing mainly with the diaphragm might suggest a chest wall problems (e.g. pleural pain or ankylosing spondylitis). Breathing mainly with the rib cage suggests diaphragm paralysis, peritonitis,

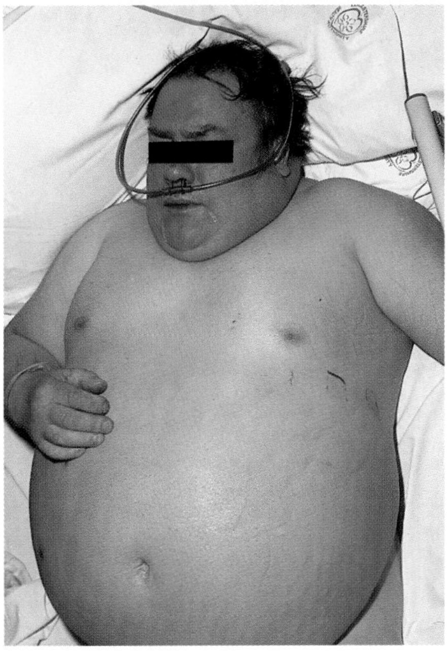

Fig. 6.48 A 'blue bloater' showing ascites from marked cor pulmonale.

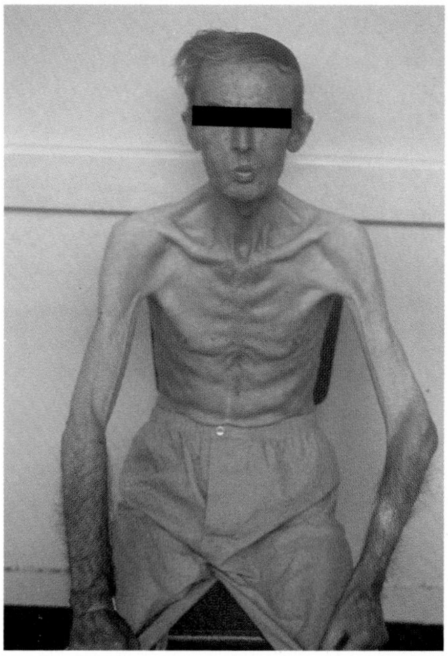

Fig. 6.49 The 'pink puffer'. Note the pursed-lip breathing.

or abdominal distension. Normally, as the diaphragm descends in inspiration the anterior abdominal wall will move outwards. If it moves inwards (abdominal paradox) then the diaphragm is probably paralysed. Similarly, in tetraplegia, when the chest wall muscles are paralysed, descent of the diaphragm produces in-drawing of the chest wall (chest wall paradox).

Is the patient distressed by his breathing? Can he carry on a normal conversation or does he have to break up his sentences, even perhaps to single words at a time? Patients with severe respiratory distress use their accessory muscles of respiration. They fix the position of the shoulder girdle by pressing the hands on the nearest fixed object and throw back their heads. This gives a purchase for accessory muscles of respiration, mainly the sternomastoids.

Does the patient breathe more comfortably in certain positions? Can he lie flat or does he have to be propped up? Patients with pulmonary oedema and severe airflow limitation will be unable to lie down for long but then most patients with breathing difficulty are more comfortable sitting up. Is breathing audible? Wheeze is a prolonged expiratory noise often audible to the patient as well as the doctor and implies airflow limitation. Stridor is a harsh, chiefly inspiratory noise and implies obstruction in the central airways. This may be at laryngeal level when the voice is usually hoarse but otherwise implies tracheal or major bronchial obstruction. In children, croup and foreign bodies are the usual causes, in adults, carcinoma, or extrinsic compression.

Pink puffers and blue bloaters

The terms 'pink puffers' and 'blue bloaters' are applied to the overall appearances of some patients with chronic airflow limitation. They describe polar groups and most patients are in between. 'Blue boaters' (Fig. 6.48) are cyanosed from hypoxia and bloated from right heart failure. Further investigation shows features of chronic obstructive bronchitis. Cough and sputum are common but breathlessness less so. Carbon dioxide retention is a feature. 'Pink puffers' (Fig. 6.49) are not cyanosed and are thin. Investigation shows features associated with emphysema. Cough and sputum are less common, but the patients are breathless. Carbon dioxide levels in the blood are normal or low.

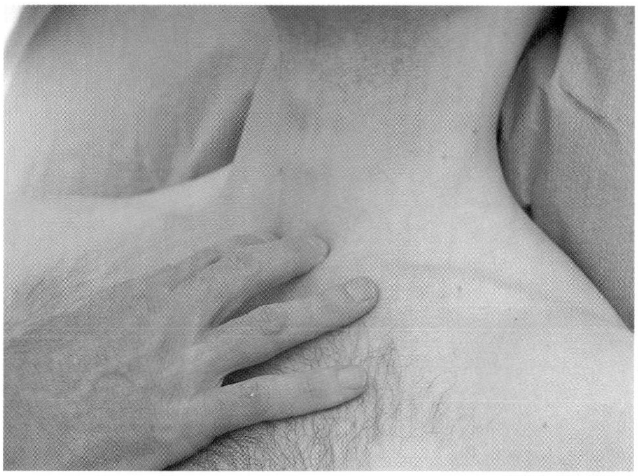

Fig. 6.50 Palpation of the trachea.

PALPATION

The trachea and mediastinum

Start palpation by feeling for the position of the trachea. Do this from the front by placing two fingers either side of the trachea and judging whether the distances between it and the sternomastoid tendons are equal on the two sides (Fig. 6.50). An alternative is to examine the patient from behind and hook your fingers round the tendons to meet the trachea. The trachea may be displaced by masses in in the neck such as thyroid enlargement; nonetheless, it gives an indication about the position of the mediastinum, although often you will only be confident about tracheal displacement after you have seen the radiograph!

The position of the apex beat also gives information about the position of the mediastinum so long as the heart is not enlarged. The trachea moves with the upper part of the mediastinum, the apex beat with the lower. The mediastinum may be pushed or pulled to either side. Large effusions push the position of the apex beat, but very large effusions are needed to displace the trachea. Pneumothorax pushes the mediastinum even though the lung collapses. This is because the pressure in the pleural space approaches or even exceeds atmospheric pressure, i.e. increases. Lung collapse and fibrosis pull the mediastinum (Fig. 6.51). Tumor, especially the pleural tumor mesothelioma, may 'fix' the mediastinum so that it cannot move despite these changes.

Chest wall

If the patient complains of chest pain, then you should gently palpate the chest for local tenderness. If present, this usually indicates disease of bones, muscles, or cartilage. As indicated earlier, one variety is called Tietze's syndrome where there is pain and swelling of one or more of the upper costal cartilages, but much more commonly than this syndrome there is merely pain and tenderness of the cartilage but no swelling. Chest wall tenderness may

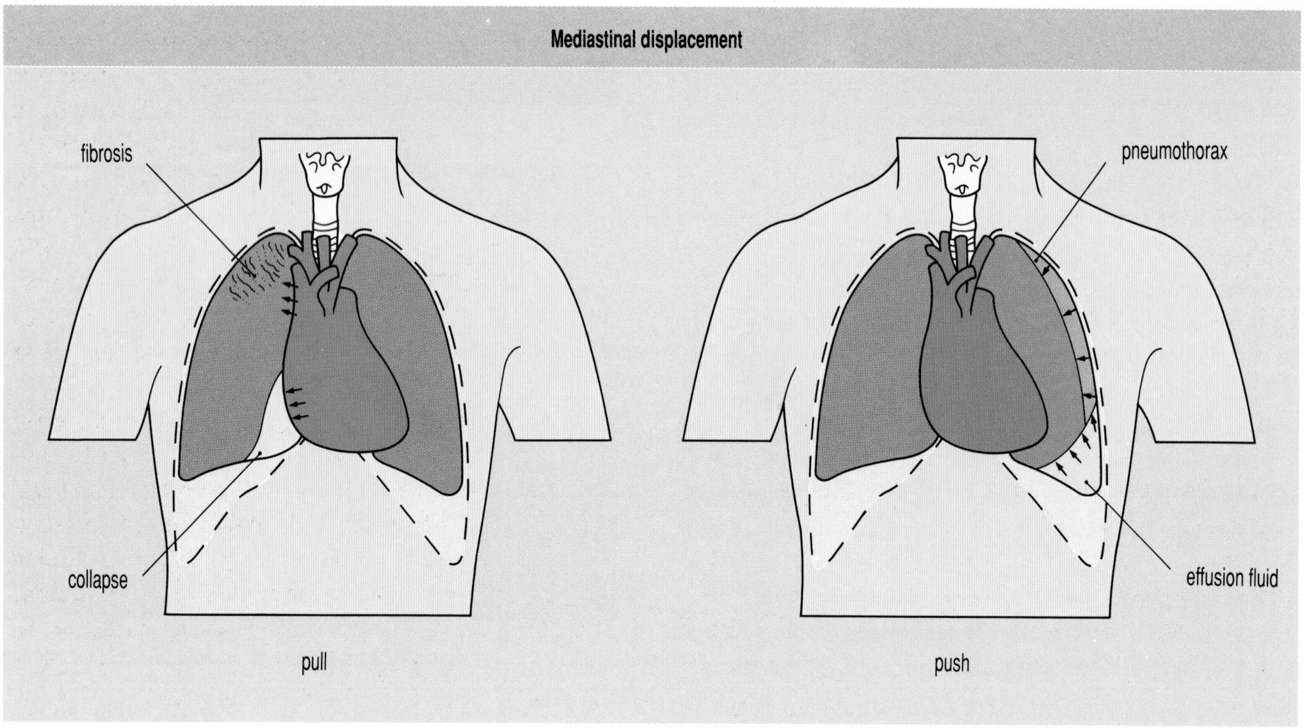

Fig. 6.51 Mediastinal displacement.

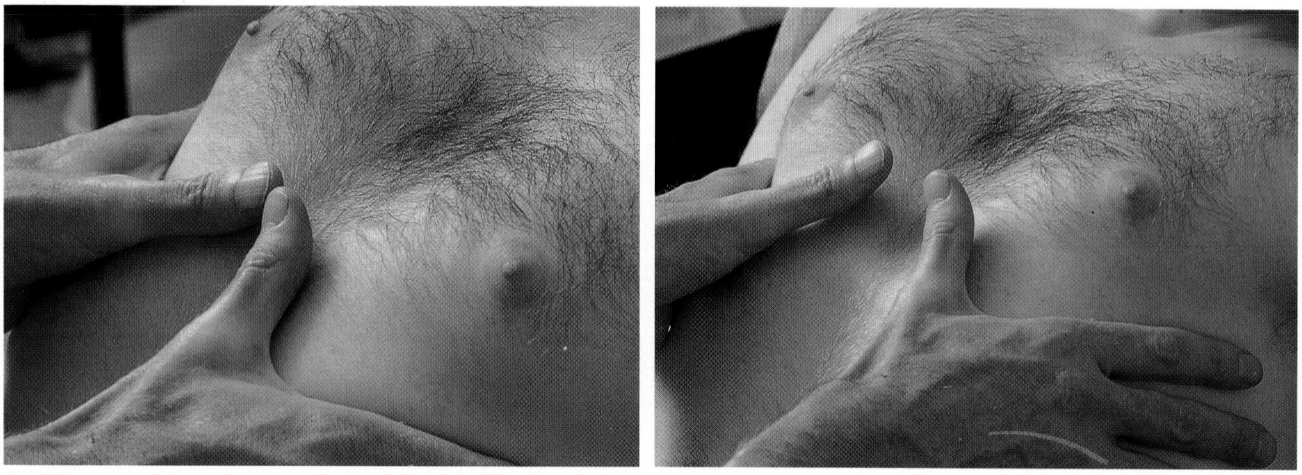

Fig. 6.52 Assessing chest expansion in expiration (left) and inspiration (right).

also be present in pleurisy; point tenderness over a rib or cartilage is almost always due to benign local disease and the worried patient can be reassured.

A systematic approach

From this point on, as with most parts of the physical examination, comparison is made between the two sides of the body as abnormality is likely to be confined to one side. Start from the front at the apex and work downwards comparing each side immediately with the other. Remember that the heart will influence the result on the left. Do not forget the lateral sides and the axillae. Then sit the patient forwards and examine the back. Sometimes you will need an assistant to help a sick patient to lean forwards. When examining from the back, place the arms of the patient forwards in the lap. This will move the scapulae laterally and uncover more of the chest wall.

Vocal fremitus

This is performed by placing either the edge or the flat of your hand on the chest and asking the patient to say '99' or count '1,2,3'. The vibrations produced by this manoeuvre are transmitted through the lung substance and are felt by the hand. The test is crude, and the mechanism and the alterations in disease are the same as for vocal resonance (see page 6.29).

Chest expansion

The purpose of this test is to determine if both sides of the chest move equally. Students often have difficulty with this examination. A good method is to put the fingers of both your hands as far round the chest as possible and then to bring the thumbs together in the midline but to keep the thumbs off the chest wall. The patient is then asked to take a deep breath in, the chest wall by moving outwards moves the fingers outwards and the thumbs are in turn distracted away from the midline (Fig. 6.52). The thumbs must be free, if they are also fixed to the chest wall they will not move. It is important to keep your fingers and thumbs in the same relationship to each other, for it is easy to move the thumb the way you think it ought to go! Examination can be performed on both the front and the back.

Expansion can be reduced on both sides equally. This is difficult to detect as there is no standard of comparison, but is produced by severe airflow limitation, extensive generalized lung fibrosis, and chest wall problems (e.g. ankylosing spondylitis).

Unilateral reduction implies that air cannot enter that side, and is seen in pleural effusion, lung collapse, pneumothorax, and pneumonia.

PERCUSSION

The purpose of percussion is to detect the resonance or hollowness of the chest. Use both hands, placing the fingers of one on the chest with the fingers separated and strike one of them with the terminal phalynx of the middle finger of the other hand (Fig. 6.53); it must be removed again immediately, like the clapper inside a bell, otherwise the resultant sound will be damped. The striking movement should be a flick of the wrist and the striking finger should be at right angles to the other finger. As well as hearing the percussion note, vibrations will be felt by your hand on the chest wall. Again, each side is compared with the equivalent area on the other from top to bottom. Do not forget the sides.

The finger on the chest should be parallel to the expected line of dullness (e.g. in an effusion, parallel to the floor). This will then produce a clearly defined change in note from normal to dull; a finger straddling the demarcation will not do this. It should be placed in the intercostal spaces. Do not percuss more heavily than is necessary, it gives no more information and can be distressing to patients. The apex of the lung can be examined by tapping directly on the middle of the clavicle (Fig. 6.54). Remember the lung extends much further down posteriorly than anteriorly (see Fig. 6.4).

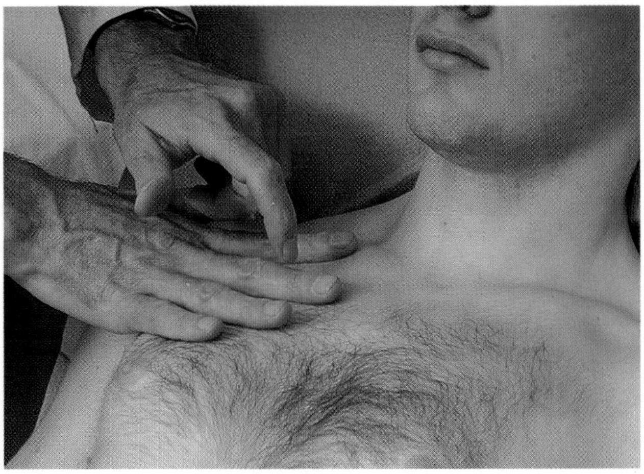

Fig. 6.53 Percussion over the anterior chest.

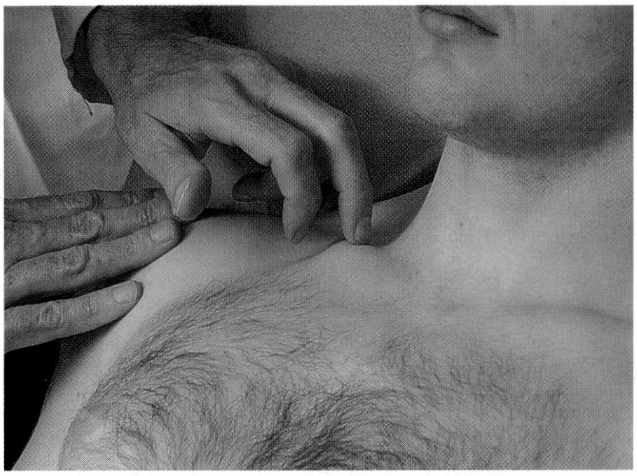

Fig. 6.54 Direct percussion of the clavicles for disease in the lung apices.

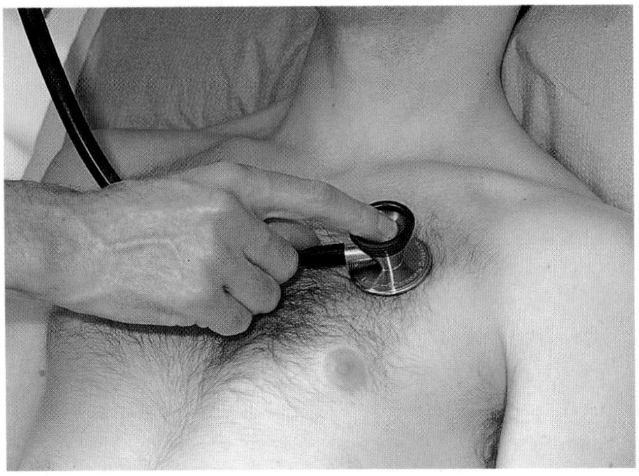

Fig. 6.55 Auscultation of the chest using the diaphragm.

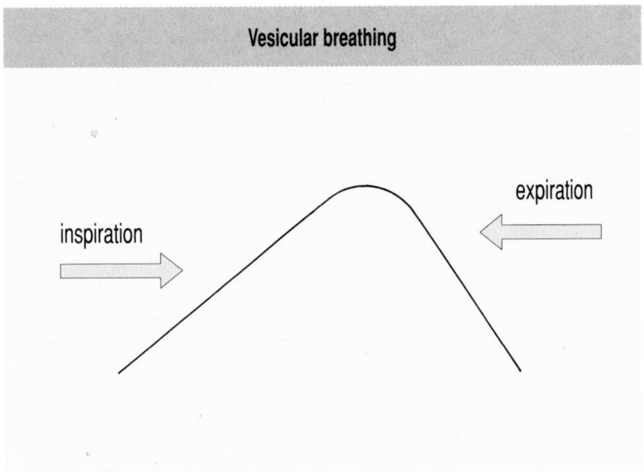

Fig. 6.56 The timing of vesicular breathing.

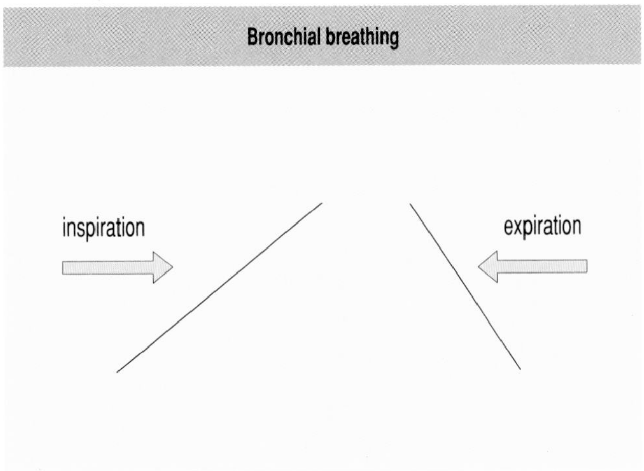

Fig. 6.57 The timing of bronchial breathing.

The degree of resonance depends on the thickness of the chest wall and on the amount of air in the structures underlying it. The possibilities are increased resonance, dullness, and so called 'stony dullness'. Obese patients and those with thick chest walls show less resonance, yet it is equal on the two sides. By contrast patients with overinflated lungs, particularly those with emphysema, have increased resonance; however, it is generalized and without a reference point is difficult to grade. It might be thought that air in the pleural space (pneumothorax) would increase resonance, but the difference is often insufficient to identify from percussion alone which is the affected side.

Resonance is decreased moderately in consolidation and fibrosis of the lung and markedly if there is fluid of any kind between the lung and the chest wall, i.e. stony dullness. A collapsed lobe can compress to a very small volume and compensatory overinflation of the other lobe fills the space. Percussion note may then be normal. A whole lung cannot collapse completely (unless there is also a pneumothorax) so the chest will be dull. Percussion can also be used to determine movement of the diaphragm as the level of dullness will descend as the patient breathes in (tidal percussion). Dullness is to be expected over the liver which anteriorly reaches as high as the sixth costal cartilage, and over the heart. Resonance in these areas, again a subjective finding, implies increased air in the lungs and is common in overinflation and emphysema. Bilateral basal dullness is more usually due to failure or inability to take a deep breath, to obesity, or to abdominal distension, as to bilateral pleural effusions. The right diaphragm is normally higher than the left so expect a slightly higher level of dullness.

AUSCULTATION

Many doctors prefer to use the diaphragm of the stethoscope for auscultation of the chest (Fig. 6.55). In thin bony chests, the bell may give a more airtight fit and is less likely to trap hairs underneath, which produces a crackling sound.

Ask the patient to take deep breaths through the mouth, then listen in sequence over the chest as before. Start at the apices and compare each side with the other. Some patients fail to understand the instruction to breathe through the mouth, but the sounds are much clearer if they do. To help them you may have to press gently on the jaw to open it. Some take enormous slow deep breaths which although otherwise satisfactory do prolong the examination. A quick demonstration of what you want will resolve any problems.

The breath sounds are produced in the large airways, transmitted through the airways, and then attenuated by the distal lung structure through which they pass. The sounds you hear at the lung surface are therefore quite different from the sounds heard over the trachea and are modified further if there is anything obstructing the airways, lung tissue, pleura, or chest wall. When reporting on auscultatory changes, you must distinguish between the breath sounds and the added sounds. Breath sounds are termed either vesicular or bronchial and the added sounds are divided into crackles, wheezes, and rubs.

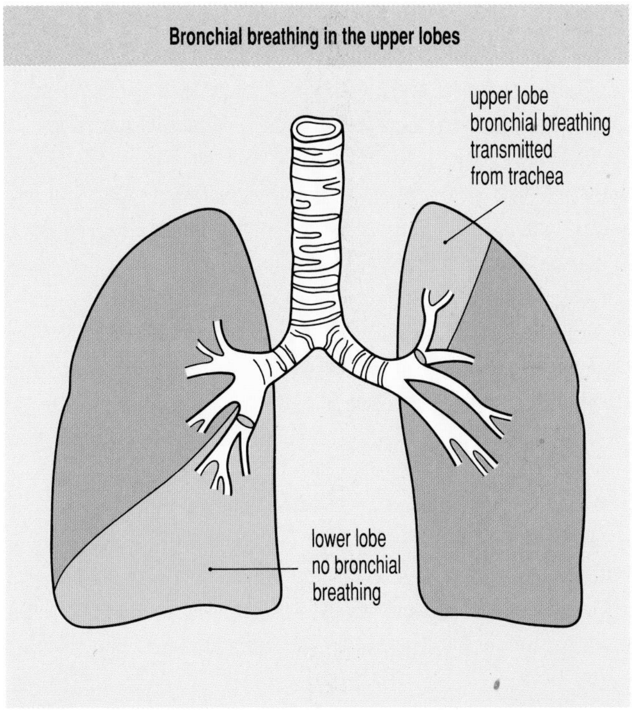

Fig. 6.58 Bronchial breathing may be heard over the upper lobes even if the bronchus is blocked.

Vesicular breath sounds

This is the sound heard over normal lungs, it has a rustling quality and is heard in inspiration and the first part of expiration (Fig. 6.56). Reduction in vesicular breath sounds can be expected with airway obstruction as in asthma, emphysema, or tumor. The so-called 'silent chest' is a sign of severe asthma: so little air enters the lung that no sound is produced. The breath sounds can be strikingly reduced in emphysema, particularly over a bulla. Generalized reduction in breath sounds also occurs with a thick chest wall or obesity.

Anything interspersed between the lung and the chest wall (air, fluid, or pleural thickening) will reduce the breath sounds; this is likely to be unilateral and therefore more easily detected.

Avoid the term 'diminished air entry' when you mean diminished breath sounds. The two are not necessary synonymous.

Bronchial breathing

Bronchial breathing causes much confusions because the essential feature of bronchial breathing, the quality of the sound, is difficult or impossible to put into words. Traditionally, it is described by its timing as occuring in both inspiration and expiration with a gap in between (Fig. 6.57). In this way it is contrasted with vesicular breathing. These features are undoubtedly true but lead to the confusion in the mind of the student that if anything is heard in mid or late expiration it must be bronchial breathing. Many normal people, and those with airways obstruction, have prolonged expiratory component to the breath sounds (this is sometimes designated 'bronchovesicular' but this term increases confusion rather than diminishes it). It is best to forget about the timing and concentrate on the essential feature, the quality of the sound. It can be mimicked to some extent by listening over the trachea with the stethoscope, though a better imitation can be obtained by putting the tip of your tongue on the roof of your mouth and breathing in and out through the open mouth.

Bronchial breathing is heard in situations where sound generated in the central airways is transmitted more or less unchanged through the lung substance. This occurs when the lung substance itself is solid as in consolidation, but the air passages remain open. Sound is conducted normally to the small airways but then instead of being modified by air in the alveoli, the lung conducts it better to the lung surface and hence to the stethoscope. If the central airways are obstructed by say a carcinoma, then no transmission of sound will take place and no bronchial breathing will occur even though the lung may be solid. An exception is seen in the upper lobes. Here, if the bronchi to either lobe are blocked, sounds from the central airways can still be transmitted directly from the trachea through the solid lung to the chest wall (Fig. 6.58).

The main cause of bronchial breathing is consolidation particularly from pneumonia, so much so that in the minds of most clinicians the three terms are synonymous. Lung abscess, if near the chest wall, can cause bronchial breathing probably because of the consolidation around it. Dense fibrosis is an occasional cause. Breath sounds over an effusion will be diminished, but bronchial breathing may be heard over its upper level perhaps because the effusion compresses the lung.

Bronchial breathing is only heard over a collapsed lung if the airway is patent. This is rare as the collapse is usually due to an obstructing carcinoma. Nevertheless, there is an exception with the upper lobes (see above).

Bronchial breathing has been divided into tubular, cavernous, and amphoric but attempts to score points on ward rounds by using these terms are best left to others!

Vocal resonance

This is the auscultatory equivalent of vocal fremitus. Place the stethoscope on the chest and ask the patient to say '99'. Normally the sound produced is 'fuzzy' and seems to come from the chest piece of the stethoscope. The changes in disease should by now be predictable. The sound is increased in consolidation (better transmission through solid lung) and decreased if there is air, fluid, or pleural thickening between the lung and the chest wall. The changes of vocal fremitus are the same. Both tests are of little value in themselves, yet a refinement of vocal resonance can be very useful. Sometimes the increased transmission of sound is so marked that even when the patient whispers the sound is still heard clearly over the affected lung (whispering pectoriloquy). When this is well-developed there is a striking difference between the normal side, where the sound appears to come from the end of the stethoscope, and the abnormal side where the syllables are much clearer and seem as if they are being whispered into your ear.

Bronchial breathing and whispering pectoriloquy often occur together; consequently, if you are in doubt about the presence of bronchial breathing then whispering pectoriloquy may confirm it. Like bronchial breathing, whispering pectoriloquy is characteristic of consolidation but can also occur with lung abscess and above an effusion.

Added sounds

There are three types of added sounds: wheezes, crackles, and pleural rubs. Much confusion has been generated in the past by other terms such as rhonchi, which are equivalent to wheezes, and crepitations and rales which are equivalent to crackles. Further subdivision is often attempted but is of very limited value.

Wheezes

These are prolonged musical sounds largely occurring in expiration, sometimes in inspiration, and are due to localized narrowing within the bronchial tree. They are caused by the vibration of the walls of a bronchus near to its point of closure. Most patients with wheeze have many, each coming from a single, narrowed area. As the lung gets smaller in expiration so the airways get smaller too, each narrowed airway reaches a critical phase when its produces a wheeze then ceases to do so; thus, during expiration numerous narrowings produce numerous wheezes in sequence and together. A single wheeze can occur and may then suggest a single narrowing often due to a carcinoma or foreign body (fixed wheeze).

Wheezes are typical of airway narrowing from any cause. Asthma and chronic bronchitis are the commonest and the narrowing is due to a combination of smooth muscle contraction, inflammatory changes in the walls, and increased bronchial secretions. Sometimes patients with these conditions have few or no wheezes. If so, ask the patient to take a deep breath and then to blow out hard. This may produce marked wheeze. Occasionally, wheeze is heard in pulmonary oedema, presumably because of bronchial wall oedema.

The term bronchospasm suggests narrowing due only to smooth muscle contraction and should be avoided as the bronchial narrowing is usually multifactorial

Wheeze like breath sounds can disappear in severe asthma and emphysema because of low rates of airflow. The amount of wheeze is not a good indicator of the degree of airways obstruction. Peak expiratory flow measurement is much better.

Stridor

Stridor may be heard better without a stethoscope by putting your ear close to the patient's mouth and asking him to breath in and out. As indicated earlier, it is a sign of large airway narrowing either in the larynx, trachea, or main bronchi.

Crackles

In a sense the term crackles if self-explanatory. Problems arise because of various descriptions that are often added such as coarse, medium, fine, wet, or dry. These add little to our understanding; nonetheless, it is possible to distinguish two main types. The first occurs where there is fluid in the larger bronchi when a coarse bubbling sound can be heard which clears or alters as the secretions causing the sound are shifted on coughing or deep breathing.

The sound of other 'fine' crackles can be imitated by rolling the hairs of your temple together between your fingers. They occur in inspiration and are high pitched, explosive sounds. The mechanism of their production is thought to be as follows. Many conditions lead to premature closure of the small airways by the end of expiration. During the succeeding inspiration these units can only be reopened by overcoming the surface tension that keeps them closed. When they eventually 'pop open' crackles are produced. During inspiration, larger bronchi will open before smaller ones so crackles from chronic bronchitis and bronchiectasis, tend to occur early.

Conditions which largely involve the alveoli, such as left ventricular failure, fibrosis, and pneumonia tend to produce crackles later in inspiration. This distinction is of clinical value. Note whether the crackles are localized. This would be expected in pneumonia and mild cases of bronchiectasis. Pulmonary oedema and fibrosing alveolitis typically affect both lung bases equally.

Normal people, especially smokers, may have a few basal crackles, these often clear with a few deep breaths.

Pleural rub

This is caused by the inflamed surfaces of the pleura rubbing together. The sound has been likened to new leather when it is bent or more vividly to the creaking noises made in a sailing ship heeling to the wind which you may have experienced from films if not in reality. Some idea of the quality of the sound can be obtained by placing one hand over the ear and rubbing the back of that hand with the fingers of the other. Pleural rubs are usually heard in both inspiration and expiration. At first you may think that you are moving the stethoscope on the chest. Sometimes coarse crackles can sound like rubs; a cough will shift the former. If there is any pain ask the patient to point to the site of the pain, this often localizes the rub too. Rubs are heard in all varieties of pleural inflammation such as in pneumonia and pulmonary embolism. Any effusion will separate the pleura and the rub may well go but sometimes remain above the effusion.

COMMON PATTERNS OF ABNORMALITY

This section summarizes what has been said before but from the perspective of the disease process. The diagnosis itself will need the integration of the history and any other information. Those considered are consolidation, pleural fluid, pneumothorax, chronic airflow limitation, lung or lobar collapse, and fibrosis. Not all the signs are present in every case and often there is more than one disease process at a time. The radiograph often illustrates the anatomical nature of the process, so examples are shown.

Consolidation

Consolidation is a confusing term as it means different things to different specialists. To a radiologist it means an alveolar-filling process with no presumption about aetiology. To a pathologist it means a heavy airless lung, and to a clinician it means bronchial breathing which he usually equates with pneumonia. To use pneumonia as an example, the affected lung or lobe is the same size or very slightly larger than normal lung. The alveoli are full of exudate, yet the air passages are open. The pleura is inflamed. Figure 6.59 lists some causes. Note that not all are infections.

Inspection of the chest may show diminished movement on the affected side, palpation shows no shift of the mediastinum but expansion is reduced, vocal fremitus may be increased, percussion note will be moderately impaired, breath sounds will be bronchial over the affected area with whispering pectoriloquy, and there may be a pleural rub. Early and late in the disease process there may also be crackles and these may be the only auscultatory change in mild cases. In lobar pneumonia, the changes are localized to a lobe which means that the signs are detected either anteriorly or posteriorly but not usually both. More widespread changes suggest 'bronchopneumonia', a complication of chronic bronchitis, or 'atypical pneumonia' due to viruses, mycoplasma, and other organisms. Radiology may show an 'air bronchogram', air in the bronchi outlined by fluid in the alveoli (Fig. 6.60).

Some causes of pneumonia
Streptococcus pneumoniae
Mycoplasma pneumoniae
Haemophilus influenzae
Influenza virus
Legionella pneumophilia
Psitticosis
Q fever
Chemical (i.e. aspiration of vomit)
Radiation

Fig. 6.59 Some causes of pneumonia.

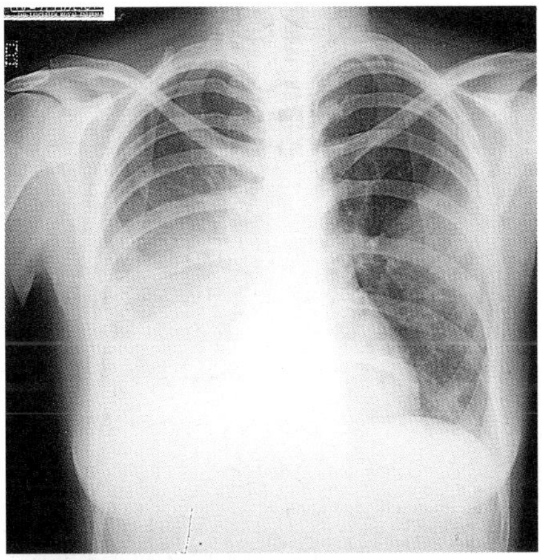

Mediastinum central
Expansion ↓
Percussion note ↓
Breath sounds bronchial
Whispering pectoriloquy
Crackles
Pleural rub

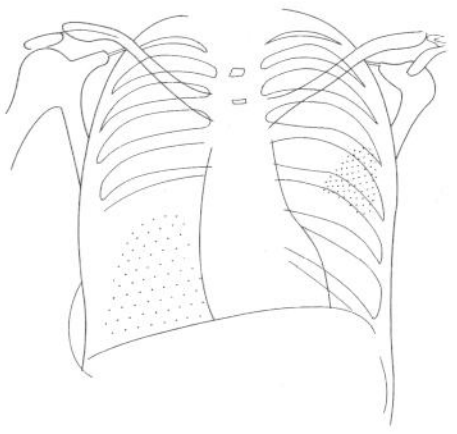

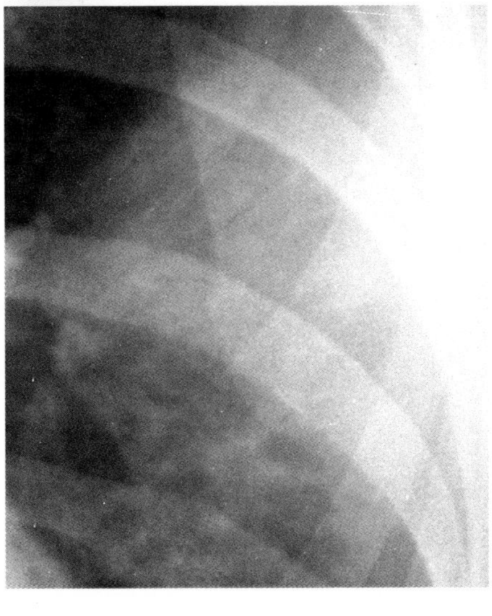

Fig. 6.60 Consolidation (unusual as it affects both lungs). Enlarged view showing air broncogram.

Pleural fluid

Whether this be from an increase in pleural transudate, pleural exudate from inflammation, blood, pus, or lymph (Fig. 6.61) the signs are the same. A large amount of fluid is needed to displace the heart and an even larger amount, filling most of the hemithorax, to displace the trachea. The displacement is away from the fluid. Expansion is diminished on the affected side, vocal fremitus is reduced, percussion note is markedly reduced –'stony dullness' – and breath sounds are absent or markedly reduced. Bronchial breathing and a rub may be heard at the upper level of the effusion. An effusion, if large enough, is detected both anteriorly and posteriorly (Figs 6.62 and 6.63).

Some causes of pleural fluid
Transudates
Congestive cardiac failure Cirrhosis Nephrotic syndrome
Exudates
Tumors – primary, secondary, and lymphomas Pneumonia Tuberculosis Rheumatoid arthritis and other connective tissue disease Pulmonary embolism and infarction
Blood
Trauma Pulmonary embolism Tumors
Pus
Pneumonia Trauma
Lymph
Tumours, especially lymphomas

Fig. 6.61 Some causes of pleural fluid.

Pneumothorax

The pressure in the pleural space is normally negative with respect to atmospheric pressure. In a pneumothorax the affected side is at a higher pressure, i.e. less negative. This pressure tends to displace the mediastinum to the opposite side and if there is a flap valve effect producing a tension pneumothorax, this can be extreme and dangerous. The affected side moves less well, vocal fremitus is reduced, and the percussion note is normal. The expected increased resonance can be difficult to detect and it is the conjunction of diminished breath sounds with a normal percussion note that distinguishes it from other causes of diminished breath sounds when there is also dullness to percussion. Vocal resonance is reduced and there are no added sounds. (Fig. 6.64). Some causes of pneumothorax are given in Figure 6.65.

Chronic airflow limitation

This term covers the entities of chronic obstructive bronchitis, emphysema, and asthma which are not always readily distinguishable. There may be hyperinflation of the chest, pursed lip breathing, and use of accessory muscles of respiration. Expansion may well be reduced but usually equally so. The mediastinum is not displaced. Vocal fremitus is normal, percussion is usually normal, but there may be increased resonance and reduced hepatic and cardiac dullness. Breath sounds are vesicular and sometimes reduced, presumably from low flow rates; the added sounds are wheezes and often crackles. The radiograph is usually normal, but sometimes shows overinflation with low flat diaphragms (Fig. 6.66).

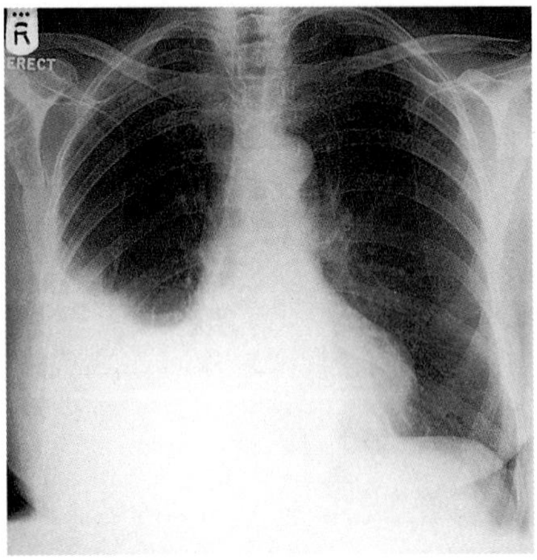

Mediastinum usually central

Expansion ↓

Percussion ↓

Breath sounds ↓

Sometimes bronchial breathing or a pleural rub at upper level

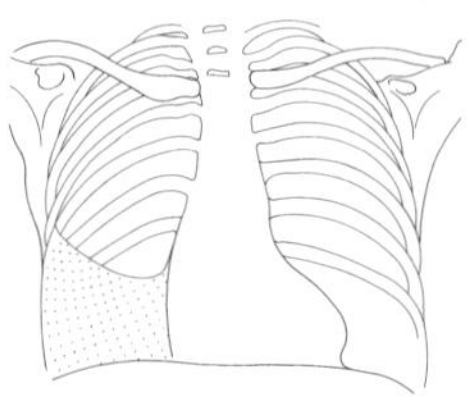

Fig. 6.62 Small effusion.

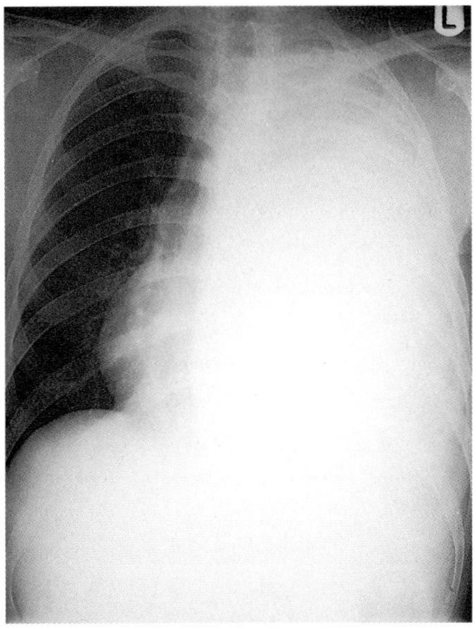

Mediastinum displaced

Expansion ↓

Percussion ↓

Breath sounds ↓

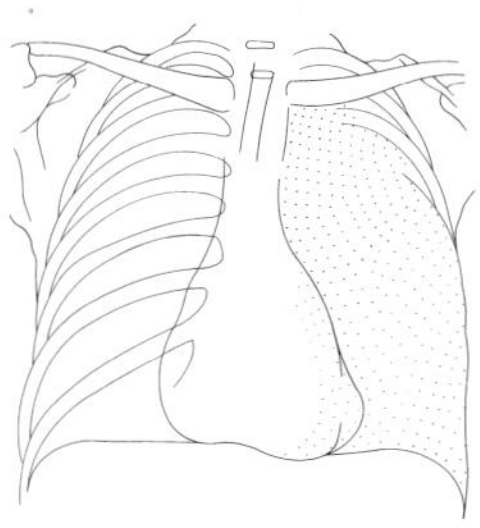

Fig. 6.63 Large effusion with mediastinal displacement.

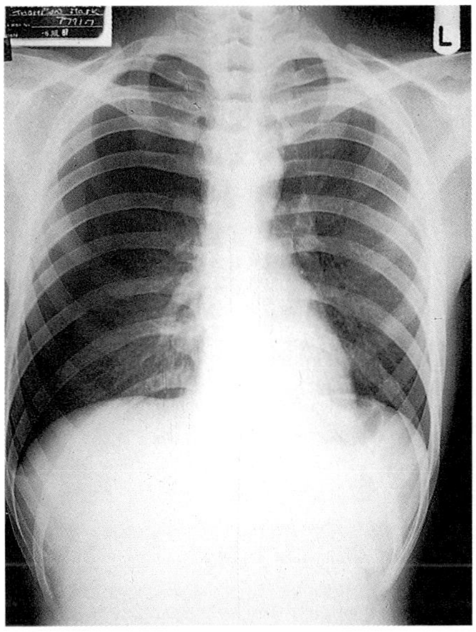

Mediastinum sometimes displaced

Expansion ↓

Percussion normal or ↑

Breath sounds ↓

No added sounds

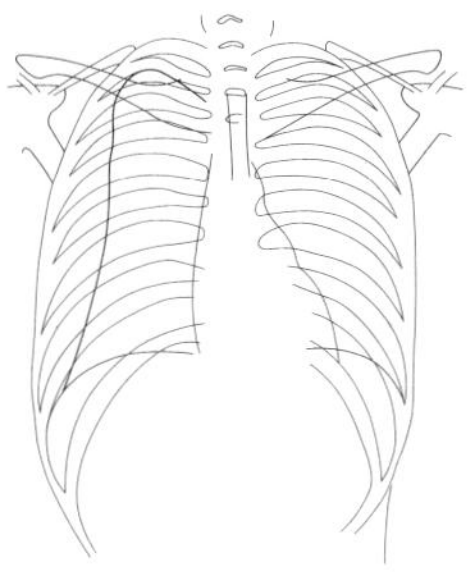

Fig. 6.64 Pneumothorax on right.

Lung and lobar collapse

The usual cause is a central bronchial carcinoma, although a foreign body has the same effect. If the lung or lobe is not ventilated the air within it is absorbed by the blood and the lung collapses. If the whole lung is involved then the degree of collapse is limited by the capacity of the chest to shrink, but if a lobe is involved then the other lobe can fill the space and the affected lung may come to occupy only a very small area. Lung collapse can also follow infection; tuberculosis and bronchiectasis are good examples. Here the airways remain open.

On examination there is diminished movement on the affected side, with the mediastinum deviating to that side. Percussion note is reduced but can be difficult to detect if only a lobe is involved and has shrunk to a small space; breath sounds are diminished but

Some causes of pneumothorax
No cause found
Apical blebs
Chronic bronchitis and emphysemsa
Staphlococcal pneumonia
Asthma
Tuberculosis
Cystic fibrosis
Trauma

Fig. 6.65 Some causes of pneumothorax.

generally remain vesicular. Vocal resonance is decreased. As indicated above, bronchial breathing, increased vocal resonance, and whispering pectoriloquy can be heard in upper lobe collapse because of direct transmission of sound from the trachea. Bronchial breathing is also heard in collapse of other lobes if the airways remain patent (Fig. 6.67). Crackles and wheeze may be present if the cause is damage from an old infection.

Lung fibrosis

This may be the end result of many lung conditions and minor degrees are undetectable clinically. Localized changes produce similar signs to lung collapse. Generalized disease is best illustrated by cryptogenic fibrosing alveolitis. The lungs are stiff, expansion may be reduced, but equally, and the mediastinum is central. Vocal fremitus is normal, percussion note is normal, or slightly reduced, breath sounds are vesicular though occasionally bronchial, yet there are marked crackles initially confined to the bases but later extending up the chest (Fig. 6.68).

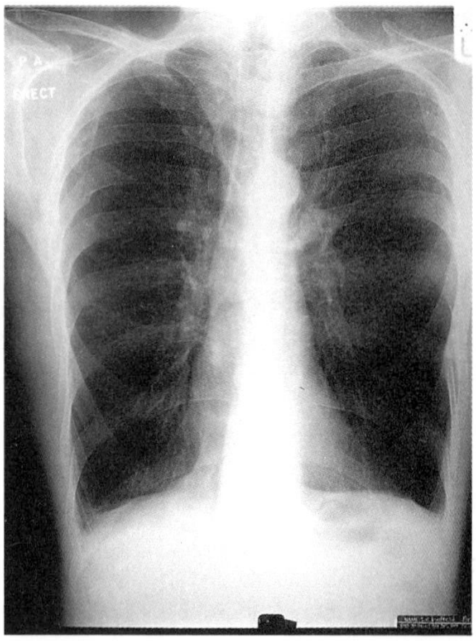

Hyperinflation

Mediastinum central

Hepatic and cardiac dullness ↓

Vesicular breath sounds

Wheezes and crackles

Radiograph often normal but here shows overinflation and low flat diaphragms

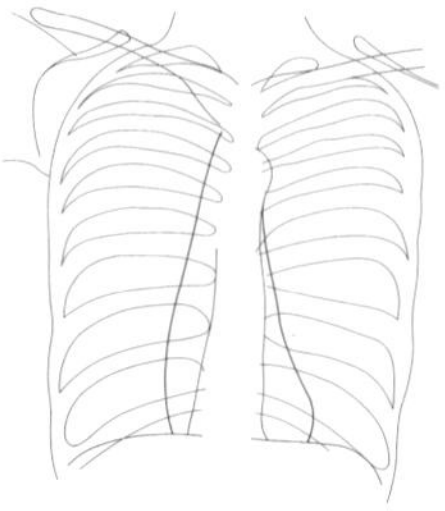

Fig. 6.66 Chronic airflow limitation. Radiograph often normal but here shows overinflation and low flat diaphragms.

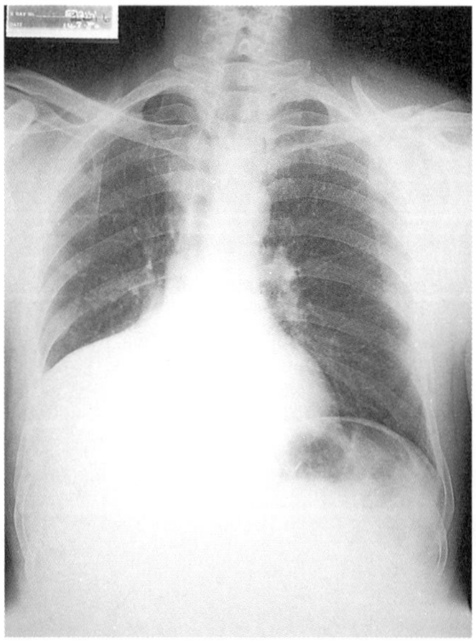

Mediastinum displaced

Expansion reduced

Percussion normal or ↓

Breath sounds vesicular but ↓

or sometimes bronchial

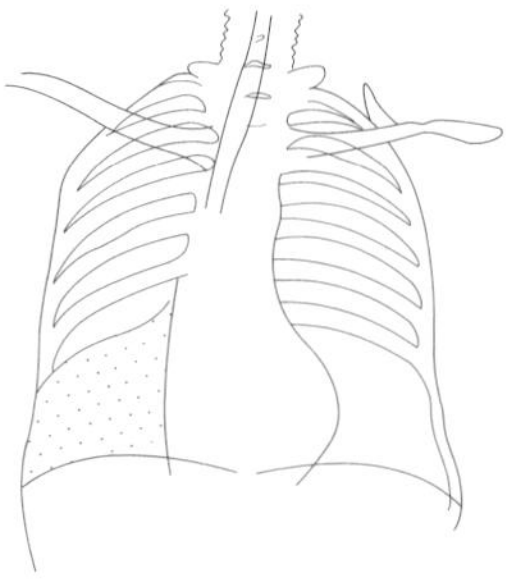

Fig. 6.67 Collapse of the right middle and right lower lobes.

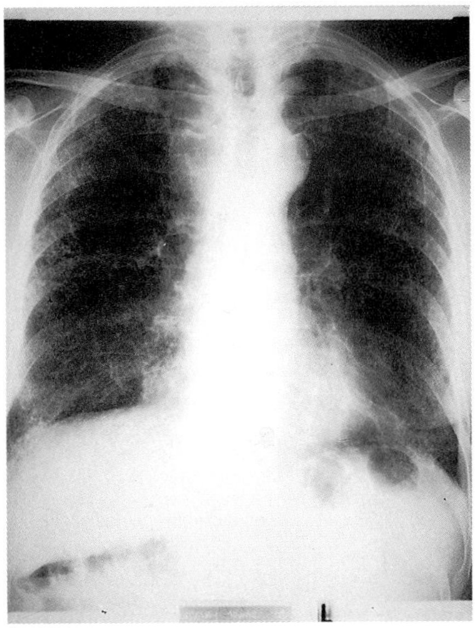

Mediastinum central

Expansion equally ↓

Percussion normal or ↓

Breath sounds vesicular (occasionally bronchial)

Crackles

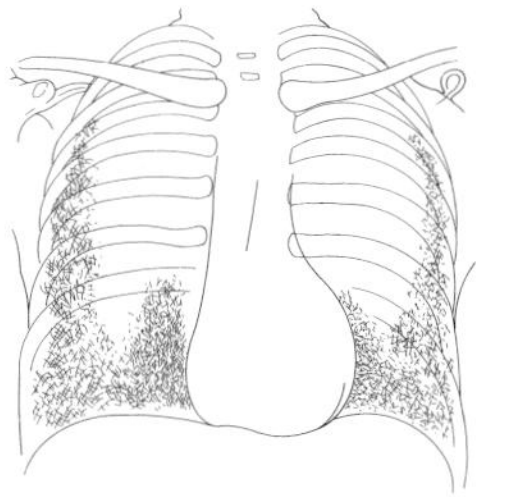

Fig. 6.68 Lung fibrosis.

THE HEART AND CARDIOVASCULAR SYSTEM

7

The cardiovascular system is fundamental to the functioning of almost every other organ system. Despite the availability of many sophisticated imaging techniques which will be discussed later, the fundamental simplicity and accessibility of the structure and function of the heart and vascular system make its physical examination both important and extremely rewarding.

STRUCTURE AND FUNCTION

The adult heart (Fig. 7.1) consists of two pumps working in series. The 'right heart' comprising the right atrium, tricuspid valve, right ventricle, pulmonary valve, and pulmonary artery is a low pressure pump receiving blood from the systemic veins pumping it to

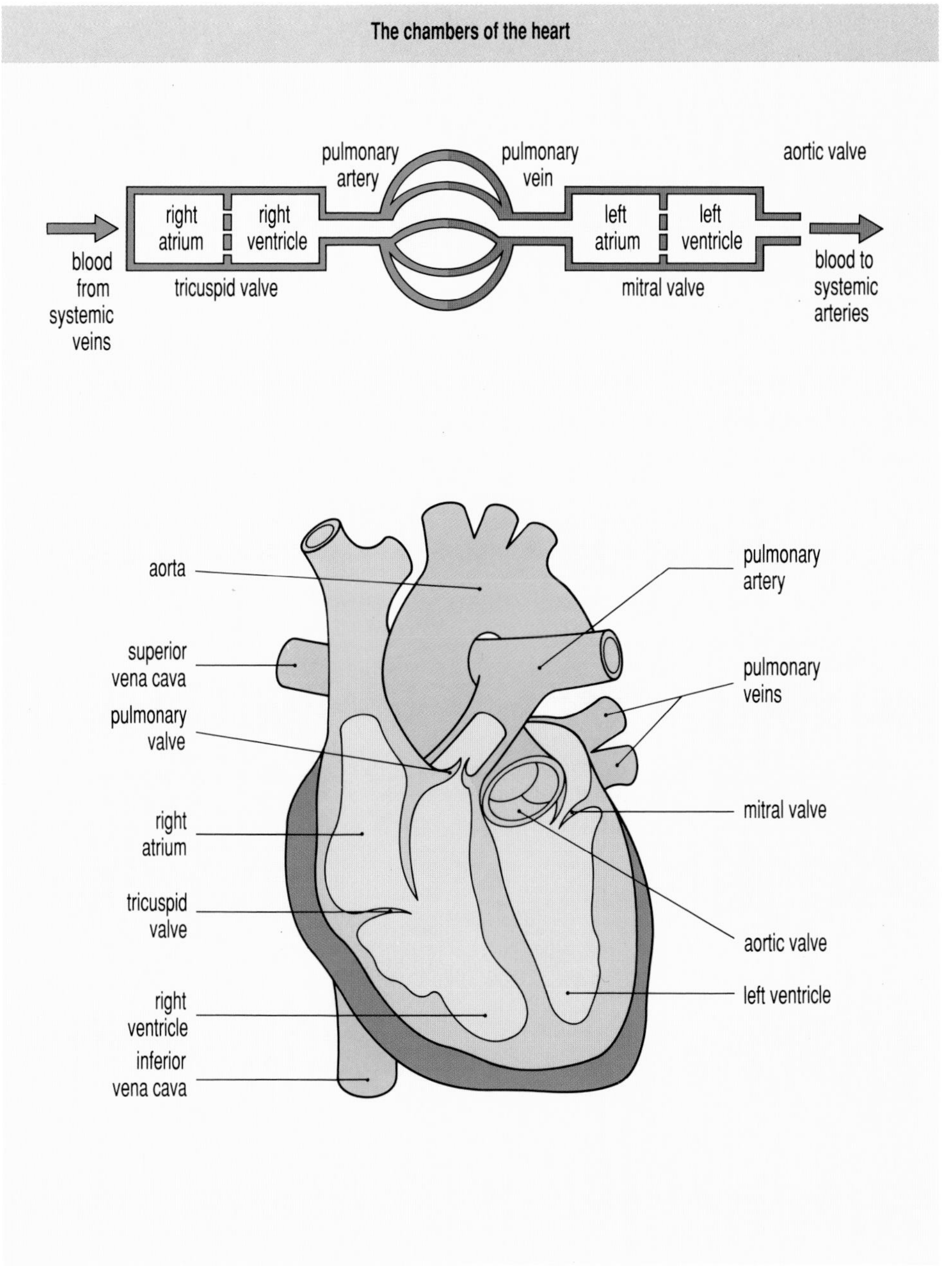

Fig. 7.1 Arrangement of the heart chambers as a 'flow diagram' (above) and in their approximate anatomical positions (below).

the lungs. The left heart comprising the left atrium, mitral valve, left ventricle, aortic valve, and aorta is a high pressure pump receiving blood from the lungs and pumping it round the body. In the early embryo, the heart forms as a simple tube down the midline of the body. As the embryo grows, the tube elongates more rapidly than the tissues around it and thus develops a loop and a twist. It also becomes divided into left and right chambers by the growth of a septum down the middle. In the ninth week of gestation, the foetal heart rotates in a clockwise direction until the right ventricle comes to rest anteriorly behind the sternum. Most of the

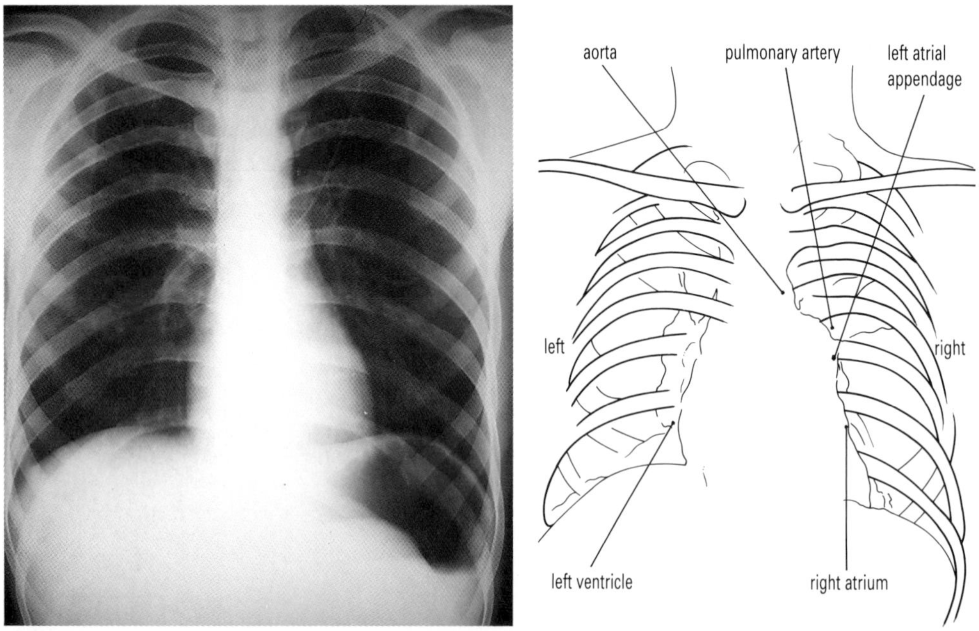

Fig. 7.2 Most of the anterior surface of the heart is in fact formed by the right ventricle and pulmonary artery. The tip of the left ventricle and the left atrial appendage also appears on the left border of the heart.

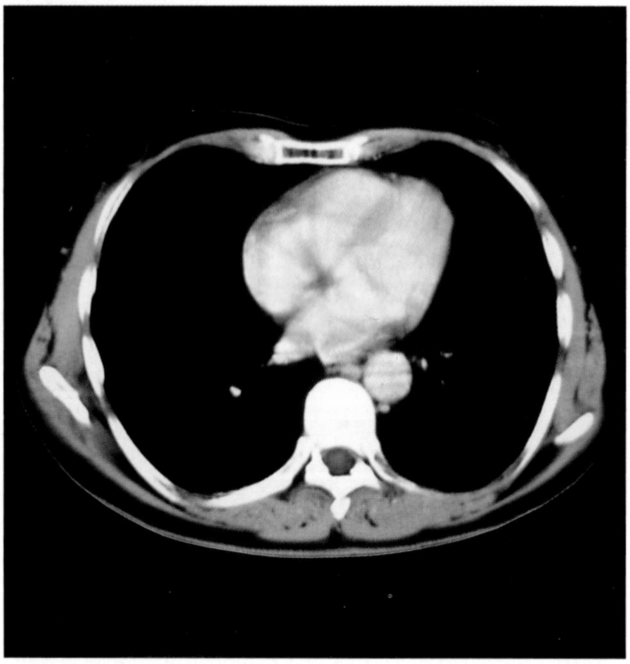

Fig. 7.3 Computerized tomography. CT scan of the heart to show the way the heart lies within the chest cavity.

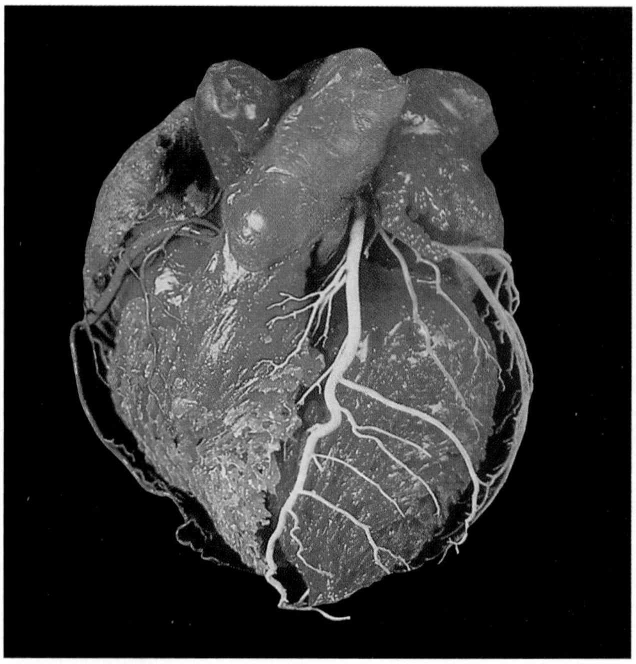

Fig. 7.4 A 'corrosion cast' of the chambers of the heart, made by filling the chambers with wax or plastic and dissolving away the muscle.

left ventricle comes to lie posteriorly apart from a small portion of left ventricular muscle which forms the left heart border when seen from the front and the extreme tip or apex of the heart (Fig. 7.2). The way the heart is situated within the chest cavity is also well shown on the computerized tomographic X-ray scan of the chest shown in Figure 7.3. Note that the heart lies obliquely in the chest and that its long axis, the planes of the interatrial and interventricular septum, and the planes of the various valves are not aligned with any of the conventional anatomic planes. The chambers of the heart can be examined after death by injecting wax or plastic and dissolving away the muscle (Fig. 7.4). They can also be examined during life by injecting radio-opaque dye through catheters placed in the various chambers of the heart and taking cine X-ray pictures. By tilting the X-ray tube and image detector appropriately, it is possible to obtain detailed pictures of the full extent of the ventricular cavities (Fig. 7.5).

HEART MUSCLE

The ventricles

Heart muscle or myocardium is a special type of muscle which is extremely resistant to fatigue. Because of the higher pressures which it normally generates, the wall of the left ventricle is much thicker than the wall of the right ventricle. In a section taken through both ventricles, left ventricular myocardium, including the intra-ventricular septum, has a roughly circular outline with the right ventricle appearing to be wrapped around one side of it (Fig. 7.6). The muscle fibres of the heart are arranged in a complicated spiral arrangement so that when they contract (systole) not only is blood forced out of the ventricles, but the heart also elongates and rotates on the fixed base provided by the attachment of the major blood vessels. It is this movement which is felt as the beating of the heart by a hand placed on the chest. The heart normally lies in its own serous cavity, the pericardium, which allows it to move without friction. Apart from moving with each heart beat, the position of the pericardium and the heart can be altered by the phase of respiration, or by rolling from one side to the other.

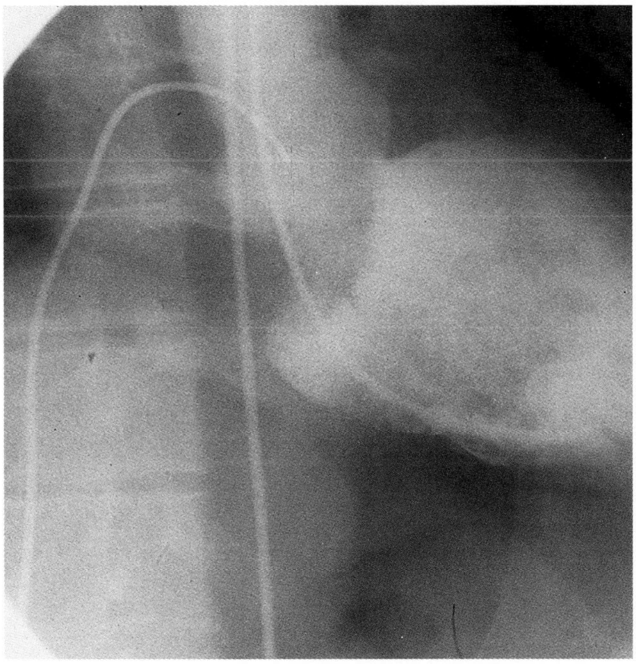

Fig. 7.5 Left ventricular cine-angiogram made by injecting radio-opaque dye into the heart through a catheter passed via the femoral artery and aorta. The X-ray tube and image intensifier are tilted into the 'right anterior oblique' positions to outline the full extent of the left ventricle.

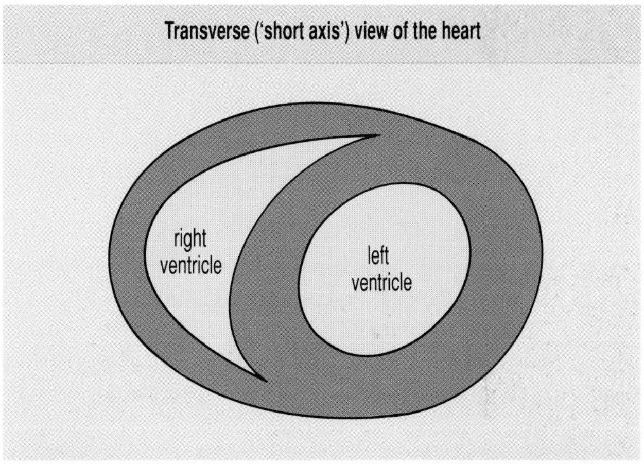

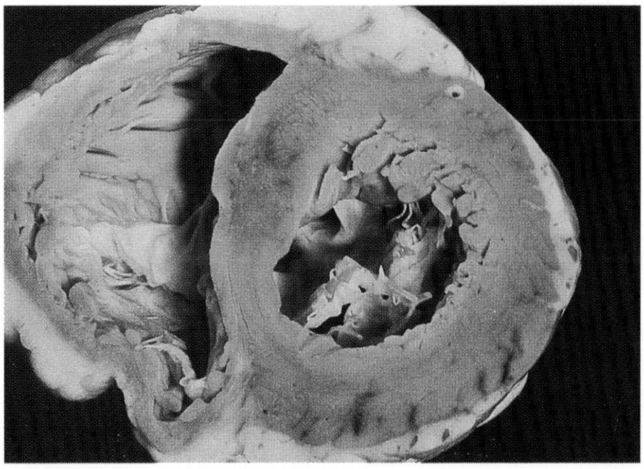

Fig. 7.6 'Short axis' view of the heart. In the short axis or transverse section, the thinner (low pressure) right ventricle is 'wrapped around' the left ventricle.

The atria

The atria of the heart are also muscular but are much thinner walled than the ventricles (Fig. 7.7). They contract a fraction of a second before the ventricles, and in doing so, they assist in the filling of the ventricles particularly when there is a need for increased cardiac output. Patients in whom, as a result of disease, the atria are paralyzed or are beating out of synchrony with the ventricles are usually comfortable at rest but may become short of breath on exercise.

Cardiac hypertrophy and dilatation

Like any muscle, cardiac muscle responds to an increased workload by growth. The heart responds in different ways to pressure load and volume load. Pressure load is caused by an increased resistance to ejection of blood from the heart (Fig. 7.8). The response to pressure load is cardiac hypertrophy, initially without dilatation of the chamber involved. Thus, for example, in aortic stenosis the left ventricular wall becomes excessively thickened, but the left ventricular cavity remains of normal size. Eventually, when the pressure load is extreme, or growth of the heart muscle has outstripped its blood supply, failure of the muscle occurs and the cavity begins to enlarge.

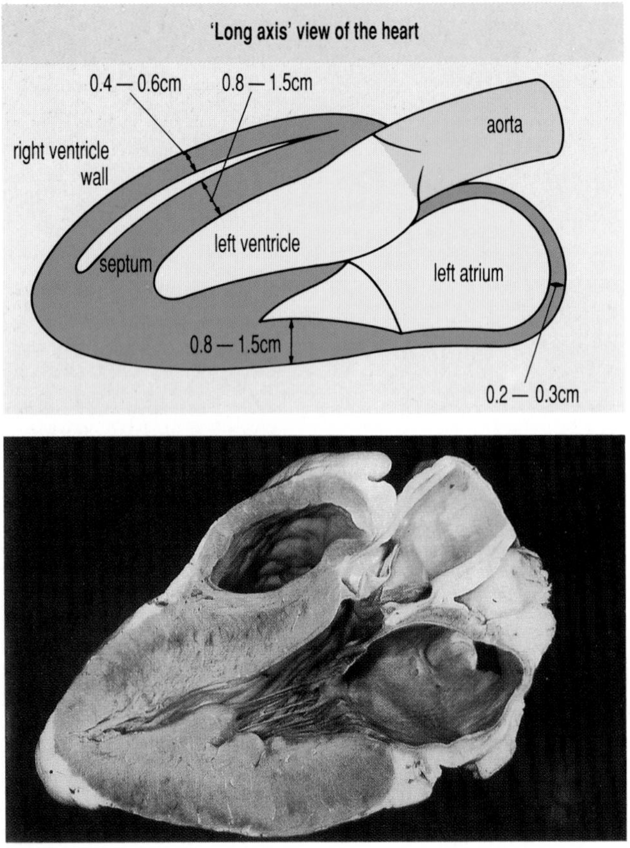

Fig. 7.7 To show the relative thickness of muscle in different parts of the heart.

The heart responds to a volume load, for example, a leaking mitral or aortic valve, or an arterior venous fistula, or left to right shunt by both hypertrophy of the myocardium and also dilatation of the chamber involved. This is to accompany the increased stroke volume which is required to deal with the volume load. The chest X-ray shows cardiac enlargement (Fig. 7.9) and this is also found on echocardiography. Both hypertrophy and dilatation produce characteristic ECG changes, and it is possible to identify the cardiac chamber involved from the ECG appearances.

HEART VALVES

There are four heart valves which fall anatomically and functionally into two groups: the atrioventricular valves and the outflow or 'semilunar' valves. The tricuspid and mitral separate right atrium and right ventricle and left atrium and left ventricle, respectively. Both develop from the endocardial cushions of the embryonic heart and are composed of thin flexible leaflets which are prevented from prolapsing back into the atrium when the ventricle contracts by being attached via chordae tendineae to specialized portions of

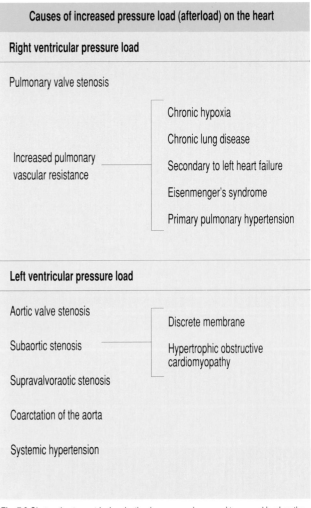

Causes of increased pressure load (afterload) on the heart

Right ventricular pressure load	
Pulmonary valve stenosis	
Increased pulmonary vascular resistance	Chronic hypoxia
	Chronic lung disease
	Secondary to left heart failure
	Eisenmenger's syndrome
	Primary pulmonary hypertension
Left ventricular pressure load	
Aortic valve stenosis	
Subaortic stenosis	Discrete membrane
	Hypertrophic obstructive cardiomyopathy
Supravalvoraotic stenosis	
Coarctation of the aorta	
Systemic hypertension	

Fig. 7.8 Obstruction to ventricular ejection imposes an increased 'pressure' load on the heart.

ventricular muscle, the papillary muscles (Fig. 7.10). The hydrodynamic efficiency of the mitral and tricuspid valves is very high. Their pliable edges smoothes out eddies and turbulence in blood flow and allow the rapid transfer of blood from atrium to ventricle with a very small pressure differential. The aortic and pulmonary valves develop from two spiral ridges which divide the single great vessel leaving the embryonic heart into aortic and pulmonary trunks. Each normally has three cusps whose arrangement reflect their embryonic origin (Fig. 7.11). Because each cusp is shaped like a half moon, they are sometimes called the semilumar valves.

HEART SOUNDS

Closure of the heart valves at different stages of the cardiac cycle gives rise to sounds which are readily audible through a stethoscope. The sounds are normally described as 'lub-dup' . The first heart sound (lub) is due to the closure of the mitral and tricuspid valves, and the second heart sound, the rather higher pitched (dup) is due to the closure of aortic and pulmonary valves. The relationship between the heart sound, the electrocardiogram, and the arterial pulse wave is shown in Figure 7.12. In children or in young

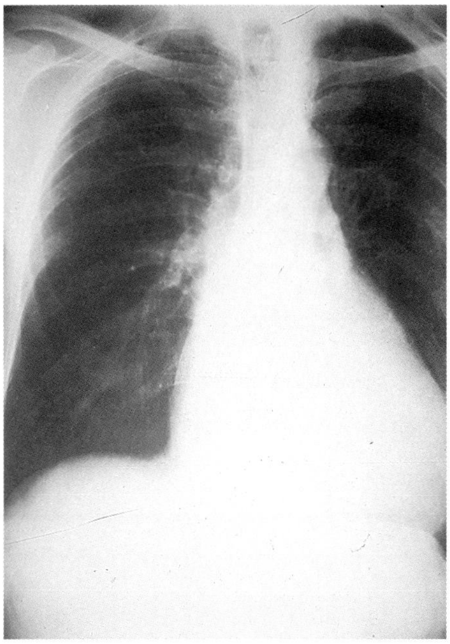

Fig. 7.9 Chest radiograph showing cardiac enlargement in response to a volume load chronic mitral regurgitation. (Compare with Fig. 7.2.)

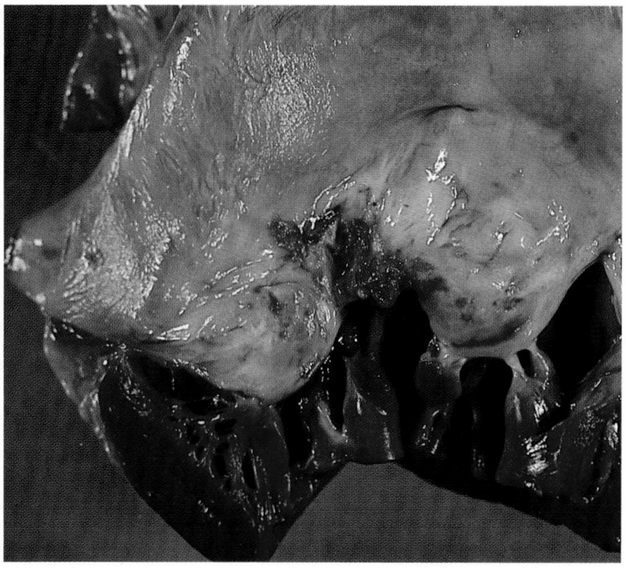

Fig. 7.10 Postmortem specimen showing attachment of valve cusps to papillary muscles via chordae tendineae.

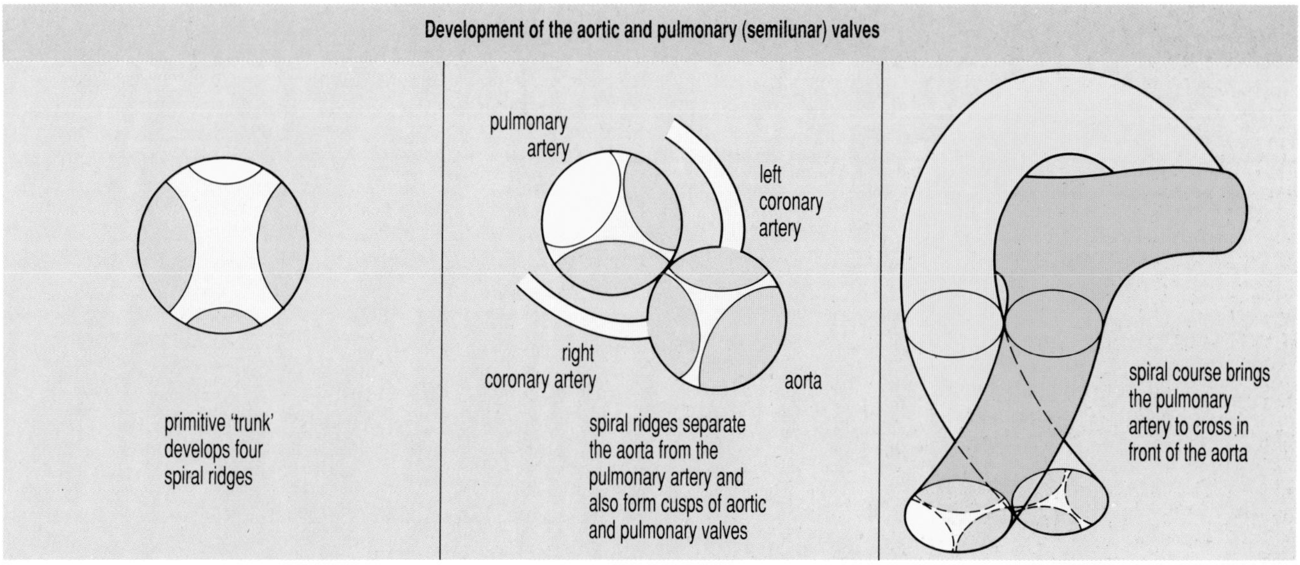
Development of the aortic and pulmonary (semilunar) valves
primitive 'trunk' develops four spiral ridges
pulmonary artery
left coronary artery
right coronary artery
aorta
spiral ridges separate the aorta from the pulmonary artery and also form cusps of aortic and pulmonary valves
spiral course brings the pulmonary artery to cross in front of the aorta

Fig. 7.11 The common 'great vessel' of the foetal heart is divided into aorta and pulmonary artery by the growth of the spiral ridges

adults, the second heart sound splits into two components during inspiration ('lub da-dup') and comes together again in expiration. This physiological splitting of the second heart sound is due to minor changes in the stroke volume of left and right ventricles during the normal respiratory cycle.

During inspiration, venous return to the right side of the heart is increased, thus increasing right ventricular stroke volume and delaying closure of the pulmonary valve. At the same time, pooling of blood in the pulmonary veins reduces filling of the left ventricle and makes aortic valve closure slightly earlier than in expiration. The split may be widened by other factors which delay right ventricular contraction, such as right bundle branch block or pulmonary valve stenosis. Conversely, anything which delays left ventricular contraction such as left bundle branch block or hypertrophic obstructive cardiomyopathy may so delay the aortic component of the second heart sound that the normal relationship is reversed and there is increasing splitting of the second heart sound on expiration with the sounds coming together on inspiration. Finally, in atrial septal defect there is characteristically fixed splitting of the second heart sound because the hole in the intra atrial septum means that left and right atrial pressure remains equal throughout the respiratory cycle (Fig. 7.13).

THE ELECTRICAL ACTIVITY OF THE HEART

The signal for contraction of each heart muscle cell is the electrical depolarization of its membrance. The electrical signal is transmitted from cell to cell in an orderly way so that under normal circumstances, the heart contracts in an orderly fashion. The physiological cardiac pacemaker is a small group of cells in the sino-atrial node situated close to where the right atrium joins the superior vena cava. These cells normally undergo cyclical repolarization and depolarization at a faster rate than cells in other parts of the heart. The electrical impulse spreads out from the sino-atrial node (Fig. 7.14) through the cardiac muscle of the atria. The atria and the ventricles are separated by a fibrous ring of tissue to which the tricuspid and mitral valves are attached and which does not support conduction of the cardiac impulse. The only way through this ring is normally through the atrioventricular node, a small area of specialized conducting tissue lying between the tricuspid valve and the aorta. There is normally a delay of 0.12–0.20 seconds while the impulse passes through the atrioventricular node, ensuring the correct delay between atrial and ventricular contraction. Once through, the atrioventricular node electrical impulse is rapidly conducted to ventricular tissue through specialized conducting fibres which form the bundle of His and its branches.

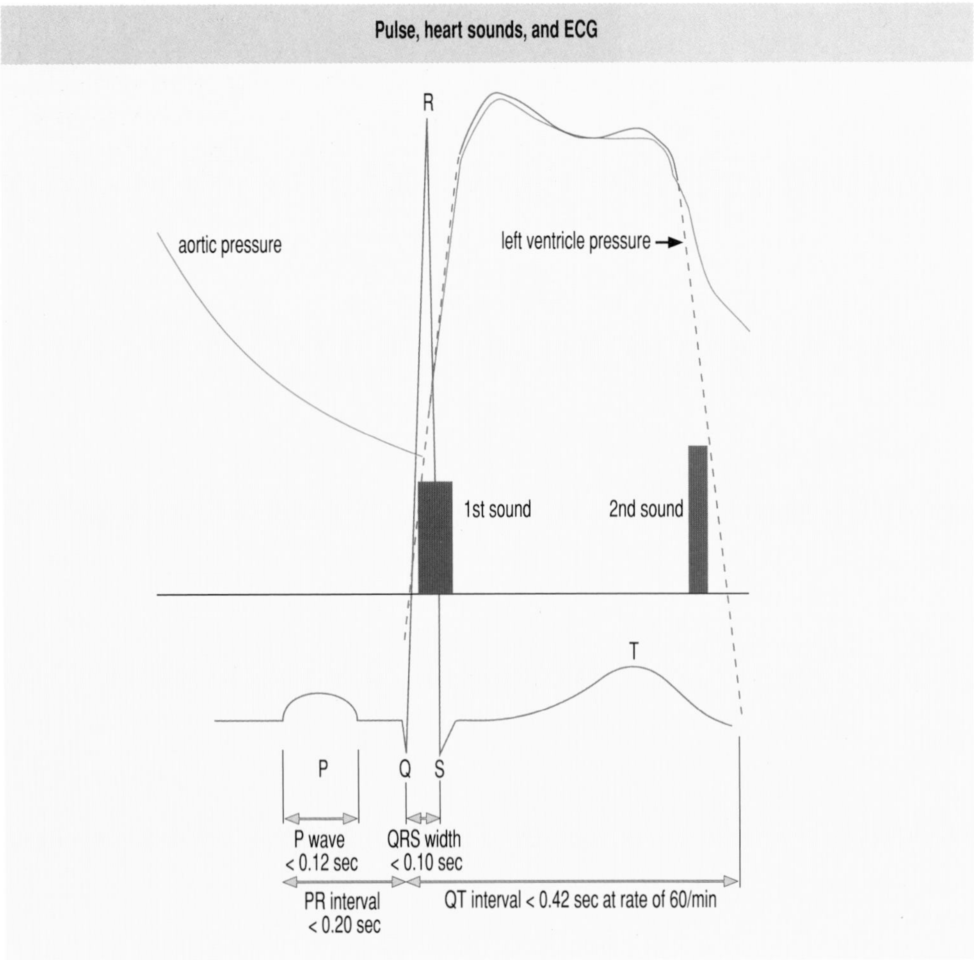

Fig. 7.12 Relationship between heart sounds, electrocardiogram, and arterial pulse.

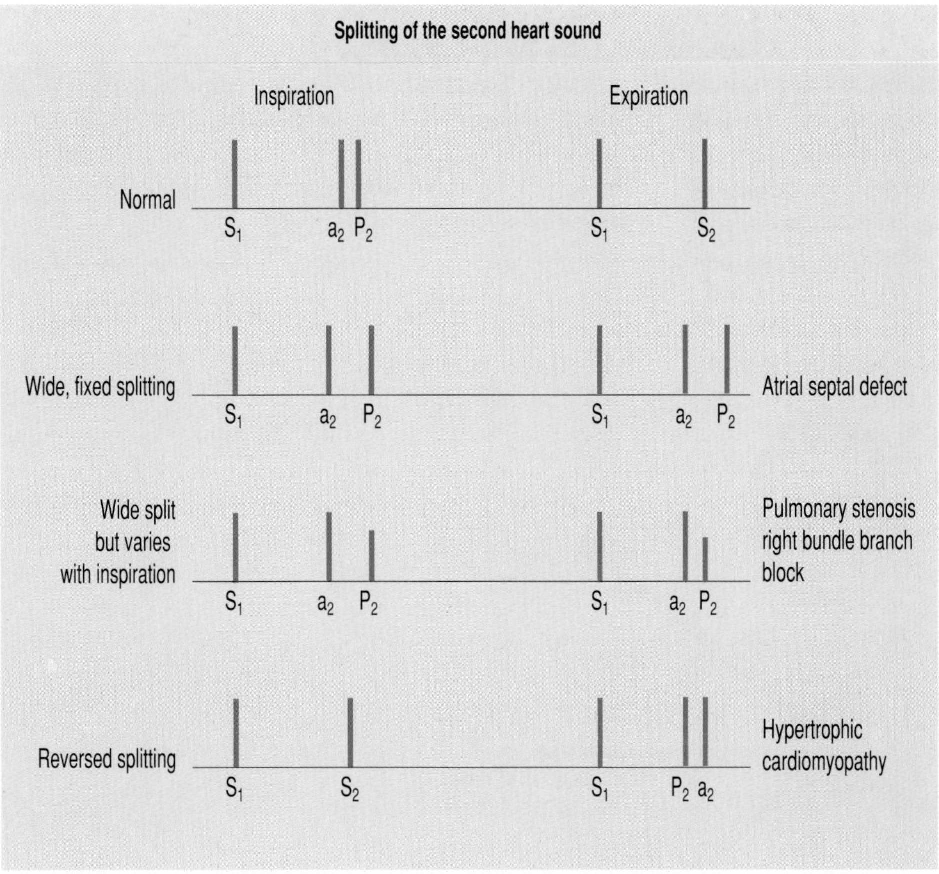

Fig. 7.13 Beat to beat variations in left and right ventricular stroke volume cause splitting of the second heart sound in phase with breathing. Splitting of the second sound inspiration is normal. Other patterns may indicate cardiac abnormalities.

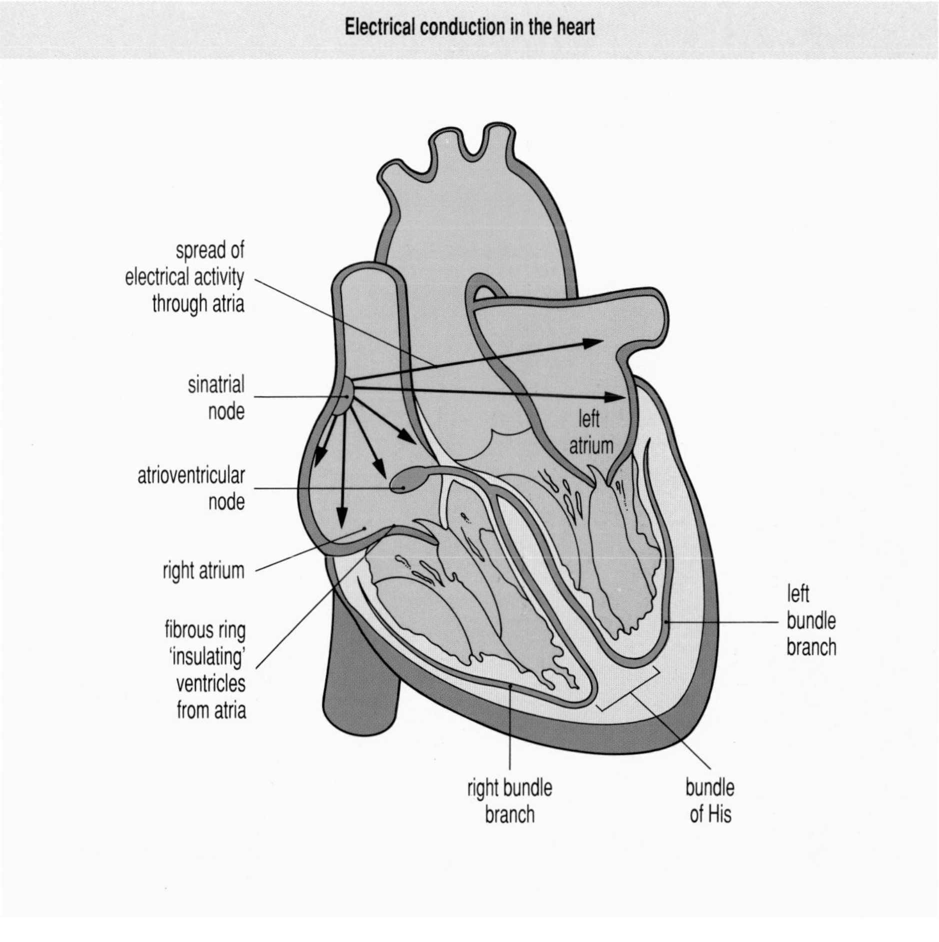

Fig. 7.14 The paths of the spread of electrical impulses in the heart. (Note that there are no specific electrical pathways in the atria.)

THE ELECTROCARDIOGRAM

The electrocardiogram is an invaluable aid to studying heart rhythm. It works by picking up and amplifying the very small electrical potential changes between different points on the surface of the body caused by the cyclical depolarization and repolarization of the heart cells. Electrical potentials are picked up by electrodes which are attached to the skin. The points at which the electrodes are attached and the conventional ways in which they are connected enables the electrocardiogram to 'look at' the heart from a series of different directions (Fig. 7.15). The cycle of electrical changes during a single heart beat is termed an ECG complex. Different parts of the ECG complex reflect the activation of different parts of the heart. The p-wave indicates atrial activity; the QRS complex indicates ventricular activity (Fig. 7.16).

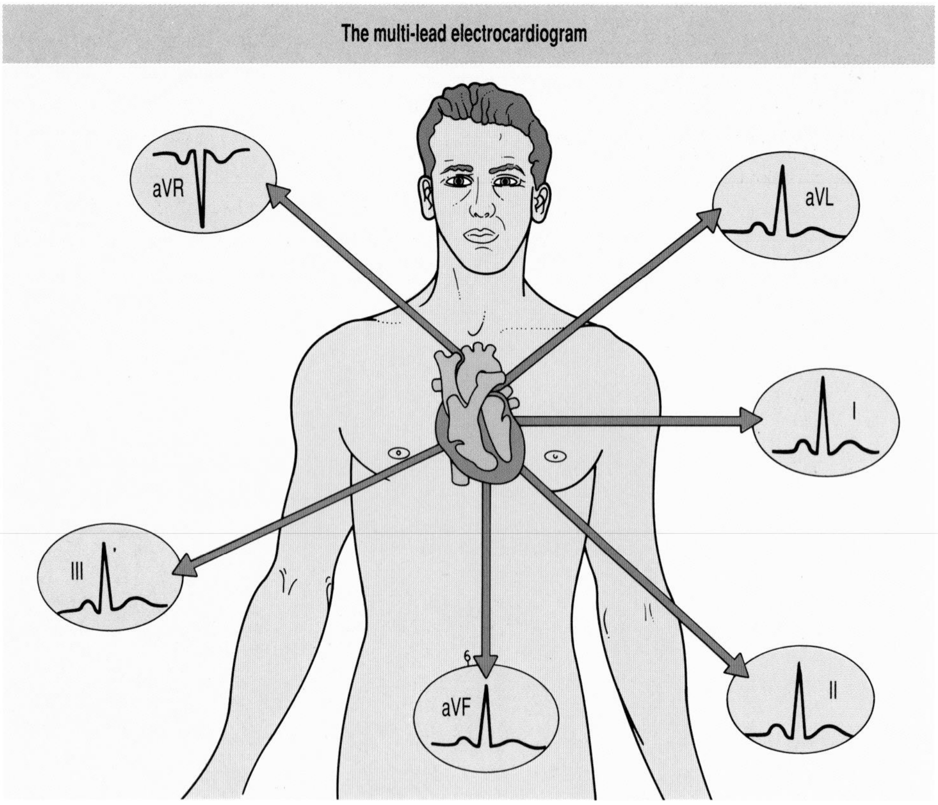

Fig. 7.15 How the electrocardiogram 'looks at' the heart from different directions (a concept due to Goldberger and Wilson).

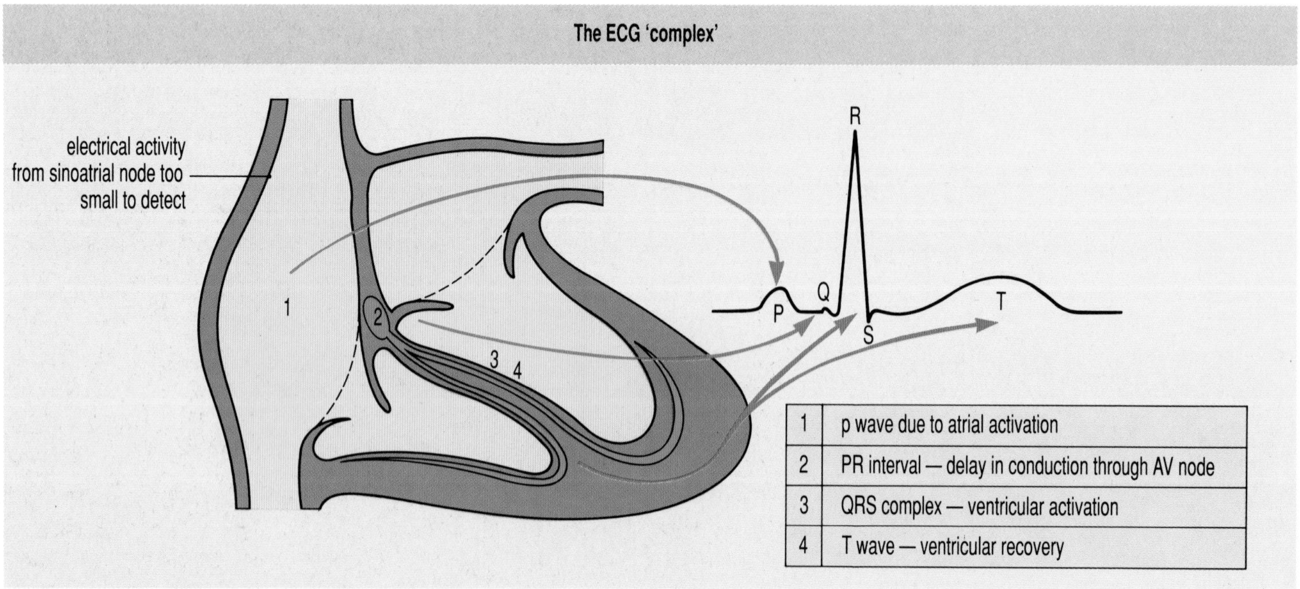

Fig. 7.16 The different parts of an electrocardiographic 'complex'.

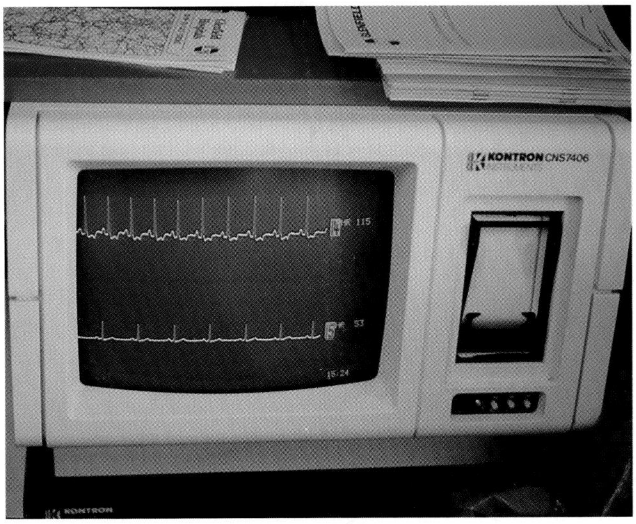

Fig. 7.17 Electrocardiogram trace displayed on monitor at nursing station or bedside.

In patients suspected of intermittent arrhythmias, the electrocardiogram may be displayed as a continuous monitor trace (Fig. 7.17). In patients outside hospital, the electrocardiogram can be recorded continuously on magnetic tape for periods of 24–48 hours and then played back to analyze any rhythm disturbances. This process is sometimes called 'Holter monitoring'. The ECG can be used to detect hypertrophy of the different chambers of the heart (Fig. 7.18), to detect abnormal rhythms, or to detect cardiac damage.

CARDIAC ARRHYTHMIAS

Abnormalities of heart rhythm can be divided into those where the heart goes too slowly (bradycardia) and those where the rate is abnormally rapid (tachycardia). Physiologically, heart rate can vary in a normal young adult from 40 beats per minute during sleep to 180 beats per minute or more during vigorous exercise.

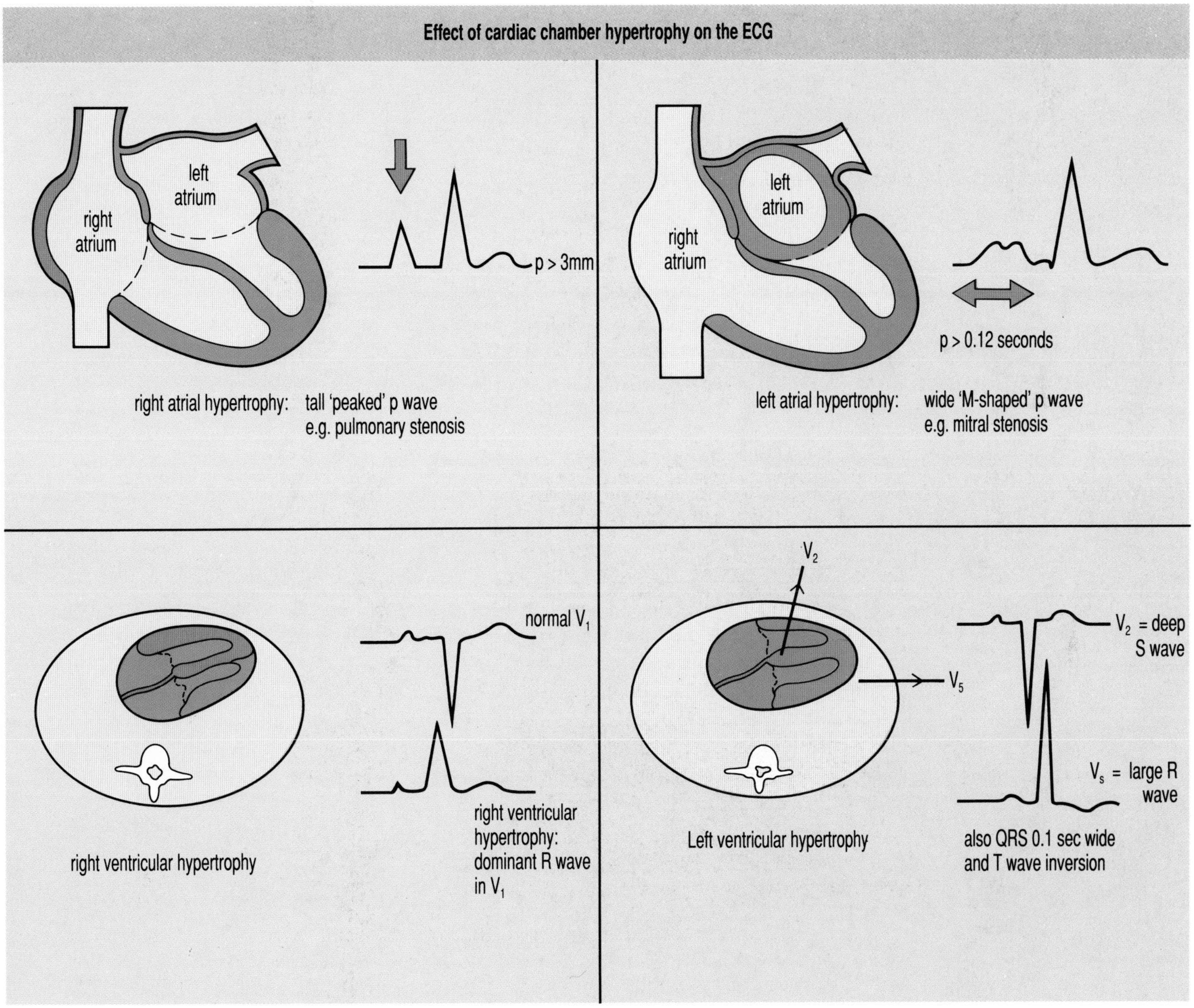

Fig. 7.18 Electrocardiographic changes can be used to identify hypertrophy of the cardiac chambers.

The physiological control of heart rate is due to a balance between sympathetic nervous activity which speeds the heart rate and vagal activity which slows it down (Fig. 7.19).

Bradycardia

Bradycardia may be due to drugs, particularly ß-adrenoceptor blocking drugs ('beta-blockers'); moreover, it may also be a physiological finding in young athletes with a high vagal tone. Extreme bradycardia may be due to *heart block* where there is failure of conduction of the electrical impulse, usually as it passes through the atrioventricular node or bundle of His (Fig. 7.20)

Tachycardia

Ectopic beats

Because all heart muscle, and not just the sino-atrial node, retains the capacity for spontaneous depolarization, it is not uncommon to find an 'ectopic focus' of electrical activity which can initiate extra beats out of time with the normal cardiac cycle. These extra beats or extrasystoles may be generated in the atrium or in the ventricle. In otherwise healthy people, extrasystoles are usually benign and harmless; nevertheless, they may act as markers for metabolic damage and, consequently, excessive irritability of the heart muscle (e.g. following myocardial infarction or during a virus infection of the heart) (Fig. 7.21).

Sustained tachycardia

A persistent tachycardia may be caused by several ectopic beats occuring in sequence (e.g. as the manifestation of a particularly irritable ectopic focus). This is called a 'focal tachycardia'.

A more common mechanism for sustained tachycardia however, is the phenomenon of re-entry (Fig. 7.22). The basic principle of a re-entry tachycardia is that there are two alternative pathways for the conduction of the electrical impulse; these pathways differ both

Autonomic effects on the heart	
Vagal tone (slows the heart)	
Increased in children, athletes	
Stimulated by:	Carotid sinus baroreceptors, pain, trauma, (via hypothalamus). Ventricular stretch receptors (fainting reflex).
Excessive in:	Malignant vasovagal syncope Carotid sinus syncope
Blocked by:	Atropine
Sympathetic tone (speeds up the heart)	
Increased by:	Fear, pain, hypovolaemia, heart failure, physical activity
Decreased:	During sleep
Blocked by:	β-adrenoceptor

Fig. 7.19

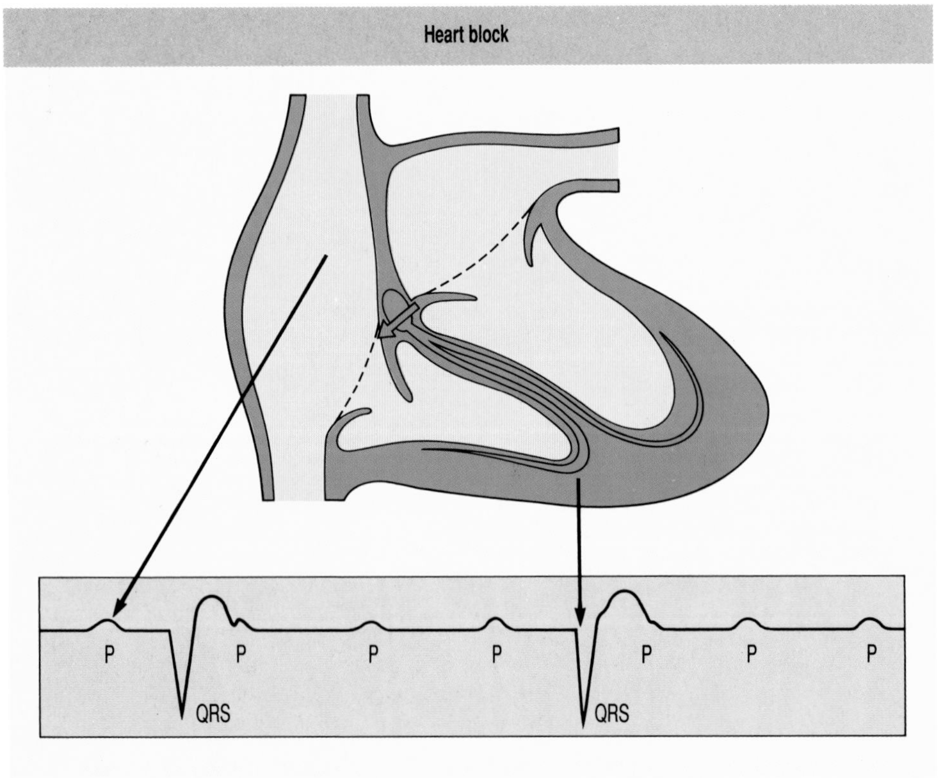

Fig. 7.20 Heart block is one cause of bradycardia: there is failure of conduction of the electrical impulses from atrium to ventricle.

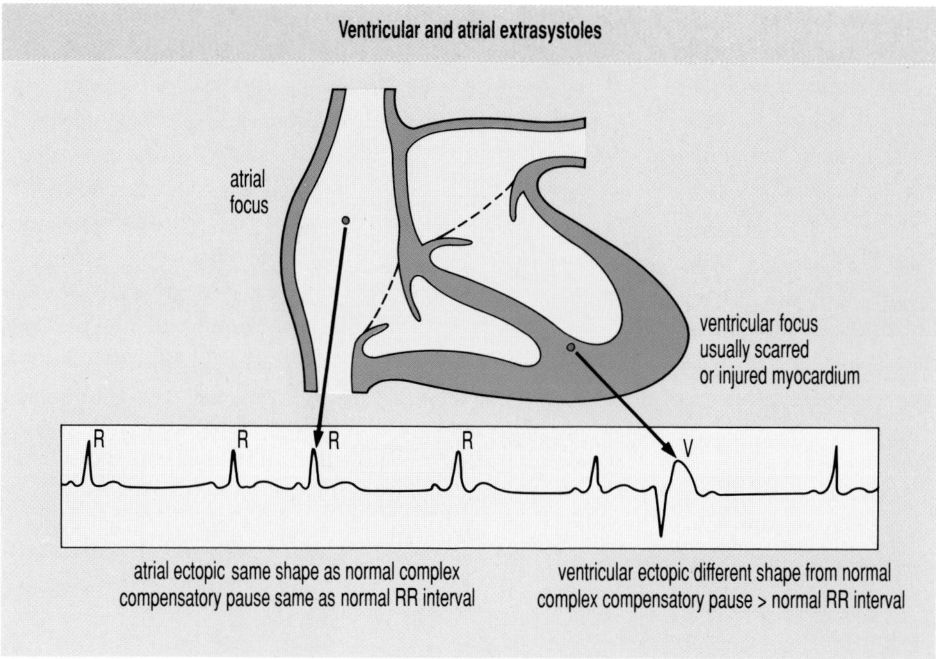

Fig. 7.21 Extrasystoles are due to an ectopic focus of electrical activity.

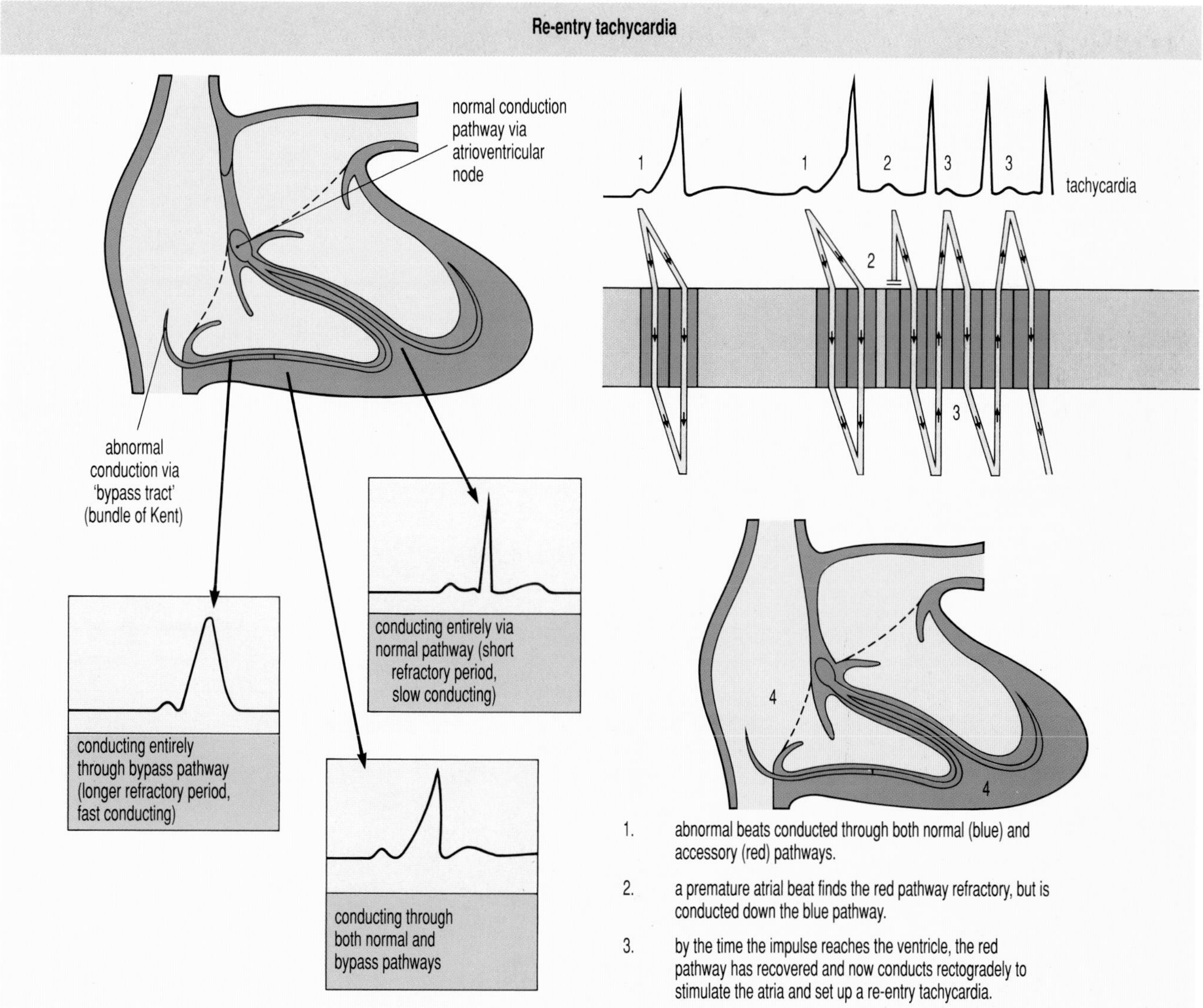

Fig. 7.22 The mechanism of a re-entry tachycardia, based on the 'paradigm' of the Wolf-Parkinson-White syndrome.

in their speed of conduction and in their refractory period. Under normal conditions, the cardiac impulse will be conducted by both pathways, but an exceptionally early beat may find one pathway still refractory to conduction and therefore be conducted down the other one alone. However, by the time it reaches the end of this pathway, the other pathway will have recovered and be able to conduct the impulse in the reverse direction. This sets up the possibility of a 'circus movement' or oscillation, and the re-entry circuit can act as a focus for generating a tachycardia. This tachycardia may continue until one of the pathways fatigues and cannot conduct fast enough to maintain the circuit or until the process is interrupted by an electrical stimulus which breaks the circuit and re-establishes normal conduction (Fig. 7.23).

Fibrillation

The most extreme form of arrhythmia occurs when the co-ordinated conduction of impulses between cells completely breaks down and individual cells contract haphazardly. This process is termed fibrillation. Atrial fibrillation is common but not particularly hazardous because the atrioventricular node acts as a filter preventing the ventricles from being stimulated at too rapid a rate. Ventricular fibrillation is, however, rapidly lethal because the ventricles are unable to pump any blood into the circulation. The only effective treatment for ventricular fibrillation is to pass a large electric current through the heart (defibrillation). This transiently wipes out all electrical activity, and allows the whole system to become reset (Fig. 7.24).

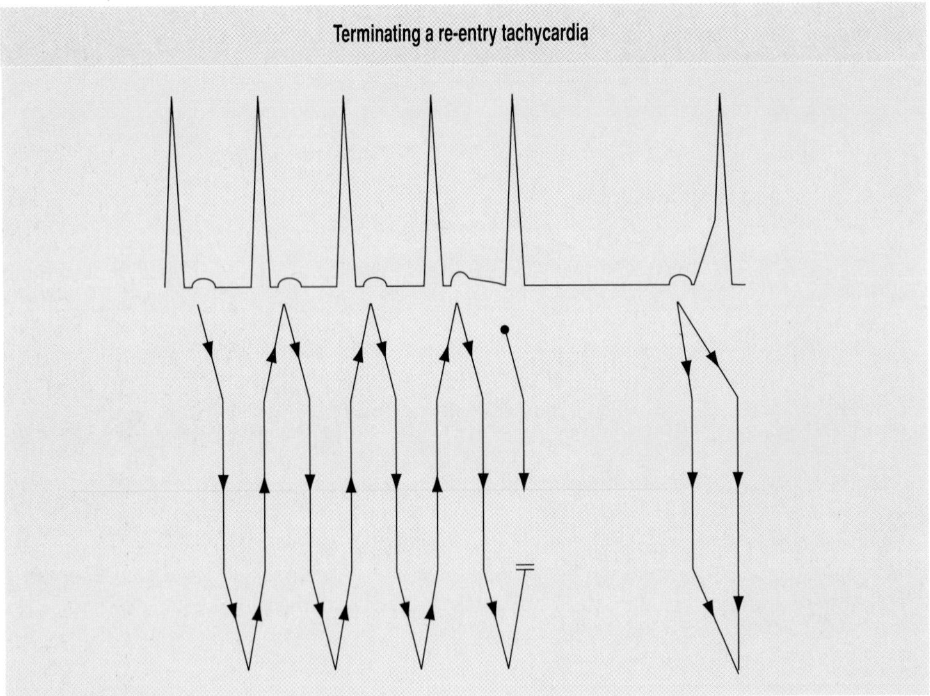

Fig. 7.23 A critically-timed extra stimulus can terminate a re-entry tachycardia by making both pathways refractory

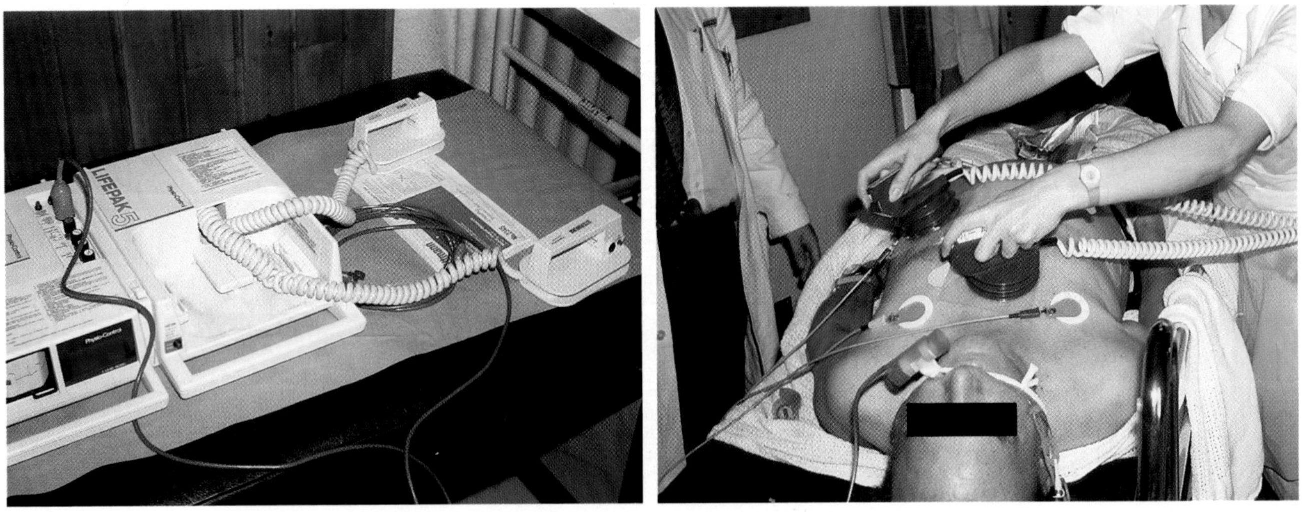

Fig. 7.24 A defibrillator (left). An electrical charge is built up within the machine and discharged through paddles applied to the patient's chest (right).

THE BLOOD SUPPLY TO THE HEART

Heart muscle needs a supply of blood to support both its basal metabolic needs and the increased oxygen requirements of exercise. The blood supply must be capable of increasing to meet the heart's demands during exercise because heart muscle, unlike skeletal muscle, can only work aerobically. The arterial blood supply to the heart is provided by the right and left coronary arteries. The right coronary artery supplies mainly the right ventricle and the inferior surface of the left ventricle. The left coronary artery divides soon after its origin into the left anterior descending coronary artery, which supplies the interventricular septum, the anterior surface and the apex of the left ventricle, and the circumflex coronary artery which supplies the lateral part of the left ventricle (Fig. 7.25).

Like other arteries in the body, coronary arteries are prone to atheroma and this in turn may lead to thrombosis which causes coronary artery obstruction. The clinical features of coronary thrombosis, and the myocardial infarction which may result, are described below.

Intracardiac shunting

In the foetus, the lungs do not participate in respiratory gas exchange (this is done by the placenta), and the unexpanded lungs offer a high resistance to blood flow. Both sides of the foetal heart work to pump a mixture of deoxygenated blood from the systemic veins and oxygenated blood from the placenta into the aorta and thus to the rest of the body. Blood collecting in the right atrium may pass either through the tricuspid valve into the right ventricle or through the foramen ovale (a hole in the intra-atrial septum) into the left atrium. Blood which enters the right ventricle is pumped into the pulmonary artery, with only a small proportion of it entering the lungs. The remainder passes via the ductus arteriosus into the aorta (Fig. 7.26).

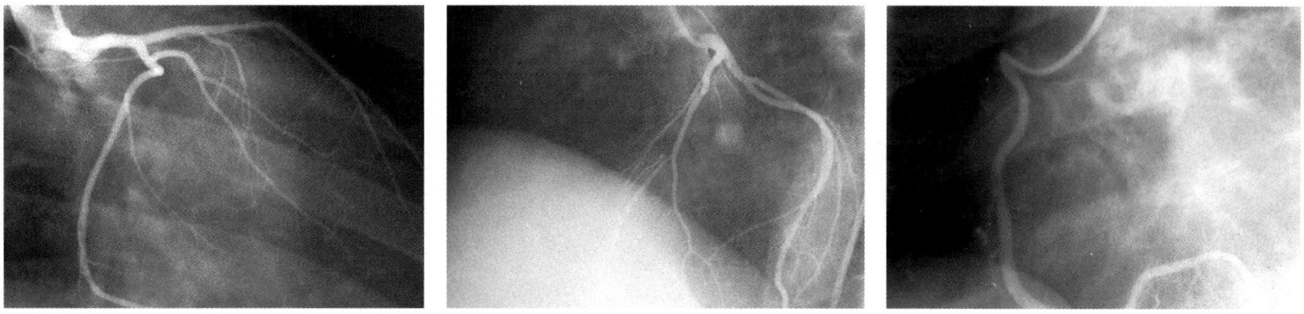

Fig. 7.25 Diagrams and cine-angiograms to show (left and middle) the left coronary artery and (right) right coronary artery.

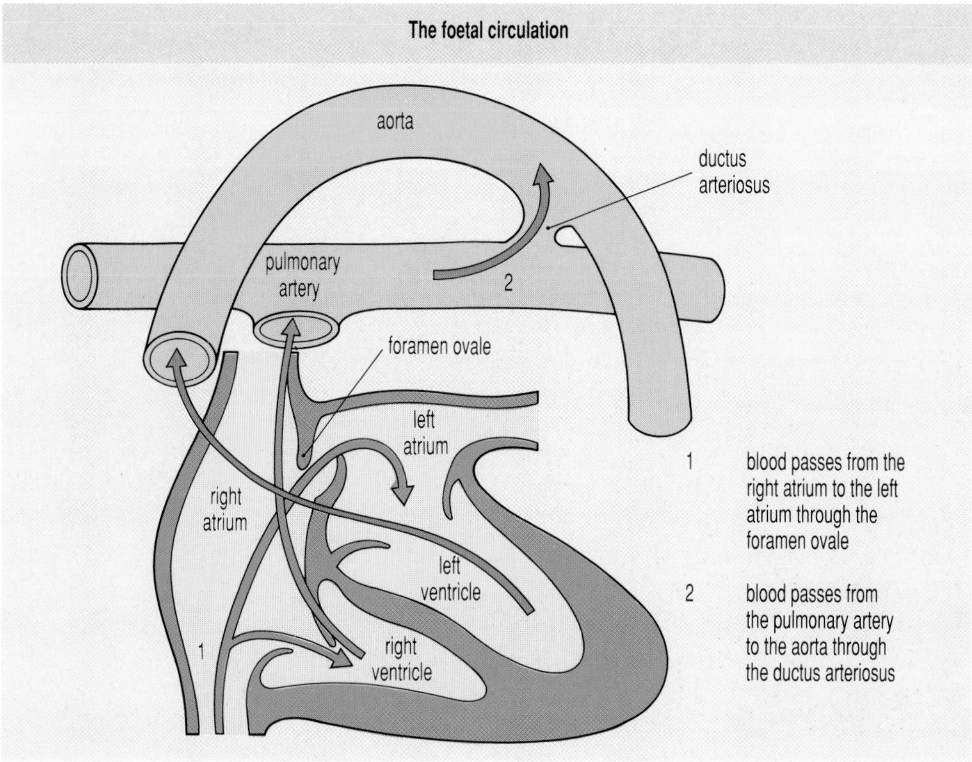
The foetal circulation
aorta
ductus arteriosus
pulmonary artery
2
foramen ovale
left atrium
right atrium
left ventricle
right ventricle
1
1 blood passes from the right atrium to the left atrium through the foramen ovale
2 blood passes from the pulmonary artery to the aorta through the ductus arteriosus

Fig. 7.26 In the foetal circulation, oxygenated blood from the umbilical vein bypasses the liver through the ductus venosus; a portion is shunted from right to left atrium through the foramen ovale, and a further portion passes through the ductus arteriosus.

After birth, the vascular resistance of the lungs falls rapidly as they are inflated with air. This causes a fall in right atrial pressure and a rise in left atrial pressure, thus closing the valve-like foramen ovale. At the same time, the ductus arteriosus constricts and closes (Fig. 7.27). This normally separates the work of the right and left sides of the heart and causes them to work in series rather than in parallel. Abnormalities in the process of transition from foetal to adult circulation, or anatomical defects in the partitions or 'septa' dividing the right and left sides of the heart, may however lead to short-circuits or 'shunts'.

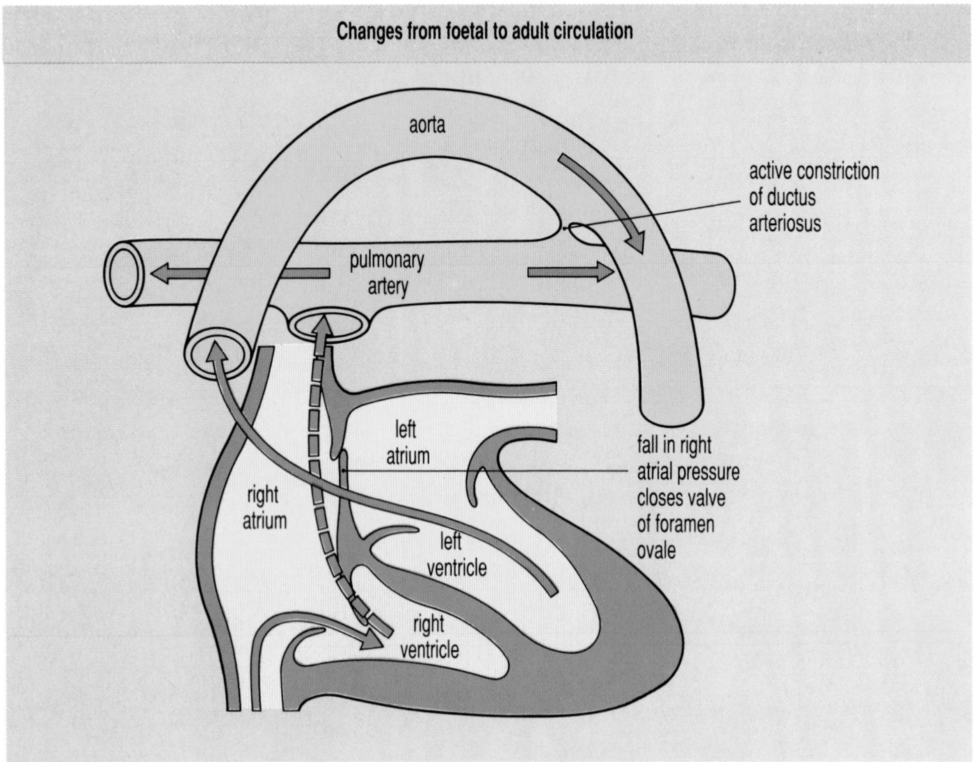

Fig. 7.27 Changes which occur in the foetal circulation at birth. The ductus arteriosus constricts and the fall in right arterial pressure as the lungs expand closes the foramen ovale.

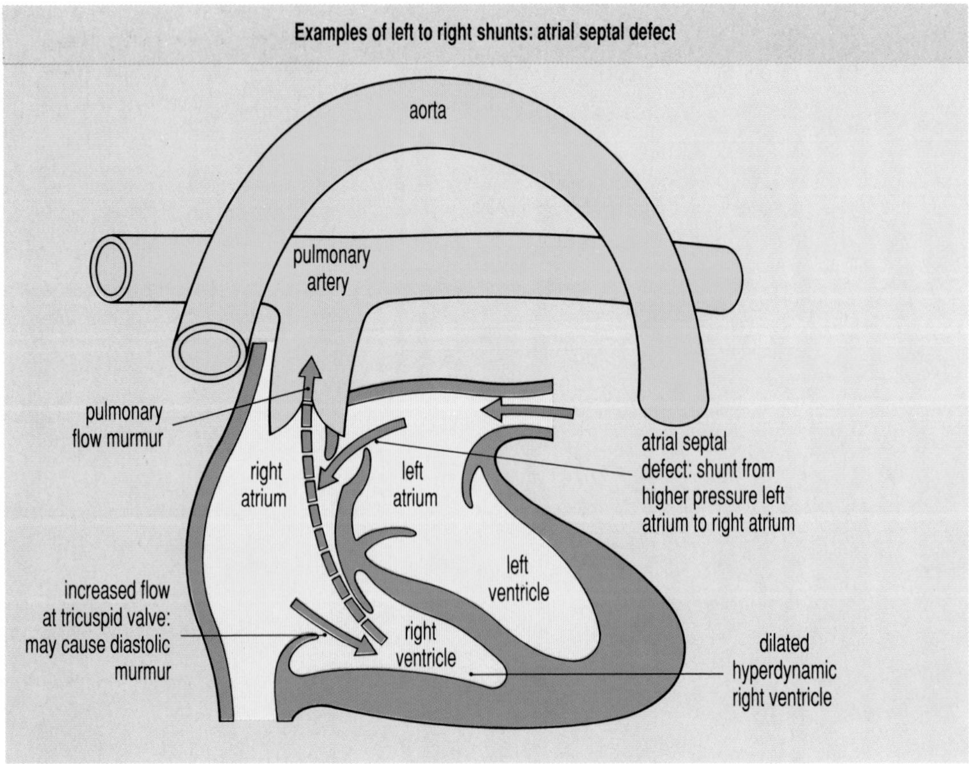

Fig. 7.28a Left to right shunt atrial septal defect. Blood passes from left atrium to right atrium. Overall result is an increase in pulmonary blood flow.

Left to right shunt

A congenital or acquired defect in the interatrial septum, the interventricular septum, or the failure of closure of the ductus arteriosus without other associated abnormality will produce a left to right shunt. Blood follows the path of least resistance from the high pressure left-sided chamber to the lower pressure right-sided chamber. The result is that instead of the left and the right sides of the heart having exactly identical outputs, the right side of the heart has to cope not only with its normal output but also with the extra load of blood transferred from the left. Atwo-to-one shunt means that the output at the right side of the heart is twice that of the left side of the heart. Eventually, the increased workload on the right side of the heart may lead to heart failure, or alternatively the excessively high blood flow through the lungs may lead to damage to the lung blood vessel and the development of pulmonary hypertension. Examples of left to right shunts are shown in Figure 7.28.

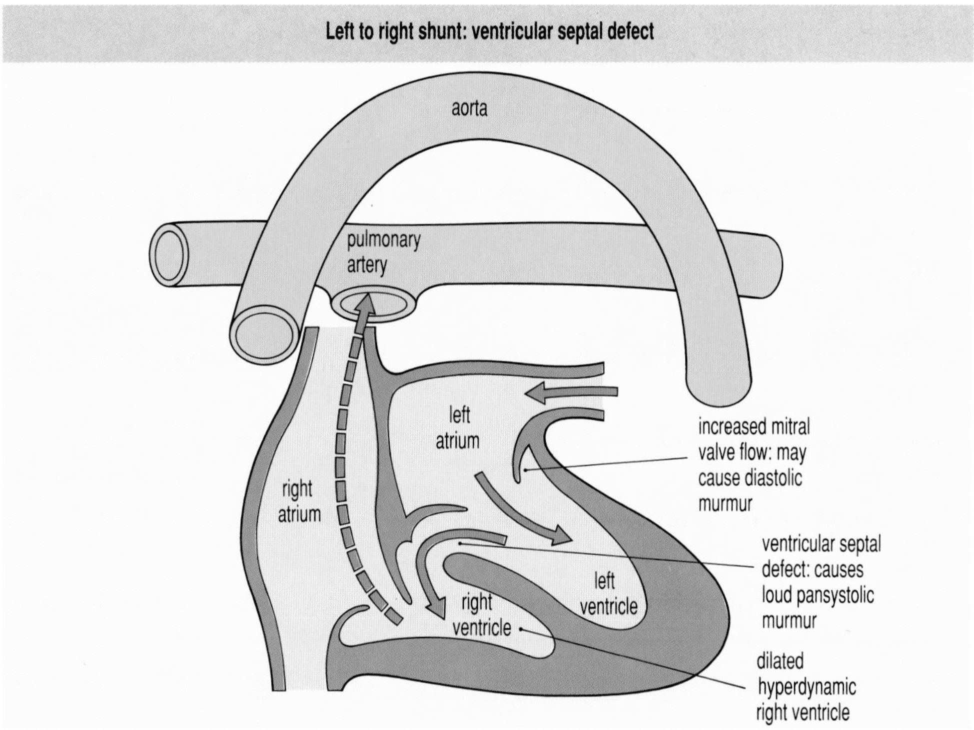

Fig. 7.28b Left to right shunt: ventricular septal defect. Blood passes from high pressure left ventricle to low pressure right ventricle.

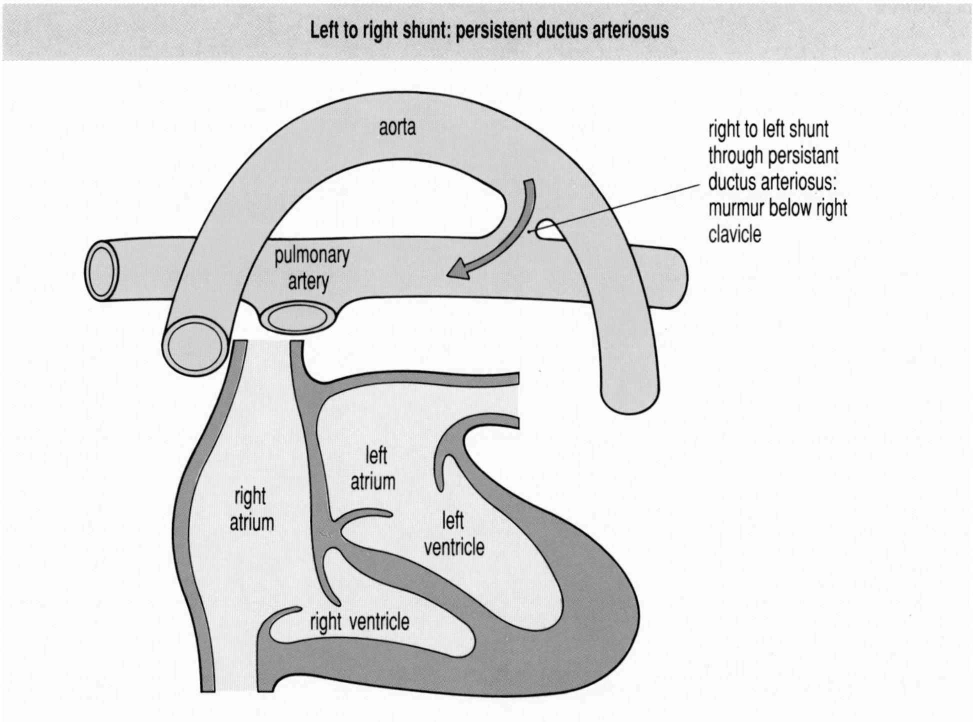

Fig. 7.28c Left to right shunt: persistent ductus arteriosus., Blood passes from high pressure aorta to lower pressure pulmonary artery.

Right to left shunt

If a septal defect or persistent ductus arteriosus is *combined* with another lesion which raises the pressure on the right side of the heart then instead of blood flowing from the left-sided chamber to the right-sided chamber, it will flow in the opposite direction, from the right side of the heart to the left. The commonest example of congenital heart disease causing a right to left shunt is Fallot's Tetralogy (Fig. 7.29) which is physiologically equivalent to a ventricular septal defect *plus* pulmonary valve stenosis. A right to left shunt can sometimes occur when pulmonary vascular damage in a patient with a severe left to right shunt causes the resistance offered by the pulmonary arteries to rise, thus leading to increased pressure on the right side of the heart and a reversal of the shunt. This is called Eisenmenger's syndrome (Fig. 7.30).

The striking clinical feature about patients with right to left shunts is that they are centrally cyanosed. This cyanosis is due to the admixture of desaturated venous blood with saturated blood coming from the pulmonary vein. It differs from the cyanosis which is due to lung disease or to pulmonary oedema in that it is not corrected by giving the patient oxygen to breathe, because the blood leaving the pulmonary veins is already fully saturated with oxygen, so giving the patient a higher concentration of oxygen to breathe will not make any difference.

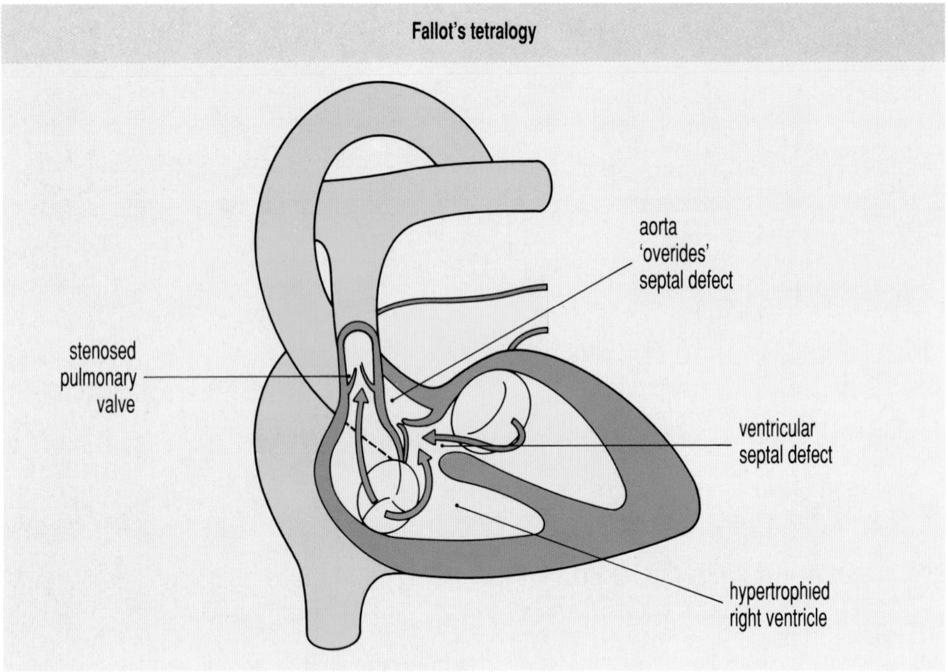

Fig. 7.29 Fallot's tetralogy is the commonest 'congenital' cause of a right to left shunt. (The 'Tetralogy' comprises pulmonary stenosis, ventricular septal defect, over-riding aorta and right ventricular hypertrophy. Note that cyanosis sometimes develops several weeks after birth, as dynamic hypertrophy of muscle in the right ventricular outflow tract worsens the obstruction.)

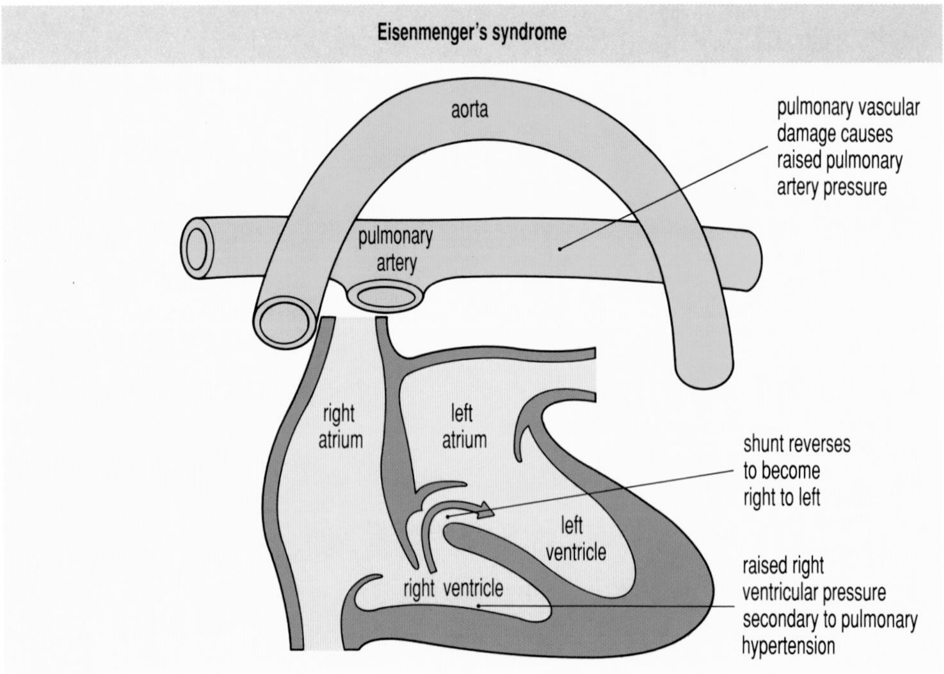

Fig. 7.30 Eisenmenger's syndrome is due to a secondary rise in pulmonary vascular resistance as a consequence of pulmonary damage from increased bloodflow initially due to a left to right shunt. (In some children, the pulmonary vasculature may never develop normally in the presence of such a shunt).

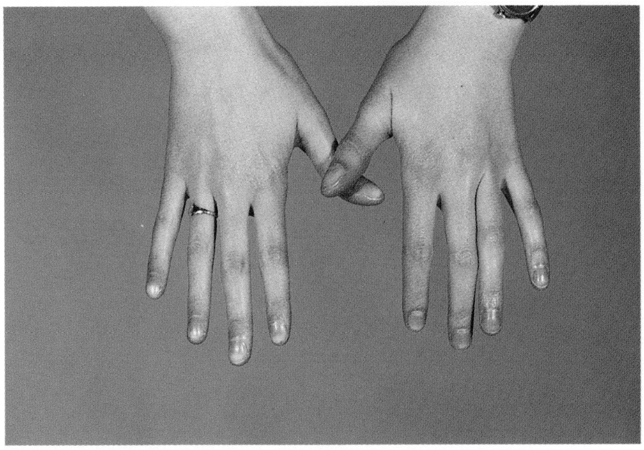

Fig. 7.31 Cyanosis and finger clubbing in a girl with Eisenmenger's syndrome.

Features of long term adaptation to a reduction in systemic arterial oxygen saturation which are seen in patients with right to left shunts include finger clubbing (Fig. 7.31), polycythemia (increased production of red blood cells), and acne (particularly in adolescent children).

THE ARTERIAL SYSTEM

The arterial system exists to distribute oxygenated blood from the heart to the tissues and organs of the body. Where arteries pass close to the surface of the body, or can be compressed against the bony skeleton they can be felt as 'pulses' (Fig. 7.32). During each cardiac cycle, the left ventricle ejects blood into the aorta and

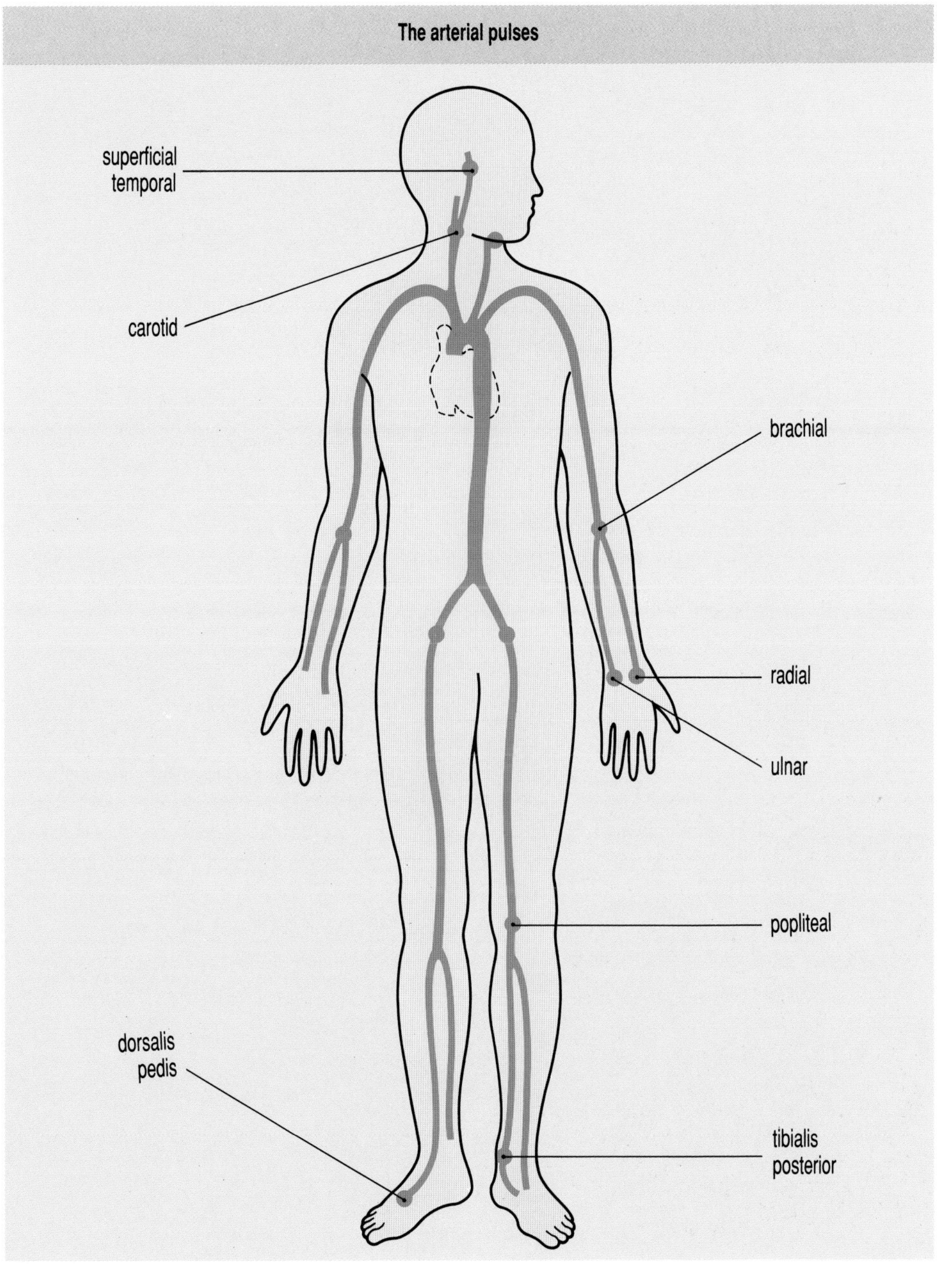

Fig. 7.32 Some of the points at which arterial pulsation can be felt. (Note the similarity to first-aiders' 'pressure points'!)

initiates a pulse wave which is transmitted to the periphery. It is important to remember that the pulse wave travels to the periphery much more rapidly than the actual flow of blood. An intra-arterial recording of pressure against time indicates the shape of the pulse wave which approximates to that which would be felt by a finger on the arterial wall (Fig. 7.33). The shape of the arterial pulse wave depends on many factors (Fig. 7.34). Some of the normal and abnormal pulse waves which can be generated are shown in Figure 7.35. The most important way in which individual organs can adjust their blood supply according to their metabolic needs is by decreas-

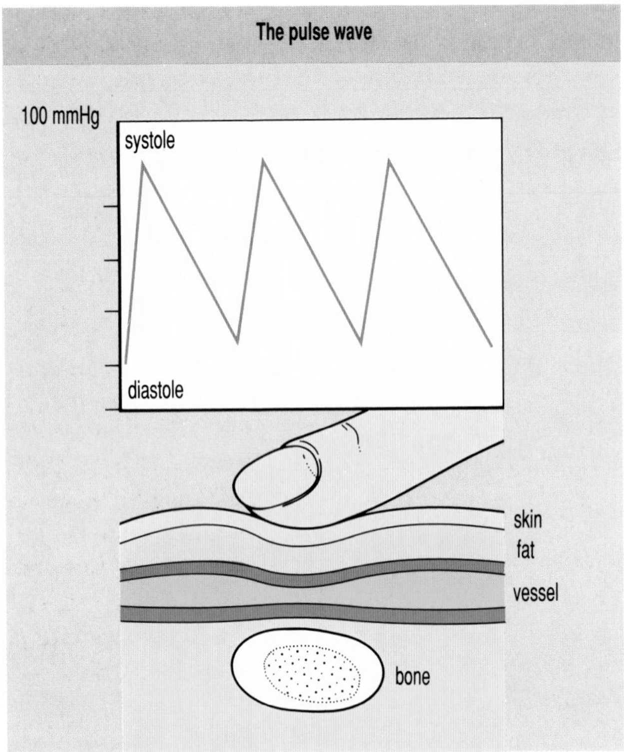

Fig. 7.33 Relationship between the pulse and the arterial waveform.

Factors which affect the shape of the pulse

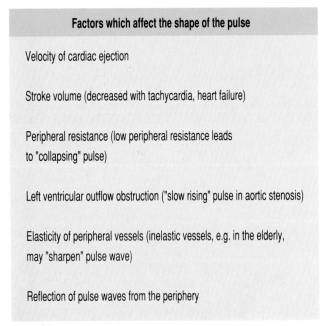

Velocity of cardiac ejection

Stroke volume (decreased with tachycardia, heart failure)

Peripheral resistance (low peripheral resistance leads to "collapsing" pulse)

Left ventricular outflow obstruction ("slow rising" pulse in aortic stenosis)

Elasticity of peripheral vessels (inelastic vessels, e.g. in the elderly, may "sharpen" pulse wave)

Reflection of pulse waves from the periphery

Fig. 7.34 Factors which affect the shape of the pulse wave.

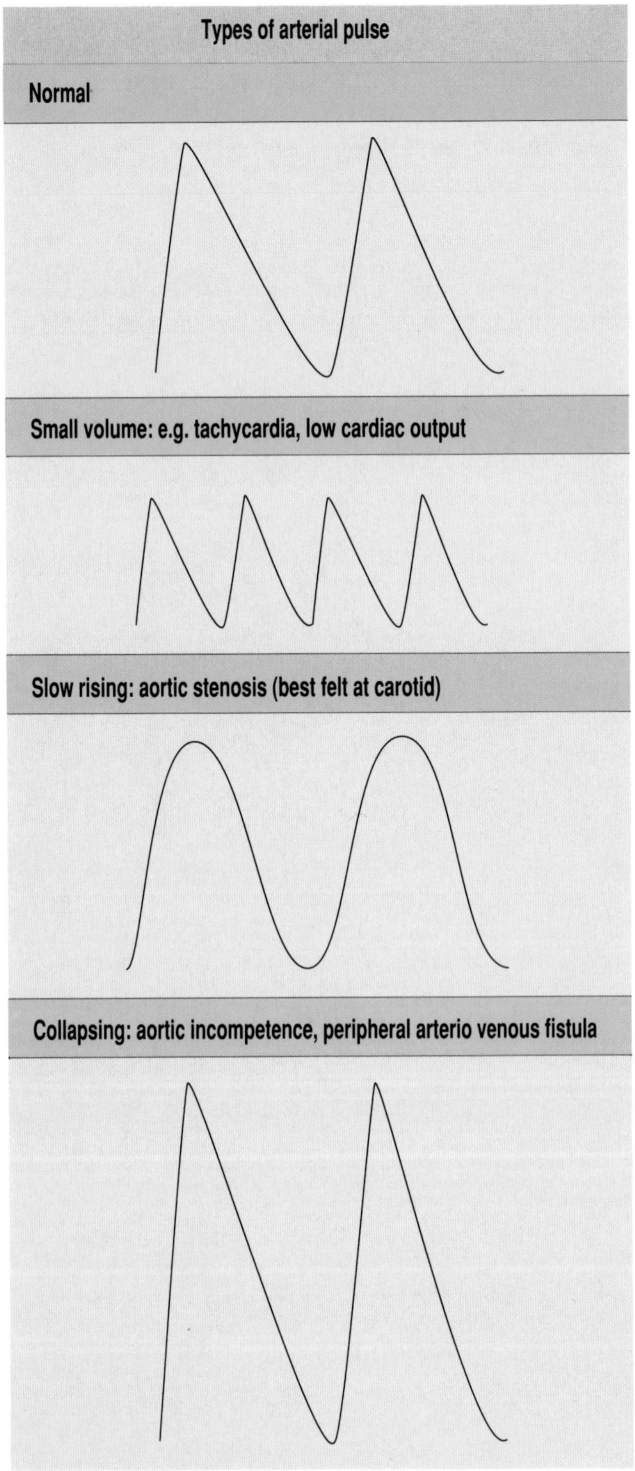

Fig. 7.35 Normal and abnormal arterial pulses in different clinical conditions.

ing or increasing the resistance of the arterioles (very small arteries 200–300mm in diameter) which supply them. Thus, the act of eating food considerably reduces vascular resistance in the gut and increases gut blood flow. Similarly, exercising skeletal muscle strikingly reduces its vascular resistance, thereby increasing local blood flow. Alteration of blood flow to the skin is one of the important mechanisms whereby the body loses or conserves heat. The arteriolar resistance in the skin and the gut is also under the control of the sympathetic nervous system as part of the general body response to 'fight, fright, or flight'. Sympathetic nervous system stimulation causes arteriolar constriction and as a result tends to raise the blood pressure. The most important blood vessels for the control of peripheral vascular resistance are the small muscular arteries and arterioles; larger blood vessels such as the femoral, carotid, or radial arteries simply act as conduits and play little or no role in the control of blood pressure.

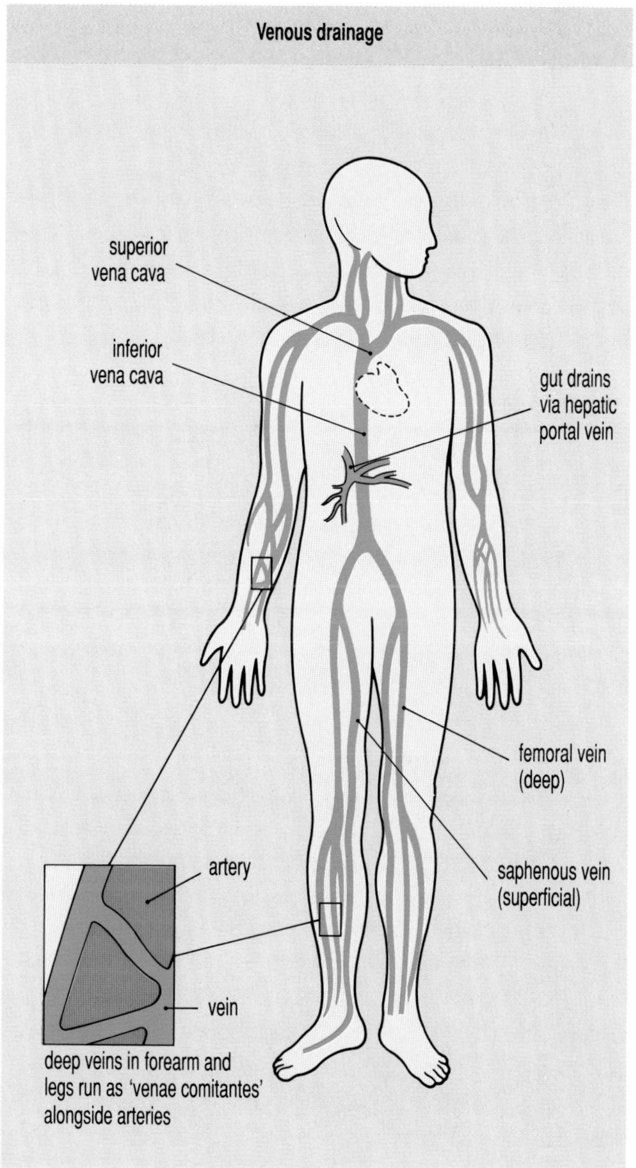

Fig. 7.36 The principal veins of the body.

THE VENOUS SYSTEM

The principle veins of the body are shown in Figure 7.36. Systemic veins collect blood from the tissues and return it to the right atrium of the heart. The venous return from the gut is a special case because it is collected by the hepatic portal vein, and carried first of all to the liver. The venous system operates at a much lower pressure than the arterial system. Veins draining the chest and abdomen drain passively into the vena cava, either directly or via the azygos vein. In the upright position, venous drainage from the head and neck is assisted by gravity. Passive venous drainage alone is inadequate for the limbs and, in particular, for the legs. Here, the venous system is divided into superficial and deep veins (Fig. 7.37) separated by one way valves. Contraction of the arm and leg muscles during normal activities massage the deep veins and actively propel blood back towards the heart. Flow of blood in the wrong direction in the leg veins is prevented by venous valves.

THE CLINICAL HISTORY

Carefully taking the history greatly enhances the efficacy of the subsequent physical examination. On the other hand, you must beware of what the great medical teacher, Maurice Pappworth, called the crime of Procrustes, namely making your physical signs fit with a preconceived diagnosis by inventing findings which do not exist or suppressing those which conflict with your hypothesis. Particular features which need to be asked about in the history with relevance to the cardiovascular system are breathlessness, chest pain, palpitation, and claudication.

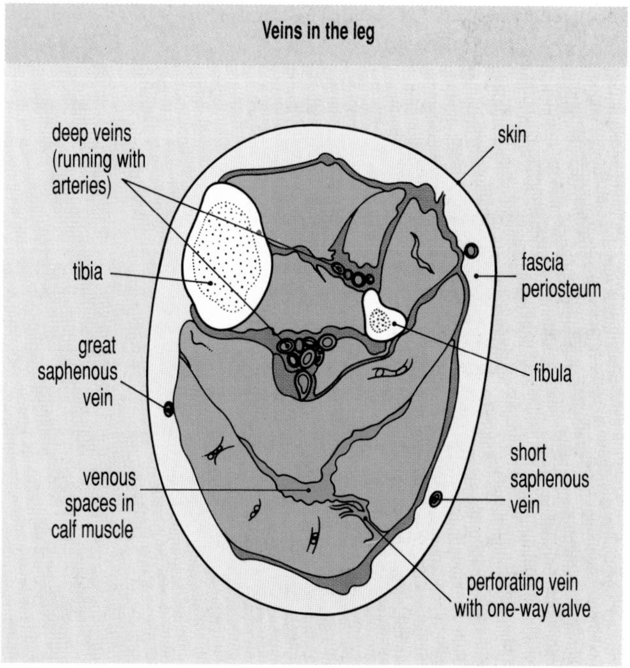

Fig 7.37 Veins in the leg form a 'muscle pump' in conjunction with the calf muscles. Muscle contraction forces blood from superficial to deep veins, and from periphery to centre

BREATHLESSNESS

Patients with heart disease which causes breathlessness characteristically experience it during physical exertion (exertional dyspnoea) and sometimes when they lie flat in bed (positional dyspnoea or orthopnoea). There is evidence that orthopnoea is caused by stimulation of fine nerve endings in the lungs as a consequence of a rise in pulmonary capillary pressure which is due to a redistribution of fluid between peripheral tissues and the lungs when the patient lies flat. Sometimes, the patient awakes from sleep extremely breathless and has to sit up gasping for breath. This is often accompanied by a cough and white frothy sputum (paroxysmal nocturnal dyspnoea).

Breathlessness

Do you ever feel short of breath?

Does this happen on exertion?
How much can you do before getting breathless?

Do you ever wake up gasping for breath?

If so, do you have to sit up or get out of bed?

How many pillows do you sleep on?

Do you cough or wheeze when you are short of breath?

New York Heart Association classification of heart failure	
Grade	
I	No symptoms at rest, dyspnoea only on vigorous exertion
II	No symptoms at rest, but dyspnoea on moderate exertion
III	May be mild symptoms at rest, dyspnoea on mild exertion, severe dyspnoea on moderate exertion
IV	Significant dyspnoea at rest, severedyspnoea even on very mild exertion. Patient often bed bound

Fig. 7.38 A useful grading system for the severity of heart failure.

The mechanism of exercise associated dyspnoea is controversial. It may partly be due to the same sort of mechanism as orthopnoea, with increased venous return from exercising muscles raising left atrial pressure. However, in exercising patients, the sensation of breathlessness does not always correlate well with directly measured left atrial pressure. Other factors such as reduced oxygen content of arterial blood and some alteration of muscle function in chronic heart failure may also be involved.

A widely used classification of exercise tolerance in heart disease is that proposed by the New York Heart Association (Fig. 7.38) which is used widely in clinical trials. For practical purposes, when taking and recording the history, it is often helpful to record the patients symptoms as much as possible in their own words and perhaps with reference to local landmarks. This can subsequently be very useful in assessing a patients progress. Breathlessness associated with wheezing may sometimes be due to heart disease but should raise the suspicion of obstructive airways disease .

Patients who feel that they suddenly have to take a deep breath unrelated to any physical exertion, who find themselves sighing excessively, or who have a constant feeling of not being able of get enough breath in are not describing common features of heart disease. These may, however, be features of anxiety.

It can sometimes be difficult to decide whether a patient's breathlessness is due to heart or lung disease. Paroxymal nocturnal dyspnoea or orthopnoea point towards heart disease, and wheezing as a prominent feature to lung disease, but the distinction can often only be made after the clinical examination.

CHEST PAIN

Chest pain caused by myocardial ischaemia

Over 50 per cent of patients presenting to cardiology clinics in the UK do so with the predominant symptom of chest pain. The commonest type of chest pain associated with heart disease is called *angina pectoris* and is due to an imbalance between the actual blood supply to a portion of heart muscle and the blood supply which this muscle needs for normal metabolism. Most patients with angina have a narrowing or stenosis in one or more coronary arteries, and the pain is precipitated when the metabolic needs of the heart are increased by physical or emotional exertion. Less often, angina is a symptom of aortic stenosis or hypertrophic cardiomyopathy.

The characteristic features of anginal pain are listed in Figure 7.39 and its distribution is illustrated in Figure 7.40. The single most characteristic feature of angina is chest pain which comes on during exertion and which goes away again as soon as, or very shortly after, the exertion stops. It is usually described as a crushing, squeezing, or constricting pain (the Greek word from which it is derived means choking).

Pain which is similar in nature to angina but comes on at rest may be due to unstable angina or to myocardial infarction. The pain of myocardial infarction is severe, persistent, and often accom-

Angina

Do you get pain in your chest on exertion (e.g. climbing stairs)?

Whereabouts in the chest do you feel it?
Is it worse in cold weather?

Is it worse if you exercise after a big meal?

Is it bad enough to stop you from exercising?

Do it go away when you rest?

Do you ever get similar pain if you get excited or upset?

panied by nausea and a feeling of impending death ('angor animi').

Pericarditis

Pericarditis is an inflammation of the pericardium, the serous sac which surrounds the heart. It may be a complication of myocardial infarction, or it may result from a viral or bacterial infection. Another important cause is uraemia (see page 7.00). The patient characteristically complains of pain which is usually described as a constant soreness behind the breast bone and which often gets much worse if the patient takes a deep breath. Unlike the pain of angina or myocardial infarction, pericarditic pain is related to movement (e.g. turning over in bed) but not to physical exertion. It sometimes radiates to the tip of the left shoulder.

Musculoskeletal chest pain

Pain arising in the chest wall or thoracic spine is often mistaken for cardiac pain. Characteristically, it tends to be an aching pain whose onset may relate to a particular twist or movement: the pain persists at rest. There is often localized tenderness, particularly over the costal cartilages. A variant of musculoskeletal pain is the precordial catch syndrome, in which the patient describes a sudden, sharp needle-like jabbing pain in the precordium. The pain is short lasting but may recur; the prognosis is benign.

Dissecting aortic aneurysm

Dissecting aneurysm of the thoracic aorta causes a rare but characteristic form of chest pain which usually starts as a 'tearing' sensation, often felt most between the shoulder blades or in the back. The pain is usually severe and persistent and may be mistaken for the pain of myocardial infarction.

Other chest pains

Other chest pains which may masquerade as cardiac pain include the pain of pleurisy, of an acute pneumothorax or of shingles.

Characteristic features of anginal pain
Brought on by physical or emotional exertion
Relieved by rest
Usually crushing, squeezing or constricting in nature
Usually retrosternal (but see Fig. 7.40)
Often worse after food or in cold winds
Often relieved by nitrates

Fig. 7.39 Clinical features of pain due to clinical ischaemia.

Sites of anginal pain

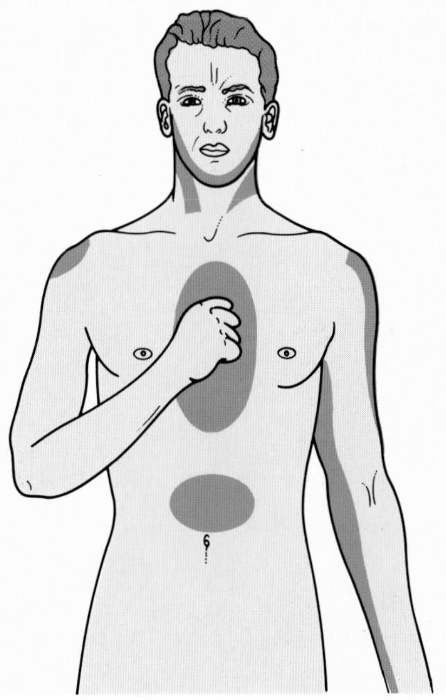

Fig. 7.40 The characteristic distribution of anginal pain.

Palpitation

Palpitation is defined as abnormal awareness of the heart beat. This may be because the heart is beating abnormally fast or irregularly as the result of an arrhythmia, or because the cardiac impulse is more forceful, perhaps as a result of excessive vasodilatation. It is important to find out which of these the patient means. It is often helpful to ask the patient to tap out the heart rhythm on the table. In patients with extrasystoles, it is often not the extra beat itself which the patient perceives, but the one following it, which is characterized by a longer than usual pause, and an excessively forceful beat. The patient may say that their heart jumps, or that it feels that it is about to stop. Ask about the circumstances when the patient feels the palpitation. Ectopic beats are often more apparent when the background heart rate is slow (e.g. when the patient lies down to rest); whereas, paroxysmal tachycardias are often precipitated by exercise or by particular movements (e.g. stooping down to open a drawer or reaching to remove something from a high shelf).

Palpitation

Please could you tap out on the table the rate you think your heart goes at during an attack?

Is the heart beat regular or irregular?

Is there anything which sets attacks off?

Can you do anything to stop an attack? What do you do when you have an attack?

Are there any foods which seem to make symptoms worse?

What medicines are you taking?

The need to treat an arrhythmia is often determined by the haemodynamic effects it is having. Find out whether the arrhythmia is simply a transient inconvenience to the patient or whether the patient has to stop working and lie down. Some arrhythmias actually cause the patient to lose consciousness. Ask how long the palpitations last and whether they stop abruptly. Many patients with paroxysmal tachycardia have learnt some trick such as the Valsalva maneouvre (forceably breathing out with the nose and the mouth held shut) which will terminate an attack.

In some patients, palpitation is precipitated by certain foods, in particular, tea, coffee, wine, and chocolates. You should also ask carefully about any medication, particular decongestants and 'cold cures' which often contain sympathomymetic drugs.

Claudication

Claudication is derived from a Latin word meaning limping. Intermittent claudication is the name given to a condition in which the patient experiences pain in one or both legs on walking which eases up when the patient rests. Just as angina is the usual initial symptom of atheromatous disease affecting the coronary arteries, so intermittent claudication is usually the earliest symptom of narrowing in the arteries supplying the legs. The pain is usually an aching pain felt in the calf, thigh, or buttocks. Intermittent claudication is more common in men, and much more common in smokers than in non-smokers. More advanced symptoms of peripheral arterial disease are discussed on pages 7.45 and 7.46.

The occupational and family history

A family history is very important in evaluating patients with heart disease, because many cardiac diseases involve an underlying genetic predisposition (e.g. towards hyperlipidaemia). Sometimes it is more helpful to ask whether specific famly members are still alive, or about the circumstances of their death, as the significance of this may not be apparent to the patient. For example, early death from stroke may indicate a family susceptibility to hypertension. The patient's occupation may be very relevant to the significance of the disease: coronary artery disease or arrhythmias may be incompatible with a continuing career as an airline pilot or truck driver.

Do not forget to enquire specifically about smoking, alcohol intake, and any medication the patient may be taking.

Family history

Is there any heart disease in the family?

Are your parents still alive?

Did they live to a good age?

Do you know what they died from?

Have you any brothers or sisters?

Do any of them have a heart problem?

Framework for routine examination of the cardiovascular system

1. While taking the history, watch the patient's face for features of anxiety, distress, breathlessness, or features of specific diseases.
2. Take the patient's hand, and assess warmth, sweating, peripheral cyanosis, and examine the nails for clubbing or splinter haemorrhages.
3. Palpate the radial pulse and assess its rate and rhythm.
4. Locate and palpate the brachial pulse and assess its character. Measure the blood pressure. If there is any suspicion of a problem with the aortic arch, compare pulses in both arms.
5. With the patient lying supine at 45°, assess the jugular venous pressure and the jugular venous pulse form.
6. Take an opportunity for a closer look at the face, the conjunctivae, the tongue, and the inside of the mouth.
7. Palpate the carotid pulse and assess its character.
8. With the patient's chest exposed, inspect the precordium and assess the breathing pattern and the presence of any abnormal pulsation.
9. Palpate the precordium, locate the apex beat and assess its character. Assess the feel of the rest of the precordium and the presence of any abnormal vibrations or thrills.
10. Listen with the stethoscope and assess heart sounds and murmurs. If appropriate, listen over the carotid artery for radiating murmurs or bruits.
11. Percuss and auscultate the chest both front and back looking for pleural effusions. Listen for crepitations at the lung bases.
12. Lie the patient flat and palpate the abdomen, feeling in particular for the liver and any dilatation of the abdominal aorta.
13. Assess the femoral pulses and the popliteal and foot pulses. Look for ankle or sacral oedema.
14. If appropriate, assess the patient's exercise tolerance by taking him for a short walk.
15. Test the urine.

Fig. 7.41 Suggested schedule for cardiovascular examination.

CLINICAL EXAMINATION OF THE CARDIOVASCULAR SYSTEM

There are three interlinking facets to the examination of the cardiovascular system. First, the student will wish to establish an examination routine which will ensure that all important aspects of the cardiovascular system are examined smoothly and efficiently and that nothing important is forgotten. Second, he or she will wish to concentrate on certain specific points to confirm or to refute a working diagnosis based on the clinical history. Third, it will frequently happen that routine clinical examination will disclose an unexpected abnormality such as a heart murmur whose differential diagnosis must then be considered.

A FRAMEWORK FOR THE ROUTINE PHYSICAL EXAMINATION OF THE CARDIOVASCULAR SYSTEM

The author's schedule for the routine examination of the cardiovascular system is set out in Figure 7.41. It is not the only possible schedule, nor necessarily the best one, and it is constantly being modified in the light of increasing experience. It will, however, serve as a framework for discussion.

The hands in heart disease

The temperature of the hands gives a guide to the extent of peripheral vasodilatation. Patients in heart failure are usually vasoconstricted, and their hands feel cold and sometimes sweaty from increased adrenaline secretion. The fingernails may show splinter haemorrhages (Fig. 7.42) in subacute infective endocarditis, and finger clubbing in endocarditis or cyanotic congenital heart disease.

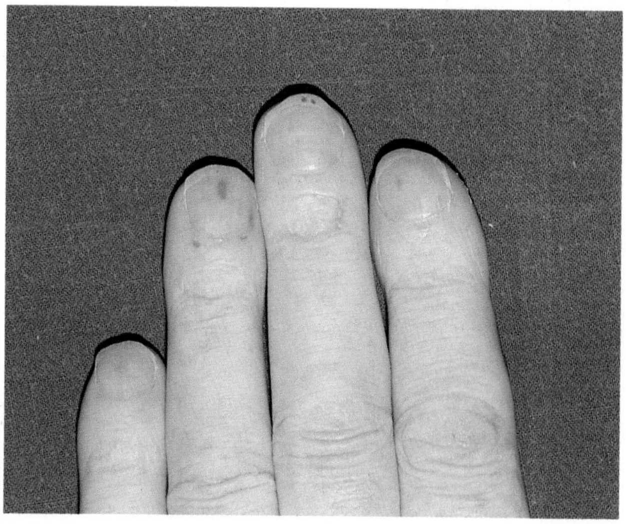

Fig. 7.42 Splinter haemorrhage in the ring finger of a man with infective endocarditis. There is an older, fading 'splinter' under the nail of the index finger. Splinter haemorrhages are often smaller and darker than this.

Feeling the peripheral pulses

The right radial pulse is usually best felt with the fingers of the examiner's left hand (Fig. 7.43). It is used to assess heart rate and rhythm. Because the radial pulse is a relatively long way from the heart, it is not a good pulse from which to attempt to assess pulse character. If there is any suspicion of an abnormality in the aortic arch or of some abnormality in the brachial artery on either side, it may be helpful to feel both radial pulses and compare their volume and timing simultaneously. In patients with suspected coarctation of the aorta, it is helpful simultaneously to feel the radial and the femoral pulse. In the presence of coarctation not only is the volume of the femoral pulse diminished, but it is also appreciably delayed compared to the radial pulse (Fig. 7.44).

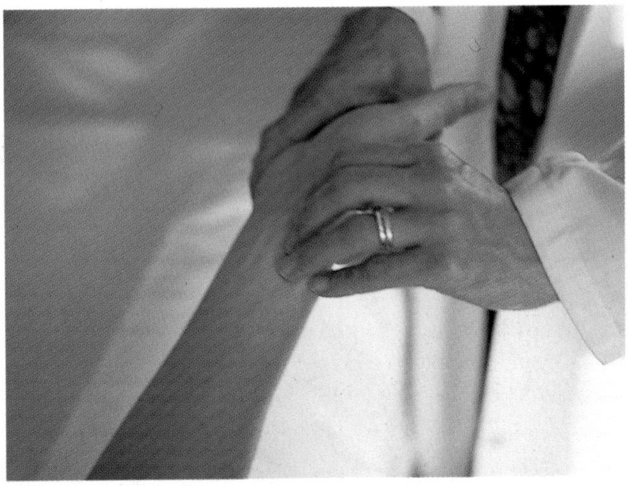

Fig. 7.43 Feeling the right radial pulse.

Brachial pulse

The best way to feel the patient's right brachial pulse is to use the thumb of the examiner's right hand, applied to the front of the elbow just medial to the biceps tendon with the fingers cupped round the back of the elbow (Fig. 7.45). Students are sometimes taught never to use the thumb for feeling a pulse because pulsation in the examiner's own thumb may lead to mistakes in the detection of very faint peripheral pulses in patients with peripheral arterial disease. However, in most patients we are not actually concerned with whether or not the brachial pulse is present but with its character (Fig. 7.46), and here the extreme kinaesthetic sensitivity of the examiner's thumb compared to the other fingers is a distinct advantage.

Carotid pulse

The carotid pulse is even closer to the heart than the brachial pulse and therefore even better for assessing pulse character as a reflection of the way the left ventricle is working. The best way to feel the patient's right carotid artery is to locate the tip of the examiner's left thumb against the patient's larynx and then gently but firmly press directly backwards so that the carotid artery is felt the precervical muscles (Fig. 7.47). Alternatively, the carotid pulse can be felt from behind by curling the examiner's fingers around the side of the neck (Fig. 7.48). In severe aortic stenosis, there is characteristically a slow rising carotid pulse, often with a palpable shudder. If the carotid pulse is difficult to feel in a patient whose radial and brachial pulses are easily felt, the cause may be aortic stenosis, as the pulse form becomes more 'normal' the nearer the periphery

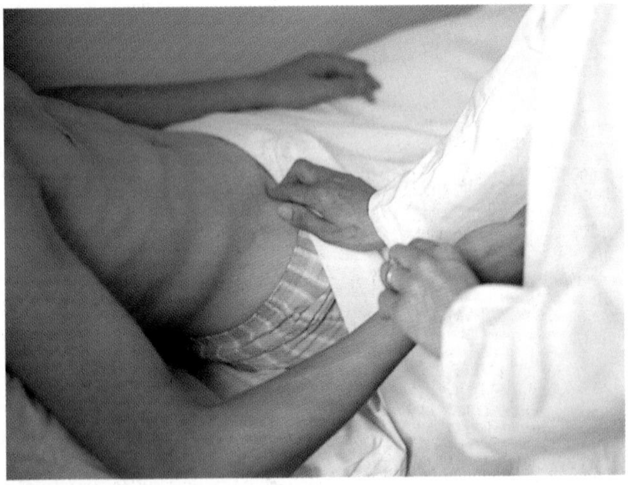

Fig. 7.44 Simultaneous palpation of the radial and femoral pulses: a delayed femoral pulse is a feature of aortic coarctation.

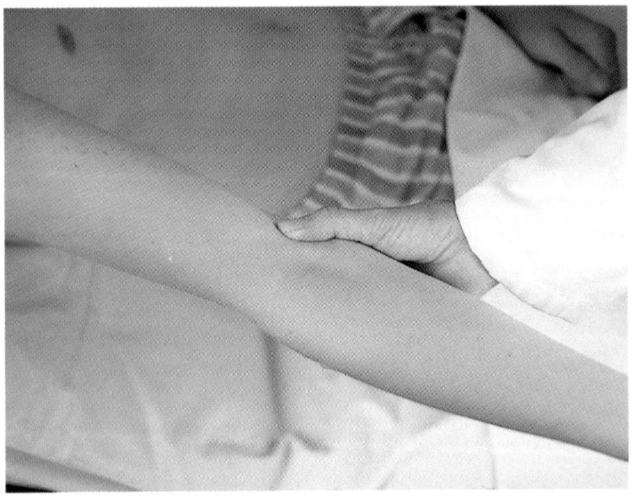

Fig. 7.45 Using the thumb to assess the character of the brachial pulse. The artery lies just medial to the tendinous insertion of the biceps muscle, and deep the fascial insertion of this muscle — fascia called the 'Grâce à dieu' (thanks be to God) fascia by medieval barber surgeons, because it saved them from fatally damaging the artery when bloodletting at the elbow!

Pulse abnormalities (felt at brachial pulse)

Name	Feels like	Associated with
Normal	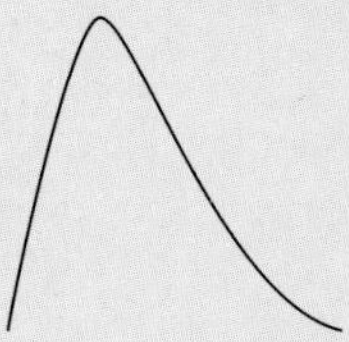	—
Slow rising	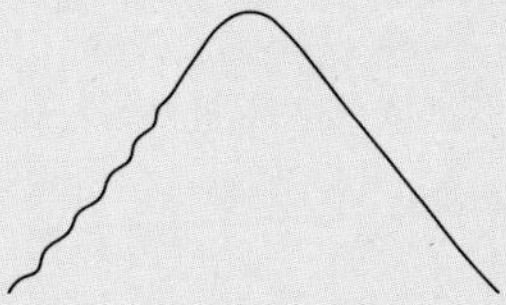	Aortic stenosis
Bisferiens ('two peaks')	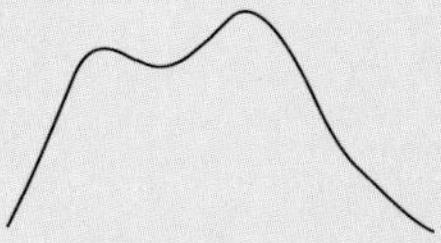	Mild aortic stenosis plus reflux
Collapsing	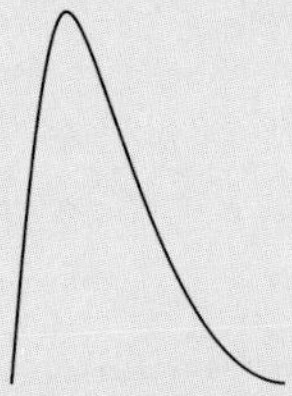	Aortic reflux Persistent ductus arteriosus
No pulse		Occluded bronchial or axillary artery

Fig. 7.46 Different pulse waveforms are associated with different cardiac or vascular abnormalities.

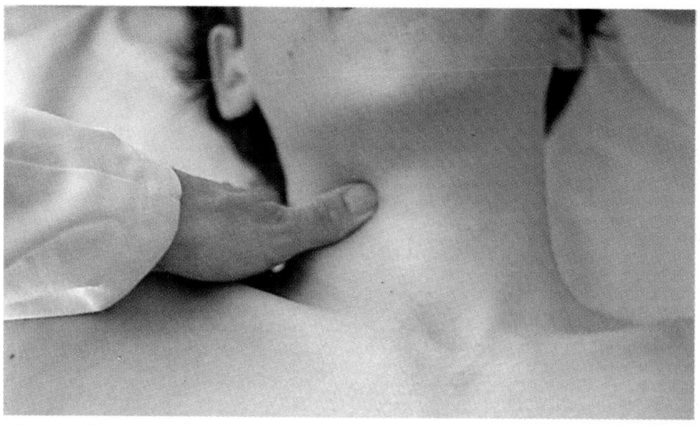

Fig. 7.47 Palpating the carotid artery using the examiner's thumb.

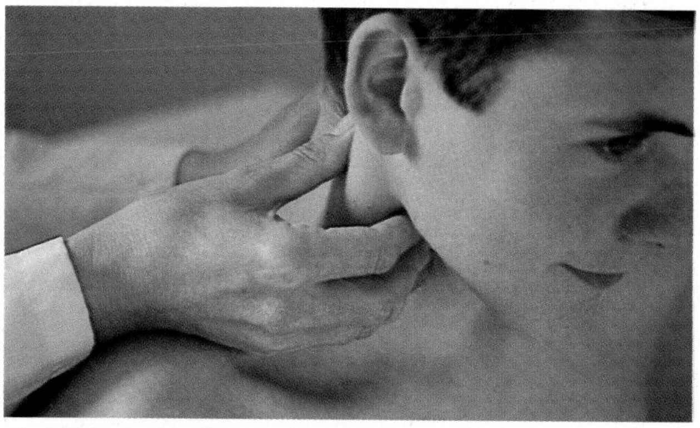

Fig. 7.48 Another way of palpating the carotid artery.

it is felt! (Fig. 7.49). Another sign best appreciated at the carotid is the jerky pulse of hypertrophic cardiomyopathy. This starts normally and then suddenly peters out as the contracting left ventricular outflow tract obstructs ejection (Fig. 7.50).

Femoral pulse

The femoral pulse is almost as valuable as the carotid pulse in assessing cardiac performance. It is more likely to be weak or absent in patients with disease of the aorta or iliac arteries. It is best examined with the patient unclothed and lying flat, by placing the thumb or finger of the examiner directly above the superior pubic ramus and midway between the pubic tubical and anterior superior iliac spine (Fig. 7.51).

Methods for assessing the popliteal and foot pulses are given here for completeness, but their main use lies in assessing peripheral arterial disease (see pages 7.45 and 7.46).

Popliteal pulse

The popliteal pulse lies deep within the popliteal fossa but is readily felt by compressing it against the posterior surface of the distal end of the femur. The patient lies flat with the knee slightly flexed. The examiner uses the fingers of one hand to press the tips of the fingers of the other hand into the popliteal fossa to feel the popliteal artery against the back of the knee joint (Fig. 7.52). Palpating the popliteal artery is mainly useful in evaluating patients with peripheral vascular disease, in particular those presenting with intermittent claudication.

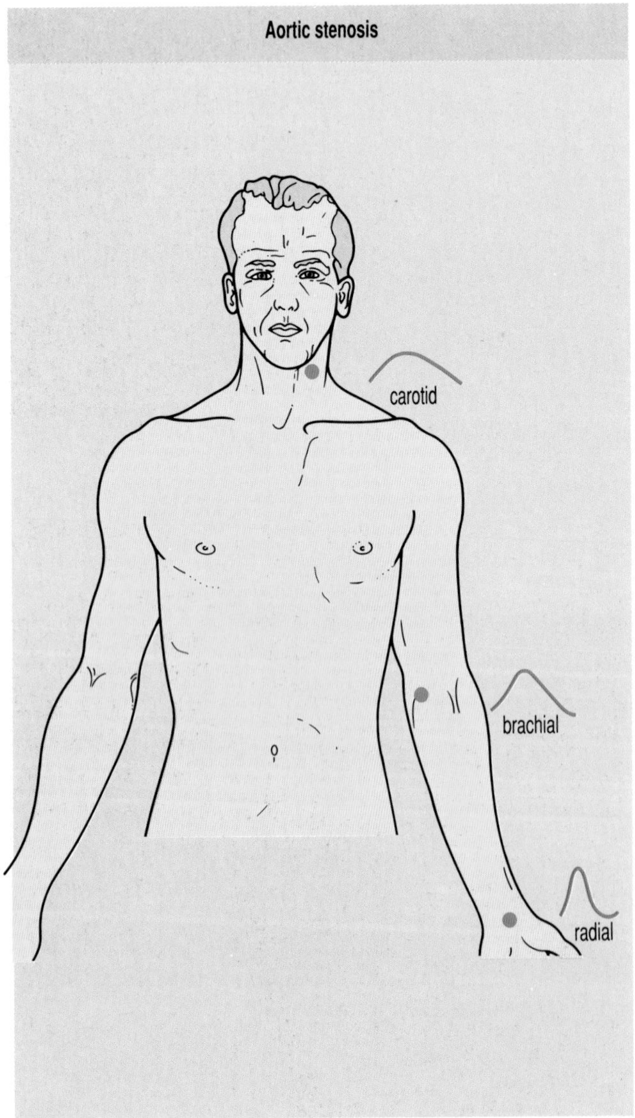

Fig. 7.49 The pulse-wave changes in aortic stenosis.

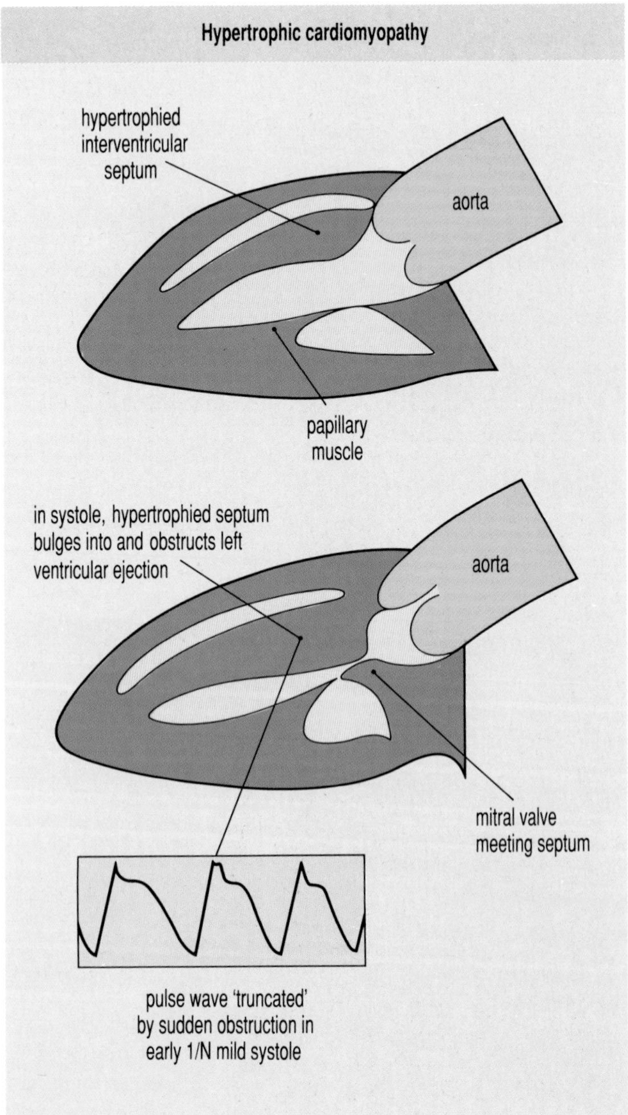

Fig. 7.50 Hypertrophic cardiomyopathy. A 'jerky' carotid pulse may result from dynamic left ventricular outflow obstruction.

Dorsalis pedis and tibialis posterior artery

Palpation of these pulses is mainly used for assessing peripheral vascular disease, although they can sometimes be used for monitoring pulse rate and rhythm during anaesthesia or recovery. The dorsalis pedis pulse is felt with the fingers aligned along the dorsum of the foot lateral to the extensor hallucis longus tendon (Fig. 7.53); the tibialis posterior pulse is felt with the fingers cupped round the ankle just posterior to the medial malleolus (Fig. 7.54).

MEASURING BLOOD PRESSURE

The most convenient way of measuring blood pressure in the clinic is with a stethoscope and sphygmomanometer. The sphygmomanometer is placed around the upper arm (Fig. 7.55) and air is pumped into the cuff. As the pressure in the sphygmomanometer cuff increases above the systolic pressure in the brachial artery, the artery is compressed, and the radial pulse becomes impalpable. As the pressure in the cuff is gradually lowered, blood can force its way past the obstruction for part of the cardiac cycle, creating

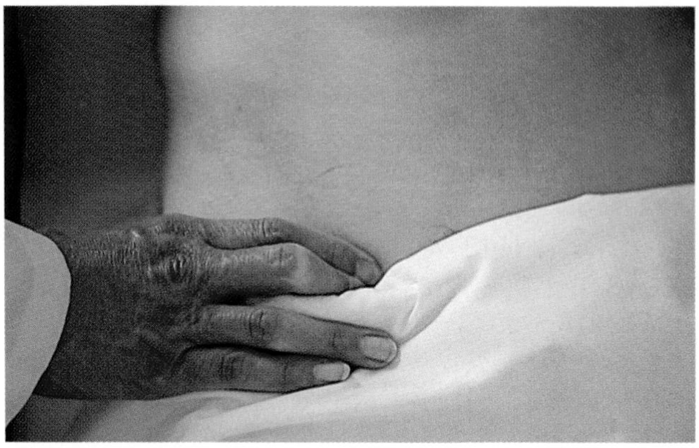

Fig. 7.51 Palpating the femoral artery.

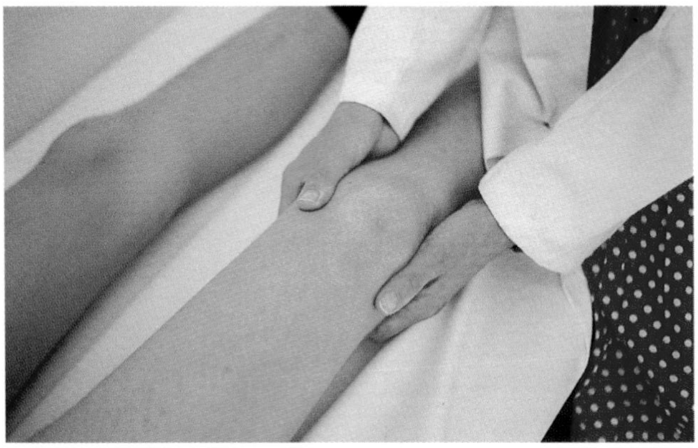

Fig. 7.52 Palpating the popliteal artery.

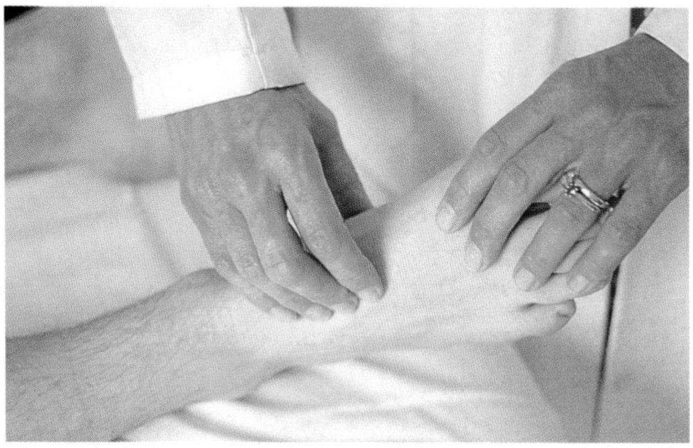

Fig. 7.53 Palpating the dorsalis pedis pulse.

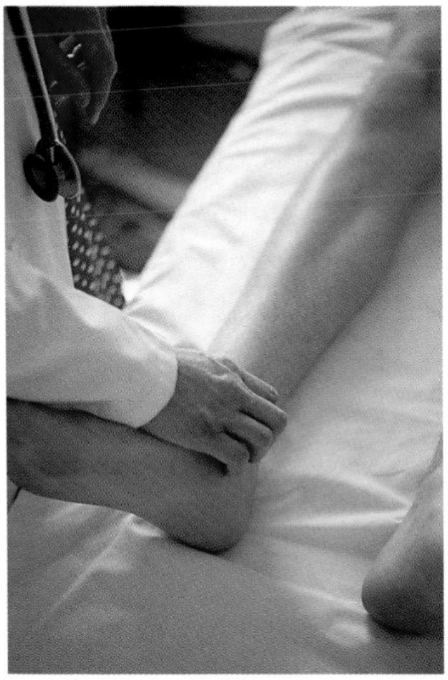

Fig. 7.54 Palpating the tibialis posterior pulse.

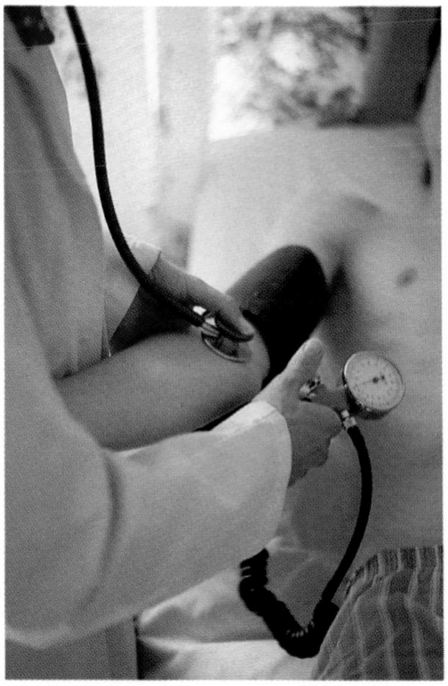

Fig. 7.55 Measuring blood pressure using a sphygmomanometer and stethoscope. The sphygmomanometer cuff is smoothly applied around the unclothed upper arm, and the examiner is supporting the patient's arm at 'heart height'.

sounds which can be heard with a stethoscope placed over the brachial artery at the elbow. These sound are called the Korotkoff sounds after the Russian physician who first described them. As pressure in the cuff is lowered, the Korotkoff sounds become louder and more ringing in nature, and then suddenly become muffled. Very shortly afterwards, the sounds usually disappear altogether. It is this point of *disappearance* of the Korotkoff sounds (sometimes called phase 5) which is now used to define diastolic pressure for clinical and epidemiological purposes. In fact it is the point of muffling of the sounds (phase 4) which corresponds most closely to the diastolic pressure as measured by an indwelling arterial cannula, but phase 5 readings have proved to be more reproducible among different observers. The generation of the Korotkoff sounds is shown diagramatically in Figure 7.56.

To measure the blood pressure reliably in the clinic, all clothing must be removed from the arm and the sphygmomanometer cuff smoothly applied. The patient's arm should be supported at heart level by an arm rest or by the examiner. It is good practice to check the systolic pressure roughly by palpation of the radial artery before applying the stethoscope. This is because in some patients with very high blood pressure the Korotkoff sounds may disappear and then reappear again as cuff pressure is lowered, a phenomenon called the auscultatory gap. For accurate measurement, pressure in the cuff should be reduced slowly, ideally at about 1mm Hg/second. Mercury manometers must be upright and not tilted. Aneroid manometers invariably become inaccurate with time and should be regularly recalibrated against mercury manometers. Most people consciously or unconsciously round off the blood pressure reading to the nearest 5–10 mm. This is frowned on by Purists. If really accurate results are needed for research purposes, it is best to use a random zero sphygmomanometer in which the operator presses levers to indicate when he thinks systolic and diastolic pressures have been reached, and then opens the back of the instrument to read the results off a concealed scale.

Patients with very high blood pressure often have other evidence of hypertensive disease in the form of retinal changes, left ventricular hypertrophy, and proteinuria. In patients without these features, it is important not to make a definitive diagnosis of hypertension on the basis of a single casual blood pressure recording. Repeated blood pressure measurements will nearly always show

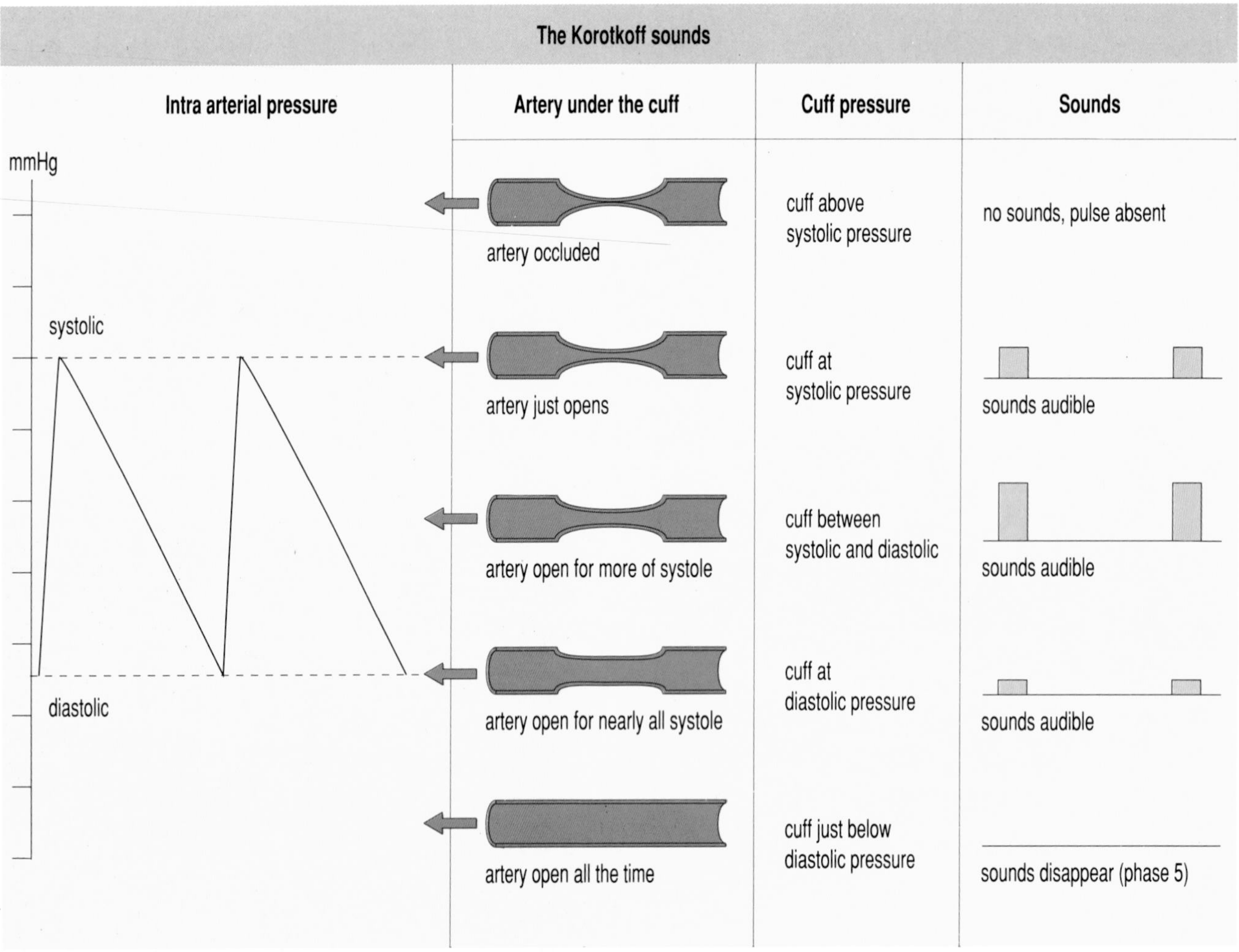

Fig. 7.56 Diagram to show the relationship between cuff pressure, Korotkoff sounds, and arterial pressure.

some tendency to revert towards normal. Some patients have high blood pressure when this measured in a hospital clinic, yet measurements in their own home or by continuous blood pressure monitoring show a much more normal pattern. The definition of what constitutes higher blood pressure has long been a subject for controversy. In any given population, the distribution of systolic and diastolic blood pressures tends to be continuous. In Western populations, there is a tendency for both systolic and diastolic pressures to increase with age, though this does not necessarily apply to other populations, particularly those where there is a low salt intake. Most authorities would accept a phase 5 diastolic pressure of over 100mm Hg on repeated measurement as defining a hypertensive population. A diastolic pressure of greater than 120mm Hg and/or evidence of end organ damage would define patients with severe hypertension. Important points about the measurement of blood pressure are summarized in Figure 7.57.

The converse of hypertension is hypotension or low blood pressure. Although a systolic blood pressure of less than 100mm Hg is part of the definition of shock, hypotension is usually defined by its consequences (e.g. impaired cerebral or renal function rather than by some arbitrary pressure level). Some patients have postural hypotension, which most commonly manifests itself as dizziness when the patient attempts to stand upright (Fig. 7.58). The diagnosis is made by measuring the blood pressure with the patient lying and standing.

Important points about measuring blood pressure
Remove all clothing from arm
Support arm comfortably at heart level
Use correct size of cuff – wide cuff for obese arms, paediatric cuff for children
Check systolic pressure by palpitation
Release pressure no faster than 1mmHg per second
Take phase V (disappearance of sounds) as diastolic pressure
Check aneroid monometers regularly against mercury monometer
If using a mercury monometer, it must be absolutely upright

Fig. 7.57 Do's and Don'ts in measuring blood pressure.

Causes of hypotension
Impaired cardiac output
Myocardial infection Pericardial tamponade Massive pulmonary embolism Acute valve incompetence
Hypovolaemia
Haemorrhage Diabetic pre-coma Dehydration from diarrhoea/vomiting
Excessive vasodilation
Anaphylaxis Gram negative septicaemia Drugs Autonomic failure

EVALUATION OF THE JUGULAR VENOUS PULSE

The evaluation of the jugular venous pulse is a key factor in assessing the performance of the 'input' side of the heart. The internal jugular vein is in direct communication, without intervening valves, with the superior vena cava and the right atrium. The normal pressure in the right atrium is equivalent to that exerted by a column of blood about 10–12cm tall. Therefore, when the patient is standing or sitting upright, the internal jugular vein is collapsed, and when he is lying flat, it is completely filled. If the patient lies supine at about 45°, the point at which jugular venous pulsation becomes visible is usually just above the clavicle; therefore, this is the position usually chosen for examination of the jugular venous pulse (Fig. 7.59). It is best if the patient rests his head comfortably against a pillow, with the neck slightly flexed and looking straight ahead. It is important not to tense the sternomastoid muscles as the

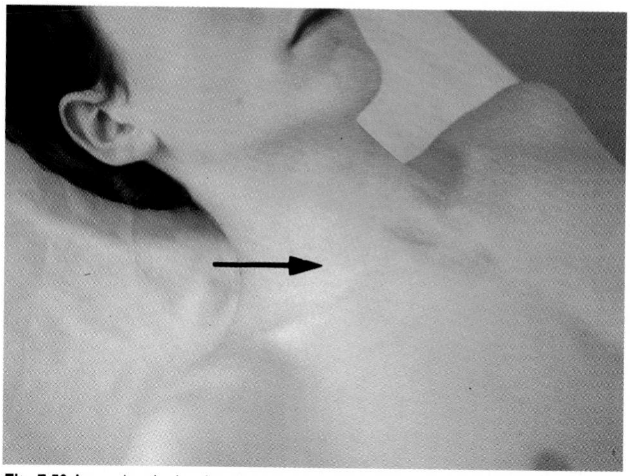

Fig. 7.59 Assessing the jugular venous pressure. With the patient lying supine at 45°, jugular pulsation is normally just visible above the clavicle.

internal jugular vein lies directly beneath them. Reliable ways of telling the jugular venous pulse from the carotid arterial pulse are listed in Figure 7.60. It is sometimes said that jugular venous pulsation can be obliterated by gentle pressure with the finger, and the jugular pulse is never palpable, but these two statements are incorrect, particularly in the presence of tricuspid regurgitation.

Once the jugular venous pulse has been identified, the examiner must try to assess first, the mean height of pulsation above right atrial level and second, the wave form of jugular venous pulsation. Because it is not actually possible to see or feel the right atrium, it is usual to express the height of jugular venous pulsation above the manubriosternal angle (Fig. 7.61). The height of the manubriosternal angle above the mid-right atrium is roughly constant irrespective of whether the patient is lying, sitting, or standing. A normal jugular venous pressure is less than 4cm above the manubriosternal angle.

In patients with a very high jugular venous pressure (e.g. those with pericardial tamponade or constrictive pericarditis), the internal jugular vein may be completely filled with the patient lying at 45° and it is necessary to sit the patient bolt upright to see the top of the pulsation. As a quick rule of thumb, if jugular venous pulsation is visible above the clavicle with the patient sitting bolt upright then the jugular venous pressure must be raised.

Distinction between jugular venous and carotid pulses

Venous	Arterial
Most rapid movement inward	Most rapid movement outward
Two peaks per cycle (in sinus rhythm)	One peak per cycle
Affected by compressing abdomen	Not affected by compressing abdomen
May displace earlobes (if venous pressure raised)	Never displaces earlobes

Fig. 7.60 How to tell the carotid from the jugular venous pulse.

Measuring the height of the JVP

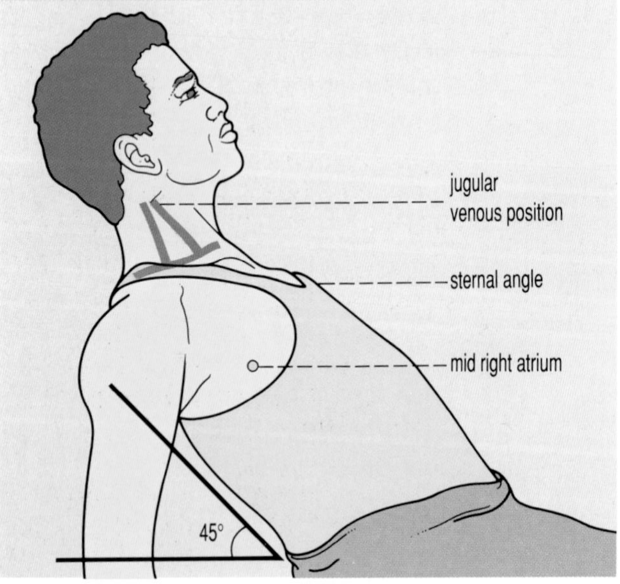

Fig. 7.61 The relationship of the jugular venous pulsation, left atrium, and manubriosternal angle.

Venous pressure waveforms

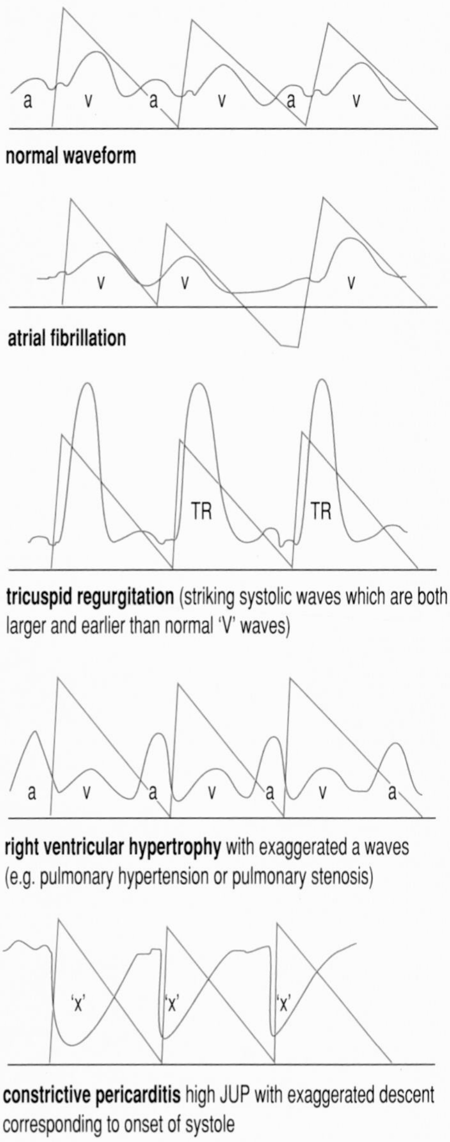

Fig. 7.62 Examples of different jugular pressure wave forms.

Even sitting the patient upright is sometimes not adequate to assess a very high venous pressure. A rough estimate can sometimes be made in these patients by raising the hand until the veins on the back of the hand collapse and by assessing the difference in height between the hand and the right atrium or sternal angle.

Examples of different jugular pressure wave forms are shown in Figure 7.62. In practice, by far the commonest and most important abnormal wave form to recognize is that of tricuspid regurgitation, which is characterized by large systolic waves which are often palpable and cannot be obliterated by pressing with a finger.

Causes and characteristics of raised jugular venous pressure	
Common	
Congestive heart failure	Normal wave pattern usually preserved
Tricuspid regurgitation	Large 'V' waves
Less common	
Pericardial tamponade Massive pulmonary embolism	Grossly elevated venous pressure, wave pattern difficult to assess as patient becomes hypotensive when sitting upright
Rare	
Superior caval obstruction	No pulsation seen
Constrictive pericarditis	Sharp pre-systolic descent
Tricuspid stenosis	Slow pre-systolic descent

Fig. 7.63 Some of the causes of a raised jugular venous pressure.

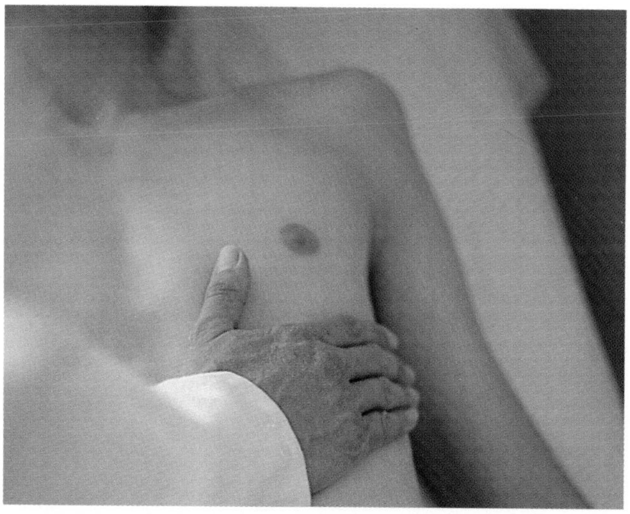

Fig. 7.64 Palpating the precordium. For locating the apex beat, the patient should be flat on his back; but to assess the quality of the impulses he may be rolled onto his left side.

By far the commonest cause of a raised jugular venous pressure is congestive heart failure (Fig. 7.63), where the raised venous pressure reflects the right ventricular failure component (see page 7.00). A raised but nonpulsatile jugular venous pressure should bring to mind the possibility of superior vena cava obstruction.

PALPATION OF THE PRECORDIUM

Palpate the precordium by laying the flat of the hand and the outstretched fingers on the chest wall to the left of the sternum (Fig. 7.64). You are literally trying to feel how the heart is working. The first thing to do is to locate the 'apex beat'. This is the furtherest outward and downward point at which pulsation is easily palpable. Its site is usually expressed in terms of fixed landmarks such as the intercostal spaces, the clavicle, and the axilla. The normal adult apex beat with the patient lying supine at 45° is in the fifth or sixth left intercostal space, in the mid-clavicular line. Remember that the heart has some mobility within the chest, so if you roll the patient onto, for example, his left hand side, the apex beat will move further outwards. Sometimes, particularly in an obese individual or one with an emphysematous chest, you will actually need to roll the patient onto his left side in order to feel cardiac pulsation properly. Do not attempt, however, to describe the position of the apex beat in these patients.

Just as important as the position of the apex beat is the quality of the impulse that you feel (Fig. 7.65). The quality of the normal apex

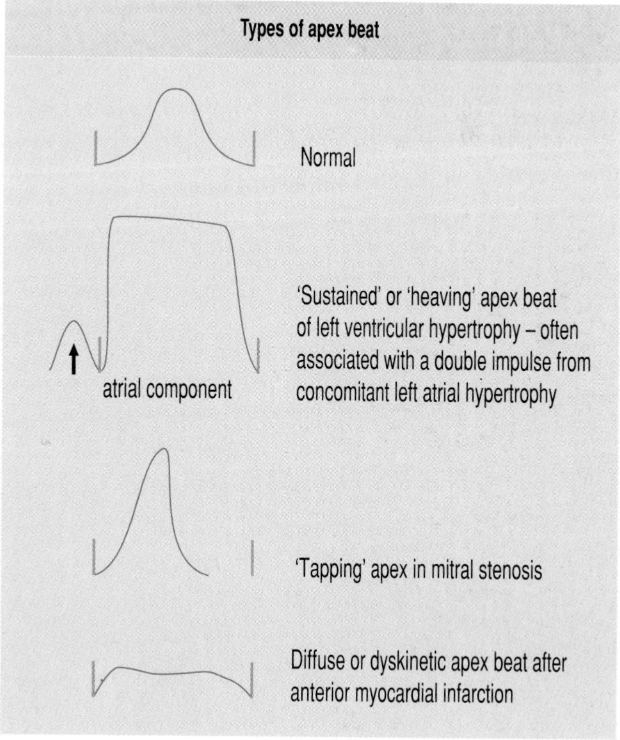
Types of apex beat
Normal
atrial component
'Sustained' or 'heaving' apex beat of left ventricular hypertrophy – often associated with a double impulse from concomitant left atrial hypertrophy
'Tapping' apex in mitral stenosis
Diffuse or dyskinetic apex beat after anterior myocardial infarction

Fig. 7.65 Types of apical impulse.

beat, and the range which this encompasses, must be learnt by experience. A forceful apex beat usually indicates increased cardiac output (e.g. in a patient with a fever, or after exercise). A diffuse poorly localized apex beat is commonly found after damage to the ventricular muscle, either by myocardial infarction or as a result of cardiomyopathy. This diffuse impulse can often be seen by inspecting the precordium as well as felt. The character of the cardiac impulse in left ventricular hypertrophy is very distinctive, being a sustained and forceful heave rather than a short sharp impulse. In mitral stenosis, the cardiac apex is often described as tapping. To some extent, this is due to displacement of the left ventricle nearer to the examining hand by an enlarged left atrium, and partly it is due to a loud first heart sound which is palpable as well as audible. Right ventricular hypertrophy or dilatation is felt as a heave close to the left sternal order.

While palpating the heart, the examining hand will sometimes detect a vibration or 'thrill'. Thrills are really 'palpable murmurs' and are always accompanied by an easily heard murmur on auscultation. A diastolic thrill (which feels very like the sensation of stroking a purring cat) may sometimes be felt in patients with mitral stenosis. Systolic thrills may accompany aortic stenosis, ventricular septal defect, or mitral reflux.

AUSCULTATION OF THE HEART

Cardiac auscultation is easier with a good quality stethoscope. The stethoscope was originally introduced into medical practice by the French physician Laennec at the beginning of the 19th century. In its original form it consisted of a wooden cylinder with a small hole drilled from end to end. In addition to introducing a decorous distance between the head of the physician and the chest of the patient, the stethoscope has two principle functions. First, it transmits sounds from the chest of the patient and helps to exclude extraneous noise; and second, it selectively emphasizes sounds of certain frequencies, thus enabling the examiner to concentrate on them.

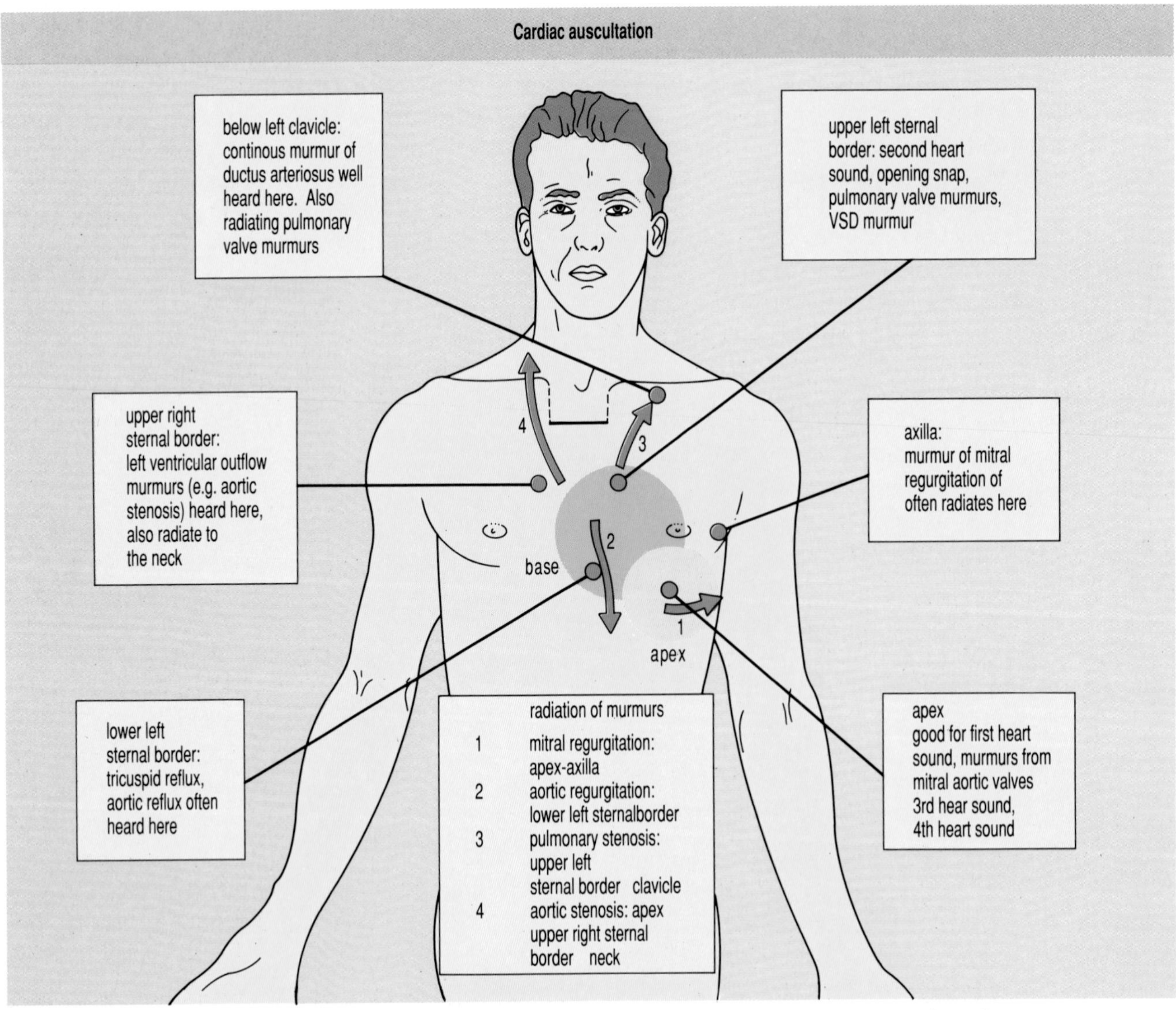
Cardiac auscultation
below left clavicle: continous murmur of ductus arteriosus well heard here. Also radiating pulmonary valve murmurs
upper left sternal border: second heart sound, opening snap, pulmonary valve murmurs, VSD murmur
upper right sternal border: left ventricular outflow murmurs (e.g. aortic stenosis) heard here, also radiate to the neck
axilla: murmur of mitral regurgitation of often radiates here
base
apex
4
3
2
1
lower left sternal border: tricuspid reflux, aortic reflux often heard here
radiation of murmurs
1 mitral regurgitation: apex-axilla
2 aortic regurgitation: lower left sternalborder
3 pulmonary stenosis: upper left sternal border clavicle
4 aortic stenosis: apex upper right sternal border neck
apex good for first heart sound, murmurs from mitral aortic valves 3rd hear sound, 4th heart sound

Fig. 7.66 Cardiac auscultation; the best sites for hearing sounds and murmurs depend on where the sound is produced and where turbulent blood flows radiate to.

An indiscriminate amplification of the sound coming from the chest, as would be produced by a sensitive high fidelity microphone, actually produces a signal which is very hard for the human ear to intrepret. A modern stethoscope consists of two ear pieces connected by tubing to a chest piece which usually has both diaphragm and bell attachments. The ear pieces should be angled forwards to match the direction of the examiner's external auditory meati. They should fit snugly but comfortably. The tubing should not be too long (cardiologists seldom wear their stethoscopes round their collars). The bell and diaphragm chest pieces selectively emphasize sounds of different frequencies. The bell is central for listening to low pitched sounds such as the mid-diastolic murmur of mitral stenosis or the third hear sound of cardiac failure. In contrast, the diaphragm filters out low pitched sounds and, therefore, emphasizes high pitched ones. The diaphragm is best for analyzing the second heart sound, for ejection and mid-systolic clicks, and for the soft but high pitched early diastolic murmur of aortic regurgitation.

It is worthwhile buying a good stethoscope, taking good care of it, and making use of every opportunity to appreciate the normal range of heart and chest sounds, both at rest and after exertion.

When auscultating the heart, you should as a minimum listen at the apex, at the base (the part of the heart between the apex and the sternum), and in the aortic and pulmonary areas to the right and left of the sternum, respectively (Fig. 7.66). Obviously, if anything abnormal is found, the stethoscope should be moved around until it is heard most clearly. It is good practice to relate the auscultatory findings to the cardiac cycle by simultaneously palpating the carotid artery while listening to the heart (Fig. 7.67).

It is helpful when learning or when confronted with a difficult problem, to analyze your oscillatory findings under three headings, namely first and second heart sounds, murmurs, and any additional heart sounds. In practice, as you gain experience, particular auscultatory patterns will be recognized as a whole, just as one recognizes speech.

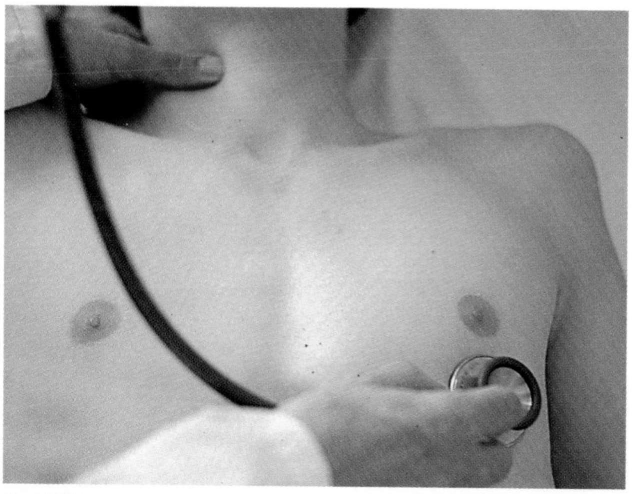

Fig. 7.67 Simultaneously listening to the heart sounds and timing them against the carotid pulse.

THE HEART SOUNDS

First and second heart sounds

The mechanism of the first and second heart sounds and the mechanism and physiology of splitting the second heart sound have already been described. The first heart sound can usually be heard easily with both the bell and the diaphragm, but the diaphragm is invaluable for analyzing the second heart sound, with the stethoscope usually best placed at the mid-left sternal edge. It is usual to record the heart sounds in a shorthand notation which derives from the records made by phonocardiography (Fig. 7.68)

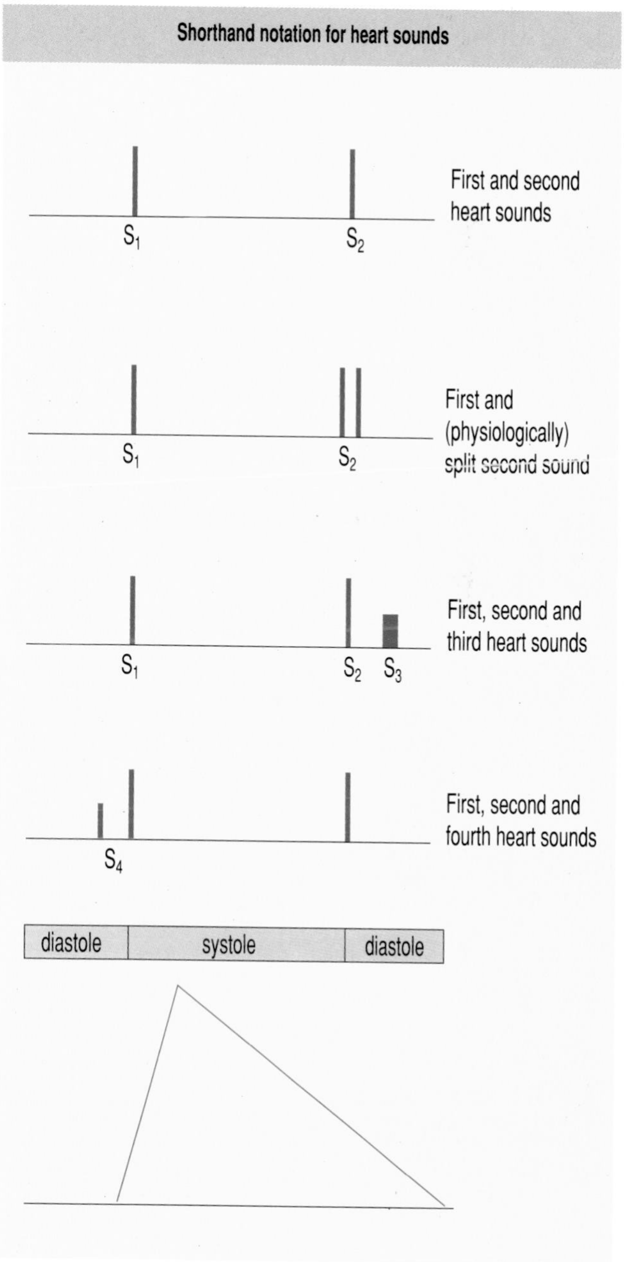

Fig. 7.68 Shorthand notation (derived from phonocardiography) for recording the heart sounds.

Factors which may cause a change in the intensity of the heart sounds are shown in Figure 7.69. The commonest causes of a loud first heart sound are an increased cardiac output or mitral stenosis. The commonest causes of an abnormally quiet first heart sound are reduced cardiac output and either a thick chest wall or emphysema. A loud ringing second heart sound may be a feature of systemic hypertension or occasionally of pulmonary hypertension.

Third and fourth heart sounds

These are abnormal heart sounds which are heard in addition to the normal ones in patients with certain specific conditions. The third heart sound is a low-pitched, thudding sound which occurs in diastole and coincides with the end of the rapid phase of ventricular filling. It occurs in two quite distinct sets of circumstances, one of which is physiological, the other pathological. A physiological third heart sound occurs in young fit adults under circumstances of increased cardiac output (e.g. in athletes, in the presence of a fever, or during pregnancy). It is of no pathological significance. A pathological third heat sound is usually a marker for severe impairment of left ventricular function. It can be heard in dilated cardiomyopathy, after acute myocardial infarction, or (in this case, coming from the right ventricle) in acute massive pulmonary embolism. In patients with a pathological third heart sound, there is nearly always a tachycardia, and the first and second heart sounds are relatively quiet. The cadence of first, second, and third heart sounds therefore sound something like 'da-da-boom, da-da-boom' and has been given the name of a gallop rhythm. (The doctor who gave it this name, Phillippe Potain, served in Napoleon's Cavalry, so presumably knew a gallop when he heard one.)

A fourth heart sound is an extra heart sound which coincides with atrial contraction. It is usually best heard in patients where the left atrium is hypertrophied (e.g. as a consequence of systemic hypertension or hyertrophic cardiomyopathy). It is not, however, heard in mitral stenosis. A fourth sound sounds a little like 'da-lub-dup da-lub-dup' (Fig. 7.70).

Other extra heart sounds

Ejection click

This is a high pitched ringing sound which usually follows very shortly after the first heart sound (Fig. 7.71). It is a feature of aortical pulmonary valve stenosis, where it is probably due to the sudden opening of the deformed valve. Sometimes, patients with a dilated pulmonary artery or an ascending aorta may have an ejection click without a stenotic valve.

The intensity of the heart sounds

Loud first sound:
Hyperdynamic circulation (fever, exercise)
Mitral stenosis
Atrial myxoma (rare!)

Soft first sound:
Low cardiac output (rest, heart failure)
Tachycardia
Severe mitral reflux (due to destruction of valve)

Variable intensity of first sound:
Atrial fibrillation
Complete heart block

Loud aortic component of second sound:
Systemic hypertension
Dilated aortic root

Soft aortic component of second sound:
Calcific aortic stenosis

Loud pulmonary component of second sound:
Pulmonary hypertension

Fig. 7.69 Factors which may influence the intensity of the heart sounds.

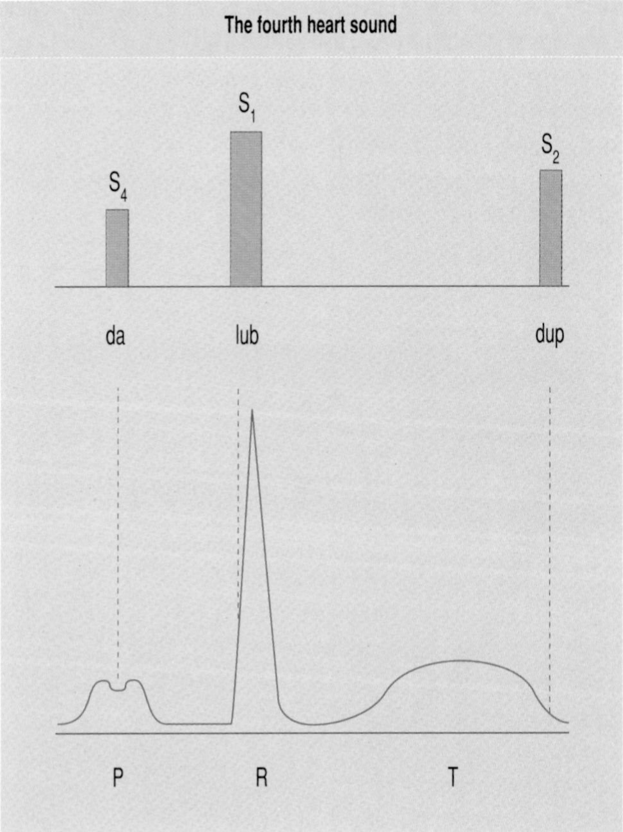

Fig. 7.70 The fourth heart sound.

Opening snap

This is a diastolic sound heard in mitral stenosis and associated with the tensing of the diaphragm formed by the stenosed mitral valve. It is best heard to the left of the sternum and sounds rather like the second part of a widely split second heart sound.

Mid-systolic clicks

These are usually associated with mitral valve prolapse and are due to the tensing of the long and redundant chordae tendineae of these valves. The clicks may or may not be associated with a late systolic murmur (see pages 7.36–7.37).

Sounds from artificial heart valves

The ball, disc, or poppet in an artificial heart valve usually makes a noise both when it opens and when the valve closes. The closing sound is usually louder than the opening sound. Thus, an aortic prosthesis will have a soft opening click just after the first heart sound and a loud closing click which contributes to the second heart sound. Conversely, a mitral valve will give a soft opening click in a similar position to the opening snap of mitral stenosis and a loud closing click which contributes to the first heart sound.

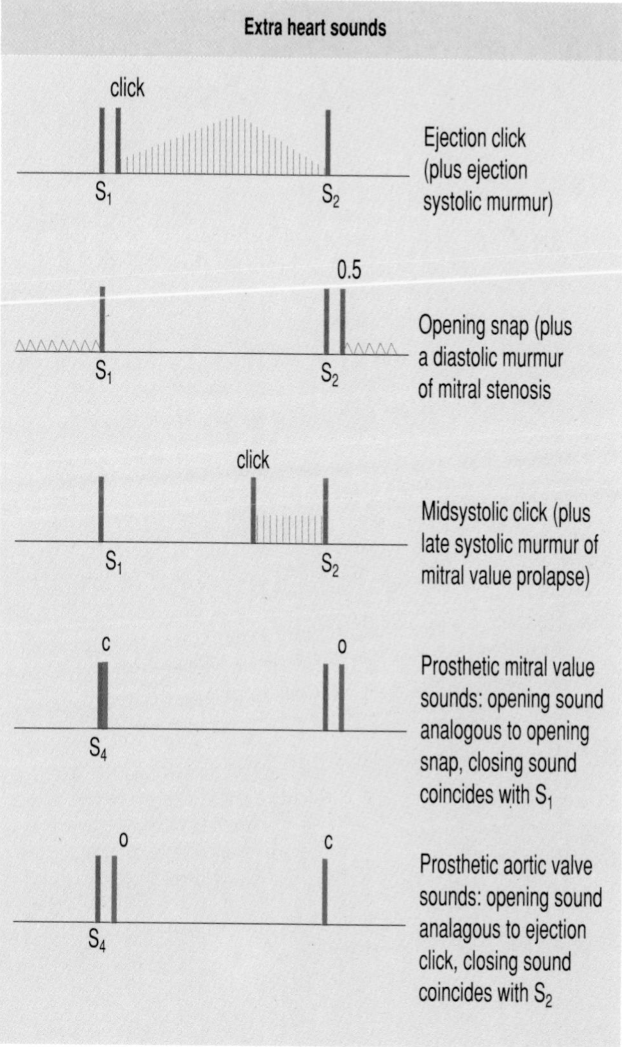

Fig. 7.71 'Extra heart sounds', o.s = opening snap, o.c = opening and closing sounds.

Murmurs

Murmurs are more or less musical sounds occuring at specific points in the cardiac cycle and resulting from turbulent blood flow. The important points in analyzing a murmur are: where is occurs in the cardiac cycle, what it sounds like, where it is best heard, where it radiates to, and what happens to manoeuvres like deep breathing (Fig. 7.72).

Systolic murmurs

Systolic murmurs are due to one of three things: leakage of blood through a structure which is normally closed during systole, i.e. mitral or tricuspid valves, or the interventricular septum, blood flow through a valve normally open in systole but which has become abnormally narrowed (e.g. aortic or pulmonary stenosis), or increased blood flow through a normal valve, i.e. a flow murmur.

Grading the intensity of murmurs

Grade 1 just audible with a good stethoscope in a quiet room

Grade 2 quiet but readily audible with a stethoscope

Grade 3 easily heard with a stethoscope

Grade 4 a loud, obvious murmur

Grade 5 very loud, heard not only over the precordium but elsewere in the body

Fig. 7.72 Summary of heart murmurs.

Murmurs that are due to leakage of blood through an incompetent mitral or tricuspid valve or a ventricular septal defect are usually of similar intensity throughout the length of systole. They are called pansystolic or holosystolic murmurs (Fig. 7.73). Occasionally, a valve is competent at the start of systole but starts to leak half way through. This is common in patients with mitral valve prolapse.

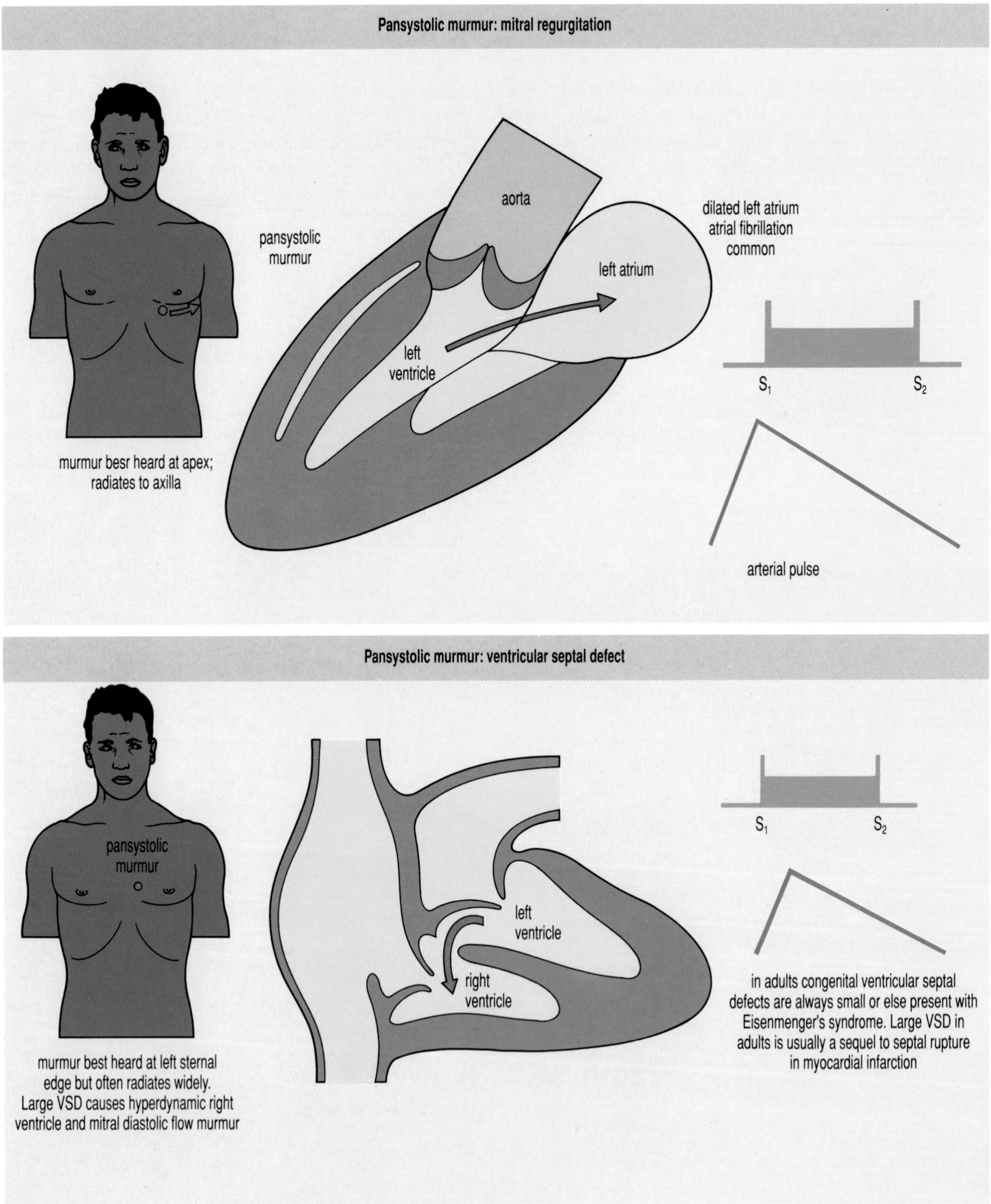

Fig. 7.73 Pansystolic (holosystolic) murmurs: mitral regurgitation (above), ventricular septal defect (below).

The result is a murmur which starts in mid or late systole, and is called a mid-systolic or late systolic murmur (see Fig. 7.71).

Murmurs which are due to blood being forced through a narrow aortic or pulmonary valve or to increased blood flow through a normal aortic or pulmonary valve tend to start quietly at the beginning of systole, rise to a crescendo in mid-systole, and then become quiet again towards the end of systole. Such murmurs are called ejection systolic murmurs (Fig. 7.74).

Innocent murmurs

Innocent murmurs are murmurs which are not associated with any major structural abnormality in the heart nor with any haemodynamic disturbance. They are common in children and young adults. They have the following characteristics: always systolic and always quiet (<grade 3); usually best heard at the left sternal edge; no associated ventricular hypertrophy; normal heart sounds, pulses, chest radiograph, and electrocardiogram.

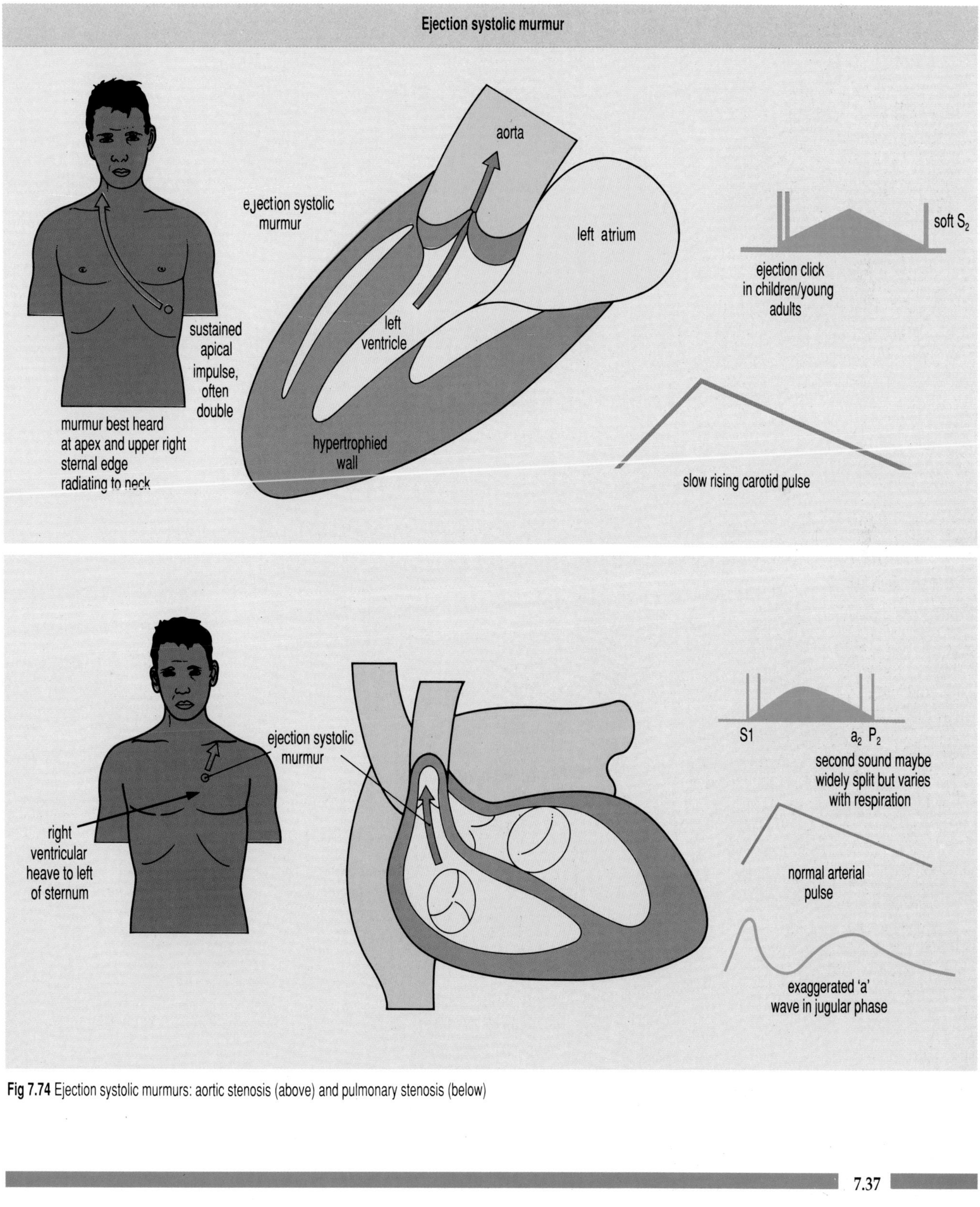

Fig 7.74 Ejection systolic murmurs: aortic stenosis (above) and pulmonary stenosis (below)

Diastolic murmurs

Diastolic murmurs can be divided into early diastolic murmurs and mid-diastolic murmurs. An early diastolic murmur is nearly always due to incompetence of either the aortic or the pulmonary valve. It is maximum at the beginning of diastole when aortic or pulmonary pressure is highest, and rapidly becomes quieter (decrescendo) as pressure in the great vessel falls. The sound of an aortic diastolic murmur has aptly been described as like a whispered letter 'r' (Fig. 7.75).

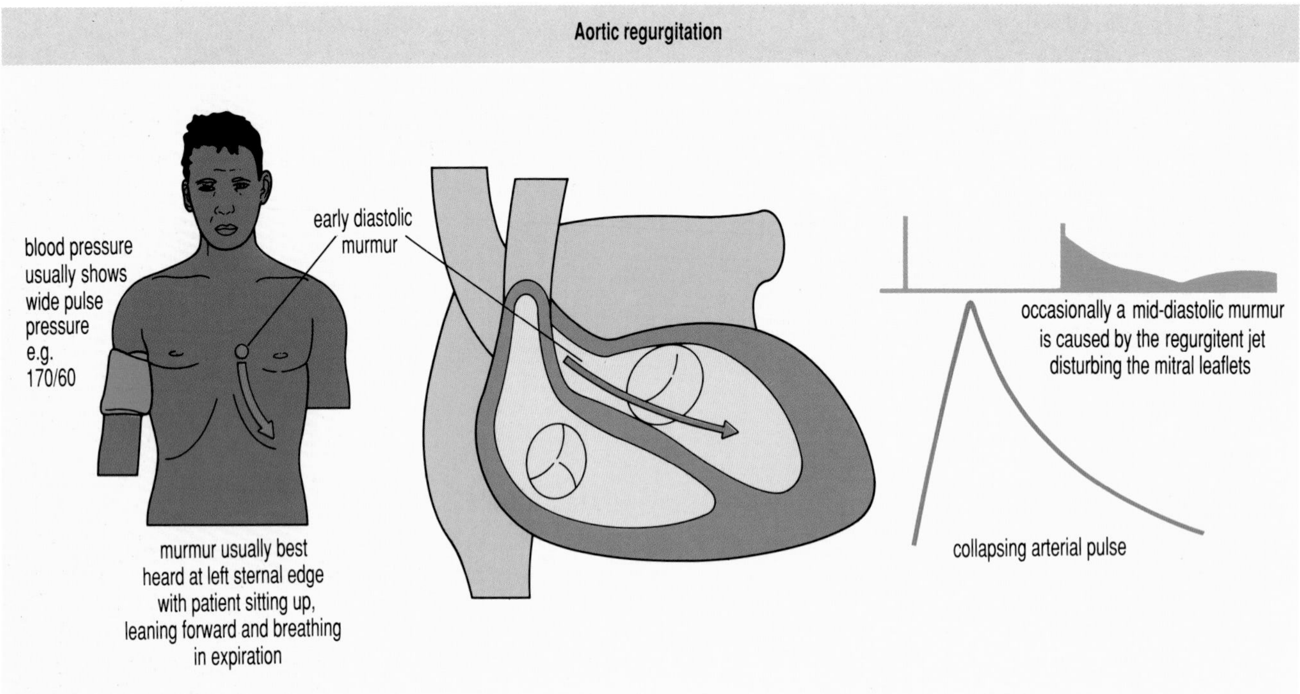

Fig. 7.75 Aortic regurgitation as an example of an early diastolic murmur.

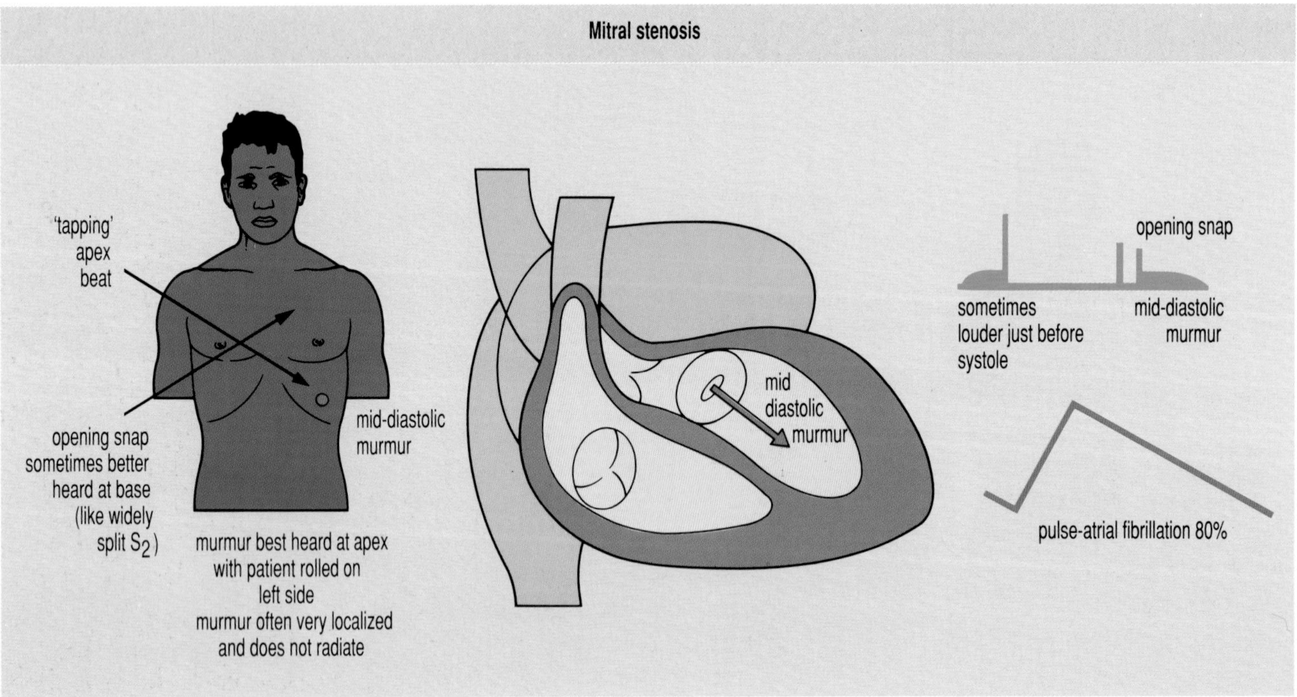

Fig. 7.76 Mitral stenosis as an example of a mid-diastolic murmur.

A mid-diastolic murmur is usually due to either blood flow through a narrowed mitral or tricuspid valve, or occasionally to increased blood flow through one of these valves (e.g. in children with atrial septal defect). The characteristic murmur of mitral stenosis is a low pitched rumbling murmur heard throughout diastole (Fig 7.76). Sometimes in patients in sinus rhythm, it gets louder just before the onset of systoles as a result of atrial contraction increasing blood flow through the narrowed valve. Sometimes patients with aortic reflux have a mid-diastolic murmur. This is caused by the regurgitant blood from the incompetent aortic valve setting up a vibration of the anterior leaflet of the mitral valve (Austin Flint murmur).

Murmurs tend to be heard best over the site of the lesion (Fig. 7.77) which is causing them, and in the direction of the turbulent blood stream which is producing the sound. It is sometimes possible to make murmurs easier to hear by putting the patient into special positions. The murmur of mitral stenosis is best heard if the patient is rolled onto his or her left hand side and the stethoscope bell applied to the cardiac apex (Fig. 7.78). The murmur of aortic reflux is sometimes best heard if the patient is made to sit up, lean forward, and breathe out fully while the stethoscope is applied at the left side of the lower part of the sternum (Fig. 7.79).

Sites of radiation of murmurs		
Cause	**'Primary site'**	**Radiation**
Tricuspid regurgitation	Lower left sternal edge	Lower right sternal edge, liver
Pulmonary stenosis	Upper left sternal edge	Towards left clavicle, beneath left scapula
Mitral regurgitation	Apex	Left axilla, beneath left scapula
Aortic regurgitation	Left sternal edge	Down left sternal edge towards apex
Aortic stenosis	Apex	Towards upper right sternal edge, over carotids
Ventricular septal defect	Left sternal edge	All over precardium
Mitral stenosis	Apex	Does not radiate

Fig. 7.77 Sites of radiation of murmurs.

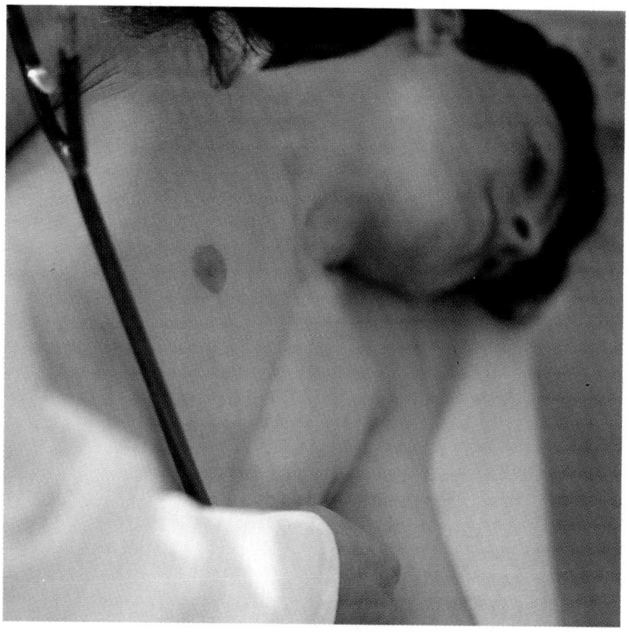

Fig. 7.78 Mitral diastolic murmurs are best heard using the bell, with the patient rolled onto the left side.

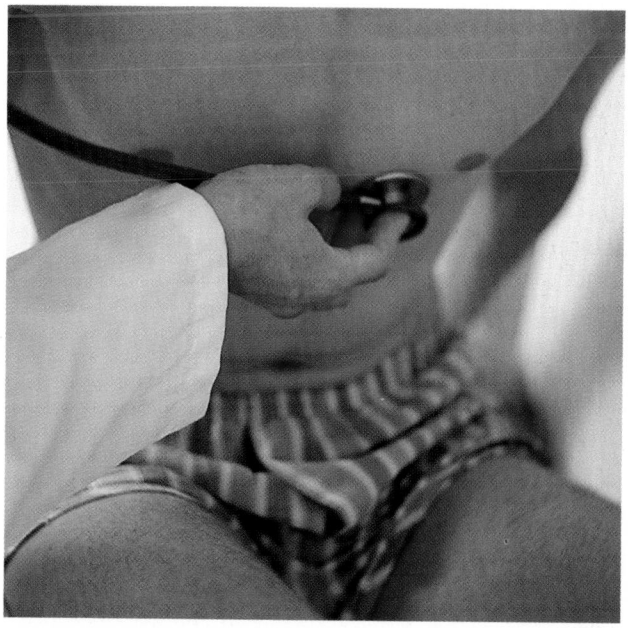

Fig. 7.79 Aortic diastolic murmurs may be heard more easily if the patient sits up, leans forwards, and holds his breath in expiration.

The behaviour of murmurs during respiration sometimes gives a clue to their nature (Fig. 7.80). Systolic murmurs arising at the pulmonary valve (i.e. pulmonary stenosis flow murmurs) tend to get louder during inspiration and quieter during expiration. Conversely, murmurs arising on the left side of the heart tend to get quieter during inspiration. Making the patient perform a Valsalva maneouvre (forceful expiration against a closed glottis) makes most murmurs quieter, for cardiac output is diminshed, whereas the murmur of hypertrophic obstructive cardiomyopathy (an ejection systolic murmur arising from the left ventricular outlet tract) tends to get louder as the degree of obstruction increases. The murmur of mitral stenosis is often easier to hear if the patient is made to exercise before listening for it.

Behaviour of murmurs during respiration
Louder immediately on inspiration
Pulmonary stenosis Pulmonary valve flow murmurs
Quieter immediately on inspiration (may become louder later)
Mitral regurgitation Aortic stenosis
Louder during Valsalva manoeuvre
Hypertrophic obstructive Cardiomyopathy
The murmer of mitral prolapse may become louder or softer during inspiration

Fig. 7.80 Behaviour of murmurs during respiration.

THE CARDIOVASCULAR SYSTEM AND CHEST EXAMINATION

The most important feature to look for in a patient with primarily cardiac disease is the presence of crepitations at the lung bases. These are crackling sounds during inspiration, and they are an early sign of pulmonary oedema. In mild heart failure crepitations are confined to the lung bases, but in severe failure they may be heard all over the chest. Patients with severe heart failure and peripheral oedema may also develop pleural effusions. The examination of the chest is discussed in detail in Chapter 6.

THE CARDIOVASCULAR SYSTEM AND ABDOMINAL EXAMINATION

Abdominal examination (see Chapter 8) also plays an important part in the examination of patients with suspected cardiovascular disease. The principle points to check for are the presence of ascites, of an enlarged or pulsatile liver, of an aortic aneurysm, and particularly in patients with high blood pressure, the presence of enlarged kidneys or a renal artery bruit.

The liver is a very vascular organ and will enlarge in response to any rise in right atrial pressure. Sometimes, particularly if the enlargement is rapid, this leads to acute discomfort in the right upper quadrant of the abdomen. The liver edge is characteristically firm and even. In patients with tricuspid reflux, there is a marked hepatic pulsation in time with the regurgitation waves in the jugular venous pulse and with the arterial pulse.

In severe heart failure, the spleen may also become passively enlarged; however, this is less common and less prominent than hepatic enlargement. Enlargement of the spleen in its role as part of the immune system is seen in subacute bacterial endocarditis.

Aneurysm of the abdominal aorta is common, particularly in men over the age of 60. It is important to detect because early elective surgery carries a much lower mortality than emergency surgery. The characteristic finding on examination is pulsation at about the level of the umbilicus. It is easy to feel the normal aorta at this level, yet the characteristic features of an aneurysm are that it is enlarged in comparison with a normal aorta and that the pulsation it generates is expansile (Fig. 7.81). Abdominal ultrasound examination is a good way of confirming the diagnosis of aortic aneurysm and of measuring its size.

Enlarged kidneys caused by polycystic disease sometimes present as hypertension, even heart failure. Another cause of hypertension is renal artery stenosis. In this condition, it is sometimes possible to hear a murmur or bruit with the stethoscope applied to one side or other of the umbilicus.

THE PERIPHERAL VASCULAR SYSTEM

Assess the skin temperature in the feet, and feel and record the popliteal and dorsalis pedis pulses. The features of peripheral arterial disease are described on page 7.45. Look for varicose veins and venous ulcers, and for the presence of oedema.

Oedema

Oedema is the collection of an abnormal amount of tissue fluid. This fluid accumulates in the extra cellular spaces between cells, and leads to local swelling. Tissue fluid is normally in dynamic equilibrium with plasma, so that the amount of fluid escaping from blood vessels is normally exactly balanced by the quantity of fluid being returned to the blood vessels plus that which is drained away by the lymphatic vessels (Fig. 7.82). Heart failure (see pages 7.42–7.43) is an important cause of oedema. The oedema of heart failure is largely due to increased venous pressure, but factors such as a slightly reduced plasma albumin concentration and abnormal capillary permeability may also play a role.

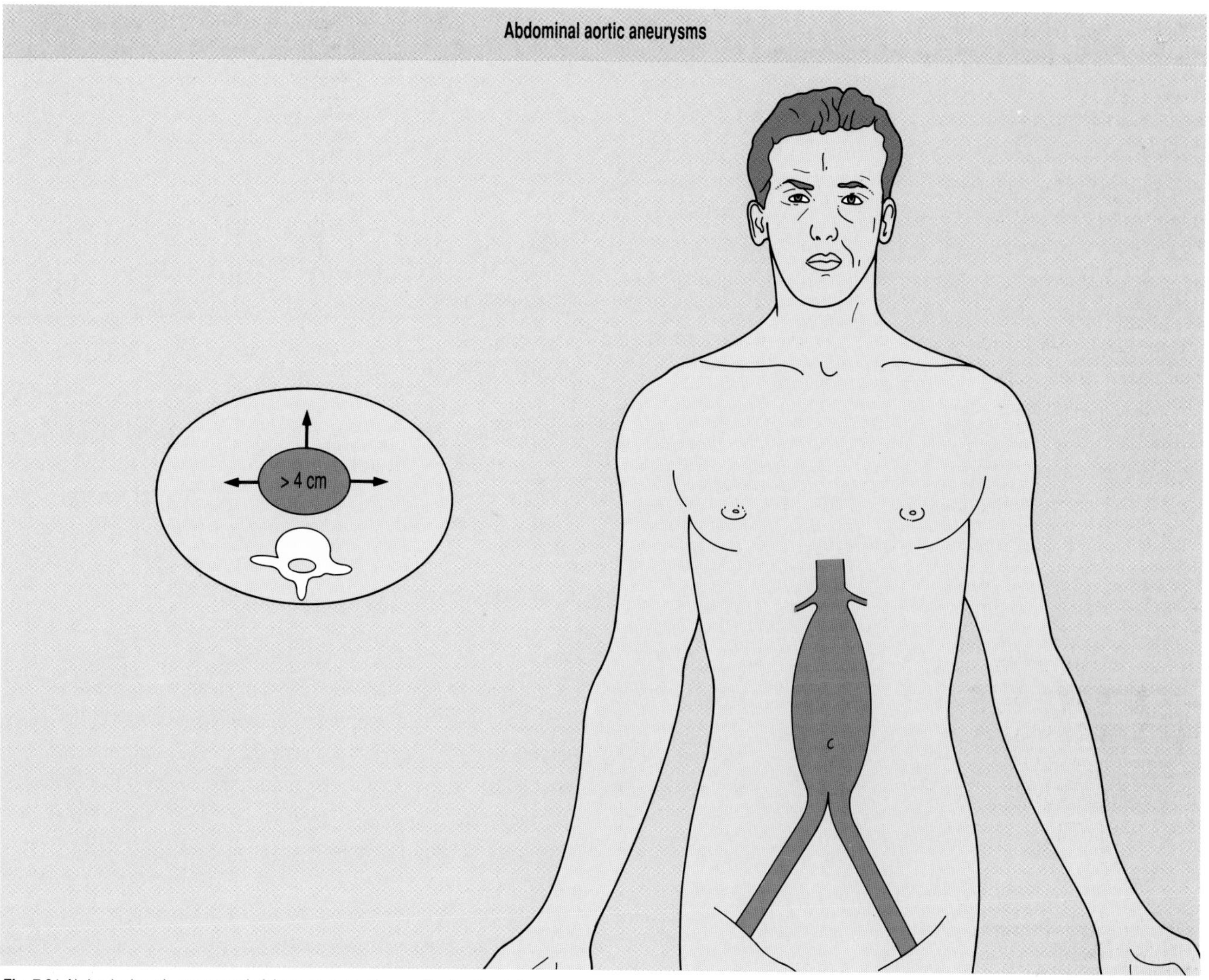

Fig. 7.81 Abdominal aortic aneurysm is felt as an 'expansive swelling' in the abdomen.

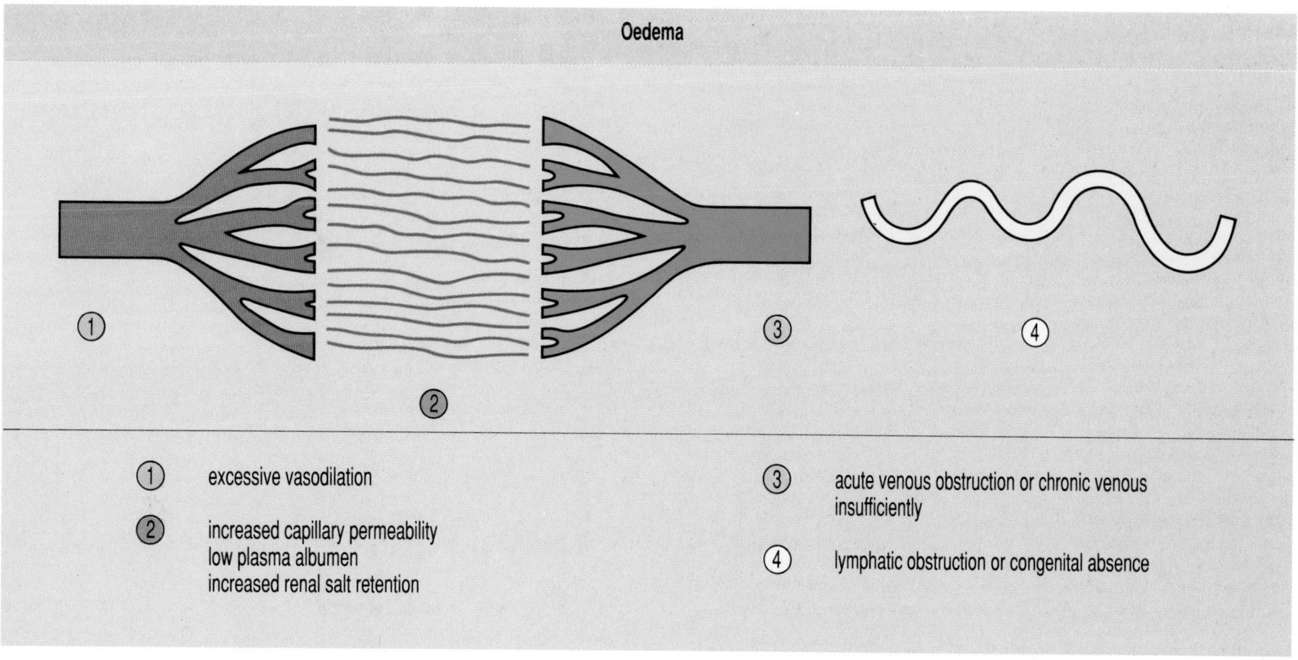

Fig. 7.82 Diagram to show the factors contributing to oedema formation.

The oedema of heart failure can be divided into pulmonary oedema and peripheral oedema. Peripheral oedema is usually a feature of right-sided heart failure or congestive heart failure. It characteristically accumulates at the lowest part of the body ('dependent oedema') namely the feet and ankles in ambulant patients, and the sacrum in patients confined to beds. The more severe the oedema the further up the leg it tends to extend. In neglected patients, it may involve the thigh, the scrotum, and the lower part of the abdominal wall. Severe oedema is frequently accompanied by increased leakage of fluid into the serous cavities, and may be accompanied by ascites and pleural effusions. Cardiac oedema virtually never involves the face.

Clinically, oedema is detected in peripheral tissue by swelling which can be displaced by firm finger pressure and which leaves a pit when the finger is removed. The main differential diagnosis of cardiac oedema is stasis oedema which occurs in elderly or immobile patients. This is caused by lack of muscle pump activity, in addition to chronic damage to venous valves and possibly a degree of lymphatic obstruction. The distinction is best made by looking for other signs of cardiac failure. In a patient who has a normal jugular venous pressure peripheral oedema is seldom due to heart failure.

Features of acute heart failure
Acute dyspnoea (pulmonary oedema)
Hypotension (may be masked by general vasoconstriction)
Cold clammy skin (peripheral vasoconstriction)
Anxiety
Confusion (impaired cerebral blood flow, hypoxaemia)
Oliguria

Fig. 7.83 Features of acute heart failure.

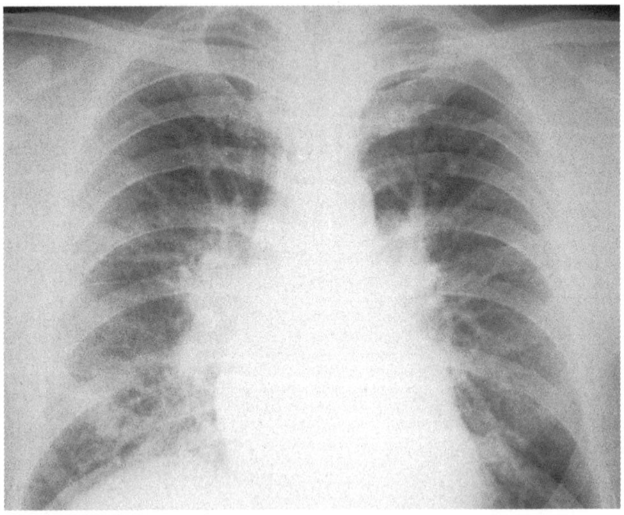

Fig. 7.84 Chest radiograph in acute left heart failure caused by mitral stenosis (Note, left heart failure does not equate with left ventricular failure: the left ventricle in mitral stenosis is fine!)

CLINICAL FEATURES OF SPECIFIC CARDIAC CONDITIONS

HEART FAILURE

Heart failure can be crudely defined as an inability to produce a cardiac output adequate to satisfy the body's needs. It can be subdivided into acute and chronic heart failure, and also into left-sided, right-sided, or mixed heart failure depending on the cause.

Acute heart failure

One of the commonest manifestations of acute heart failure is a low systemic blood pressure (Fig. 7.83), but sometimes intense peripheral vasoconstriction supports a normal or even increased blood pressure despite a very much reduced cardiac output. Acute *left* heart failure is accompanied by pulmonary oedema. This is due to a rise in pulmonary venous pressure to a point where there is net movement of fluid out into the alveolar spaces of the lungs. The patient becomes extremely breathless, develops a cough, and may produce frothy pink stained sputum. The characteristic clinical sign of pulmonary oedema is the presence of widespread crepitations or crackling sounds usually best heard at the basis of the lungs. The chest X-ray (Fig. 7.84) shows white fluffy shadows in both lungs. In severe cases, both lung fields become almost opaque. With acute right heart failure, for example, as a consequence of acute massive

Features of chronic heart failure
Tiredness on minimal exertion
Exertional dyspnoea
Peripheral oedema
Abdominal discomfort (from hepatic distention)
Nocturia (reversal of diurnal rhythm)
Weight loss and cachexia

Fig. 7.85 Features of chronic heart failure.

pulmonary embolism, there is no pulmonary oedema, but the jugular venous pressure is massively elevated and blood pressure is very low.

Chronic heart failure

In chronic heart failure, the body does its best to compensate for the cardiac problems (Fig. 7.85). In chronic left heart failure, there is very often a reflex rise in pulmonary vascular resistance, thus protecting the patient from pulmonary oedema at the cost of precipitating secondary right heart failure. This combination is sometimes called mixed or *congestive* heart failure (Fig. 7.86).

Another important compensatory mechanism is fluid retention mediated by increased renal salt and water reabsorption. This has the effect of increasing cardiac filling pressure (manifested by a raised jugular venous pressure) at the cost of increased oedema.

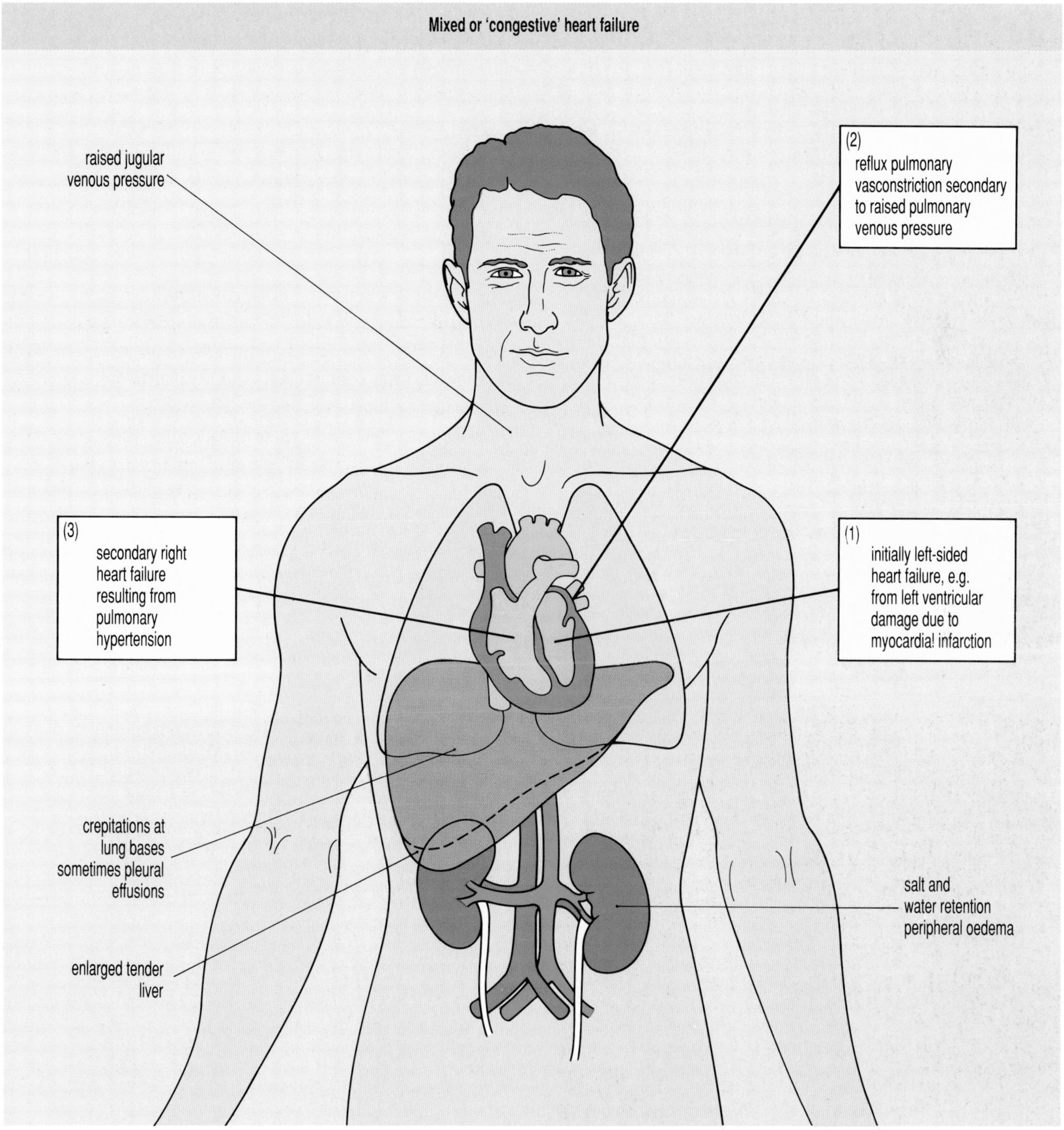

Fig. 7.86 Mixed or 'congestive' heart failure starts as left heart failure, but secondary pulmonary vasoconstriction then causes right heart failure.

CORONARY ARTERY DISEASE

Angina

Coronary artery disease is the commonest form of heart disease in the Western world. It has three principle manifestations: angina, acute myocardial infarction, and chronic heart failure. The characteristic features of angina have already been described in the section on taking a cardiac history. Physical examination of the angina patient is frequently entirely normal; nonetheless, the examiner should be alert for features of hyperlipidaemia such as corneal arcus, thickened achilles tendons, and xanthelasma (Fig. 7.87). Confirmation of angina is usually made by ECG exercise testing (Fig. 7.88), as the resting electrocardiogram is frequently entirely normal. Further information can be provided by exercise thallium scanning, and by coronary arteriography (Fig. 7.89).

Features of hyperlipidaemia
Common
Corneal arcus (nonspecific in patients over 50)
Xanthelasma (nonspecific in patients over 50)
Tendon xanthomas (mainly in familial hypercholesterolaemia)
Less common
Palmar xanthomas
Eruptive xanthomas
Ejection systolic murmur (familial hypercholesterolaemia)
Lipaemia retinalis

Fig. 7.87 Features of hyperlipidaemia.

Myocardial infarction

Acute myocardial infarction is nearly always caused by coronary thrombosis. The coronary thrombosis occurs on the basis of a cracked atheromatous plaque. The patient may previously have suffered from angina, but frequently this is not the case. The most characteristic symptom of myocardial infarction is chest pain which is similar in distribution to the pain of angina but is usually much more severe and persists even when the patient rests. In a small proportion of patients, particularly the elderly and those with diabetes mellitus, myocardial infarction can be relatively painless.

On physical examination, there is nearly always marked evidence of sympathetic nervous system activation, the blood pressure tends to be low with a narrow pulse pressure, there may be a third heart sound, and there are frequently ventricular extrasystoles (Fig. 7.90). The diagnosis of myocardial infarction is usually confirmed by electrocardiography (Fig. 7.91) and by characteristic changes in the plasma level of cardiac enzymes.

The main risk in the early stages of acute myocardial infarction is of ventricular fibrillation. This requires constant observation of the patient and treatment if necessary with a defibrillator. Later complications include arrhythmias, cardiac rupture, and occasionally the development of ventricular septal defect or mitral reflux.

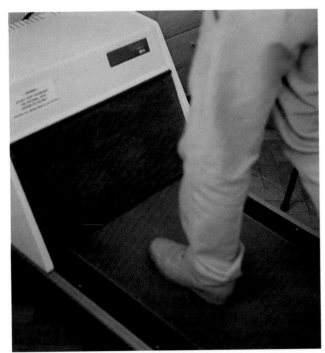

Fig. 7.88 Treadmill exercise testing is best used to confirm a clinical diagnosis of angina and to get an objective estimate of exercise tolerance.

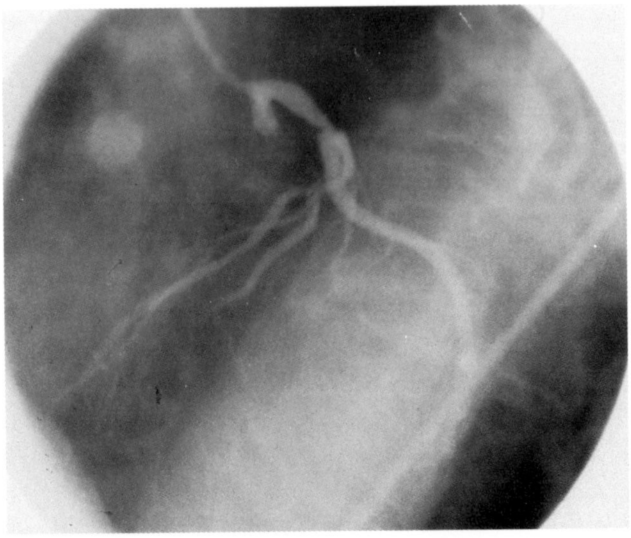

Fig. 7.89 Coronary artercogram showing left main coronary stenosis. (Compare with Fig. 7.25b.)

Features of acute myocardial infarction
Symptoms
Severe pain Pain persists despite rest
Physical signs
Signs of sympathetic activation (pallor, sweating) Narrow pulse pressures May be extrasystoles May be added (3rd) heart sound

Fig. 7.90 Features of acute myocardial infarction.

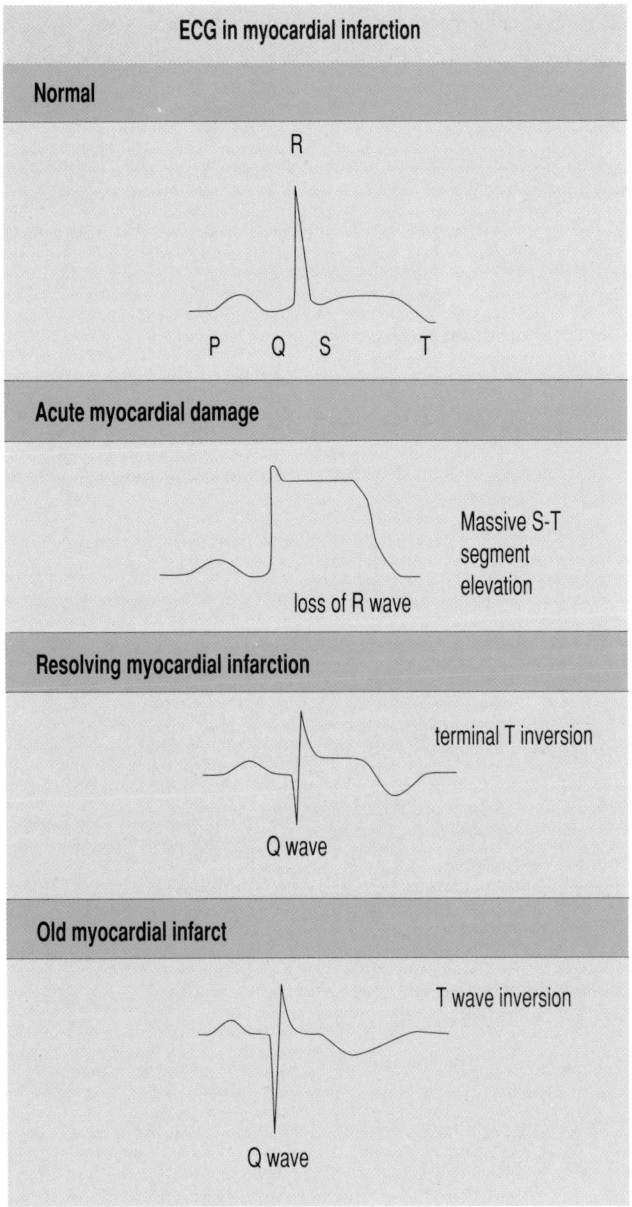

Fig. 7.91 Electrocardiogram showing features of acute myocardial infarction.

Chronic heart failure due to ischaemic heart disease has the clinical features of any other form of chronic heart failure, but diagnosis is usually made on the basis of the history.

PERIPHERAL VASCULAR DISEASE

This can be considered under two headings: disease of the peripheral arterial system and of the peripheral venous system. Peripheral arterial disease is mainly to do with acute or chronic impairment of the blood supply to a limb. This may result from atheromatous narrowing of the artery, from thrombosis, or much more rarely from embolism from the heart.

Acute arterial obstruction presents with a cold, white, painful, pulseless limb. The sight of obstruction is usually obvious from examining the pulses, but confirmation by ultrasound or by angiography before surgery is generally necessary. It is important to check pulses in the other limbs as well even if they are not obviously ischaemic. Thromboembolism to multiple sites may be the first clue to a cardiac disease such as atrial myxoma.

Chronic arterial insufficiency is much commoner in the lower limb, and usually presents as intermittent claudication. The patient is aware of pain either in the leg, the thigh, or the buttock which comes on with walking and goes away when stopping to rest. Examination of the leg reveals weak or absent foot, knee, and sometimes femoral pulses. There may be a murmur or bruit over the femoral artery because of turbulence due to narrowing upstream in the internal or external iliac arteries. As the disease progresses, pain comes on with progressively less exertion until finally the patient experiences pain at rest. Pain is often worse at night. Patients with severe chronic arterial insufficiency in the legs often gain partial relief by hanging their leg over the side of the bed outside the bedclothes. Paradoxically, this often makes perfusion of the foot worse. The skin tends to become discoloured and shiny, and hair is lost from the foot. Infection which often starts with a small injury such as one derived from paring the toenails spreads rapidly. Eventually, gangrene may affect the toes and foot (Fig. 7.92).

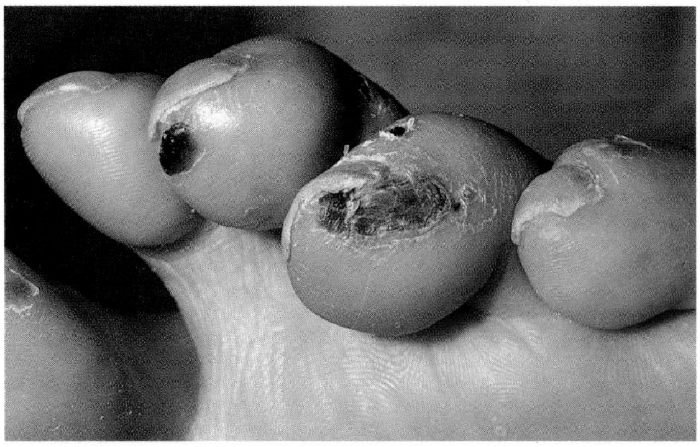

Fig. 7.92 Gangrene of toes in peripheral vascular disease.

Patients with diabetes mellitus are particularly susceptible to peripheral arterial disease. Because diabetes affects both large and small blood vessels, and also the intercellular matrix of the tissues, peripheral tissue damage tends to be more severe than would be expected from the large vessel pulses alone. The position is made worse by diabetic neuropathy which means that patients may sustain injuries giving rise to infection without noticing much discomfort until the infection is well-established.

The main aids to clinical diagnosis in peripheral arterial disease are ultrasound examination, which can detect both vessel diameter and blood flow, and angiography.

DISEASE OF THE PERIPHERAL VEINS

The principal diseases of the peripheral veins are varicose veins, thrombophlebitis, and deep venous thrombosis.

Varicose veins

Varicose veins are excessively dilated superficial leg veins. They usually result from defects in the 'muscle pump' system which normally pumps venous blood from the legs via the deep veins against the force of gravity. In adopting an upright posture, the human race has considerably increased the difficulty of securing adequate venous drainage from the legs. The two major causes of varicose veins are defective valves in the 'perforating veins' which connect the deep and superficial venous systems in the calf (Fig. 7.93) and defective valves in the upper part of the long saphenous vein where it joins the the femoral vein at the thigh. Commonly, the problem is initiated by incompetent valves in the perforating veins, and saphenofemoral incompetence is secondary to the resulting dilatation of the superficial venous system.

Causes of varicose veins
Obesity
Stasis from sitting or standing (position)
Pregnancy
Pelvic venous obstruction
Damage to deep veins from thrombosis
Trauma to short or long saphenous vein
Hereditary

Fig. 7.93 Causes of varicose veins.

Varicose veins are always most apparent when the patient is standing upright, and empty completely when the legs are raised above heart level. By elevating the legs to empty the veins and then watching the veins fill as the leg is lowered, it is often possible to see the sites of incompetent perforating veins and to control them by local finger pressure. If the saphenofemoral junction is incompetent, it may be necessary first to prevent blood flowing back from the femoral vain by tying a tourniquet around the upper thigh. Identification of the site of perforating veins is an important step in treating varicose veins by injecting a sclerosant solution around incompetent perforators. Very advanced varicose veins may still need to be treated by ligating and stripping the long (and sometimes the short) saphcnous vein. The importance of the long saphenous vein as a conduit in coronary bypass surgery makes it important to preserve this vessel if possible.

Chronic venous insufficiency

Failure or inadequacy of the 'muscle pump' mechanism may also lead to chronic oedema of the legs and feet, with or without obvious varicose veins. This is more common in elderly, obese, and sedentary patients, and tends to become self-perpetuating as the legs are often painful to walk on. The oedema is often relatively firm, and pits only reluctantly on pressure; it is usually least apparent in the morning, and gels worse as the day goes on. The condition is distinguished from heart failure because the jugular venous pressure is normal. Sometimes chronic venous insufficiency is associated with obstruction of the inferior vena cava, but in this case there are usually grossly distended veins on the abdominal wall.

Varicose ulceration and eczema

Chronic venous insufficiency results in a rise in tissue pressure in the skin and subcutaneous tissues which can interfere with adequate nutrient blood flow. This may lead to skin necrosis and ulceration, most commonly at the ankle just above the malleoli. The skin is often dusky and indurated. Scarring as part of the healing process tends to impair the microcirculation further, and the condition may become self-perpetuating.

Thrombophlebitis

Superficial thrombophlebitis is inflammation and thrombosis of a superficial vein. This commonly results either from local trauma or from an intravenous infusion, but may occur spontaneously. There is local pain, redness, and tenderness over the course of the vein. The condition is usually benign and self-limiting, but septic thrombophlebitis from a drip site infection can lead to septicaemia.

Deep vein thrombosis

Thrombosis of the deep veins in the calf or the pelvis usually occurs as a result of a combination of damage to the endothelium lining of the vein, with stasis of the blood within them as a consequence of physical inactivity. Until measures were taken to prevent it by encouraging early mobilization and using low dose heparin, it was a common complication of any form of major surgery. In some patients, deep vein thrombosis occurs in the absence of any obvious external cause; it is important that these patients should be investigated for abnormalities of the blood clotting and fibrinolytic systems.

The characteristic clinical features of deep vein thrombosis in the leg are pain, swelling, and occasionally redness. The pain is a deep aching pain which is worse on activity but persists at rest. Sometimes it is absent. The leg may be swollen (compare it with the other one) and there is often dilatation of the superficial veins and a warm skin as a result of blood flow diversion from the deep to the superficial veins. Pain in the calf can sometimes be produced by dorsiflexing the foot but since this can sometimes cause the detachment thrombus in the form of an embolism it is not recommended. If pain and swelling are mainly below the knee, then it is likely that the thrombosis is in the calf veins. If however, the swelling and tenderness extend to the thigh or the groin, then the thrombosis may involve the femoral or iliac veins: this is potentially more serious because thrombo-embolism from these sites is frequently massive.

The main differential diagnosis of deep vein thrombosis (Fig. 7.94) in legs is from spontaneous rupture of the gastrocnemius muscle and rupture of an arthritic Baker's cyst from the knee joint. The diagnosis of deep vein thrombosis needs to be confirmed with either ultrasound scanning or phlebography. It is important to remember that deep vein thrombosis, particularly in the elderly, may be accompanied by very few clinical signs and often goes unnoticed until it presents as pulmonary embolism.

The intact endothelium in the veins of the body normally prevents thrombus formation, and any small quantity of thrombus that does form is dealt with by the body's own thrombolytic mechanisms. If extensive thrombus does form in veins, it may become detached and travel through the great veins to the heart, where it may either lodge in the right ventricle or in the pulmonary artery. Clinically, pulmonary embolism may present in three ways: pulmonary infarction, acute massive pulmonary embolus, and chronic thrombo-embolic pulmonary hypertension.

Differential diagnosis of deep vein thrombosis

Pain and swelling in the leg may be due to:

- Deep vein thrombosis
- Ruptured head of gastrocnemius muscle
- Ruptured osteoarthritic cyst (Baker's cyst) of knee joint
- Anterior compartment syndrome (skin splints)

Fig. 7.94 Differential diagnosis of deep vein thrombosis.

Acute pulmonary infarction

This is usually the consequence of a relatively small pulmonary embolus that lodges in a branch of the pulmonary artery. As a result of spasm and reduced air entry, a wedge-shaped section of the lung downstream of the block becomes necrotic. This induces pleural inflammation over the infarct and the resulting pleurisy causes pain. The clinical presentation is with the relatively sudden onset of pleuritic chest pain. The patient may be moderately breathless but is seldom hypotensive. Arterial blood gas measurements often show quite marked hypoxemia, but $pC0_2$ is normal. The chest X-ray may show a wedge-shaped opacity based on the pleura. A perfusion lung scan often shows other perfusion defects besides that causing the infarct. It is important to look for other evidence of deep vein thrombosis both by clinical examination and by phlebography because the pulmonary infarction may be a warning of a possible massive pulmonary embolus later on.

Acute massive pulmonary embolism

This is most common in postoperative patients. The patient suddenly becomes extremely short of breath, severely hypotensive, and may not be able to sit upright. There is often an urge to evacuate the bowels. The jugular veins are markedly distended and the liver may also be enlarged. Heart sounds are usually quiet because of the reduced cardiac output; nonetheless, there may be a third sound best heard to the left of the sternum. The chest X-ray is usually unhelpful, but the ECG shows characteristic features of acute right ventricular strain. Echocardiography shows a dilated, poorly contracting, right ventricle and a small under-filled left ventricle. Definitive diagnosis is by pulmonary angiography.

Chronic thrombo-embolic hypertension

Chronic pulmonary hypertension is a result of multiple pulmonary emboli over a period of time. The clinical feature are those of chronic pulmonary hypertension. The causal diagnosis can sometimes be made on the basis of recurrent history of deep vein thrombosis, but sometimes has to be made on the basis of pulmonary angiography and/or lung biopsy.

INFECTIVE ENDOCARDITIS

Infective endocarditis is an infection of the endocardial lining of the heart. There are three principal clinical types: acute endocarditis, subacute endocarditis, and postoperative endocarditis.

Acute endocarditis

Acute endocarditis is the result of infection of a normal or abnormal heart with a virulent organism such as *Staphylococcus aureus* or *Streptococcus pneumoniae*. The infection usually involves one of the heart valves, but may involve the endocardium next to a defect such as a ventricular septal defect. The infection may cause *destruction* of valve tissue, *abscess formation*, or the formation of large *vegetations* which are composed of masses of bacteria, platelets, and thrombin. The patient is nearly always severely ill with a fever and marked systemic symptoms. One of the characteristic clinical findings is that heart murmurs develop, or change rapidly, as the destructive process goes on. There may also be *systemic emboli* as portions of vegetation break off and are carried away by the bloodstream. There may be finger clubbing and splinter haemorrhages, but often they do not have time to develop, so rapid is the course of the disease.

Subacute endocarditis

Subacute endocarditis may result either from infection of a diseased heart valve or septal defect with a rather indolent organism, such as *Streptococcus sanguis*, or from the partial treatment of acute endocarditis with inadequate doses of antibiotics. The time course of the illness is much more insidious. Patients present with unexplained fever, excessive tiredness, depressive symptoms, or with the consequences of valve destruction or systemic embolization. There is nearly always a heart murmur: the combination of fever and a heart murmur should always lead to suspicion of endocarditis. As in acute endocarditis, the murmurs may change, but this is usually over a time course of days or weeks rather than hours. Finger clubbing and splinter haemorrhages are common. In neglected cases there may be anaemia and a brown pigmentation of the skin. There is often splenomegaly. There may be localized subconjunctival haemorrhages, tender swellings (Osler's nodes) in the finger pulps, and haemorrhaic spots (Roth spots) in the retina. All these are features of a systemic vasculitis (Fig. 7.95).

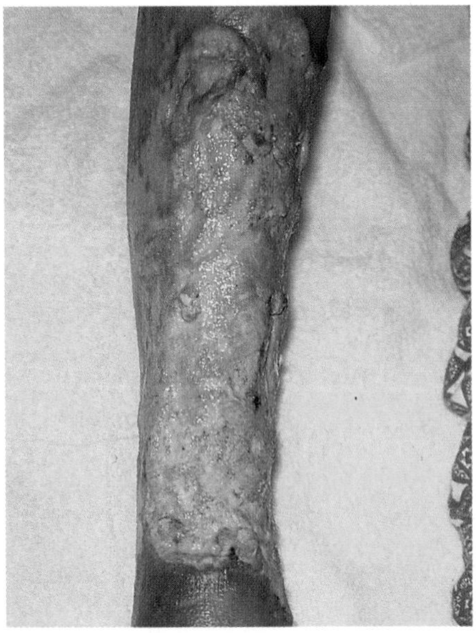

Fig. 7.95 Severe varicose ulceration of the leg.

Postoperative endocarditis

Postoperative endocarditis occurs in patients who have had open heart surgery, and may involve artificial heart valves or other implanted material. The most common organism is a coagulase-negative staphylococcus. The clinical features may resemble those of acute or subacute endocarditis.

MYOCARDITIS

Myocarditis is an inflammatory infection of heart muscle, usually the result of a virus infection. Clinically, this may present with heart failure or an arrhythmia. There may be cardiac dilatation, a third heart sound , or a systolic murmur from 'functional' mitral incompetence resulting from dilatation of the ventricle.

CARDIOMYOPATHY

Cardiomyopathy is a general term meaning 'heart muscle disease'. Clinically, cardiomyopathy can be classified into hypertrophic, dilated, and restrictive types.

Hypertrophic cardiomyopathy

Hypertrophic cardiomyopathy is characterized by excessive cardiac muscle hypertrophy in the absence of a stimulus such as hypertension. The hypertrophy may be 'asymetrical', i.e. it specifically affects the interventricular septum, which bulges into the left ventricular outflow tract and causes obstruction to bloodflow. This variant is called hypertrophic obstructive cardiomyopathy (HOCM). Some patients with HOCM die suddenly, often when engaged in sport or exercise. The clinical features of hypertrophic cardiomyopathy are summarized in Figure 7.96.

Dilated Cardiomyopathy

Dilated cardiomyopathy is characterized by a global impairment of left ventricular function, leading to progressive dilatation of the ventricles. The basic cause is unknown, but similar patterns can be reproduced in association with excessive alcohol intake, or systemic diseases (e.g. sarcoidois). Clinical presentation is usually with heart failure. There is a displaced apex beat, a gallop rhythm, and possibly secondary mitral or tricupid regurgitation.

Restrictive cardiomyopathy

This is a rare condition in Western countries. The clinical presentation mimics constrictive pericarditis.

ACUTE RHEUMATIC FEVER

Acute rheumatic fever is a consequence of an autommune response to heart tissue precipitated by exposure to certain strains of streptococcus. It is now very uncommon in Western countries, although its long term consequences are still seen as an important cause of chronic valvular heart disease. Clinically, acute rheumatic fever presents in children or young adults either with an acute, migratory (i.e. flitting from joint to joint) polyarthritis, or with chorea.

Cardiac involvement is usually signalled by the development of a murmur: either a pansystolic murmur of mitral regurgitation, or a soft mid-diastolic murmur which resembles that of mitral stenosis. The latter is called a Carey Coombs murmur, and is probably due to oedema of the mitral valve cusps, and to small platelet vegetations. There is commonly a skin rash, which again is often fleeting and variable. Rheumatic nodules are not seen in all cases, but are virtually pathognomic; they consist of firm subcutaneous nodules, often on the extensor surfaces of knees and elbows.

PERICARDIAL DISEASE

The heart normally contracts within a smooth, closely fitting serous cavity, the pericardium. The principal pericardial diseases are acute pericarditis, pericardial effusion, and chronic constrictive pericarditis.

Acute pericarditis.

The symptoms of acute pericarditis have already been discussed under chest pain. The most characteristic physical finding is the pericardial rub. This is often mistaken for a murmur, but it usually has a distinct scratchy quality. In patients in sinus rhythm, there are often three components to the pericardial rub, corresponding to atrial contraction, ventricular contraction, and ventricular relaxation. Pericardial rubs are often best heard if the patient is made to sit up, lean forward, and breathe out fully (similar to the position for hear-

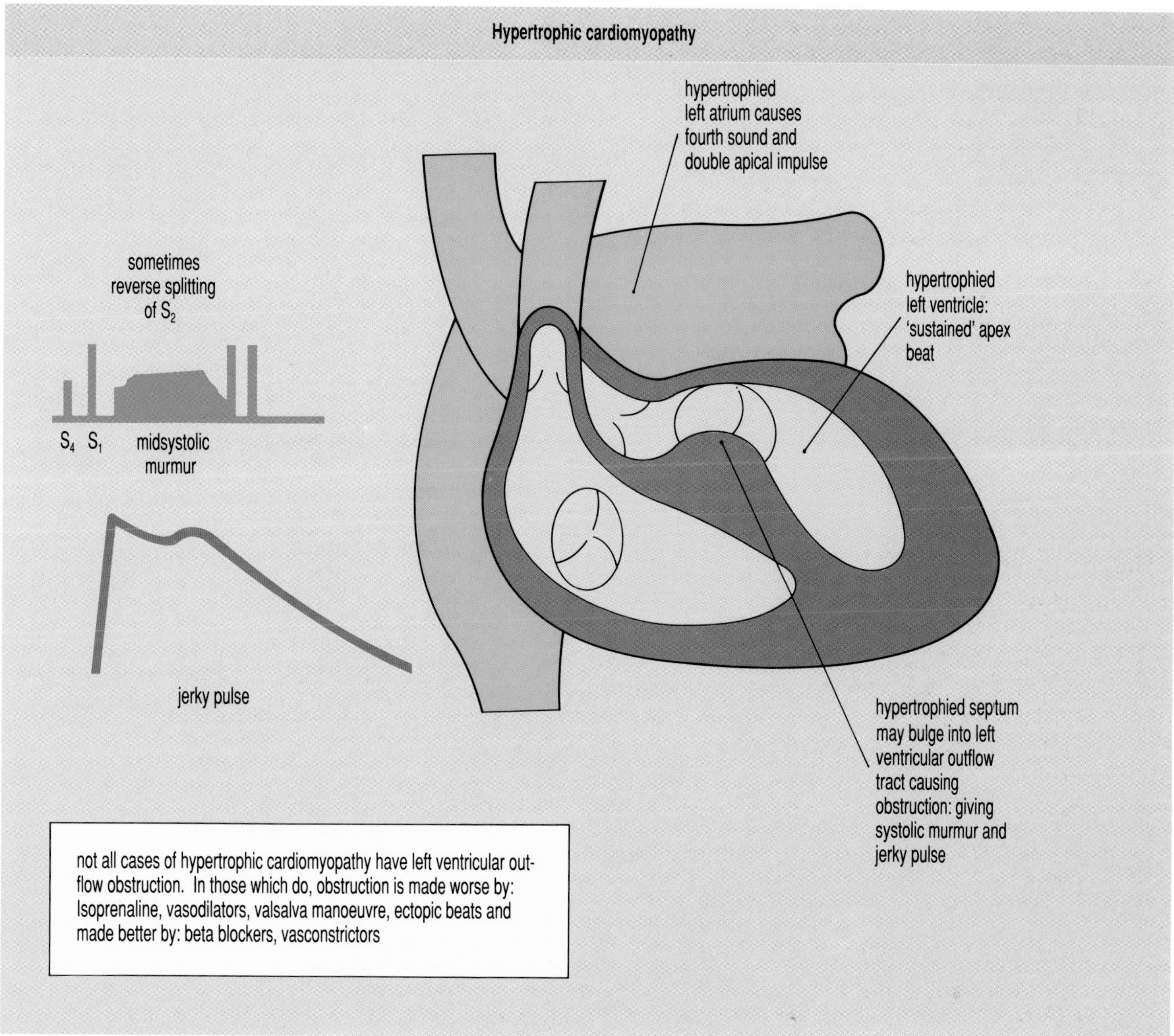

Fig. 7.96 Findings in hypertrophic cardiomyopathy.

ing aortic diastolic murmurs). It is characteristic of a pericardial rub that it comes and goes over a period of a few hours. Patients with acute pericarditis are often parexial, and may feel systemically unwell.

Pericardial effusion

Normally, there is only just sufficient fluid in the pericardial cavity to lubricate the heart in its movements. An excess of accumulation of pericardial fluid is called a pericardial effusion (Fig. 7.97).

The clinical features of a pericardial effusion depend both on the amount of fluid and the speed with which it accumulates. A large amount of fluid, or the very rapid accumulation of fluid, causes compression of the heart, particularly the right ventricle and can cause a substantial reduction in cardiac output. This is cardiac tamponade (Fig. 7.98) and is a medical emergency. The patient is often very ill, hypotensive, and peripherally constricted. They may be pulsus paradoxus: a variation in pulse volume with respiration (Fig. 7.99). The jugular venous pressure is very high, but this may be hard to see as the patient may be too hypotensive to sit upright. Because even a small amount of fluid if it accumulates rapidly can cause cardiac tamponade, signs such as cardiac enlargement on a chest radiograph or an increased area of dullness to percussion in the front of the chest are unreliable in diagnosing cardiac tamponade. The best way of confirming the diagnosis is by bedside echocardiography, which can be followed immediately by pericardiocentesis.

If fluid accumulates slowly in the pericardium over days or weeks, then it is often accommodated by stretching of the pericardium rather than cardiac tamponade. The chronic pericardial effusion may be picked up by accident, or (more commonly) it presents as chronic predominantly right-sided cardiac failure, often with very marked peripheral oedema and perhaps ascites. There may or may not be a pericardial rub. There is often an enlarged area of dullness on percussion to the left of the sternum. The jugular venous pressure is usually markedly elevated. There may be a paradoxical pulse, but it is often less prominent than in acute cardiac tamponade. Chest X-ray shows cardiac enlargement. Again, echocardiography is the simplest investigation to confirm the diagnosis.

Chronic constrictive pericarditis

Chronic, as opposed to acute, inflammation of the pericardium may lead to a thickened fibrotic pericardial membrane which as a long term result of scarring, constricts and compresses the heart. Worldwide, the commonest cause of this is chronic tuberculous pericarditis, but it may also follow acute viral pericarditis or cardiac surgery.

The clinical features of chronic constrictive pericarditis are quite

Causes of pericardial effusion
Infection
Viral pericarditis Bacterial pericarditis (streptococcus, pneumococcus) Tuberculous pericarditis
Myocardial Infarction
Peri-infarct pericarditis Cardiac rupture Dressler's syndrome
Malignant pericarditis
Secondary (common) or primary (rare) tumors Leukaemia
Auto-allergic
Acute rheumatic fever Rheumatoid arthritis
Other
Myxaedema Trauma (stab wounds) Post-cardiac surgery

Fig. 7.97 Pericardial effusion: causes.

Cardiac tamponade
Causes
Any cause of pericardial effusion (see Fig. 7.94) Pneumonia Trauma
Clinical presentation
Hypotension Oliguria Raised JVP Paradoxical pulse
Diagnosis
Chest X-ray – enlarged heart shadow ECG – small voltages, 'electrical alternons' Echo – effusion with collapse of right ventricle
Treatment
Pericardiocentesis Surgical drainage

Fig. 7.98 Cardiac tamponade.

similar to those of chronic pericardial effusion. There tends to be predominantly right-sided heart failure often with massive oedema. The jugular venous pressure is elevated, and often has a characteristic pulse wave form, with a very rapid dip in the pulse as the tricuspid valve opens followed by an equally abrupt termination as filling of the ventricle is curtailed. In long standing severe constrictive pericarditis, pericardium may become adherent to the ribcage and the examiner can feel a tugging on the posterior ribs in time with the heart beat.

Pulsus paradoxus

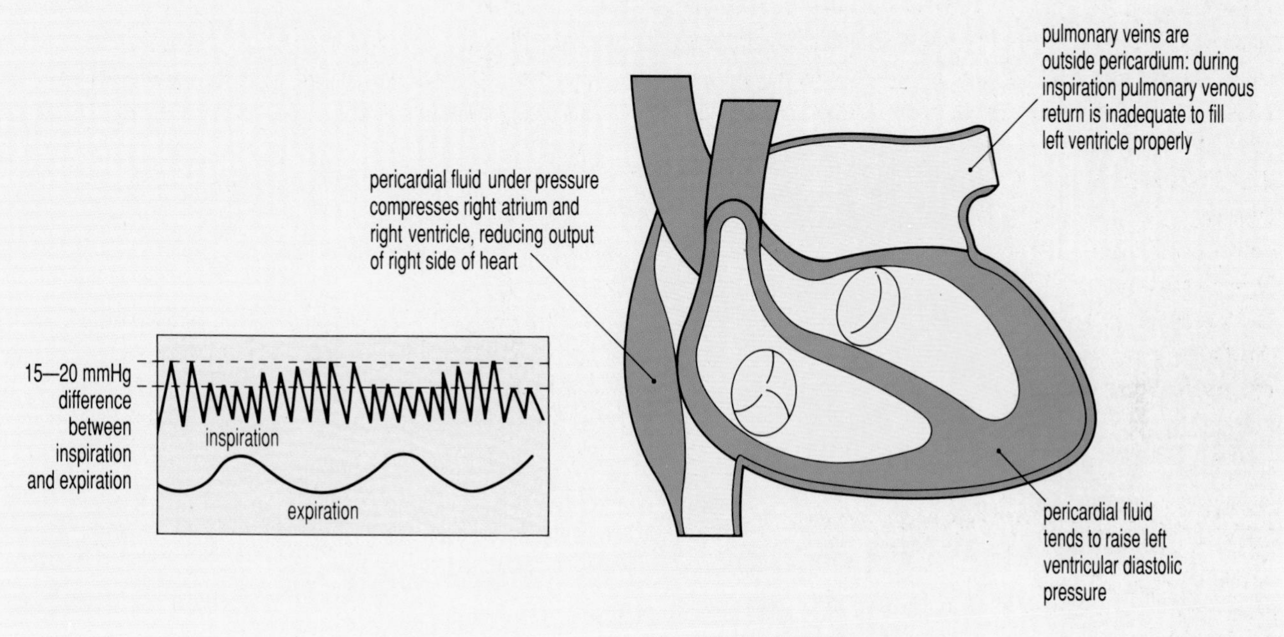
pulmonary veins are outside pericardium: during inspiration pulmonary venous return is inadequate to fill left ventricle properly
pericardial fluid under pressure compresses right atrium and right ventricle, reducing output of right side of heart
15–20 mmHg difference between inspiration and expiration
inspiration
expiration
pericardial fluid tends to raise left ventricular diastolic pressure

Fig. 7.99 Pulses paradoxus , or the apparent diminuition of the pulse on inspiration, is a feature of pericardial tamponade.

The abdominal examination follows that of the heart and lungs. Diseases of the abdominal organs may already be apparent from the general examination. For example, you may have noticed jaundice when examining the skin or eyes, and in patients with obstructive jaundice scratch marks may be apparent. You may have been aware of abnormal weight loss, signs of malnutrition, or anaemia. Underlying iron deficiency may be revealed by a smooth, atrophic tongue and by cracks at the angles of the mouth (cheilosis), which may also suggest a vitamin B group deficiency.

STRUCTURE AND FUNCTION

The symptoms and signs of abdominal disease reflect disorder in the anatomy and physiology of the major abdominal organs. These organs are packed neatly into the abdominal cavity (Fig. 8.1). The liver, gallbladder, and spleen lie protected under cover of the lower thoracic ribs, whilst the stomach, 6m of small intestine and 1.5m of large bowel cover and cushion the pancreas, kidneys, and ureters. The urinary bladder, and in women the ovaries and adnexae, lie hidden deep in the protective wall of the pelvis.

THE GASTROINTESTINAL TRACT

The mouth and oesophagus

Digestion begins in the mouth where food is chewed and moistened with saliva. The salivary fluid is a cocktail of enzymes, including amylase and lingual lipase, plus bicarbonate and lysozyme. It is secreted by the parotid, submandibular, and sublingual glands, with a small contribution from the labial glands on the inner aspects of the lips.

Swallowing is controlled by a medullary centre in the brain stem which relays to and from the pharynx and oesophagus via the glossopharyngeal and vagus nerves (Fig. 8.2). There is also an intrinsic innervation within the smooth muscle of the oesophagus. There are three phases to the swallowing reflex: the oral, pharyngeal, and oesophageal phases. During the oral phase, the tongue presses the bolus up against the hard palate and drives the food into the pharynx. In the pharyngeal phase, the respiratory tract closes off, the upper pharyngeal sphincter (cricopharyngeus) relaxes, and the upper, middle, and lower pharyngeal constrictors propel the food into the oesophagus. In the oesophageal phase, a powerful peristalitic

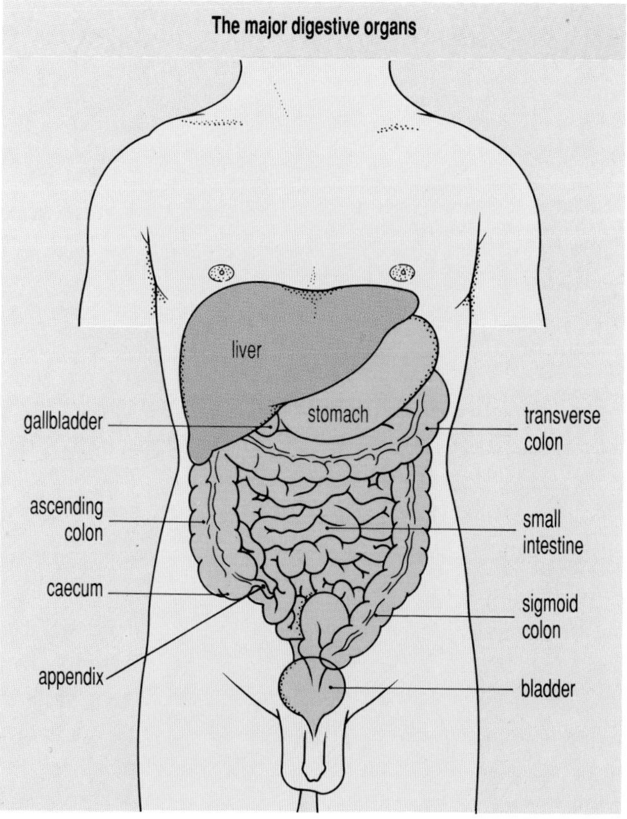

Fig. 8.1 The anatomical relationships of the major digestive organs.

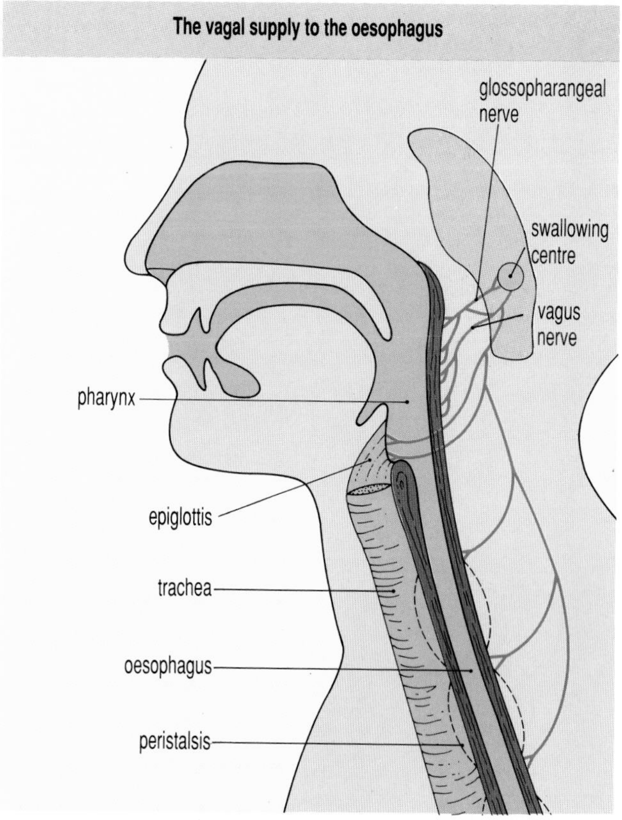

Fig. 8.2 The innervation of the oesophagus.

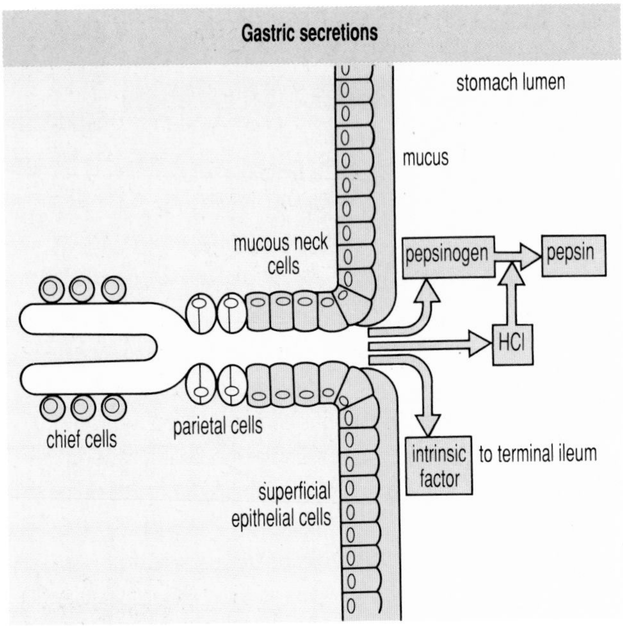

Fig. 8.3 Cells found in the mucosa of the stomach body are responsible for the principal gastric secretions.

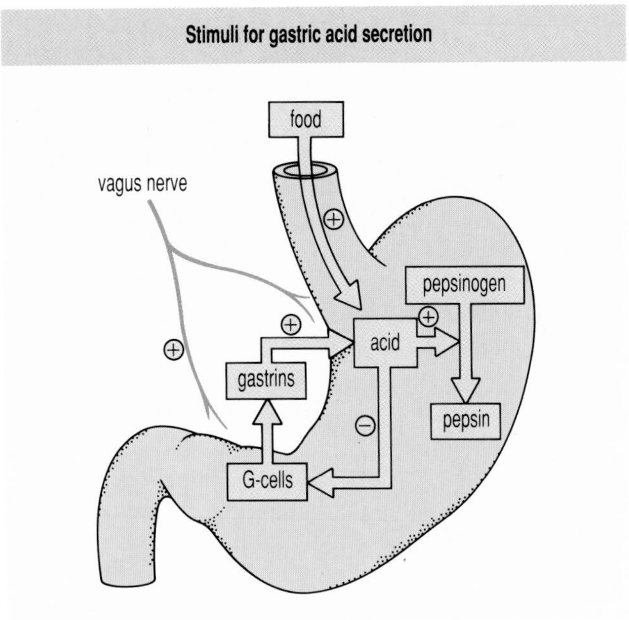

Fig. 8.4 The control of gastric acid secretion by food, vagal stimulation, and gastrin. Pepsinogen is activated to pepsin at low pH.

wave propels the bolus towards the stomach. The lower oesophageal sphincter has intrinsic tone which prevents regurgitation of the gastric contents: it relaxes in advance of the peristaltic wave and remains relaxed for a few seconds after the wave has passed.

Difficulty swallowing (dysphagia) may be caused by damage to the neural control, abnormalities of the oesphageal muscle, or obstruction of the lumen.

The stomach

The churning action of the stomach continues the mixing process started in the mouth and prepares food for its journey into the duodenum. The parietal cells in the body of this muscular organ (Fig. 8.3) secrete hydrochloric acid, which sterilizes the meal, and intrinsic factor, which is necessary for the absorption of vitamin B_{12} in the terminal ileum. The Chief cells secrete pepsinogen which is converted to the proteolytic enzyme pepsin by the low pH of the stomach lumen. The secretion of acid is stimulated by the vagus nerve, distention of the stomach with food, and the secretion of the hormone gastrin from the G-cells of the gastric antrum (Fig. 8.4). A mucous layer coats the stomach mucosa, protecting it from self-inflicted injury by acid and pepsin.

Regurgitation of gastric contents into the oesophagus is prevented by an anti-reflux mechanism at the gastro-oesophageal junction. This includes the intrinsic tone of the lower oesophageal sphincter, the flap-valve effect of the angle of His, and the squeezing effect of intra-abdominal pressure on the small segment of oesophagus which protrudes through the diaphragm into the abdomen (Fig. 8.5). If one or more of these anti-reflux mechanisms breaks down, gastric contents may regurgitate into the lower oesophagus, damaging the mucosa and causing heartburn.

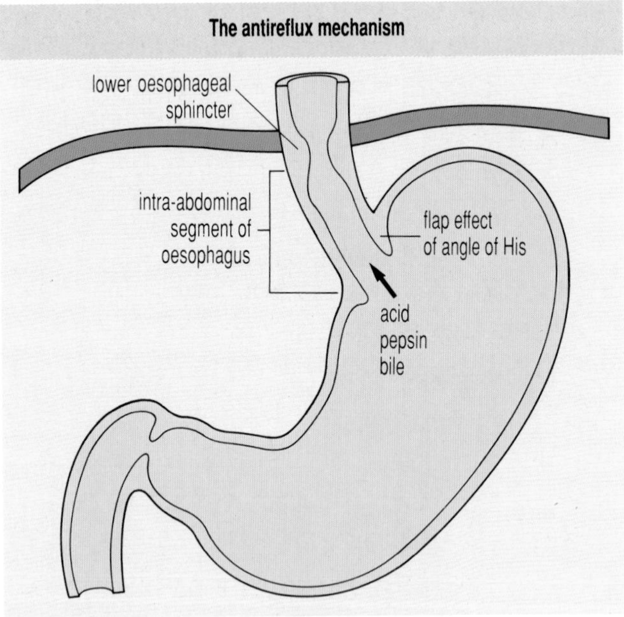

Fig. 8.5 The antireflux mechanism comprises the intrinsic tone of the lower oesophageal sphincter, the acute angle formed at the oesophago-gastric junction (angle of His), and the pressure on the intra-abdominal oesophagus.

The small intestine

The small intestine comprises the duodenum, the jejunum and the ileum. It fills most of the anterior abdomen and is framed by the ascending, transverse, and descending colon. Blood is supplied by the superior mesenteric vessels (Fig. 8.6). The principal role of the small intestine is digestion and absorption, with a vast absorptive area presented by a combination of macroscopic and microscopic folds (Fig. 8.7).

Blood supply to the intestine

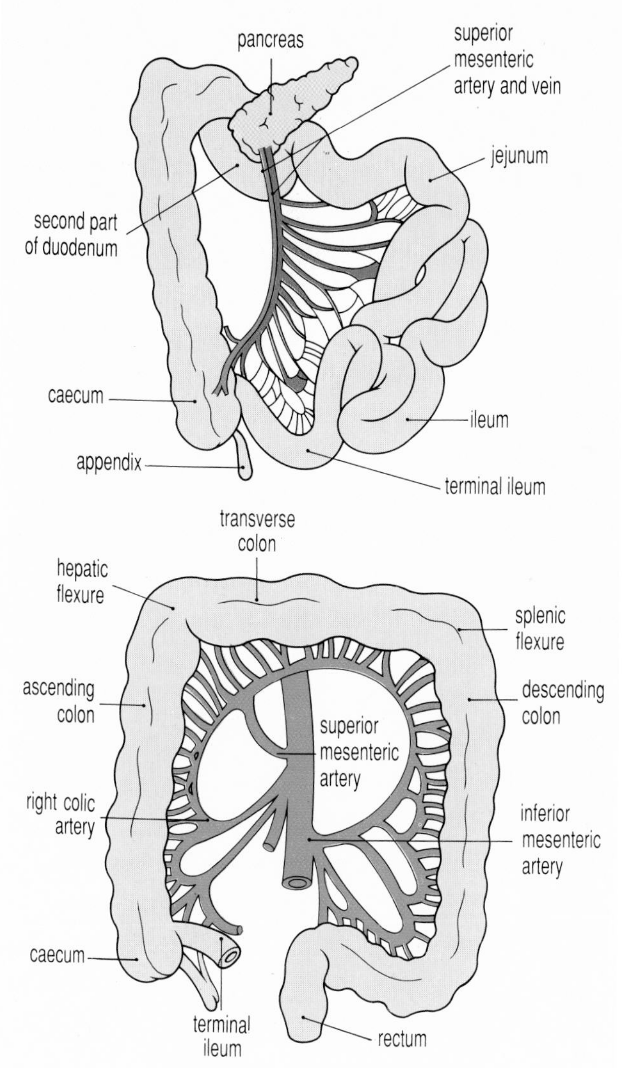

Fig. 8.6 The blood supply of the small intestine, colon, sigmoid and rectum.

The folds forming the surface of the bowel

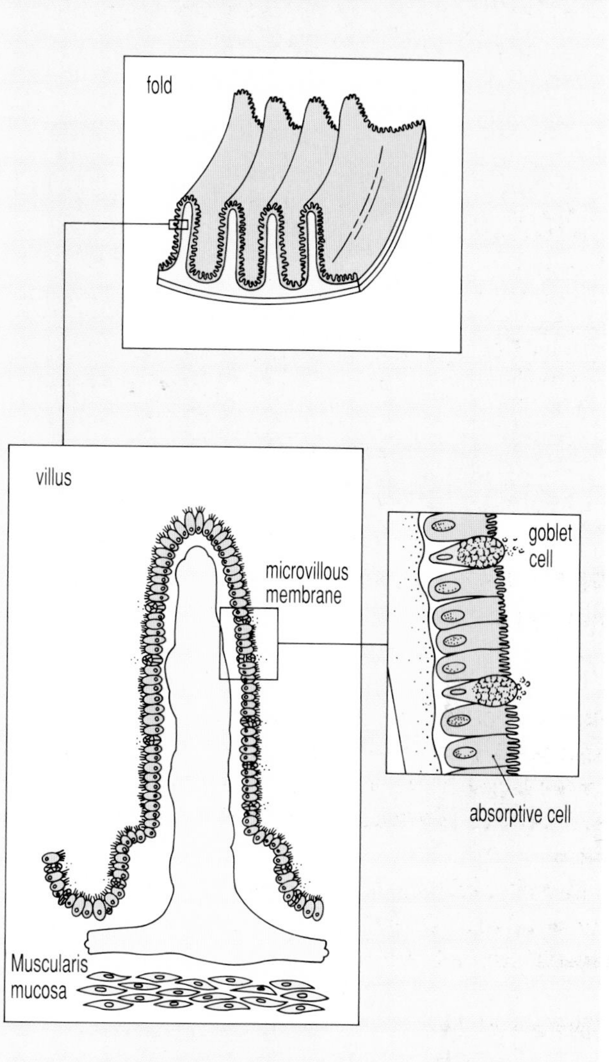

Fig. 8.7 The large surface area of the small intestine is formed by the duodenal folds, the villi, and the microvillous membrane of the enterocyte.

Most of the enzymes necessary for the digestion of fat, protein, and carbohydrate are present in the duodenum. Enterocytes develop in the base of the crypts of Lieberkuhn and migrate to the tip of the finger-shaped villus (Fig. 8.8). Both its capacity to produce specialized digestive enzymes on the brush border membrane and the absorptive properties of an enterocyte develop progressively as the cell migrates towards the villous tip, at which point these functions are maximally developed.

Carbohydrate digestion is initiated by salivary and pancreatic amylase. Enzymes, such as lactase and sucrase, on the brush border membrane of the enterocytes complete the digestion of complex polysaccharides and disaccharides to monosaccharides, which are then transported through the enterocyte by specialized transporters on the brush border and basolateral membranes (Fig. 8.9).

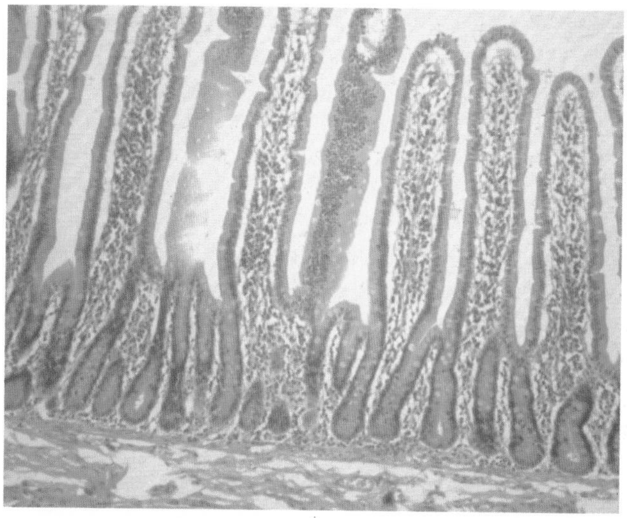

Fig. 8.8 Duodenal enterocytes develop in the crypts and migrate towards the villous tip.

Digestion of carbohydrate, fat, and protein

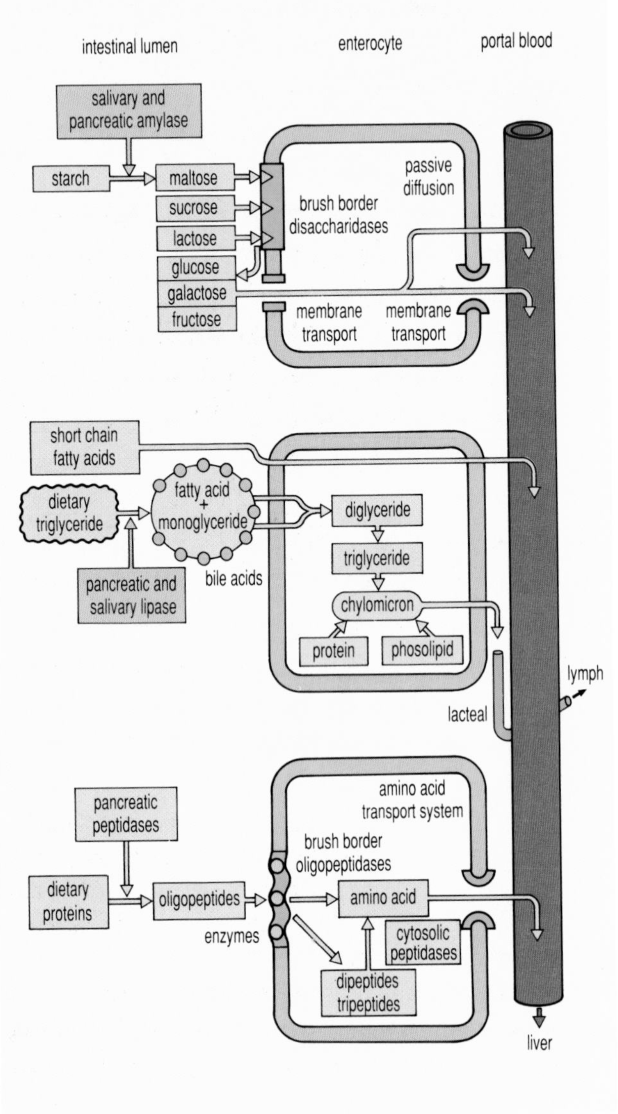

Fig. 8.9 Digestion in the small intestine. Digestion of complex carbohydrates occurs in the lumen and at the brush border membrane. Monosaccharides can then be absorbed through the brush border membrane into the portal circulation. Fat digestion occurs in the lumen and triglyceride is reconstituted in the enterocyte prior to absorption. Proteins are digested in the lumen and at the brush border membrane. Amino acids are then absorbed into the enterocyte and portal circulation.

Pancreatic lipase hydrolyzes triglycerides to fatty acids and monoglycerides. These products are emulsified by bile acids which help form micelles, which are then taken up at the brush border and diffuse passively into the enterocyte where the triglyceride is reconstituted (see Fig. 8.9). These triglycerides, as well as absorbed cholesterol, are formed into fat aggregates (chylomicrons) which are absorbed into the lymphatics and discharged into the circulation through the thoracic duct. The fat-soluble vitamins A,D,K, and E are absorbed in a similar manner to other lipids.

Gastrointestinal hormones

Gastrin	stimulates gastric acid secretion
Cholecystokinin	stimulates gallbladder contraction and pancreatic enzyme secretion, relaxes sphincter of Oddi
Secretin	stimulates secretion of pancreatic fluid and bicarbonate
Gastric inhibitory polypeptide	potentiates the insulin response to glucose
Enteroglucagon	trophic to small intestine
Vasoactive intestinal polypeptide (VIP)	secretin-like effect on pancreas, affects intestinal motility and mesenteric blood flow
Motilin	stimulates intestinal motility between meals
Somatostatin	inhibits secretion of gastrin, other gut hormones and pepsin, stimulates gastric mucus production
Insulin	lowers blood glucose, stimulates glycogen synthesis protein and fat anabolism
Pancreatic glucagon	promotes glucogenolysis, lipolysis, gluconeogenesis. Slows intestinal motility
Pancreatic polypeptide	inhibits pancreatic secretion and relaxes the gallbladder

Fig. 8.10 The gastrointestinal hormones and their principal effects.

Proteolysis is initiated in the stomach by pepsin, yet the bulk of protein digestion is mediated by trypsin and other pancreatic peptidases in the small intestine (see Fig. 8.9). The action of these enzymes produces small peptides with 4–6 amino acids which undergo further processing to amino acids, dipeptides, and tripeptides by oligopeptidases on the enterocyte brush border membrane. These are absorbed into the enterocytes where the final digestion to single amino acids occurs. The amino acids are transported to the liver by the portal blood.

The addition of pancreatic juice and bile which are secreted through the ampulla of Vater modifies and enriches the chyme entering the duodenum from the stomach.

Absorption of nutrients occurs in the jejunum and ileum, along with the production and secretion of a range of hormones (Fig.

The lobes of the liver

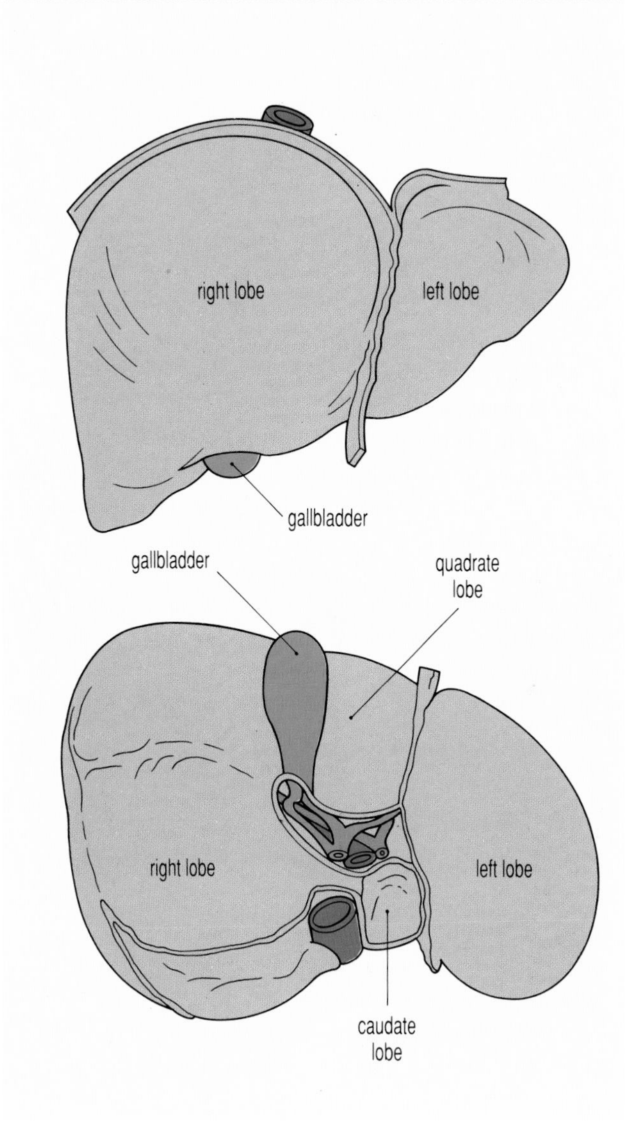

Fig. 8.11 The gross anatomy of the liver.

The portal venous system

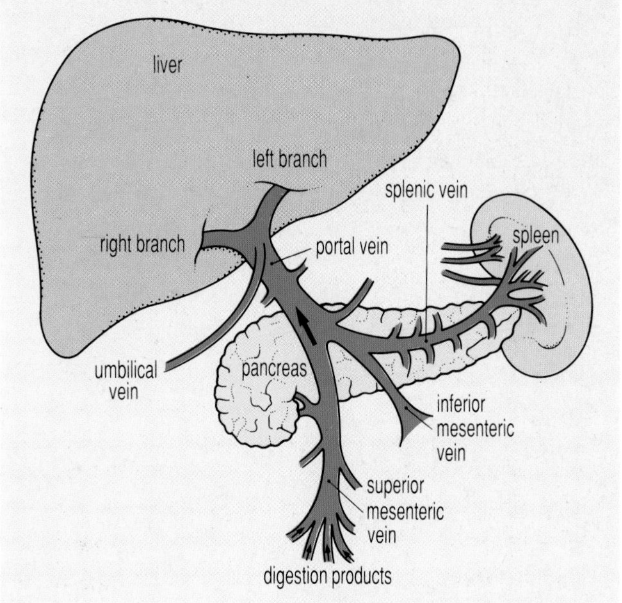

Fig. 8.12 The anatomy of the portal venous system. The vessels drain into the liver sinusoids carrying nutrients from the intestine, pancreatic hormones from the islets of Langerhans and antibodies from the spleen.

8.10) The terminal ileum absorbs vitamin B_{12} and bile acids.

The small intestine has a considerable functional reserve and only fails when 80–90 per cent of its length is diseased or surgically resected.

The colon

The ileum enters the caecum through the ileocaecal valve, which prevents reflux of colonic contents into the small intestine. Whereas the small intestine is relatively microbe free, the colon is heavily colonized by bacteria. Approximately 1.5 litres of ileal fluid empties into the caecum each day. Most of this effluent is reabsorbed as it passes through the ascending, transverse, and descending colon. The colon concentrates the ileal outflow so that the daily stool output on a Western diet averages 200g; 75 per cent of stool weight is water and the remainder comprises unabsorbed food and bacteria. The colonic mucosa is rich in glands producing mucus, which provides constant lubrication for the passage of faeces and protects the mucosa from bacterial enzymes.

Infection or inflammation of the colonic mucosa may provoke fluid and electrolyte secretion and interfere with absorption, causing diarrhoea and dehydration. Diarrhoea may also occur in small bowel disease when the volume of ileal effluent exceeds the colon's absorptive capacity.

THE LIVER

The liver is the largest intra-abdominal organ. The falciform ligament divides the organ into a larger right lobe and a smaller left lobe (Fig. 8.11). Two smaller lobes, the anterior quadrate and posterior caudate, are squeezed between the left and right lobes on the visceral surface of the liver.

The liver is the focal point of intermediary metabolism and energy production, and it lies in a strategic position between the gut and the systemic organs. The products of digestion are absorbed into the mesenteric veins which drain into the portal vein and ultimately into the hepatic sinusoids (Fig. 8.12). Specialized macrophages (Kupffer cells) straddle the sinusoids and mount an almost impenetrable defence against unwanted microbes or matter which escapes the first line of defence in the bowel. Nutrient-rich plasma filters through the small holes (fenestrae) in the endothelial cells lining the sinusoids and passes into the space of Disse which lies between the endothelial cells and hepatocytes (Fig. 8.13). The plasma filtrate bathes these highly adapted cells, which are enriched with a range of enzymes able to metabolize the wide variety of incoming digestion products. Three hepatic veins collect the sinusoidal outflow and deliver it into the inferior vena cava.

Hepatocytes perform a remarkable array of synthetic and catabolic functions, with many clinical features of liver disease resulting from derangement of these processes. They convert glucose to glycogen, which can be stored and later reconverted on demand to glucose, synthesize a range of proteins (including albumin and the clotting factors), degrade protein to amino acids, synthesize urea from ammonia, and manufacture cholesterol and bile acids. The lateral borders of hepatocytes are modified to form bile canaliculi which interconnect and eventually converge as the left and right main hepatic ducts at the liver hilum. The liver cells secrete bile into the canaliculi. Bile is a fluid comprising bile salts, cholesterol, and bilirubin, a pigment derived from haemoglobin released from dead erythrocytes. Bilirubin cannot be excreted in bile until it has been rendered water-soluble by conjugation with glucuronic acid in the liver (Fig. 8.14).

The liver is an important storage site for iron and vitamins and plays a central role in the hydroxylation of vitamin D. Other functions include the conjugation and excretion of steroid hormones, the detoxification of drugs, and the conversion of fat-soluble waste products to water-soluble substances for excretion by the kidneys.

THE GALLBLADDER

The gallbladder is a pear-shaped organ with a fundus, a body, and a neck which narrows to give rise to the cystic duct. It lies protected beneath the lower surface of the liver in the gallbladder fossa which separates the right and quadrate lobes. The gall bladder concentrates and stores bile, and under the influence of cholecystokinin it pumps bile through the cystic duct into the common bile duct and through the ampulla of Vater into the duodenum, where it blends with the other products of digestion (Fig. 8.15).

THE PANCREAS

The pancreas is an elongated retroperitoneal organ which lies in the transpyloric plane with its head tucked into the C-shaped loop of the duodenum and its tail abutting the spleen (Fig. 8.16). Its posterior position places the organ well out of reach of the examining hand, and diagnosis of pancreatic disease is largely dependent on the use of special imaging techniques such as CT scanning and endoscopic retrograde cholangiopancreatography (ERCP) (Fig. 8.17).

The pancreas has mixed exocrine and endocrine functions. The duct cells secrete bicarbonate which protects the duodenum from gastric acid and ensures an optimum pH for digestive enzyme activity. The exocrine acinar cells secrete lipase, phospholipase, amylase, and peptidases (trypsinogen, chymotrypsinogen, elastase, and carboxypeptidase). All the pancreatic enzymes are secreted in an inactive precursor form and are only cleaved to their active forms in the duodenum by enterokinase, which is fixed on the ente-

Microanatomy of the liver

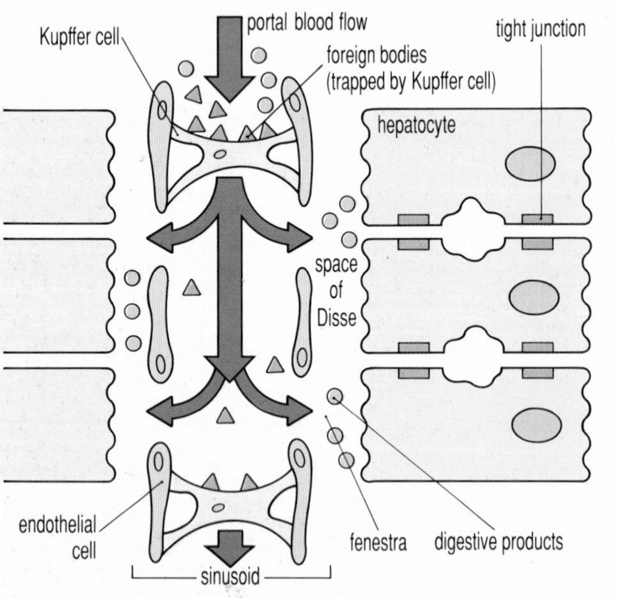

Fig. 8.13 Microanatomy of the liver sinusoids, the space of Disse, and hepatocytes. Tight junctions adjacent to the bile canaliculi bind the hepatocytes together.

Bilirubin metabolism

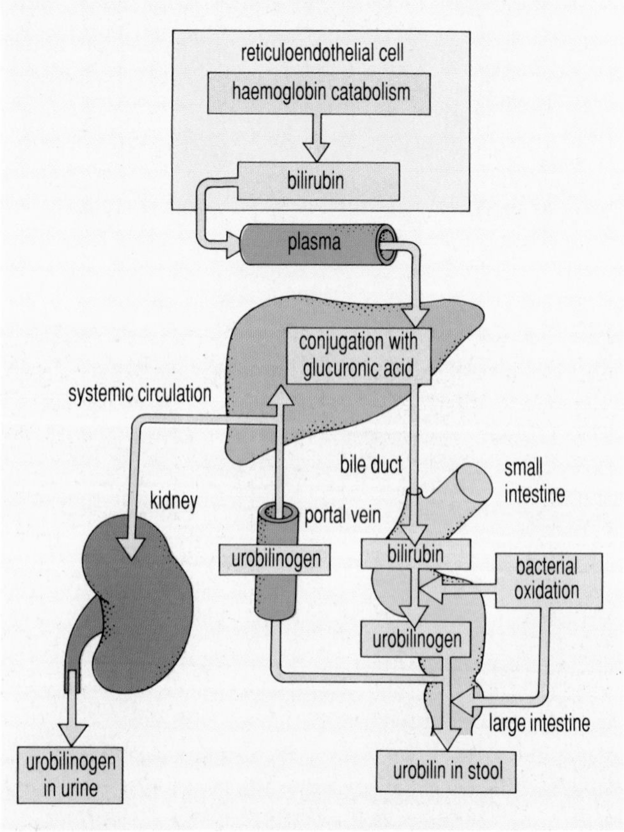

Fig. 8.14 Bilirubin is a product of haemoglobin catabolism.

rocyte brush border membrane. The hormone cholecystokinin mediates pancreatic enzyme secretion, while secretin promotes the secretion of fluid and bicarbonate from duct cells. The mucosa of the duodenum synthesizes both these hormones. The endocrine secretion of the pancreas arises from the islets of Langerhans which secrete insulin, glucagon, somatostatin, and pancreatic polypeptide into the pancreatic and portal veins.

Blockage of the main pancreatic duct by a carcinoma or diffuse damage caused by pancreatitis may cause maldigestion of protein, fat, and carbohydrate. Patients with pancreatic exocrine failure pass pale, fatty stools which are difficult to flush (steatorrhoea).

THE SPLEEN

The spleen is a highly modified lymphoid organ which also regulates the destruction of red cells. Reticuloendothelial cells populate the bulk of the spleen, forming the white pulp. These cells provide an important line of defence, and the organ is a major site of antibody production. The remainder of the spleen, the red pulp, consists of capillaries and venous sinuses which act as a sump for the storage of red cells, white cells, and platelets. When the spleen enlarges, excessive pooling of these cells may occur, causing a fall in the peripheral blood count. The splenic venous outflow drains into the portal vein, adding a rich supply of antibodies to the portal blood entering the liver.

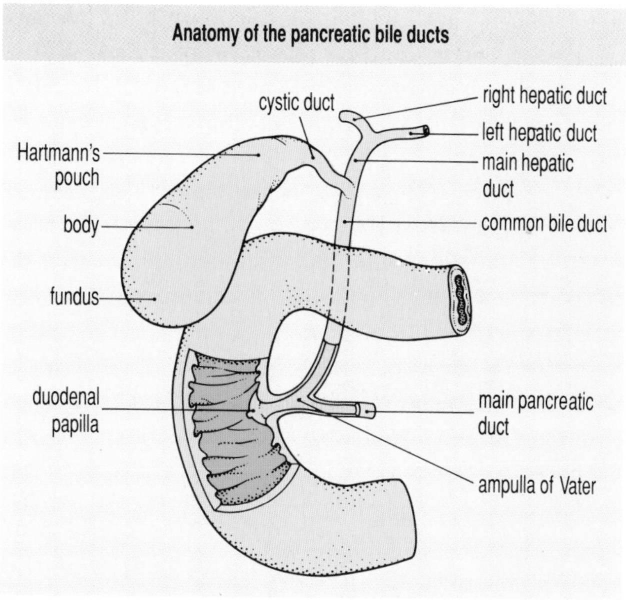

Fig. 8.15 The gallbladder and related ducts. Both bile and pancreatic juice enter the duodenum through the ampulla of Vater.

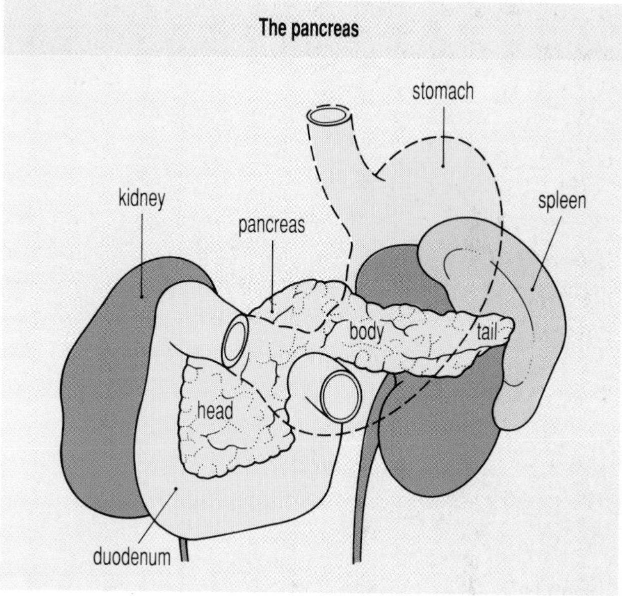

Fig. 8.16 The anatomical relationships of the pancreas.

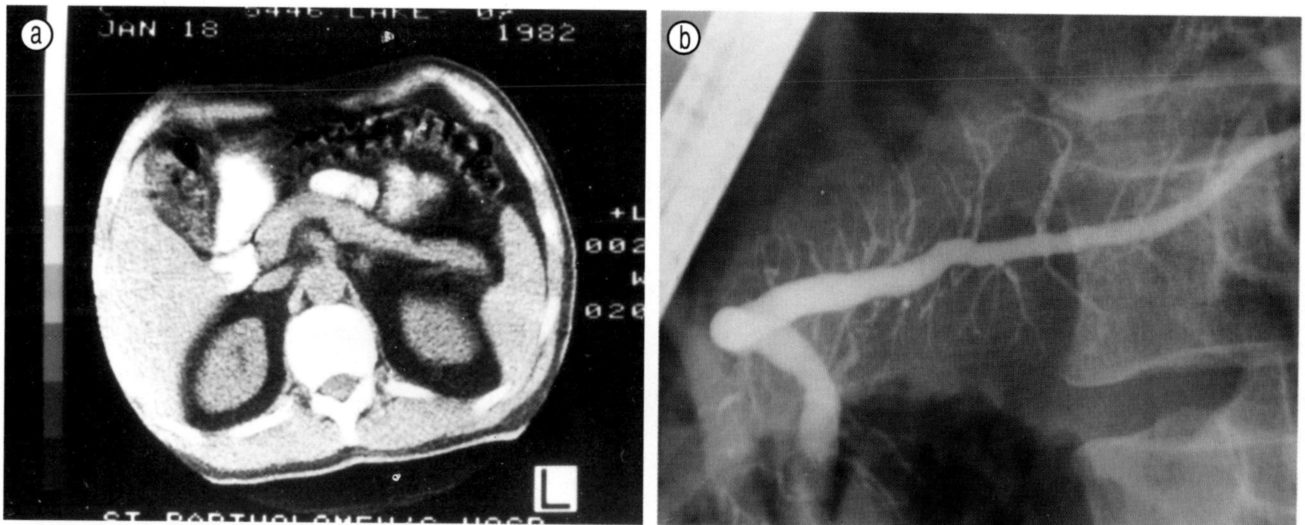

Fig. 8.17 (a) CT scan showing a normal pancreas and the surrounding structures, and (b) the pancreatic duct visualized after ERCP injection of radio-opaque contrast medium through the ampulla of vater (b).

THE KIDNEYS

The kidneys control fluid electrolyte balance and produce the hormones erythropoietin and renin. Each kidney contains about 1.2 million nephrons. The structural and functional arrangement of a typical nephron is shown in Fig. 8.18.

The capillary loops of the glomerulus form between the afferent and efferent arterioles supplying each glomerulus; the capillary tuft is embedded in the mesangium, which consists of a matrix and specialized mesangial cells. The basement membrane of the capillary tuft impinges on the epithelium of Bowman's capsule via foot processes (podocytes) which arise from the visceral cells. This complex anatomical relationship allows a protein-free fluid to filter under pressure from the blood into the proximal convoluted tubule, where specialized epithelium allows the reabsorption of sodium, water, bicarbonate, glucose, and amino acids into the efferent arteriole. Approximately two-thirds of the glomerular filtrate is reabsorbed in the proximal convoluted tubule.

The fluid entering the descending limb of the loop of Henle is isosmotic. The proximal and distal limbs of this loop are highly differentiated in their ability to secrete water, chloride, and sodium, and this, together with the spatial orientation of the loop, is responsible for the progressive increase in the NaCl concentration gradient between the cortex and medulla. This medullary hyperosmolality is vital for the further reabsorption of water. The thin descending limb of the loop of Henle is permeable to the outflow of water but not to that of sodium and chloride, so as the filtrate approaches the hairpin bend in the loop it becomes hypertonic. The thick ascending limb of the loop is impermeable to the efflux of water, yet permeable to the efflux of sodium which follows the active secretion of chloride ions. In the ascending limb, the tubular fluid becomes hypotonic, whilst the medullary interstitium becomes hypertonic. More sodium is reabsorbed from the distal convoluted tubule in exchange for potassium under the modulating influence of aldosterone.

The final composition of urine is determined by the collecting ducts which course through the medulla. The collecting ducts are normally impermeable to water, but they are rendered permeable by the action of antidiuretic hormone (ADH), which is secreted by the pituitary. This allows water to be reabsorbed passively down the osmotic gradient which exists between the duct lumen and interstitial fluid. The permeability of the collecting duct is modified in response to body water requirements and is important for the fine tuning of fluid balance. Failure to produce ADH or insensitivity of the renal tubule to ADH causes inappropriate loss of water through the kidneys, and excess urine secretion (polyuria), a syndrome known as diabetes insipidus. Sodium is also actively reabsorbed in the collecting tubules under the influence of aldosterone.

The nephron

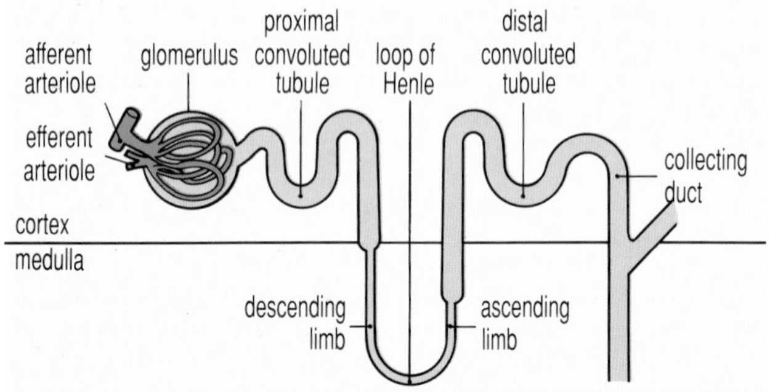

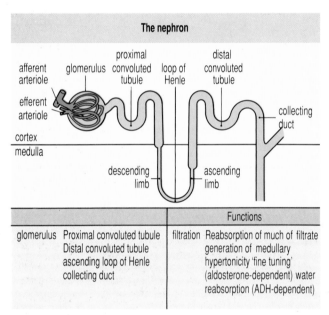

	Functions
glomerulus Proximal convoluted tubule Distal convoluted tubule ascending loop of Henle collecting duct	filtration Reabsorption of much of filtrate generation of medullary hypertonicity 'fine tuning' (aldosterone-dependent) water reabsorption (ADH-dependent)

Fig. 8.18 The structure and function of a typical nephron.

Distinguishing features of reflux and myocardial ischaemic pain

	Position	Character	Associated features	Aggravating factors	Relieving factors
Reflux	radiates towards the chest from the epigastrium	burning, scalding	water brash	bending, lying down eating	antacids
Myocardial ischaemia	radiates across the chest, into the jaw and down the left arm	gripping vice-like pressure	nausea, shortness of breath	exercise	ceasing exercise, nitrates

Fig. 8.19 The features characteristic of pain arising from oesophageal reflux compared to those of pain caused by myocardial ischaemia.

THE SYMPTOMS OF ABDOMINAL DISORDERS

GASTROINTESTINAL DISEASE

The principal symptoms of gastrointestinal disease include dysphagia, heartburn, abdominal pain, loss of appetite, nausea and vomiting, weight loss, constipation or diarrhoea, and rectal bleeding.

Dysphagia

Difficulty in swallowing the principal symptom of oesophageal disease. Patients can usually indicate the level of obstruction, but this does not always correspond to the actual level. Determine whether the dysphagia developed suddenly or gradually over weeks or months. Enquire whether the symptom is constant or intermittent and whether the dysphagia occurs with both solids and liquids. Associated symptoms such as weight loss and pain or cough with swallowing may help you construct a differential diagnosis.

The more common causes of dysphagia include oesophageal cancer, benign stricture caused by long-standing acid reflux, and excessive tone of the lower oesophageal sphincter (achalasia of the cardia). The history may indicate the underlying cause, although special tests such as barium swallow and oesophagoscopy are required to make a definitive diagnosis.

Dysphagia caused by carcinoma usually progresses rapidly over 6-10 weeks and is worse for solids than liquids. Profound weight loss results from reduced food intake and the wasting effect of the cancer.

Patients with a benign 'peptic' stricture often have a long history of heartburn, a slower rate of progression and less marked weight loss. Achalasia of the cardia may be particularly difficult to distinguish as the cause from the history, although some patients report that the symptom fluctuates in intensity and that the dysphagia is equal for liquids and solids.

When dysphagia is caused by disease of the swallowing centre in the brain stem (e.g. pseudobulbar palsy) or damage to the vagus nerve (e.g. bulbar palsy caused by polio), the symptom is accompanied by coughing and spluttering as food spills into the larynx and trachea.

Dysphagia

At what level does food stick?

Has the symptom developed over weeks, months, or longer?

Is the dysphagia intermittent or progressive?

Do both food and drink get held up equally?

Is there a past history of reflux symptoms?

Heartburn

Malfunction of the anti-reflux mechanism of the gastro-oesophageal junction allows gastric acid, pepsin, and bile to reflux into the oesophagus, causing damage to the mucosa, muscle spasm, and pain felt behind the sternum. Most people have experienced heartburn: the pain is a scalding or burning sensation which wells up behind the sternum and radiates towards the throat. An acid or bitter taste may develop in the mouth and reflex salivation may cause it to fill with saliva (water brash). The patient's description is often accompanied by a hand gesture which illustrates the upward radiation of the pain behind the sternum. Heartburn is rapidly relieved by antacids. Retrosternal chest pain caused by reflux may occasionally mimic the pain of myocardial ischaemia (Fig. 8.19).

A common cause of heartburn is an hiatus hernia, where the oesophagogastric junction prolapses into the chest through the oesophageal hiatus (Fig. 8.20). The heartburn is often provoked by postures which raise intra-abdominal pressure such as stooping,

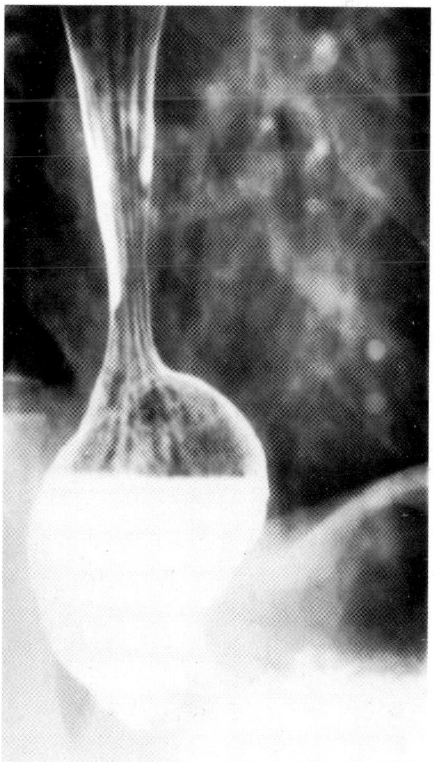

Fig. 8.20 Barium meal showing a sliding hiatus hernia with the gastro-oesophageal junction and a segment of stomach prolapsing into the chest.

bending, or lying down. This diagnosis may be suspected in overweight patients, but confirmation relies on visualizing the hernia, either by barium meal or endoscopy, and assessing the response to treatment.

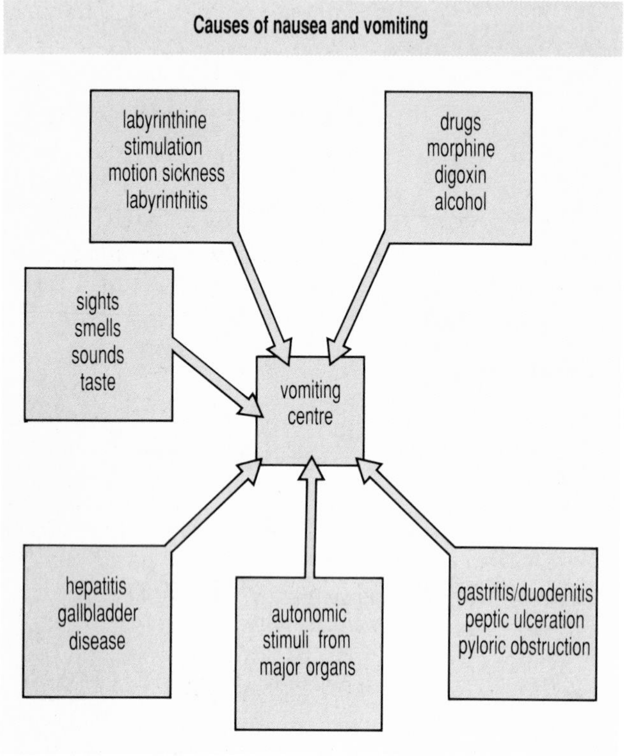

Fig. 8.21 The causes of nausea and vomiting.

Causes of gastrointestinal bleeding

Cause	Frequency (%)
Gastric ulcer	30
Duodenal ulcer	21
Gastritis/erosions	9
Oesophagitis/oesophageal ulcer	8
Duodenitis	4
Varices	3
Tumours	2
Mallory–Weiss tear	1
Others	22

Fig. 8 22 The different causes of gastrointestinal bleeding and their relative frequencies.

Heartburn may result from a particular diet and lifestyle; chocolate and alcohol consumption and cigarette smoking relax the lower oesophageal sphincter allowing reflux to occur. It is a common symptom in the later months of pregnancy. This is due both to the increase in intra-abdominal pressure and the loss of sphincter tone caused by high oestrogen levels.

Pain on swallowing (odynophagia)

Chest pain caused by swallowing has a deep 'boring' quality which differs from heartburn, although both may occur together. The symptom suggests intense spasm of the oesophagus; it may be provoked by obstruction or an intrinsic motor disorder causing abnormal, intense, and uncoordinated contraction ('nutcracker' oesophagus).

Loss of appetite (anorexia)

Loss of appetite is a nonspecific symptom which commonly accompanies both acute and chronic ill health. Return of appetite usually heralds recovery, and prolonged or unexplained anorexia, especially when accompanied by weight loss, should alert you to a serious

Weight loss

Is your appetite normal, increased, or decreased?

Over what timespan has the weight been lost?

Do you enjoy your meals?

Describe your usual breakfast, lunch, and supper.

Is the weight loss associated with nausea, vomiting, or abdominal pain?

Are your motions normal in colour and consistency?

Has there been a fever?

Do you pass excessive volumes of urine?

Have you noticed a recent change in

underlying disease. Anorexia may be a prominent feature of digestive diseases, failure of the major organs (kidneys, liver, heart and lungs) and generalized debilitating illnesses (e.g. cancer and tuberculosis).

Profound anorexia occurs in anorexia nervosa, a psychiatric disorder occurring mainly in young women. Anorexia in these patients results in marked weight loss, malnutrition, and cessation of menstruation (amenorrhoea). Suspect anorexia nervosa in teenagers and young adults, otherwise healthy, who present with an eating disorder associated with depression, vomiting, or purgative abuse.

Weight loss

Weight loss is an important, but rather nonspecific, symptom of gastrointestinal and other diseases. Enquire about appetite, eating habits, and average daily diet. When eating causes pain (as in gastric ulceration, mesenteric angina, or pancreatitis) the inclination to eat is suppressed. Weight loss may be caused by inappropriate wastage of calories due to steatorrhoea, thyrotoxicosis, or diabetes mellitus. Marked weight loss accompanies serious diseases such as advanced malignancy, chronic infections and failure of the major organs.

Dyspepsia and indigestion

Most people have experienced 'indigestion' or 'dyspepsia'. Patients and doctors use these terms rather loosely and interchangeably to describe a range of subjective abdominal symptoms. Most often these terms apply to a sensation of pain, discomfort or fullness in the epigastrium, frequently accompanied by belching, nausea, or heartburn. Determine the character and timing, the aggravating and relieving factors, and the associated symptoms. Dyspepsia should focus your attention on foregut disorders (e.g. peptic ulcer, gastritis, duodenitis, pancreatitis, pancreatic cancer, and gallstones).

Nausea

This term describes the sensation experienced prior to vomiting, although it often occurs without vomiting. Nausea may last hours or days, usually comes in waves, and is often associated with belching. It may be relieved by vomiting. The symptom may be provoked by unpleasant sights, smells and tastes, or by abnormal stimulation of the inner ear labyrinths (motion sickness). Nausea may be accompanied by other complaints such as abdominal pain and diarrhoea (Fig. 8.21). It is a characteristic of the prodromal phase of viral hepatitis and often accompanies biliary diseases such (e.g. cholecystitis). Drugs causing gastric irritation (e.g nonsteroidal analgesics) or those stimulating the vomiting centre (e.g digoxin, morphine and anti-cancer drugs) cause nausea. Early morning nausea commonly occurs during the first trimester of pregnancy.

Vomiting and haematemesis

A wave of nausea usually heralds vomiting, and the causes of nausea and vomiting are similar. Vomiting may occur in diseases of the gastrointestinal and biliary tracts, as well as in a variety of systemic and metabolic disorders. It may also be the presenting symptom of psychological disorders such as anorexia nervosa, bulaemia and fear. Suspect an iatrogenic cause in patients taking digoxin or morphine and in those undergoing cancer treatment with cytotoxic drugs. Try to establish whether the vomit is bile-stained, as this indicates patency between the stomach and duodenum. The presence of undigested food and a lack of bile suggest pyloric obstruction. Early morning nausea and vomiting are characteristic of early pregnancy and alcoholism.

Vomiting

Is the vomiting worse in the mornings?

Does the vomiting occur in relation to meals?

Is there associated abdominal pain?

Is the vomit blood- or bile-stained?

Is there recognizable food or coffee-grounds in the vomit?

What drugs are being taken?

Vomiting blood (haematemesis) indicates bleeding from the oesophagus, stomach or, duodenum (Fig. 8.22). If the bleeding is brisk the vomit may be heavily blood-stained, but if bleeding is slower, or vomiting delayed, gastric acid reacts with haemoglobin turning it a dark brown or 'coffee ground' colour. The patient's history often yields clues to the cause of haematemesis. If the bleeding is preceded by repeated bouts of retching or vomiting, consider as the cause a Mallory–Weiss tear, which results from mechanical disruption of the mucosa at the gastro-oesophageal junction. Enquire about ingestion of alcohol or other gastric irritants (e.g. aspirin). If there is evidence of coincident liver disease consider oesophageal varices to be the cause of bleeding. Weight loss may suggest bleeding from a gastric cancer, and a history of epigastric pain or heartburn suggests bleeding from a peptic ulcer or ulcerated oesophagus.

Diagnostic features of abdominal pain

Disorder	Localization	Character	Aggravating factors	Relieving factors	Visceral symptoms	Major physical signs	Diagnostic test
Acute pancreatitis	Epigastric and left hypochondrium radiating to back	Severe, constant pain		May improve when sitting forward	Nausea, vomiting	Tachycardia, shock, tender upper abdomen with guarding. Bruising in flanks	Raised serum and urinary amylase
Acute cholycystitis/ biliary colic	Right hypocondrium/ epigastrium radiating to right scapula and shoulder	Initially colicky, becomes continuous. Patient writhes			Nausea, vomiting, may have fever and rigors	Tender right hypochondrium, positive Murphy's sign, may be jaundiced	Biliary tract ultrasound, ERCP
Renal colic (ureteric stones)	Loin pain radiating to groin, and in males the scrotum	Very intense colicky pain. Patient writhes			Nausea, vomiting, frequency	Microscopic or obvious haematuria	Abdominal X-ray (90% stones visible), ultrasound intravenous urogram
Intestinal obstruction	Large bowel:lower abdomen Small intestine: periumbilical	Colic	Food, drink		Large bowel: constipation, vomiting occurs later Small intestine: vomiting, constipation occurs later	Abdominal distension, empty rectum	X-ray of abdomen shows air-fluid levels in bowel
Acute appendicitis	Initially, periumbilical pain, later localizes to right iliac fossa	Initally dull, later severe	Movement, hip extension		Nausea, anorexia, vomiting	Fever, tenderness and guarding in the right iliac fossa	
Perforated peptic ulcer	Sudden onset of epigastric pain. May radiate to the shoulder and extend to whole abdomen	Severe, persistent	Movement	Lying still	Nausea, vomiting	Fever, tachycardia, hypotension, shock, rigid abdomen with rebound tenderness	Chest X-ray reveals air under the diaphragm
Ruptured ectopic pregnancy	lower abdomen	Sudden onset, severe pain	Movement	Lying still		Tachycardia, hypotension, shock. Lower abdominal tenderness may become generalized. Guarding and rebound tenderness, tender cervix	Positive pregnancy test, anaemia, ultrasound
Ruptured aortic aneurysm	Pain radiating to the back	Moderately severe				Pulsatile tender mass, hypotension, shock, oliguria/ aneuria	Abdominal X-ray (calcification), ultrasound angiography

Fig. 8.23 The characteristics of abdominal pain which may help in making a differential diagnosis.

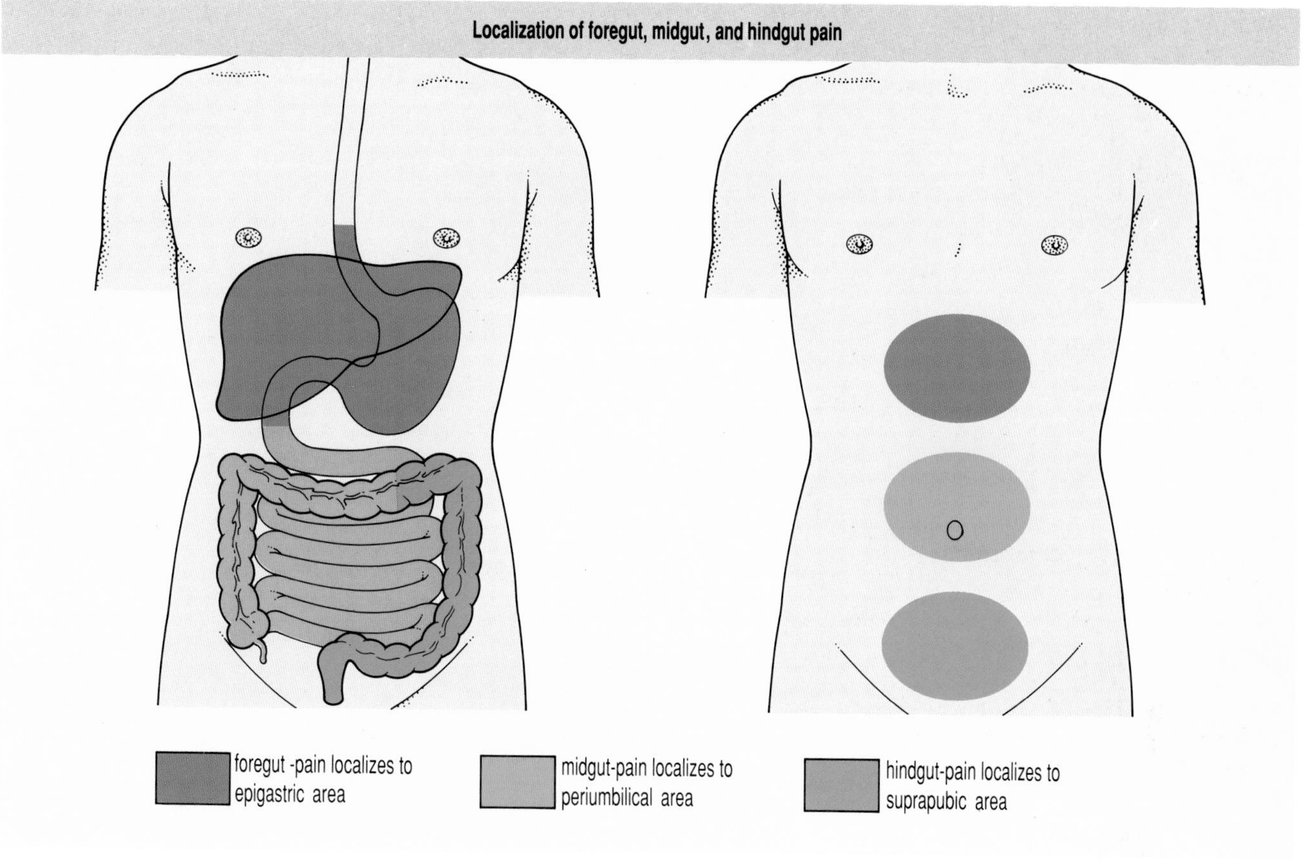

Fig. 8.24 Perception of visceral pain is localized to the epigastric, umbilical or suprapubic region according to the embryological origin of the diseased organ.

Abdominal pain

Pain is an important symptom of abdominal disease which may present in various shades, ranging from a dull ache to cramp, colic, and peritonitis. A differential diagnosis can often be constructed from the position, character and timing, the aggravating and relieving factors, and other distinctive or associated features (Fig. 8.23). When taking a history of abdominal pain, aim to distinguish between visceral, parietal, and referred pain.

Visceral pain is caused by stretching or inflammation of a hollow muscular organ (gut, gallbladder, bile duct, ureters, uterus). It is often described as a 'dull ache', or a 'gnawing' or 'cramping' sensation which is perceived near the midline, irrespective of the location of the organ. The pain can usually be localized to the epigastric, periumbilical or suprapubic areas depending upon whether the affected organ is derived from the embryological foregut, midgut or hindgut (Fig. 8.24). Pain arising from foregut is usually felt in the epigastrium, midgut pain is perceived around the umbilicus, and pain arising from the hindgut is felt in the suprapubic area. Visceral pain may also radiate to specific sites, and this helps to establish its origin (Fig. 8.25). It is commonly accompanied by nonspecific, 'visceral' symptoms (e.g. anorexia, nausea, pallor, and sweating).

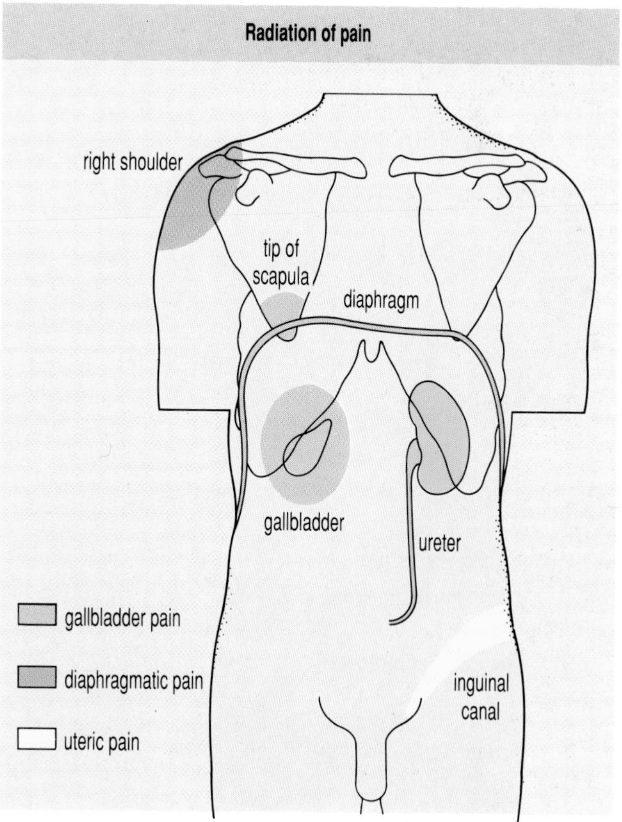

Fig. 8.25 Characteristic radiation of pain from the gallbladder, diaphragm, and ureters. The pain is not always felt in the organ concerned.

Colic is a characteristic manifestation of visceral pain and is caused by concerted and excessive smooth muscle contraction. It signifies obstruction of a hollow, muscular organ, such as the intestine, gallbladder, bile duct, or ureter, and consists of recurring bouts of intense, cramping, visceral pain which build to a crescendo and then fade away. When the smaller organs such as the gallbladder, bile duct, or ureters are acutely obstructed by a stone, the cyclical nature of colic soon gives way to a continuous visceral pain caused by the inflammatory effect of the impacted stone or secondary infection. Movement does not aggravate visceral pain, so the patient may writhe or double-up in response to it.

Abdominal pain

Describe the position, character, and radiation of the pain.

Has the pain been present for hours, days, weeks, months, or years?

Is the pain constant or intermittent?

Have you noted specific aggravating or relieving factors?

Is the pain affected by eating or defecation?

Does the pain wake you from sleep?

Is there associated nausea or vomiting?

Has there been associated weight loss?

Is there a history of ulcerogenic drugs?

Has there been a change in bowel habit?

Unlike the visceral peritoneum, the parietal peritoneum is innervated by pain-sensitive fibres. Therefore, pain arising from the parietal peritoneum is well-localized to the area immediately overlying the area of inflammation or irritation. Parietal pain is aggravated by stretching or moving the peritoneal membrane; the patient lies as still as possible. Palpation over the area is exquisitely painful, with the overlying muscles contracting to protect the peritoneum (guarding). When the pressure of the examining hand is suddenly released the pain is further aggravated and the patient winces. This sign is known as 'rebound tenderness'.

Abdominal pain may progress from a visceral sensation to parietal pain. Acute appendicitis provides an excellent example of this transition. When this midgut structure becomes inflamed and obstructed, a dull pain localizes to the periumbilical area, and the patient may feel nauseous and sweaty. As the inflammation advances through the visceral covering to the parietal peritoneum, the pain appears to shift to the right iliac fossa where it localizes over McBurney's point. The character of the pain also changes from dull to sharp. The area overlying the appendix is exquisitely tender, and palpation causes reflex guarding and rebound tenderness.

Mesenteric Angina

When the mesenteric arteries are stenosed by atherosclerosis the blood supply to the bowel may be impaired. The collateral supply to the bowel is well-developed, and the pain of bowel ischaemia usually becomes apparent only upon eating, when the metabolic demands of digestion and absorption require an increase in the blood supply. Patients complain of a severe visceral periumbilical pain occurring soon after meals (mesenteric angina). The pain causes anorexia, which, together with damage to the bowel mucosa, results in considerable weight loss.

Wind

Most gas in the gastrointestinal tract is swallowed, with a smaller contribution arising from fermentation of cellulose in the colon. Small, imperceptible amounts of gas constantly escape from the bowel via the mouth and anus. Excessive belching (flatulence) or the passage of wind through the anus (flatus) are common symptoms which cause considerable distress. These symptoms are rather nonspecific and occur in both functional and organic disorders of the gastrointestinal tract. Flatulence is usually caused by excessive air swallowing (aerophagy) and often occurs with an hiatus hernia, peptic ulceration, and chronic gallbladder disease. The symptom may be accompanied by a feeling of abdominal distention. Intestinal gas is produced by fermentation of certain foods, especially legumes, in the colon, and your history should seek to identify a possible dietary cause of excessive flatus and flatulence.

Change in bowel habit

Constipation

Most people on a Western diet expect bowel actions once to twice daily. Consequently, constipation usually implies failure to produce a stool over 24 hours. However, normal expectations vary between individuals and cultures; some healthy individuals evacuate every other day or even only three times a week, whilst others, particularly those on high roughage diets, expect up to three bulky bowel actions daily. Constipation is described more precisely as a disorder of bowel habit characterized by straining and the infrequent passage of small, hard stools. Constipated patients often complain that

Constipation

What is the normal stool frequency?

Do you strain at stool?

How long have you been constipated?

Is there associated abdominal pain, distention, nausea, or vomiting?

Are the stools large or small and pellet-shaped?

Have you noted intercurrent diarrhoea (spurious diarrhoea)?

Are any constipating drugs, such as codeine or other opiates, being used?

they are left dissatisfied, with a sensation of incomplete evacuation (tenesmus). Patients with troublesome constipation often seek medicinal relief, and a history of laxative use may be a helpful guide to the severity of the condition.

When constipation has troubled a patient for years, or even decades, the cause is likely to be functional rather than obstructive, and it may be attributed to diet, lifestyle, or psychological makeup. Lack of exercise, inadequate fluid and fibre intake, irritable bowel syndrome, and depression may all cause constipation.

When constipation presents as a recent change, and especially if it is associated with colic, suspect an organic cause such as malignancy or stricture formation. Enquire about constipating drugs, (e.g. codeine-containing analgesics and aluminium-containing antacids), and about rectal bleeding, which raises the suspicion of cancer. Consider hypothyroidism or electrolyte abnormalities. Anal pain caused by a fissure or a thromosed pile may cause profound constipation due to the patient's fear of pain at stool.

Constipation due to chronic partial obstruction may be punctuated by periods of loose or watery stool. This 'spurious diarrhoea' occurs in elderly patients with faecal impaction and also when colon cancer causes a partial obstruction. The proximal bowel dilates and fills with fluid which then seeps around the obstruction, presenting as liquid diarrhoea.

Diarrhoea

Diarrhoea implies increased stool volume and frequency and a change in consistency from formed to semi-formed, semi-liquid, or liquid. Always enquire about the presence of blood and mucus, and establish whether or not there is accompanying pain or colic. There is a wide differential diagnosis and the history may give some leads. Functional diarrhoea caused by anxiety, stress, or the irritable bowel syndrome does not wake the patient from sleep nor is it associated with rectal bleeding. Recent travel abroad, eating out, or an outbreak amongst people living in close proximity suggests an infective cause. Enquire about colour; in fat malabsorption, the stool is pale, malodorous, poorly formed, and difficult to flush. Blood and mucus mixed in the stool suggests an infective colitis or inflammatory bowel disease. When a cause is not readily apparent, consider laxative abuse and recent broad-spectrum antibiotic treatment, both of which may precipitate diarrhoea. Thyrotoxicosis may present with increased stool frequency and weight loss.

Diarrhoea

What is the normal stool frequency?

How many stools daily?

How long have you had diarrhoea?

Are you woken from sleep to open the bowels?

What is the colour and consistency of stools?

Are blood and mucus present?

Any travel abroad, or contacts with diarrhoea?

Is there associated nausea, vomiting, weight loss, or pain?

Any purgative abuse?

Any antibiotics?

Rectal bleeding

Rectal bleeding is a symptom common to several disorders (Fig. 8.26), and the history is not of much diagnostic value. Bright red rectal bleeding usually arises from the sigmoid colon or rectum, and more proximal colonic bleeding is often a darker red or maroon colour. The blood usually coats the stool, although in

Gastrointestinal bleeding

Is there a past history of abdominal pain or other GI symptoms?

Is there a history of chronic alcoholism or excessive intake?

Is there a past history of haematemesis, melena, or anaemia?

Are any nonsteroidals, steroids, or proprietary medicines being taken?

Was the bleed preceded by intense retching?

Has there been ingestion of iron or bismuth which may stain the stools

haemorrhoidal bleeding the blood may be most noticeable on the toilet paper. Colon cancer and polyps often present with intermittent rectal bleeding, whilst patients with inflammatory bowel disease pass blood, often mixed with mucus, with most stools. Torrential haemorrhage may occur from diverticular disease, and quite marked bleeding may occur in mesenteric vascular disease when the ischaemic colonic mucosa ulcerates and bleeds. Microscopic blood loss, (occult bleeding) usually presents with symptoms of anaemia. Always consider a diagnosis of gastric, caecal, or colon cancer in patients with unexplained iron deficiency anaemia. Haemorrhoids are common, so always consider other causes of bleeding in patients with piles, especially in those patients aged 40 and over.

The passage of sticky, black stools with the colour and consistency of tar (melena) usually indicates bleeding from the oesophagus, stomach, or duodenum. The characteristic appearance and smell is attributed to the denaturing effect of gastric acid and enzymes on blood. Treatment with iron and certain drugs (e.g. bismuth-containing preparations) also blackens the stool, and this cause must be distinguished from melena.

LIVER DISEASE

The background symptoms of liver disease may reflect damage to the parenchymal liver cells (hepatocellular disease) or obstruction

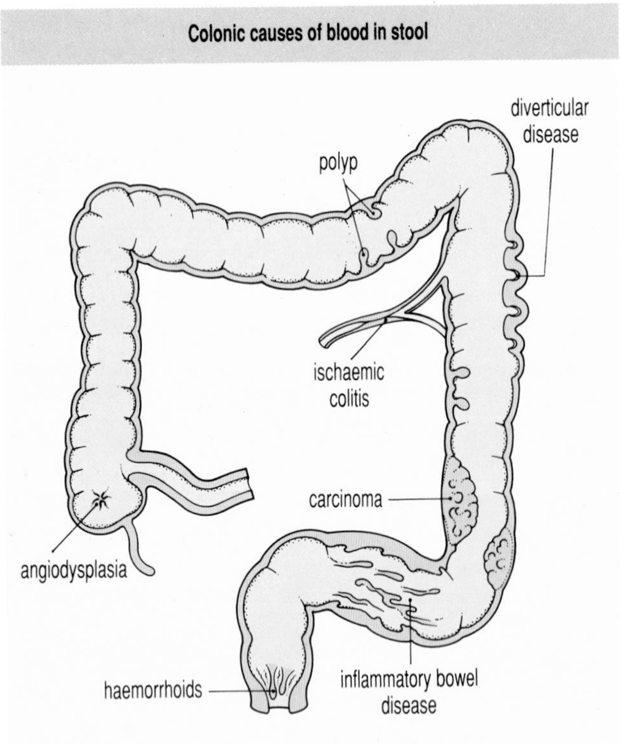

Fig. 8.26 Potential causes of bright red/maroon coloured rectal bleeding.

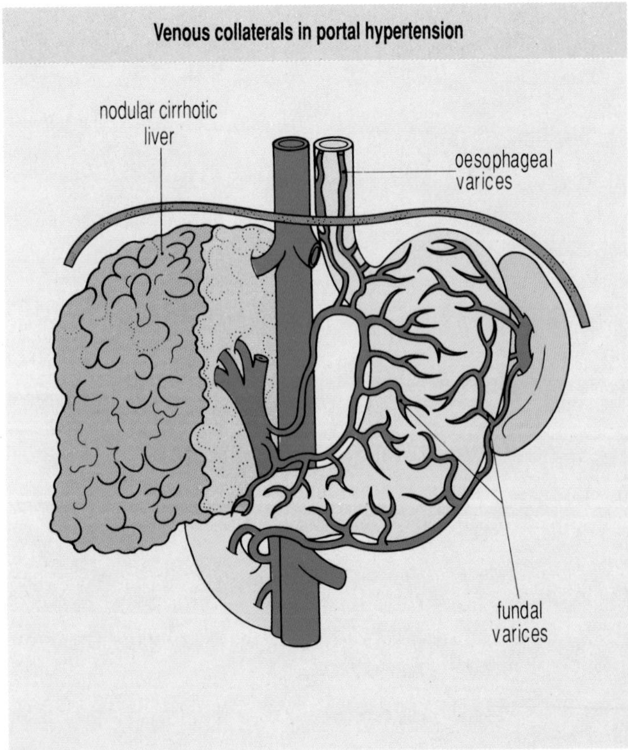

Fig. 8.27 Cirrhosis of the liver. When portal pressure rises, collateral veins open and blood bypasses the liver through dilated fundal and oesophageal varices which eventually drain into the azygos vein and superior vena cava.

of the biliary tree (intra- or extrahepatic cholestasis). Patients may also complain of symptoms related to the development of portal hypertension. Both liver cell damage and obstruction of the bile duct have numerous clinical consequences, the most striking of which are jaundice, pale stools, and darkening of the urine. When sufficient hepatocyte damage occurs, glycogen storage and glucose secretion are impaired, albumin levels fall, clotting is deranged, fat absorption is impaired, and the patient becomes jaundiced as bilirubin excretion fails and the pigment deposits in tissues. When hepatocytes are damaged or dead, enzymes leak into the blood where they can be measured. The high plasma activity of these enzymes is the basis of biochemical tests for liver damage.

In cirrhosis, liver architecture is severely disturbed, with regenerating nodules distorting and compressing the sinusoids and intrahepatic portal venous radicals. In addition, collagen is deposited between the sinusoidal lining cells and the hepatocytes, causing gradual obliteration of the space of Disse. Blood flow through the liver is partially obstructed and pressure rises in the portal vein. Resistance to blood flow through the liver encourages diversion of portal blood through collaterals (Fig. 8.27). A collateral circulation is established through the veins of the oesophagus. At endoscopy these abnormally dilated oesophageal veins are seen as tortuous, dilated veins (varices). Oesophageal varices are prone to rupture and may cause torrential haemorrhage.

Gut bacteria metabolize unabsorbed protein, releasing potentially neurotoxic breakdown products into the portal blood. The liver normally detoxifies these gut-derived products, but in patients with portal hypertension, portal blood bypasses the liver (portasystemic shunting) and the brain is exposed to gut-derived products which depress brain function, causing a characteristic neurological syndrome known as hepatic encephalopathy.

A further clinical consequence of portal hypertension is fluid retention in the abdominal cavity (ascites). The combination of high portal pressure and low serum albumin allows fluid to escape and to accumulate in the abdominal cavity.

Causes of biliary obstruction
Intrahepatic
Drug-induced cholestasis Primary biliary cirrhosis
Extrahepatic
Bile duct cancer Common bile duct stone Sclerosing cholangitis Cancer of the head of pancreas

Fig. 8.28 Causes of intra- and extrahepatic biliary obstruction.

Liver cell damage

The earliest symptoms of liver damage are rather nonspecific and include malaise, fatigue, anorexia, and nausea. Viral hepatitis is preceded by prodromes such as fatigue, nausea, and a profound distaste for alcohol and cigarettes. Before the onset of jaundice the patient may notice darkening of the urine and lightening of stool colour. This is caused by failure of the liver cells to excrete conjugated bilirubin.

Enquire about the principal causes of liver damage. Calculate the number of units (or grams) of alcohol consumed in a week as this provides a good guide to the risk of liver damage (see Chapter 2). Ask about any foreign travel, intravenous drug abuse, or exposure to blood products, and establish the patient's sexual orientation. Enquire about drugs which may cause liver damage and ask about a family history of liver disease.

The principal complications of chronic liver cell damage are cirrhosis and portal hypertension. The patient may notice increasing girth and weight gain. This is caused by the accumulation of ascites. If encephalopathy occurs, the sleep pattern may be reversed and the patient may undergo a change in personality.

Biliary obstruction

The principal symptom is itching (pruritus) and this may occur long before the patient becomes jaundiced. The cause of pruritus is unknown, although the deposition of bile acids in the skin has been suggested. As with viral hepatitis, lightening of the stools and darkening of the urine often precedes jaundice. The history may not help distinguish between the different causes of intra- and extrahepatic obstruction (Fig. 8.28). Severe epigastric and right hypochondrial pain accompanied by fever and jaundice suggests impaction of a gallstone in the common bile duct, whereas 'painless' jaundice suggests either a more chronic obstruction of the common bile duct (e.g. cancer of either the bile duct or head of the pancreas) or damage to the intrahepatic biliary tree (e.g. primary biliary cirrhosis, sclerosing cholangitis, and drugs). Impaired bile flow into the duodenum causes fat malabsorption and steatorrhoea; marked weight loss may occur.

PANCREATIC DISEASE

Acute pancreatitis presents with the acute onset of upper abdominal pain which is most prominent in the epigastrium and left upper quadrant. The pain may radiate through to the back, with its intensity varying from mild to severe. It is persistent and often lasts a

Jaundice

Have you travelled to areas where hepatitis A is endemic?

Is there a history of alcohol or intravenous drug abuse?

Have you ever had a blood transfusion?

Have you had contact with jaundiced patients?

Have you experienced skin itching?

What medication has been used recently?

Occupational contact with hepatotoxins?

Is there pain and weight loss?

Stool and urine colour?

Is there a family history of liver disease?

few days before abating. The pain` is commonly accompanied by nausea and vomiting; some relief may be obtained by sitting forward. Ask about alcohol intake and drugs (e.g. azathioprine, furosemide, corticosteroids) and consider underlying gallstones which may precipitate acute pancreatitis.

Recurrent attacks of acute pancreatitis may result in chronic pancreatitis. This is often characterized by persistent, severe upper abdominal pain which may radiate to the back. Progressive loss of exocrine function eventually leads to steatorrhoea and weight loss. Endocrine failure with diabetes is a late manifestation. Occasionally, chronic pancreatitis develops insidiously and presents with weight loss and steatorrhoea. Progressive fibrosis may occlude the lower bile duct causing thereby jaundice.

KIDNEY AND BLADDER DISEASE

The principal symptoms of diseases affecting the kidneys, ureters and bladder are pain and an alteration in the volume and frequency of bladder emptying. These symptoms and their underlying causes are summarized in Figure 8.29.

Frequency and urgency

Frequency refers to the desire to pass urine more often than normal, although there is not necessarily an increase in the volume of voided urine. Urgency, may accompany by frequency (i.e. a strong urge to urinate even though only small amounts of urine are present in the bladder).

Nocturia

It is fairly unusual to be woken from sleep to pass urine (nocturia), but this may occur in patients with daytime frequency or those pro-

Some renal symptoms and their causes
Frequency

Irritable bladder
  Infection, inflammation, chemical irritation
Reduced compliance
  Fibrosis, tumour infiltration
Bladder outlet obstruction
  In prostatism, detrusor failure may limit the volume voided

Polyuria
Ingestion of large volumes of water, beverages or alcohol Chronic renal failure (loss of concentrating power) Diabetes mellitus (osmotic effect of glucose in urine) Diabetes insipidus (due to lack of ADH or tubules insensitive to circulating ADH) Diuretic treatment
Dysuria
Bacterial infection of the bladder (cystitis) Inflammation of the urethra (urethritis) Infection/inflammation of the prostate (prostatitis)
Incontinence
Sphincter damage/weakness following childbirth Sphincter weakness in old age Prostate cancer Benign prostatic hypertrophy Spinal cord disease, paraplegia
Oliguria/anuria
Hypovolaemia (dehydration/shock) Acute renal failure due to acute glomerulonephritis Bilateral ureteric obstruction (retroperitoneal fibrosis) Detrusor muscle failure (bladder outlet obstruction or neurological disease)

Fig. 8.29 Symptoms of renal disease.

ducing excessive quantities of urine (polyuria). Incomplete bladder voiding due to prostatism often presents with nocturia.

Incontinence

Incontinence is an involuntary leakage of urine. If the symptom is provoked by increased intra-abdominal pressure (coughing, sneezing, or laughing), it is referred to as 'stress incontinence'.

Diseases causing excessive bladder filling (e.g. bladder outlet obstruction or damage to the nervous supply of the bladder) may cause 'overflow incontinence' which reflects spill-over from an over- filled, hypotonic bladder.

Hesitancy

Hesitancy is a delay between attempting to initiate urination and the actual flow of urine. It is a characteristic sign of bladder outlet obstruction, (e.g. due to prostatic hypertrophy).

Oliguria and anuria

Patients may complain of passing only small volumes of urine. The term oliguria is used if less than 500ml of urine is passed over 24 hours. The subjective assessment of urine volume is often inaccurate and requires confirmation by 24-hour urine collection and measurement. Apparent oliguria may occur in patients with bladder muscle (detrusor) failure; consequently it may be necessary to pass a catheter to confirm true oliguria.

Pain

Pain may originate in the kidneys, ureter, bladder, or urethra. Infection of the kidneys (pyelonephritis) causes pain and tenderness in the renal angles, usually associated with fever, anorexia, and nausea. Obstruction of the ureters by stones, sloughed papillae, or blood may cause intense pain in the renal angle. This pain may radiate towards the groins and, in males, into the testes. Renal 'colic' due to stones in the ureters is extremely painful, often causing the patient to double-up or roll around in a futile effort to find relief. Bladder pain may occur in severe cystitis. The pain is of moderate severity, localized to the suprapubic region, and associated with urgency and frequency.

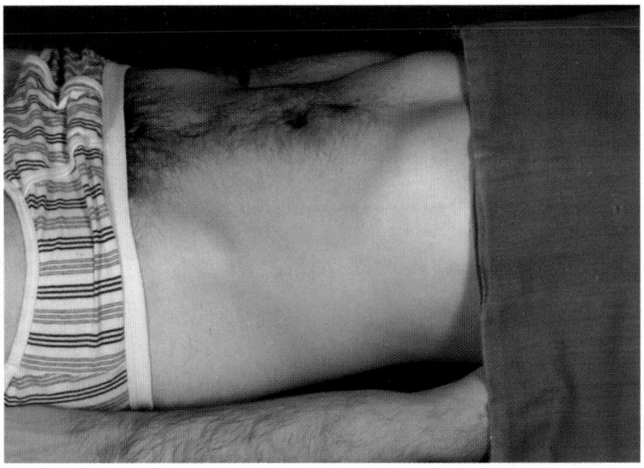

Fig. 8.30 The patient should be exposed as little as possible during your examination.

Dysuria

Dysuria describes a stinging or burning sensation which occurs when passing urine. It is often accompanied by frequency and urgency. The most common cause of dysuria is cystitis.

EXAMINATION OF THE ABDOMEN

Before beginning your examination ask the patient to lie flat, with their head resting comfortably on a pillow, arms lying loosely on either side. According to the demands of the particular procedure you are performing, try to expose the patient as little as possible. The 'classical' arrangement is shown in Figure 8.30, but until you gain experience it will help to have the visual clues provided by the landmarks of the entire abdomen and lower chest; subsequent illustrations reflect this.

The abdominal examination depends largely upon palpation and percussion of organs which normally lie out of reach of the examining hand. As with all other examinations it is important to become completely familiar with the clinical anatomy of the abdomen.

The costal margin demarcates the superficial boundary between the chest and abdomen, though the domes of the diaphragm rise behind the ribs to accommodate the liver and spleen, so a full abdominal examination also includes examination of the lower half of the chest (Fig. 8.31). Familiarize yourself with the bony land-

Examination of the liver and spleen

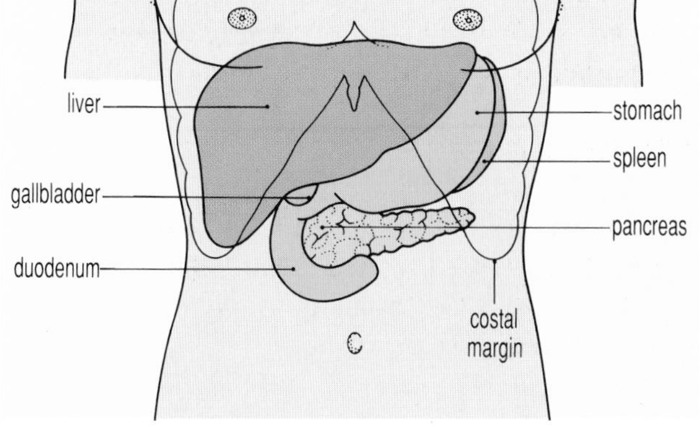

Fig. 8.31 The liver and spleen lie protected under the ribs and so the lower half of the chest must be exposed in order to examine them.

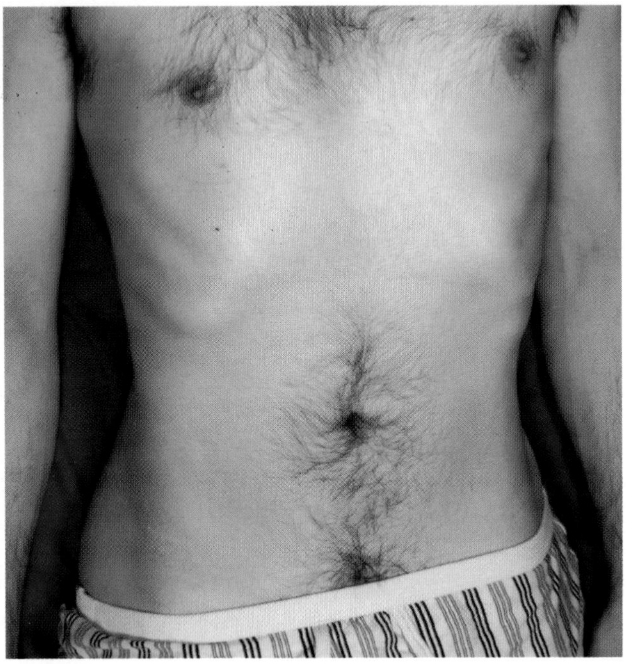

Fig. 8.32 The bony landmarks of the anterior abdominal wall.

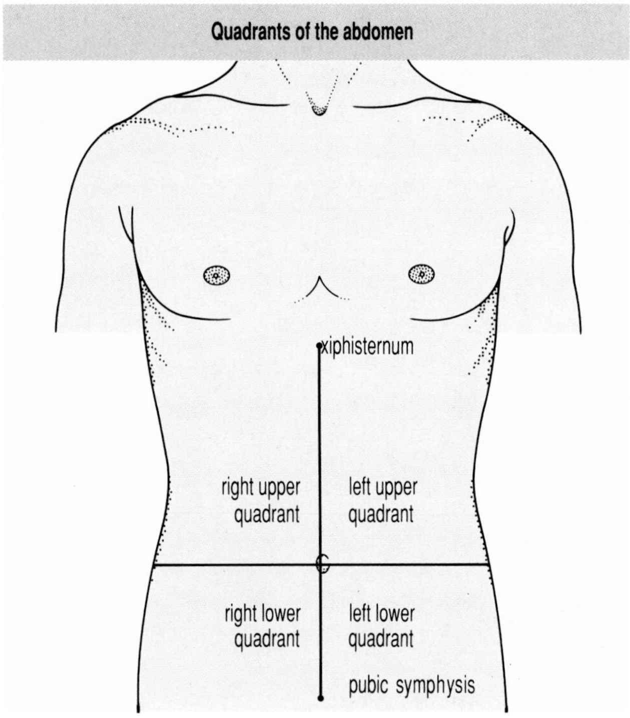

Fig. 8.33 The quadrants of the anterior abdominal wall.

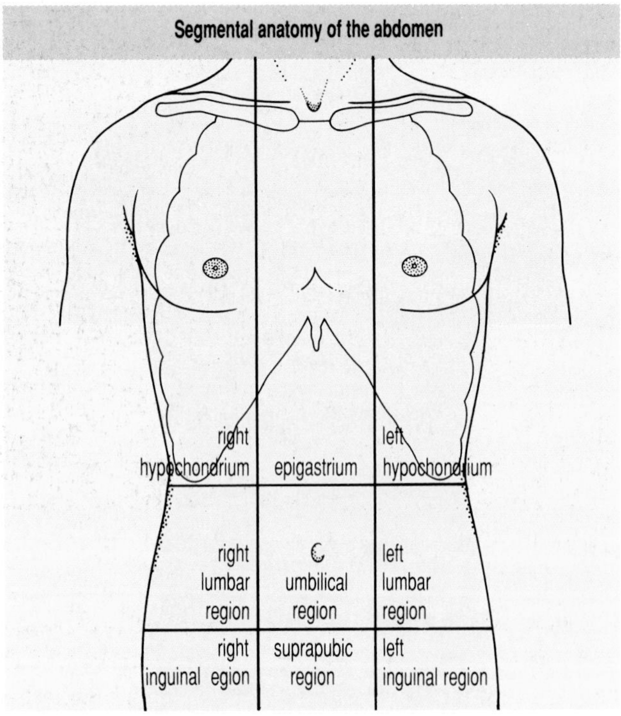

Fig. 8.34 The nine segments of the anterior abdominal wall.

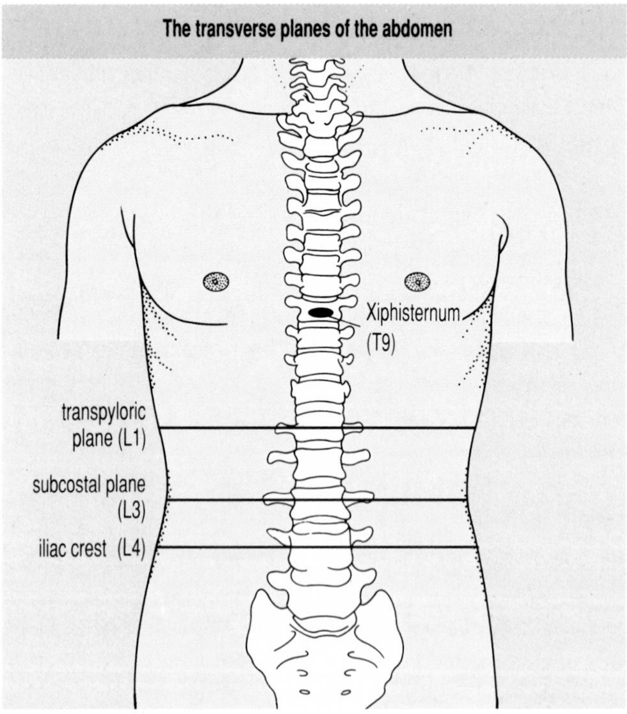

Fig. 8.35 The transverse planes and their equivalent vertebral levels.

marks of the abdomen (Fig. 8.32). Feel the xiphisternum at the lower end of the sternum, then trace the outline of the costal margin formed by the seventh costal cartilage at the xiphisternum to the tip of the twelfth rib. Note a distinct step in the costal margin which provides a useful landmark, as it coincides with the tip of the tenth rib. Turn your attention to the bony margins of the lower abdomen. The iliac crest has a distinct anterior prominence, the anterior superior iliac spine, from which the inguinal ligament runs downward and medially to attach to a lateral prominence on the pubic bone (the pubic tubercle).

For descriptive purposes the anterior abdominal wall may be divided into four quadrants (Fig. 8.33). Trace the imaginary lines demarcating the left and right upper and lower quadrants. A vertical line extends from the xiphisternum to the pubic symphysis in

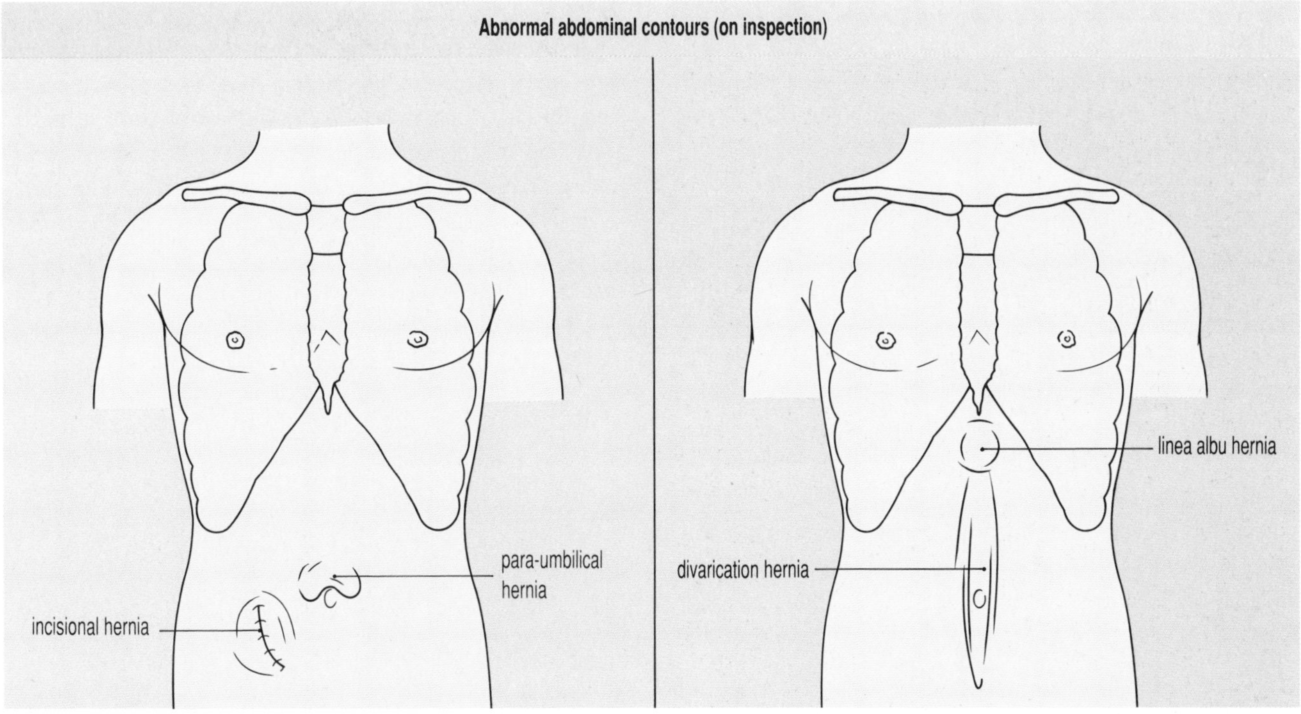

Fig. 8.36 Some abnormal abdominal contours.

the midline, whilst a horizontal line is drawn through the umbilicus. The abdomen may also be divided into nine segments resembling a 'noughts and crosses' matrix (Fig. 8.34). These segments are useful landmarks for ensuring a complete and systematic examination of the abdomen. A vertical line is dropped from the midclavicular points on either side, and these are crossed by a horizontal line drawn in the subcostal plane and by a line joining the anterior superior iliac spines.

When locating or describing the position of the abdominal organs it is useful to recognize the anterior anatomical planes and their correlation with vertebral levels (Fig. 8.35). The xiphisternum corresponds to the level of T9. The transpyloric plane lies midway between the suprasternal notch and the pubis, approximately a hand's breadth below the xiphoid cartilage. This plane corresponds to the vertebral level of L1 and passes through the pylorus, the long axis of the pancreas, the duodeno-jejunal flexure, and the hila of the kidneys. The subcostal plane coincides with the level of L3 and is defined by a line joining the lowest point of the thoracic cage on either side. A line joining the highest points of the iliac crest corresponds to the level of L4.

INSPECTION OF THE ABDOMEN

Contours

Expose the patient to the groins and observe the symmetry of the abdomen from the foot of the bed. The normal abdomen is concave and symmetrical and moves gently with respiration. Next, move to the patient's right and view the abdomen tangentially. From this position it is easier to pick out more the subtle changes of contour and shadow. In thin individuals you may notice the pulsation of the abdominal aorta in the midline above the umbilicus. Ask the patient to raise their head a few inches off the pillow. This tenses the rectus abdominis which becomes firm and prominent on either side of the midline.

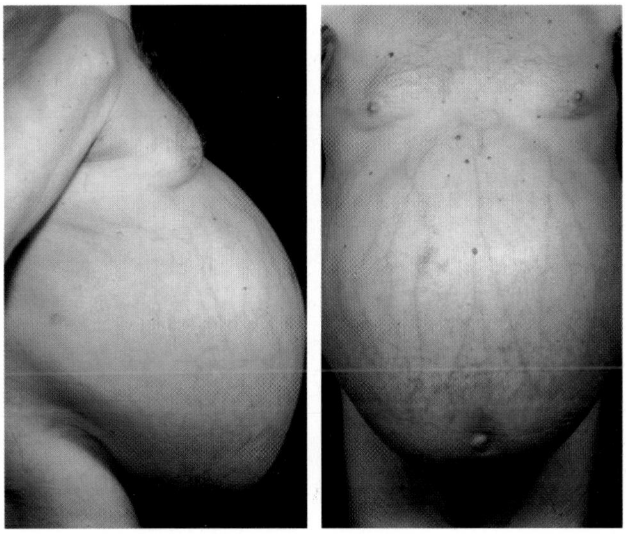

Fig. 8.37 The characteristic appearance of gross ascites.

Abnormal contours and distention of the abdomen may be caused by a number of mechanisms (Fig. 8.36). Establish whether the swelling is generalized or localized. Fluid and gaseous distention is generalized and symmetrical (Fig. 8.37). Fluid gravitates towards the flanks causing the loins to bulge, and the umbilicus, which is normally inverted, may become everted when massive ascites distends the abdomen beyond its normal compliance. In thin individuals the contour of an enlarged liver may be visible below the right costal margin. A midline fullness in the upper abdomen may indicate disease of the stomach (e.g. carcinoma), pancreas (e.g. pancreatic cysts) or an abdominal aortic aneurysm. Suprapubic fullness may reflect an enlarged uterus (pregnancy or fibroids), ovaries (cysts or carcinoma), or a full bladder. The periodic rippling movement of bowel peristalsis may be observed in intestinal obstruction, especially in thin individuals.

Abnormal bulges may appear when intra-abdominal pressure is raised and may be revealed by tensing the abdominal muscles. If the muscles of the recti are abnormally separated on either side of the midline (divarication of the recti), tensing the abdominal muscles causes a longitudinal bulge to appear in the midline (see Fig. 8.36). The appearance of a more localized bulge just above or below the umbilicus occurs with a para-umbilical hernia (see Fig. 8.36). Direct and indirect inguinal herniae may also become prominent when intra-abdominal pressure is raised by coughing. Surgical scars are potential points of weakness in the abdominal wall and incisional herniae may develop under the scar.

Skin

During pregnancy the abdominal wall skin is stretched and after childbirth many women are left with tell-tale stretch lines (striae gravidarum) which arc across the mid and lower abdominal wall on either side of the midline (Fig. 8.38). Stretch marks similar to those occuring after pregnancy may occur in patients successfully treated for ascites. In Cushing's syndrome, excessive adrenal corticosteroid secretion thins the skin and purplish striae appear on the abdominal wall even in the absence of a pregnancy. In acute haemorrhagic pancreatitis there may be a bluish discolouration of either the flanks (Grey Turner's sign) or the periumbilical area (Cullen's sign) which results from seepage of blood-stained ascitic fluid along the fascial planes and into the subcutaneous tissue. A similar appearance may occur following rupture of an ectopic pregnancy.

Look for veins coursing over the abdominal wall: they are rarely prominent in health. If veins are visible map the direction of flow by emptying the vein with the index finger of one hand whilst simultaneously attempting to prevent refilling by applying occlu-

Fig. 8.38 Striae gravidarum appear following pregnancy

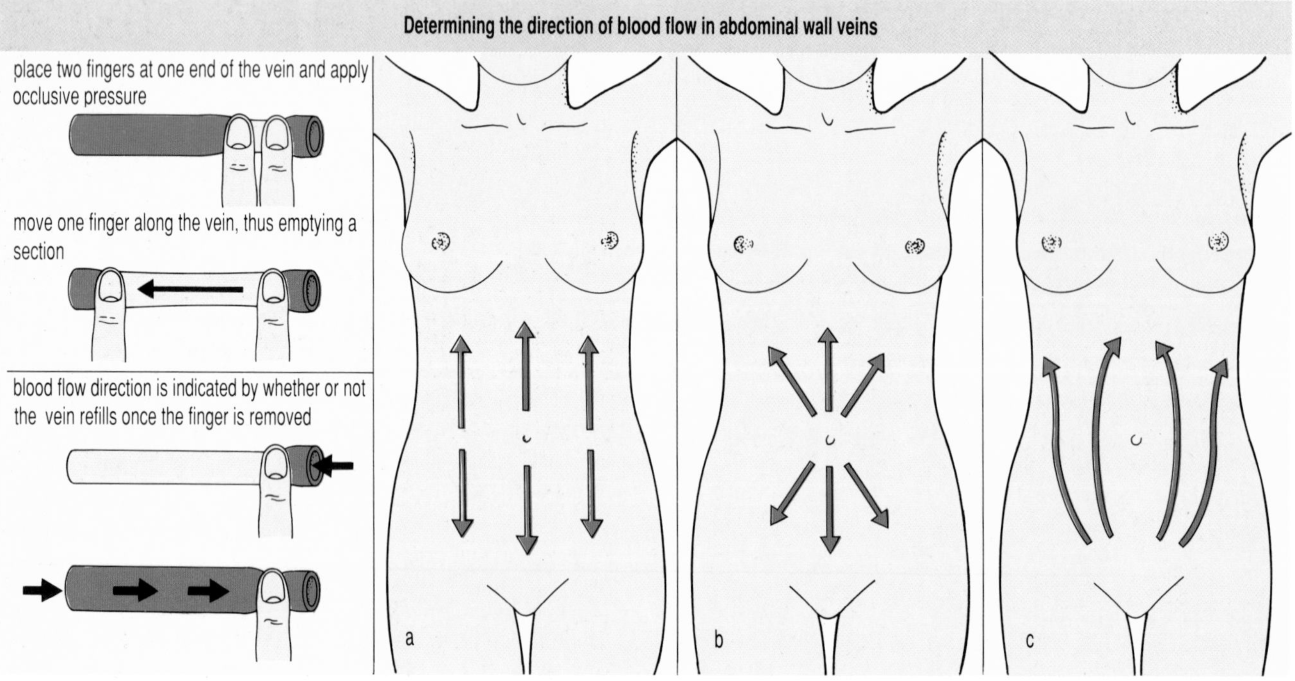
Determining the direction of blood flow in abdominal wall veins
place two fingers at one end of the vein and apply occlusive pressure
move one finger along the vein, thus emptying a section
blood flow direction is indicated by whether or not the vein refills once the finger is removed
a
b
c

Fig. 8.39 Determining the direction of blood flow in abdominal veins. (a) Normal blood flow pattern and those characteristic of (b) portal hypertension and (c) obstruction of the inferior vena cava.

sive pressure more proximally over the vein. The direction of flow helps distinguish normal from abnormal flow patterns (Fig. 8.39). In portal hypertension and inferior vena caval obstruction, the venous return to the liver or vena cava is redirected through abdominal wall collaterals which provide an alternative route to the right atrium. These veins dilate and may be seen coursing across the abdominal wall. It is possible to distinguish collaterals caused by portal hypertension from those caused by inferior vena caval obstruction by mapping the direction of flow in these vessels.

Look for surgical scars, which should have a fleshy red or pink colouring in the first year after an operation, becoming white as the scar tissue matures. Common locations of surgical scars are shown in Figure 8.40.

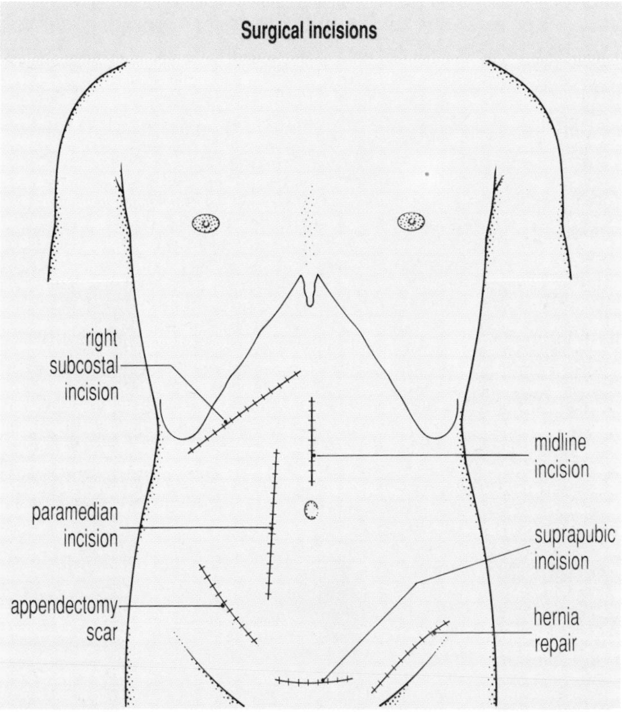

Fig. 8.40 Surgical scars commonly seen on the abdomen.

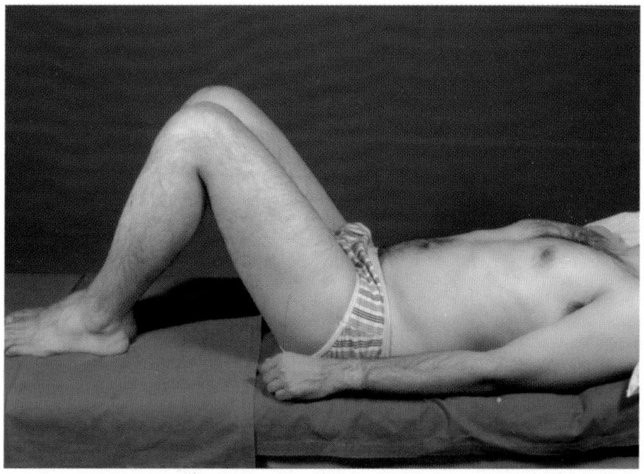

Fig. 8.41 Palpation of the abdomen may be aided if the patient is asked to flex their hips. This helps to relax the anterior abdominal wall muscles.

PALPATION OF THE ABDOMEN

Although the intra-abdominal organs are normally impalpable, in diseased states palpation and percussion provide substantial clinical information. These procedures are difficult to perform if the patient is not relaxed. If the abdominal wall muscles are tense, ask the patient to bend the knees and to flex the hips (Fig. 8.41). This helps to relax the abdomen. Always warm your hands before palpating the abdomen, and use the fingertips and palmar aspects of the fingers; a single-handed technique may be used, but you may prefer to use both hands, the upper hand applying pressure, whilst the lower hand concentrates on feeling (Fig. 8.42).

Light palpation

Before laying a hand on the abdomen ask the patient to localize any areas of pain or tenderness. If these are present, begin the examination in the segment furthest from the discomfort. Start light palpation by gently pressing your fingers into each of the nine segments, sustaining the light pressure for a few seconds whilst gently exploring each area with the fingertips. Tenderness may be reflected by grimacing, so with every move of your hand briefly look to see the patient's facial response.

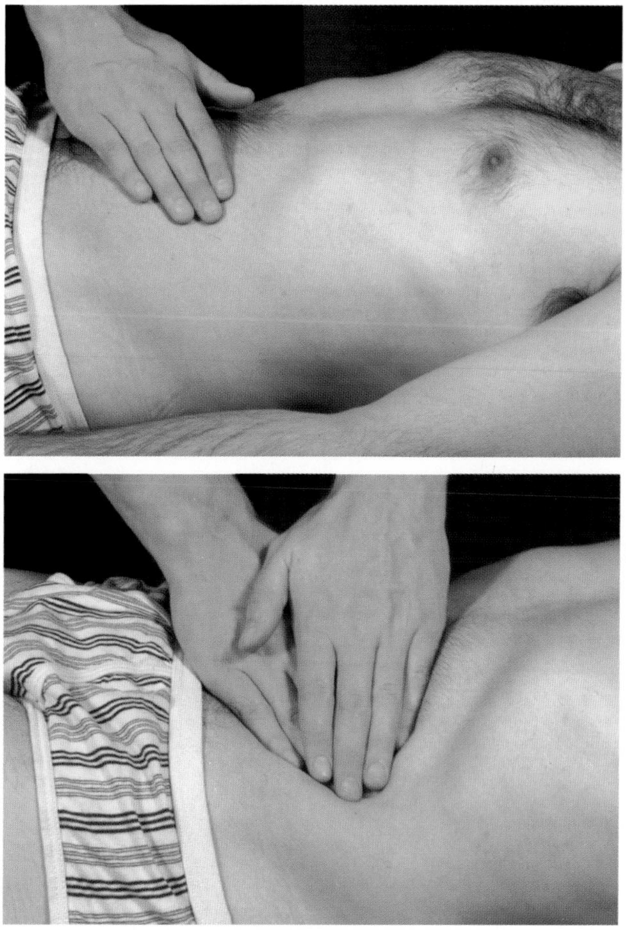

Fig. 8.42 Light abdominal palpation is performed using one hand (upper) or both (lower).

Structures which may be felt on deep palpation

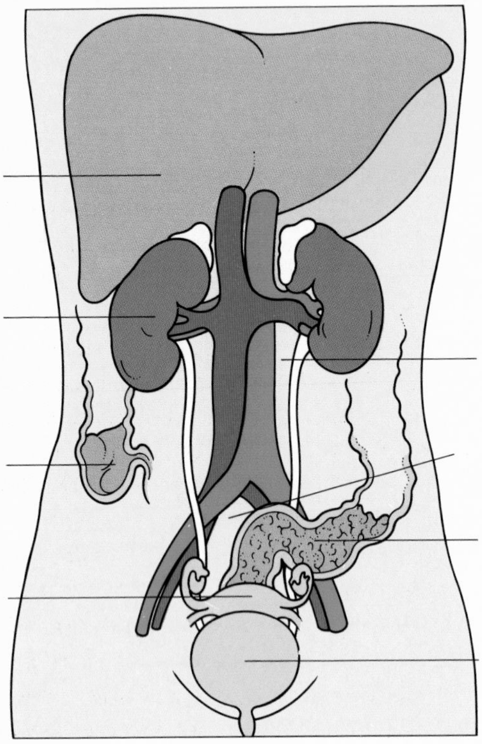

Fig. 8.43 Upon deep palpation of the abdomen, these structures may be palpated.

Gentle palpation will detect tenderness caused by inflammation of the parietal peritoneum. In peritonitis, the patient flinches on even the lightest palpation and there is reflex rigidity, guarding, and rebound tenderness. Light palpation may localize an area of peritoneal inflammation, thereby helping to establish a differential diagnosis. It is unusual to feel the abdominal organs or large masses on light palpation unless they are grossly enlarged.

Deep palpation

Once you have used light palpation to explore for areas of tenderness and muscle tension, the sequence is repeated using firm but gentle deep pressure with the palmar surface of the fingers. If the patient is relaxed it is usually possible to press deeply into the abdomen. Whilst doing so try to imagine the anatomy underlying your hand (Fig. 8.43). In thin individuals the descending and/or sigmoid colon may be felt as an elongated tubular structure in the left loin and lower quadrant. The sigmoid is mobile and can readily be rolled under the fingers. The colon can usually be distinguished from other structures because of its firm stool content. It has a putty-like consistency and can be indented with the fingertips. The 'mass' also becomes less obvious after the passage of stool. In thin individuals, the abdominal aorta may be felt as a discrete pulsatile structure in the midline, above the umbilicus. The rectus muscles may be mistaken for an abnormal fullness or the edge of a mass. Tensing the abdominal muscles causes the rectus to become more prominent, whereas intra-abdominal masses are less easy to feel.

Abdominal masses and enlargement of the liver, spleen, and kidneys may also be felt upon deep palpation. Any abnormal fullness,

Distinction between aortic pulsation and movement of an overlying structure

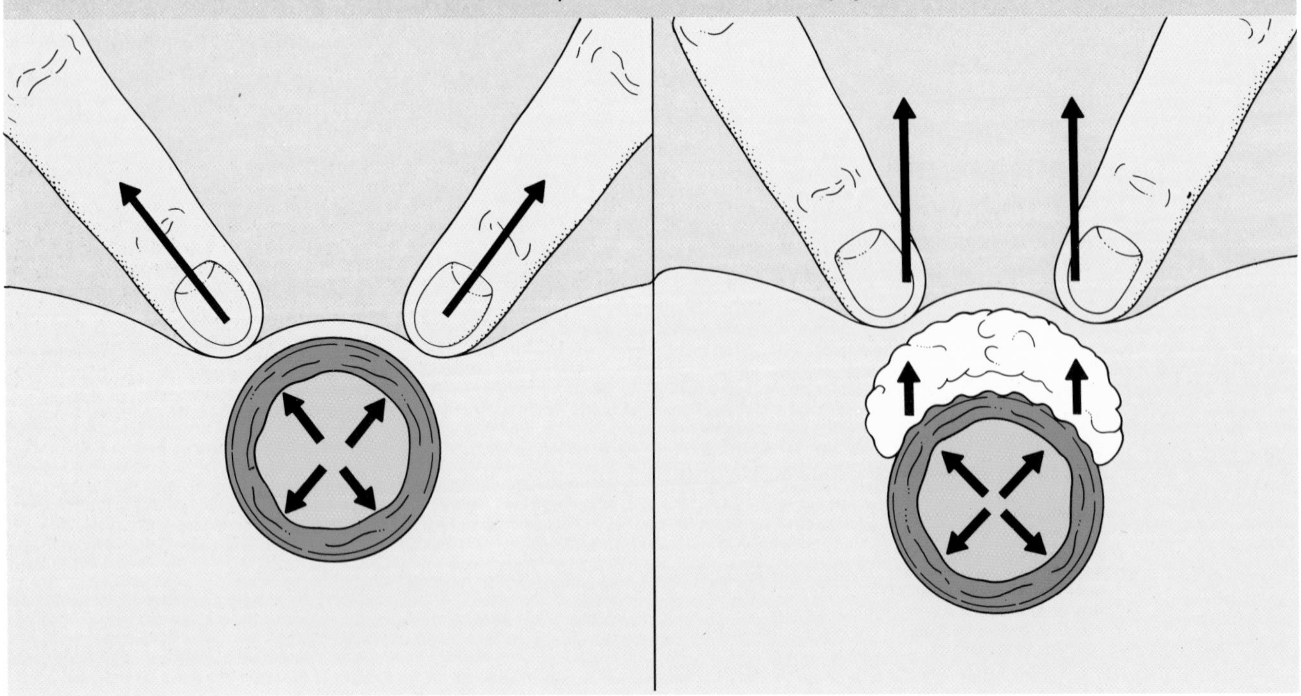

Fig. 8.44 Palpating the aorta. The direction of the pulsation indicates whether it arises directly from the aorta (left) or is transmitted by a mass overlying the tissues (right).

firmness or discrete mass should be localized by careful palpation of shape, mobility, consistency, and movement with respiration. Localization helps determine which organ might be involved. Determine whether there is any deep tenderness, suggesting stretching of the capsule of either the liver or kidney, or early peritoneal inflammation or infiltration. A large pulsatile structure in the midline above the umbilicus indicates an aortic aneurysm or a transmitted impulse to a mass overlying the aorta. These can usually be distinguished using the index finger of either hand to sense whether the movement is pulsatile or transmitted (Fig. 8.44).

ORGAN PALPATION

The solid organs (liver, pancreas, kidneys, and spleen) are normally out of reach of the examining hand. The stomach, small intestine, and colon are soft, pliable, and usually impalpable. In chronic fibrosing diseases of the liver (e.g. micronodular cirrhosis) or kidneys (e.g. chronic glomerulonephritis), these organs shrink even further from reach. However, they may become palpable when enlarged.

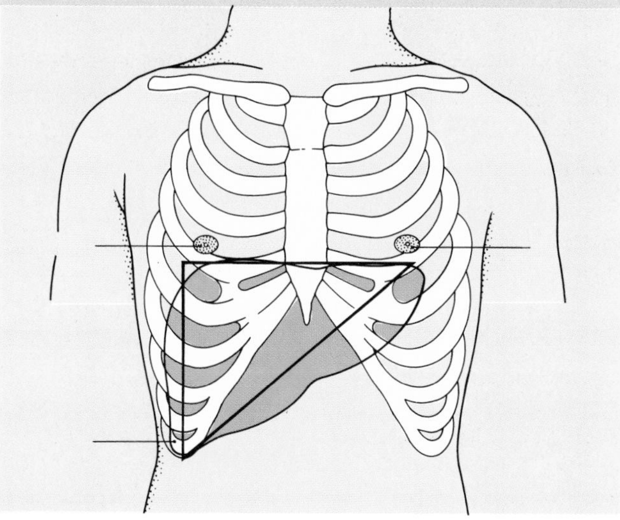

Fig. 8.45 The clinical anatomy of the liver.

Palpating the liver

Examine the liver with the surface anatomy in mind. Visualize its upper margin as a line passing just below each nipple on either side, and imagine the lower margin spanning a line from the tip of the tenth rib on the right to a point just below the left nipple (Fig. 8.45). The upper surface of the organ is tightly apposed to the under surface of the diaphragm and examination takes advantage of the movement of the liver with respiration. The initial aim of the examination is to define the outline of the lower edge of the right lobe, which is normally tucked along the inner surface the right costal margin. The edge of the smaller left lobe nestles under the lower left rib cage and is often impalpable even when the organ is generally enlarged.

Examine from the patient's right and use either the fingertips or the radial side of the index finger to explore for the liver edge under the costal margin. Point the ends of the index, middle, and ring fingers in an upward position, facing the liver edge, at a point midway between the costal margin and iliac crests, lateral to the rectus muscle (Fig. 8.46). Press the fingertips inwards and upwards and hold this position whilst the patient takes a deep inspiration. Near the height of inspiration relax the inward pressure slightly but maintain upward pressure. As the fingers drift upwards feel for the liver edge slipping under them as the organ descends. If no edge is felt repeat the manouevre in a stepwise fashion, each time moving the starting position a little closer to the costal margin. If the liver is impalpable at this point you should repeat the procedure more laterally in line with the anterior axillary line. In patients of thin or medium build a normal liver edge may be palpable just below the right costal margin at the

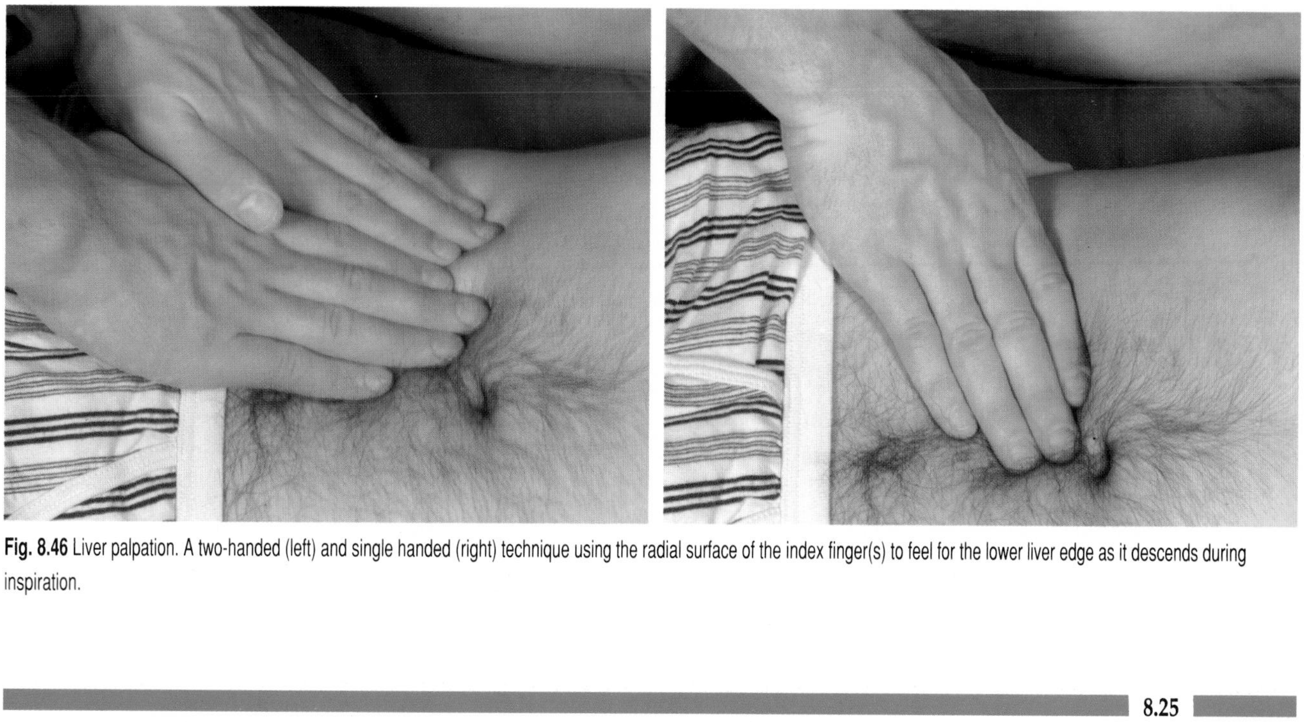

Fig. 8.46 Liver palpation. A two-handed (left) and single handed (right) technique using the radial surface of the index finger(s) to feel for the lower liver edge as it descends during inspiration.

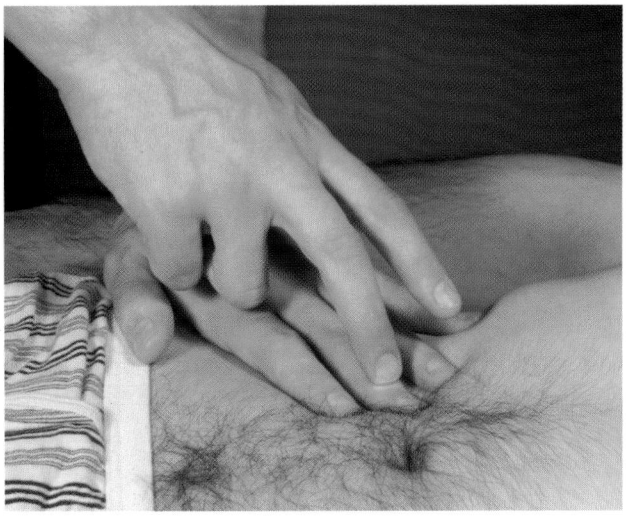

Fig. 8.47 Positioning of the hand when percussing for the lower border of the liver.

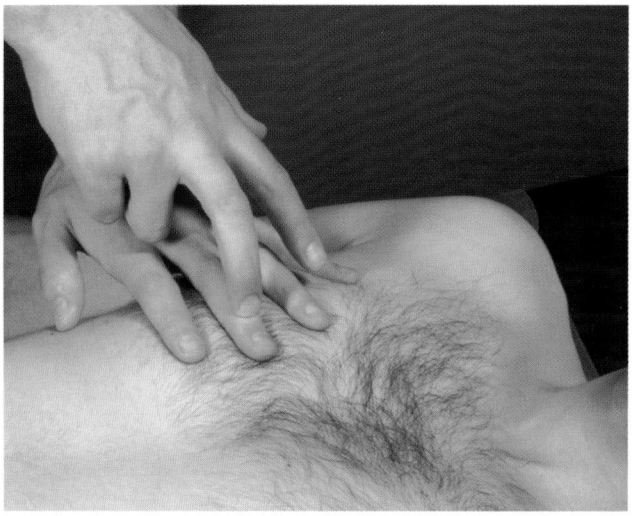

Fig. 8.48 Percussion of the upper border of the liver.

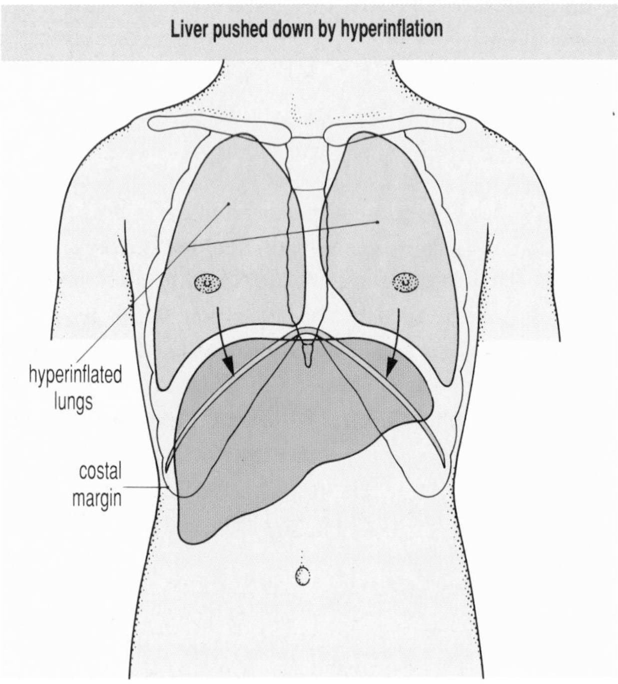

Fig. 8.49 When the lung fields are markedly hyperinflated, the liver is pushed down and the lower border may be readily palpable although the span is normal.

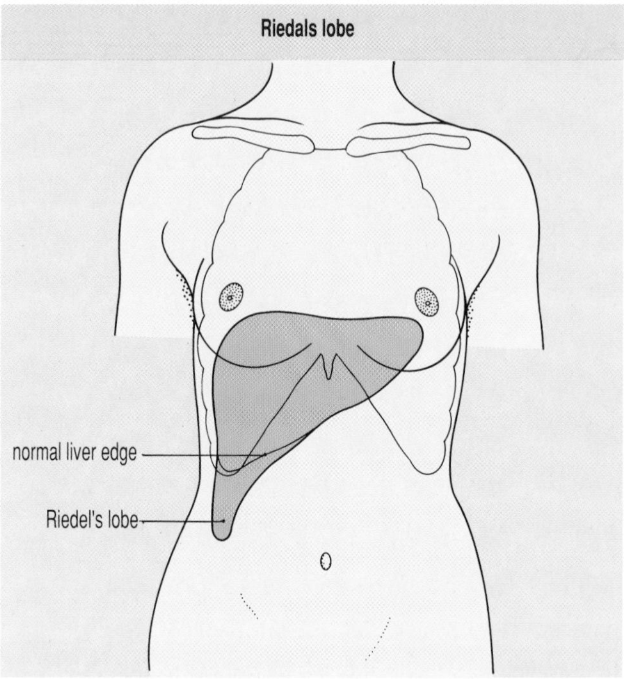

Fig. 8.50 A Riedels lobe is a normal variant of shape. The elongated 'tongue' is palpable and must be distinguished from a mass.

height of inspiration. Repeat the palpation in the midline and below the left costal margin where the lower edge of the middle and left lobes should not be palpable. A single-handed technique may also be used (Fig. 8.46). The radial surface of the index finger is positioned below and parallel to the costal margin and this surface is used to explore for the lower liver edge as it descends during inspiration.

At this point in the examination it is useful to percuss for the lower liver edge. With the long axis of your middle finger positioned parallel to the right costal margin, percuss from the point where you started palpating for the liver (Fig. 8.47). This point normally overlies bowel and should sound resonant. Repeat the percussion in a stepwise manner, each time moving the finger closer to the costal margin until the note becomes duller. This should coincide with the the costal margin. Ask the patient to inspire deeply; the dullness should move down as the liver descends.

Next find the position of the upper margin of the liver so that you can assess the liver span. The upper margin cannot be palpated because it lies high in the dome of the diaphragm, but it can be located by noting the change in percussion note from the resonance of the lungs to the dullness of the liver. The upper margin of the liver usually lies deep to the fifth or sixth intercostal space. Percuss the third space and then percuss each succeeding interspace until you detect the transition from resonance to dullness (Fig. 8.48). On deep inspiration the percussion interface should descend by either one or two interspaces as the lungs

Smooth and irregular liver surface

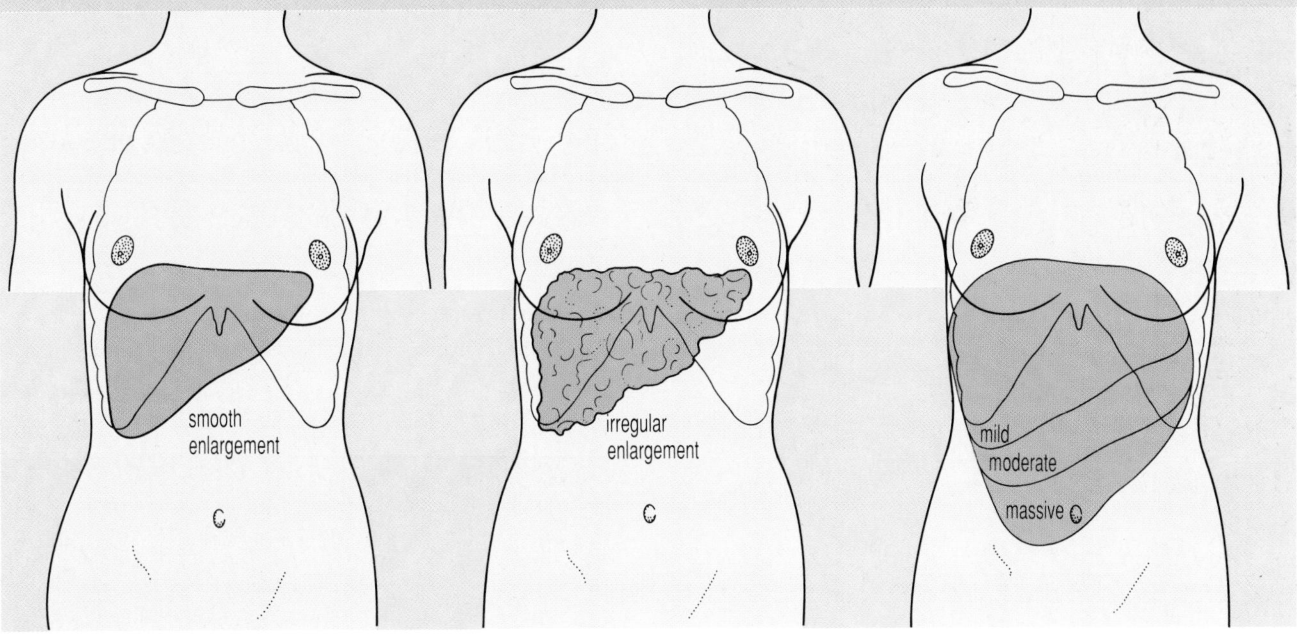

Fig. 8.51 Liver enlargement. Enlargement of the liver can be smooth (e.g, fatty liver) or irregular (e.g, macronodular cirrhosis, tumor infiltration).

expand and the liver descends. Liver size is proportional to body size. Measure the liver span in the midclavicular line; in women this should measure 8–10cm, whilst in men, the span is 10–12cm.

Downward displacement of the liver.

In patients with hyperinflated lungs (e.g. emphysema), the diaphragms are flattened and the liver is pushed down so that the edge may be easily palpable below the costal margin (Fig. 8.49). Percussion reveals that the upper border of the liver is depressed and that the liver span is within normal limits.

Abnormal liver shape

The right lobe of the liver may be abnormally shaped, with an elongated tongue-like projection pointing towards the right iliac crest (Fig. 8.50). This anatomical variant, known as a Riedel's lobe, is more common in women and feels like a mobile mass on the right side of the abdomen arising from under the costal margin and moving with respiration. A Riedel's lobe is commonly mistaken for an enlarged right kidney, and if in doubt this can be resolved by ultrasound scanning.

Enlargement of the liver.

Liver enlargement is usually described as mild, moderate, or massive (Fig. 8.51). If the liver is enlarged trace the shape of the liver edge decide whether it is smooth or irregular, whether the consistency is soft, firm or hard and whether or not the organ is tender. The presence of a palpable spleen suggests cirrhosis with portal hypertension or infiltrating diseases of the reticuloendothelial and haemopoietic systems.

Small livers

The lower margin of the liver may not be palpable because of fibrosis or atrophy of the organ. This may be difficult to detect clinically, but should be suspected if the liver edge is not palpable and if , on percussion, the dullness of the lower liver margin is detected well above the costal margin (Fig. 8.52). Atrophy of the liver may be a result either of severe acute liver damage, perhaps caused by fulmi-

Percussion of shrunken liver

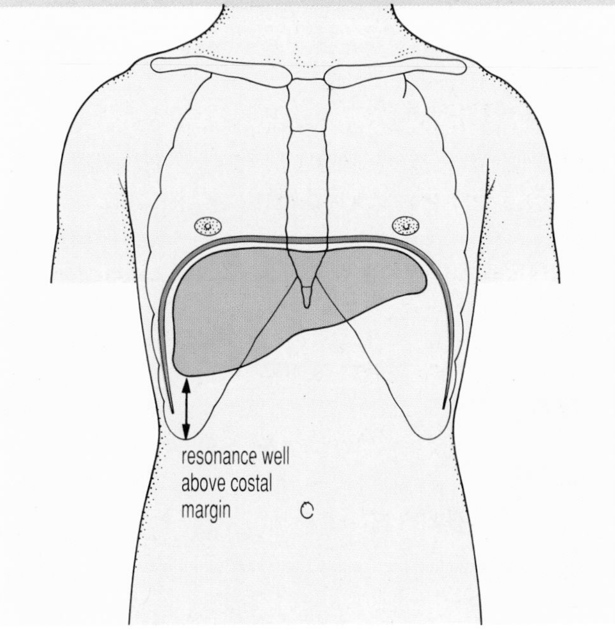

Fig. 8.52 Atrophy of the liver may be detected by percussing the lower border. The area of resonance will extend above the costal margin.

Signs of liver disease
Head and neck
Jaundice Xanthelasma (cholestasis) Foetor hepatis Parotid swelling Spider naevi
Trunk/abdomen
Gynaecomastia Splenomegaly Dilated abdominal veins Ascites Easy bruising
Groin
Testicular atrophy
Hands
Flapping tremor (arterixis) Finger clubbing White nails (hypoproteinaemia) Dupuytren's contracture Palmar erythema

Fig. 8.53 Signs of chronic liver disease.

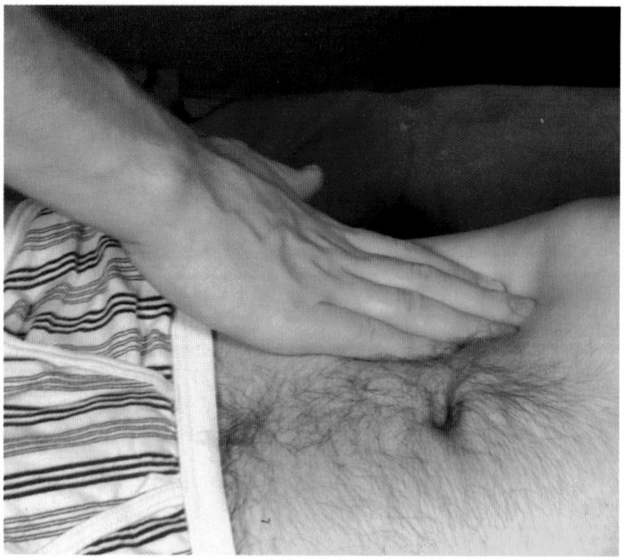

Fig. 8.55 Palpating the gallbladder.

nant viral hepatitis or hepatotoxic poisons, or chronic disease causing fibrosis and micronodular cirrhosis (e.g. alcoholic cirrhosis).

General signs of liver disease

The liver has considerable functional reserve, but as this is exhausted the patient develops characteristic signs of liver failure (Fig. 8.53). Look for jaundice in the sclerae which are normally a brilliant white colour. Mild jaundice may be difficult to discern in artificial light, and in dark-skinned patients the sclerae may be slightly pigmented. With deepening jaundice the skin becomes yellow, and in chronic, severe obstructive jaundice the skin may appear almost green in colour.

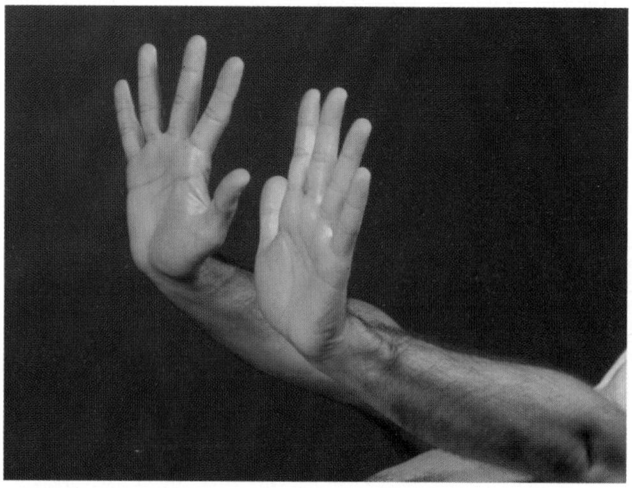

Fig. 8.54 To elicit a flapping tremor in hepatic encephalopathy, ask the patient to outstretch their arms with the hands extended at the wrist and metacarpophalangeal joints. This position is held for 20 seconds.

Courvoisier's 'law'

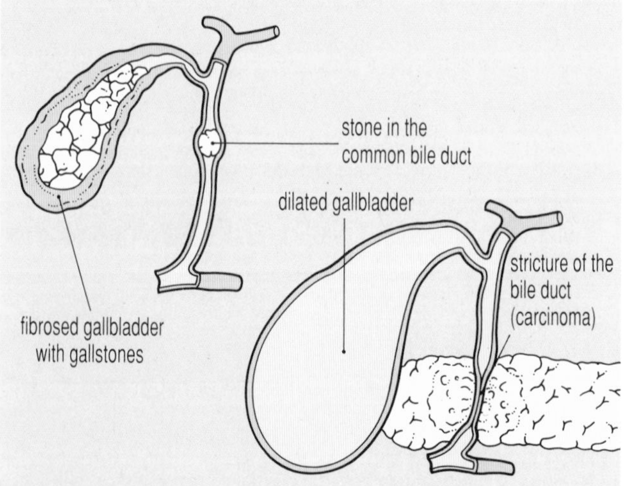

Fig. 8.56 If jaundice is caused by impaction of a gallstone in the bile duct, the fibrosed, stone-filled gallbladder does not dilate. However, if jaundice is caused by a bile duct stricture the healthy gallbladder dilates and can be palpated as a soft mass arising from behind the ninth right rib anteriorly.

In patients with chronic liver disease, localized vascular dilatation results in the appearance of vascular spiders (spider naevi). These consist of a central arteriole from which branch a series of smaller vessels, in a pattern resembling spider legs. Spider naevi are found in the territory drained by the superior vena cava, and common sites include the neck, face, and dorsa of the hands. The central arteriole can be occluded with a pencil tip, and on release of the pressure the vessels rapidly refill from the centre.

Severe hepatocellular disease associated with portasystemic shunting can result in hepatic encephalopathy. Often there are accompanying signs of portal hypertension, such as splenomegaly and ascites, but the physical sign characteristic of hepatic encephalopathy is a 'flapping tremor'. Ask the patient to stretch out both arms and hyperextend the wrists with the fingers held separated (Fig. 8.54). A coarse, involuntary flap occurs at the wrist and metacarpophalangeal joints. A further sign is sleepiness, and this may progress to coma. Encephalopathic patients often have difficulty copying a picture of a five-pointed star, and they may struggle to complete a simple 'dot-to-dot' diagram.

Palpating the gallbladder

Conclude the liver palpation by feeling for the gallbladder. Imagine the position of the fundus which lies under the point where the rectus abdominis muscle intersects the costal margin. This surface marking coincides with the tip of the right ninth rib.

Using gentle but firm pressure palpate the gallbladder area by pointing the tips of the fingers towards the organ whilst the patient inspires deeply (Fig. 8.55). When the gallbladder is inflamed (cholecystitis), the most striking physical sign is tenderness and guarding over the gallbladder region. The patient experiences intense pain, winces, and interrupts the breath as your fingers make contact with the descending organ (Murphy's sign).

The normal gallbladder is impalpable and only becomes palpable when obstructed and distended with bile. The distended organ is contiguous with the lower border of the liver and moves with respiration. In the absence of jaundice, a palpable gallbladder suggests obstruction of the cystic duct with the formation of a mucocele. Obstruction of the bile duct by a stone causes jaundice, but the gallbladder is rarely palpable because stone formation is associated with chronic cholecystitis and the thickened, fibrosed gallbladder wall does not distend. Jaundice associated with a palpable gallbladder usually implies biliary obstruction due to a carcinoma of either the head of the pancreas or the common bile duct. In this case the organ is not diseased and is able to dilate (Courvoisier's 'law') (Fig. 8.56). Remember, however, that exceptions to this rule do occur.

Palpating for the spleen

The normal spleen cannot be felt and only becomes palpable once it has doubled in size. The spleen enlarges from under the left costal margin towards the right iliac fossa in a downward and medial direction. Often only a tip of spleen can be felt as it enlarges, although in moderate and massive splenomegaly the organ can be felt well below the costal margin (Fig. 8.57).

Before palpating for the spleen, wrap the palmar surface of your left hand around the back and side of the lower rib cage to provide support. Start the examination from the region of the umbilicus. Position the fingers of the right hand obliquely across the

Distinction between left kidney and enlarged spleen

Kidney	Enlarged spleen
Moves late in inspiration	Moves early in inspiration
Possible to 'get above' upper pole	Impossible to 'get above' a spleen
Smooth shape	Notched leading edge
Resonant to percussion	Dull to precussion in Traub's space
	Enlarges towards umbilicus

Fig. 8.57 Differentiation between splenomegaly and palpation of the left kidney.

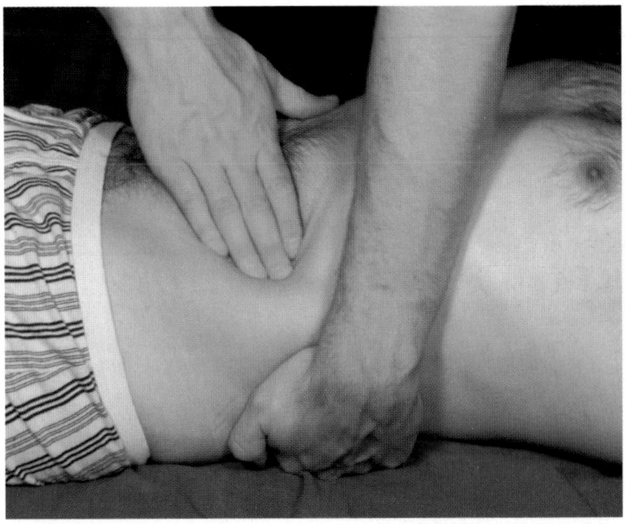

Fig. 8.58 When palpating the spleen use your left hand to support the ribcage posteriorly, whilst the fingertips of your right hand explore for the leading edge of the organ.

Percussion of spleen

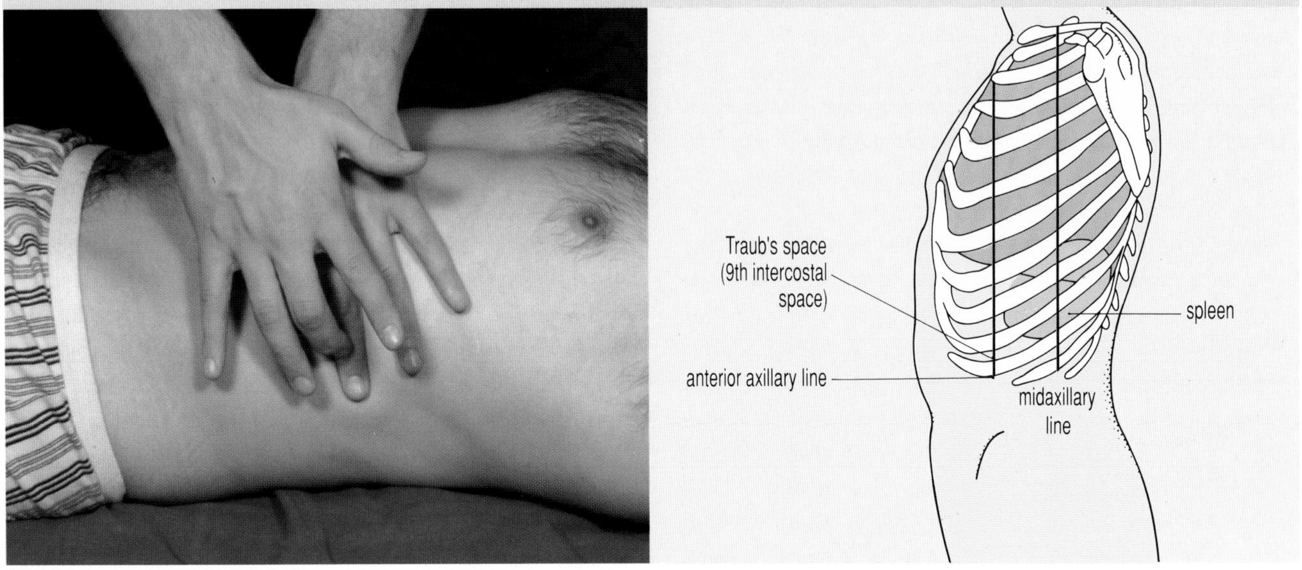

Fig. 8.59 After palpating for the spleen, percuss for the enlarged organ in the ninth intercostal space anterior to the midclavicular line.

Description of splenomegaly

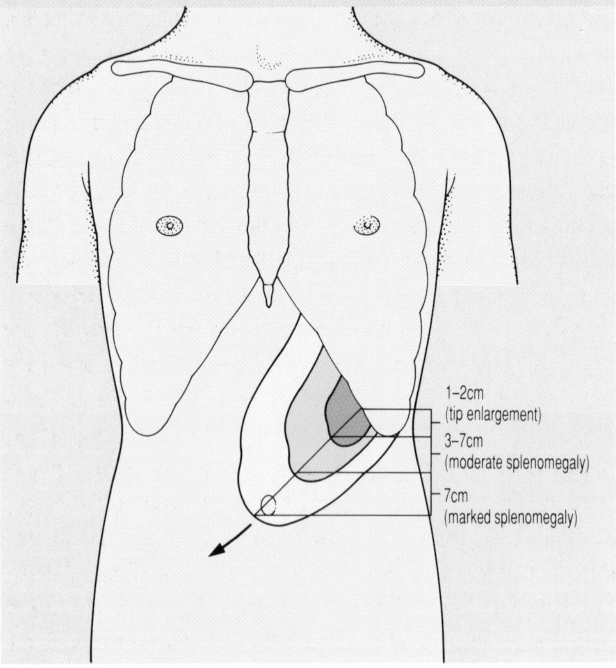

Fig. 8.60 The different degrees of splenomegaly.

Surface markings of the kidney

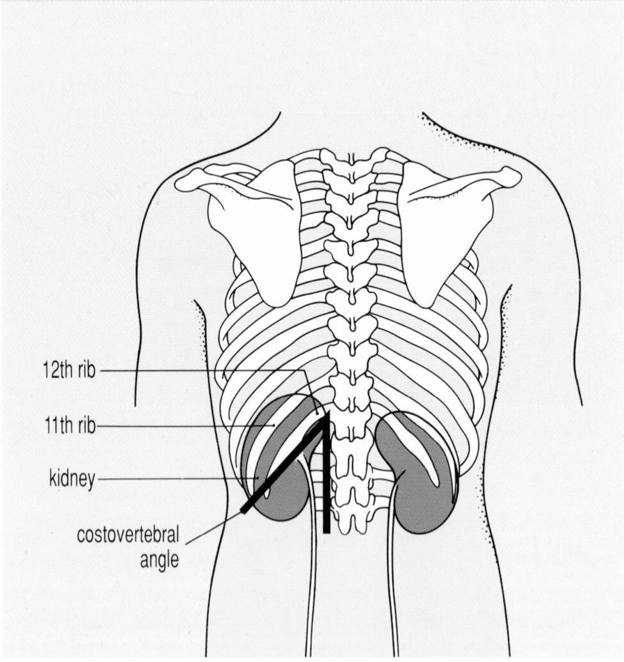

Fig. 8.61 The clinical anatomy of the kidneys.

abdomen, with the fingertips pointing at the left costal margin and towards the axilla (Fig. 8.58). The general technique is similar to that described for the liver. Using a moderate amount of pressure, press the index and middle fingers inwards and upwards and hold this steady whilst asking the patient to breathe in deeply. At the midpoint of the inspiratory effort lessen the inward pressure but maintain the upward pressure, allowing the fingers to drift in the direction of the descending spleen. The notched leading edge of an enlarged spleen can be felt passing under the fingers and glancing off at the height of inspiration.

If the spleen is impalpable at the starting point of the examination, move the fingertips progressively closer to the left lower rib cage. Make a final pass at the lower costal margin with the fingers probing just under the rib cage. Some clinicians prefer to palpate the spleen with the patient rolled into the right lateral position, with their knees drawn up to relax the abdominal muscles.

At this point in the examination it is useful to percuss for splenic dullness. The tip of a normal spleen lies posterior to the anterior axillary line and is bounded anteriorly by the gas-filled stomach and colon. Percuss the ninth intercostal space anterior to the anteri-

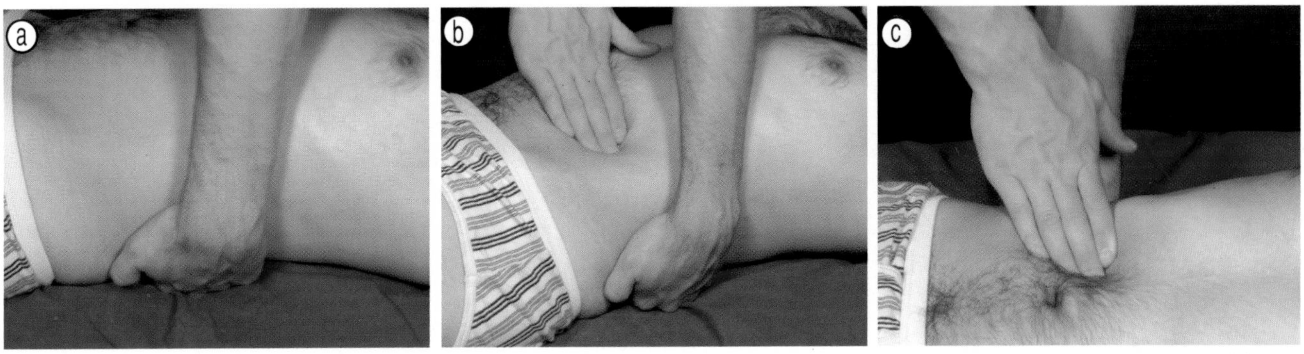

Fig. 8.62 (a) When palpating the kidney tuck the left hand behind the patient's back with your fingers positioned in the renal angle. Positioning the hands when palpating (b) the left and (c) the right kidney.

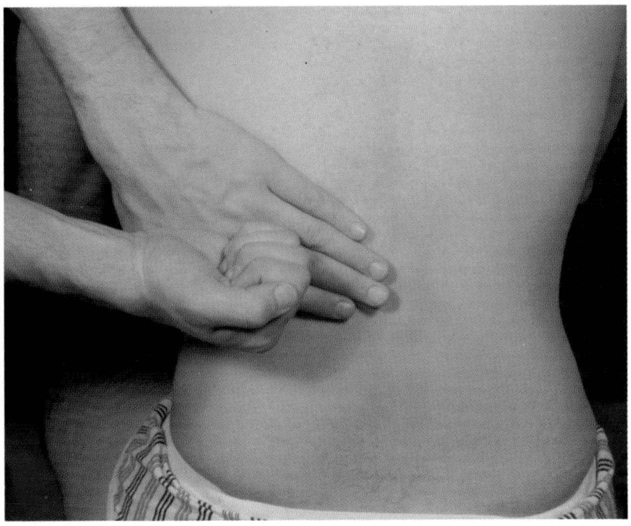

Fig. 8.63 Assessing punch tenderness over the renal angles.

or axillary line (Traub's Space)(Fig. 8.59). This space overlies bowel and is normally tympanitic, but as the solid spleen enlarges this area becomes less resonant, eventually sounding dull with more marked splenomegaly.

An enlarged spleen is readily distinguished from other organs in the region, such as the left kidney (Fig. 8.57). Note whether there is tenderness and assess the degree of enlargement, using a ruler to measure the distance from the left costal margin to the tip of the spleen (Fig. 8.60). Splenomegaly may be caused by stimulation and hypertrophy of the reticuloendothelial elements (e.g. infection), congestion with blood (e.g. portal hypertension) or by infiltration by abnormal cells (e.g. haematological malignancies).

Palpating for the kidneys

Pole to pole the kidneys extend from the vertebral level of T12 to L3, and the larger right lobe of the liver displaces the right kidney 2cm lower than the left. Viewed from the rear the kidneys lie in the renal angle formed by the twelfth rib and the lateral margin of the vertebral column (Fig. 8.61). The adrenal glands perch on the upper pole of each kidney.

The kidneys are not usually palpable through the thickness of the abdominal wall and abdominal contents, though in thin individuals a normal sized kidney may be felt. The right kidney is easier to palpate because it lies lower than the left. A normal kidney has a firm consistency and a smooth surface.

When examining the kidneys position the patient close to the edge of the bed, and examine each kidney from the patient's right, bearing in mind the surface anatomy. The kidneys are retroperitoneal organs and deep bimanual palpation is required to explore for them. When examining the left kidney, tuck the palmar surfaces of the left hand posteriorly into the left flank, and nestle the fingertips in the renal angle (Fig. 8.62a). Position the middle three fingers of the right hand below the left costal margin, lateral to the rectus muscle and at a point opposite the posterior hand (Fig. 8.62b). To examine the right kidney tuck your left hand behind the right loin and position the fingers of your right hand below the right costal margin, lateral to rectus abdominis. Palpate for the lower pole of each kidney in turn. The aim of the manoeuvre is to briefly trap the lower pole of the kidney between the fingers of both hands as the organ moves up and down with deep respiration. The spleen is closely associated with the diaphragm, and thus moves early in respiration, but the kidneys lie lower down and they only descend towards the end of inspiration. Ask the patient to inspire deeply and press the fingers of both hands firmly together, attempting to capture the lower pole as it slips through the fingertips (ballotting the kidney) (Fig 8.62c). If the kidney is palpable the rounded lower pole can be felt slipping between the opposing fingers as the patient breathes in and out.

The kidney may be tender, especially when acutely infected (pyelonephritis) or obstructed (hydronephrosis). This may be apparent on bimanual palpation, although a more specific sign is 'punch' tenderness over the renal angles. To test this response sit the patient forward and place the palm of the left hand over the renal angle. Then, using moderate force, punch the dorsal surface of the hand with the ulnar surface of the clenched right fist (Fig. 8.63). Perform this test for each kidney in turn and assess the patient's reaction.

It is important to distinguish kidney enlargement from splenomegaly on the left (see Fig. 8.59) and hepatomegaly on the right. The principal cause of bilateral enlargement is polycystic disease of the kidney, whilst unilateral enlargement suggests a malignant tumour (e.g. hypernephroma).

Palpating the aorta

The descending aorta emerges through the aortic hiatus in the diaphragm and hugs the vertebral bodies until it bifurcates into the common iliac arteries at the level of L4, which approximates to a point just below the umbilicus. It lies adjacent to the inferior vena cava and gives off a number of major tributaries which feed the major abdominal organs (Fig. 8.64). The aorta can be palpated between the thumb and fingers of one hand or by positioning the fingers of both hands on either side of the midline at a point midway between the xiphisternum and the umbilicus (Fig. 8.65). Press the fingers posteriorly and slightly medially and feel for the pulsation of the abdominal aorta against your fingertips. This pulsation can be felt in thin individuals, but it is usually impalpable in muscular or obese patients.

An abdominal aortic aneurysm may be felt as a large pulsatile mass above the level of the umbilicus. The abdominal aorta may also become abnormally prominent in the elderly when marked curvature of the spine displaces it anteriorly and laterally.

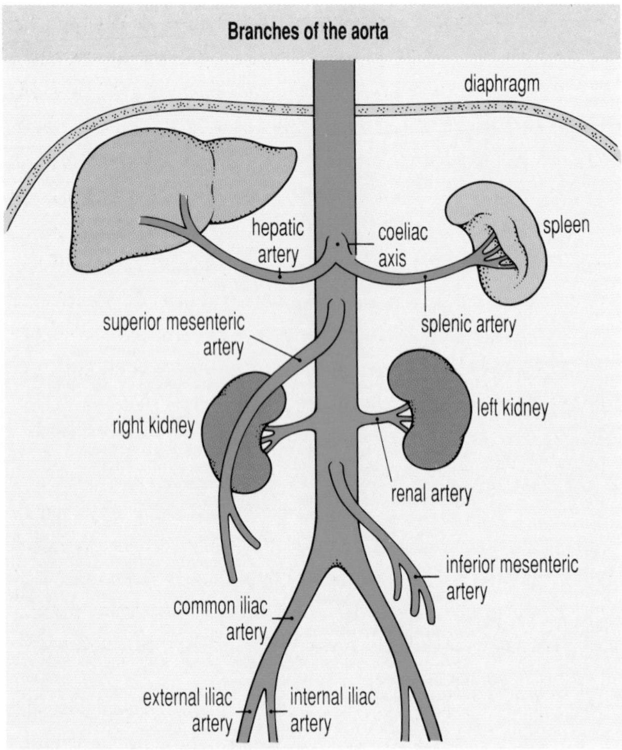

Fig. 8.64 The abdominal aorta and its branches.

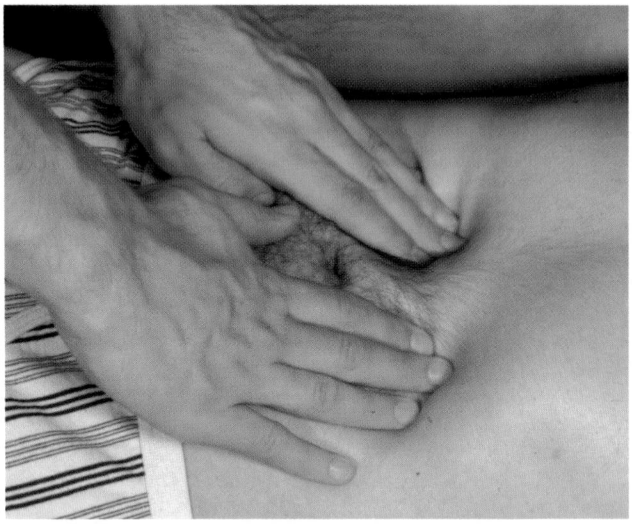

Fig. 8.65 Palpation of the aorta at a point midway between the umbilicus and the xiphisternum.

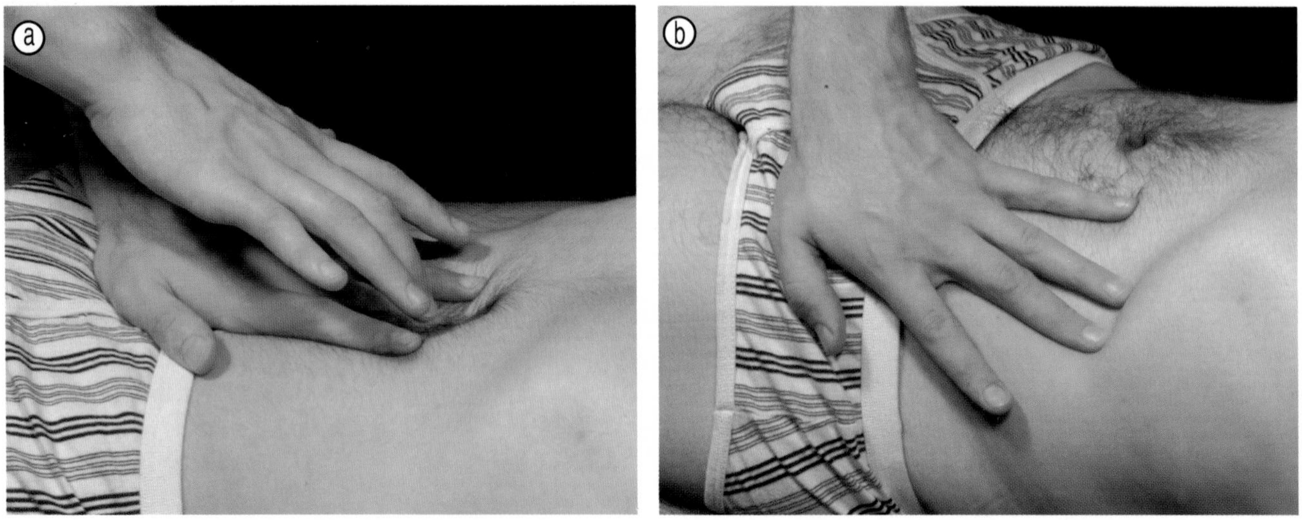

Fig. 8.66 When percussing for ascites, (a) begin in the midline with your finger parallel to the lateral wall of the abdomen (b) and continue towards the left flank. A change in the percussion note indicates a gas -fluid interface.

PERCUSSION OF THE ABDOMEN

At this stage of the examination you will have percussed the liver and spleen. General percussion of the abdomen is used to establish whether abdominal distension is caused by gas or fluid. Percussion is also used to detect an over-filled urinary bladder. The stomach, small bowel, and colon fill the entire anterior abdomen, and the percussion note of the anterior abdominal wall between the costal margins and iliac crests is normally tympanitic.

Percussion to detect ascites

Abdominal distension is usually caused either by gaseous dilatation of the bowel or abnormal accumulation of fluid. In the supine position gas accumulates more centrally, whereas fluid gravitates into the flanks. The gas-filled normal bowel tends to float above ascites, so the gas-fluid interface characteristic of ascites is detected by a change in the percussion note from the resonance overlying bowel to the dullness of fluid. The presence of ascites can be confirmed by altering the patient's posture and demonstrating a change in the position of the gas-fluid interface.

A change in percussion note (shifting dullness) is easiest to assess by percussing from an area of resonance to an area of dullness. With the patient supine, percuss in the midline at the level of the umbilicus with the fingers parallel to the lateral wall of the abdomen (Fig. 8.66a). This point overlies gas-filled bowel and the percussion note should be tympanitic. Progressively reposition your hand about 2cm to the left and repeat the percussion towards the left flank (Fig. 8.66b). The note should remain tympanitic until you reach the lateral abdominal wall. A distinct transition zone between tympany and dullness, a gas-fluid interface, should be marked lightly with a water-soluble marking pen. Now ask the patient to roll into the right lateral position. This allows the fluid to gravitate to the right flank and the gas-filled bowel to rise into the left flank (Fig. 8.67). Repeat the percussion from the midline towards the left flank. The tympany should extend well lateral to the interface marked in supine examination.

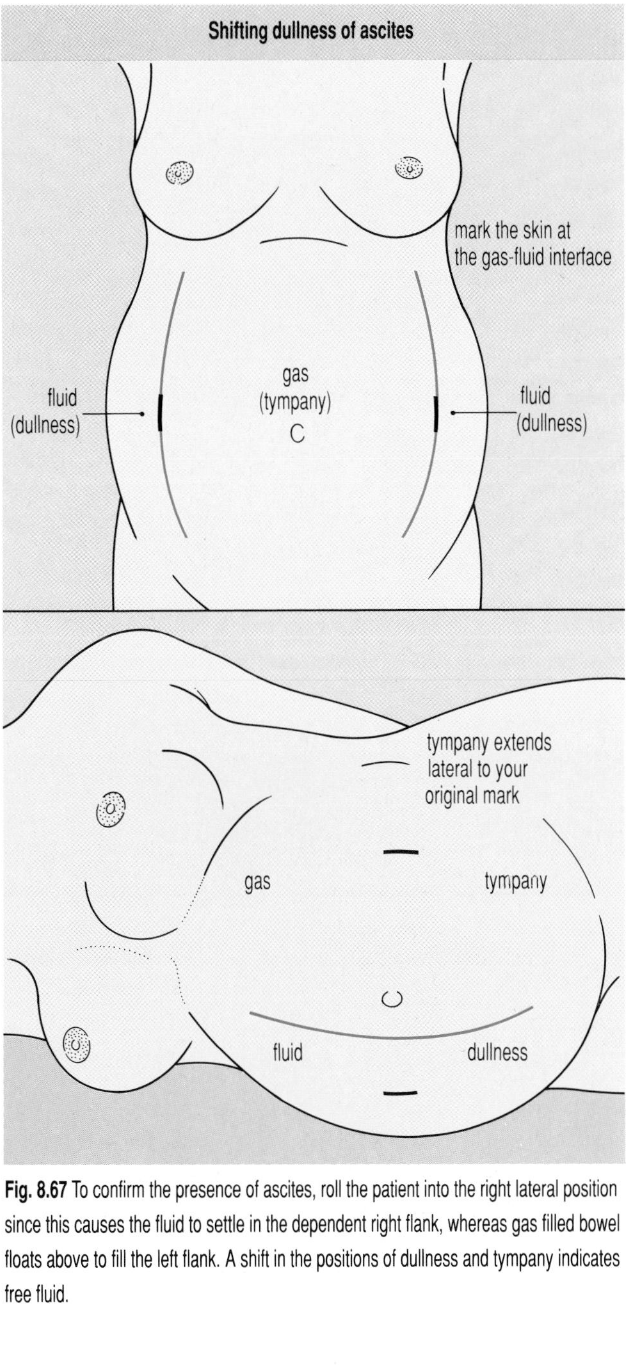

Fig. 8.67 To confirm the presence of ascites, roll the patient into the right lateral position since this causes the fluid to settle in the dependent right flank, whereas gas filled bowel floats above to fill the left flank. A shift in the positions of dullness and tympany indicates free fluid.

Percussing for a distended bladder

If the bladder outlet is obstructed and the detrusor muscle fails, the organ distends and emerges above the pubic bone from its usual position deep within the pelvis. The suprapubic area is usually tympanitic, and a dull sound upon percussion here is a useful clinical sign of bladder distention.

Use the general principle of percussing from resonance to dullness to check for bladder enlargement. Percuss from the level of the umbilicus, parallel to the pubis (Fig. 8.68), and progress down the

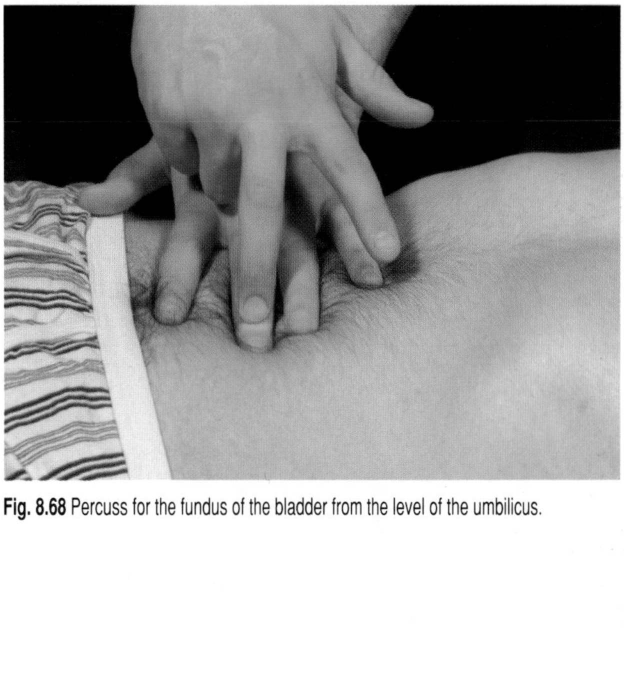

Fig. 8.68 Percuss for the fundus of the bladder from the level of the umbilicus.

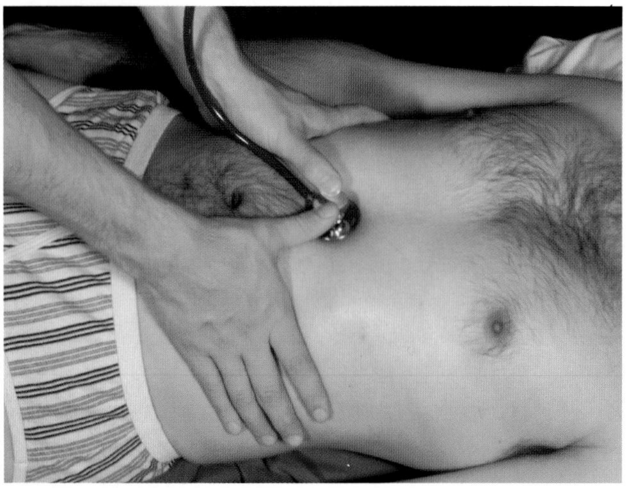

Fig. 8.69 If you suspect obstruction of the pyloric outlet check for a 'succussion splash' by simultaneously listening in the epigastrium and shaking the upper abdomen from side to side.

midline towards the pubic bone. The note should remain tympanitic to the pubic bone. A level of dullness above this landmark indicates the upper margin of a distended bladder, or possibly enlargement of the uterus. An enlarged bladder is felt as a rounded fullness, whereas an enlarged uterus is felt as a more distinct solid structure.

AUSCULTATION OF THE ABDOMEN

The sounds generated by the abdomen are gurgling noises caused by intestinal peristalsis moving gas and fluid through the bowel lumen. These are best assessed by auscultation.

Listening for bowel sounds

Place the diaphragm of the stethoscope on the mid-abdomen and listen for intermittent gurgling sounds (borborygma). These peri-

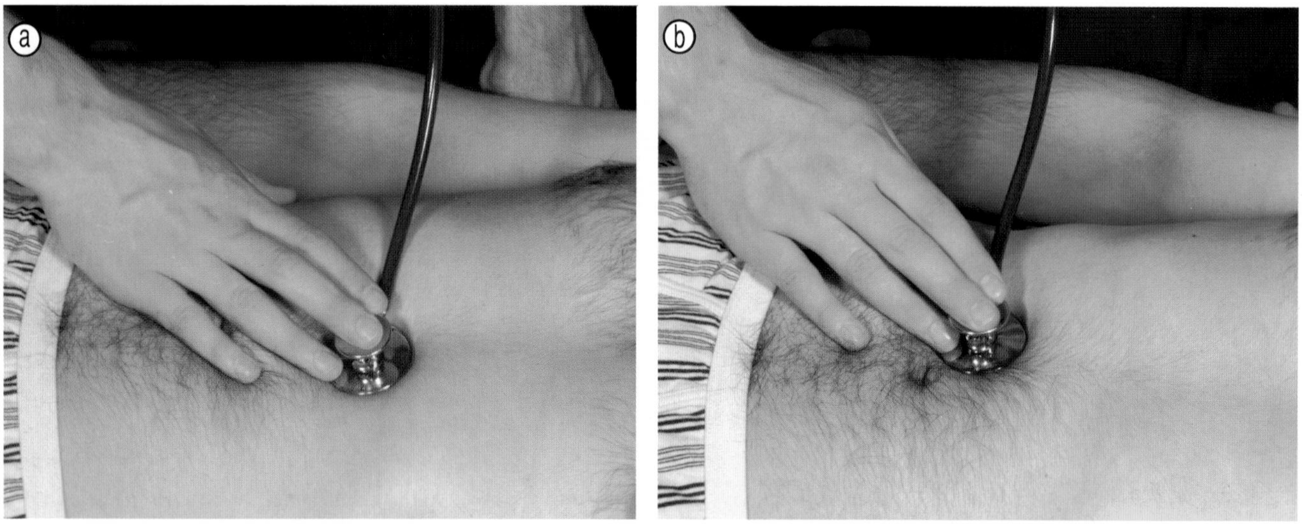

Fig. 8.70 Position of the stethoscope when listening for bruits in (a) the aorta and (b) the renal artery.

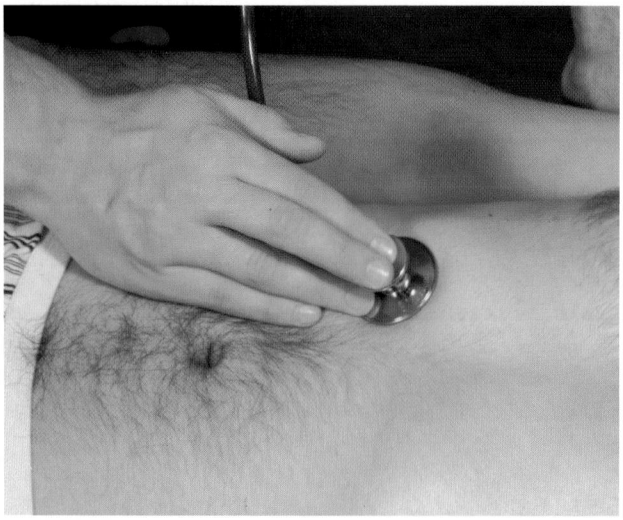

Fig. 8.71 Position of the stethoscope when listening for a liver bruit.

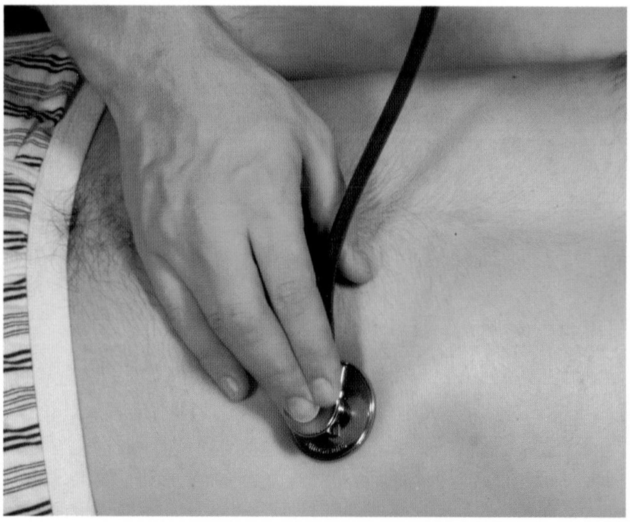

Fig. 8.72 Position of the stethoscope when listening for a splenic rub.

staltic sounds occur episodically at 5–10 second intervals, although longer silent periods may occur. Keep listening for about 30 seconds before concluding that bowel sounds are reduced or absent.

The absence of bowel sounds indicates intestinal paralysis (paralytic ileus) and is always associated with abdominal distension. Rapidly repetitive bowel sounds (often termed 'active' bowel sounds) may be normal, but they may be an early sign of mechanical obstruction if associated with colicky abdominal pain. In progressive bowel obstruction, large amounts of gas and fluid accumulate and the sounds change in quality to a higher pitched 'tinkling'. This is an ominous sign of impending bowel paralysis.

Auscultation may also be helpful when diagnosing obstruction of gastric outflow. In pyloric obstruction the stomach distends with gas and fluid; this can be detected by listening for a 'succussion splash'. Steady the diaphragm of the stethoscope on the epigastrium and shake the upper abdomen from side to side, listening simultaneously for the splashing sound characteristic of gastric outflow obstruction (Fig. 8.69).

Listening for arterial bruits

Position the diaphragm of the stethoscope over the abdominal aorta and apply moderate pressure (Fig. 8.70a). The heart sounds may be transmitted to this area, but aortic flow should be silent. A distinct systolic murmur (a bruit) indicates turbulent flow and suggests arteriosclerosis or an aneurysm.

Listen for renal arterial bruits at a point 2.5cm above and lateral to the umbilicus (Fig. 8.70b). The presence of a renal bruit suggests congenital or arteriosclerotic renal artery stenosis or narrowing due to fibromuscular hyperplasia.

Auscultation over the liver and spleen

Conclude the auscultation by listening over the liver (Fig. 8.71) and spleen (Fig. 8.72). A soft and distant bruit heard over an enlarged liver is always abnormal, suggesting either a primary liver cell carcinoma or acute alcoholic hepatitis. Secondary liver tumors do not transmit bruits. Occasionally, a creaking 'rub' may be heard over the liver or spleen. This indicates inflammation of the outer capsule of the organ and adjacent peritoneum, perhaps caused by perihepatitis or perisplenitis. More rarely, carcinomatous infiltration of the capsule and surrounding structures may be the underlying cause.

EXAMINING THE GROINS

The spermatic cord, inguinal lymph nodes, and femoral artery occupy the groin. A swelling in the groin is usually due either to an inguinal or femoral hernia, or to enlarged lymph nodes.

The inguinal canal and femoral sheath

During male foetal development the testis and spermatic cord migrate from the abdomen into the scrotum through the inguinal canal. This passage occludes after the descent of the testis, but it remains a potential route through which bowel can herniate in later life, causing an inguinal hernia.

The inguinal canal passes downward and medially from the internal to the external ring, running above and parallel to the inguinal ligament which forms its lower border (Fig. 8.73). The internal ring lies immediately above the point at which the inguinal ligament and femoral artery intersect. The femoral artery lies at the mid-femoral point, which is located midway between the anterior superior iliac spine and the symphysis pubis. The external ring lies immediately above and medial to the pubic tubercle. The femoral artery enters the femoral triangle from beneath the inguinal ligament and is enclosed in a fascial sheath. This sheath also accommodates the femoral vein, which lies medial to the artery, and the femoral canal, which is a small gap immediately adjacent and

Anatomy of the inguinal region

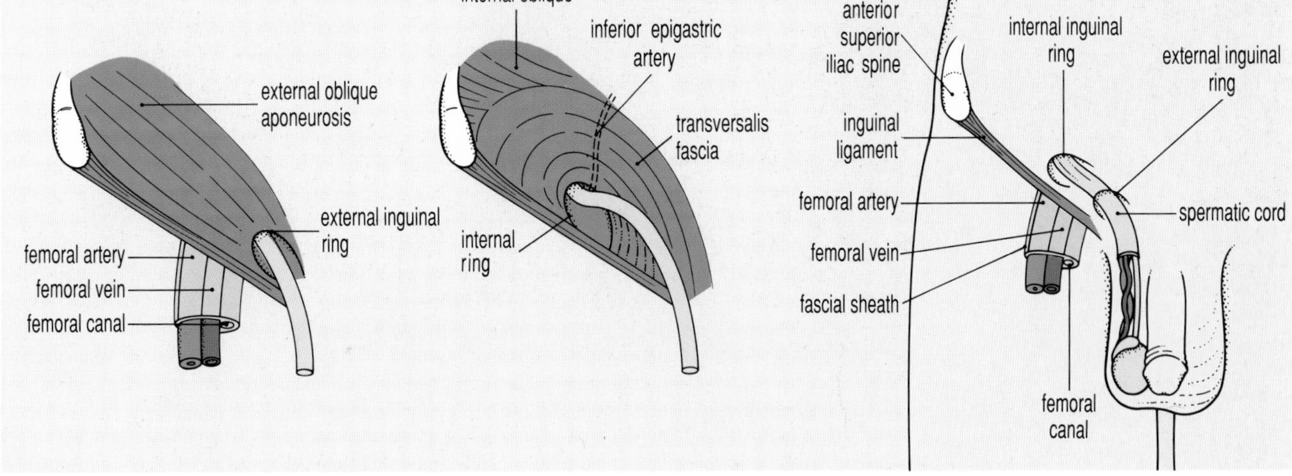

Fig. 8.73 The anatomy of the inguinal canal and femoral sheath.

medial to the vein. The femoral canal is plugged with fat and a lymph node (Cloquet's gland), and it is a potential pathway for the formation of a direct femoral hernia.

Examining herniae

An indirect inguinal hernia forms when bowel or omentum protrudes through a lax internal ring and finds its way into the inguinal canal. Bowel may force its way through the external ring and even slip into the scrotum (Fig. 8.74).

An inguinal hernia usually presents as a lump in the groin or the scrotum which is most prominent when the intra-abdominal pressure is raised (e.g. when standing or coughing). The hernia may reduce spontaneously when the patient lies down, so it is best to examine the hernia with the patient standing. Place two fingers on the mass and ascertain whether or not an impulse is transmitted to your finger tips when the patient coughs. Most herniae can be reduced manually, so attempt this by gently massaging the mass towards the internal ring. Once the hernia is fully reduced occlude the internal ring with a finger pressing over the femoral point. Ask the patient to cough. An indirect inguinal hernia should not reappear until you release the occlusion of the internal ring.

A direct inguinal hernia develops through a weakness in the posterior wall of the inguinal canal. These herniae seldom force their way into the scrotum, and, once reduced, their reappearance is not controlled by pressure over the internal ring.

When an inguinal hernia extends as far as the external ring it may be confused with a femoral hernia. The distinction is made by establishing the relationship of the hernia to the pubic tubercle: an inguinal hernia lies above and medial to the tubercle, whilst a femoral hernia lies below and lateral.

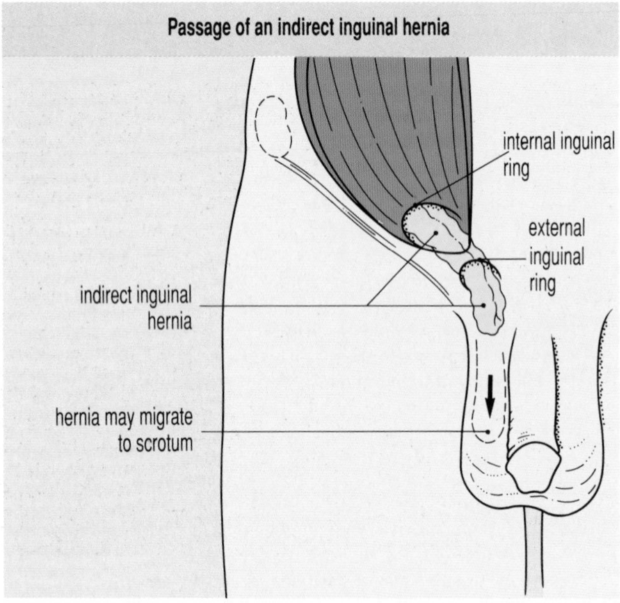

Fig. 8.74 An indirect hernia enters through the internal ring and exits through the external ring

EXAMINING THE ANUS, RECTUM, AND PROSTATE

The rectum and anus

The rectum is a curved segment of bowel, around 12cm long, lying in the concavity of the mid and lower sacrum (Fig. 8.75). The upper two-thirds of the anterior rectum, but not the posterior surface, is covered by peritoneum. The anterior rectal peritoneum reflects onto the bladder base in men, it forms the rectouterine pouch (known as the pouch of Douglas) in women, and is filled with loops of bowel. Anterior to the lower third of the rectum lie the prostate, bladder base and seminal vesicles in men and the vagina in women. The anus is 3–4cm long and joins the rectum to the per-

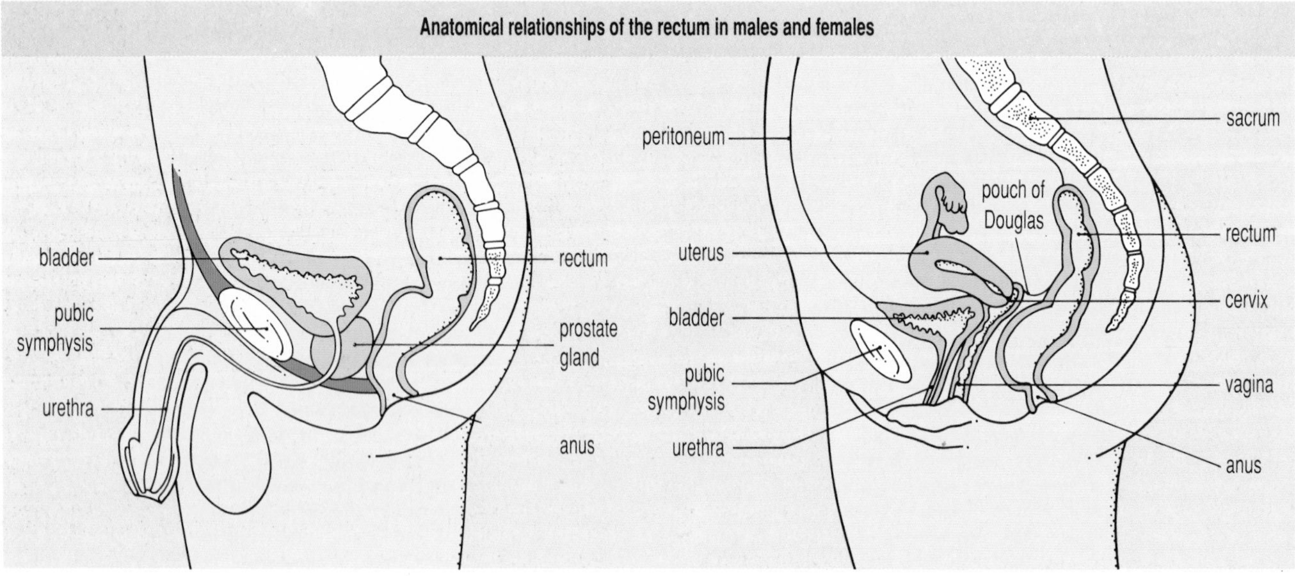

Fig. 8.75 The relationship of the anterior rectum to the prostate gland and bladder base in men (left) and the posterior vaginal wall and uterine cervix in women (right).

ineum. The anal wall is supported by powerful sphincter muscles, the voluntary external and involuntary internal sphincters, which constrict to provide tone and continence (Fig. 8.76). The rectal mucosa can be directly visualized through a proctoscope or sigmoidoscope, but a great deal may be learned by palpation of the anus, rectum, and prostate.

Rectal examination should not be unduly painful, and it is important to explain this to the patient, along with your reasons for performing it. The examination will promote a feeling of rectal fullness, and it may stimulate a desire to evacuate. Tell the patient to expect this, and always work with an assistant. Always glove both hands.

Position the patient in the left lateral position with the hips and knees well flexed and the buttock positioned at the edge of the bed (Fig. 8.77). The positions around the anal opening are described by the positions of the clock face (Fig. 8.78). Gently separate the buttocks to expose the natal cleft and anal verge (Fig. 8.79). Inspection of the natal cleft and anal verge may reveal skin tags, pilonidal sinuses, warts, fissures, fistulas, external haemorrhoids, or prolapsed rectal mucosa (Fig. 8.80). A bluish discolouration of the perianal skin suggests Crohn's disease. The anal skin is innervated with pain fibres, and anal pain and tenderness are suggestive of infection (e.g. perianal abscess), fissure and fistula in ano, or thrombosis of an external haemorrhoid.

Lubricate your index finger with a clear, water-soluble gel (e.g. K-Y jelly), and press the finger tip against the anal verge with the pulp facing the 6 o'clock position (see Fig. 8.79). Slip your finger into the anal canal and then insert it into the rectum, directing the

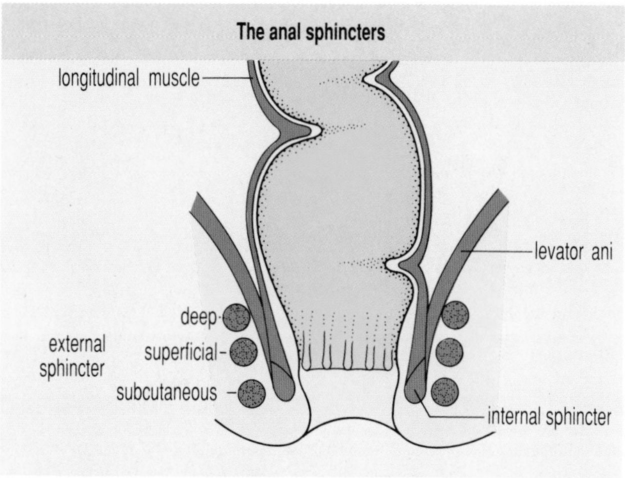

Fig. 8.76 The internal and external anal sphincters.

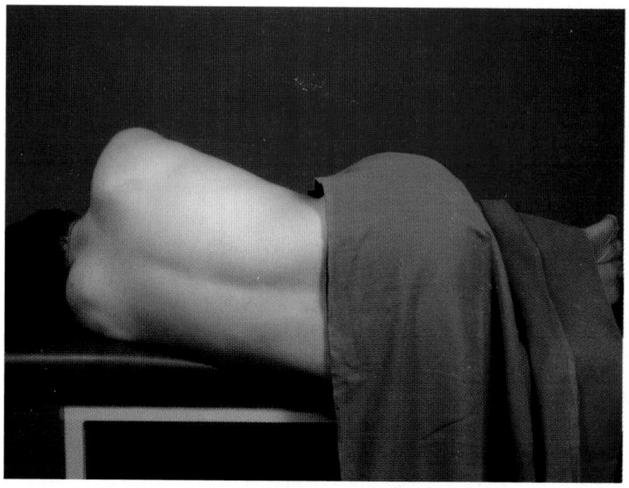

Fig. 8.77 The correct position of the patient prior to a rectal examination.

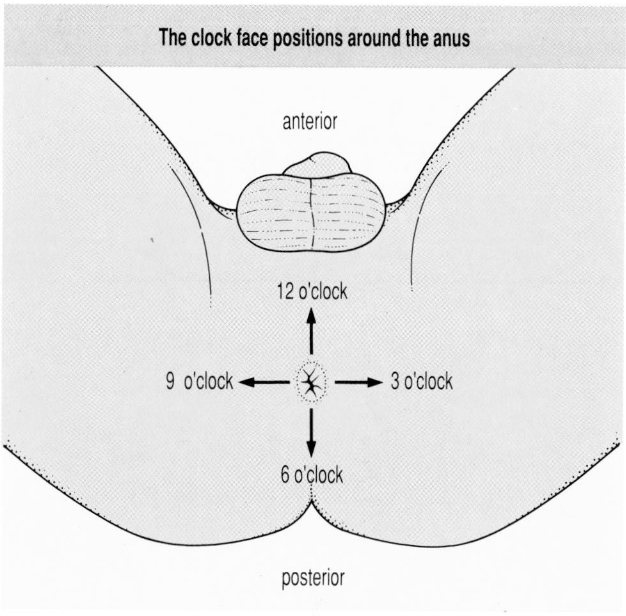

Fig. 8.78 The positions of the clock face are used to describe positions around the anus.

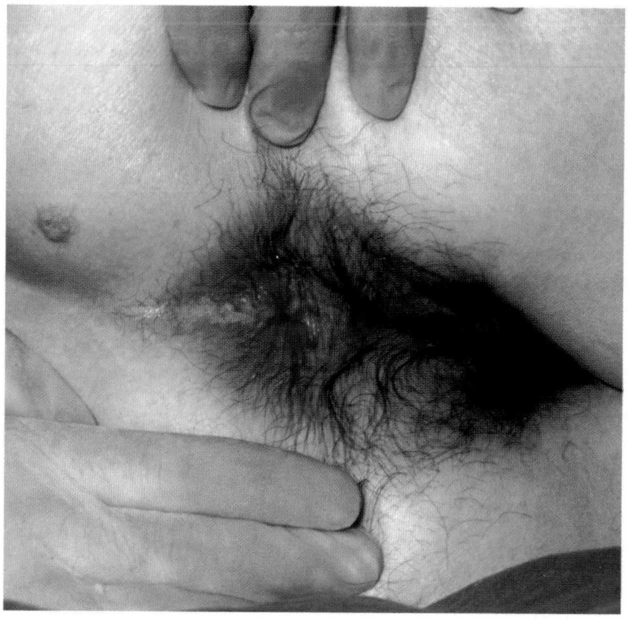

Fig. 8.79 Exposing the anus.

tip posteriorly to follow the sacral curve (Fig. 8.81). With your finger fully introduced, check on anal tone by asking the patient to squeeze your finger with the anal muscles. Then gently sweep the finger through 180° using the palmar surface of the finger to explore the posterior and postero-lateral walls of the rectum. Rotate the finger round to the 12 o'clock position. This is accomplished more easily by adopting a half-crouched position and simultaneously pronating your wrist. This position allows you to sweep the finger across the anterior and anterolateral walls of the rectum. The normal rectum feels uniformly smooth and pliable. In men, the prostate can be felt anteriorly, and in women it may be possible to feel the cervix as well as a retroverted uterus.

Upon rectal palpation you may feel an intrinsic tumor caused by a carcinoma or polyp. Perirectal sepsis causes marked rectal wall tenderness, and an abscess may be felt pointing into the lumen. The anterior rectal peritoneal reflection straddles both the anterior rectum itself and the structures lying in front of it. Consequently, malignant or inflammatory lesions of the peritoneum may be felt through the anterior wall of the rectum.

Withdraw your finger from the rectum and anus and check the glove tip for stool. There may be melena, blood, or pus and you may notice the pale, greasy stools characteristic of malabsorption.

The prostate

The prostate gland is examined during the rectal examination. The normal prostate measures about 3.5cm from side to side and protrudes lcm into the rectum (Fig. 8.82a). The gland has a rubbery, smooth consistency, and a shallow longitudinal groove separates the right and left lobes. It should not be tender to palpation, but the patient may experience the urge to urinate.

Palpation of the prostate aims to assess size, consistency, nodularity, and tenderness. The assessment of prostatic size is learnt through experience. Benign hypertrophy of the prostate is common in patients over 60 years old. The enlargement is smooth and symmetrical and the gland feels rubbery or slightly boggy (Fig. 8.82b). A cancerous prostate may feel asymmetric, with a stony hard consistency, and discrete nodules may be palpable (Fig. 8.82c). Marked prostatic tenderness suggests acute prostatitis, a prostatic abscess or inflammation of the seminal vesicles. If prostatic infection is suspected attempt to massage the organ from within the rectum in order to squeeze prostatic fluid towards the urethral meatus, where it can be collected for microscopy and culture.

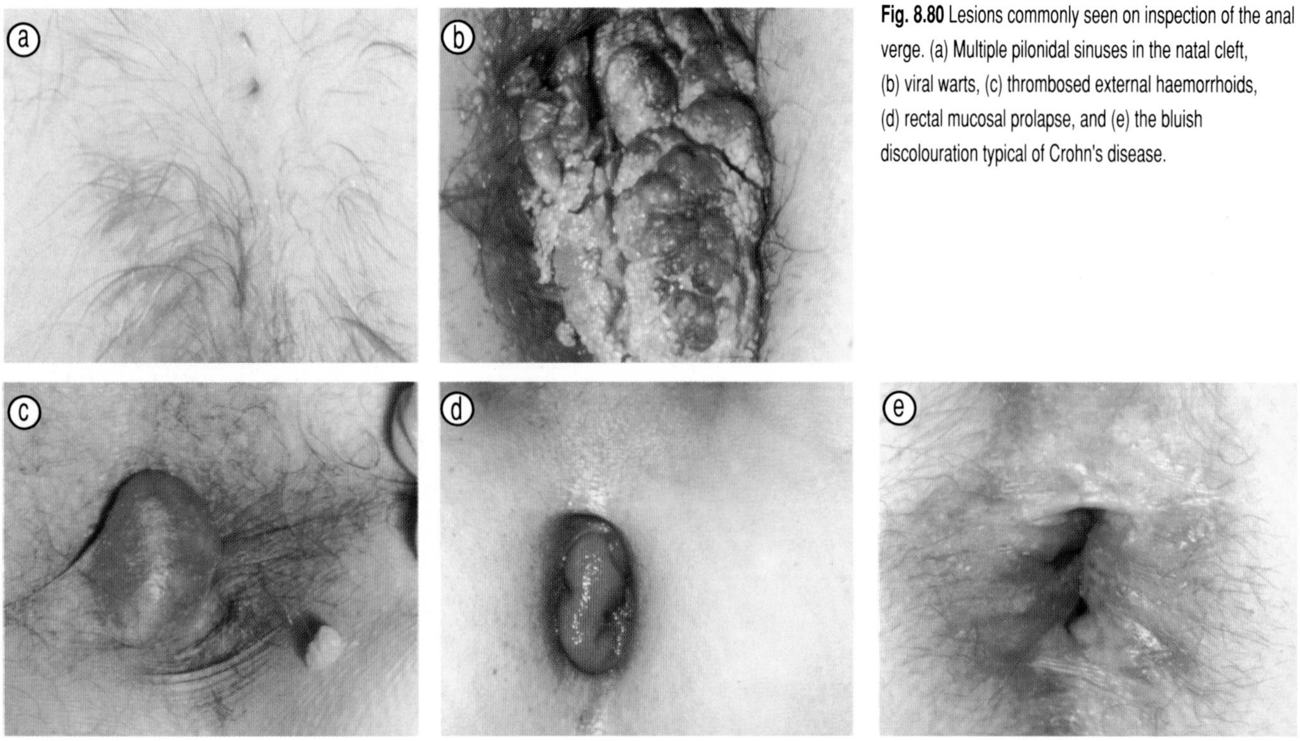

Fig. 8.80 Lesions commonly seen on inspection of the anal verge. (a) Multiple pilonidal sinuses in the natal cleft, (b) viral warts, (c) thrombosed external haemorrhoids, (d) rectal mucosal prolapse, and (e) the bluish discolouration typical of Crohn's disease.

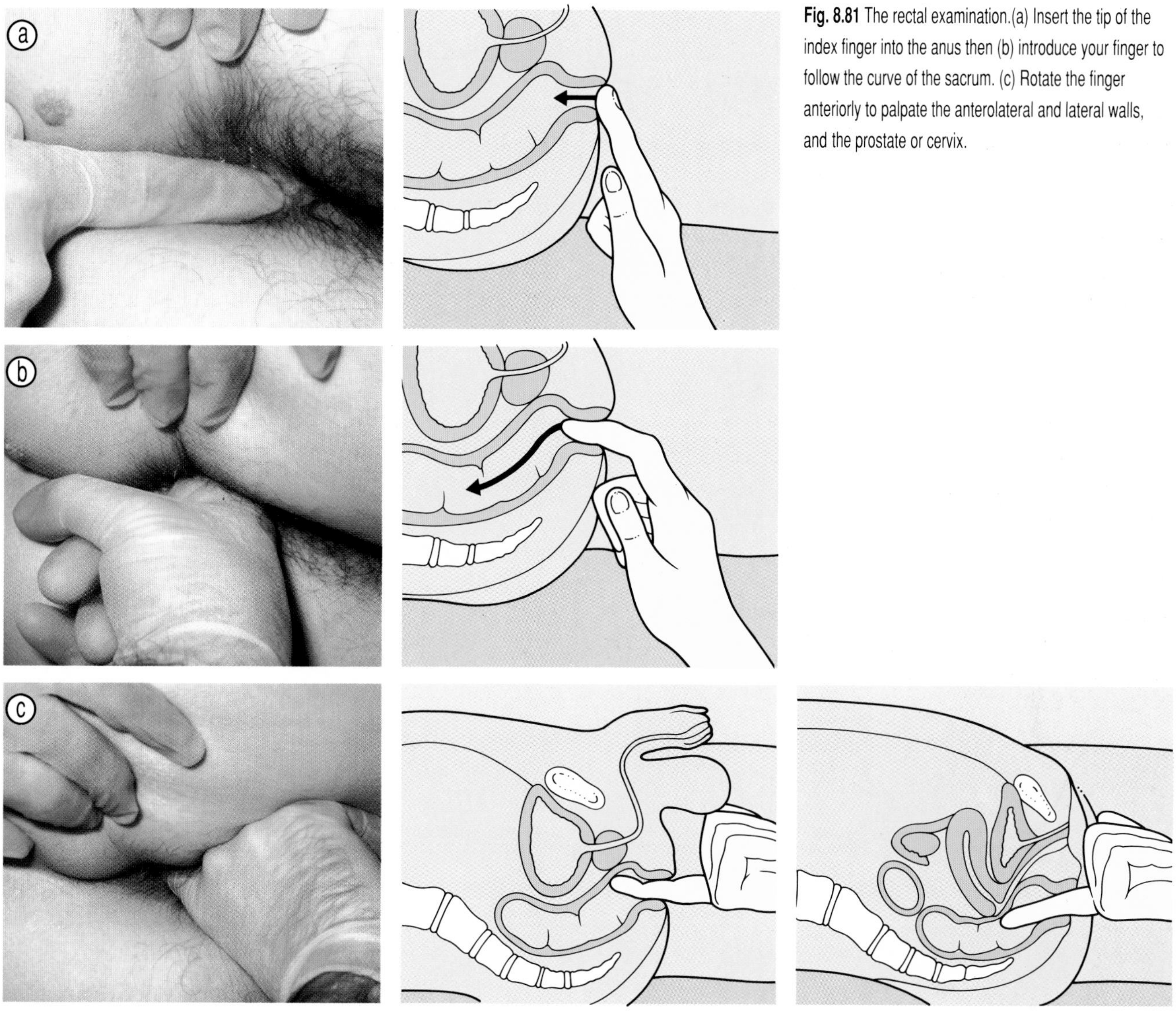

Fig. 8.81 The rectal examination.(a) Insert the tip of the index finger into the anus then (b) introduce your finger to follow the curve of the sacrum. (c) Rotate the finger anteriorly to palpate the anterolateral and lateral walls, and the prostate or cervix.

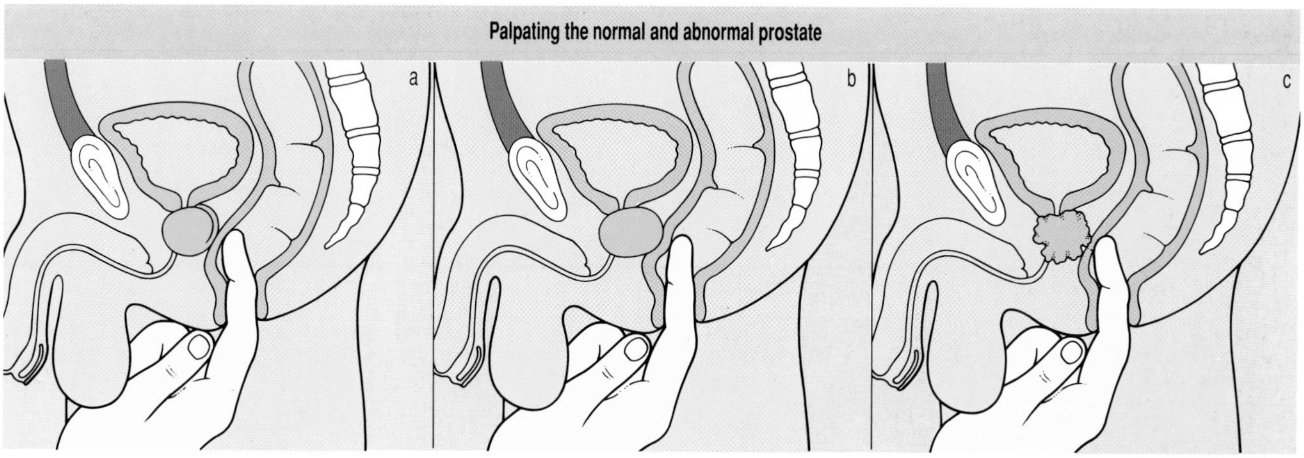

Fig. 8.82 (a) The normal prostate felt through the anterior rectal wall has a median sulcus separating the two lateral lobes. (b)The median sulcus may become indistinct in a benign hypertrophied prostate, and the gland feels firm and smooth and bulges more than 1cm into the lumen. (c) A carcinomatous prostate feels hard and irregular and the median sulcus is obliterated.

FEMALE BREASTS AND GENITALIA

9

The clinical assessment of the reproductive system is often neglected in routine examinations because of the patient's discomfort and embarrassment, and due to the doctor's reluctance to conduct the genital examination as a routine procedure. The case history and examination intrude into the patient's most intimate boundaries, so careful scripting is necessary to reassure the patient. The sensitivity associated with the examination is further heightened when dealing with patients of the opposite sex. A chaperone should always be close at hand when the opposite sex is examined.

It is reassuring to remember that most patients feel reasonably comfortable discussing sexual problems with their doctor; this stems from a cultural acceptance that doctors deal with all aspects of bodily function and an understanding that the doctor-patient relationship is confidential and professional. It is important to establish trust and competence when assessing the genital tract. Undergraduate courses in gynaecology, obstetrics, and genitourinary medicine provide the opportunity to learn the examination techniques required for a thorough examination.

STRUCTURE AND FUNCTION

With the onset of puberty, the child begins the rapid physical evolution from childhood through adolescence to adulthood. This is a grey zone between paediatric and adult medicine and it is important to appreciate the variability of growth during this period. Understanding the physiological events of puberty, the menstrual cycle, normal sexual function and anatomy, and the menopause should help you to deal confidently with the sexual history and examination of the genitalia.

PUBERTY

The transition from childhood to adolescence is regulated by hormones secreted by the hypothalamic-pituitary axis. During puberty there is a rapid spurt in growth, accounting for about 25 per cent of the final adult height. Secondary sexual characteristics develop and sexual awareness is aroused.

The age of puberty varies and parents and teenagers often worry about what they perceive as a delayed growth spurt. A number of factors determine the onset of puberty. Over the past 150 years there has been a progressive fall in the age of the first menstrual period (menarche). This is thought to reflect the effects of improving nutrition and general health on the onset of puberty. There is evidence that body weight is an important trigger for puberty: moderately overweight girls tend to enter puberty earlier than their lean contemporaries. Abnormal weight loss (such as occurs with anorexia nervosa or a debilitating illness) causes delay of the menarche or cessation of established periods altogether (amenorrhoea).

Adolescent development can be assessed using pubertal milestones defined by Tanner (Fig. 9.1). In girls this is based on breast development and the growth of pubic hair. Puberty in girls begins

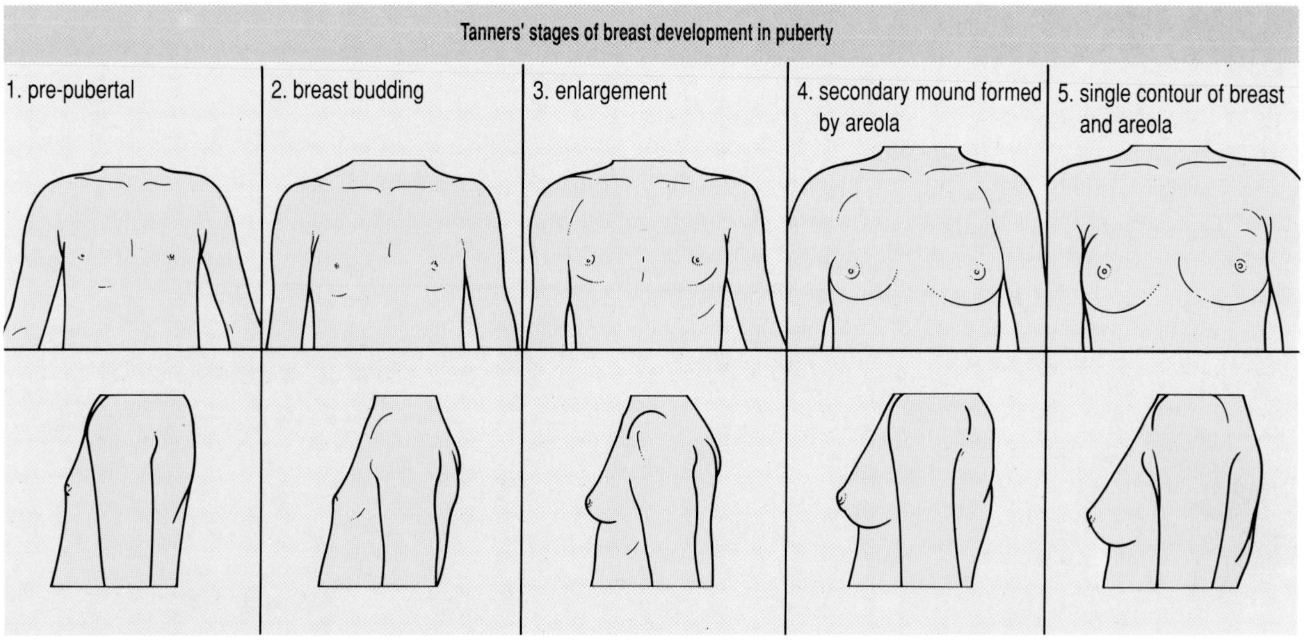

Fig. 9.1 Stages of breast development. Development from the preadolescent stage (1) begins initially with a widening of the areola and the development of subareolar tissue (2). Progressive expansion occurs (3–4) until adult size is attained (5).

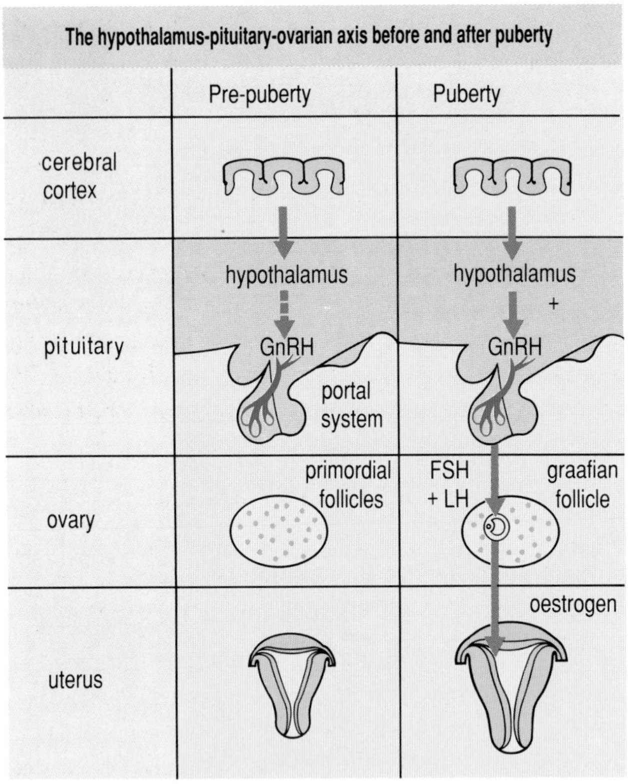

Fig. 9.2 The hypothalmo-pituitary-gonadal axis. In childhood gonadotrophin-releasing hormone (GnRH) secretion is inhibited (left). Loss of GnRH inhibition induces puberty and provides the signal for the release of follicle stimulating hormone (FSH) and luteinizing hormone (LH). FSH and LH stimulate the gonads and exert cyclical changes in the uterine endometrium (right).

between 8 and 13 years of age. The average age of the menarche is 12.5 years and most girls will have menstruated by the age of 14.5 years.

Hormonal changes in puberty

Puberty is established by the activation of the neuro-endocrine axis. The cerebral cortex plays a central role in the initial activation of the hypothalamus which stores gonadotrophin-releasing hormone (GnRH). This hormone is released into the hypothalamo-hypophyseal portal system and carried to the anterior lobe of the pituitary gland where it stimulates the release of sex hormones. During childhood, GnRH secretion is inhibited and loss of this inhibition signals the onset of puberty (Fig. 9.2). Pulsatile release of GnRH provides the signal for the pulsatile release of follicle stimulating hormone (FSH) and luteinizing hormone (LH) from the pituitary gland which, in turn, stimulates the gonads. The hormonal products of the female gonads then exert their specific influences on the reproductive organs and induce the development of secondary sexual characteristics. Breast growth (telarche) in women is followed by the menarche and the establishment of the menstrual cycle.

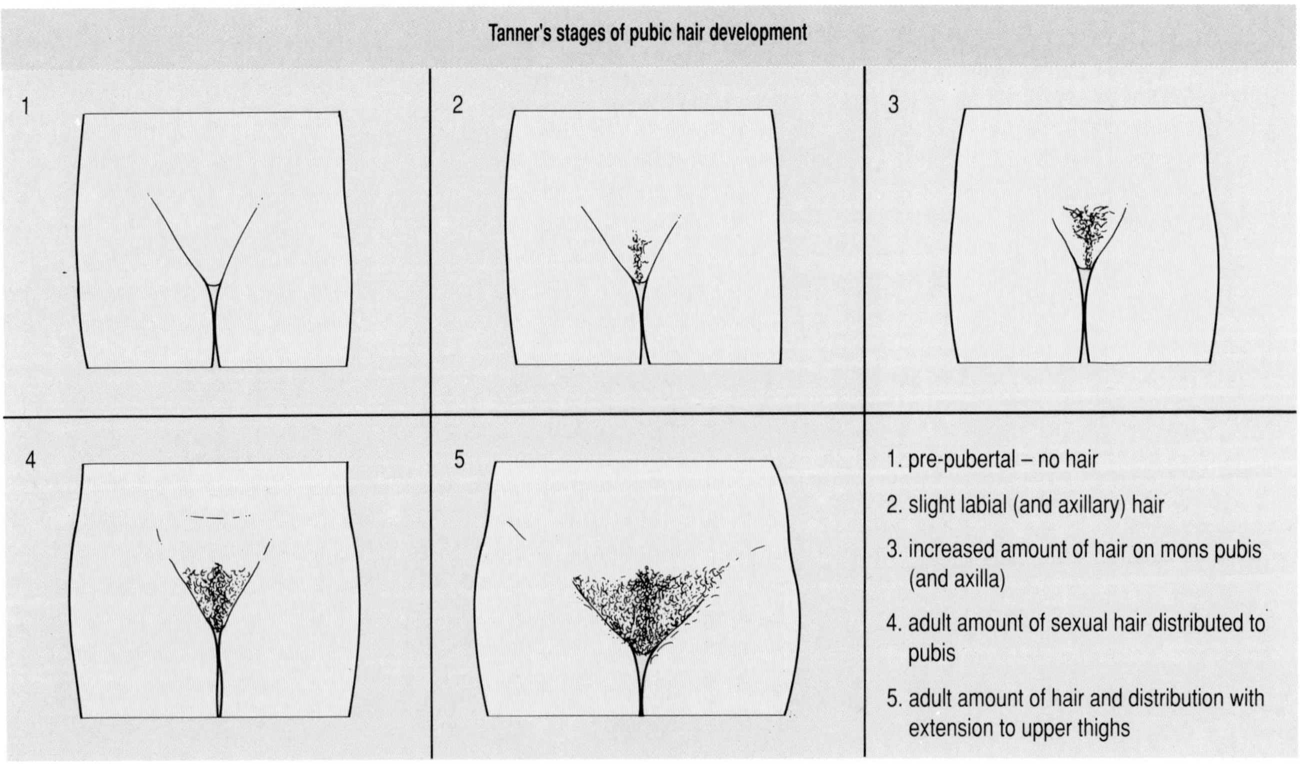

Fig. 9.3 Pubic hair development. Development from the preadolescent (1) begins with the growth of sparse straight hair along the medial borders of the labia (2). Further growth of darker coarser curlier hair continues (3–4) until the typical inverted triangular distribution of the adult female is seen (5).

Breast development

Oestrogen secretion from the developing ovaries is the prime stimulus for breast development. Initially, there is widening of the areola with a small mound of breast tissue developing beneath it. This is followed by progressive enlargement of the breasts until the full adult size is attained (see Fig. 9.1).

Pubic hair growth

In both males and females, growth of the pubic hair is regulated by adrenal androgens, with an additional contribution of testicular androgen in the male. In females the pattern of pubic hair growth has a characteristic inverted triangular appearance (Fig. 9.3).

The ovarian and menstrual cycle

The cyclical release of FSH and LH from the pituitary are reflected in serum concentration changes. Ovulation occurs in response to these changes, and this in turn, regulates cyclical changes in the uterine endometrium (Fig. 9.4). In each cycle, a few 'selected' dormant ovarian follicles become responsive to FSH, with usually only a single dominant follicle maturing to the point of ovulation (Fig. 9.5). The primordial follicle consists of a large oocyte surrounded

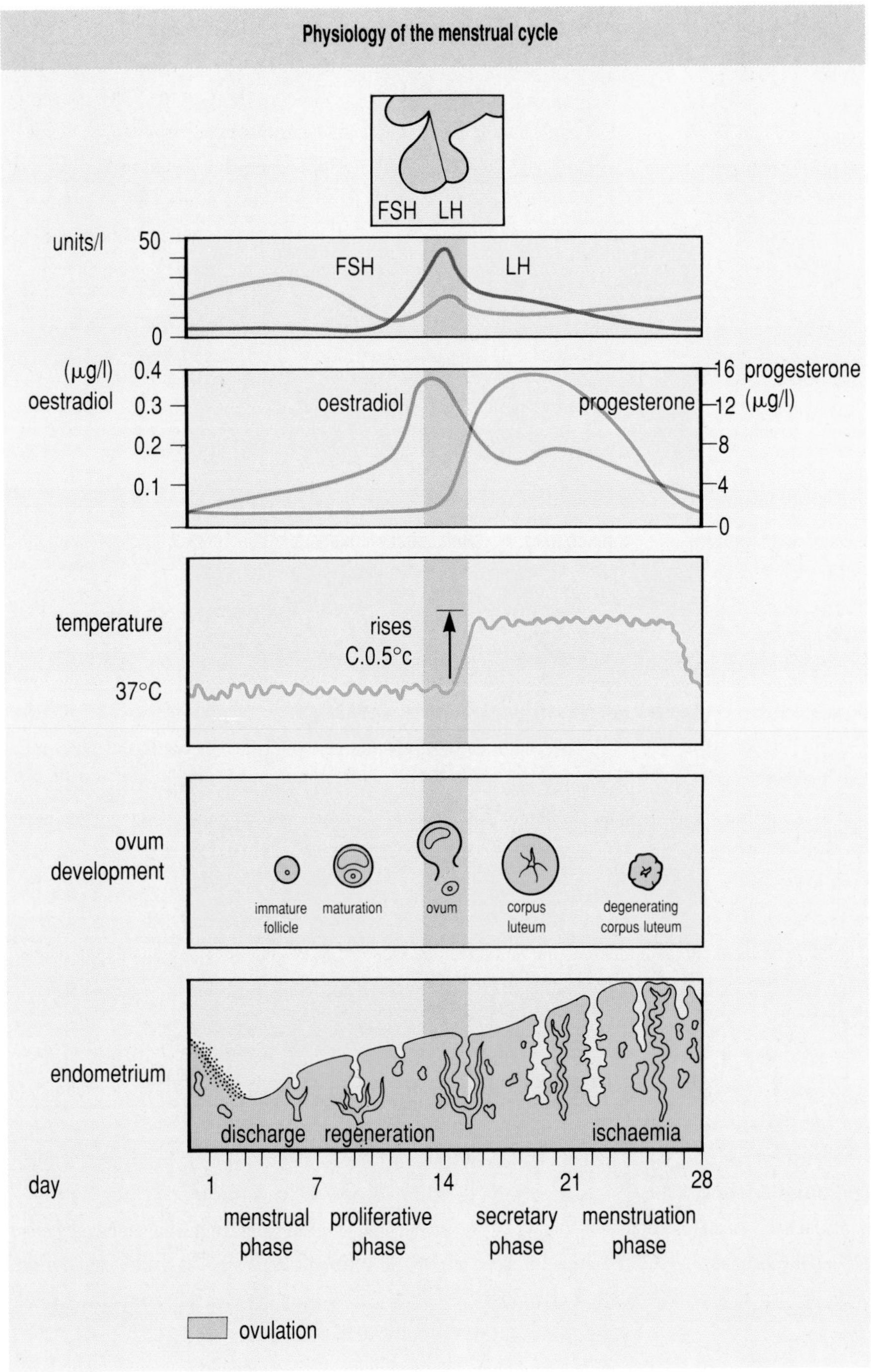

Fig. 9.4 Physiological changes associated with the menstrual cycle.

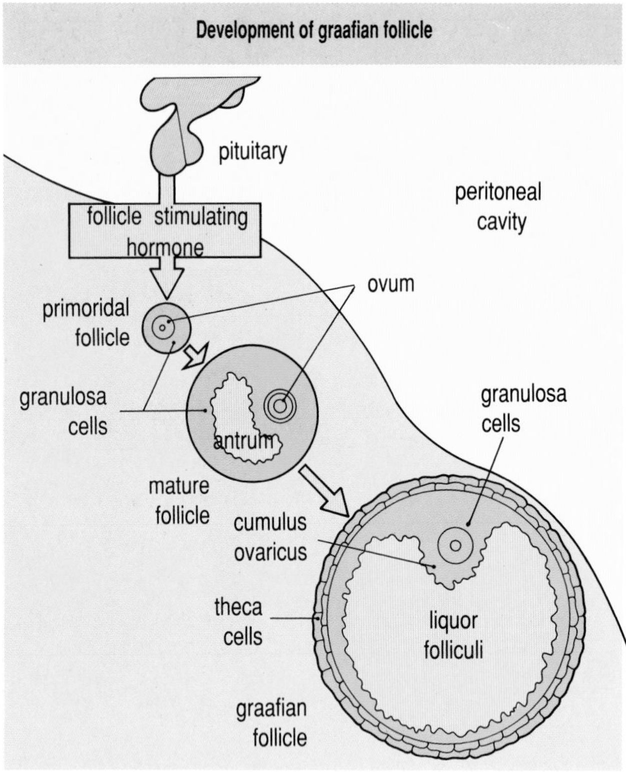

Fig. 9.5 Development of mature ovarian follicle.

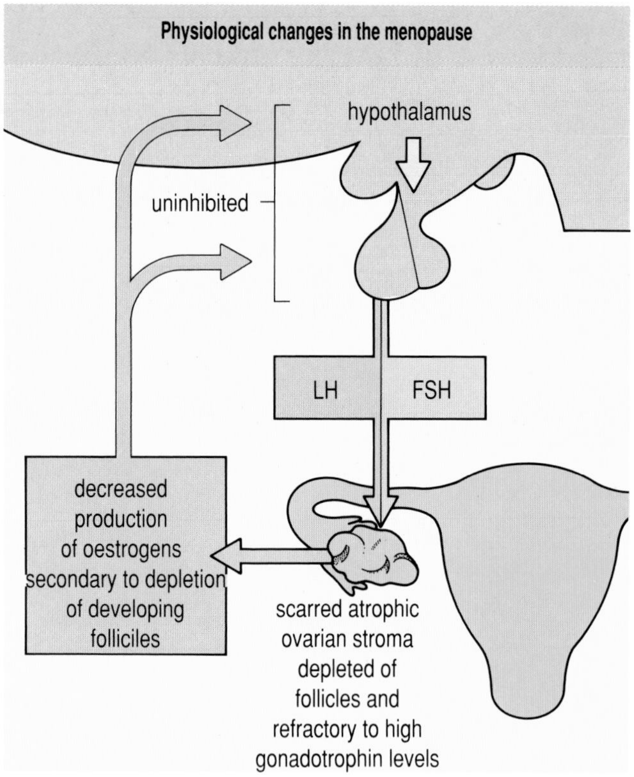

Fig. 9.6 Loss of hormonal feedback in the menopause. The hypothalmus tries to compensate for the falling oestrogen level by increasing production of FSH and LH.

by a flattened follicular epithelium. In the few responsive follicles, FSH stimulates the proliferation of granulosa cells which secrete an oestradiol-rich fluid that accumulates in the follicle (the antrum). As the follicle grows, it is surrounded by a specialized layer of thecal cells which are derived from the ovarian stroma. The responsive follicle grows to attain a pre-ovulatory size of 2–3cm. In mid-cycle there is a surge of both FSH and LH (see Fig. 9.4); the LH surge is thought to trigger the events leading to the extrusion of the ovum from the ovary.

Extrusion of the ovum leaves behind the corpus luteum (see Fig. 9.4), which secretes progesterone, the dominant sex hormone in the second phase of the ovulatory cycle. The granulosa cells of the corpus luteum express LH receptors which are also capable of binding human chorionic gonadotrophin (HCG), a hormone secreted by the foetal syncytiotrophoblast. In the absence of fertilization, HCG does not appear in the circulation, and by about the 23rd day of the cycle, the corpus luteum starts to atrophy. Progesterone levels fall, allowing the re-expression of FSH secretion and the initiation of another cycle. If conception has not occurred, menstruation commences. This is caused by an intense vasospasm in the arterioles feeding the superficial layers of the endometrium which causes hypoxic necrosis of this tissue. The tissue is then expelled through the vagina.

The climacteric and menopause

By about the age of 40, the number of functional oöcytes has fallen to the point where sex hormone synthesis is reduced. This signals the onset of the climacteric, which over a period of years culminates in the cessation of menstruation (the menopause). Initially, FSH levels increase in an attempt to stimulate follicular ripening; later, anovulatory cycles develop with irregular menstrual bleeding; finally, at about the age of 50 years, menstruation ceases. Loss of hormonal feedback results in high serum levels of FSH and LH (Fig. 9.6). Serum levels of these hormones are used as a test for the climacteric and menopause. The decline in oestrogen production results in atrophy of the breasts, genital organs, and bone. Vasomotor instability may result in hot flushes.

BREAST STRUCTURE AND FUNCTION

The breasts overly the pectoralis major and serratus anterior muscles, and extend from the second to sixth ribs (Fig. 9.7). It is convenient to divide the breast into 4 quadrants by horizontal and vertical lines intersecting at the nipple (Fig. 9.8). A lateral extension of breast tissue (the axillary tail of Spence) extends from the upper outer quadrant towards the axilla.

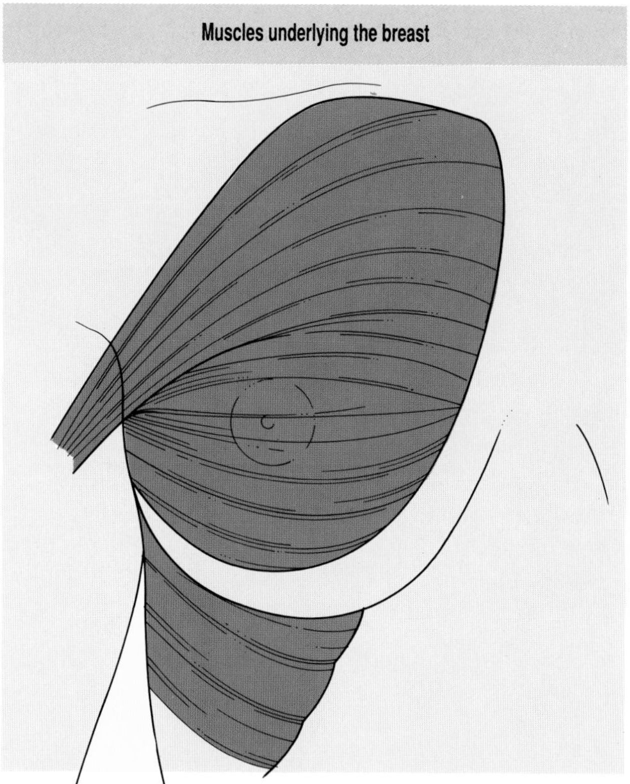

Fig. 9.7 The breast overlies pectoralis major and serratus anterior muscles.

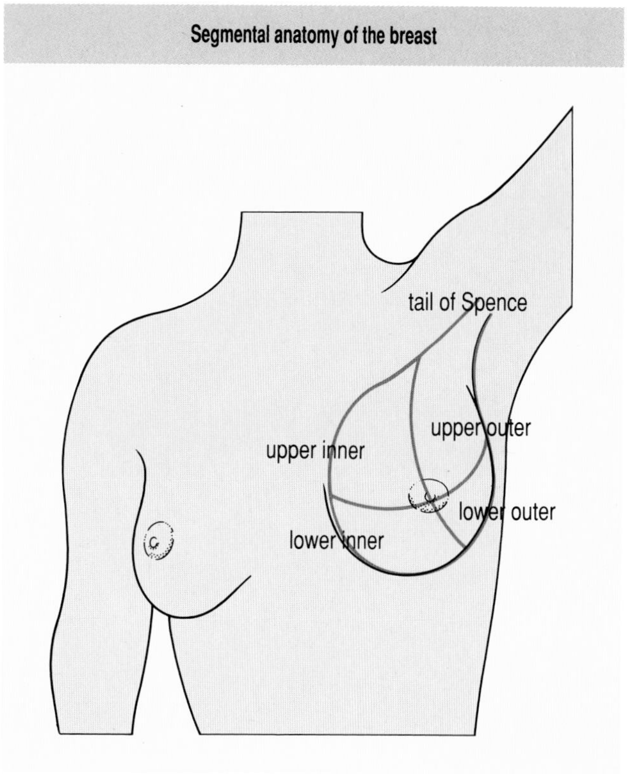

Fig. 9.8 For descriptive purposes, the breast is divide into 4 quadrants and a tail (of Spence).

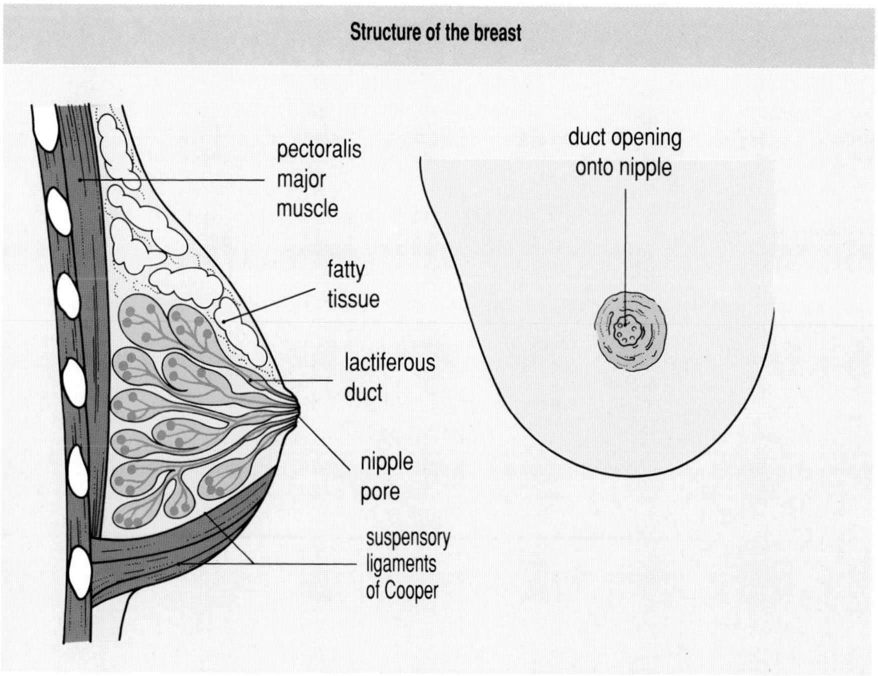

Fig. 9.9 The breast is formed by glands with their ducts opening individually through the nipple. Fatty tissue shapes the breast and the fibrous ligaments (of Cooper) provide support.

Each breast is formed by 15–20 glandular lobules embedded in a supporting bed of fatty and fibrous tissue which gives shape to the organ (Fig. 9.9). Fibrous septa known as Cooper's (suspensory) ligaments separate the lobules and provide support by attaching between the subcutaneous tissue and the fascia of the muscles. Each glandular lobule drains into the nipple through a lactiferous duct. This duct is surrounded by myoepithelial cells which can contract to eject milk into the nipple. The nipple is infiltrated with smooth muscle which contract in response to sensory and tactile stimuli, causing the nipple to become erect. Surrounding the nipple is the pigmented areola. Sebaceous glands (the glands of Montgomery) provide local secretion. Extra nipples with breast

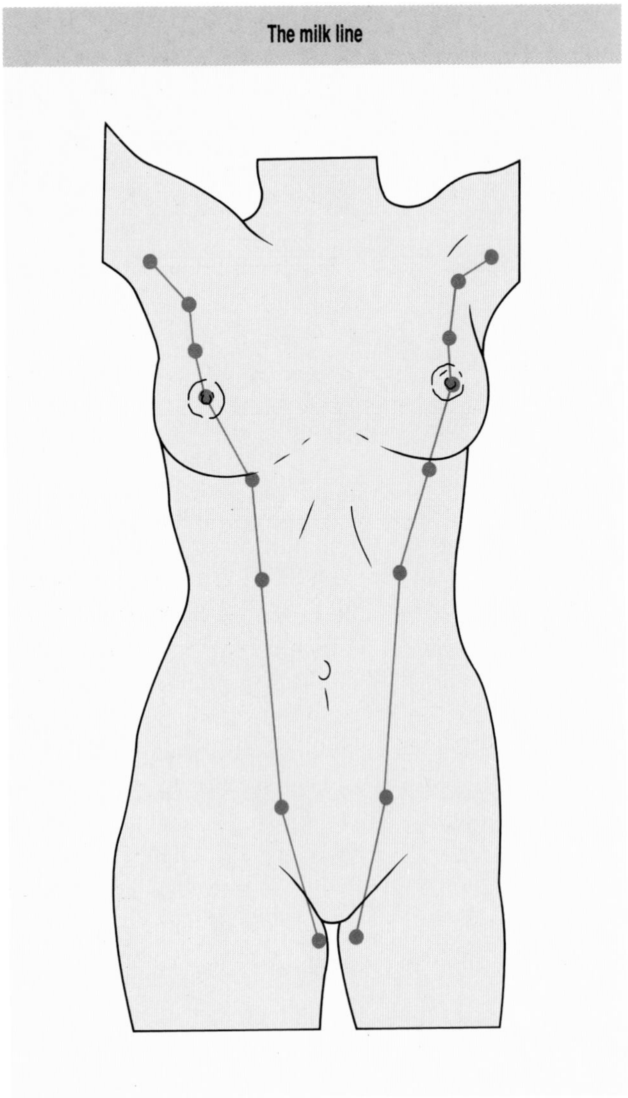

Fig. 9.10 Supernumerary nipples and breast tissue may appear along the milk line.

breast tissue may occur along a primordial 'milk line' which extends from the axilla to the groin (Fig. 9.10).

Lymphatic drainage of the breast

Because breast cancer spreads to regional lymph nodes, it is important to appreciate lymphatic drainage the discovery of affected nodes implies a more serious prognosis and influences the mode of treatment. In general, the lymphatics follow the blood supply, there is yet a free connection between the lymphatics of the one breast, and sometimes with the other. Nonetheless, the lateral part of the breast usually drains towards the axillary group of nodes and the medial half towards the internal mammary chain. The axillary nodes are arranged into 5 groups, each of which must be examined (Fig. 9.11). The vast interconnection of lymphatics predisposes to widespread metastatic proliferation, with nodes in the opposite axilla becoming affected. Even the abdominal nodes may be involved.

Function of the breast

During puberty, glandular growth is primarily under the trophic influence of oestrodiol and progesterone. Throughout pregnancy, the breasts enlarge further under the influences of rising concentrations of oestrogens, progesterone, placental lactogen, and prolactin secreted by the anterior pituitary. A darkish ring (secondary areola) appears around the areola during pregnancy. Suckling by the newborn child stimulates a neuro-endocrine reflex which causes further release of prolactin as well as oxytocin (from the posterior pituitary). Oxytocin (which also has a uterine-contracting action) stimulates contraction of the myoepithelial cells surrounding the lobules and lactiferous ducts causing the expression of milk (Fig. 9.12).

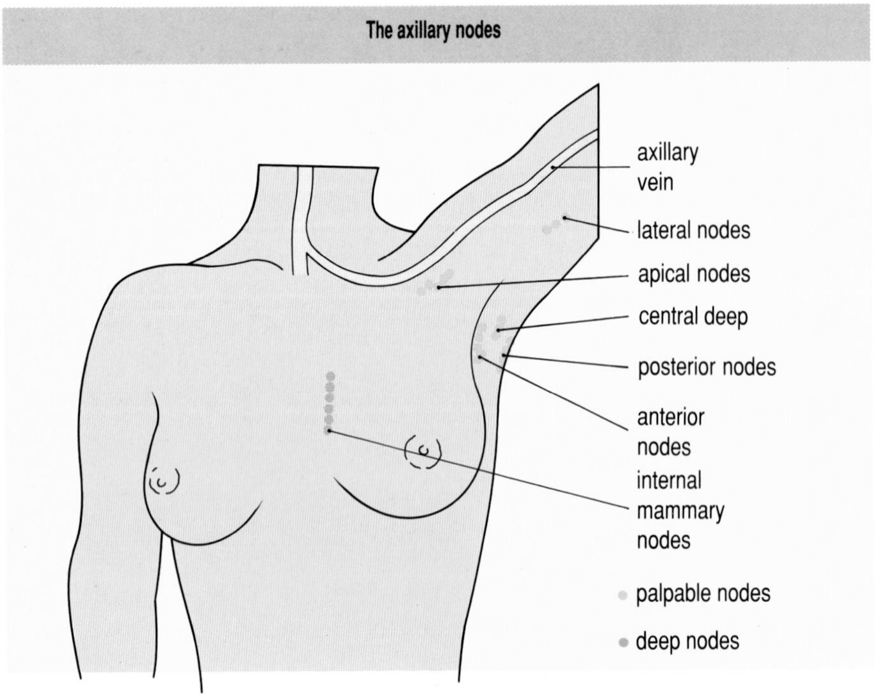

Fig. 9.11 Diagramatic representation illustrating the position of the axillary lymph nodes.

The effect of sucking on the nipple sustains lactation. Feeding mothers produce about one litre of milk daily. When the child is weaned, the sucking reflex is lost and lactation dries up.

SYMPTOMS OF BREAST DISEASE

Pain

Throughout the menstrual cycle there are cyclical, trophic, and involutional changes in the glandular tissue. This dynamic response of the tissue to changes in hormones may cause breast pain and tenderness which fluctuates predictably with the menstrual cycle, usually more towards the end of a cycle. A painful breast in the first few months of lactation is almost always due to a bacterial infection of the gland and is characterized by fever as well as redness and tenderness over the infected segment. Ask about local trauma, as fat necrosis may cause pain, and consider thrombophlebitis of the veins (Mondor's disease).

Discharge

Patients may present with an abnormal nipple discharge. Determine whether the fluid is clear, opalescent, or blood-stained.

The sucking reflex in lactation

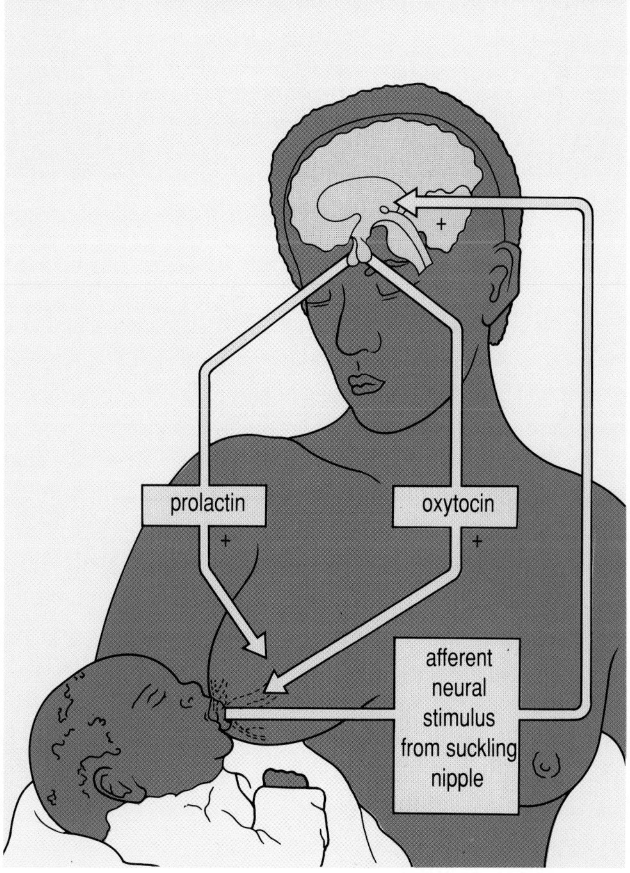

Fig. 9.12 Sucking sends an afferent stimulus to the anterior and posterior pituitary, resulting in the release of prolactin and oxygtocin.

In men, and women who have never conceived, a discharge is always abnormal; however, after childbearing, some women continue to discharge a small secretion well after lactation has stopped. The inappropriate secretion of milk (galactorrhoea) is due to a deranged prolactin physiology. A blood discharge should always alert you to the likelihood of an underlying breast cancer.

Breast lumps

A patient may present after discovering a breast lump on self-examination. This discovery causes great alarm as your patient will usually associate the lump with breast cancer.

EXAMINATION OF THE BREAST

You will usually examine the breast in the course of the chest examination. In asymptomatic women, you will need to decide whether to include a full breast examination as part of your routine examination. Male doctors must always examine in the presence of a female nurse or chaperone. The aim of examination is to check for breast lumps, and it is reasonable to recommend a formal breast examination in asymptomatic women over the age of forty. Before examining the patient, suggest to her that the general examination of the chest offers a good opportunity to check the breasts for lumps. Remember to inform her of your findings (reassurance is the best of all medicines). Many techniques have been described, yet the principles remain similar.

Inspection

The patient should undress to the waist. Position yourself in front of the patient who should be sitting comfortably with her arms at her side (Fig. 9.13). Note the size, symmetry, and contour of the breasts, and the colour and venous pattern of the skin. Observe the nipples and note whether they are symmetrically everted, flat, or inverted. If there is unilateral flattening or nipple inversion, ask

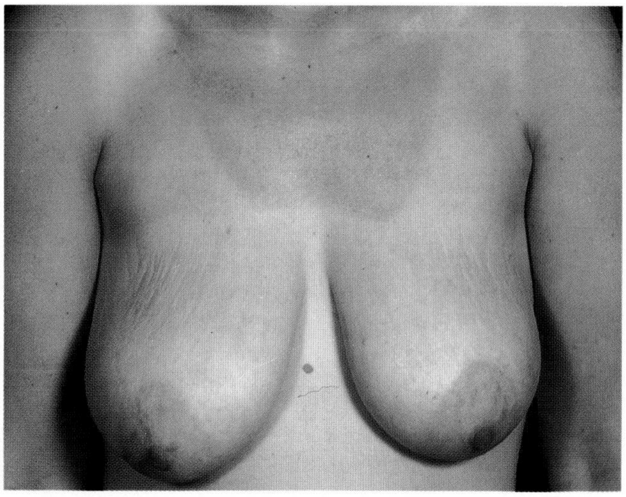

Fig. 9.13 Initially, inspect the breast from the front with the patient sitting with her arms comfortably resting at her sides.

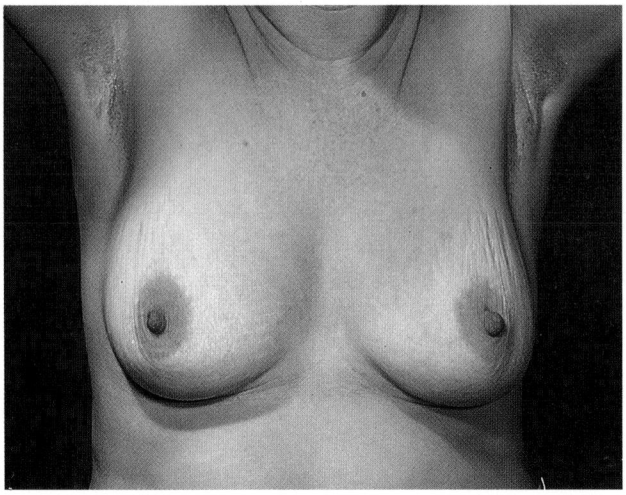

Fig. 9.14 To accentuate any asymmetry of the breast ask the patient to raise her arms above the head.

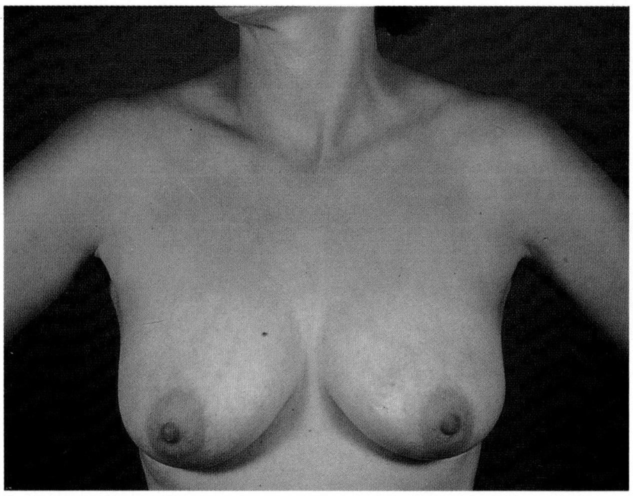

Fig. 9.15 Another technique for accentuating the breast contours is by pressing the hands against the hips.

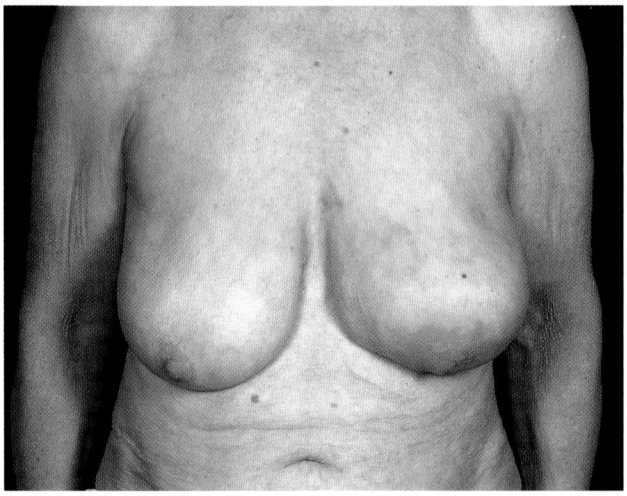

Fig. 9.16 Asymmetry of the breast.

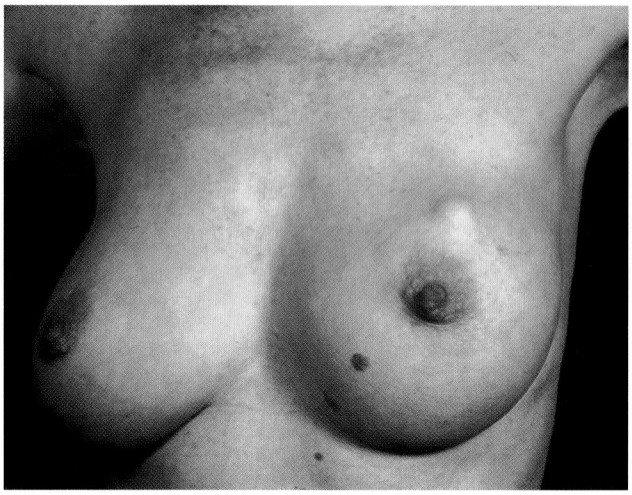

Fig. 9.17 An obvious breast lump.

whether this is a recent or longstanding appearance. In fair-skinned women, the areola has a pink colour but darkens and becomes permanently pigmented during the first pregnancy. Ask the patient to raise her arms above her head and then press her hands against the hips (Figs 9.14 and 9.15). These movements tighten the suspensory ligaments exaggerating the contours and highlighting any abnormality. In men the nipple should lie flat on the pectoralis muscle.

Abnormalities on inspection

In normal women there may be some asymmetry of the breast and nipples, ranging from unilateral hypoplasia to a mild but obvious asymmetry (Figs. 9.16). You may be struck by an obvious lump (Fig. 9.17), retraction or gross deviation of a nipple (Fig. 9.18), prominent veins, or oedema of the skin with dimpling like an orange skin (*peau d'orange*). Abnormal reddening, thickening, or ulceration of the areola should alert you to the possibility of Paget's disease of the breast, a specialized form of breast cancer (Fig. 9.19). Male gynaecomastia is an important physical sign and may be spotted on inspection as a swelling of the areola , or in more florid cases, the development of obvious breasts (see Chapter 10).

Breast palpation

During the chest examination the patient will be lying on the examination couch with her arms resting comfortably at her side or held above her head. Palpate the breast tissue with the palmar surface of the middle three fingers, using an even rotary movement to compress the breast tissue gently towards the chest wall (Fig. 9.20). Examine each breast by following a concentric or parallel trail which effects a systematic path that always begins and ends at a constant spot (Fig. 9.21). An obsessive and systematic exploration of all the breast tissue ensures that small lumps which could be easily missed are not. If the breasts are abnormally large or pedulous,

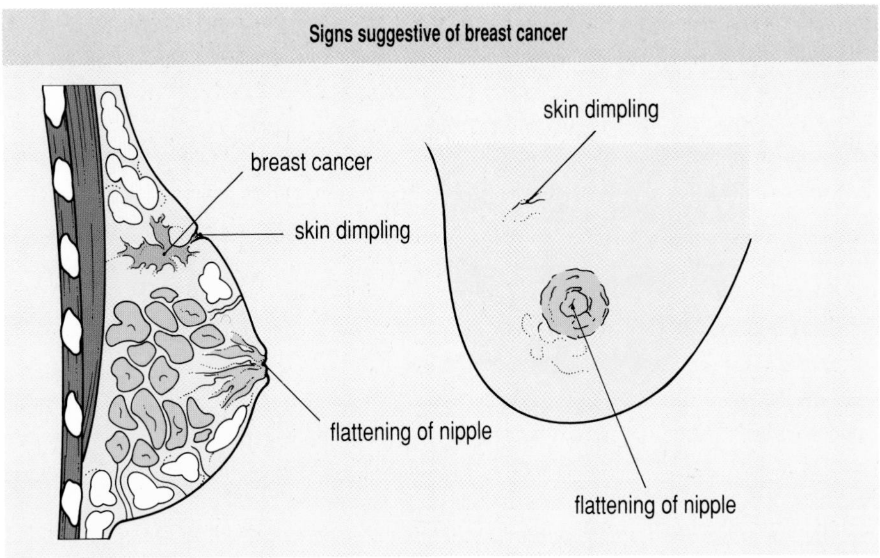

Fig. 9.18 Nipples may be everted, flat or retracted.

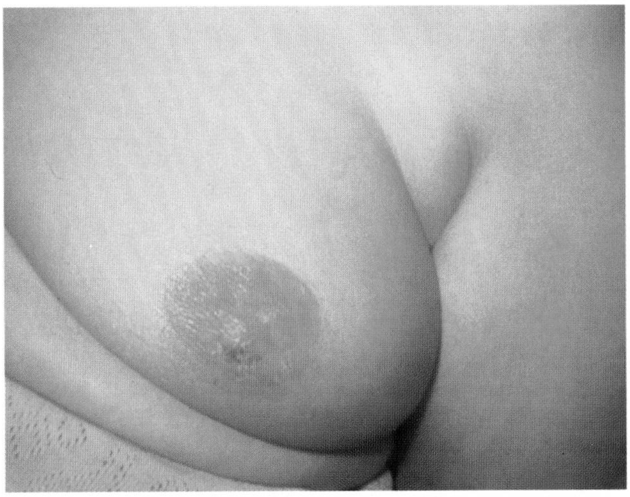

Fig. 9.19 Typical appearance of Paget's disease of the breast with reddening and scaling of the areolar skin.

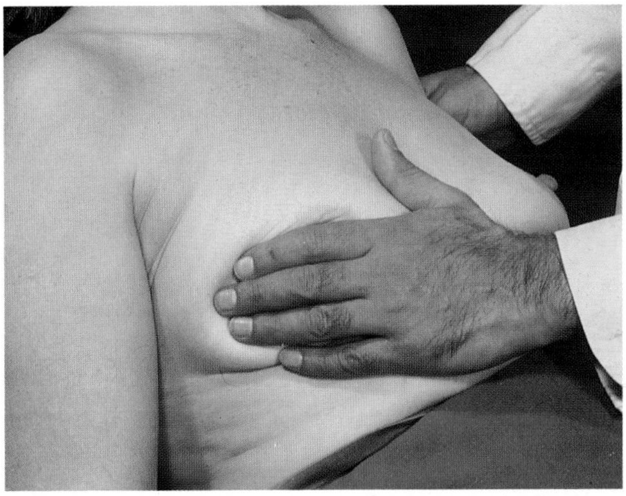

Fig. 9.20 Palpate the breast with the middle 3 fingers, rotating around the point of contract whilst pressing firmly but gently towards the chest wall.

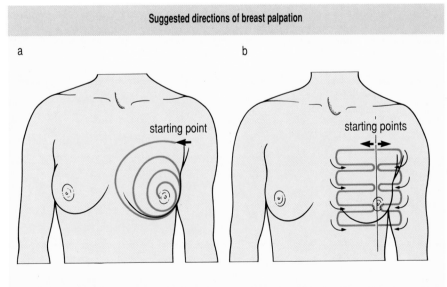

Fig. 9.21 Trace a systematic path either by following a concentric circular pattern (left) or examining each half of the breast sequentially from above down (right).

use one hand to steady the breast on its lower border whilst palpating with the other. The texture of normal breast tissue varies from smooth to granular, even knotty, and only experience will teach you the spectrum of normality. Texture may also vary with the menstrual cycle; nodularity and tenderness often increases towards the end of a cycle and during menstruation. Remember that breast texture is normally symmetrical and a comparison of the two breasts may help you to judge whether an area is abnormal or not.

To examine the axillary tail of Spence, ask the patient to rest her arms above her head. Feel the tail between your thumb and fingers as it extends from the upper outer quadrant towards the axilla (Fig. 9.22). If you feel a breast lump, examine the mass between your fingers and assess its size, consistency, mobility, and whether or not there is tenderness.

In men, palpation helps distinguish true from 'pseudo' gynaecomastia (obesity with fatty breast). In true gynaecomastia a disc of breast tissue can be felt under the areola. Unlike fat, breast tissue has a distinctly lobular texture which may be tender to palpation.

Nipple palpation

Hold the nipple between thumb and fingers and gently compress and attempt to express any discharge (Fig. 9.23). If fluid appears, note its colour, prepare a smear for cytology and send a swab for microbiology.

Lymph node palpation

The axillae can be palpated with the patient lying or sitting. When examining the left axilla in the sitting position, the patient may rest her (or his) left hand on your right shoulder whilst you explore the axilla with your right hand. Alternatively, there are different tech-

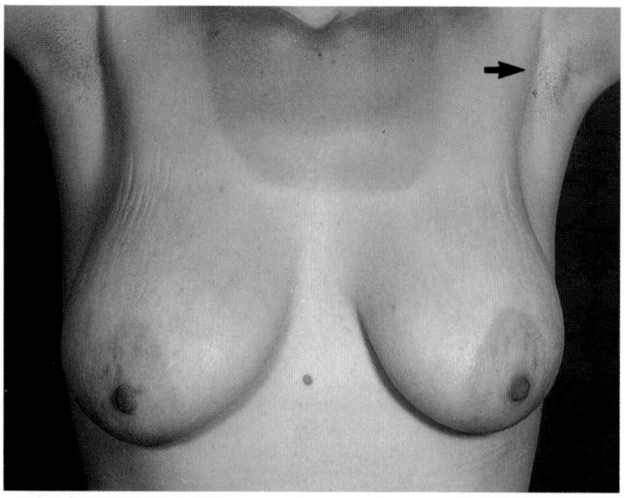

Fig. 9.22 Examine the tail of Spence with the patient's arms resting above the head. Use your thumb and first two fingers to trace the extension of breast tissue between the upper-outer quadrant and the axilla.

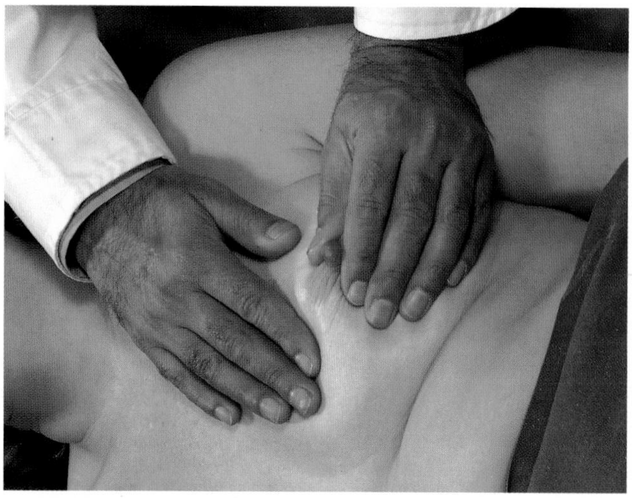

Fig. 9.23 Inspection of the nipple.

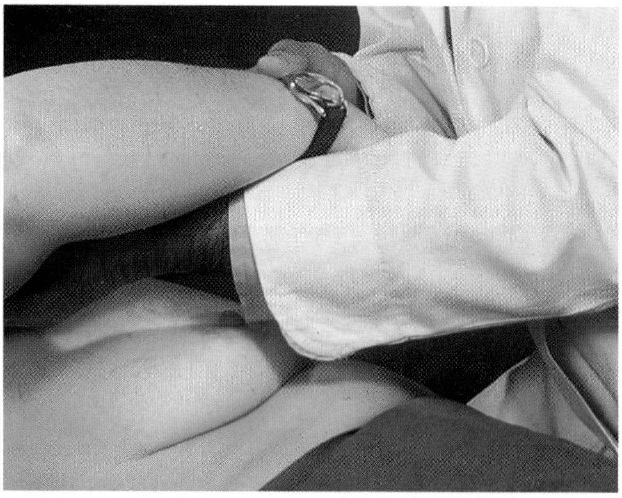

Fig. 9.24 Exposing the axilla by abductiong the arm and supporting it at the wrist.

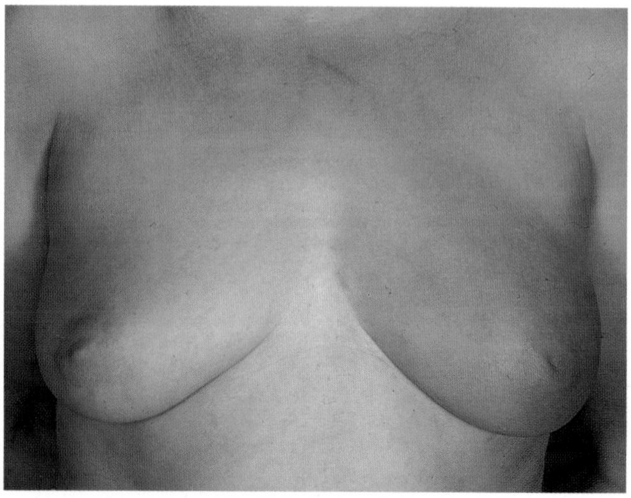

Fig. 9.25 Erythema of the skin overlying an area of mastitis.

niques for exposing the axilla. You may choose to abduct the arm gently by supporting the patient's wrist with your right hand and examining with the other hand (Fig. 9.24). The opposite hands are used to examine the other axilla. Slightly cup your examining hand and palpate into the apex of the axilla for the apical group of nodes. Small nodes may only be felt by rotating the exploring fingertips quite firmly against the chest wall. Next, feel for the anterior group of nodes along the posterior border of the anterior axillary fold, the central group against the lateral chest wall, and the posterior group along the posterior axillary fold. Finally, palpate along the medial border of the humerus to check for the lateral group of nodes and inspect the infra- and supraclavicular spaces for lymphadenopathy. If you feel nodes, assess size, shape, consistency, mobility, and tenderness.

Abnormal palpation

Breast lumps

Although there are clinical features which may favour a benign lesion rather than malignancy, all breast lumps should be investigated for possible malignancy. Common benign lumps include fibroadenomas, fibroadenosis, benign breast cysts, and fat necrosis. A fibroadenoma is usually felt as a discreet, firm and smooth lump which is quite mobile in its surrounding tissue (endearingly referred to as a 'breast mouse'). Fibroadenosis is a bilateral condition characterized by 'lumpiness' of the breasts, which may be tender, especially in the premenstrual and menstrual phases of the cycle. Cancerous lesions usually feel hard and irregular, and unlike benign lesions may be fixed to the skin or the underlying chest wall muscle. Special tests such as mammography, needle aspiration, and biopsy may be necessary to differentiate benign from malignant diseases.

Breast abscess (mastitis)

This usually occurs during lactation and is generally caused by blockage of a duct. The temperature is raised and the skin of the infected breasts inflamed (Fig. 9.25). Palpation may reveal an area of tenderness and induration. If an abscess forms, you usually feel an extremely tender fluctuant mass.

Abnormal nipple and areola

A blood-stained nipple discharge suggests an intraductal carcinoma of benign papilloma. Unilateral retraction or distortion of a nipple should also alert you to the possibility of malignancy, especially if the abnormality is relatively recent. A unilateral red, crusty, and scaling areola suggests Paget's disease of the breast (see Fig. 9.19). This disorder should alert you to a likely ductal carcinoma underlying the areola. Blockage of the sebaceous glands of Montogomery may cause retention cysts.

Palpable lymph nodes

If you detect axillary lymphadenopathy, suspect malignancy if the nodes are hard, non-tender, and/or fixed. Infection of axillary hair follicles or breast tissue may cause tender lymphadenitis. Look carefully for a local primary site of infection such as an abrasion caused by shaving the axilla. Occasionally patients with longstanding fibrocystic disease may have mild axillary node enlargement.

STRUCTURE OF THE GENITAL TRACT

The female reproductive organs include the ovaries, fallopian tubes, uterus, and vagina. These organs lie deep in the pelvis (Fig. 9.26), occupying the space between the rectum posteriorly, and the

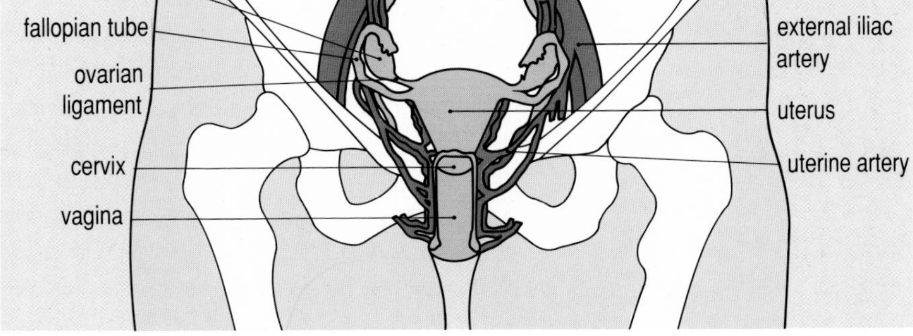

Fig. 9.26 The female pelvis and internal genitalia.

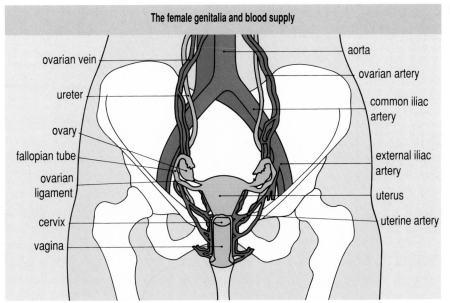

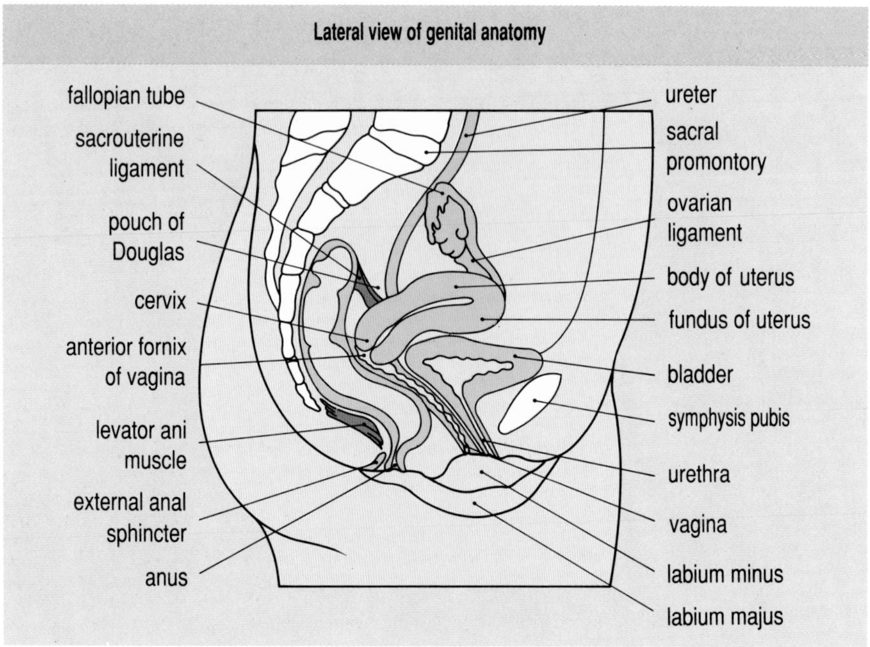

Fig. 9.27 Lateral view of the female internal genitalia showing the anatomical relationship to the rectum and bladder.

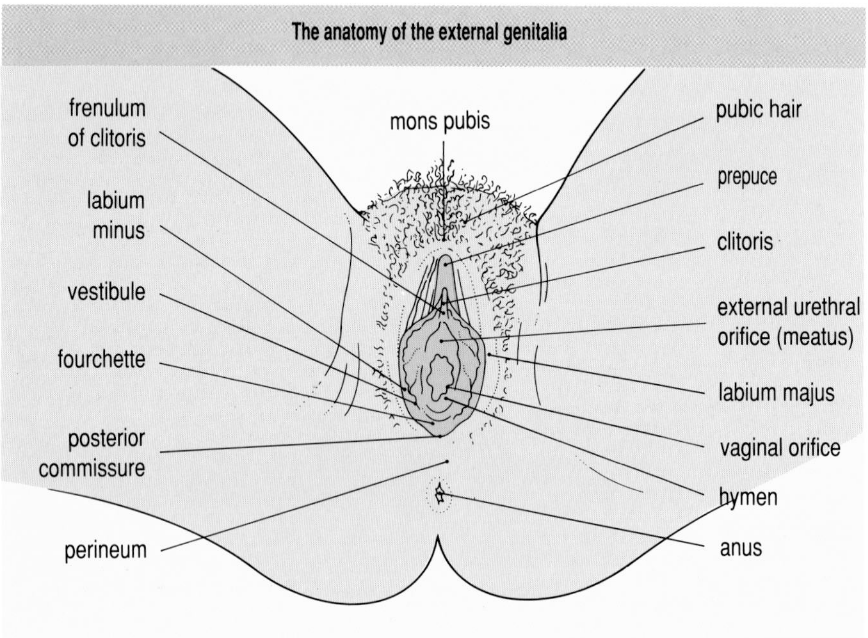

Fig. 9.28 The external female genitalia.

bladder and ureter anteriorly (Fig. 9.27). The female internal genitalia can be inspected through the vagina; the cervix can be palpated directly or through the anterior rectal wall; and the uterus, fallopian tubes, and ovaries can be examined using the technique of bimanual palpation.

The vulva

The external genitalia in the female is termed the vulva (Fig. 9.28). This comprises a fat pad which overlies the symphysis pubis (the mons pubis), a pair of prominent hair-lined skin folds extending on either side from the mons to meet posteriorly in the midline in front of the anal verge (the labia majora), and a pair of hairless, flat folds lying adjacent and medial to the labia majora (the labia minora). The labia minora converge anteriorly in front of the vaginal orifice, with each splitting into two small folds which meet in the midline. The anterior folds from either side merge to form the prepuce; the posterior folds form the frenulum. A nub of erectile tissue (the clitoris) lies tucked between the frenulum and prepuce. Posteriorly, the labia minora fuse to form a distinct ridge known as the fourchette. The labia minora demarcate the vestibule which contains the urethral meatus and vaginal orifice. Bartholin's glands are

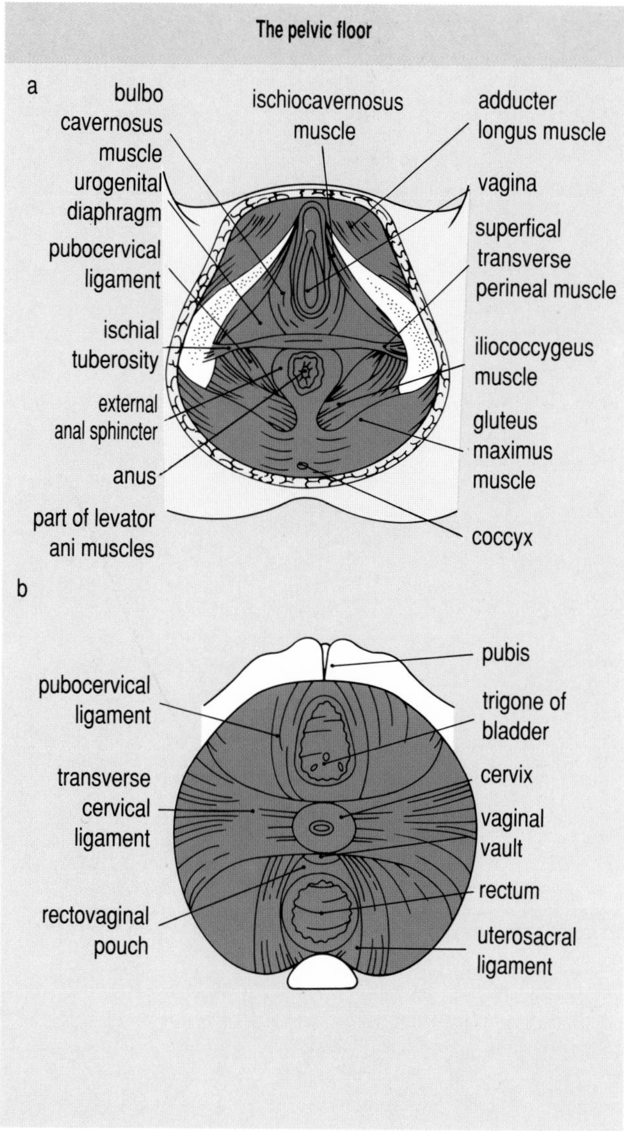

Fig. 9.29 The pelvic floor muscles support the pelvic organs. (a) Superficial perineal muscles. (b) Fascia and ligaments.

a pair of pea-sized mucus glands which lie deep to the posterior margin of the labia minora and empty through a duct into the vestibule, providing lubrication of the introitus. Bartholin's glands may become infected if the ducts are obstructed, resulting in painful swelling and abscess formation.

The vulva rests on the pelvic floor which is formed by a complex arrangement of muscles which supports the rectum, vagina, and urethra (Fig. 9.29).

The vagina

The vagina is a tube-shaped passage connecting the vulva to the cervix of the uterus. Its opening in the vulva (the introitus) lies between the urethra and anus. The vagina is inclined in an upward and posterior direction. A connective tissue septum separates the vagina anteriorly from the bladder base and urethra, and posteriorly from the rectum. The uterine cervix pouts through the upper vault of the vagina and divides the blind end of the vagina into the anterior, posterior, and lateral fornices (Fig. 9.30). These thin-walled fornices provide a convenient access point for examining the pelvic organs.

The uterus

The uterus is a muscular, pear-shaped organ consisting of the cervix, body, and fundus (Fig. 9.31). The adult uterus is usually angled forward from the plane of the vagina (anteverted) and bends forward on itself at the junction of the internal os and the

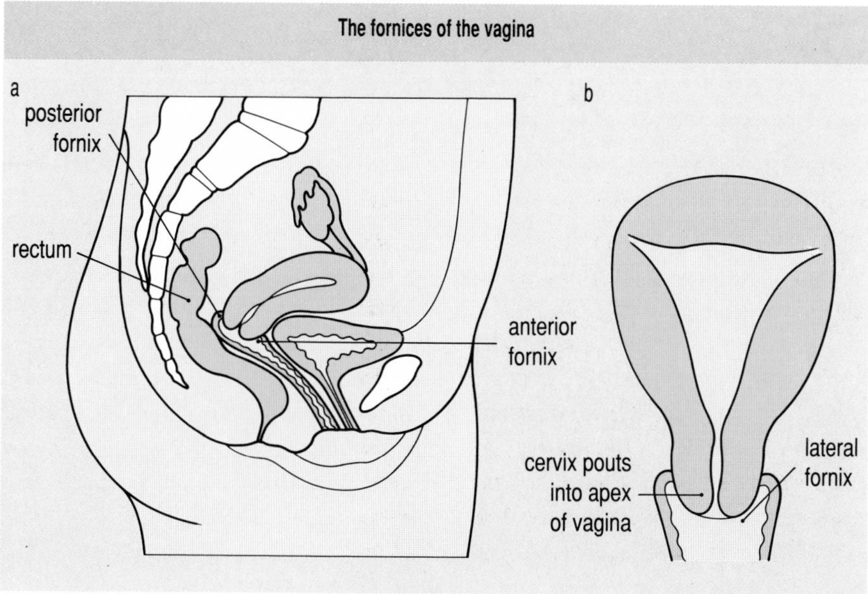

Fig. 9.30 The cervix projects into the vagina creating the anterior, posterior, and lateral fornices.

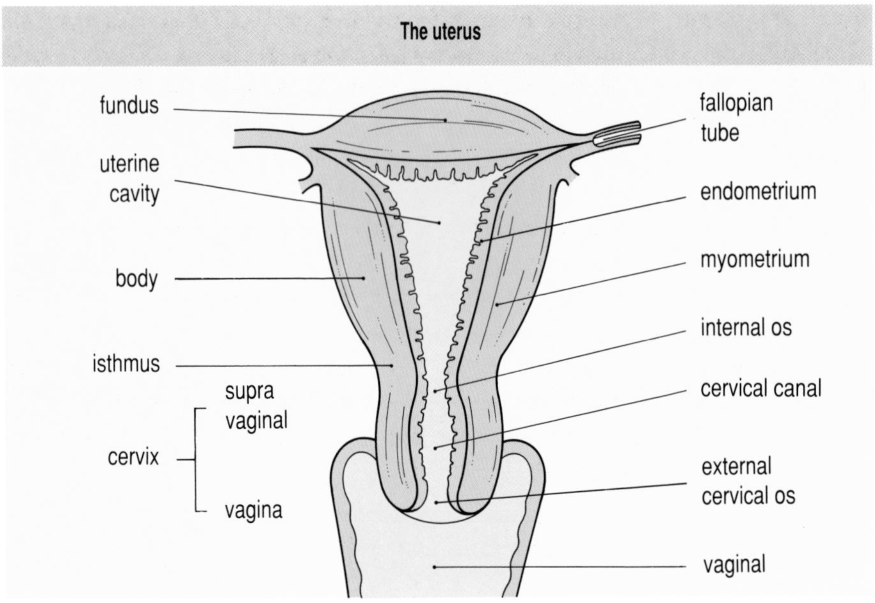

Fig. 9.31 Section through the pear-shaped, muscular uterus showing the cervix, isthmus, body (corpus), and fundus. The mucosa is called the endometrium. The cervical canal has an internal and external os.

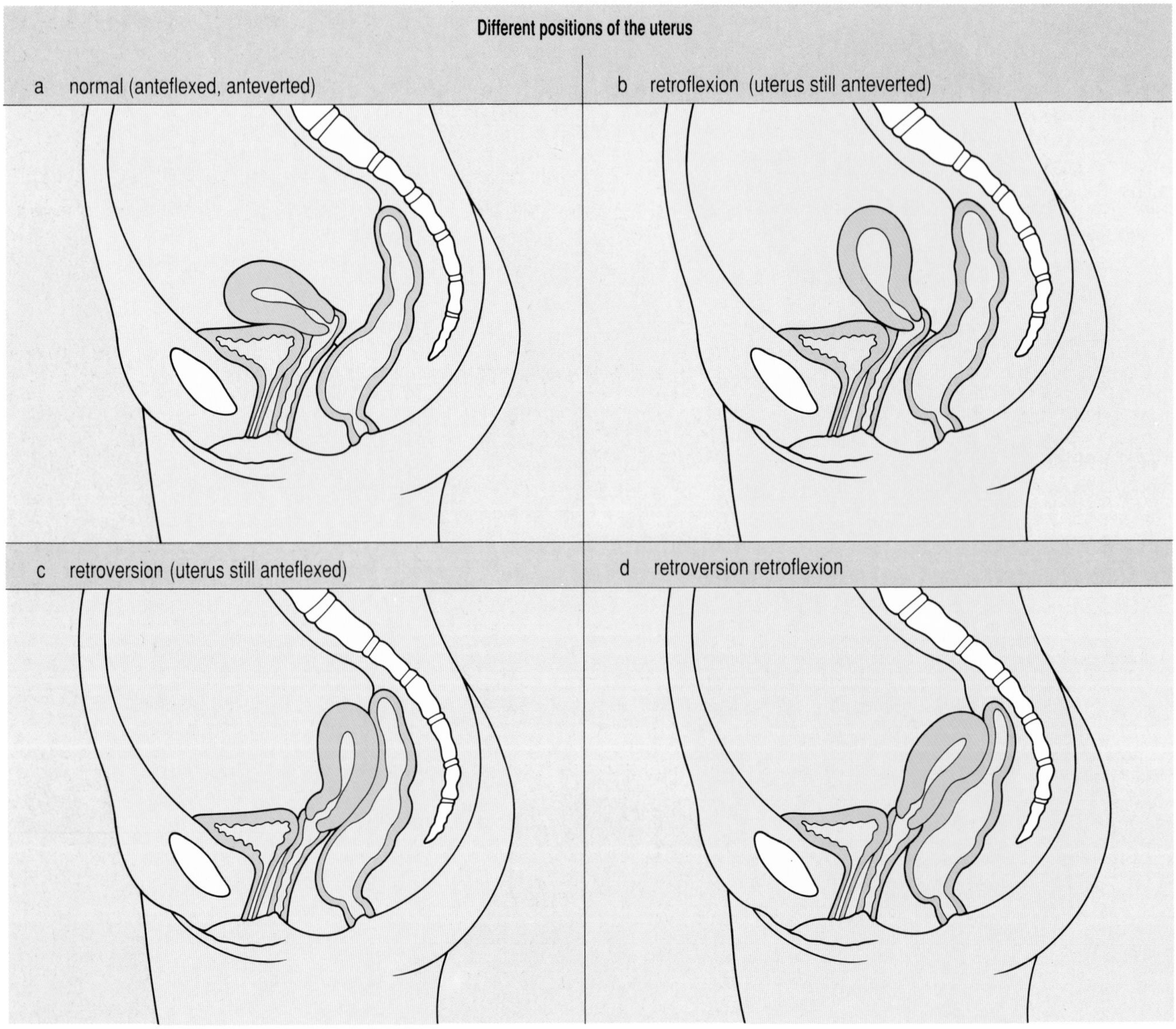

Fig. 9.32 The different anatomical positions of the uterine body within the pelvis. (a). The normal uterus is angled forward from the plane of the vagina (anteverted) and bends forward on itself (anteflexed). In some women the uterus assumes different positions: (b) retroflexed, anteverted; (c) retroverted, anteflexed; or (d) retroverted, retroflexed.

body (anteflexion) (Fig. 9.32a). In some women the uterus assumes different positions: an anteverted uterus may lie retroflexed (Fig. 9.32b), and a retroverted uterus may be anteflexed (Fig. 9.32c), or retroflexed (Fig. 9.32d).

The vaginal surface of the cervix is covered by stratified squamous epithelium. The uterus is covered with peritoneum which reflects anteriorly onto the bladder, posteriorly onto the rectum, and laterally to form the broad ligaments. The peritoneum covering the posterior uterus and upper vagina reflects onto the anterior rectal wall forming a blind pocket known as the Pouch of Douglas. The cuboidal cells lining the uterine cavity (the endometrium) respond to the hormonal changes of the menstrual cycle.

The adnexae

The adnexae refers to the fallopian tubes, ovaries, and their connective tissue attachments.

The fallopian tubes

The fallopian tubes insert into the upper outer uterus (the cornu) and project laterally along the free edge of the broad ligaments curving around the ovaries (Fig. 9.33). The tubes vary in length from 8–14cm and open into the peritoneum through the trumpet-shaped infundibulum. The entrance to the fallopian tube (the ostium) is bounded by fringe-like fimbria which overlie the ovary and help to capture the ovum when it is expelled in mid-cycle. The ovum moves along the fallopian tube by a combination of peristalsis and the wafting action of the cilia on the mucosal lining cells.

The ovaries

There are two ovaries. Each is oval in shape and usually rests in a slight depression in the side wall of the pelvis. The ovary is not lined by peritoneum and measures 3cm long, 2cm wide and 1cm thick. The ovarian ligament connects the ovary to the cornu of the uterus. The connective tissue stroma of the ovary contains Graafian follicles at various stages of development, the corpus luteum which develops after ovulation, and the corpus albicans, a relic of a degenerating corpus luteum.

The pelvic fascia and ligaments

The connective tissue overlying the muscular floor of the pelvis condenses into ligaments which stabilize and support the pelvic organs by attachments to the pelvis. The cardinal ligaments (Mackenrodt's ligaments) span laterally, connecting the cervix and upper vagina to the bony pelvis. The uterosacral ligaments pass posteriorly and backwards from the posterolateral cervix, attaching to the periosteum overlying the sacro-iliac joints and the mid-sacrum. The pubocervical fascia extends forward from the cardinal ligament, joining to the pubic bone on either side of the bladder.

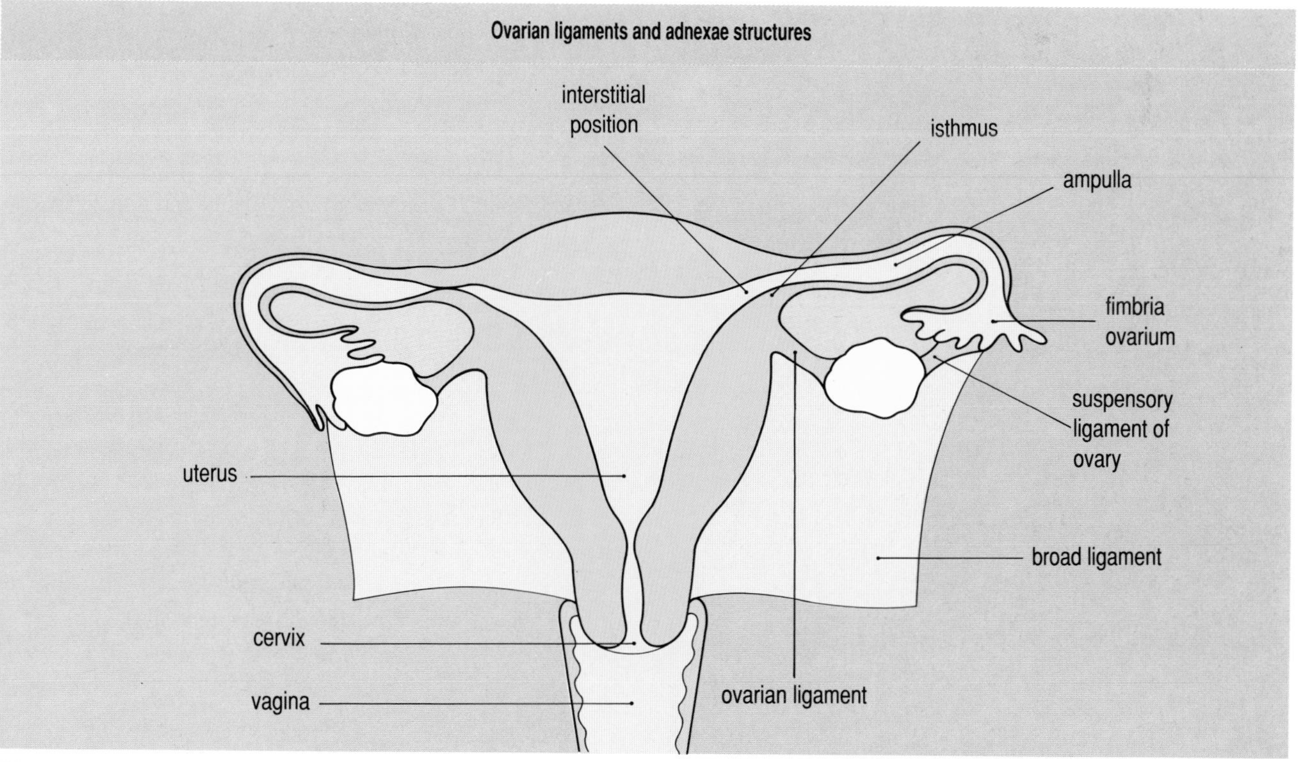

Fig. 9.33 Coronal section of the uterus and fallopian tubes showing the ligamentous attachments of the ovary.

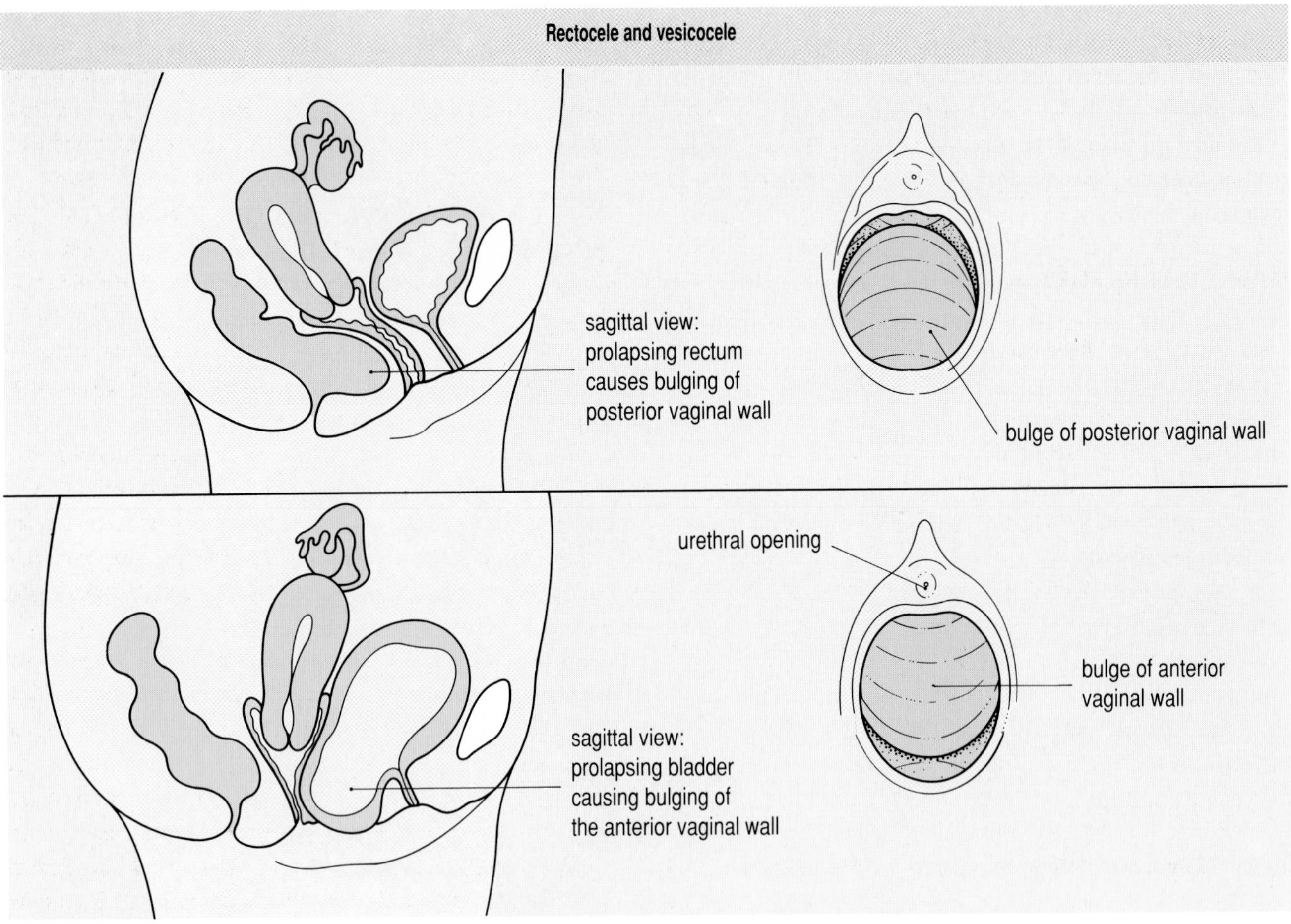

Fig. 9.34 Pelvic floor examination. Prolapsing rectum causes bulging of posterior vaginal wall (top). Prolapsing bladder causing bulging of the anterior wall (bottom).

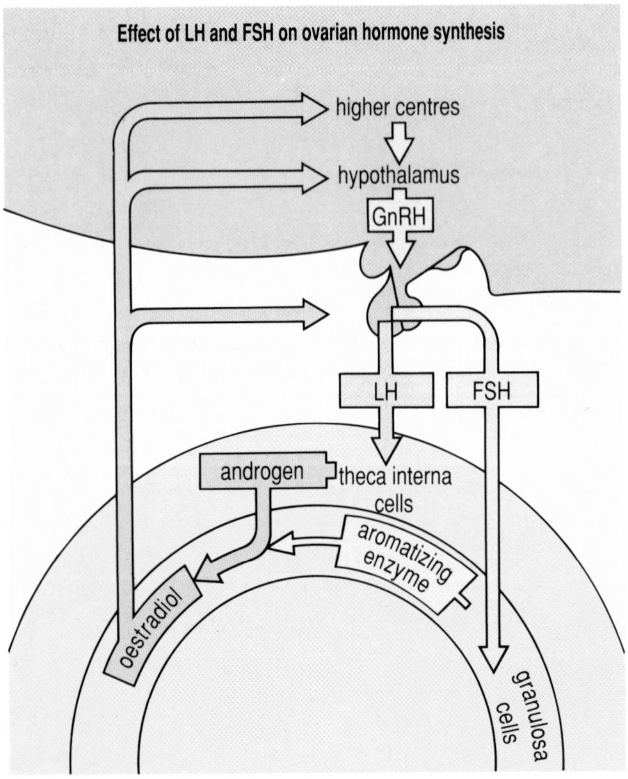

Fig. 9.35 Effect of.gonadotrophins on the theca interna and granulosa cells which produce the ovarian hormones.

These pelvic ligaments and the muscular floor of the pelvis may become lax and weaken allowing the uterus to drop and prolapse (Fig. 9.51).

The broad ligament is formed from peritoneum which suspends from the lateral wall of the uterus to the lateral wall of the pelvis. The fallopian tubes, ovarian ligament, uterine and ovarian vessels, and lymphatics run in the broad ligament.

SYMPTOMS OF GENITAL TRACT DISEASE

There may be initial reluctance to discuss genital and sexual disorders, but with gentle coaxing you should be able to lead the patient towards a frank account of their sexual history. The degree to which you pursue the history depends on the relevance to the patient's problems. Organic and psychological disorders may affect sexual function and this may be important, although not central, to the presenting disease. Cardiac and respiratory disease may interfere with normal sexual activity; after a myocardial infarct there is often concern about recommencing a normal sex life. Reduction or loss of libido is common in acute and chronic illness. Patients with psychological disorders such as anorexia nervosa or depression may present with a primary complaint of loss of libido or a menstrual disorder. In contrast, patients suffering from primary sexual problems may present with physical symptoms such as abdominal pain which may camouflage the underlying sexual problem.

The genital-sexual history commonly follows the urinary history. You might find that asking about previous pregnancies or the pattern of the menstrual cycle provides a suitable platform for more detailed questioning.

MENSTRUAL HISTORY

Establish the age of the menarche

Because of the wide variation in the age of the menarche, parents and children may be unduly concerned about delay. Most European and North American girls start menstruating by the age of 14.5 (range 9–16 years old). Body weight appears to play a role and the menarche occurs at an average weight of 48kg. If there is anxiety about delayed menarche or primary amenorrhoea, ask whether or not pubic and axillary hair growth and breast development have commenced. By the age of 14, secondary sexual characteristics should have appeared. If the menarche has not occurred and there are no other signs of sexual development, it is reasonable to consider organic causes of primary amenorrhoea, such as gonadal dysgenesis (Turner's syndrome), congenital anatomical abnormalities of the genital tract (e.g. its absence, or uterine or vaginal hypoplasia), polycystic ovaries, or pituitary/hypothalamic tumors in childhood. If secondary sexual characteristics have appeared, reassure the patient that investigation is usually only necessary if the menarche has not occurred by the age of 16.

The menstrual cycle

Age of menarche.

Age of telarche.

Do you use the contraceptive pill or HRT?

Length of cycle.

Days of blood loss.

Number of tampons/pads used per day.

Are there clots?

Determine the pattern of the menstrual cycle

Throughout the child-bearing years, women should be encouraged to specify the starting date of each menstrual period (i.e. the date when bleeding commences). Record the starting date of the most recent period. The duration of the menstrual cycle is calculated from the first day of bleeding to the first day of bleeding in the next menstrual cycle. This cycle may vary in normal women from 21–35
menstrual cycle. This cycle may vary in normal women from 21–35
days, but the average duration is 28 days. Most healthy, fertile women have regular, predictable cycles which vary in duration to within 1 to 2 days. Once regular periods are established concern is soon aroused if there is deviation from the norm.

Blood loss from menstruation averages about 70ml (range from yet there are indicators: women with heavy periods saturate rather than stain tampons or pads, whilst the passage of large and frequent clots suggests excessive bleeding. The only accurate method for assessing menstrual loss is to weigh absorbant pads before and after each change.

Attempt to classify any change or abnormality in the menstrual cycle. First establish whether the cycles are regular and if so, calculate the cycle length and attempt to assess whether the periods are scanty or heavy. Bear in mind contraceptive practices as the patient's intrinsic rhythms will be masked if she is taking a cyclical contraceptive pill or undergoing hormone replacement therapy (HRT). The most common irregularities include failure to menstruate at the expected time (secondary amenorrhoea). Cycles may be infrequent and scanty (oligomenorrhoea), unusually frequent (polymenorrhoea), excessively heavy (menorrhagia), or frequent and heavy (polymenorrhagia). Bleeding after intercourse is termed post-coital bleeding. If regular cycles are interrupted by days of spotting or blood-tinged discharge, this is known as intermenstrual bleeding.

Secondary amenorrhoea

Develop the case history by considering possible causes of secondary amenorrhoea (Fig. 9.36). Pregnancy and lactation are the most common cause. The patient may suspect a pregnancy: there may be clues such as early morning nausea and vomiting, urinary frequency, and tender enlargement of the breasts. Stress, anxiety, depression, bereavement, and a change of environment may interrupt the cyclical release of sex hormones by the hypothalamic-pituitary. Consider fear of pregnancy which is a common cause of delayed menstruation. Not only do patients with excessive weight loss due to anorexia nervosa present with amenorrhoea but highly-trained long distance athletes may also stop menstruating. Enquire about contraceptive practices as 'post pill' amenorrhoea is well-recognized. Consider the menopause in women entering the climacteric years. This is often heralded by a change in the cyclical pattern, reduced menstrual flow, and the onset of menopausal symp-

Causes of secondary amenorrhoea
Physiological
Pregnancy
Lactation
Psychological
Anorexia nervosa
Depression
Fear of pregnancy
Hormonal
Post-contraceptive pill
Pituitary tumors
Hyperthyroidism
Adrenal tumors
Ovarian
Polycystic ovaries
Ovarian tumor
Ovarian tuberculosis
Constitutional disease
Severe acute illness
Chronic infections/illnesses
Autoimmune diseases

Fig. 9.36 Secondary amenorrhoea.

Causes of vaginal discharges
Physiological
Pregnancy
Sexual arousal
Menstual cycle variation
Pathological
Vaginal
Candidosis (thrush)
Trichomoniasis
Gardenella-associated
Other bacteria (e.g. due to retained tampon)
Post-menopausal vaginitis
Cervical
Gonorrhoea
Non-specific genital infection
Herpes
Cervical ectopy
Cervical neoplasm (e.g. polyp)
Intrauterine contraceptive device

Fig. 9.37 Vaginal discharge.

toms such as hot flushes and dryness of the introitus and vagina. In the absence of an obvious cause for amenorrhoea, consider diseases of the hypothalamus, pituitary, and ovary.

Abnormal patterns of uterine bleeding

Oligomenorrhoea

Oligomenorrhoea is the term used to describe infrequent or scanty menstrual periods. This pattern may be normal between the menarche and the establishment of a regular menstrual pattern, and is also a feature of the climacteric as the menopause approaches. In some women, the oligomenorrhoea of puberty persists into adult life. Ascertain whether the infrequent, scanty periods are a change from the normal pattern or a pattern present from puberty. If oligomenorrhoea presents as a distinct change in the menstrual pattern, consider the same factors implicated in the differential diagnosis of secondary amenorrhoea.

Dysfunctional uterine bleeding

This term is used to describe frequent bleeding or excessive menstrual loss which cannot be ascribed to local pelvic pathology (e.g. fibroids, pelvic inflammatory disease, carcinoma, polyps). Establish whether the abnormal cyclical pattern is regular or irregular. Regular dysfunctional bleeding may present as menorrhagia, epimenorrhoea, or polymenorrhoea. The predictability of these abnormal cycles usually implies that ovulation is occurring, although this needs to be confirmed. Irregular dysfunctional bleeding usually implies that ovulation has ceased; the menstrual rhythm is lost and the cyclical pattern is replaced by unpredictable bleeding of varying severity.

Intermenstrual and postmenopausal bleeding

Patients may complain of vaginal bleeding happening unexpectedly between normal periods or after the menopause. Enquire about

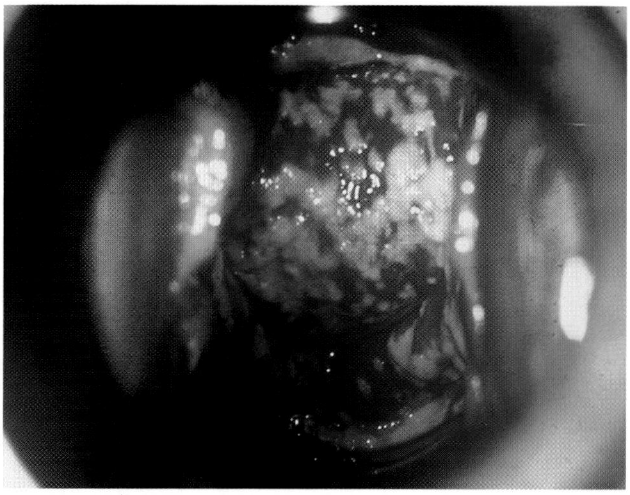

Fig. 9.38 Vaginal candidiasis has a curd-like appearance.

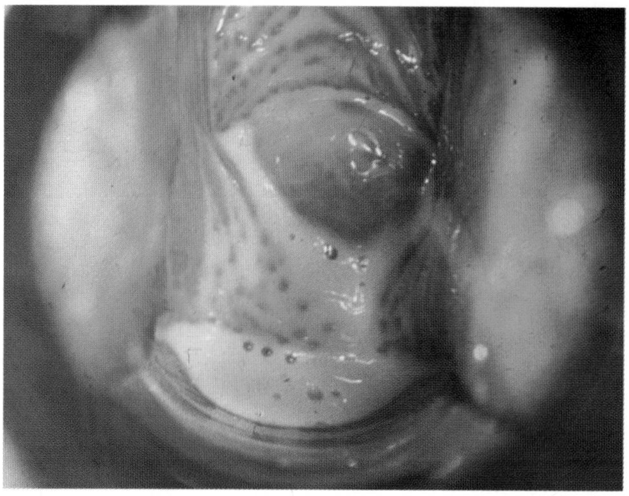

Fig. 9.39 Trichomoniasis.

sex-hormone therapy as 'breakthrough bleeding' may occur with hormone treatment. Diseases of the uterus and cervix may present with abnormal bleeding, so you should consider disorders of the mucosa (e.g. endometritis, carcinoma, or endometrial polyps) or submucosa (e.g. submucosal leiomyomas or fibroids). Post-coital bleeding usually indicates local cervical or uterine disease (carcinoma or a cervical polyp).

Vaginal discharge

Vaginal discharge is a common complaint during the child-bearing years (Fig. 9.37). Many women notice slight soiling of the underwear at the end of the day; this is a normal physiological response to the cyclical changes occurring in the glandular epithelium of the genital tract and it is likely to become more profuse in pregnancy. A physiological discharge is scanty, mucoid, and odourless. Pathological discharge is usually trichomonal or candidal vaginitis. The discharge may irritate the vulval skin causing itching (pruritus vulvae) or burning. Attempt to assess the severity of the discharge by ascertaining whether the discharge merely stains the underwear or is heavier and requires protective pads.

The nature of the discharge may be helpful. With vaginitis caused by Candida albicans the discharge is white, has a curd-like appearance and consistency (Fig. 9.38), and causes intense itching. Vaginitis caused by Trichomonas vaginalis usually presents with a profuse opaque or cream-coloured, frothy discharge which has a characteristic 'fishy' smell (Fig. 9.39). The trichomonal discharge may cause vulval irritation and is occasionally accompanied by burning upon micturition: this is caused by inflammation of the urethral meatus. If the patient complains of a profuse, foul-smelling discharge, consider a retained foreign body (e.g. a tampon). Cervical infection due to gonorrhoea, Chlamydia trachomatis, or non-specific cervicitis may present with a discharge, but unlike vaginitis, these rarely cause itching or burning of the vulva.

Vaginal discharge

How long has the discharge been present?

Is the discharge scanty or profuse?

Is extra protection necessary or does the discharge simply spot or stain?

What is the colour and consistency?

Is there an odour?

Is the discharge blood-stained?

Is there associated lower abdominal pain and fever?

Is there itching or burning of the vulval area?

Pain

Gynaecological disorders should always be considered in women presenting with lower abdominal pain. If the pain predictably occurs immediately before and during a period, the likely cause is dysmenorrhoea. This is a suprapubic, boring or cramp-like pain caused by intense pelvic congestion; it occurs a day or two before menstruation or with uterine contraction during the shedding and expulsion of the endometrium. Severe dysmenorrhoea should alert you to the possibility of endometriosis, a disorder resulting from cyclical changes (including withdrawal bleeding) occurring in endometrial tissue implanted in ectopic sites (e.g. in the fallopian tubes or peritoneum).

Ovulation may cause a unilateral iliac fossa or supra-pubic pain in mid-cycle which lasts a few hours (mittleschmertz). Severe iliac fossa pain should warm you of the possibility of a haemorrhage into an ovarian cyst or torsion of a cyst. If the pain is preceded by a missed period and especially if there is shock, you should also consider the possibility of a ruptured ectopic pregnancy. If the lower abdominal pain is accompanied by a vaginal discharge, fever, anorexia, and nausea, consider acute infection of the fallopian tubes (acute salpingitis).

Dyspareunia

Pain on intercourse (dyspareunia) may be caused by either psychological or organic disorders. Try to distinguish vaginal spasm which makes penetration difficult (vaginismus) from pain occurring once penetration has occurred. Assess whether the pain is superficial (suggesting a local vulval cause or a psychological spasm) or deep (suggesting inflammatory or malignant disease of the cervix, uterus, or adnexae). After the menopause, the vulva and vagina becomes dry and atrophic, and this may cause discomfort on intercourse.

PSYCHOSEXUAL HISTORY

A satisfactory sex life is an important component of a healthy emotional relationship. In unmarried women, ask whether she has had intercourse. Patients may complain of loss of sex drive (libido), failure to achieve orgasm, pain or difficulty with intercourse, and ambivalence about sexual preference. These symptoms and personal problems are often camouflaged behind other symptoms such as non-specific abdominal pain, depression, fatigue, or headache. It requires shrewd clinical judgment to recognize the underlying psychosexual problem. Tactfully enquire about the sexual history.

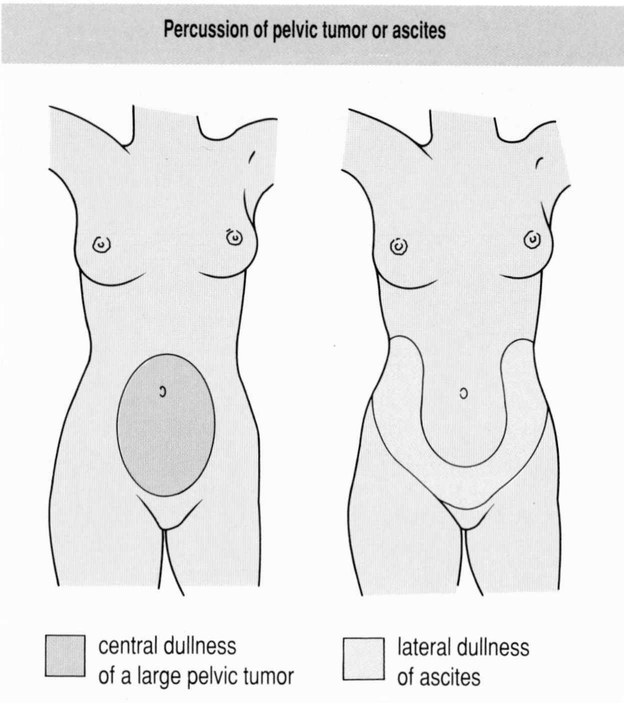

Fig. 9.40 Careful examination of the abdomen allows differentiation between large ovarian cysts and ascites. (a) An ovarian cyst displaces the bowel towards the flanks, the central abdomen is dull while the flanks are more resonant. (b) This contrasts with ascites, where the flanks are dull and the central abdomen tympanitic.

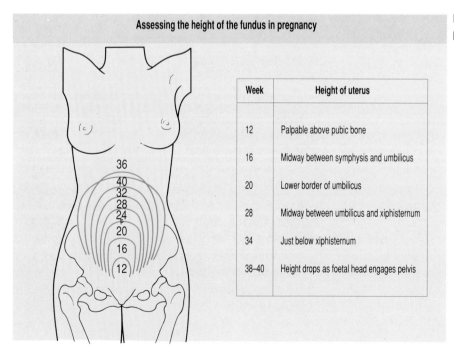

Assessing the height of the fundus in pregnancy

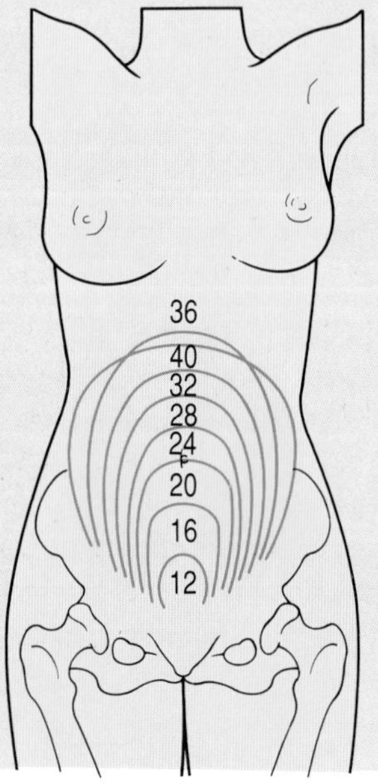

Week	Height of uterus
12	Palpable above pubic bone
16	Midway between symphysis and umbilicus
20	Lower border of umbilicus
28	Midway between umbilicus and xiphisternum
34	Just below xiphisternum
38–40	Height drops as foetal head engages pelvis

Fig. 9.41 The maturity of the pregnancy can be assessed by examining the height of the fundus.

Psychosexual history

Are you able to develop satisfying emotional relationships?

Do you have satisfying physical relationships?

Are you heterosexual, homosexual, or ambivalent?

Do you use contraception and, if so, what form?

Do you have problems achieving arousal?

Do you experience orgasm?

OBSTETRIC HISTORY

Enquire whether the patient has ever been pregnant and whether there were fertility problems. Record the number of completed and unsuccessful pregnancies. If the patient has miscarried, record the maturity of the pregnancy at the time of miscarriage. Ask about complications during pregnancy (e.g. hypertension, diabetes) and problems associated with labour and the period after delivery (the puerperium).

Obstetric history

Have you ever been pregnant and, if so, how often?

Did you have any problems falling pregnant?

How many children do you have?

Have you miscarried and, if so, at what stage of pregnancy?

Were there any complications in pregnancy (e.g. high blood pressure or diabetes)?

Was the labour normal or did you require forceps assistance or a caesarian section?

EXAMINATION OF THE FEMALE GENITAL TRACT

Examination of the genitalia is intrusive; nonetheless, most women are psychologically prepared if they are seeking attention for a gynaecological disorder. In the course of taking the history you should already have established rapport with your patient and if there are gynaecological symptoms, the examination should follow on quite naturally.

Before the examination, take the time to explain the need for the examination and procedure the examination. If you have no reason to suspect a painful examination, reassure the patient that there should be little discomfort. If there is a suggestion of vaginitis or pelvic inflammatory disease, explain that there may be a little discomfort and that the patient should inform you there is pain. Whilst ensuring the patient's comfort and privacy you should always be accompanied by a nurse who can provide reassurance for the patient and assist you with the procedure (e.g. speculum examination and cervical smears).

Before the examination, ask the patient to empty her bladder. This adds to the comfort of the examination and excludes a full bladder in the differential diagnosis of suprapubic and pelvic swellings. Ensure that a clean gown is available and that there are satisfactory facilities for the patient to undress.

THE GENERAL EXAMINATION

Before examining the genital tract you should perform a general examination. Excessive facial hair (hirsutes) may be normal but if excessive, may provide a clue to an endocrine imbalance. Anaemia may occur with menstrual disorders, and you might recognize syndromes which are commonly associated with menstrual disorders (e.g. thyrotoxicosis, myxoedema, Cushing's syndrome, anorexia nervosa, and other serious chronic diseases). You will have examined the breasts during the chest examination and assessed the development of secondary sexual characteristics.

EXAMINATION OF THE ABDOMEN

A full abdominal examination precedes the vulval and vaginal examination. Although the uterus and adnexae lie deep within the protective confines of the pelvis, abnormalities may be apparent above the pubis. Lower abdominal tenderness occurs in pelvic inflammatory disease; moreover, enlargement of the uterus or ovaries might present with a palpable lower abdominal mass. Large ovarian cysts may fill the abdomen; this presentation is readily mistaken for ascites. Careful abdominal percussion helps distinguish ascites from a cystic ovarian tumor. A large ovarian cyst displaces bowel laterally, and on percussion there is central dullness with resonance in the flanks (Fig. 9.40). This contrasts with ascites which is characterized by central resonance and dullness in the flanks.

Examination of the genitalia

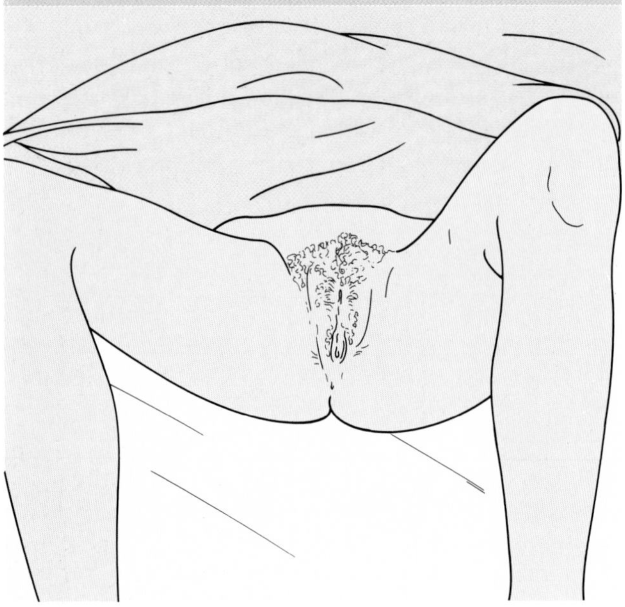

Fig. 9.42 The correct position of the patient prior to examination of the genitalia.

Labial palpation

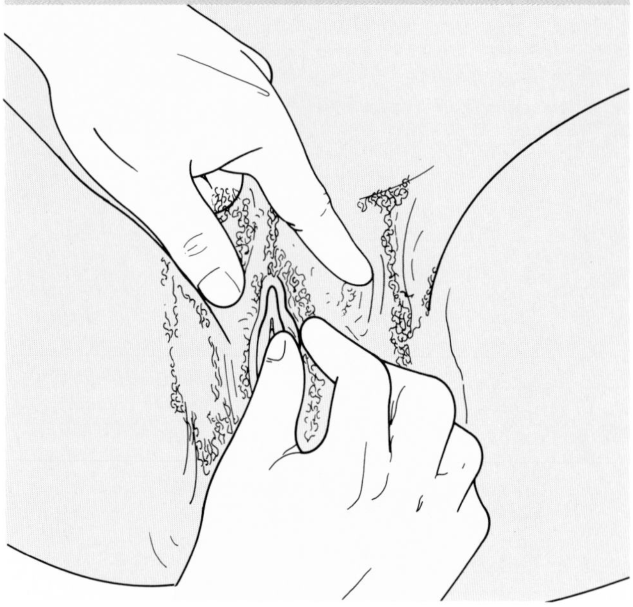

Fig. 9.43 Palpate the labia majora between the thumb and index finger.

Palpation for Bartholin's gland

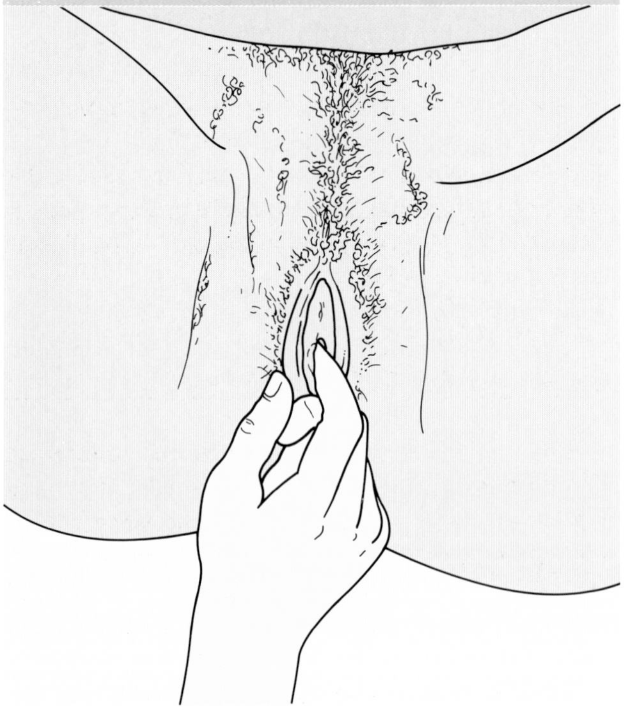

Fig. 9.44 Palpating Bartholin's gland with the index finger just inside the introitus and the thumb on the outer aspect of the labium majorus.

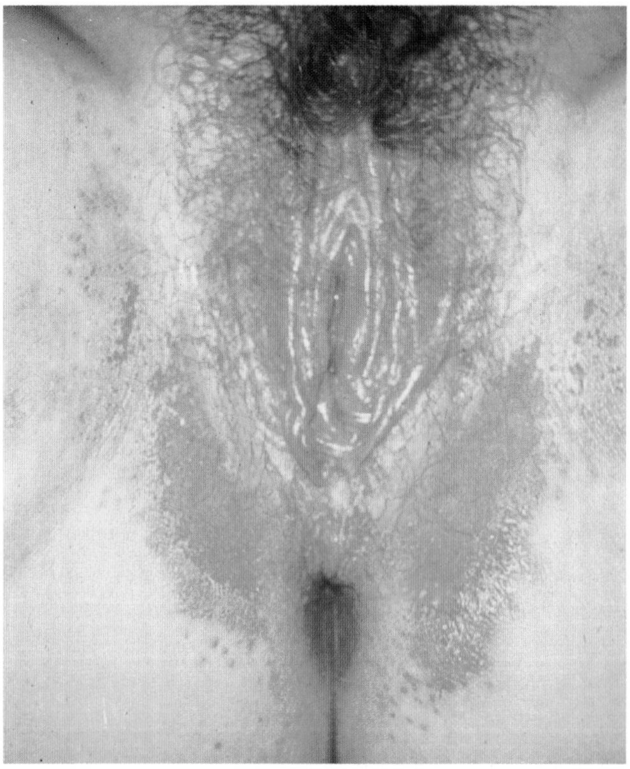

Fig. 9.45 Primary cutaneous candidosis of the vulva.

The abdomen in pregnancy

After the twelfth week of the pregnancy, the uterus becomes palpable above the symphysis pubis, so it is possible to assess the maturity of the foetus from the height of the fundus (Fig. 9.41).

EXAMINING THE EXTERNAL GENITALIA

This examination is usually performed on a conventional examination couch. The nurse should prepare and position the patient for the examination. The patient lies supine with the hips and knees

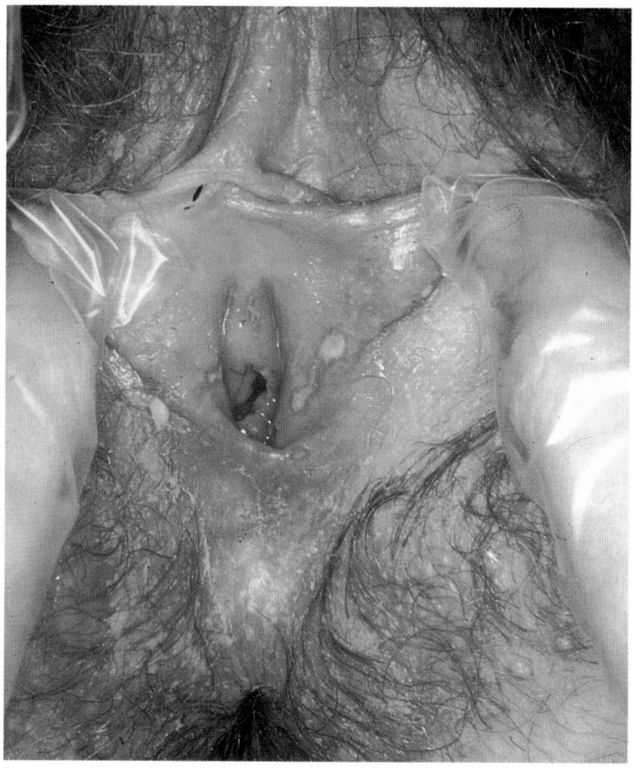

Fig. 9.46 Herpes simplex vesicles in the perianal region, fourchette and inner surface of the labia minora.

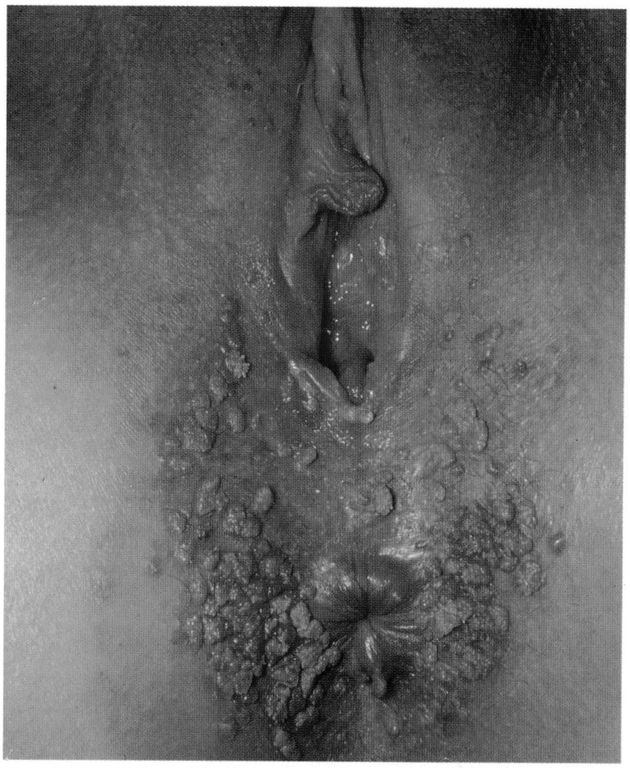

Fig. 9.47 Multiple perianal warts (*Condylomata acuminata*) encroaching onto the labia.

flexed and the heels close together. Help the patient to abduct the thighs to allow adequate access to the external genitalia (Fig. 9.42). Use a blanket or sheet to cover the abdomen and mons pubis. Ensure good general lighting; additionally, you will require a direct light source to focus on the vulva. When examining the vulva and vagina, wear disposable plastic gloves on each hand.

INSPECTION AND PALPATION OF THE VULVA

Explain that you are going to examine the labia and the area surrounding the vaginal opening. Maintain intermittent eye contact with the patient. Uncover the mons to expose the external genitalia. The pattern of hair distribution over the mons pubis provides a useful measure of sexual development. Once puberty is complete the mons and outer aspects of the labia majora should be well-covered with hair. Systematically examine the labia majora, labia minora, the introitus, urethra, and clitoris.

The labia majora on either side lie in close contact in the midline. Gently separate the labia with the fingers of your left hand and inspect the medial aspect which should be pink and slightly moist. Palpate the length of the labia majora between index finger and thumb (Fig. 9.43); the tissue should feel pliant and fleshy. Next, examine the Bartholin's gland between the index finger and thumb (Fig. 9.44). The right index finger palpates from the entrance of the vagina whilst the thumb palpates the outer surface of the labia majora posteriorly. A normal Bartholin's gland is not palpable.

To expose the vestibule, separate the labia minora. The vestibular tissue should be supple and slightly moist. Separation of the labia minora exposes the vaginal orifice and urethra.

After the menopause the skin and subcutaneous tissue of the external genitalia become atrophic and the mucosa loses its moist texture. These involutional, atrophic changes are normal and result from the loss of ovarian hormones.

ABNORMALITIES OF THE VULVA

A confluent, itchy, red rash on the inner aspects of the thighs and extending to the labia suggests candidiasis (Fig. 9.45). This is often associated with a vaginal discharge and should alert you to the possibility of diabetes or recent treatment with broad spectrum antibiotics. A vaginal discharge due to candidiasis or a trichomonal infection may irritate the vulval skin causing redness and tenderness (vulvitis).

The vulva is a common site for boils (furuncles) to appear. These are tender to palpation and should be distinguished from sebaceous cysts which are firm, rounded, yellowish, and non-tender, with an apical punctum indicating the opening of the blocked duct.

Many papular vulval lesions are caused by sexually transmitted infections. Crops of small, painful, vulval, and perianal papules, and vesicles which ulcerate suggests a herpes simplex infection (Fig. 9.46). You might notice multiple genital warts (Condylomata acuminata) which can coalesce to form large irregular tissue masses (Figs 9.47 and 9.48). Most genital warts are caused by a human papilloma virus. The lesions usually occur on the fourchette and may extend onto the labia, into the vagina, and posteriorly onto the perineum. Flat, round, or oval papules covered by a grey exudate suggests lesions of secondary syphilis (Condylomata latum) (Fig. 9.49).

Vulval ulceration has a wide differential diagnosis. The most common ulcerating lesions include carcinoma of the vulva or macerated, ulcerating herpetic warts. Acute vulval ulceration occurring in association with mouth and tongue ulcers and inflamed red eyes suggests Bechet's syndrome. A firm painless labial ulcer suggests the chancre of primary syphilis, whilst broad, moist ulcerating papules covered by grey slough suggest the secondary stage of syphilis. Suspect granuloma inguinale (caused by Chlamydia trachomatis) in women from tropical and subtropical regions presenting with vulval nodules and inguinal lymphadenopathy. The nodules coalesce and ulcerate, forming a large ulcer with rolled edges which must be distinguished from carcinoma. Chancroid, caused by Haemophilus ducreyi, is another sexually transmitted ulcerating disease affecting the vulva.

Leukoplakia is a potentially malignant, hypertrophic skin lesion, affecting the labia, clitoris, and perineum. The skin thickens, feels hard and indurated, and is distinguished from the surrounding tissue by its white colour.

Bartholin's glands become palpable if the ducts obstruct. This may result in a painless cystic mass or an acute (Bartholin's) abscess presenting as a hot, red, tender swelling in the posterolateral portion of the labia majora deep to the posterior end of the labia minora (Fig. 9.50).

EXAMINATION OF THE VAGINA

If the patient has an intact hymen, you may choose to examine the genitalia indirectly through the rectum. If the woman has an intact hymen but uses vaginal tampons, it is usually possible to perform a single digit vaginal examination.

Before proceeding with the internal examination, separate the labia to expose the vestibule and ask the patient to 'bear down' and exert a downward force on the vulva. If the pelvic floor is stable and the muscles intact, bulges and swellings should not appear through the vaginal walls below the introitus. If there is muscle weakness, the posterior bladder wall may prolapse causing a bulge (a cystocele) along the anterior vaginal wall (Fig. 9.34). If the rectum prolapses, this may cause a bulge (a rectocele) in the posterior vaginal wall.

A full vaginal examination includes inspection with a speculum, followed by a bimanual examination of the uterus and adnexae. Before continuing the examination, explain that you are about to inspect the vagina and cervix with a speculum.

THE SPECULUM EXAMINATION

The speculum is designed for inspection of the cervix and vaginal walls. In addition, the speculum provides access to the cervix and fornices for bacteriological swabs and cervical smears. If you anticipate taking samples, use water as a lubricant for your gloved fingers and the speculum, as lubricant gels may interfere with the processing and analysis of samples.

A bivalve speculum (e.g. Cusco's) is the instrument most commonly used to inspect the vagina (Fig. 9.52). Thoroughly familiarize yourself with its operation before examining a patient. The instrument is made of either stainless steel or plastic, and is available in different sizes. There are two blunt rounded elongated blades hinged at the base. In the closed position, the tips of the blades appose allowing the closed blades to slide safely into the slit-shaped introitus and into the tubular vagina. The blades open when the thumbpiece is squeezed (Fig. 9.53), and once positioned in the vagina, a hinged screw and nut arrangement fixes the blades in the open position.

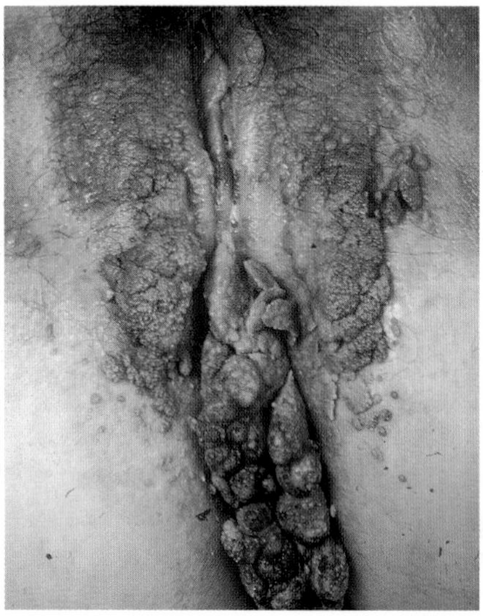

Fig. 9.48 Perianal warts.

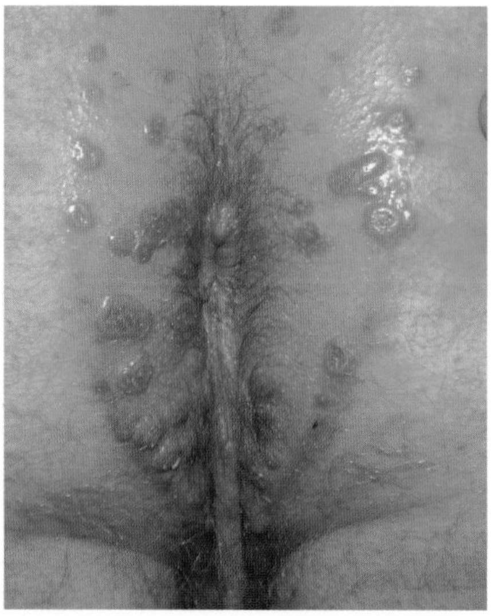

Fig. 9.49 *Condyloma latum* caused by secondary syphilis tends to occur in moist areas of the body and are particularly prevalent in the vulval and perianal areas.

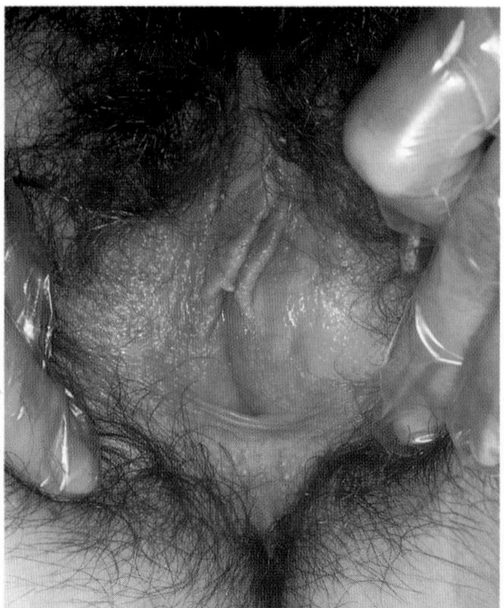

Fig. 9.50 Swelling of posterolateral perineum caused by Bartholin's abscess.

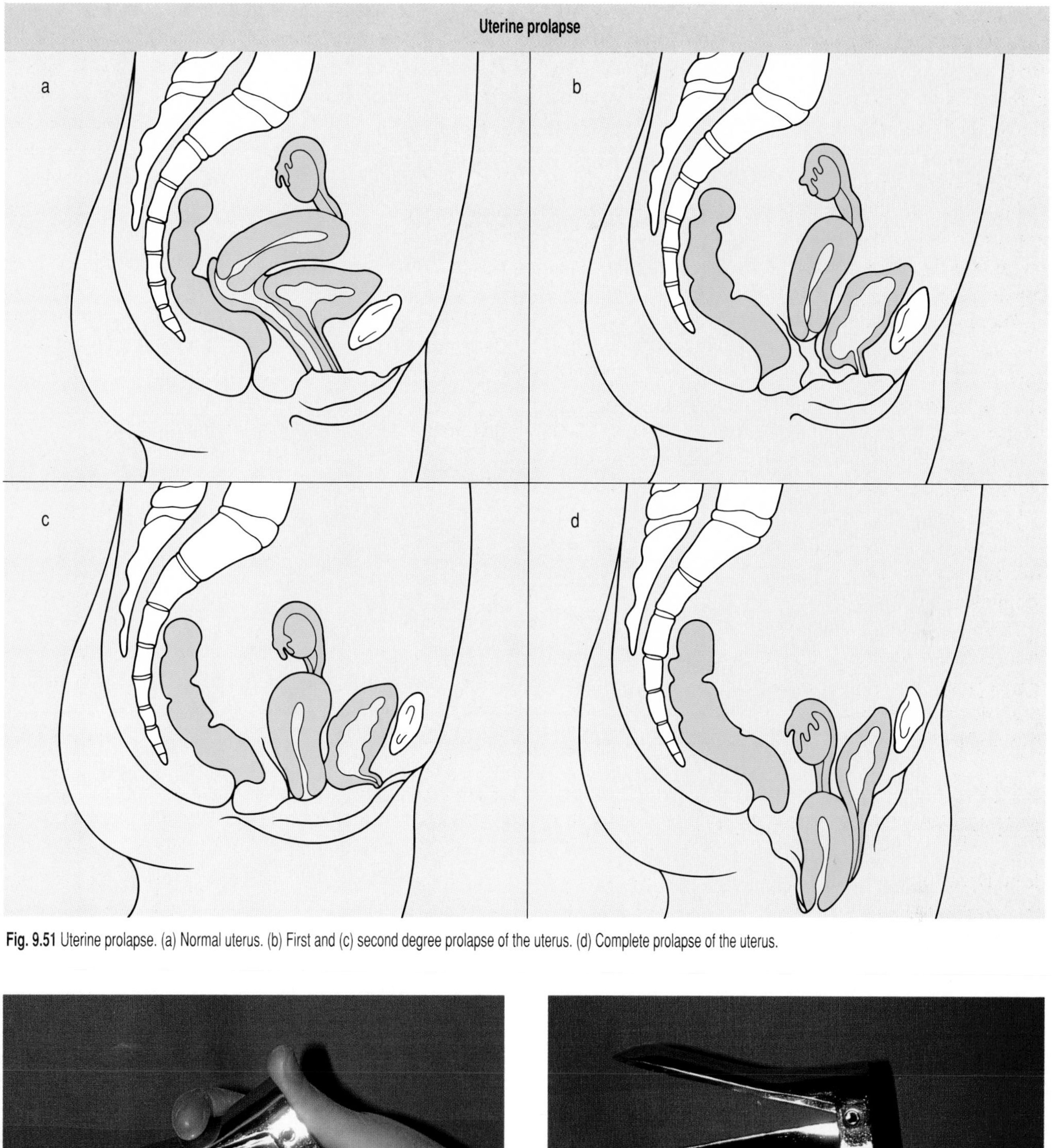

Fig. 9.51 Uterine prolapse. (a) Normal uterus. (b) First and (c) second degree prolapse of the uterus. (d) Complete prolapse of the uterus.

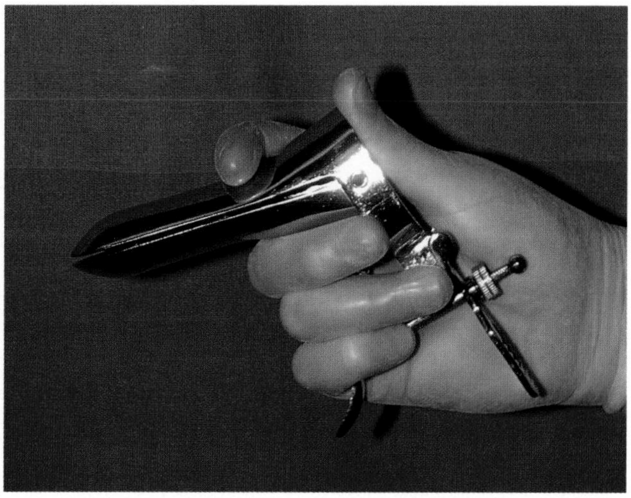

Fig. 9.52 A bivalve Cusco's speculum used for examining the vaginal walls and cervix.

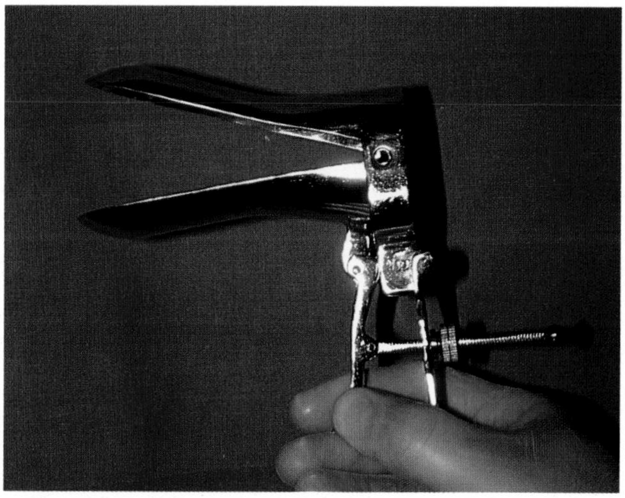

Fig. 9.53 Speculum held in the open position with a lock-nut.

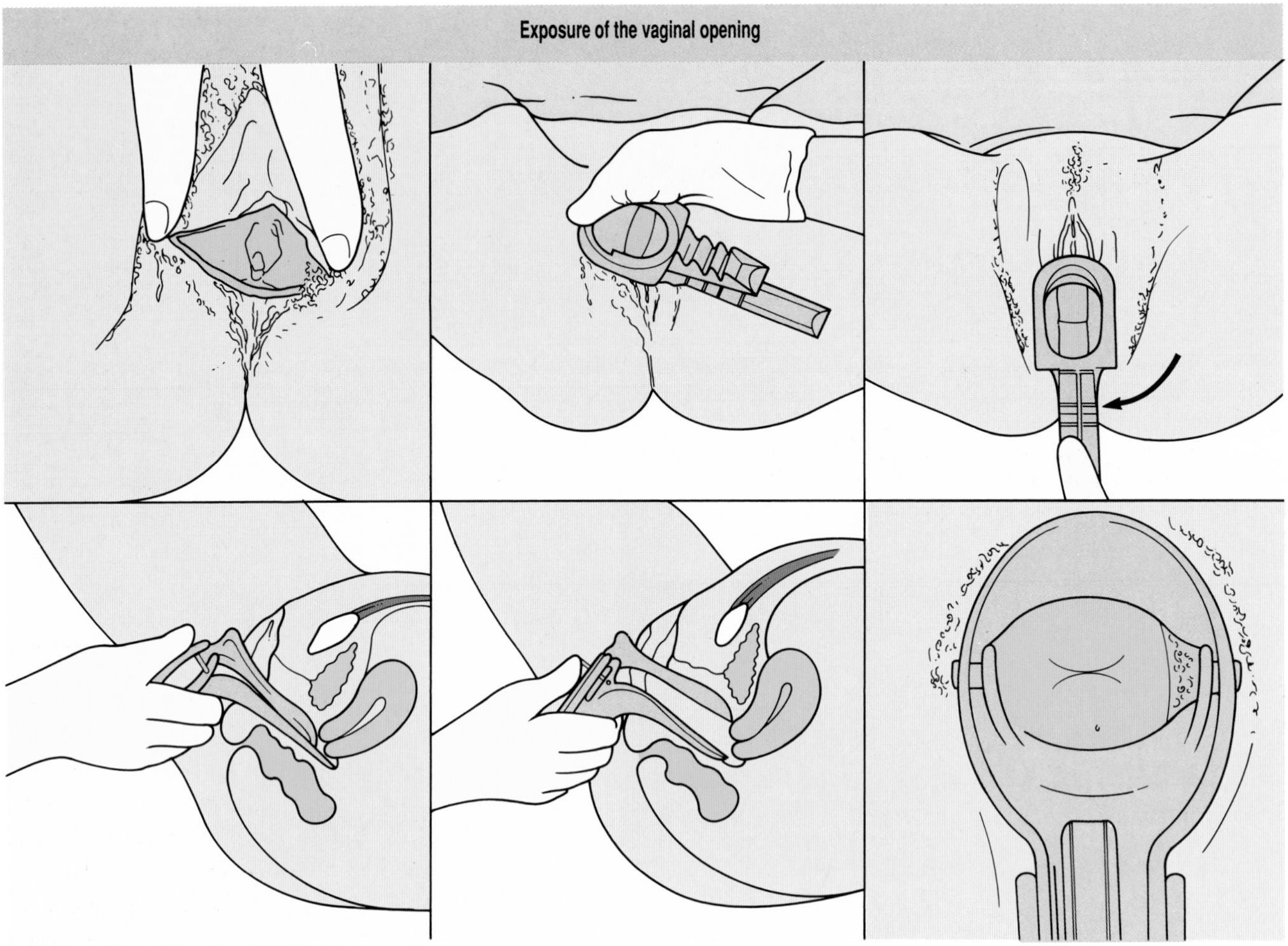

Fig. 9.54 (a) Exposing the vaginal opening; (b) direct the closed speculum into the vagina, (c) rotating it as it penetrates the long axis; and (d). The final position of the fully inserted speculum (e). Open the blades; (f) search for the cervix and os.

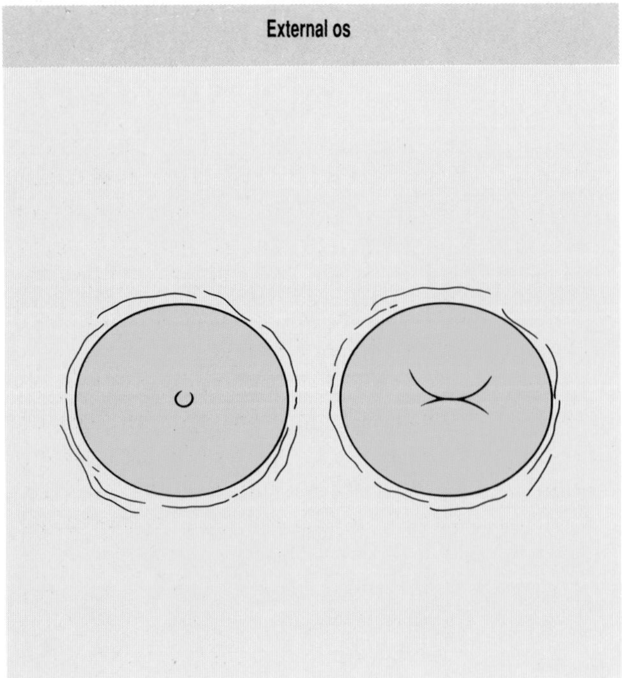

Fig. 9.55 In nulliparous women the external os is round (left); it becomes slit-shaped or stellate (right) after the birth of a child.

Warm the blades under a stream of tepid water. The most convenient hand position for holding the speculum is illustrated in Fig. 9.52. Explain to the patient that you are about to insert the instrument and reassure her that the procedure should be painless. Use the index and middle fingers of the free hand to separate the labia and expose the introitus (Fig. 9.54a). Position these two fingers just inside the introitus, pressing gently towards the perineal body. Slide the closed blades obliquely over the fingers into the introitus and introduce the instrument into the vagina, directing it to follow the line of the long axis of the vagina, maintaining a posterior angulation of about 45° (Fig. 9.54b). Whilst inserting the instrument, rotate it in a clockwise direction until the anterior and posterior blades run along the length of the anterior and posterior vaginal walls with the handles pointing towards the anus (Figs 9.54c and d). Maintain a downward pressure on the speculum and press on the thumbpiece to hinge the blades open (Fig. 9.52e) to expose the vaginal vault and cervix (Fig. 9.54f).

Adjust the light source to illuminate the vagina. If the cervix is not immediately visible, arc the blades anteriorly to bring the cervix into view. If you have difficulty finding the cervix, withdraw the blades a little and reposition the speculum in a more horizontal

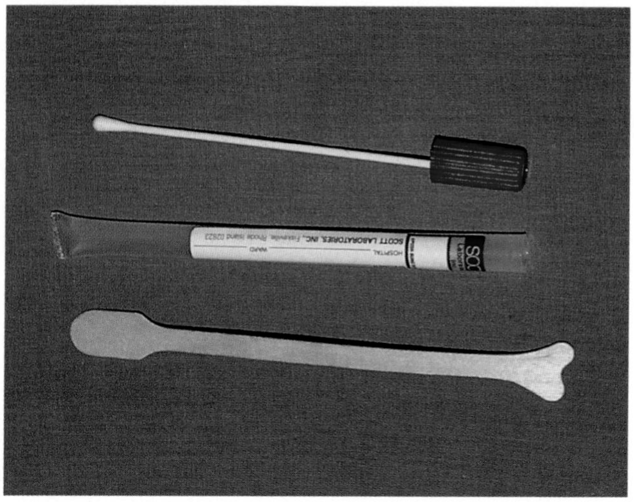

Fig. 9.56 Spatula with bifid end used for cervical cytology. Swab and transport medium for microbiology.

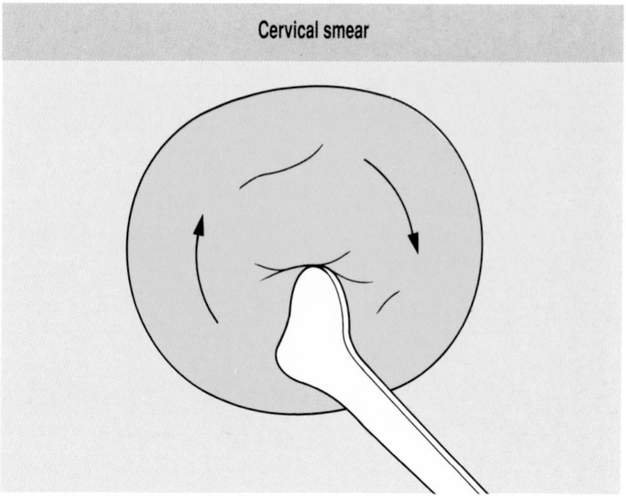

Fig. 9.57 Cervical meat. The bifid end of the spatula is advanced to the external os and the cervical cells are harvested by rotating the spatula around the circumference of the os.

plane. Make any minor adjustments necessary to establish the optimal position for visualizing the cervix, then tighten the thumbscrew to secure the position.

EXAMINATION OF THE CERVIX

The position of the cervix relates to the position of the uterus (see Fig. 9.32). The cervix usually points posteriorly and the uterus lies in an anterior plane (anteversion). Conversely, the cervix may point anteriorly with the uterus in a posterior retroverted position. There are also intermediate positions between these two. The cervix should lie centrally along the long axis of the vagina projecting 1–3cm into the vagina. The shape of the external os changes after childbirth. In nulliparous women, the os is round, whereas after childbirth, the os may be slit-like or stellate (Fig. 9.55).

Inspect the colour of the cervix. The colour varies according to the position of the meeting point, usually in the region of the external os, of the squamous epithelium covering the vaginal surface of the cervix and the mucosal lining of the cervical canal. The surface of the cervix is pink, smooth, and regular, and resembles the epithelium of the vagina. In early pregnancy the cervix has a bluish colour due to increased vascularity (Chadwick's sign). During pregnancy, the squamocolumnar junction may migrate beyond the external os and onto the cervix, retreating back, a few months after childbirth, into the cervical canal. Periodically, after pregnancy, the squamocolumnar junctions fail, to regress into the os giving the appearance of an erosion (ectopy). Failure to regress during foetal development may give rise to a congenital erosion. Cervical 'erosions' are not ulcerated surfaces, but a term used to describe the appearance of the cervix when the endocervical epithelium extends onto the outer surface of the cervix. The columnar epithelium appears as a strawberry-red area spreading circumferentially around the os or onto the anterior or posterior lips. Cervical ectopy cannot be confidently distinguished from early cervical cancer, so cytology should always be performed.

ABNORMALITIES OF THE CERVIX

An excentric cervix suggests disease of the uterus or the adnexae. Nabothian cysts may develop if there is obstruction of the endocervical glands. These are seen as small, round, raised white or yellow lesions which only assume importance if they become infected. There may be a cervical discharge. If there is a pungent odour, suspect an infective cause and swab the area. An inflamed cervix covered by a mucopurulent discharge or slough is characteristic of acute and chronic cervicitis; the mucosa looks red rather than pink and if the cervicitis follows pregnancy, you might notice laceration and pouting of the endocervical mucosa (ectropion). Cherry-red friable polyps may grow from the cervix (a source of vaginal bleeding after intercourse). Ulceration and fungating growths suggest cervical carcinoma.

The cervical smear

Cytologists can detect premalignant cells or established cervical cancer by examining a preparation of cells scraped from the surface of the cervix. The technique is routine in the course of the speculum examination. The demonstration of premalignant cells provides the opportunity for cancer prevention: the early detection of cancer allows for a higher, successful cure rate.

Before proceeding with the smear, prepare three clean glass microscope slides. Accurate labelling of the specimens is critical: slides with frosted glass at one end are preferable, for this allows you to write the patient's name and number clearly on the slide. Prepare the slide, mark with the patient's details, and label 'cervical smear'. Explain to the patient that you are about to take a smear. The cervical smear is performed after inspecting the cervix. A specially-designed disposable wooden spatula with a bifid end at one side and a rounded end at the other is used (Fig. 9.56). The bifid end is used to harvest the cervical cells. Introduce the spatula through the speculum and position the bifid end at the os (Fig. 9.57). The desquamating cells are collected by rotating the spatula around the circumference of the os and the lips of the cervix. Withdraw the spatula and spread the cervical material onto the labelled glass slide by stroking each side of the bifid end of the spatula along the glass. The cervical cells and some mucus should cling to the glass. Immediately spray the slides with fixative or fix them by immersion in 95 per cent alcohol.

Taking vaginal swabs

If the patient has a vaginal discharge, use the speculum examination to take a swab for culture. You can use a conventional throat swab; insert the cotton wool end into the secretion (e.g. the region of the cervical os and vaginal pool) and allow the tip sufficient time to soak up secretion. Remove the swab, place it in a suitable transport medium, and send the specimen immediately to the laboratory for processing.

Removing the speculum

After inspecting the cervix, undo the thumbscrew and simultaneously withdraw the speculum and rotate the open blades in an anticlockwise direction so that the anterior and posterior walls of the vagina can be inspected. Near the introitus, allow the blades to close taking care not to pinch the labia or any hairs whilst withdrawing the speculum.

INTERNAL EXAMINATION OF THE UTERUS

The speculum examination is followed by the vaginal examination. Explain that you are about to perform an internal examination of the uterus, tubes, and ovaries. Again, expose the introitus by separating the labia with the thumb and forefinger of the gloved left hand and gently introduce the gloved and lubricated right index and middle fingers into the vagina, remembering that the organ is directed backwards in the direction of the sacrum. The thumb is abducted to allow maximum use of the length of the index and middle fingers; the ring and little finger are flexed into the palm (Fig. 9.58). Palpate the vaginal wall as you introduce your fingers. The walls are slightly rugose, supple, and moist.

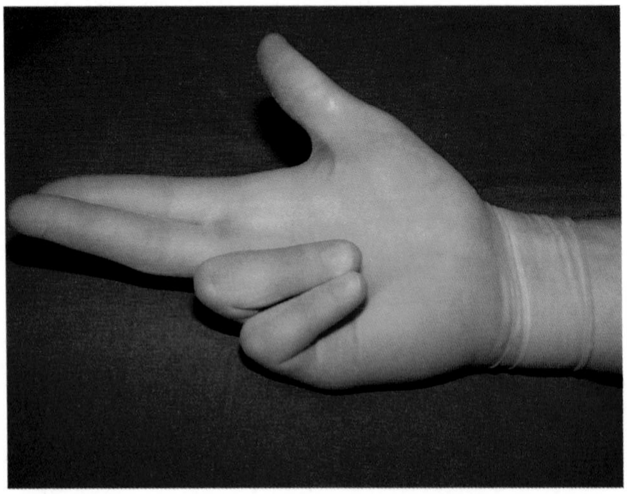

Fig. 9.58 The finger position used for performing a vaginal examination.

The cervix

Locate the cervix with the pulps of your fingertips. The cervix should feel firm, rounded, and smooth. Assess the mobility of the cervix by moving it gently and palpate the fornices. This procedure should be painless.

Abnormalities of the cervix

In pregnancy, the cervix softens (Hegar's sign). If there is tenderness on movement (known as 'excitation tenderness'), suspect infection or inflammation of the uterus or adnexae; or if the patient is shocked, suspect an ectopic pregnancy. You may palpate an ulcer or tumor already noted on the speculum examination.

The uterus

Next, palpate the uterus. A bimanual technique is used to assess the size and position of the organ (Fig. 9.59). Position the palmar

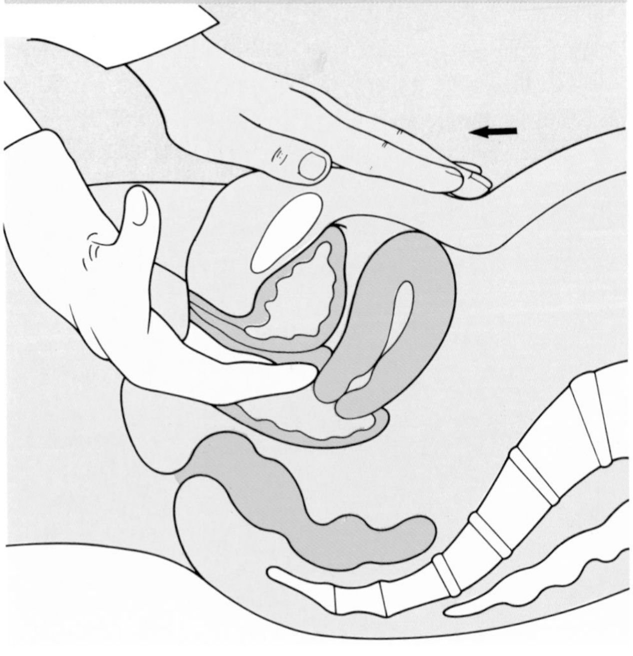

Fig. 9.59 By placing the vaginal fingers in the anterior fornix it is possible to examine the anterior surface of the uterus.

surface of your free hand on the anterior abdominal wall about 4cm above the symphysis pubis. Attempt to 'capture' the uterus gently between your apposing fingers. Use your internal fingers to elevate the cervix and uterus in the direction of the external hand whilst simultaneously pressing the fingertips of the external hand in the direction of the internal fingers. Using this displacement technique an anteverted fundus should be palpable just above the symphysis. Assess its size, consistency, and mobility, and note any masses and tenderness.

Further exploration may be helped by re-examining the uterus with your fingers positioned in the anterior fornix (Fig. 9.60); this permits the vaginal fingers to examine the anterior surface of the uterus whilst the abdominal fingers explore the posterior wall. If the uterus is retroverted, the fundus is more difficult to feel through the abdominal wall; nevertheless, it might become more readily palpable if the vaginal fingers are positioned in the posterior fornix.

Abnormalities of the uterus

If the uterus appears to be uniformly enlarged, consider a pregnancy, fibroid or endometrial tumor. Fibromyomas (fibroids) are common benign uterine tumors which may be single or multiple and may vary in size. Single, large uterine fibroids are felt on abdominal examination as a firm, non-tender, well-defined rounded mass arising from the pelvis. On bimanual palpation, the mass appears contiguous with the cervix: the two structures move together. Multiple fibroids give the uterus a lobulated feel. Occasionally, the fibroid is pedunculated and is felt as a mobile pelvic mass which is readily confused with a mass arising from the adnexae.

Examination of the adnexae

Palpate the left and right adnexae in turn. Note, the adnexae are difficult to palpate in obese women. Place the fingers of your abdominal hand over the iliac fossa whilst readjusting the vaginal fingers into the lateral fornix and positioning the finger pulps to face the abdominal fingers (Fig. 9.61). Remembering the anatomy of the ovaries and fallopian tubes, gently but firmly appose the fingers of either hand by pressing the abdominal hand inward and downward, and the vaginal fingers upwards and laterally. Feel for the adnexal structures as the interposed tissues slip between your fingers. The manouevre should be relatively painless, although palpation of the ovaries might elicit some tenderness. Yet again, reassure you patient that any discomfort she feels is normal. If you feel an adnexal structure, assess its size, shape, mobility, and tenderness. Ovaries are firm, ovoid, and often palpable. Normal fallopian tubes are impalpable.

Abnormalities of the adnexal structures

The most common causes of enlarged ovaries include benign cysts (e.g. follicular or corpus luteal cysts) and malignant ovarian tumors. Ovarian tumors are either unilateral or bilateral. Cysts feel smooth and the wall may be compressible. Occasionally, ovarian tumors are large enough to be palpable on abdominal examination and may fill the lower and mid- abdomen, creating the impression of ascites.

In acute infections of the fallopian tubes (salpingitis), there is lower abdominal tenderness and guarding, and on vaginal examination, marked tenderness of the lateral fornices and cervix. The

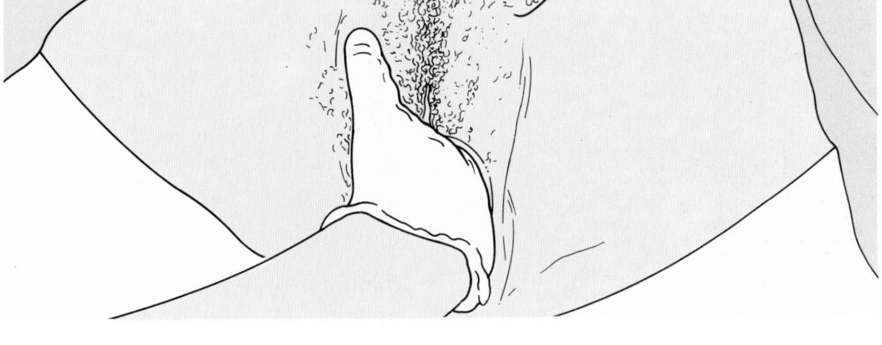

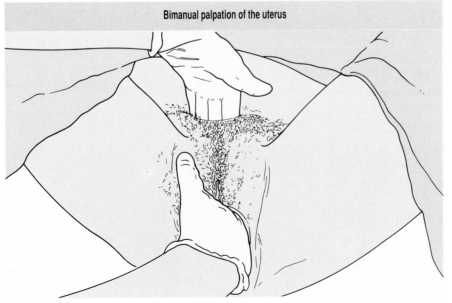

Fig. 9.60 The bimanual technique used to palpate the uterus. The vaginal fingers lift the cervix, whilst the abdominal hand dips downwards and inwards to meet the fundus.

acute pain makes palpation of the adnexae difficult. In chronic salpingitis, the lower abdomen and lateral fornices are tender, yet the uterus and adnexae may be amenable to examination. If the uterus is retroverted and fixed by adhesions, it may be possible to feel thickening and swelling of the tubes extending to the ovaries. If the tubes are blocked, there may be cystic swelling of the tubes (hydrosalpinx) or they may become infected and purulent (pyosalpinx).

After completing the bimanual examination, withdraw your fingers from the vagina and inspect the glove tips for blood or discharge. Redrape the genital area and reassure the patient that the examination is complete and that you will discuss the findings in the consulting room once she is dressed.

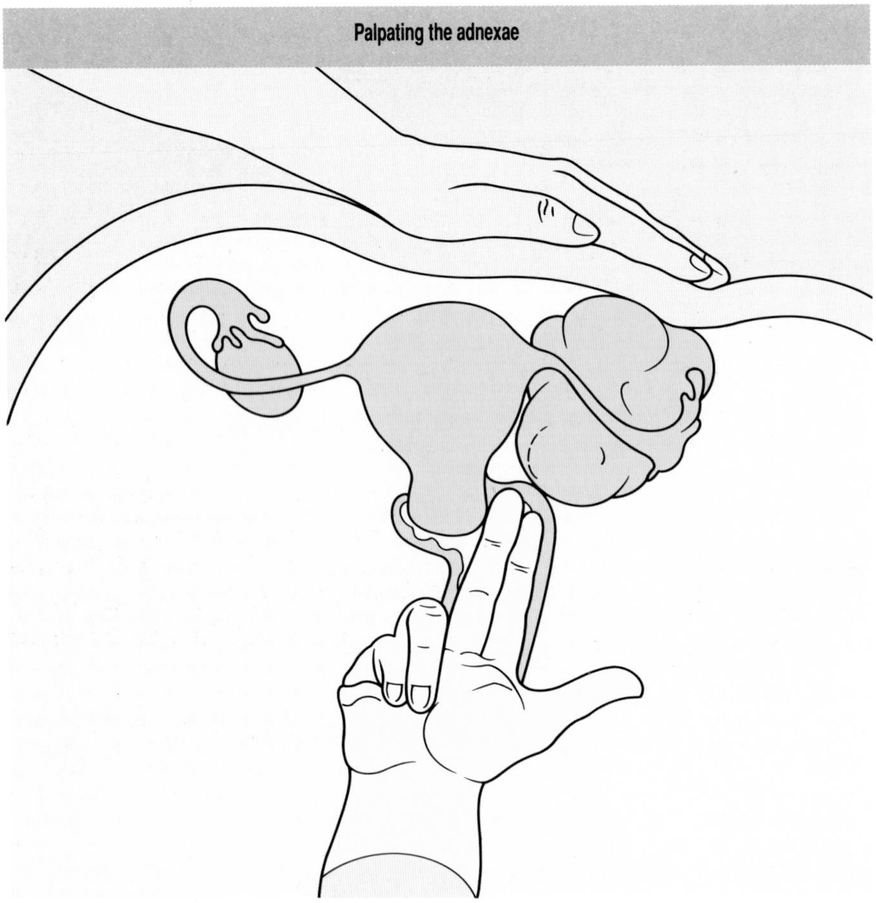

Fig. 9.61 Positioning the vaginal and abdominal fingers to palpate the adnexal structures.

Unlike the female genitalia, the male organs are readily accessible for examination. As is the case for women, taking a sexual case history and examining a male is embarrassing and intrusive, so care must be taken to ensure confidentiality, privacy, and comfort. An overview of structure and function will help you gain confidence when taking a history and examining the genitalia and will aid the interpretation of symptoms and signs.

STRUCTURE AND FUNCTION

The male genitalia includes the penis, scrotum, testes, epididymides, seminal vesicles, and prostate gland (Fig. 10.1). The penis provides a common pathway to the exterior for both urine and semen. In foetal development, the testes develop close to the kidneys and slowly migrate caudally, emerging at the external inguinal ring in the 8th month of development, and descending into the scrotum in the 9th month. The neural, vascular, and lymphatic supply to the testes also arises from near the kidney, and the migrating testes drag these structures through the inguinal canal into the scrotum. This has important clinical implications as renal pain is often referred to the scrotum and the natural route for lymphatic spread of testicular cancer is to para-aortic (rather than inguinal) nodes.

PUBERTY

In boys, puberty starts 1–2 years later than in girls. The onset of male puberty is signalled by an increase in testicular volume and this is followed about a year later by a spurt in linear growth and an increase in muscle bulk.

Hormonal changes in puberty

Testosterone feedback on the hypothalamus can inhibit the hypothalamo-pituitary axis release of luteinizing hormone (LH) and follicle-stimulating hormone (FSH). In the child, this feedback is especially sensitive and even low levels of circulating gonadal steroids are sufficient to inhibit secretion of FSH and LH. Male puberty is initiated by a fall in the sensitivity of the hypothalamus to inhibition at low levels of circulating sex hormones. By resetting the sensitivity of the feedback on hypothalamus, FSH and LH are released, thereby exerting their trophic effects on their target cells in the testes.

Throughout male puberty, LH levels increase slowly and steadily (Fig. 10.2), whereas FSH levels increase more sharply in early puberty, with a more gentle increase afterwards. FSH stimulates the Sertoli cells, regulates the growth of seminiferous tubules, and spermatogenesis. As most of the testis is formed of tubules, the

Anatomy of the male genitalia

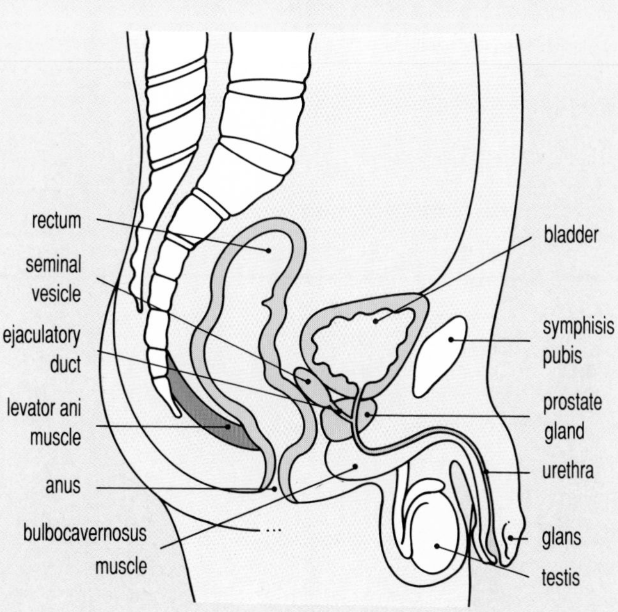

Fig. 10.1 The male genitalia includes the external organs, the seminal vesicles, and the prostate gland.

Developmental changes in LH and FSH

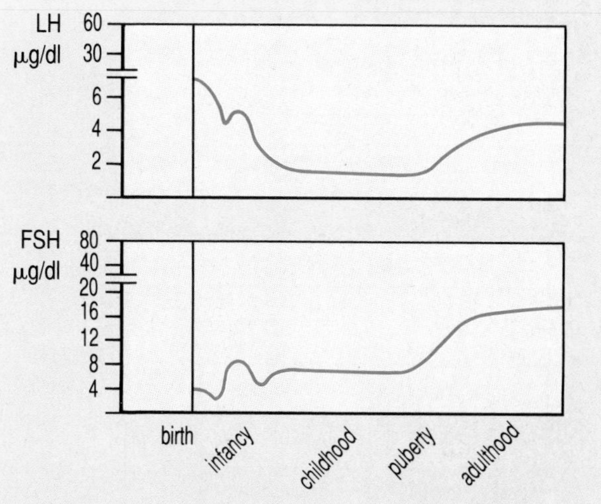

Fig. 10.2 Changes in FSH and LH secretion before, during, and after puberty.

increased testicular volume in puberty is largely under the control of FSH. LH stimulates the Leydig (interstitial) cells which synthesize testosterone from cholesterol (Fig. 10.3). Testosterone circulates bound to sex hormone binding globulin (SHBG). The linear growth spurt follows closely behind the surge of testosterone (Fig. 10.4). Some testosterone is converted to oestrodiol in the Leydig cells and other extra gonadal tissue sites. The importance of oestrogen in males remains unclear, although it does regulate the synthesis of SHBG.

Testosterone synthesis

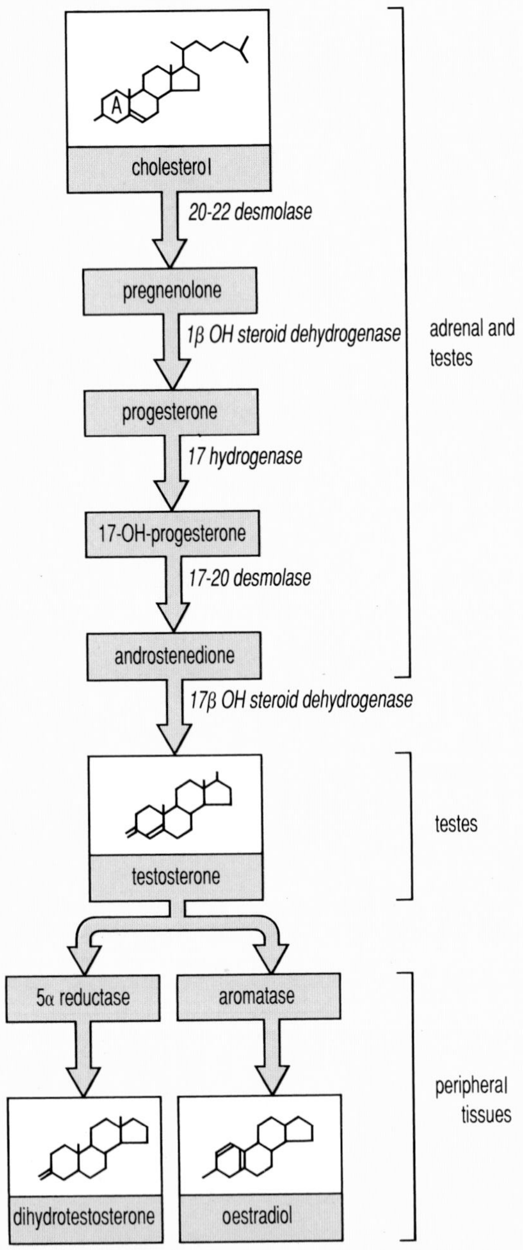

Fig. 10.3 Biochemical pathway in the synthesis of testosterone from cholesterol.

Development of secondary sexual development

Tanner has described the pubertal development of the male genitalia and pubic hair growth (Fig. 10.5). Initially the testes

Effects of testosterone

Stimulates the development of secondary sexual characteristics

Controls libido

Anabolic effect causes muscle growth and fat deposition

With growth hormone, stimulates linear growth in adolescence

With erythropoietin, stimulates red cell production

Fig. 10.4 The effects of testosterone.

Genital maturation in puberty

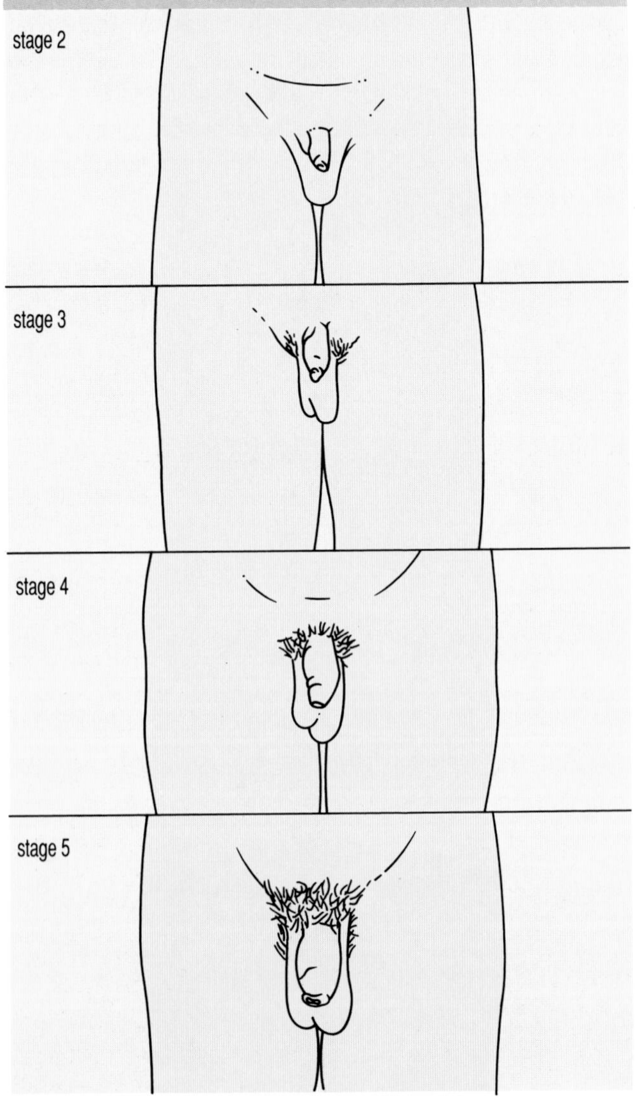

Fig. 10.5 Tanner's 5 stages of male genital maturation. Stage 1 preadolescent (not shown).

enlarge and the scrotal skin becomes thin and red (Stage 2). The enlargement of the phallus occurs later in the growth spurt and is associated with thickening, crinkling, and pigmentation of the scrotal skin (3). Increasing levels of gonadal and adrenal androgens stimulate the growth of pubic, axillary, and facial hair. Pubic hair begins to develope as sparse, long, slightly curly hair at the base of the phallus (4). Later, coarser, curlier hair extends to cover the symphysis pubis and finally extends to the inner thigh and along the linea alba (this constitutes the male escatcheon) (5).

Male fertility

The male testis is composed of a network of tightly-coiled and convoluted seminiferous tubules which drain through the rete testis into the epididymis. Spermatazoa develop from the germinal epithelium of the seminiferous tubules which lie in close contact with the Leydig and Sertoli cells (Fig. 10.6). LH binds to the Leydig cells, stimulating the production of testosterone from cholesterol. FSH binds to the Sertoli cells, stimulating the synthesis of inhibin, a peptide hormone which inhibits FSH production by the pituitary (Fig. 10.6). The development from immature spermatogonium to mature spermatozoa takes 72 days. The passage of the sperm through the epididymis to the ejaculatory ducts takes a further 14 days, during which time the spermatozoa become motile.

Spermatogenesis occurs most efficiently when the ambient testicular temperature is 36°C. The smooth muscle of the scrotum and spermatic cord alters the position of the testicles in relation to the external inguinal ring to maintain (under various conditions of heat and cold) an optimal temperature for spermatogenesis.

THE PENIS

The penis consists of the two spongelike cylinders: the corpora cavernosa forming the dorsal and lateral surfaces; and the corpus spongiosum which ends in a bulbous expansion, the glans penis (Fig. 10.8). The urethra passes through the corpus spongiosum. The skin covering the corpora extends over the glans to form the prepuce.

Tactile and psychogenic stimuli cause sexual arousal. An autonomic (parasympathetic) reflex causes increased arterial flow through branches of the pudendal artery to the penis and fills the

The hypothalamo-pituitary-gonadal axis

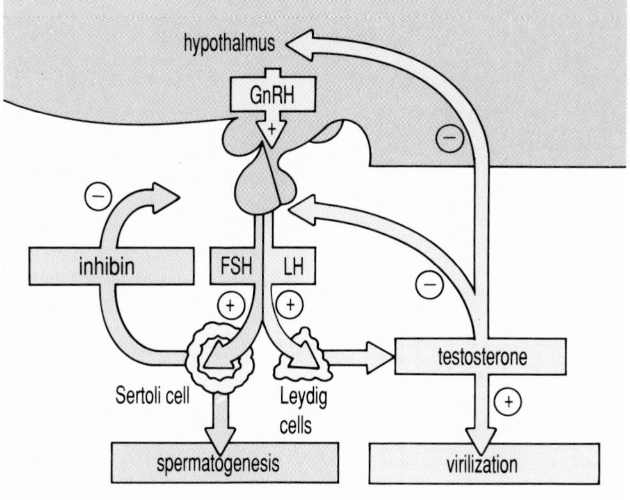

Fig. 10.6 The hypothalamo-pituitary-testicular axis. Pulsatile release of GnRH stimulates the anterior pituitary to secrete LH and FSH which stimulate the Leydig and Sertoli cells, respectively.

Histology of the testis

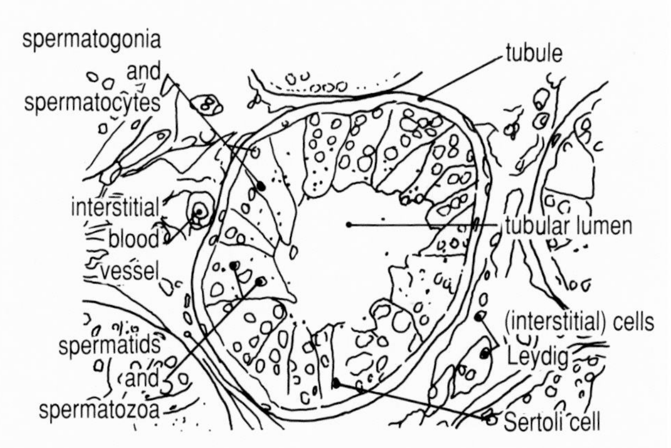

Fig. 10.7 Diagrammatic histological section through a testis showing seminiferous tubules, developing sperm. Leydig and Sertoli cells.

Anatomy of the penis

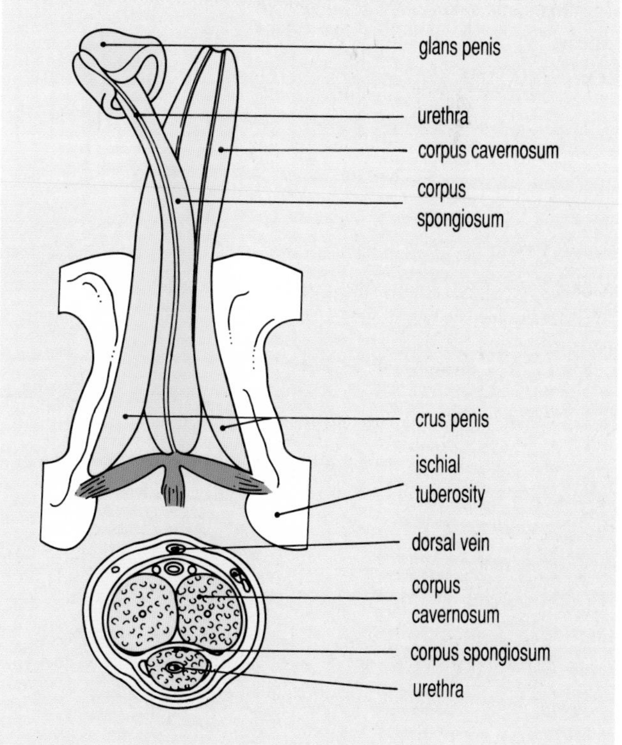

Fig. 10.8 The shaft and glans penis is formed from (a) the corpus spongiosum and (b) the corpus cavernosum.

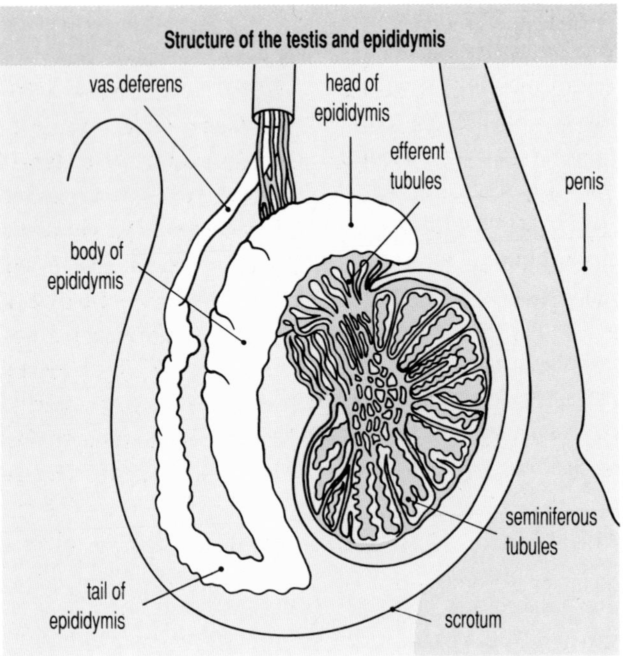

Fig. 10.9 Schematic coronal section through the testis showing the seminiferous tubules of the testis converging to form the efferent tubules which then give rise to the head, body, and tail of the epididymis and vas deferens.

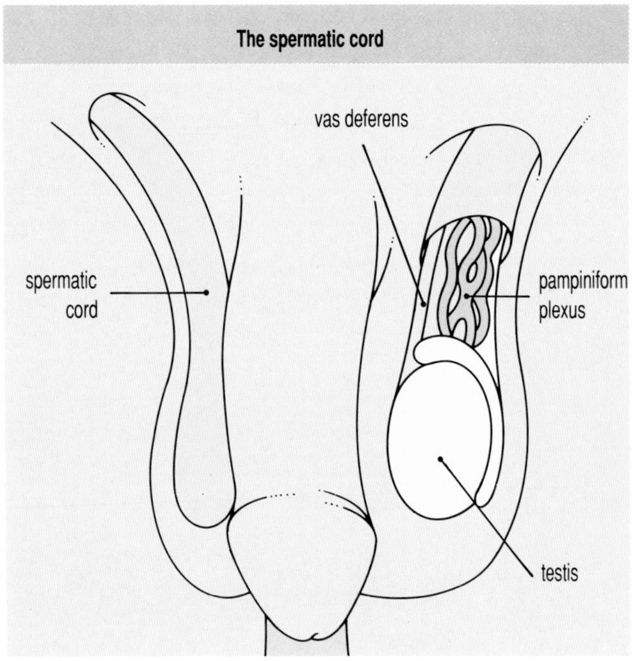

Fig. 10.10 The vas deferens passes into the inguinal canal as the spermatic cord which then converges on the seminal vesicles. The pampiniform vascular plexus surrounds the spermatic cord.

corpora spongiosum. The organ assumes the erectile position necessary for vaginal penetration. The reflex is completed by a sympathetic neural outflow which results in contraction of the ejaculatory ducts and the bladder neck, causing ejaculation of semen and orgasm. This is followed by increased tone in the arterioles and sinusoids of the corpora, diversion of blood away from the penis, and finally detumscence.

THE SCROTUM AND ITS CONTENTS

Before attempting to examine the testis and epididymis, it is important to understand the structure of these organs. The scrotum is a muscular pouch which holds the testes. A septum separates the left and right testicles. The scrotal skin is thin, pigmented, and crinkled, and lined by the dartos muscle. This permits considerable contraction and relaxation of the scrotum which helps keep the optimal temperature for spermatogenesis.

The left testis almost always lies lower than the right. Each testis is ovoid in shape, measuring approximately 4x3x2cm. A fibrous capsule, the tunica albuginea, invests the testis. The seminiferous tubules converge and anastomose posteriorly to form the efferent tubules which converge to form the head of the epididymis (Fig. 10.9). This, in turn, gives rise to the body and tail which drain into the vas deferens. The vas deferens passes through the inguinal canal (Fig. 10.10), joining the seminal vesicles which, in turn, converge to form the ejaculatory duct. The epididymis attaches along the posterior border and upper pole of the testis. Both the testis and the epididymis have vestigeal remnants of foetal development known as the appendix testis and hydatid of Morgagni, respectively. These occasionally twist and can cause severe testicular pain.

Lymphatics from the penile and scrotal skin drain to the inguinal nodes. Examination of the groin nodes is an integral part of the genital examination, especially if there is an ulcer or discharge.

THE PROSTATE

The structure of the prostate is described in Chapter 8. The organ envelops the first part of the urethra and the ejaculatory ducts from the seminal vesicles which open into the prostatic urethra. The prostates secretes a specialized fluid which provides lubrication prior to intercourse and serves also to increase the volume of the ejaculate.

SYMPTOMS OF GENITAL TRACT DISEASE

Like women, men may choose either to express their symptoms openly or to expose the problem in a less obvious manner. Moreover, the doctor may feel embarrassed to broach the sensitive issues of sexual orientation, sexual function, venereal disease, and the possible exposure to the human immunodeficiency virus (HIV). Learn to ask direct questions with sensitivity whilst maintaining the firm impression that you are both confident and decisive when talking about what is, after all, another normal bodily function.

At the outset of your history-taking, you will already have ascertained whether the patient is single or married and if he has fathered any children. The genital and sexual history follows on most naturally from the urinary tract history (see Chapter 8). Ask about penile discharge, pain or swelling of the testes, and his ability to enjoy normal sexual relations. These questions should provide the cue for a shy or inhibited patient to talk about sexual or genital problems. Depending on the nature of the presenting symptoms you may wish to ask about homosexual contact. You may feel uneasy about phrasing the question, but in societies where acquired immune deficiency syndrome (AIDS) is acknowledged as a problem, the majority of patients understand the importance of the question and most often will not take offence to a question like "have you ever had a homosexual partner?" or "do you practice safe sex?" If a genital or sexual symptom becomes apparent, assure the patient of the confidentiality of the interview and attempt to analyze the problem in greater depth.

Urethral discharge

Is there a possibility of recent exposure to a sexually transmitted disease?

How long ago might you have had such a contact (incubation period)?

Does you partner complain of a vaginal discharge?

Have you experienced joint pains or gritty, red eyes?

Have you recently suffered from gastroenteritis?

Causes of urethral discharge

PHYSIOLOGICAL - Sexual arousal

PATHOLOGICAL

- Gonococcal urethritis
- Non-gonococcal urethritis
- *Chlamydia trachomatis*
- *Trichomonas vaginalis*
- Candida
- Idiopathic non-specific urethritis
- Post-urinary catheter
- Reiter's syndrome may follow gastroenteritis, arthritis (large joints and sacro-iliacs), and conjunctivitis

Fig. 10.11 Causes of urethral discharge.

Urethral discharge

A urethral discharge is a common presenting symptom (Fig. 10.11). Remember that a discharge of smegma from a normal prepuce is quite different from a discharge caused by urethritis. In urethritis, the patient may notice staining of his underwear and complain of urinary symptoms such as burning or stinging when passing urine. Venereal disease is a common cause of urethral discharge and patients concerned about sexually transmitted disease will usually mention the fear of venereal disease. If this information is not forthcoming, ask the patient directly about the possibilty of contact with venereal disease. Ask about a recent episode of gastroenteritis, for urethritis may follow a few weeks later. Reiter's syndrome (Fig 10.12) is the most florid manifestation of this association and is characterized by a urethral discharge, balanitis, painful joints (arthritis and tendinitis), bilateral conjunctivitis, which often follow an attack of gastroenteritis.

Genital ulcers

The appearance of an ulcer or 'sore' always raises the spectre of venereal disease; consequently, this possibility is likely to alarm your patient even though ulcers are not always caused by sexual transmission. Enquire discreetly about possible contact with venereal disease or casual sexual encounters. Ask whether the ulcer is painful and try to assess a possible incubation period. Herpetic ulcers tend to recur and may be preceded by a prodrome of a prickly sensation or pain in the loins. There may be a clear history of contact with a partner infected with herpes, and sexual transmission may affect the mouth or anus as well as the penis. Exotic ulcerating venereal infections occur in the tropics and it is important to obtain a careful history of foreign travel, and also possible sexual contact.

Testicular pain

Was the pain preceded by trauma?

How rapidly did the pain develop?

Was the pain preceded by a fever or swelling of the salivary glands (mumps)?

Was the pain preceded by burning on micturition or a urethral discharge?

Testicular pain

Inflammation or trauma to the testes causes an intense visceral pain which may radiate towards the groin and abdomen. Testicular pain has a deep boring quality often accompanied by nausea. The pain may be accompanied by swelling and aggravated by movement and even light palpation. The commonest causes are trauma, infection (orchitis), and torsion. Painless swelling of the testis should alert you to the possibility of a cystic lesion or a malignancy.

Impotence

This term refers to a spectrum of sexual dysfuction ranging from loss of libido, failure to obtain or to maintain an erection, and/or inability to achieve orgasm. Impotence is often a manifestation of emotional disturbance; therefore, you should try to assess whether the patient is depressed, anxious about sexual encounters, or troubled by emotional aspects of the relationship. Fear of pregnancy and concern about a disease such as AIDS may serve to cause impotence. Take a careful drug and alcohol history; alcoholism is an important cause of impotence and many widely prescribed drugs are associated with impotence (Fig. 10.13). An obvious association with organic disease may be apparent in patients presenting with concomitant cardiovascular, respiratory, or neurological symptoms.

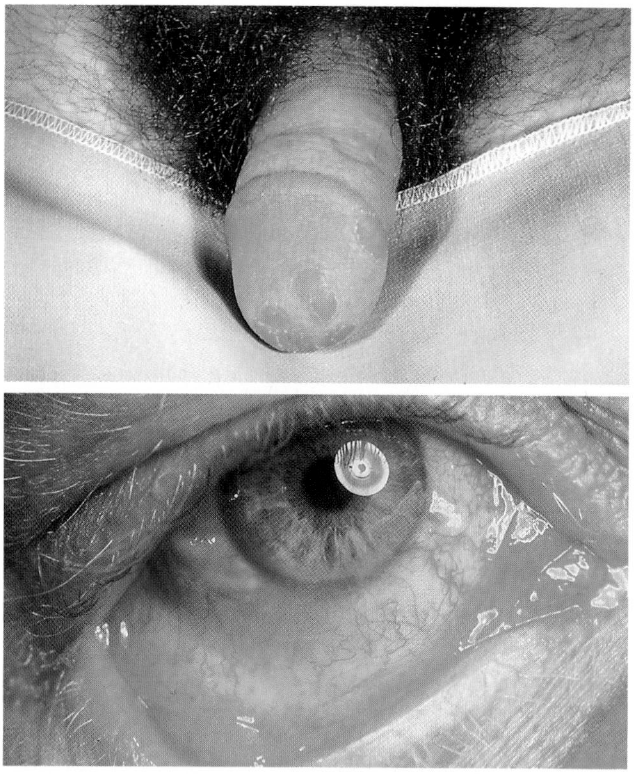

Fig. 10.12 Reiter's syndrome is characterized by (above) circinate balanitis and (below) conjunctivitis.

Infertility

Have you or your partner ever conceived?

Do you have difficulty obtaining or maintaining an erection?

Do you ejaculate?

Do you understand the timing of ovulation in your partner?

Are you on any medication which may cause impotence or sperm malfunction (e.g. salazopyrine)?

Have you noticed any change in facial hair growth?

Have you ever had cancer treatment?

Infertility

Primary infertility refers to a failure to achieve conception, whereas secondary infertility refers to a difficulty or a failure to conceive although there has been at least one successful conception in the past. Male infertility accounts for about one third of childless relationships; consequently, both partners are evaluated when couples present with infertilty. Ask about the duration of infertility and whether the patient has ever managed to conceive. Because many couples have little understanding of the timing of ovulation and conception, you should enquire into some depth about frequency and timing of intercourse and about attempts to time intercourse to coincide with the female partner's fertile period. Ask about drugs, as antimetabolites used in cancer treatment or sulphasalazine used in colitis may cause subfertility.

EXAMINATION OF THE MALE GENITALIA

This examination usually follows the abdominal examination and you will already have approached the area when examining the groin and hernial orifices. Although a detailed genital examination is usually only undertaken when the patient complains of appropriate symptoms, it is advisable to check the testes in the course of a routine examination as 'opportunistic screening' may occasionally reveal a testicular tumor. Explain that you would like to examine the penis and testes and offer reassurance that the examination will be quick and gentle. Like any other examination, your confidence, or lack of it, soon becomes apparent to the patient. If you have a good grasp of the anatomy and physiology outlined above, you will soon master a quick but thorough examination. It is advisable for women doctors to examine the genitalia with a chaperone close at hand.

Drugs associated with impotence
Major tranquilizers (phenothiazines)
Lithium
Sedatives (barbituates, benzodiazepines)
Antihypertensives (methyldopa, debrisoquine, clonidine)
Alcohol
Oestrogens
Drug abuse (heroin, methadone)

Fig. 10.13 Drugs associated with impotence.

Causes of male gynaecomastia
Physiological
Puberty
Old age
Hypogonadism
Liver cirrhosis
Drugs (spironolactone, digoxin, oestrogens)
Tumors (bronchogenic carcinoma, adrenal carcinoma, testicular tumors)
Thyrotoxicosis

Fig. 10.15 Causes of male gynaecomastia.

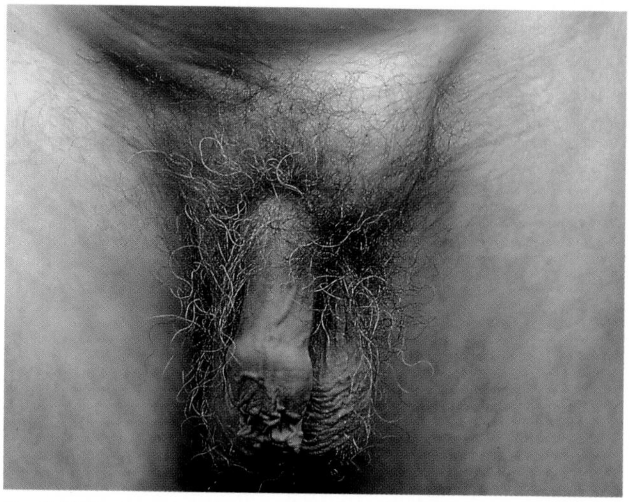

Fig. 10.14 Hernias may only become apparant when the patient stands.

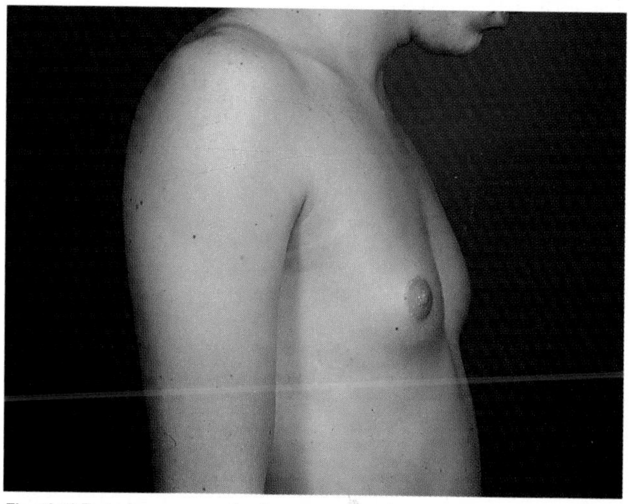

Fig. 10.16 Typical appearance of male gynaecomastasia.

It is usual practice to wear disposable plastic gloves for hygienic reasons and to emphasize the strictly clinical nature of the examination. The genitalia are usually examined with the patient lying but remember that varicoceles and scrotal hernias may only be apparent when the patient stands and it is advisable to check for scrotal swellings in the standing position if the diagnosis is unclear with the patient lying (Fig. 10.14). Avoid a feeling of total nakedness by maintaining some cover of the thighs.

THE GENERAL EXAMINATION

You will already have performed a general examination and noted the distribution of facial, axillary, and abdominal hair. In testicular malfunction (hypogonadism), there may be loss of axillary hair, the pubic hair distribution might start to resemble the distinctive female pattern, and there is a typical facial appearance with wrinkling around the mouth. You will have also checked the breast and noted whether or not gynaecomastia was evident (Figs 10.15 and 10.16).

The normal penis

The length and thickness of the flaccid penis vary widely and bear no relationship either to potency or to fertility. The dorsal vein of the penis is usually prominent along the dorsal midline. Gently retract the foreskin (prepuce) to expose the glans penis. The foreskin should be supple, allowing smooth and painless retraction. There is often a trace of odourless, curd-like smegma underlying the foreskin. Examine the external urethral meatus which is a slit-like orifice extending from the ventral pole of the tip of the glans. Use your index finger and thumb to squeeze the meatus gently open. This should expose healthy, glistening pink mucosa. If the patient has complained of a urethral discharge, try to elicit this sign. The patient may be able to 'milk' the shaft of the penis to express the secretion; if not, you may try to express a discharge by 'milking' the shaft of the penis from the base towards the glans. If you demonstrate a discharge, swab the area with a sterile bud and immerse the specimen in a transport medium for quick despatch to the microbiology laboratory.

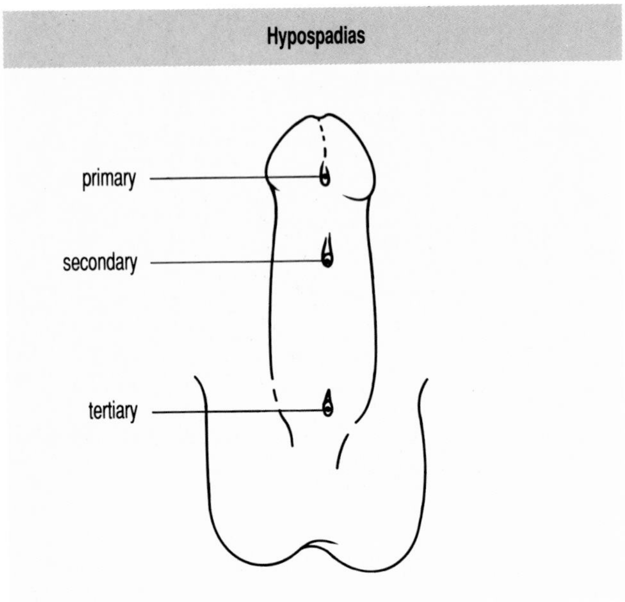

Fig. 10.17 Hypospadias, a developmental abnormality. The urethral meatus opens on the ventral surface of the penis..

Causes of genital ulcers

Infections	genital herpes syphilis (chancre, mucous patches, gumma) tropical ulcers
Balanitis	severe candida circinate balanitis (Reiter's syndrome)
Drug eruption	localized fixed drug eruption generalized (Stevens–Johnson syndrome)
Carcinoma	
Behcet's syndrome	

Fig. 10.18 Causes of genital ulcers.

ABNORMALITIES OF THE PENIS

The prepuce

The prepuce may be too tight to retract over the glans (phimosis). If the prepuce is tight but retracts and catches behind the glans, oedema and swelling may occur, preventing the return of the foreskin (paraphimosis). If left untreated, the swelling and congestion may result in gangrene.

The glans

Hypospadias (Fig. 10.17) is a developmental abnormality causing the urethral meatus to appear on the inferior (ventral) surface of the glans (primary hypospadias), penis (secondary hypospadias) or even the perineum (tertiary hypospadias). Inflammation of the glans is termed balanitis (Fig. 10.12); if there is inflammation of the glans and prepuce, the term balanoposthitis is used. Genital (herpetic) warts may be seen on the glans.

Urethral discharge

This is one of the commonest genital disorders in men and is caused by urethral inflammation (urethritis). The cause of a urethral discharge cannot be confidently predicted from appearance, though gonorrhoea is likely to cause a profuse purulent discharge. Non-gonococcal urethritis may also be caused by urethral infection or associated with Reiter's syndrome

Penile ulcers

Ulceration of the glans or, more rarely, the shaft of the penis may occur in a number of disorders. Examine the ulcer and always palpate the groins for inguinal lymph node involvement, as the skin of the penis drains to this group of nodes. The commonest cause is herpetic ulceration (Fig. 10.18). Characteristic painless vesicles occur 4–5 days after sexual contact (Fig. 10.19). The vesicles often rupture, causing painful superficial erosions with a characteristic erythematous halo. The confluence of these erosions may cause discreet ulcers which can become secondarily infected. The urethral meatus may be affected, thus causing dysuria. If there is a possible history of venereal disease, consider syphilis (primary chancre) (Fig. 10.20), and in the tropics consider chancroid,

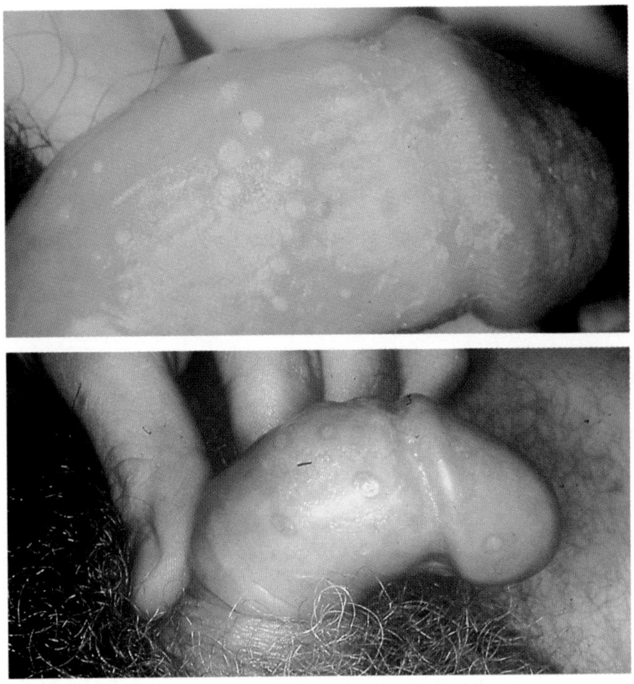

Fig. 10.19 After 4–5 days incubation, a crop of relatively painless herpetic vesicles appear on the penis (upper). Vesicles rupture with the development of painful superficial erosions with a characteristic erythematous halo (lower).

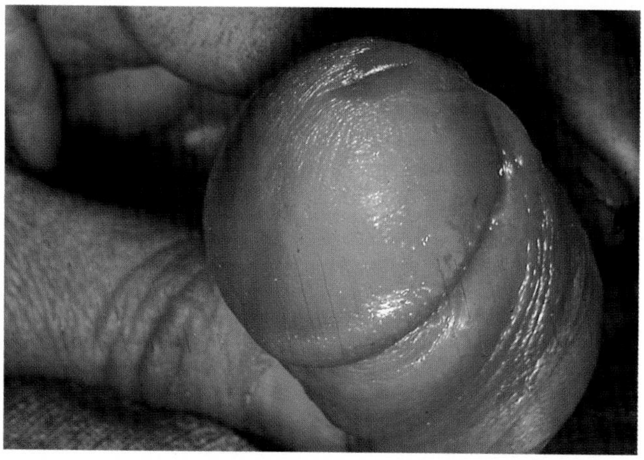

Fig. 10.20 The primary chancre of syphilis may occur on the glans, prepuce, or shaft.

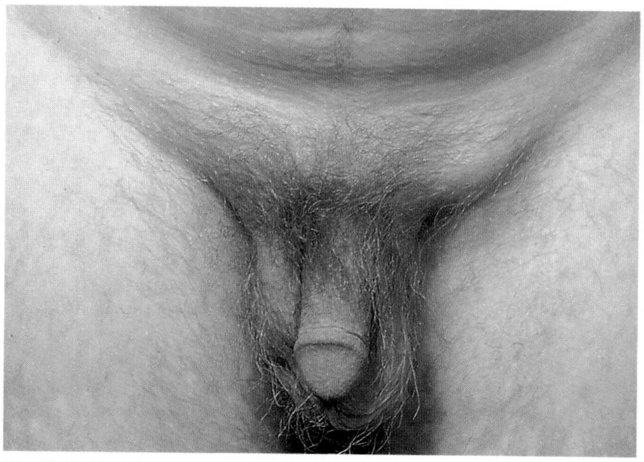

Fig. 10.21 The left testis lies lower than the right.

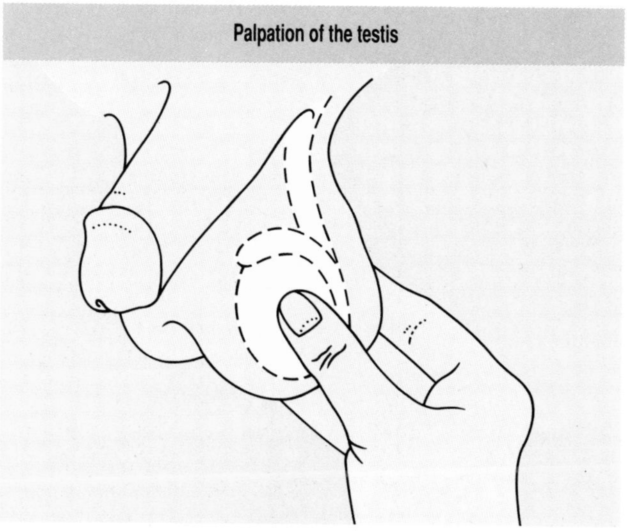

Fig. 10.22 Palpate the testis between your thumb and first two fingers.

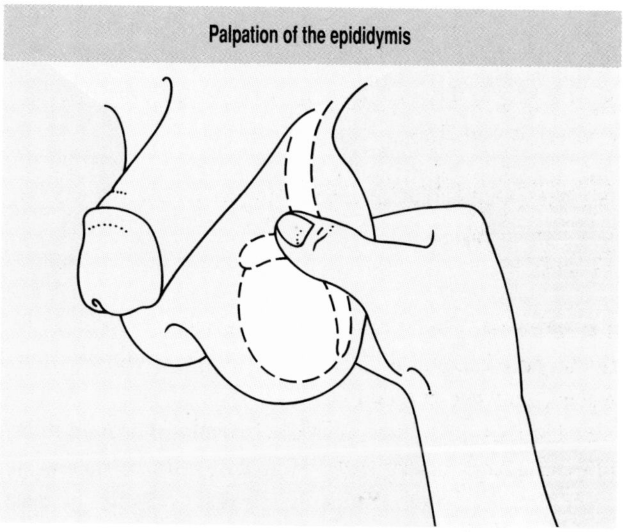

Fig. 10.23 The epididymis is felt along the posterior pole of the testis.

lymphogranuloma venereum and granuloma inguinale. Infrequently, fixed drug reactions may cause penile ulceration. Squamous cell carcinoma may present as an ulcer of the penis or the scrotum.

Priapism

Occasionally, a patient may present with a painful and prolonged erection. This pathological erection is termed priapism. Most often, there is no obvious cause, but predisposing factors such as leukaemia, haemoglobinopathies (e.g. sickle cell anaemia), and drugs (aphrodisiacs) should be considered.

EXAMINATION OF THE SCROTUM

Inspect the scrotal skin which is pigmented when compared to body skin. The left testis lies lower than the right, but the impression of both testes is readily identified (Fig. 10.21). The tone of the dartos muscle is influenced by ambient temperature; consequently, the normal scrotal appearance varies with temperature.

Ensure that your hands are warm before palpating the testis. Use gentle pressure, sufficient to explore the bulk of the tissue without causing pain. Throughout the examination, watch the patient's facial expression, for this should reassure you that the examination is not causing undue discomfort. Compare the left and right testes as many testicular disorders are unilateral. Feel the testicle between your thumb and first two fingers (Fig. 10.22). Note the size and consistency of the testis. The organ has a pliant, soft-rubbery consistency and there should not be much tenderness. Next, palpate the epididymis which is felt as an elongated structure along the posterolateral surface of the testicle (Fig. 10.23). The epididymis normally feels smooth and is broadest superiorly, at its head.

Finally, roll with the finger and thumb the vas deferens which passes from the tail of the epididymis to the inguinal canal through the external inguinal canal. This strucure is smooth and non-tender, and is felt leading from the epididymis to the external inguinal ring.

ABNORMALITIES OF THE SCROTUM

The scrotum

If one half of the scrotum appears smooth and poorly developed, consider an undescended testis (cryptorchidism). This appearance of the scrotum helps to distinguish a maldescent from a retractile testis, where the testis has descended but retracts vigorously towards the external inguinal ring. The retracted testis will be difficult to palpate.

The scrotal skin may be red and inflamed; a common cause is candidiasis (Fig. 10.24). Small yellowish scrotal lumps or nodules are quite common and usually represent sebaceous cysts.

Swellings in the scrotum

Decide whether the swelling arises from an indirect inguinal hernia or from the scrotal contents. It is possible to 'get above' a testicular swelling but not a scrotal hernia (Fig. 10.25). An intrinsic swelling may arise from enlargement of the testis, testicular appendages, epididymis, or by an accumulation of fluid in the tunica vaginalis, a double membrane which invests the testes.

Palpate the swelling between the thumb and first two fingers and decide whether the swelling is solid or cystic.

Cystic swelling

Cystic accumulations are caused by entrapment of fluid in the tunica vaginalis (a hydrocele) or accumulation of fluid in an epididymal cyst, and are typically fluctuant. Steady the mass between thumb and first two fingers of one hand and use the index finger of the other hand to invaginate the mass in a second plane (Fig. 10.26). The tense fluid-filled cyst will fluctuate between finger and thumb in response to the pressure change. Cystic lesions usually transilluminate. Darken the room and place a pentorch light up against the swelling. A fluid-filled cyst spreads a bright red glow into the scrotum, whereas this does not occur with solid tumors. Remember that if the cyst wall is abnormally thickened or the effusion is blood-stained, transillumination may not occur. Next, try to distinguish between a hydrocele and an epididymal cyst. As the epididymis lies behind the body of the testis, an epididymal cyst is felt as a distinct swelling behind the adjoining testis (Fig. 10.27). In contrast, a hydrocele surrounds and envelops the testis which becomes impalpable as a discreet organ (Fig. 10.28). The distinction between an epididymal cyst and hydrocele is not always clear and the two may occur together.

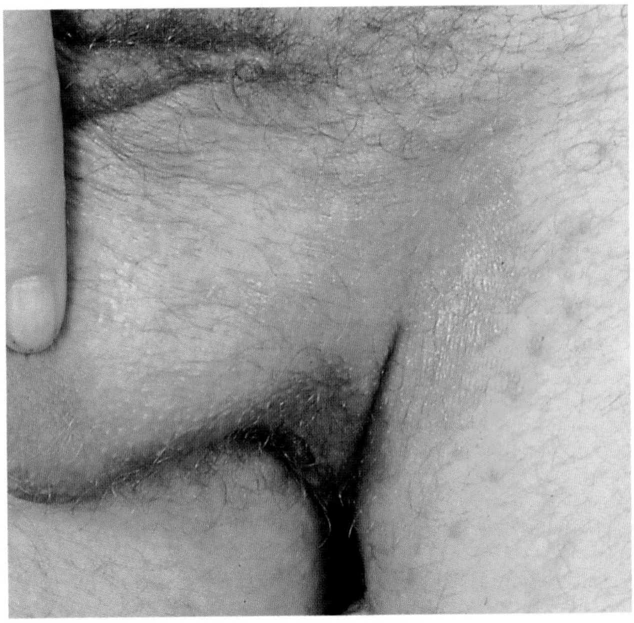

Fig. 10.24 Candida infection of the scrotum often extends to the groin and thigh.

Testing for scrotal swellings

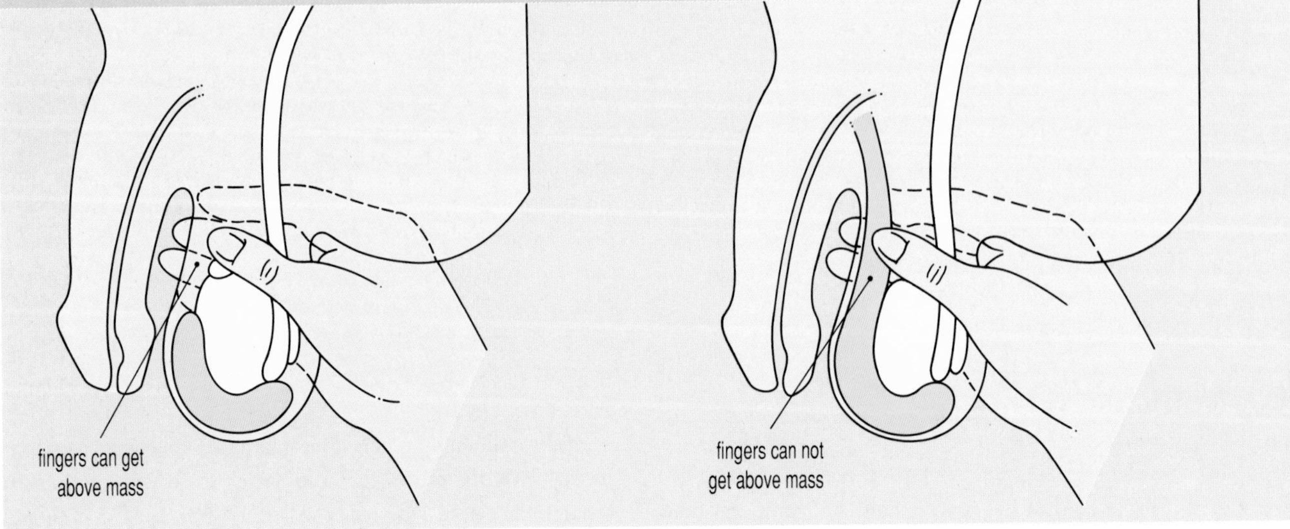

Fig. 10.25 It is possible to get above a true scrotal swelling (left), whereas this is not possible if the swelling is due to an inguinal hernia which has descended into the scrotum (right).

Varicocele

Varicoceles occur in 5–8 per cent of normal adult males and are almost always left-sided (Fig. 10.29). A varicocele results from a varicosity of the veins of the pampiniform plexus, a leash of vessels surrounding the spermatic cord, and is caused by abnormality of the valve mechanism where the left testicular vein drains into the left renal vein (the right drains directly into the inferior vena cava). Most varicoceles do not cause symptoms and are discovered as an incidental finding. However, patients may rarely present with scrotal swelling, discomfort, or infertility. Examine the patient in the standing position; the varicocele feels like a 'bag of worms'. Ask the patient to cough whilst you palpate the varicocele; a characteristic feature is transmission of the raised intra-abdominal pressure to the varicocele which is felt as a discreet cough impulse. The varicocele is separate from the testis. The ipsilateral testis is usually smaller than expected. A varicocele usually empties when the patient lies supine.

Fluctuations of the cystic swelling

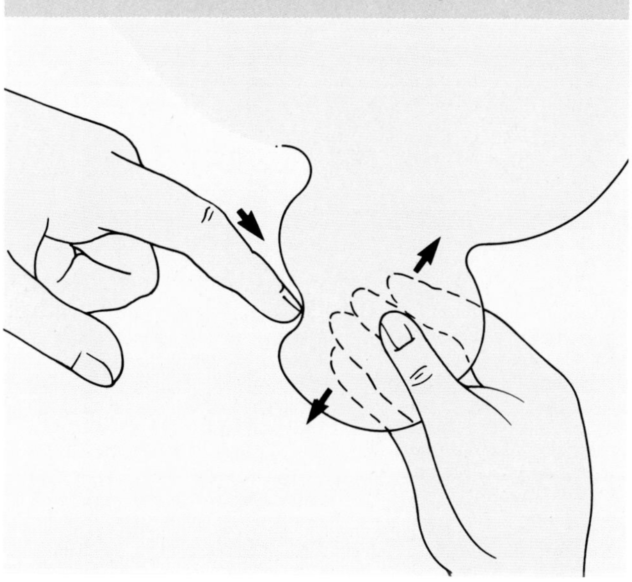

Fig. 10.26 To distinguish a solid from a cystic mass, fix the swelling between finger and thumb of one hand and use the index finger of the other hand to invaginate at right angles.

Epididymal cyst

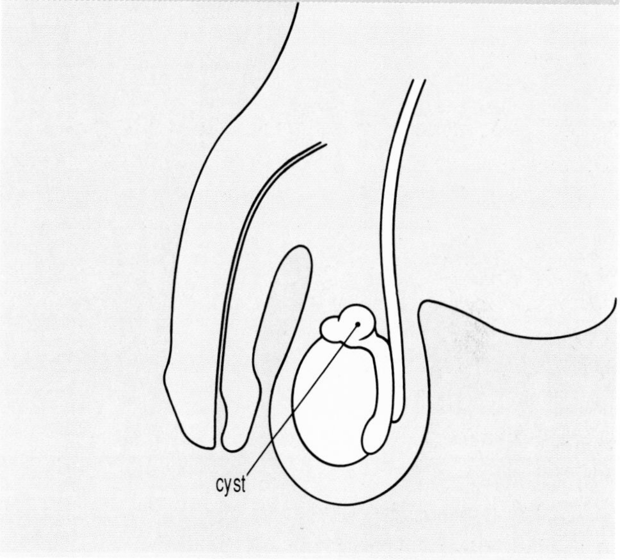

Fig. 10.27 An epididymal cyst is felt separate from the testis and lies posterior.

Hydrocele

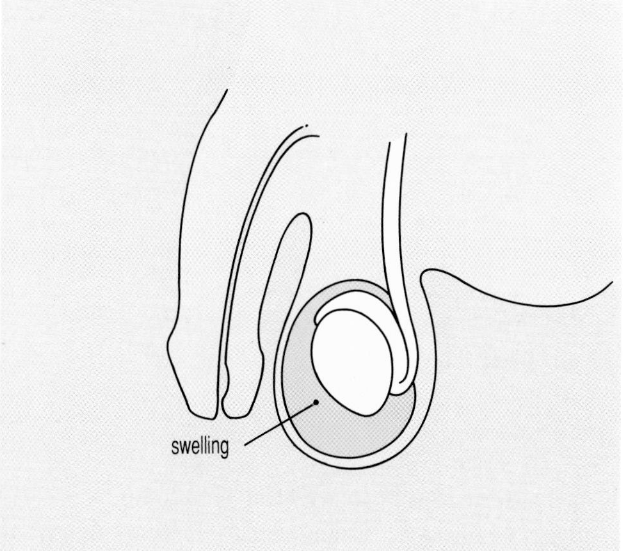

Fig. 10.28 An hydrocele surrounds the entire testis which cannot, therefore, be felt as a discreet organ.

Varicocele

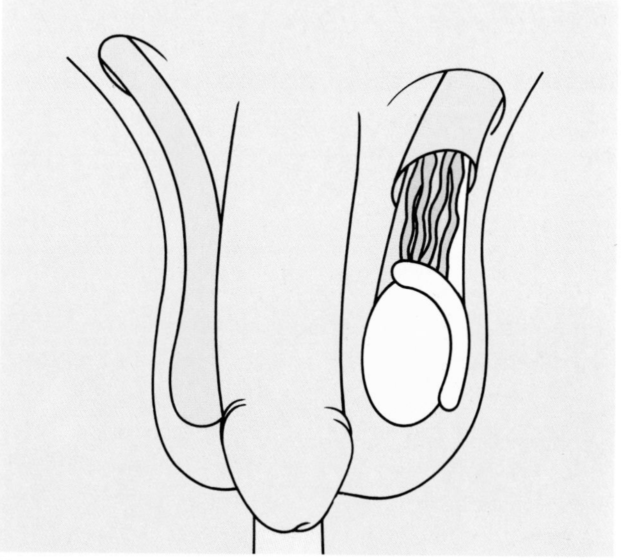

Fig. 10.29 A left-sided varicocele has the texture of a 'bag of worms' when palpated. The mass is separate from the testis and epididymis..

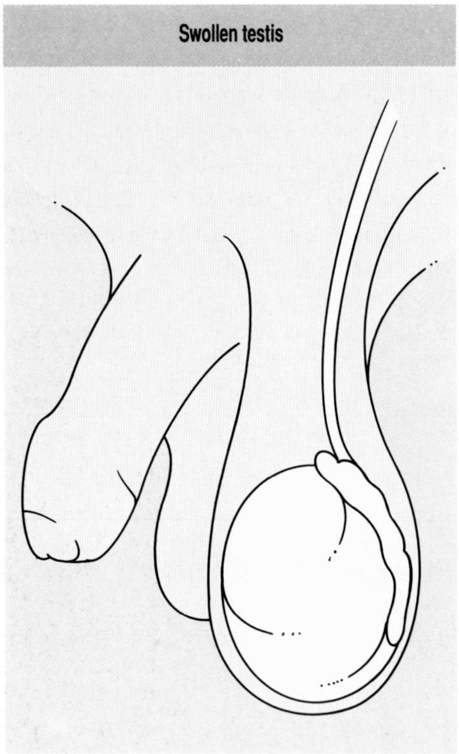

Fig. 10.30 In orchitis, the testis is swollen, tense, and very tender. Usually only one testis is involved.

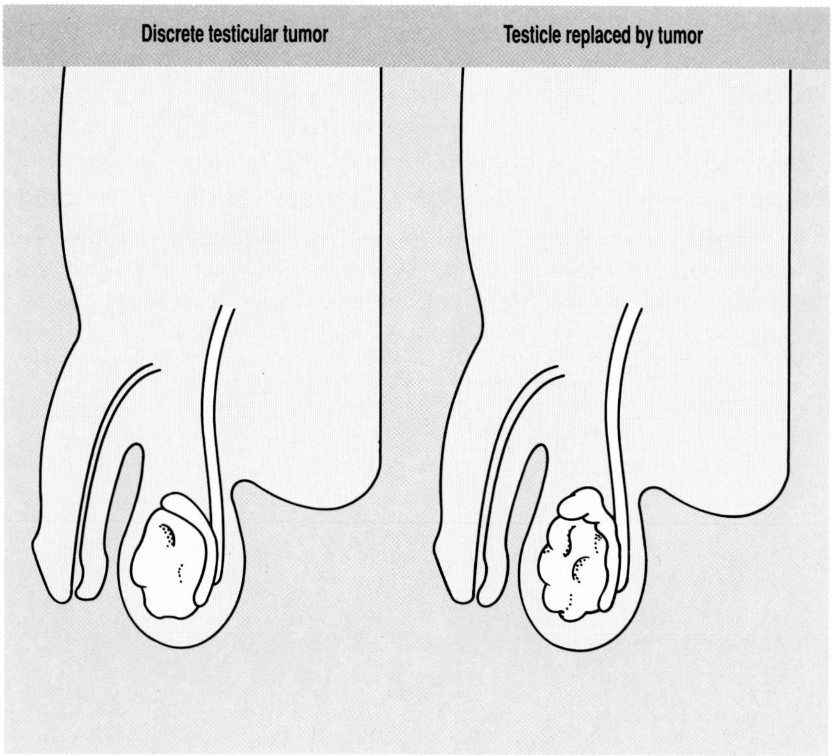

Fig. 10.31 Carcinoma may present as a discreet mass within a testis (left) or may expand to replace the entire organ (right).

Solid swellings

As with cystic swellings, use your knowledge of the anatomy to distinguish between a testicular and an epididymal mass. Diffuse, acutely painful swelling usually occurs in acute inflammatory condition such as orchitis (Fig. 10.30) or torsion of the testis. These acute emergencies are usually readily distinguished from a solid or discreet swelling of the body of the testis. Solid masses may be smooth or craggy, tender or painless, but whatever the character, carcinoma must be the first differential diagnosis (Fig. 10.31). Other solid masses include tuberculomas and syphilitic gummas. Solid tumors of the epididymis are due to chronic inflammation (usually tuberculous epididymitis) and are usually benign. The epididymis feels hard and craggy (Fig. 10.32) and is not unduly tender.

Torsion of the testis

This usually occurs in young boys and presents with severe scrotal pain which usually radiates to the inguinal region and lower abdomen. On examination, the scrotal skin overlying the affected testis may be reddened, with the affected testis lying higher than the unaffected testis (Fig. 10.33). The testis may be exquisitely tender and the spermatic cord may feel thickened and sensitive to palpation. The opposite testis may have an abnormal lie, as it is not uncommon for both testes to be abnormally positioned. The presentation and findings may be confused with orchitis and testicular torsion.

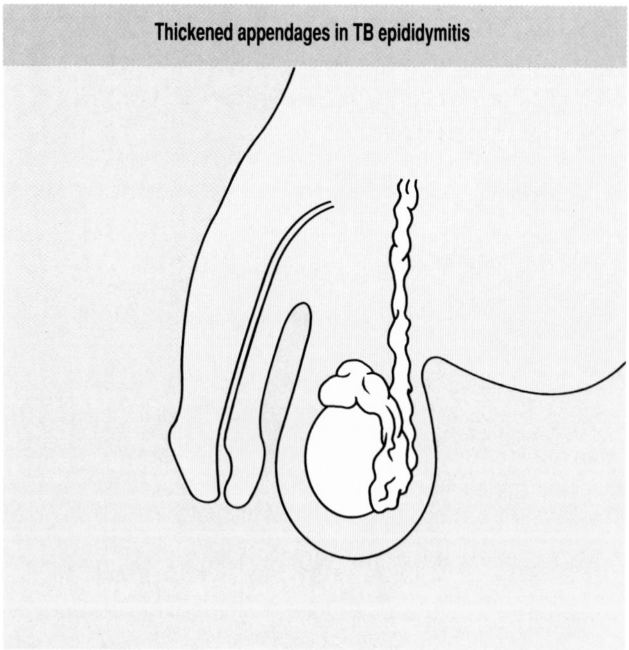

Fig. 10.32 In tuberculous epididymitis, the epididymis is firm and thickened and the cord may feel beaded.

Scrotal oedema

Scrotal oedema usually occurs when there is diffuse oedema (anasarca) caused by severe congestive heart failure or hypoproteinaemia such as nephrotic syndrome. The scrotal tissue becomes stretched and taut with pitting of the skin.

EXAMINATION OF THE LYMPHATICS

The skin of the penis and scrotum drain towards the inguinal nodes; you should complete the genital examination by feeling for nodes in the groin which are felt deep to the the inguinal crease. The testicular lymphatics drain to intra-abdominal nodes. Special tests such as CT scanning or lymphangiography are necessary to evaluate the testicular lymphatics.

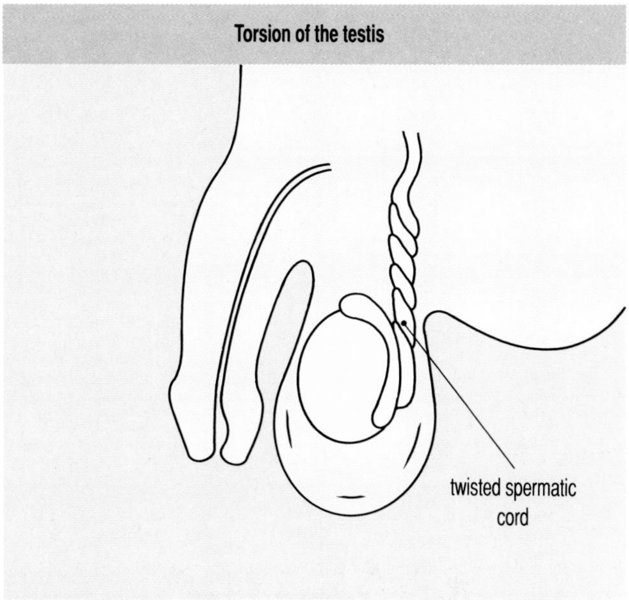

Fig. 10.33 Torsion of the testicle on the spermatic cord impairs the blood supply. The affected testis is swollen, tender, and lies higher than expected. The overlying scrotal skin is often reddened and oedematous.

Enlarged inquinal nodes

Enlarged nodes occur in infective and malignant disorders affecting the skin of the penis and scrotum. The primary chancre of syphilis is usually associated with lymphadenopathy. The nodes are typically mobile, rubbery, and non-tender. The most florid forms of inguinal lymphadenopathy occur in patients with lymphogranloma venereum (Fig. 10.34).

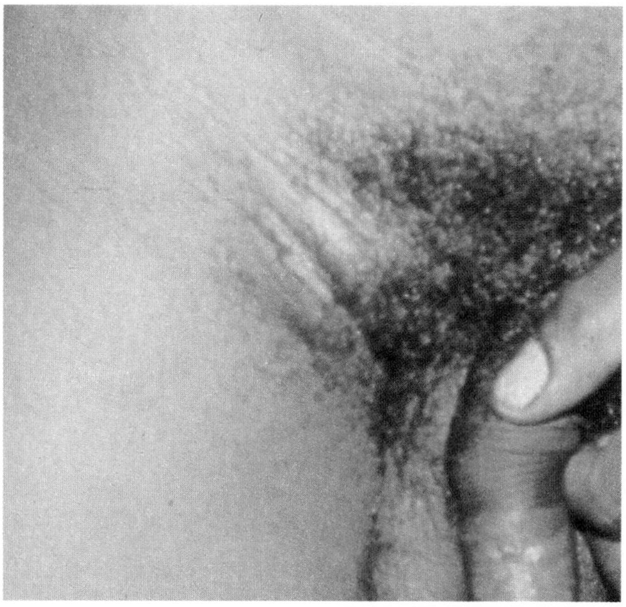

Fig. 10.34 In lymphogranuloma venereum, the inguinal lymph nodes enlarge.

BONE, JOINT, AND MUSCLE

11

The skeleton provides protection for the internal organs along with a strengthening and support system for the limbs. The presence of joints in the limbs and spine permits movement of what would otherwise be rigid structures. The cartilage interposed between the bone surfaces of a joint cushions the forces which are generated during movement. Joint strength is enhanced by ligaments which are either incorporated into the joint capsule or independent of it. Movement at the joint is achieved by contraction of the muscles passing across it.

STRUCTURE AND FUNCTION

BONE

Long bones are hollow with an outer layer of compact bone arranged, on the surface, into flat layers of lamellae and, more deeply, as concentric rings traversed by longitudinal passages (the Haversian canals) (Fig. 11.1). The central cavity of a long bone is occupied by bone marrow. At the ends of the long bones, a mesh-work (cancellous bone) forms with marrow in its interstices. The arrangement of the mesh-work is determined by the stresses to which the bone is exposed. Between adjacent Haversian canals and their surrounding concentric rings, the bony lamellae are arranged more haphazardly. In the spaces between these bony lamellae lie osteocytes.

Formation of bone is controlled by osteoblasts and its destruction by osteoclasts. The osteocytes, derived from osteoblasts, are concerned with the exchange of calcium between bone and the extracellular fluid. Collagen, synthesized by osteoblasts and fibroblasts, forms the major part of the bone matrix. The calcium content of bone is mainly composed of crystals of hydroxyapatite. About one per cent of the calcium and phosphate of bone is in equilibrium with the extracellular fluid. Only osteoclastic resorption can release the remainder. The exchange of calcium between bone and extracellular fluid is controlled by parathormone and calcitriol, a metabolite of vitamin D.

The tubular arrangement of the long bones achieves maximal resistance to a bending force while economizing on the amount of material used in its construction. The lines of the trabeculae in cancellous bone match the lines of stress encountered at those particular points. The surface markings and contours of bone are determined by external forces and the origins of tendons and ligaments.

Cartilage consists of a collection of rounded cells (chondroblasts) embedded in a matrix. There are three main types: hyaline, elastic, and fibrocartilage. Hyaline cartilage is found on the articular surface of joints, in the costal cartilages, and in the larynx, trachea and bronchi. Hyaline cartilage combines elasticity with a capacity to resist external forces. With increasing age, cartilage water content falls with a consequent deterioration in tensile stiffness, fracture strength and fatigue resistance. Fibrocartilage is predominantly composed of fibrous tissue and is a part of the tendon at the point of its insertion into bone (Sharpey's fibres). It is also found in certain joints. Elastic cartilage has a concentrated network of elastic fibres which gives its structure considerable flexibility. It is found in the pinna and in some of the laryngeal cartilages.

JOINTS

Joints can be classified into those allowing free movement (diarthroses), those that are fixed (synarthroses) and a group that permits limited movement (amphiarthroses). In diarthroses

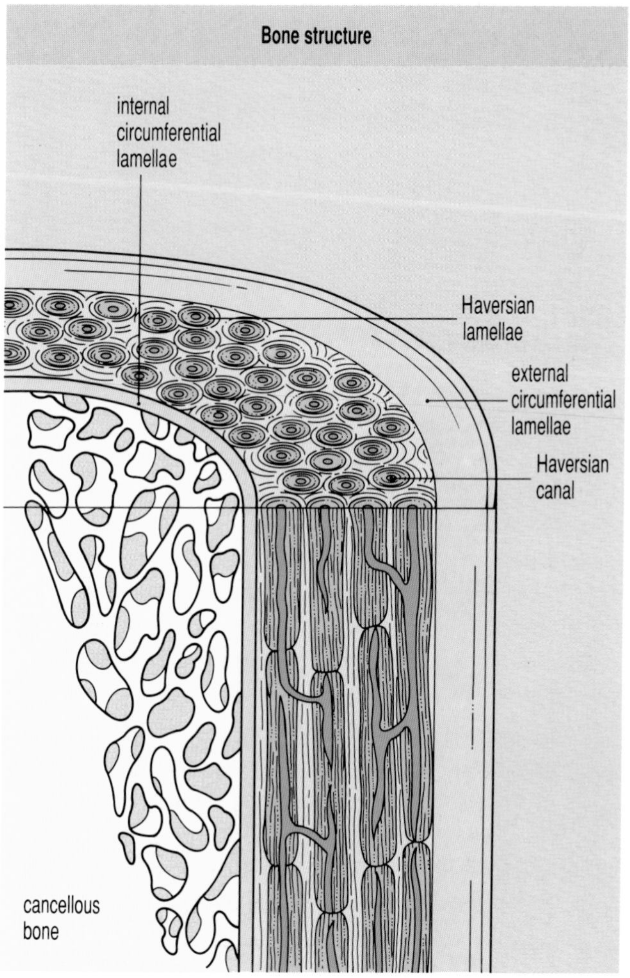

Fig. 11.1 Representation of bone structure.

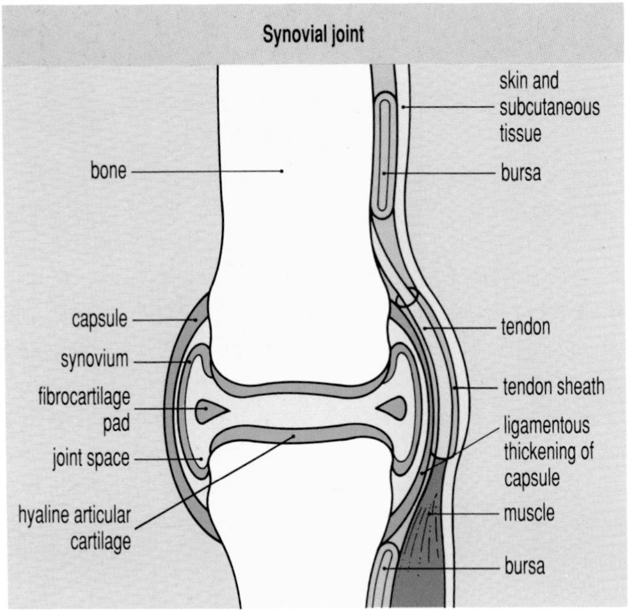

Fig. 11.2 Cross-section of a synovial joint.

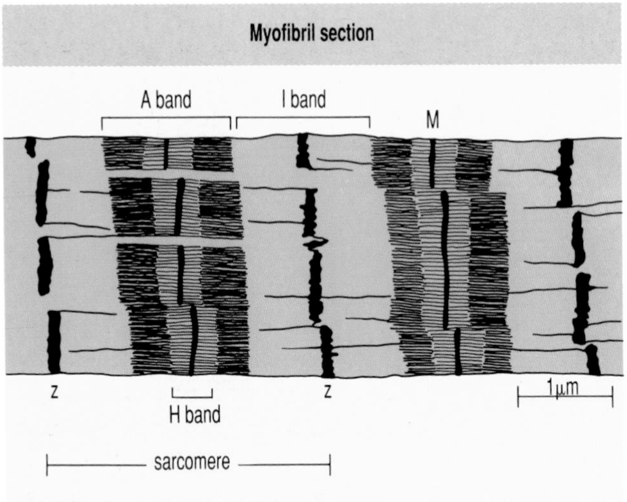

Fig. 11.4 Longitudinal section through myofibrils.

(synovial joints) a space exists between the bone surfaces allowing movement of one bone against the other (Fig. 11.2). Further classification of these joints can be made according to the type of movement which occurs (e.g. hinge, ball and socket, etc.). A synovial joint is enclosed by a collagenous capsule attached to the bone at some distance from the joint. The inner surface of the capsule is lined by a fluid-producing membrane. Localized thickenings of the capsule, the ligaments, connect the adjacent bones. Other ligaments blend into the capsule at one end but are attached to bone at the other (Fig. 11.3) or remain totally independent of the joint capsule.

The synovial membrane is one cell thick. One type of cell ingests foreign or autologous material that has entered the joint; another synthesizes and secretes the synovial fluid. Synovial fluid is a dialysate of plasma with the addition of hyaluronate proteoglycin.

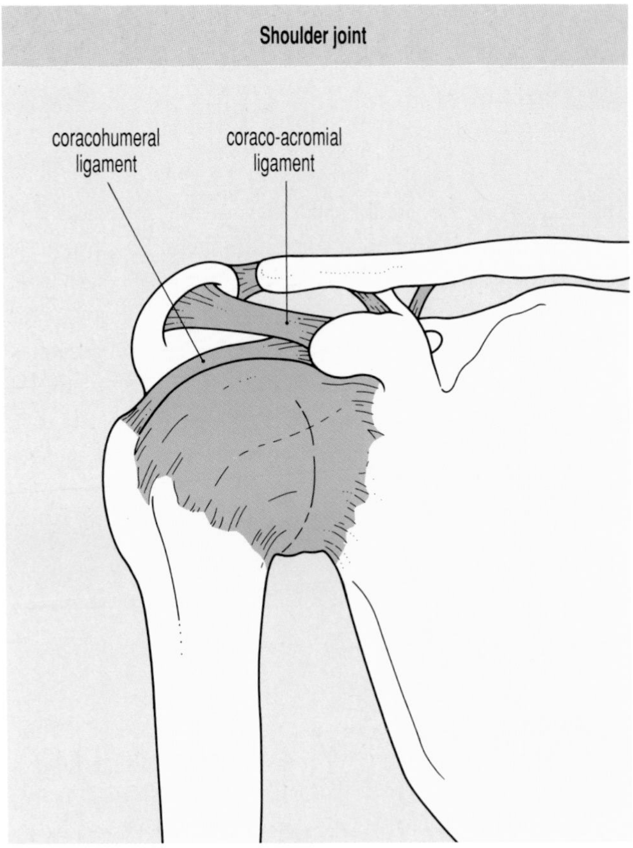

Fig. 11.3 The shoulder joint and the attachments of the coracohumeral ligament.

The ratio of the concentration of a synovial fluid protein to its serum concentration is determined by molecular size. The synovial fluid provides both nutrition for the articular cartilage and lubricates the joint surfaces.

Temporary synarthroses (synchondroses) are found at the growing points of long bones in the form of epiphysial cartilage. The sutures of the skull are synarthroses, the bony margins being joined by fibrous tissue.

Amphiarthroses are permanent joints. A good example is the intervertebral disc of the spine. An outer layer of dense concentric bundles of collagen, the annulus fibrosus, encloses a core of hydrated compact tissue, the nucleus pulposus.

MUSCLE

A motor neurone innervates 100–1000 skeletal muscle fibres. Within the muscle fibre is a recurring anatomical structure, the sarcomere, consisting of thin filaments which are composed of actin, and thick filaments based on myosin (Fig. 11.4). During contraction and relaxation of muscle, the thin and thick filaments move in relationship to one another. All the fibres of a particular motor unit have similar properties. Muscle fibres are divided into fast and slow twitch (Type I and Type II) according to their speed of contraction, though in man a continuum of twitch speed exists.

Slowly contracting motor units are innervated by slowly conducting nerve fibres with a low threshold and firing frequency.

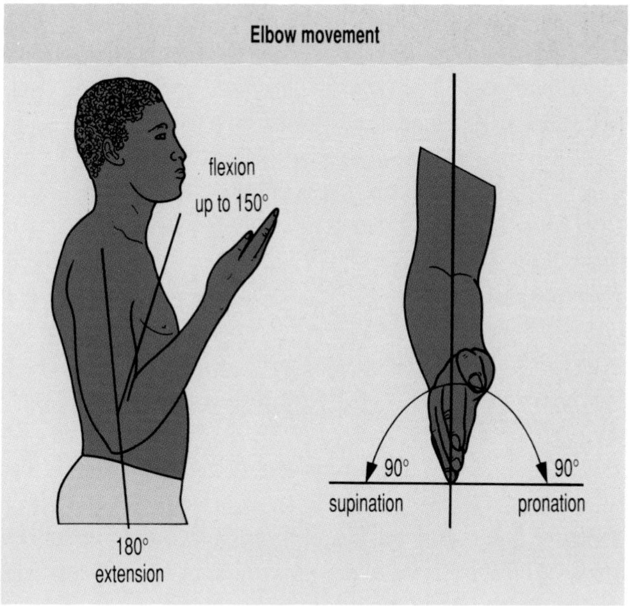

Fig. 11.5 Range of movement at the elbow.

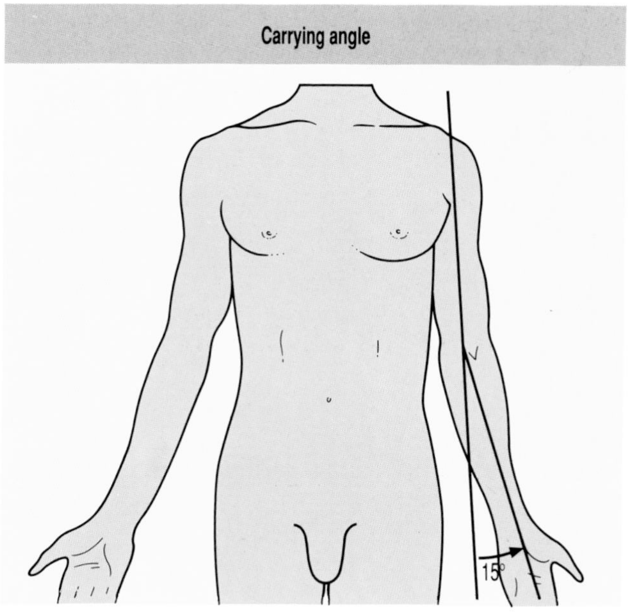

Fig. 11.6 Carrying angle of the forearm.

Rapidly contracting motor units are innervated by axons that conduct rapidly but have a high threshold. The strength of muscle contraction can be altered either by varying the number of motor units recruited or by altering their firing frequency. The recruitment process begins with smaller units and progresses to larger. Firing frequency ranges from 10–20Hz for slow units and up to 100Hz for fast units. Slow twitch muscles have a high myoglobin content, producing a reddish appearance. Slow-twitch fibres utilize oxidative mechanisms for energy formation; fast-twitch fibres employ glycolysis. The former are fatigue-resistant, the latter rapidly fatiguable. In general, slow units provide sustained muscle tension over long periods, of the sort required to maintain a particular posture, whereas fast units allow short-lived, sudden muscle contraction.

REGIONAL STRUCTURE AND FUNCTION

The spine

The primary curvatures of the spine, in the thoracic and sacral regions, are determined by differences in height of the anterior and posterior aspects of the vertebrae at these levels. The secondary curvatures of the cervical and lumbar regions depend more on the relative heights of the anterior and posterior aspects of the intervertebral discs. The nucleus pulposus allows an even distribution of applied force on to the annulus fibrosus and the hyaline laminae covering the opposing vertebral bodies.

Forward flexion and extension occur at all levels of the spine but are maximal at the junction of the atlas with the occiput, and in the lumbar and cervical regions. Lateral flexion is greatest at the atlanto-occipital junction, occurs to some extent in the lumbar and cervical regions, but minimally in the thoracic region. Rotation, other than at the atlanto-axial joints, is determined by the shape of the apophyseal joints and is maximal at the thoracic level.

The shoulder

Movement of the shoulder takes place both at the glenohumeral and the scapulothoracic joints. For abduction, the first 90° of movement takes place at the glenohumeral joint. This is achieved by contraction first of supraspinatus (0–30°) then of deltoid (30–90°). Abduction of the shoulder beyond 90° requires rotation of the scapula, which is achieved by contraction of trapezius. Adduction is principally due to pectoralis major and latissimus dorsi. Forward flexion depends mainly on pectoralis major and the anterior fibres of deltoid, extension on latissimus dorsi, teres major, and the posterior fibres of deltoid. Lateral rotation is accomplished by contraction of infraspinatus and medial rotation by pectoralis major, latissimus dorsi, and the anterior fibres of deltoid. Immediately above the glenohumeral joint lies the subacromial bursa and the rotator cuff, which is formed by the tendons of supraspinatus, infraspinatus, and subscapularis.

The elbow

There are two joints at the elbow, one involving the humerus, radius, and ulna, the other joining the upper ends of the radius and ulna. Flexion/extension movement occurs at the former through a range of about 150°. The latter joint allows the forearm to rotate (pronation-supination) through a range of 180° (Fig.11.5). In males, the forearm is only slightly abducted from the axis of the humerus. In females, the abduction is greater, forming a carrying angle of about 15° (Fig. 11.6).

Biceps flexes the elbow when the arm is supinated. Brachioradialis and brachialis flex the elbow in either the pronated or supinated position. Extension of the elbow is achieved by triceps, with a minor contribution from anconeus (Fig. 11.7). Supination is produced by contraction of supinator, and pronation by the combined action of pronator teres and pronator quadratus.

The wrist and hand

Movements of the wrist comprise flexion, extension, and ulnar and radial deviation (Fig. 11.8). Flexion-extension movements of the fingers occur at both the metacarpophalangeal and the interphalangeal joints. The former joints also allow abduction and adduction movements when the fingers are extended (Fig. 11.9). Abduction of the thumb carries it away from the plane of the palm of the hand and adduction towards it. Extension moves the thumb radially in the plane of the hand, flexion in the ulnar direction. Opposition rotates the thumb bringing its palmar surface into contact with the fifth finger (Fig. 11.10).

The major flexors of the wrist are flexor carpi radialis and ulnaris. The major extensors are extensor carpi ulnaris and extensor carpi radialis longus and brevis. The long flexors and extensors of the fingers and thumb, by virtue of passing over the wrist joint, also exert a minor effect there.

The small muscles of the hand control fine movements of the thumb and fingers. The thenar eminence muscles consist of abductor pollicis brevis, flexor pollicis brevis, and opponens pollicis. Contained in the hypothenar eminence are abductor digiti minimi, flexor digiti minimi, and opponens digiti minimi. Finally, there are the lumbrical muscles, the dorsal and palmar interossei, and adductor pollicis. The lumbricals extend the fingers at the interphalangeal joints (with additional more complex actions), the interossei principally abduct and adduct the fingers, while adductor pollicis adducts the thumb.

The hip

The hip is a ball and socket joint allowing flexion, extension, abduction, adduction, and both internal and external rotation. The neck of the femur forms an angle of approximately 130° with the shaft.

Muscles acting at the hip joint may have additional actions on the spine or knee. Psoas major passes from the lumbar spine to the lesser trochanter of the femur. In addition to flexing the hip, it

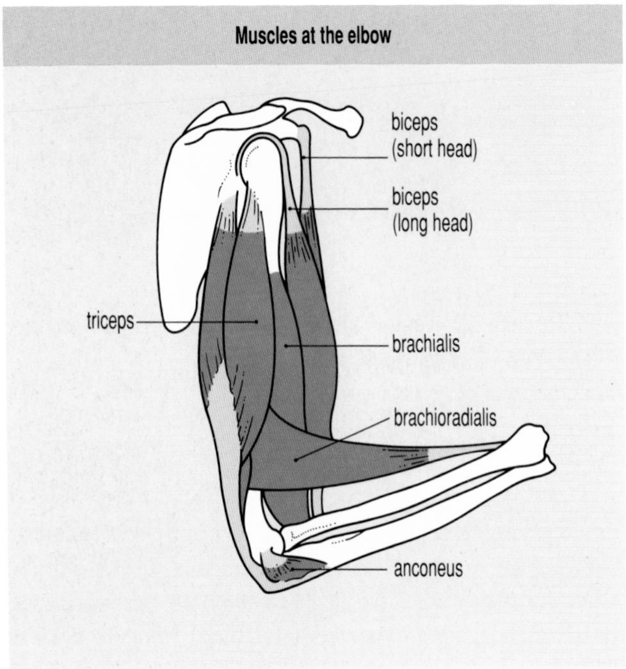

Fig. 11.7 Flexors and extensors of the elbow.

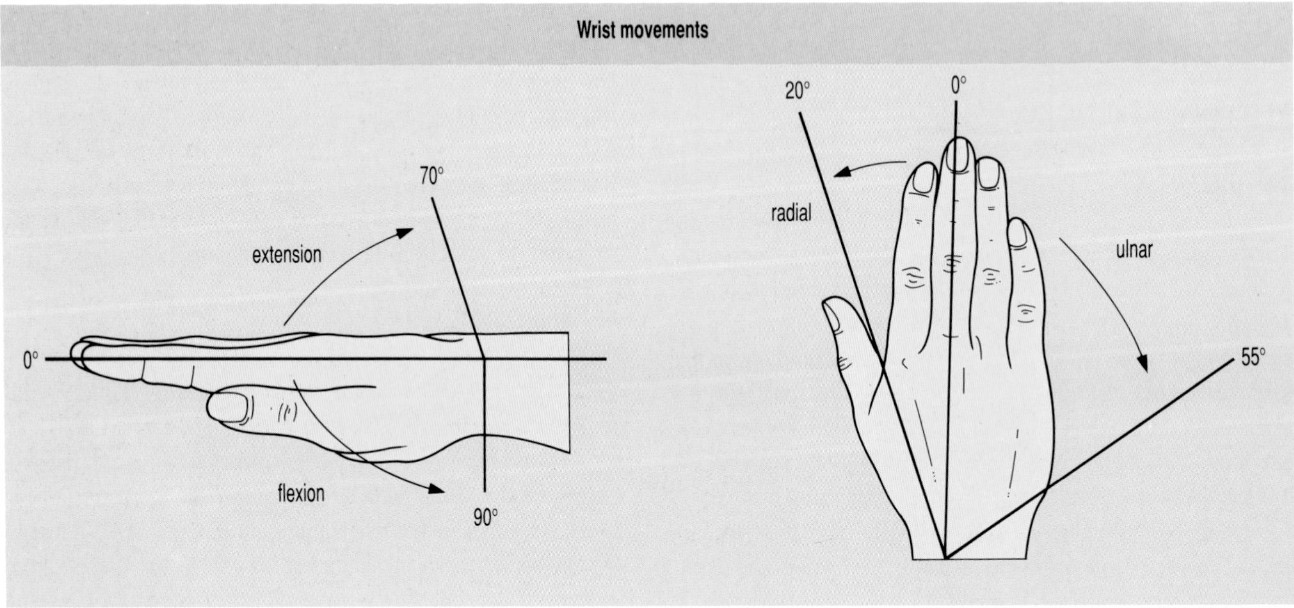

Fig. 11.8 Wrist movements.

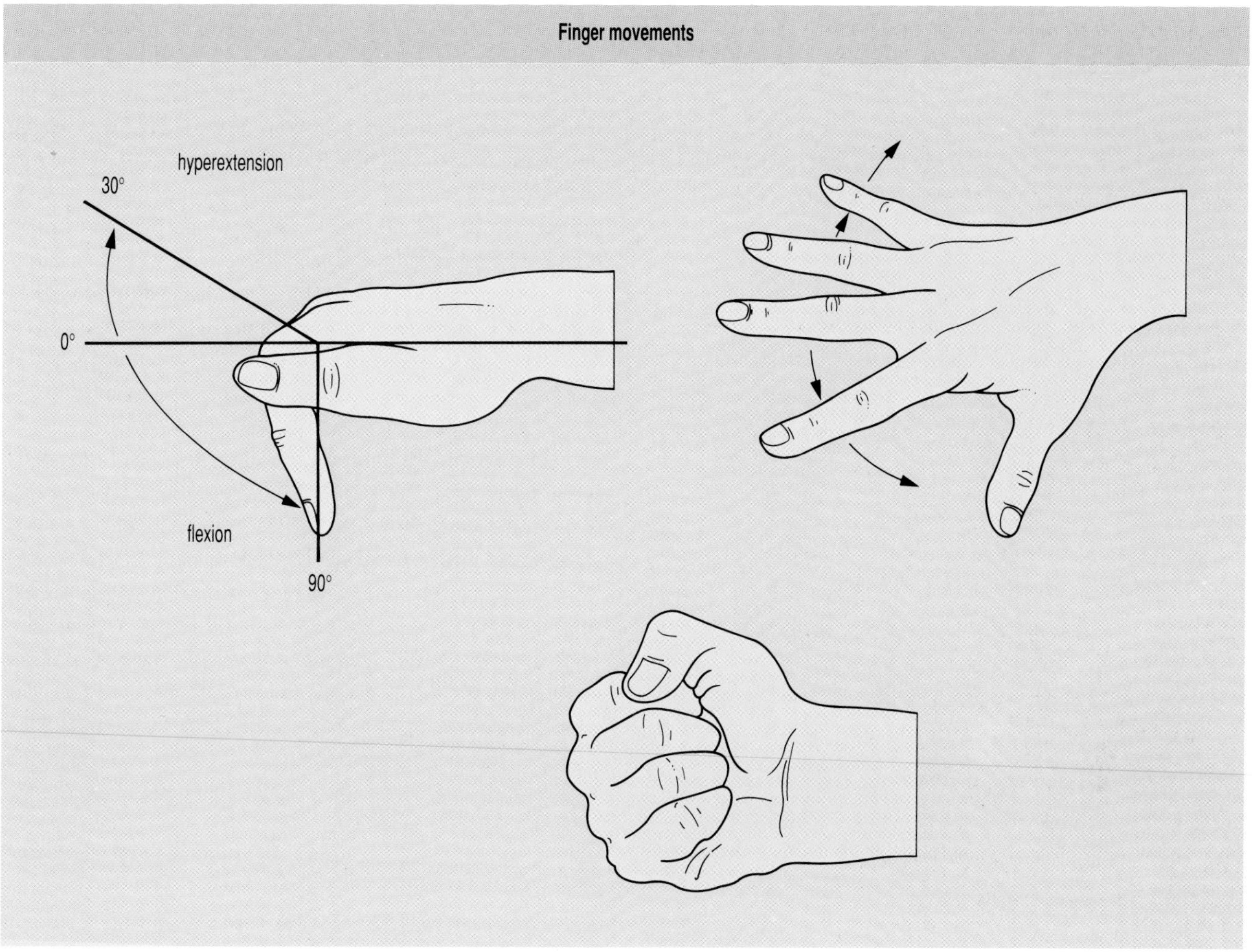

Fig. 11.9 Finger movements at the metacarpophalangeal (left and right) and at the interphalangeal joints (below).

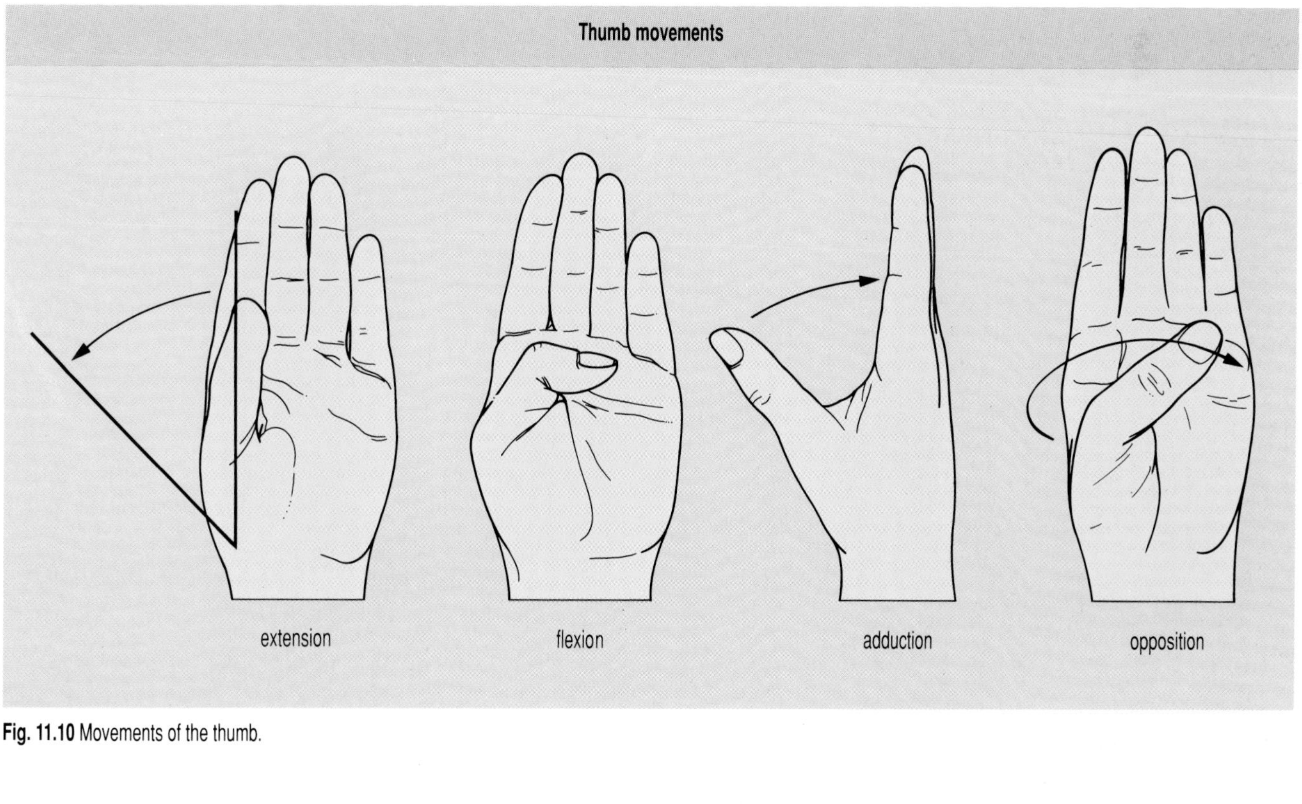

Fig. 11.10 Movements of the thumb.

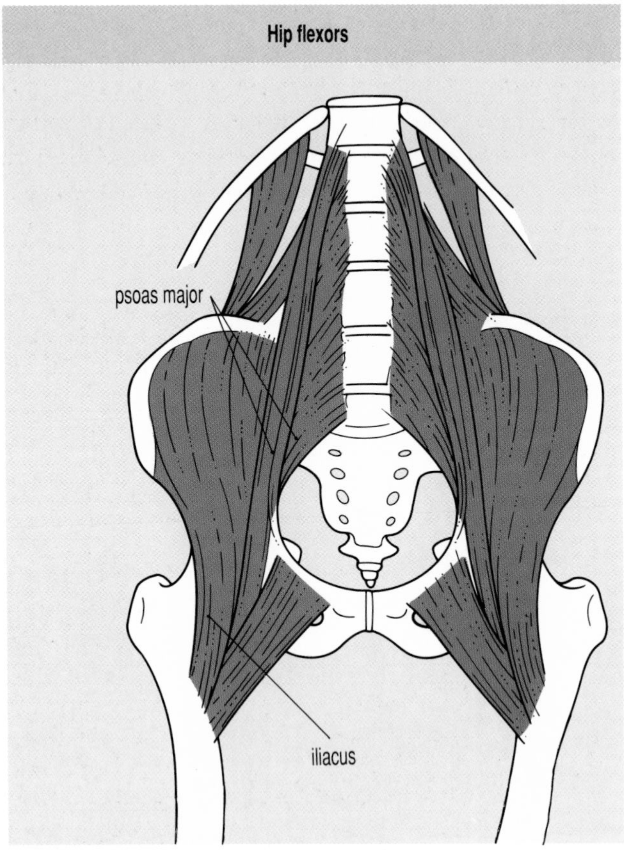

Fig. 11.11 Origin and insertion of iliacus and psoas muscles.

flexes the lumbar spine. Iliacus passes from the iliac fossa part of the hip bone and inserts principally into the lesser trochanter (Fig. 11.11). It acts as a hip flexor. The glutei arise mainly from the ileum. Gluteus maximus is a pure hip extensor; the other glutei principally act as abductors. The thigh is externally rotated by obturator and adducted by adductor majoris. Several muscles connect the pelvis with the tibia and fibula. The hamstrings comprise biceps femoris, semi-tendinosus, and semi-membranosus (Fig 11.12). They act (apart from the short head of biceps) as extensors of the hip joint and flexors of the knee joint.

The knee

Though principally a hinge joint, a limited range of rotation is possible at the knee. Anteriorly the capsule is formed by the tendon of quadriceps femoris and the patella. At the sides, the capsule is strengthened by the medial and lateral collateral ligaments. Within the joint are the anterior and posterior cruciate ligaments passing from the tibia to the lateral and medial condyles of the femur, respectively (Fig. 11.13). Interposed between the femoral condyles and the tibia are the fibrocartilagenous semilunar cartilages. The joint capsule is lined by synovium which partly surrounds the cruciate ligaments. Communicating with the synovial cavity are bursae which are related to the insertions or origins of some of the tendons around the joint (Fig. 11.14).

Flexion–extension occurs between about 0° and 135° (Fig. 11.15).

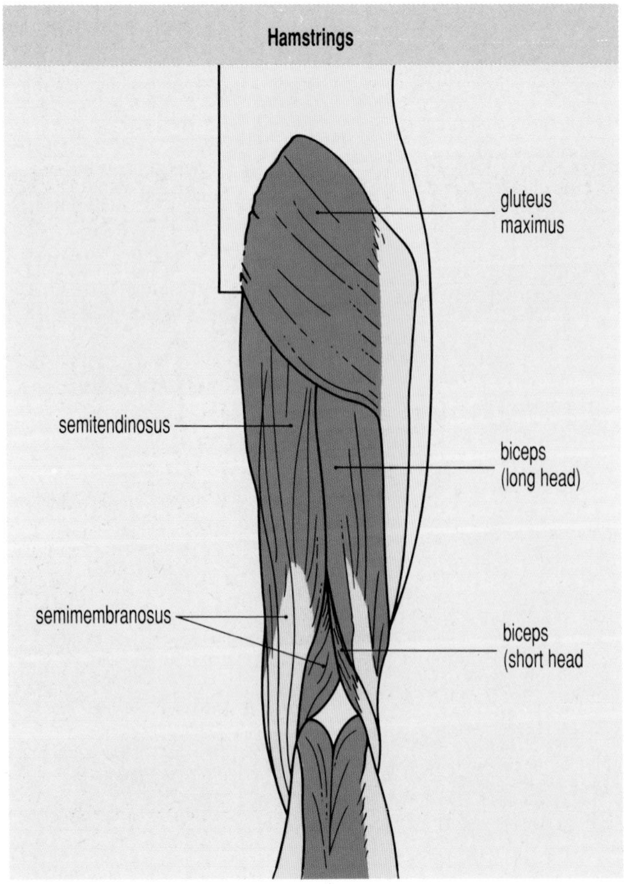

Fig. 11.12 The hamstring muscles.

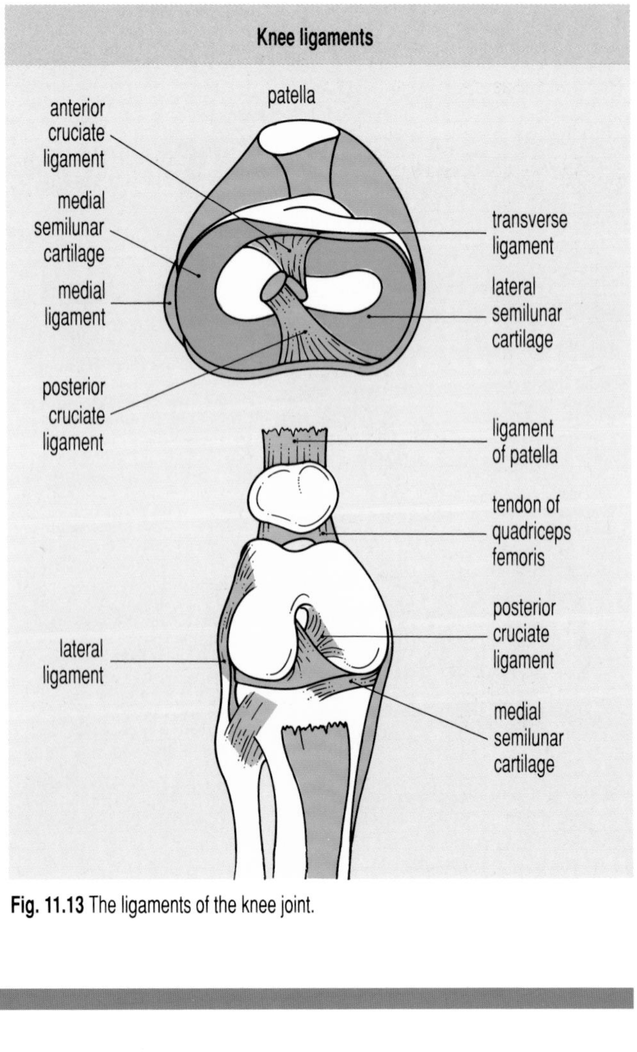

Fig. 11.13 The ligaments of the knee joint.

A minor degree of hyperextension can occur in some normal subjects. As full extension is reached, the femur rotates medially, due to the longer articular surface of the medial condyle, tightening the capsular ligaments in the process. Flexion is produced by the hamstrings and extension by the quadriceps femoris.

The ankle and foot

Movements of the ankle are essentially confined to extension (dorsiflexion) and flexion (plantar flexion). Inversion and eversion of the foot are partly achieved by movement at the subtalar joint (approximately 5°) and partly by movement at the mid-tarsal joints (20°). The predominant movements of the toes are dorsiflexion and plantar flexion (Fig. 11.16).

Knee bursae

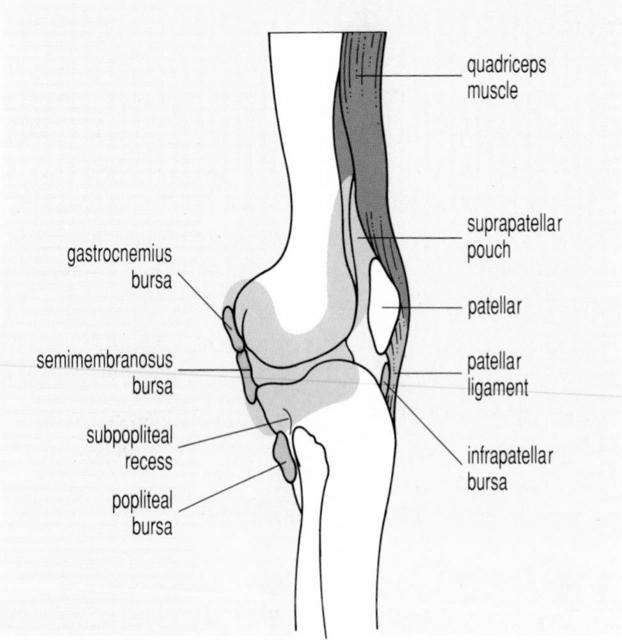

Fig. 11.14 Bursae related to the knee joint.

Knee flexion/extension

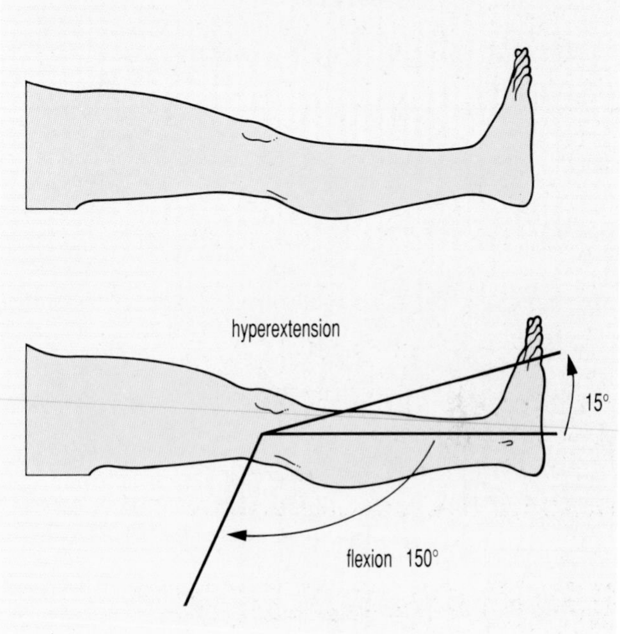

Fig. 11.15 Flexion-extension at the knee joint.

Ankle and foot movements

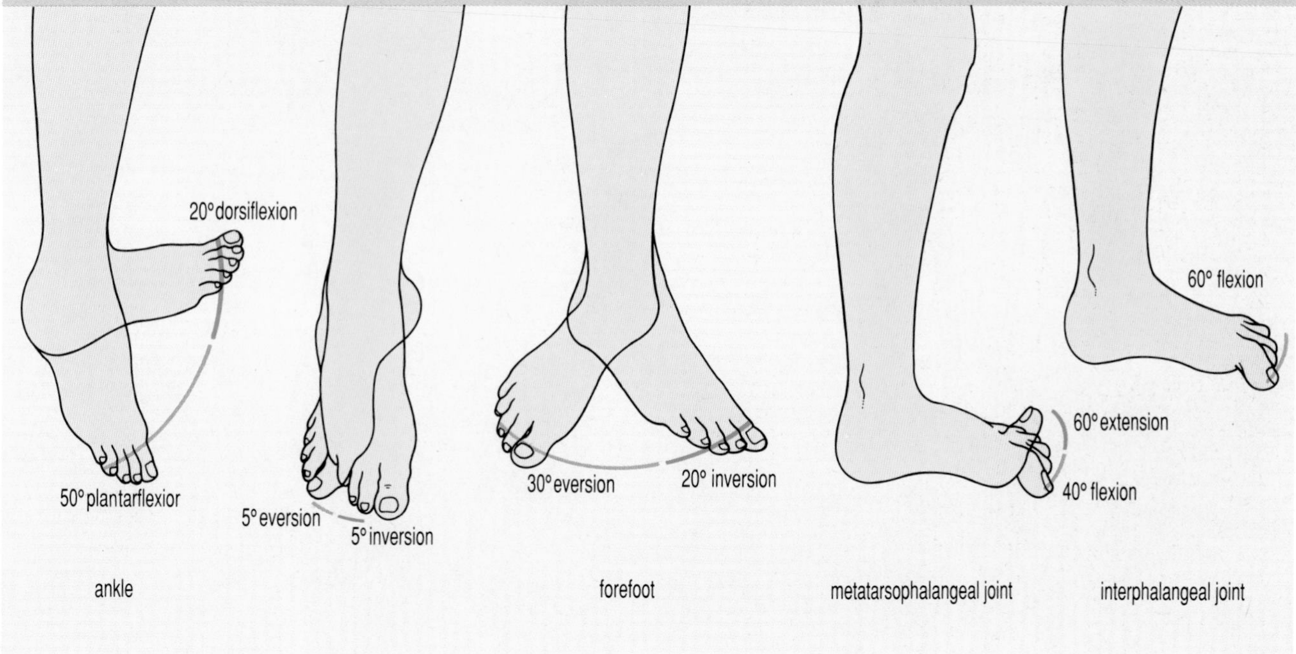

Fig. 11.16 Movements of the ankle, foot, and big toe.

The main muscles of the calf are soleus and gastrocnemius. Soleus acts purely as a flexor of the ankle, gastrocnemius flexes both the ankle and the knee. Of the other muscles in the posterior compartment, tibialis posterior inverts the foot while flexor digitorum longus and flexor hallucis longus flex the toes and big toe, respectively (Fig 11.17).

The anterior compartment muscles include tibialis anterior, extensor digitorum longus, and extensor hallucis longus (Fig. 11.18). Tibialis anterior inverts the foot and dorsiflexes the ankle. The other two dorsiflex the toes and big toe, respectively. The peronei act as evertors of the foot.

SYMPTOMS OF BONE, JOINT, AND MUSCLE DISORDERS

BONE

Pain

Bone pain has a deep, boring quality. The pain is focal in the presence of a bone tumor or infection but diffuse in generalized disorders (e.g. osteoporosis) (Fig. 11.19). The pain of a fracture is sharp and piercing, is exacerbated by movement, and relieved by rest.

JOINT

Joint symptoms include pain, swelling, crepitus, and locking.

Pain

In an arthritic disorder, pain is usually the most prominent complaint. Important aspects to determine are the site and severity of the pain, whether it is acute or chronic, how it is influenced by rest and activity and whether it appears during a particular range of movement.

Ask the patient to point to the maximal site of pain. Though irritation of structures close to the skin produces well-localized pain, disturbance of deeper structures produces pain which is poorly localized and eventually segmental in distribution. The

Calf muscles

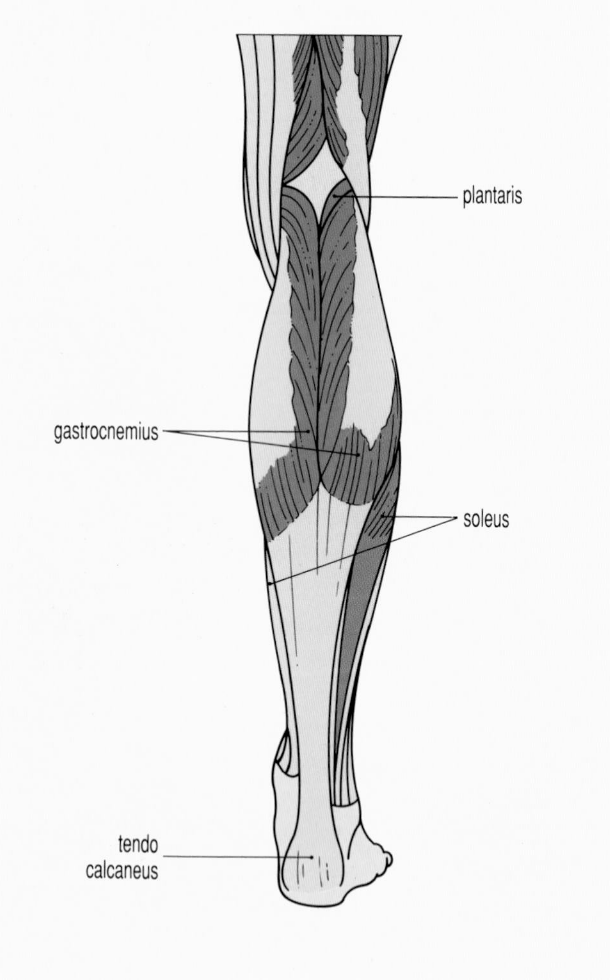

Fig. 11.17 The muscles of the calf.

Tibial compartment muscles

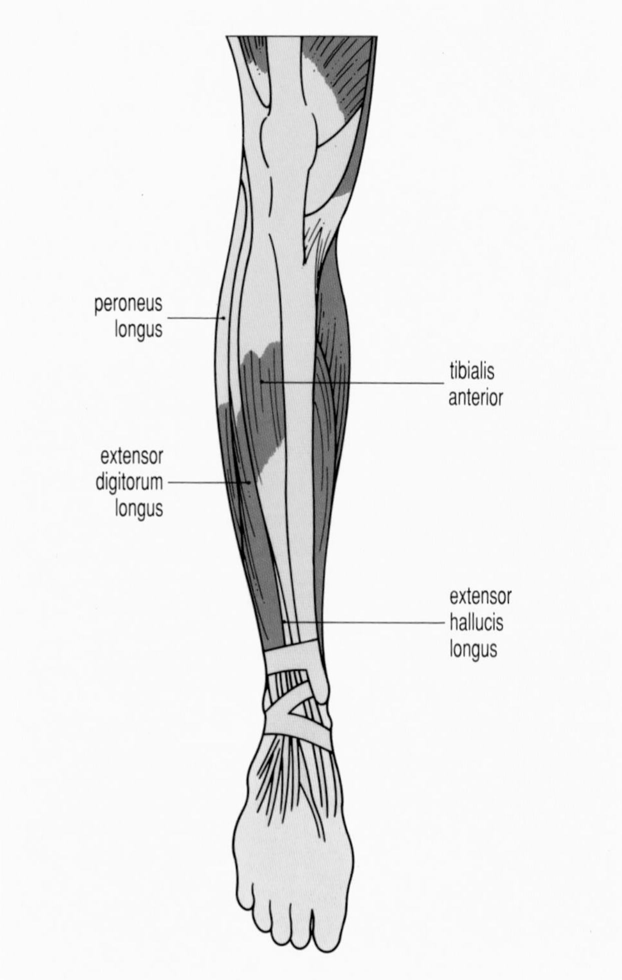

Fig. 11.18 Muscles in the anterior compartment of the leg.

Causes of bone pain	
Focal pain	**Diffuse pain**
Fracture/trauma	Malignancy
Infection	Paget's disease
Malignancy	Osteomalacia
Paget's disease	Osteoporosis
Osteoid osteoma	Metabolic bone disease

Fig. 11.19 Causes of bone pain.

Joint pain

Where is the maximal site of pain?

Does the pain change during the course of the day?

Has the pain been there for a short or long time?

Does the pain get better or worse as you move about?

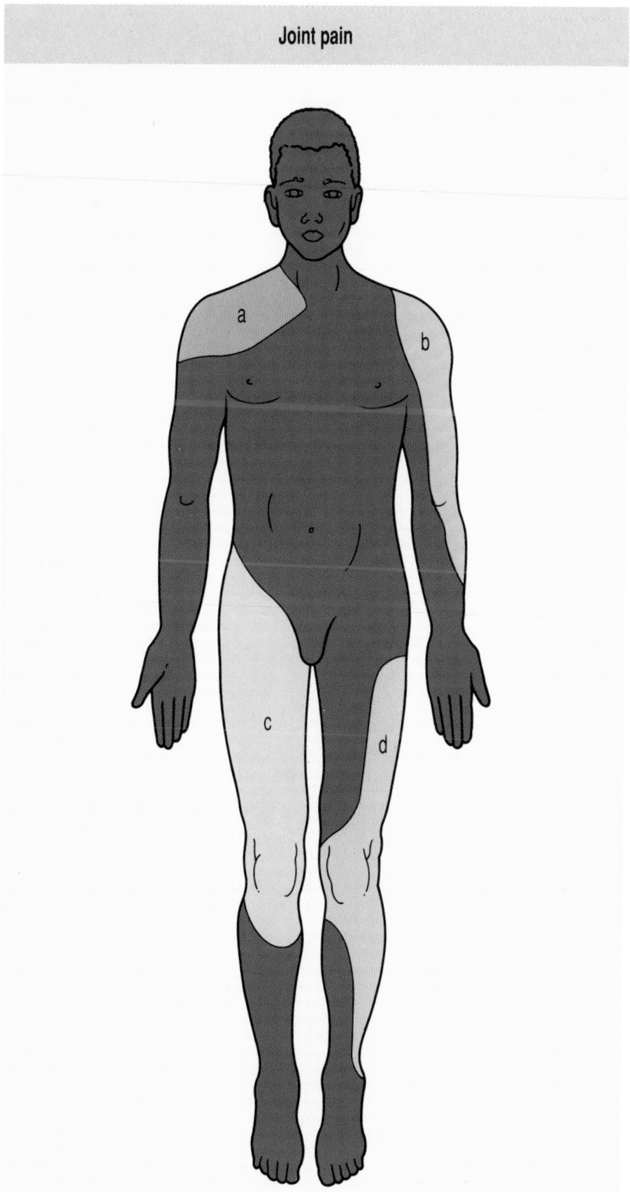

Fig. 11.20 Distribution of pain arising from: (a) acromioclavicular or sternoclavicular joints; (b) scapulohumeral joint; (c) hip joint; (d) knee joint.

segments to which the pain is referred (the sclerotomes) differ somewhat from dermatomal distributions. Consequently, deep pain can be felt at a point some distance from the affected structure, i.e. referred pain. Where joint disease exists, misinterpretation of the site of the disease process can follow (Fig. 11.20). Spinal pain can also be referred. Abnormal function in the upper cervical spine can lead to pain over the occipital region, while disorders of the lower lumbar spine may lead to upper lumbar back pain stemming from the fact that the posterior longitudinal ligament is innervated by the upper lumbar nerves.

Severity of joint pain is difficult to judge, depending, as it does, on the patient's personality. Osteo- and rheumatoid arthritis typically result in chronic pain with periodic exacerbation; septic arthritis or gout produce an acute, exquisitely painful joint.

Inflammatory joint disease tends to cause pain on waking, improving with activity, but returning at rest (Fig. 11.21). Mechanical joint disease (e.g. due to osteoarthritis) leads to pain which worsens during the course of the day, particularly with activity.

Causes of joint pain	
Inflammatory	Rheumatoid arthritis Ankylosing spondylitis
Mechanical	Osteoarthritis
Infective	Pyogenic Tuberculosis Brucellosis
Traumatic	

Fig. 11.21 Causes of joint pain.

For certain joint disorders (e.g. at the shoulder), pain is apparent only during a specific range of movement. If confirmed by examination this selectivity can be valuable in differential diagnosis.

Swelling and crepitus

If the patient has noticed joint swelling, elicit for how long it has been present, whether there is associated pain and whether the swelling fluctuates in degree. A noisy joint is not necessarily pathological. Introspective individuals are likely to interpret periodic clicking in a joint, in the absence of pain, as having pathological significance. It does not. Crepitus is a grating noise or sensation; it can have both auditory and palpable qualities. Fine crepitus is more readily felt than heard, but crepitus stemming from advanced degeneration of a large joint (e.g. the hip) is readily audible.

Locking

A joint locks if ectopic material becomes interposed between the articular surfaces. It is particularly associated with damage to the knee cartilages. Ascertain if the locking occurs at a particular point during movement of the joint.

MUSCLE

Muscle symptoms include pain and stiffness, weakness, wasting, abnormal spontaneous movements, and cramps.

Pain and stiffness

Muscle pain tends to be deep, constant and poorly localized. If due to local muscle disease, it is likely to be exacerbated by contraction of the muscle and relieved by rest (Fig. 11.22). If the patient complains more of muscle stiffness (particularly of the lower limbs) than pain, suspect the possibility of spasticity due to an upper motor neurone lesion.

Causes of muscle pain	
Inflammatory	Polymyositis Dermatomyositis
Infective	Pyogenic Cysticercosis
Traumatic	
Polymyalgia rheumatica	
Neuropathic	e.g. Guillain–Barré syndrome

Fig. 11.22 Causes of muscle pain.

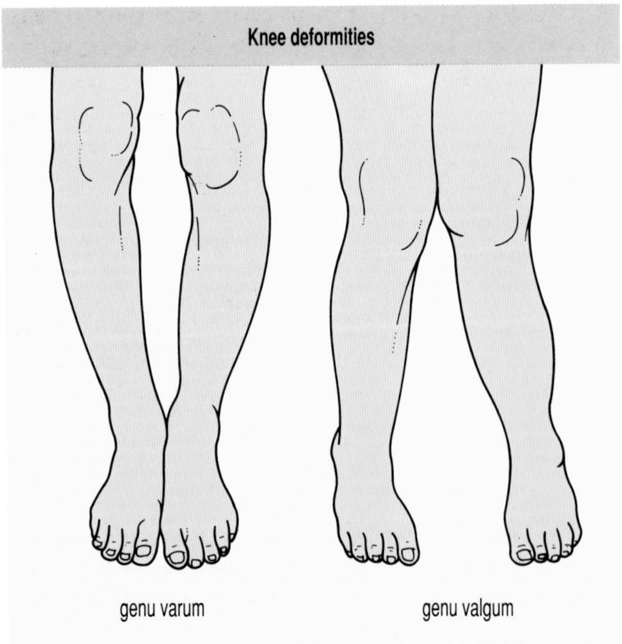

Fig. 11.23 Genu varum (left) and genu valgum (right).

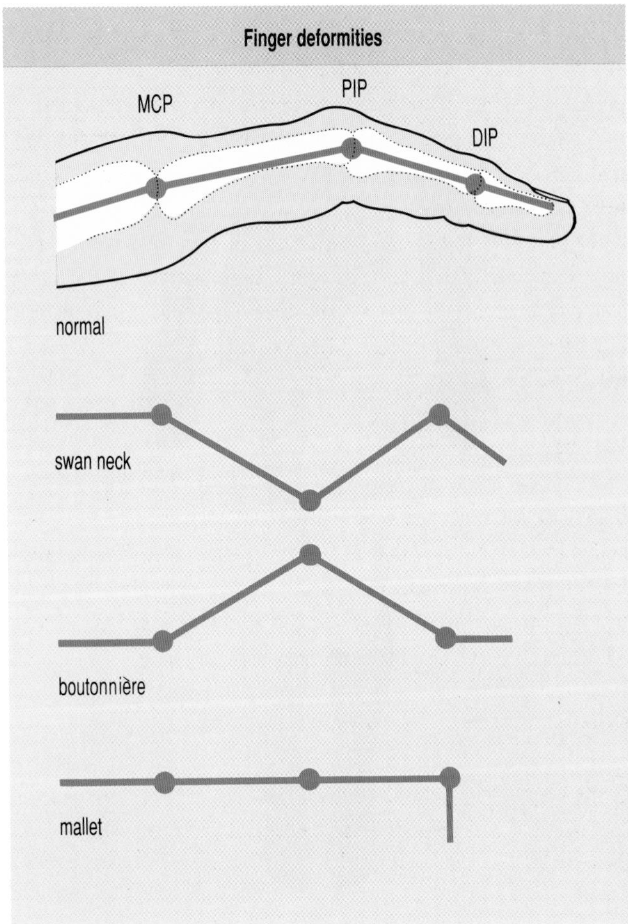

Fig. 11.24 Deformities of the finger in rheumatoid arthritis.

Weakness

A complaint of global weakness is more likely in neurotic individuals than in patients with neurological disorders.

> **Muscle weakness**
>
> Is the weakness global or focal?
>
> Is the weakness secondary to a painful limb?
>
> Does the weakness fluctuate in degree?
>
> Is the weakness increasing in severity?

Important questions to ask include the distribution of the weakness, whether it appears related to any pain in the limb, whether it fluctuates in degree, and whether it is static or progressive. A complaint of predominant proximal weakness suggests the possibility of primary muscle disease (e.g. polymyositis or myopathy). A predominantly distal weakness is more likely to be neuropathic. If the weakness is fluctuant, and particularly if it worsens during the course of activity, you will need to consider myasthenia gravis when you come to examine the patient (see also page 12.73). Weakness due to sudden entrapment of a peripheral nerve (e.g. a traumatic radial nerve palsy) will be stable or even improving by the time the patient seeks medical attention. In other conditions the weakness is progressive (e.g. motor neurone disease).

Wasting and fasciculation

Both these features form an important part of the examination, but both may have been noticed by the patient and volunteered during history taking. If the patient describes muscle twitching, ascertain whether the movement has occurred in several different muscles or whether it has been confined, most likely to the calves.

Cramps

Cramps are seldom of pathological significance. They are usually confined to the calves and can by triggered by forced contraction of the muscle.

EXAMINATION – THE GENERAL PRINCIPLES

BONE

Whichever structure is being examined, ensure that it is completely exposed and that the patient is comfortably positioned. Determine whether there is any abnormal angularity. Is there limb shortening. Look for tenderness by gently palpating those parts of the bone close to the skin surface.

JOINT

You need to follow a strict routine with joint examination incorporating inspection, palpation, and assessment of the movement of the joint.

Inspection

Things you are looking for include swelling, joint deformity, overlying skin changes and the appearance of the surrounding structures.

Swelling

Causes of joint swelling include effusions, thickening of the synovial tissues and of the bony margins of the joint. Differentiation of these causes is achieved by palpation. If you suspect joint swelling, compare it to the joint of the opposite limb. Particularly note if the swelling appears to be of the joint itself or of the adjacent structures.

Deformity

Deformity results either from misalignment of the bones forming the joint, or from alteration of the relationship between the articular surfaces. If misalignment exists, a deviation of the part distal to the joint away from the midline is called a valgus deformity, and a deviation towards the midline a varus deformity (Fig. 11.23). If a deformity exists you will need, later, to determine whether it is fixed or mobile. Partial loss of contact of the articulating surfaces is called subluxation and complete loss, dislocation. Though these are usually traumatic, they can also be seen in inflammatory joint disease, particularly rheumatoid arthritis. Swan neck, Boutonnière, and mallet are descriptive terms used for deformities in the metacarpo- and interphalangeal joints of the hand (Fig. 11.24).

Skin changes

You will want to palpate the skin over a joint to assess its temperature rather than relying simply on its colour. Redness of the skin over a joint implies an underlying acute inflammatory reaction (e.g. gout) (Fig. 11.25).

Changes of adjacent structures

The most striking change adjacent to a diseased joint is wasting of muscle. Assess muscle bulk above and below the affected joint, making a comparison with the opposite limb if that is spared. Wasting of quadriceps is particularly conspicuous in severe disease of the knee joint.

Palpation

During palpation of a joint, assess the nature of any swelling, whether there is tenderness and whether the joint is hot.

Swelling

The method of examining for an effusion will be described for the individual joints. Your first step is to determine the consistency of any swelling. Is the swelling hard, suggesting bone deformities secondary to osteoarthritis? Certain sites are particularly susceptible to osteoarthritic change (e.g. the distal interphalangeal joints of the hand) (Fig. 11.26). A slightly spongy, or boggy swelling suggests synovial thickening and is particularly associated with rheumatoid arthritis. An effusion is fluctuant, i.e. the fluid can be displaced from one part of the joint to another. Swellings may also arise adjacent to a joint. Again determine their consistency. Soft fluctuant swellings suggest enlarged bursae. Harder swellings occur in rheumatoid arthritis and gout.

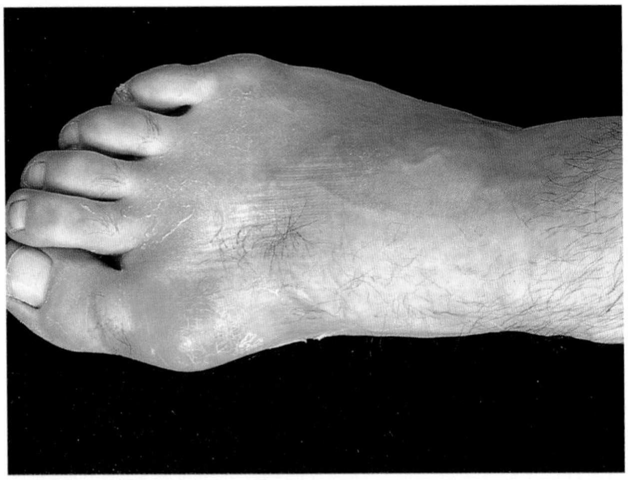

Fig. 11.25 Acute gout of the first MTP joint.

Tenderness

Carefully palpate the joint margin and adjacent bony surfaces together with the surrounding ligaments and tendons. Your task is to discover whether any tenderness is within the joint or outside it, and whether the tenderness is focal or generalized. In an acutely inflamed joint, the whole of its palpable contours will be tender. If there is derangement of a single knee cartilage, tenderness will be confined to the margin of that cartilage. In degenerative joint disease, you may find tenderness in structures adjacent to the joint. Tenderness close to the joint may reflect primary pathology in bone (e.g. osteomyelitis) or in the tendon sheath (e.g. De Quervain's tenosynovitis) (Figs 11.27 and 11.28).

Temperature

For a small joint, in the finger for example, assess temperature with the finger tips, using an unaffected joint in the same or the other hand for comparison. For a larger joint, say the knee, rub the back of your hand across the joint then compare with the other limb. If the contralateral joint is also affected, carry your hand above and below the joint margins to effect the comparison.

Joint movement

Next proceed to examine the range of movement of the joint, whether movement is limited by pain and whether there is instability.

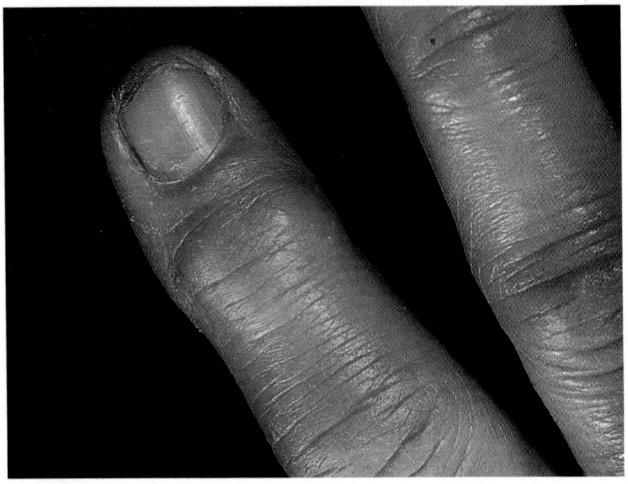

Fig. 11.26 Osteoarthritis of the DIP joint.

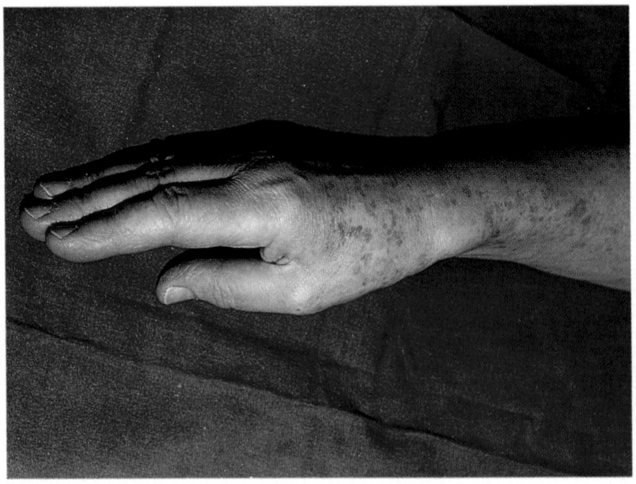

Fig. 11.27 Tendons involved in De Quervain's tenosynovitis.

To define the range of joint movement, start with the joints in the neutral position, defined as the limbs extended with the feet dorsiflexed to 90° and the upper limbs midway between pronation and supination with the arms flexed to 90° at the elbows (Fig. 11.29). For accurate measurement of joint movement you will need a goniometer (Fig. 11.30), but for routine purposes your eye should allow a reasonably true estimate. Movement of a joint is either active (i.e. induced by the patient) or passive (i.e. induced by the examiner). Sometimes you need to assess both; however, you will generally assess active movements in the spine but passive movements in the limb joints. Restriction of active compared to passive movement is usually due to muscle weakness.

From the neutral position, record the degrees of flexion and extension. If extension does not normally occur at a joint (e.g. the knee) but is present, describe the movement as hyperextension and give its range in degrees. Sometimes there is restriction of the range of movement. For example, if the knee fails by 30° to reach the extended position, describe this as either a 30° flexion deformity or as a 30° lack of extension (Fig. 11.31). For the ankle and wrist, extension is described as dorsiflexion, and flexion as plantar and

De Quervain's tenosynovitis

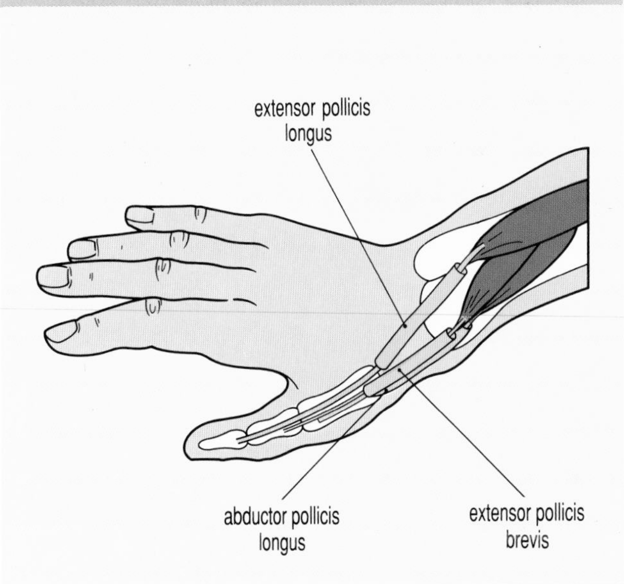

Fig. 11.28 De Quervain's tenosynovitis.

Neutral position

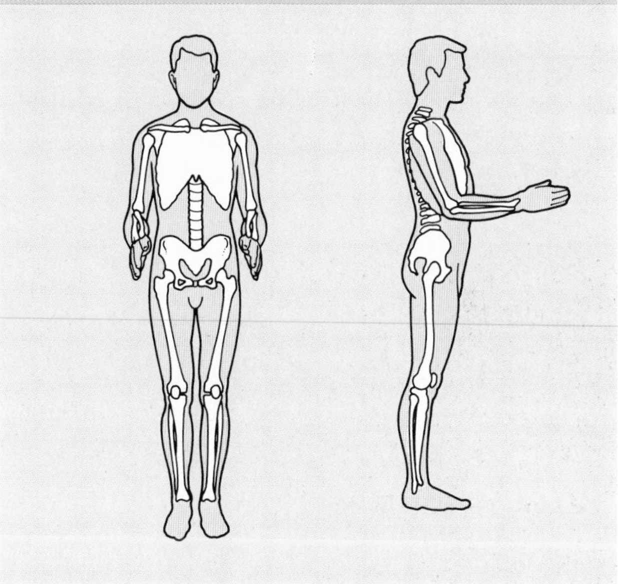

Fig. 11.29 The neutral position from which joint measurement is performed.

Range of joint movement

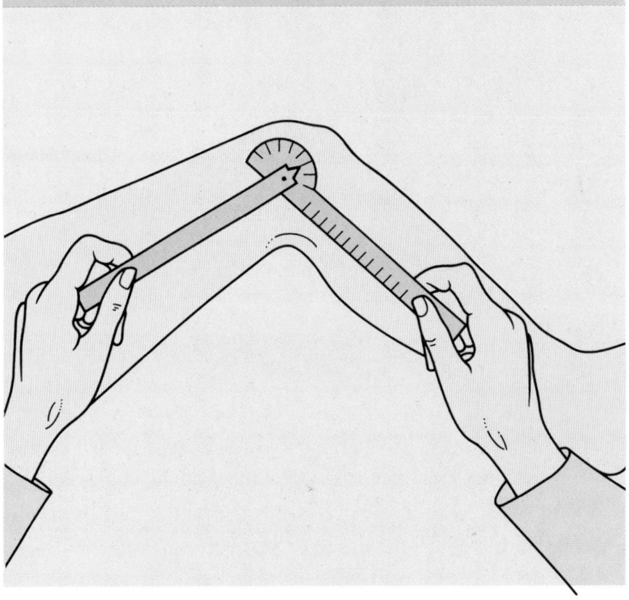

Fig. 11.30 Measuring the range of joint movement.

Flexion deformity

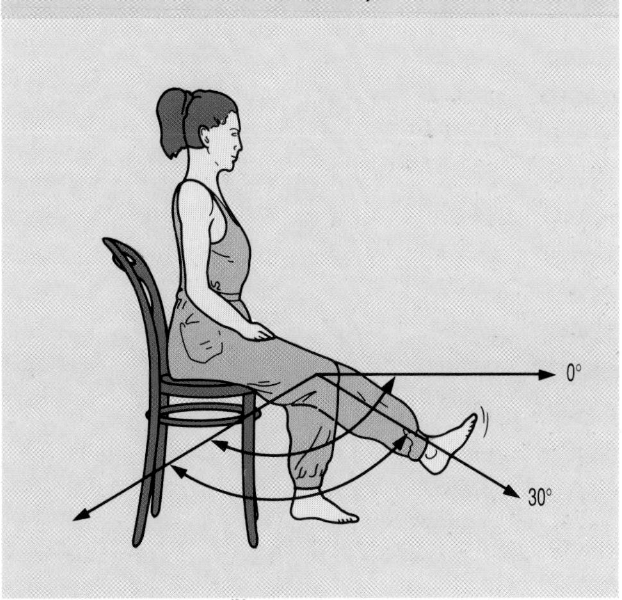

Fig. 11.31 30° flexion deformity of the knee.

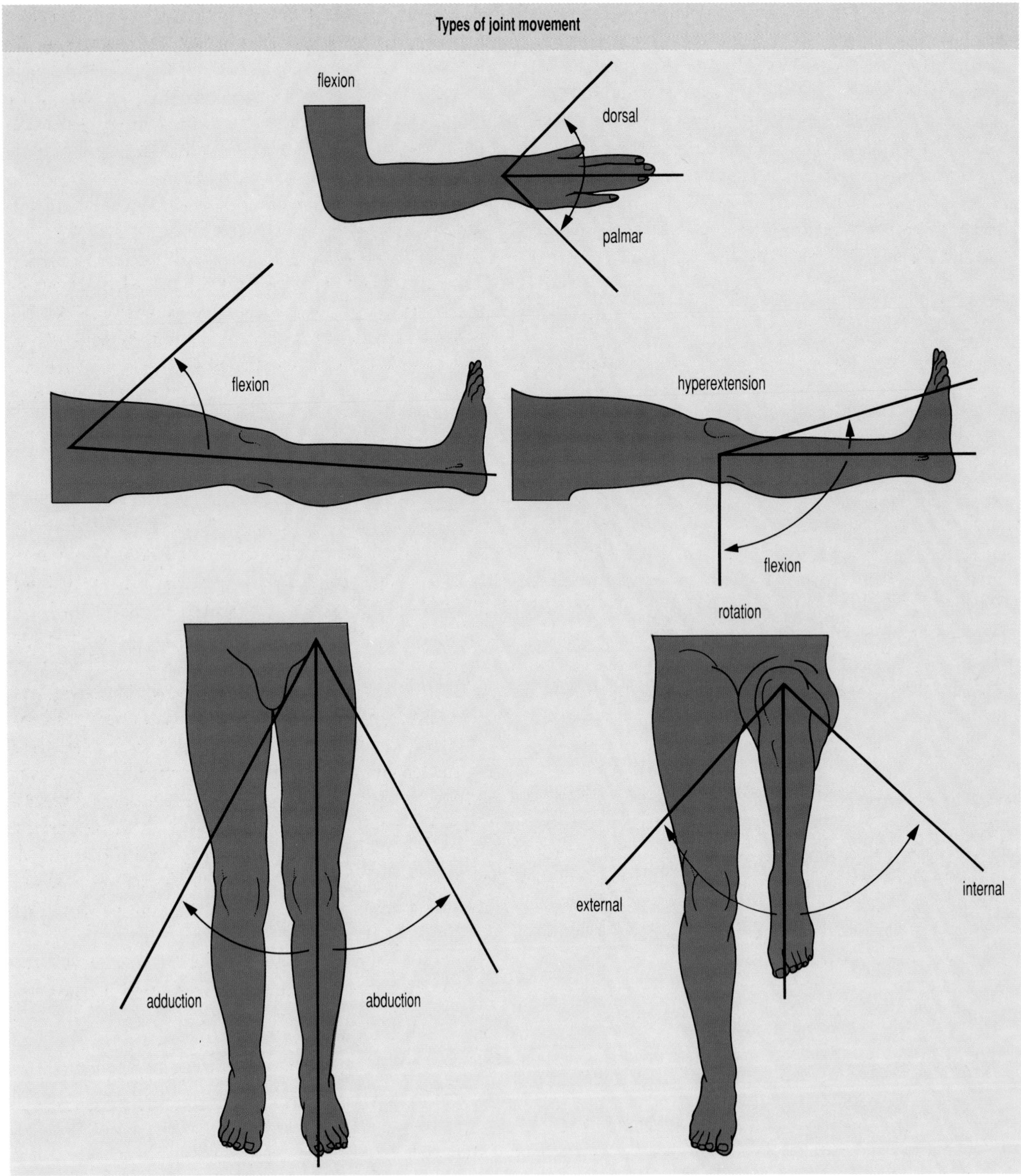

Fig. 11.32 Description of joint movement according to the type of joint.

palmar flexion, respectively. For a ball and socket joint, you will need to record the range of flexion, extension, abduction, adduction, and internal and external rotation (Fig. 11.32). The range of joint movement varies between individuals: an excessive range of movement can be constitutional as well as pathological. Carefully note if pain occurs during joint movement. In joint disease, pain is likely throughout the range of movement. In certain disease processes around the joint (e.g. the ligaments or bursae) pain can be restricted to a particular range or type of movement. Damage of either the articular surfaces or of the ligaments related to a joint can lead to instability. You will discover this partly by finding that the joint can be moved into abnormal positions and partly, particularly for the knee joint, by observing the joint as the patient walks.

MUSCLE

The methods for examining specific muscles will be given in the section on regional examination. Initially your assessment will include inspection, palpation, then testing of muscle power.

Inspection

Look for evidence of muscle wasting, for signs of abnormal muscle bulk, and for spontaneous contractions.

Wasting

Remember that quite striking muscle wasting can accompany joint disease (e.g. wasting of the small hand muscles in rheumatoid arthritis and wasting of the quadriceps in virtually any arthropathy affecting the knee joint). If there is no significant joint disease, wasting (other than due to a profound loss of body weight) reflects either primary muscle disease or disease of its innervating neurone. Make allowances for the age of the patient and his or her occupation. Some thinning of the hand muscles occurs in the elderly but is not accompanied by weakness. If you suspect wasting of one limb, measure the circumference of that limb and compare it with its fellow. For example, for the thigh, mark the line of the medial cartilage of the knee joint, measure up, say, 20cm, on each thigh and record the diameter of the legs at that point.

Increased muscle bulk

Usually abnormal muscle bulk reflects the patient's obsession with his own bodily strength (it almost always is a male). There are rare conditions which lead to muscle hypertrophy. If the enlargement is due to increase in muscle bulk, it is called true hypertrophy and is seen, for example, in congenital myotonia. If the increased bulk is due to fatty infiltration (and you will then discover the muscle is actually weak) it is called pseudo-hypertrophy. This finding is characteristic of certain of the muscular dystrophies (e.g. Duchenne's).

Spontaneous contractions

Completely expose the muscle when looking for evidence of spontaneous contraction. Make sure the patient is warm and relaxed. Shivering brought on by cold can be difficult to distinguish from fasciculation. Spontaneous movements can occur with both upper and lower motor neurone lesions. In the former, particularly at the spinal level, you may see either flexor or extensor spasms of the legs, either at the hips or knees. The movements can occur spontaneously or be triggered by attempting to move the patient and are often painful. Fasciculation produces episodic muscle twitching which can be quite subtle in small muscles. It is a feature of lower motor neurone lesions but can also be seen in normal individuals. Fasciculation is intermittent – wait for a few minutes before deciding it is absent. It is particularly important to determine whether the fasciculation is confined to a single muscle or whether it is more widely distributed. The former may reflect the result of cervical radiculopathy or be physiological (particularly if confined to the calves); the latter suggests a diagnosis of motor neurone disease.

Palpation

Muscle palpation is of limited value. If the muscle is infected or inflamed it is likely to be tender. Most myopathies are painless but there are exceptions (e.g. the acute myopathy occurring in alcoholics). Muscle tenderness can also occur in neurogenic disorders (e.g. the peripheral neuropathy of thiamine deficiency can lead to marked calf tenderness).

Testing muscle power

You should follow the MRC classification (see Fig.12.136) when testing and recording muscle power. Remember to make allowance for sex, age, and the patient's stature. If the muscle itself, or the joint which it moves, is painful, then power will be correspondingly limited. Patterns of muscle weakness are particularly important in neurological diagnosis. Is the weakness global, does it predominate distally or proximally in the limb, does its distribution fit with either a peripheral nerve or root distribution? Sometimes muscle power is decidedly fluctuant: there is a sudden give alternating with more effective contraction. Though this pattern can occur in myasthenia gravis, it is usually the reflection of a non-organic disability. If muscle fatigue is a prominent symptom assess it objectively. For example, for deltoid, ask the patient to abduct the shoulder to 90°. Test power immediately, then after the patient has held that posture for 60 seconds.

You will need to be selective when deciding which muscles to test. Your choice will partly be guided by the patient's complaints both in terms of their distribution and their quality.

REGIONAL EXAMINATION

THE TEMPOROMANDIBULAR JOINTS

Ask the patient to open and close the jaw. If the temporomandibular joints are lax, there may be considerable side-to-side movement. Now palpate the joint margins by placing your fingers immediately in front of and below the tragus. As the patient opens the jaw, palpate the head of the mandible as it moves forwards and downwards. In temporomandibular joint dysfunction the joint capsule is tender and chewing is painful. The generalized arthritic disorders seldom affect this joint.

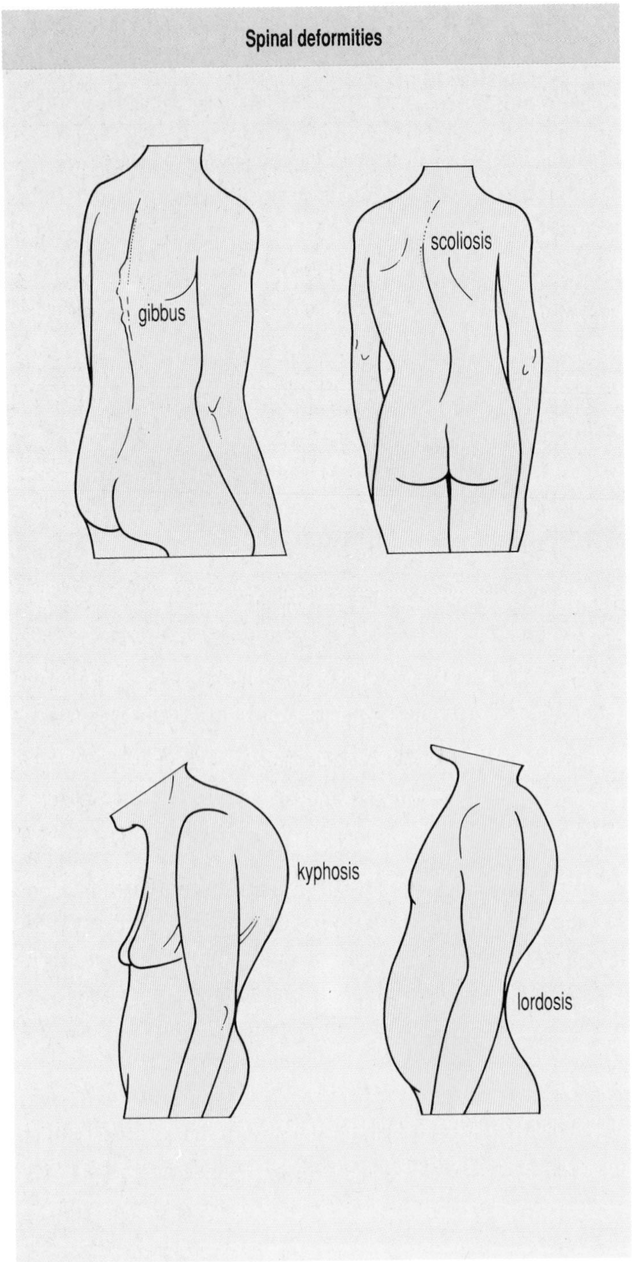

Fig. 11.33 Spinal deformities.

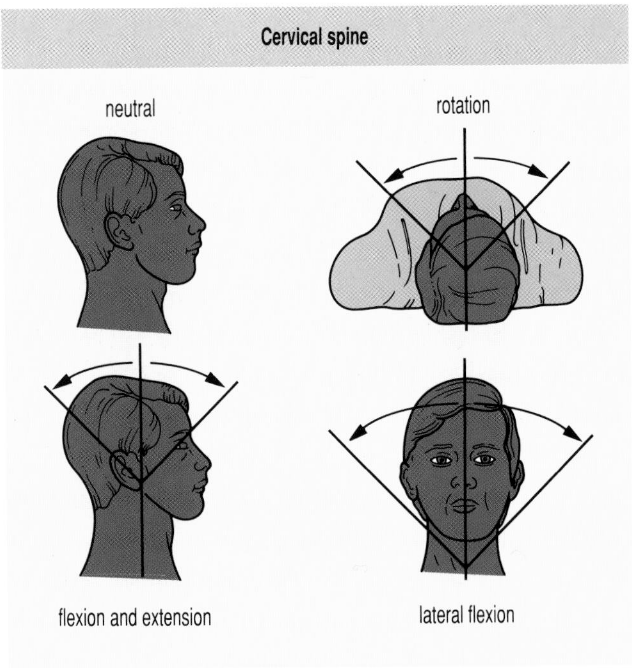

Fig. 11.34 Movements of the cervical spine.

THE SPINE

With the patient undressed to their underwear, ask them to stand upright. Assess the posture of the whole spine before examining its component parts. An increased flexion is called kyphosis, an increased extension lordosis, and a lateral curvature scoliosis. Gibbus refers to a focal flexion deformity (Fig. 11.33). Using the position of the spinous processes tends to underestimate the degree of scoliosis, as the spines rotate towards the midline. The scoliosis is accentuated when the patient bends forwards.

For each spinal level, start by inspection and follow by palpation so as to elicit any tenderness. Finally, assess the range of movement and determine whether it is restricted by pain.

Cervical spine

The examination is best achieved with the patient sitting. Note any deformity, then palpate the spinous processes. A cervical rib is sometimes palpable in the supraclavicular fossa. Obliteration of the radial pulse by downward traction of the arm does not reliably predict the presence of a cervical rib or band.

Examine active then passive movements. For flexion, ask the patient to bring the chin on to the chest and for extension ask them to bend the head backwards as far as possible. Observe both these movements from the side. For lateral flexion, stand in front of or behind the patient and ask him to bring the ear towards the shoulder first on one side, then the other. For rotation, stand in front or above the patient asking him to look over one shoulder then the other (Fig. 11.34). Note whether any movement triggers pain either locally or in the upper limb. Repeating the movements while applying gentle pressure over the vertex of the skull may trigger pain or paraesthesiae in the arm if there is a critical degree of narrowing at an intervertebral foramen (Fig.11.35).

Thoracic spine

Sit the patient with the arms folded across the chest, then ask him to twist as far as possible first to one side then to the other. The range of movement is best appreciated from above. Next measure chest expansion. A movement of at least 5cm should occur and provides an assessment of the mobility of the costovertebral junction. Palpate the spinous processes for any tenderness and assess any deformity.

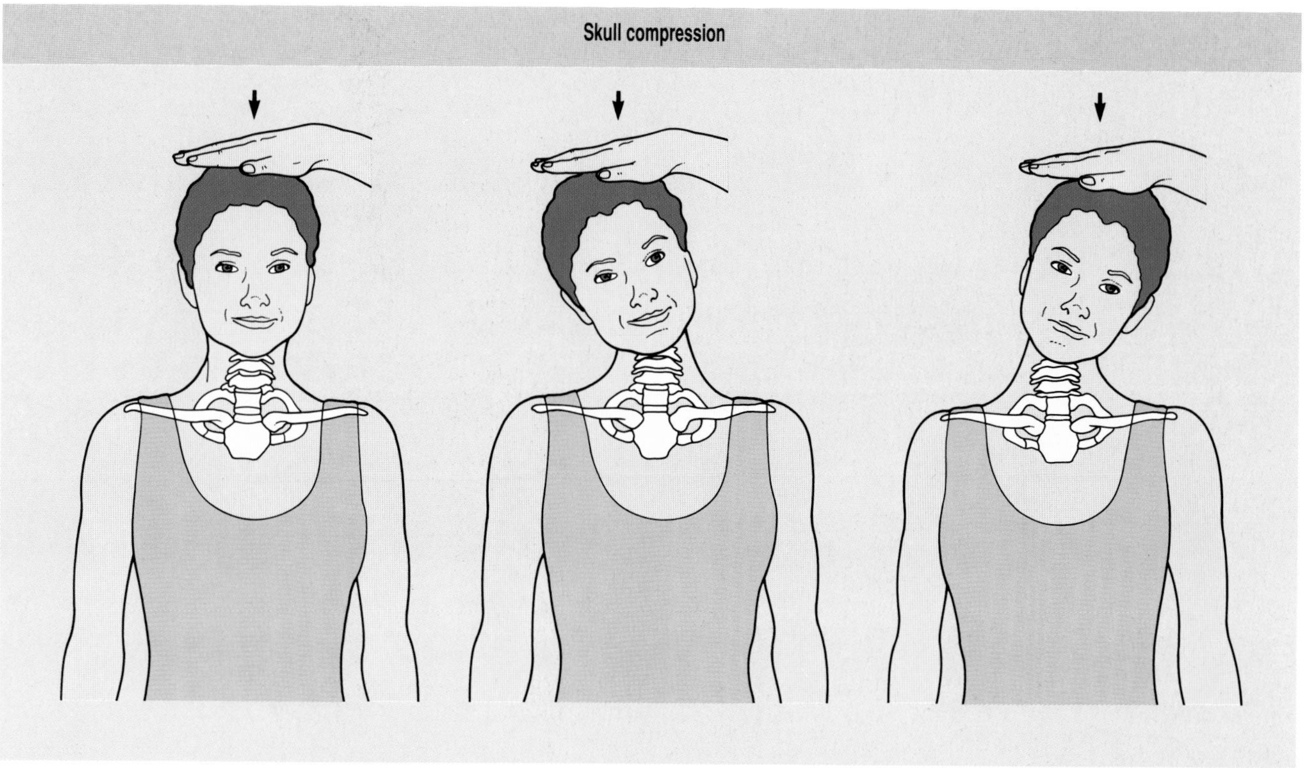

Fig. 11.35 Compression of the vertex of the skull to reproduce cervical root pain. Compression with the head in the neutral position (left) or laterally flexed to the right is painless (middle). With the neck flexed to the left (right), the side of the root compression, downward pressure is painful.

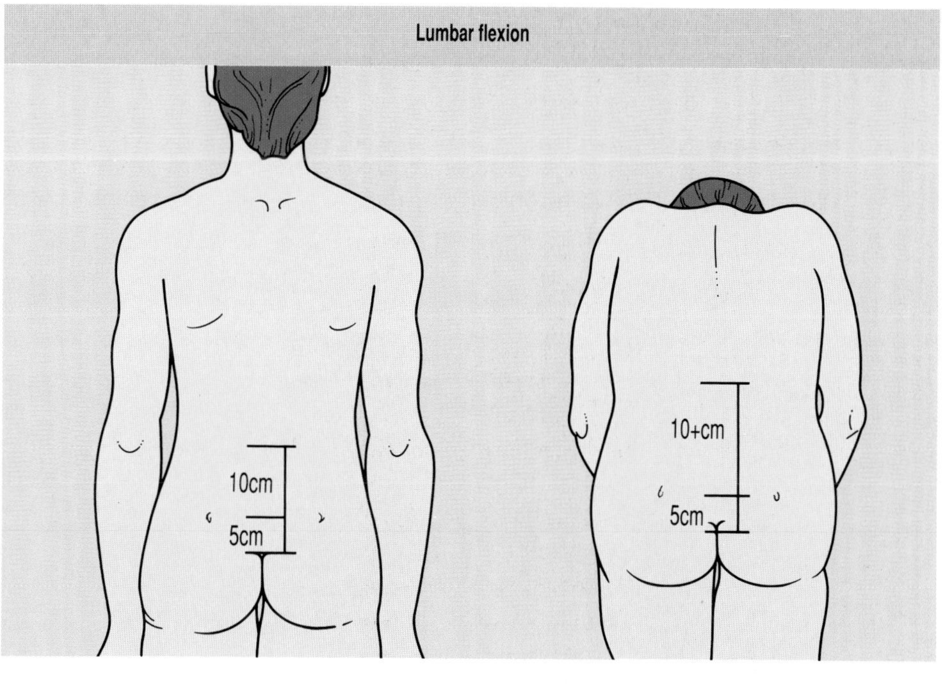

Fig. 11.36 Measuring lumbar flexion.

Lumbar spine

Having inspected the lumbar spine and tested for tenderness, assess the range of movement. While standing at the patient's side, ask him to touch his toes, keeping the knees straight. To assess the contribution made to flexion by the lumbar spine, mark the spine at the lumbosacral junction, then 10cm above and 5cm below this point. On forward flexion the distance between the two uppermarks should increase by about 4 cm, the distance between the lower two remaining unaltered (Fig. 11.36). Now assess extension, again from the side, then lateral flexion. For this, stand behind the patient and ask him to slide the hands down the outside of the leg, first to one side, then to the other (Fig. 11.37).

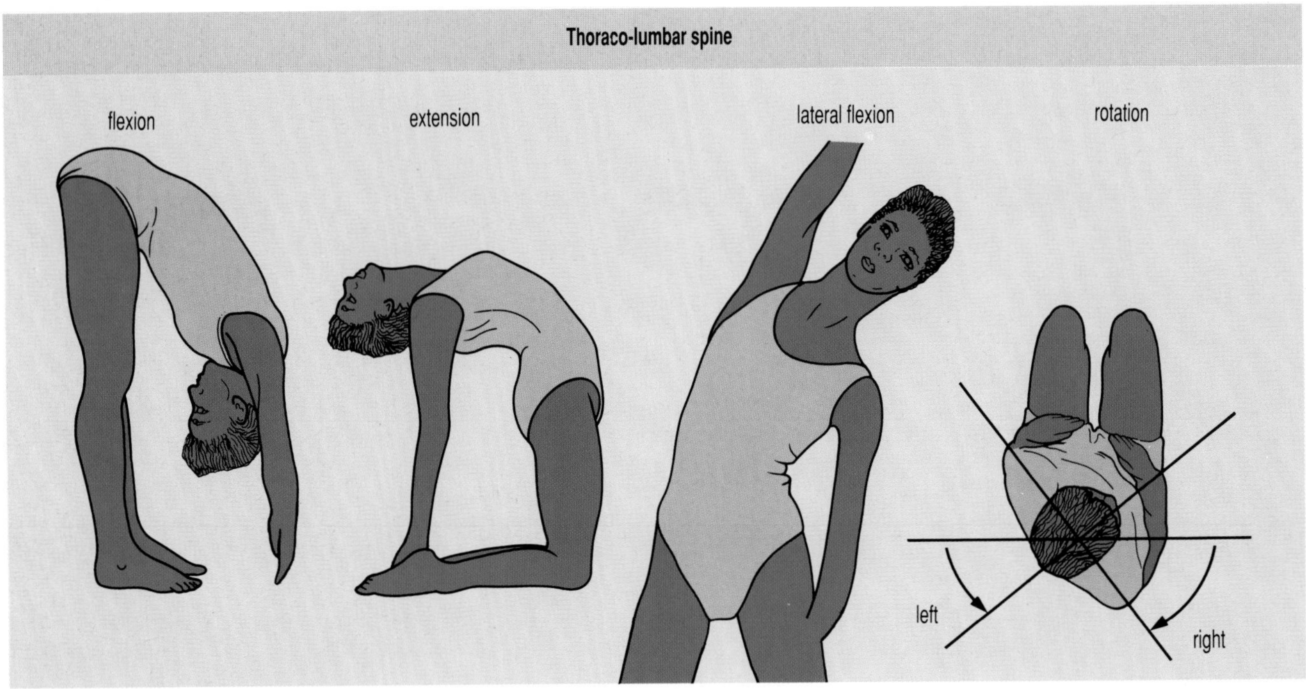

Fig. 11.37 Movements of the thoraco-lumbar spine.

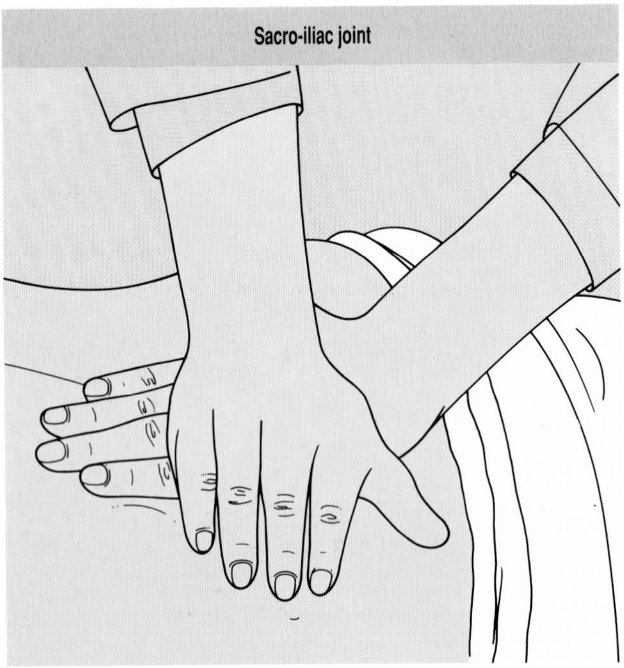

Fig. 11.38 Assessing the sacro-iliac joint.

Sacro-iliac joints

Palpate the joints, which lie under the dimples found in the lower lumbar region. To test whether movements at the joints are painful, first press firmly down over the midline of the sacrum with the patient prone (Fig. 11.38); then, with the patient supine, forcibly flex one hip while maintaining the other in an extended position.

Nerve stretch tests

Nerve stretch tests are carried out to determine whether there is evidence of nerve root irritation, usually as a consequence of prolapse of a lumbar disc.

Straight leg raising

With the patient supine, carefully elevate the extended leg at the hip. Normally some 80–90° of flexion is possible.

Restriction of movement can occur with both spinal and hip disease. In the presence of nerve root irritation at the L4 level or below, straight leg raising evokes pain as the sciatic nerve is stretched (Fig. 11.39). If the foot is now dorsiflexed, the pain increases (Bragard's test). Return the foot to the neutral position, then flex the knee. The hip can now be flexed further before pain reappears, but if the knee is then extended, the pain increases (Lasegue's test).

Femoral stretch test

Turn the patient into the prone position. First flex the knee. If this fails to trigger pain, extend the leg at the hip. A positive response, with pain in the back extending into the anterior thigh, suggests irritation of the second, third or fourth lumbar root on that side (Fig. 11.40).

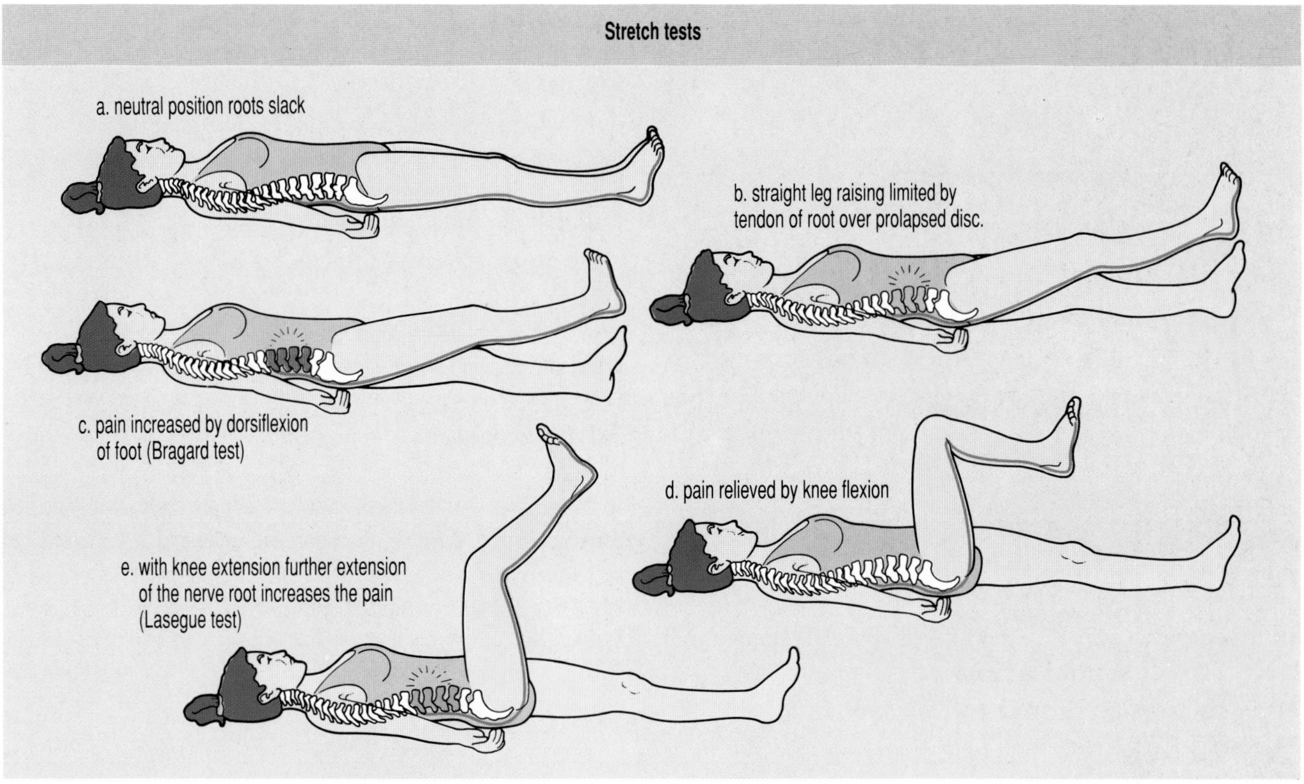
Stretch tests
a. neutral position roots slack
b. straight leg raising limited by tendon of root over prolapsed disc.
c. pain increased by dorsiflexion of foot (Bragard test)
d. pain relieved by knee flexion
e. with knee extension further extension of the nerve root increases the pain (Lasegue test)

Fig. 11.39 Stretch tests; (a) neutral position, (b) straight leg raising, (c) Bragard's test, (d) knee flexion, and (e) Lasegue's test.

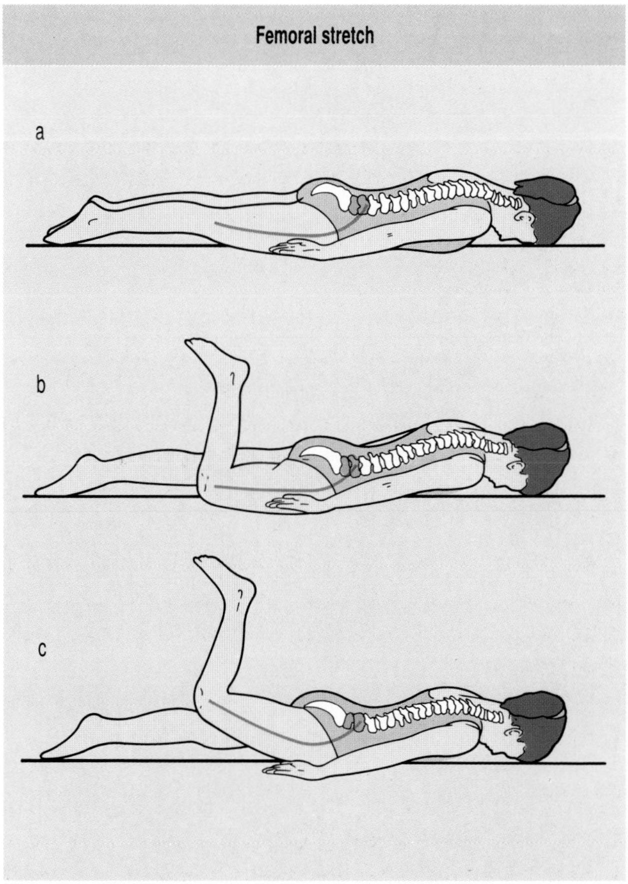
Femoral stretch
a
b
c

Fig. 11.40 (a) Femoral stretch. The pain may be triggered by (b) knee flexion alone or (c) in combination with hip extension.

Clinical application

Back pain can arise from disease processes in the vertebrae, from degenerative changes in the joints between the vertebrae, from degeneration or actual prolapse of the intervertebral disc, and from the ligaments and muscles supporting and moving the spine (Fig. 11.41).

> **Back pain**
>
> Is the pain confined to the back or does it radiate to the upper or lower limb?
>
> Is the pain exacerbated by coughing or sneezing?
>
> Did the pain begin suddenly or gradually?

Causes of back pain		
Muscle or ligamentous strain		
Degenerative intervertebral disc		
Spondylolisthesis		
Arthritis	–	Osteoarthritis Rheumatoid arthritis Ankylosing spondylitis
Bone infection		Pyogenic Tuberculous
Trauma		
Tumor		
Osteochondritis		
Metabolic bone disease		

Fig. 11.41 Causes of back pain.

Prolapsed intervertebral disc

A prolapse of disc material is most likely to occur either in the cervical (principally at C5/6) or the lumbar (principally at L5/S1) region. Once nerve root irritation occurs, likely symptoms include local and referred pain, with sensory and motor symptoms in the limb. The pattern of distribution of sensory change, weakness or reflex change allows prediction of the affected nerve root (Fig. 11.42).

Other conditions

Ankylosing spondylitis

In ankylosing spondylitis the patient, usually male, complains of spinal pain and stiffness, the latter improving with exercise. The sacro-iliac joints are affected initially. Increasing loss of spinal mobility can lead to a thoracic kyphosis combined with loss of the lumbar lordosis (Fig. 11.43).

Root syndromes

muscle

Root	Muscle
C5	spinati
C5, C6	supinator, deltoid, biceps
C6, C7	triceps
C7	finger extensors
C8	long finger flexors
L4, L5	tibialis anterior
L5	extensor hallucis longus
L5, S1	gastrocnemius, soleus

reflex

Root	Reflex
C5, C6	biceps, supinator
C6, C7	triceps
L4	knee (+ L2,3)
L5	no reflex
S1	ankle

sensory

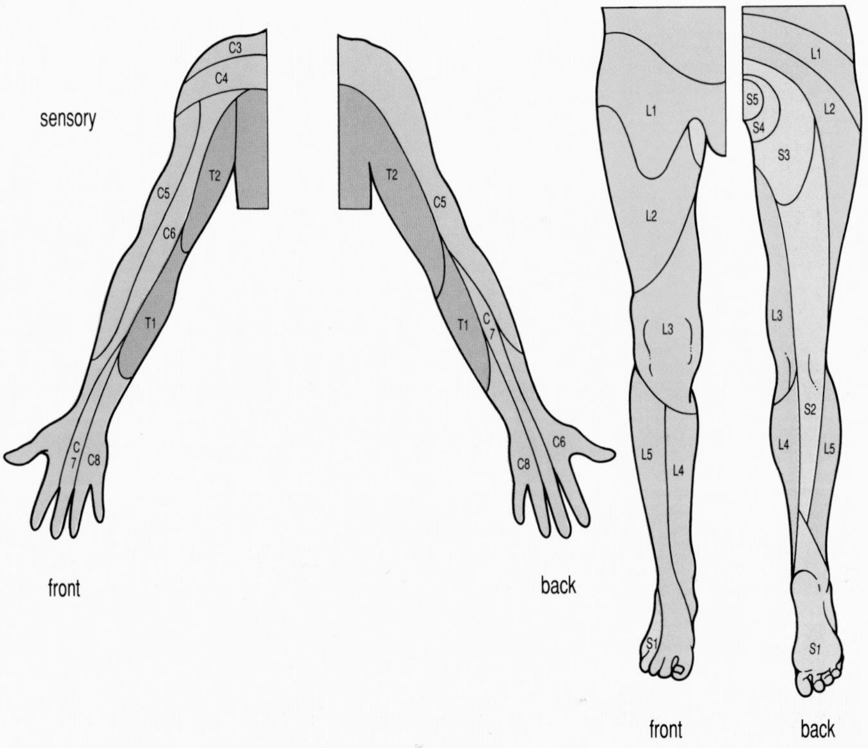

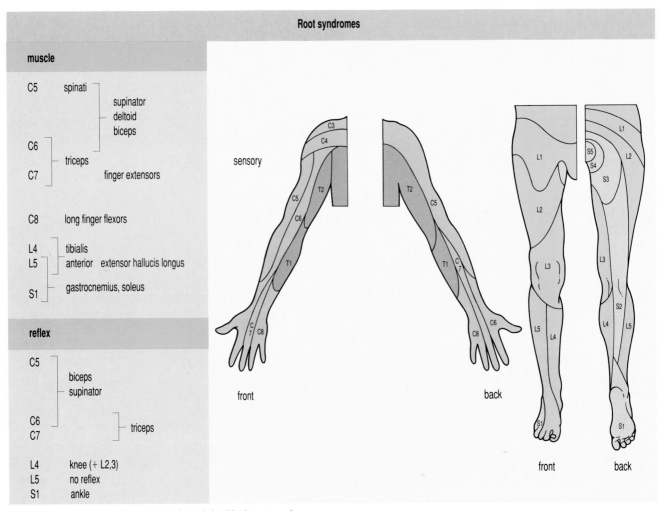

Fig. 11.42 Sensory, motor, and reflex changes in cervical and lumbar root syndromes.

Rheumatoid arthritis

This complaint commonly involves the upper cervical spine. Synovitis affecting the cruciate ligament allows posterior subluxation of the odontoid peg. Compression of the upper cervical cord is a potential hazard, producing a tetraparesis (Fig. 11.44).

Spinal tumors

Spinal tumors are usually metastatic from prostate, breast, bronchus, or kidney. Initially there is local, severe rest pain, sometimes with a referred component due to spinal root compression. Later focal neurological signs appear.

Tuberculosis

This disease most commonly involves the thoracic or lumbar spine. The infective process begins in the anterior margin of the vertebral body with early involvement of the disc space. Vertebral collapse with gibbus formation and paraspinal abscess follow. Symptoms include back pain and deformity with evidence of spinal cord compression.

THE SHOULDER

Inspection and palpation

Inspect the contour of the shoulder and its surrounding structures. Small effusions in the shoulder are difficult to detect. Anterior dislocation results in a forward and downward displacement with alteration of the shoulder contour (Fig. 11.45). Posterior dislocation is obvious. Fracture of the clavicle and anterior dislocation of the sternoclavicular joint are usually readily visible. Look at the deltoid to see if it is wasted. Then inspect the periscapular muscles. The bulk of supraspinatus and infraspinatus is easily assessed. Palpate the shoulder and sterno-clavicular joints for tenderness.

Joint movement

Remember that most movement at the shoulder involves both the glenohumeral joint and rotation of the scapula across the thorax. You will test flexion and extension, internal and external rotation,

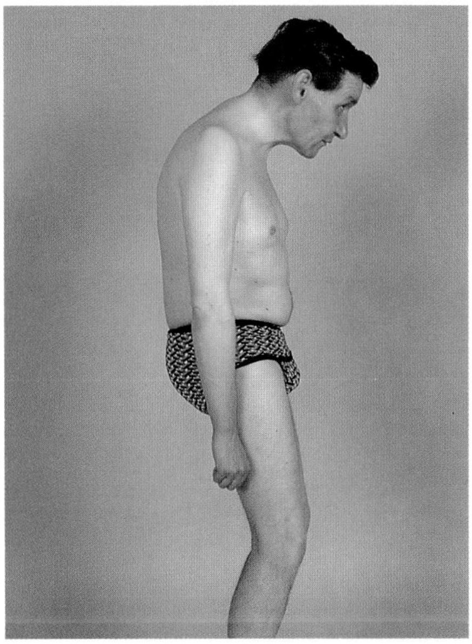

Fig. 11.43 Advanced ankylosing spondylitis.

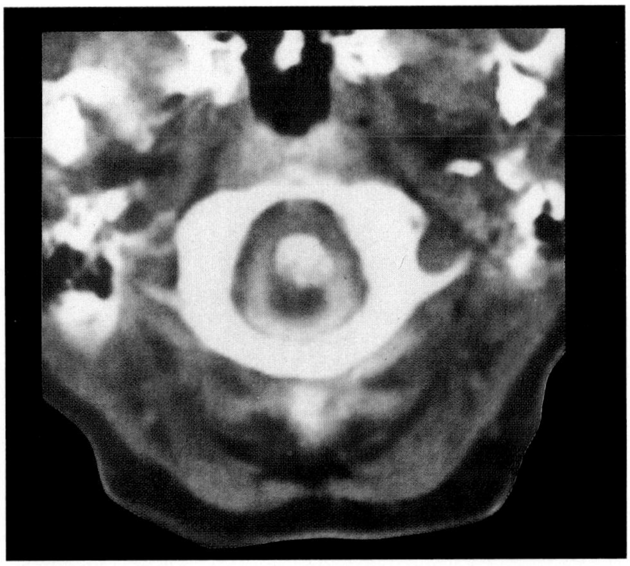

Fig. 11.44 Atlanto-axial subluxation, CT myelography demonstrating cord compression.

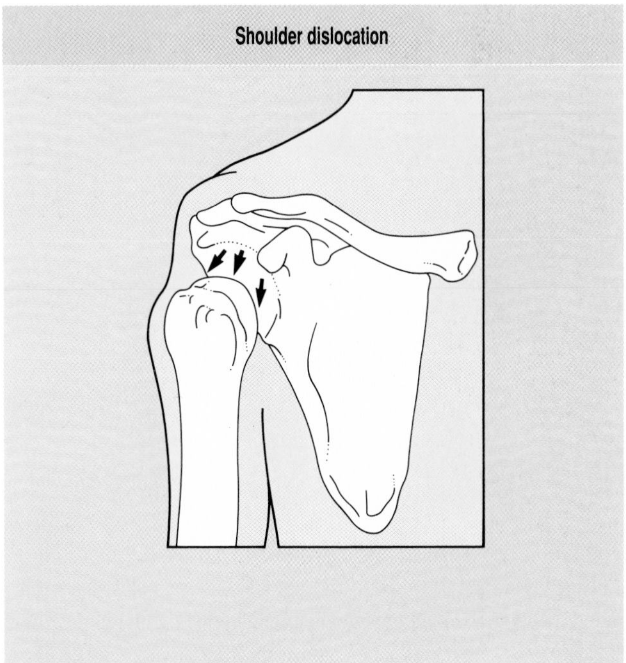

Fig. 11.45 Dislocation of the shoulder.

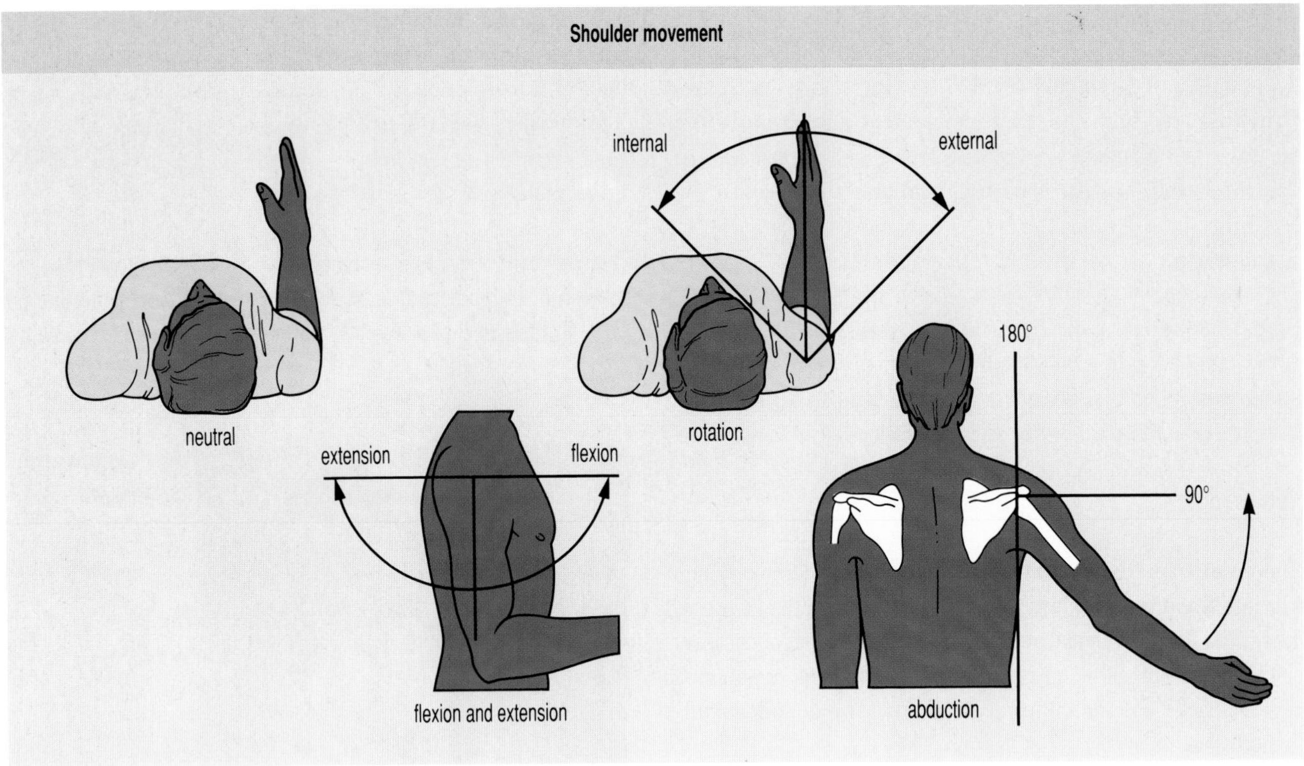

Fig. 11.46 Testing shoulder movement.

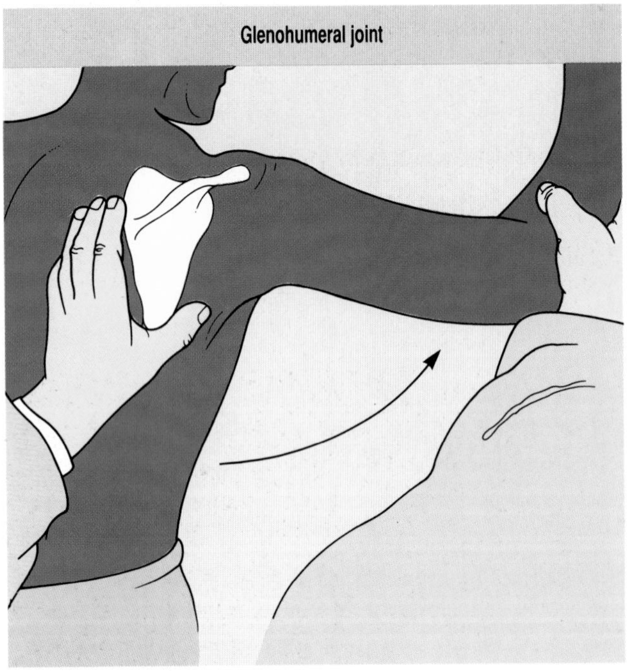

Fig. 11.47 Testing abduction at the glenohumeral joint.

abduction and adduction (Fig. 11.46). When testing abduction, anchor the scapula with your free hand, to ensure that over the first 90° only glenohumeral movement is allowed (Fig. 11.47). Test first passive then active movement. During abduction, note particularly if pain occurs. Is the pain present throughout the movement or only over a particular range? With a frozen shoulder (attributed to capsulitis of the glenohumeral joint) pain is accompanied by restriction of all glenohumeral movements.

Painful arc syndrome

The painful arc syndrome causes pain on shoulder elevation. As the arm is elevated, elements of the rotator cuff, comprising the tendons of supraspinatus, infraspinatus, and subscapularis come into contact with the under surface of the acromion. Inflammation of one of the muscles, particularly supraspinatus, or of the subacromial bursa, causes pain in the region of the shoulder, with a painful arc of movement during abduction (Fig. 11.48). Pain is absent initially, develops during abduction as elements of the cuff come into contact with the undersurface of the acromion, then disappears in the final part of abduction as the tendons fall away from the acromion.

Bicipital tendonitis

In bicipital tendonitis tenosynovitis involves the long head of biceps. The patient complains of pain in the anterior aspect of the shoulder and arm. The pain is reproduced by palpating the tendon or by contracting the muscle.

Muscle function

In the presence of any of the above conditions, muscle power is

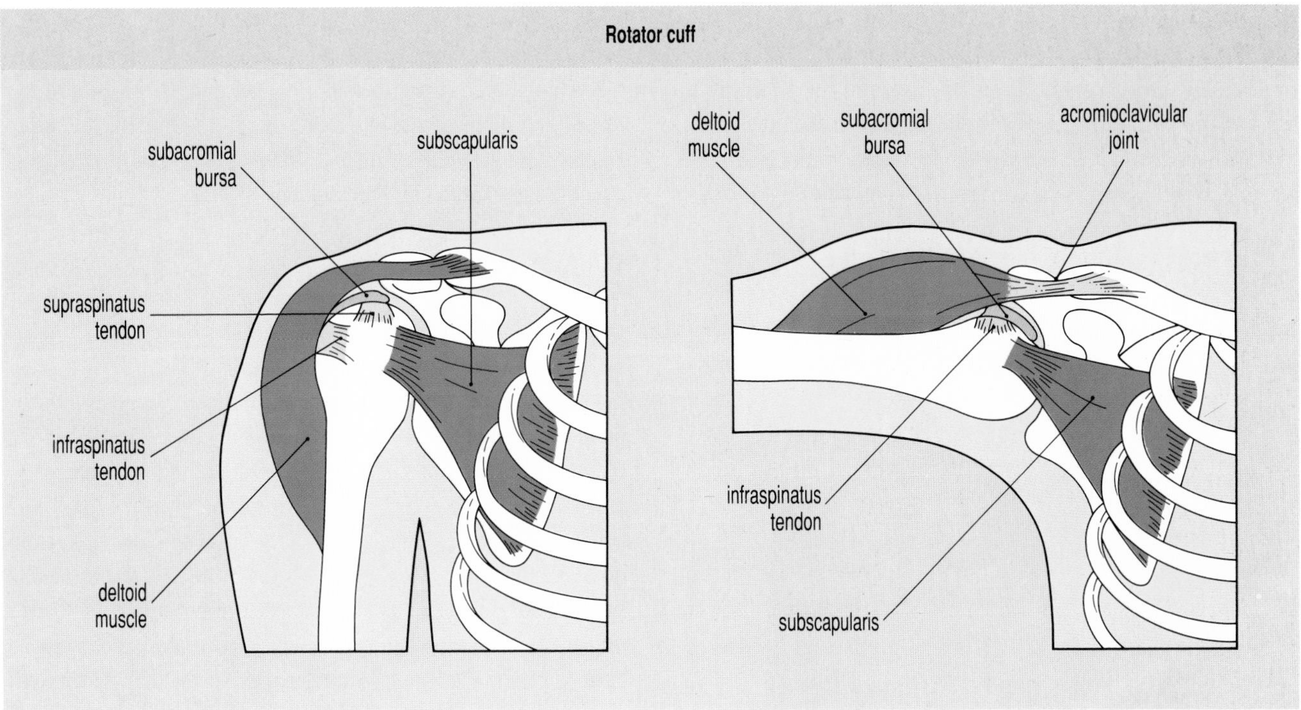

Fig. 11.48 The rotator cuff apparatus.

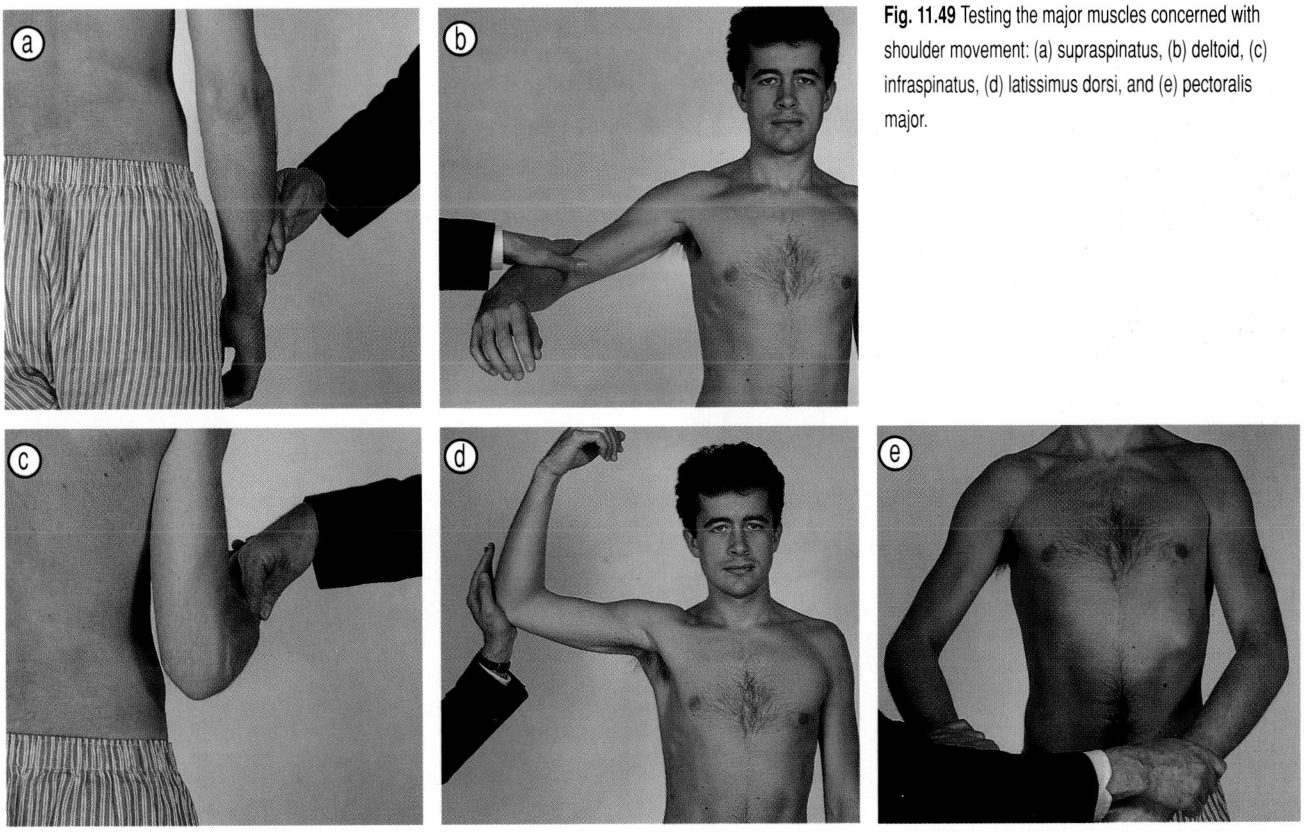

Fig. 11.49 Testing the major muscles concerned with shoulder movement: (a) supraspinatus, (b) deltoid, (c) infraspinatus, (d) latissimus dorsi, and (e) pectoralis major.

limited by concomitant pain. If shoulder movements are free and painless, the individual muscles concerned with movement around the joint can now be tested (Fig. 11.49).

Cervical radiculopathy

Cervical radiculopathy quite often affects the fifth nerve root. Weakness is found in the spinati, deltoid, and biceps. Wasting may follow (Fig. 11.50). The biceps and supinator reflexes are depressed.

Neuralgic amyotrophy

In neuralgic amyotrophy, severe pain around the shoulder is followed by patchy weakness and wasting in the shoulder girdle muscles. One form affects the long thoracic nerve, with consequent winging of the scapula as the arm is pushed forwards (Fig. 11.51).

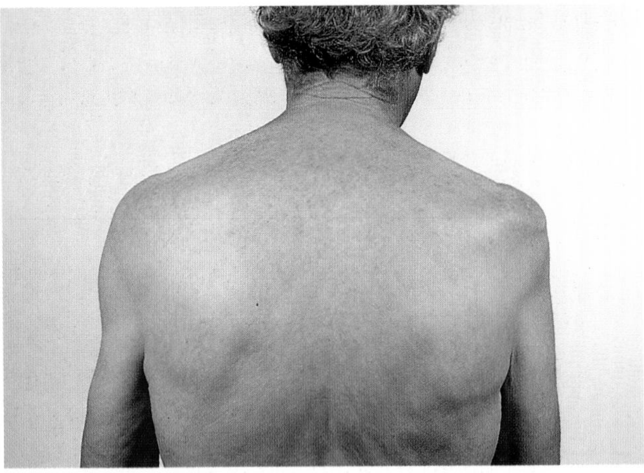

Fig. 11.50 Wasting of deltoid, infraspinatus and supraspinatus in a right C5 root lesion.

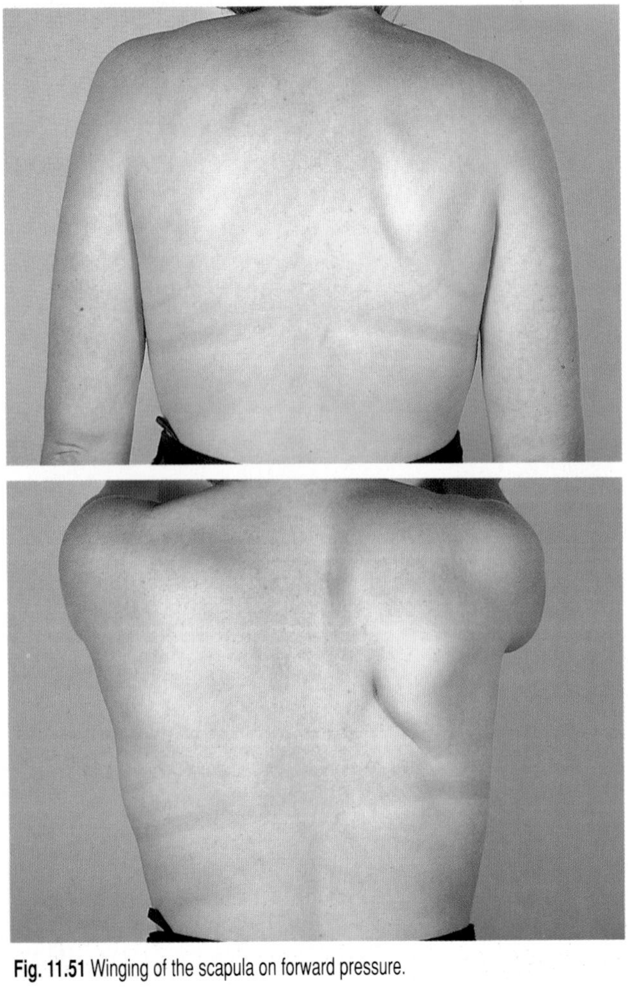

Fig. 11.51 Winging of the scapula on forward pressure.

Nerve palsies

Nerve palsies affecting the shoulder are rare. A fracture of the upper end of the humerus can damage the circumflex nerve resulting in weakness of deltoid and a small patch of numbness over the lateral aspect of the shoulder.

THE ELBOW

Inspection and palpation

Inspect the joint from behind, comparing its alignment with the other arm. An effusion produces a swelling on either side of the olecranon. Swelling of the olecranon bursa can follow trauma or in association with rheumatoid arthritis. Now palpate the subcutaneous border of the ulna, a common site for rheumatoid nodules (Fig. 11.52). Move on to palpate the lateral and medial epicondyles (Fig. 11.53). Inflammation of the extensor and flexor origins at these respective sites (tennis elbow and golfer's elbow) leads to pain in the region of the elbow exacerbated by forced wrist extension for the former, and forced wrist flexion for the latter. Immediately inside the medial epicondyle is the ulnar groove, within which you can palpate the ulnar nerve. The nerve tends to thicken at this site even in normal subjects.

Joint movement

Flexion and extension at the elbow allow a total range of movement of about 160°. Supination and pronation both occur through a range of about 90°.

Muscle function

Test the principal muscles concerned with elbow flexion and extension, together with pronation and supination (Fig. 11.54).

A *lesion of the C6 nerve root* is common (Fig. 11.55). Muscles that can be affected include biceps, brachioradialis, supinator, and

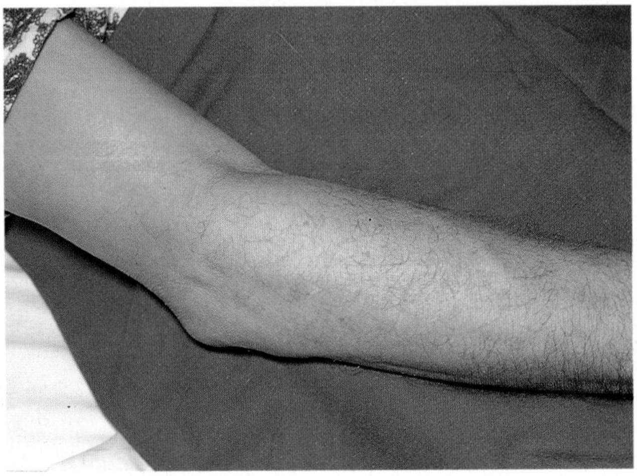

Fig. 11.52 Rheumatoid nodule.

triceps. In practice triceps weakness predominates, with depression or loss of the triceps reflex. Any loss of sensation occupies the thumb and index finger.

THE FOREARM AND WRIST

Inspection and palpation

Compare the size of the forearms, but remember that the dominant forearm tends to be rather larger. Compare the two wrists for size, and for any evidence of swelling or deviation. Malunion of a distal fracture (Colles) leads to an extension deformity. If the patient describes a wrist strain, carefully palpate in the region of the anatomical snuff box. Localized tenderness suggests a diagnosis of a fractured scaphoid. In *De Quervain's tenosynovitis*, inflammation of the tendons of abductor pollicis longus and extensor pollicis brevis causes wrist pain, with localized tenderness and crepitus as the tendon moves through its sheath (see Fig. 11.28).

Joint movement

From the neutral position test flexion of the wrist (about 90°) then extension (about 70°). A comparison of the degree of dorsiflexion between the two wrists is best achieved by asking the patient to

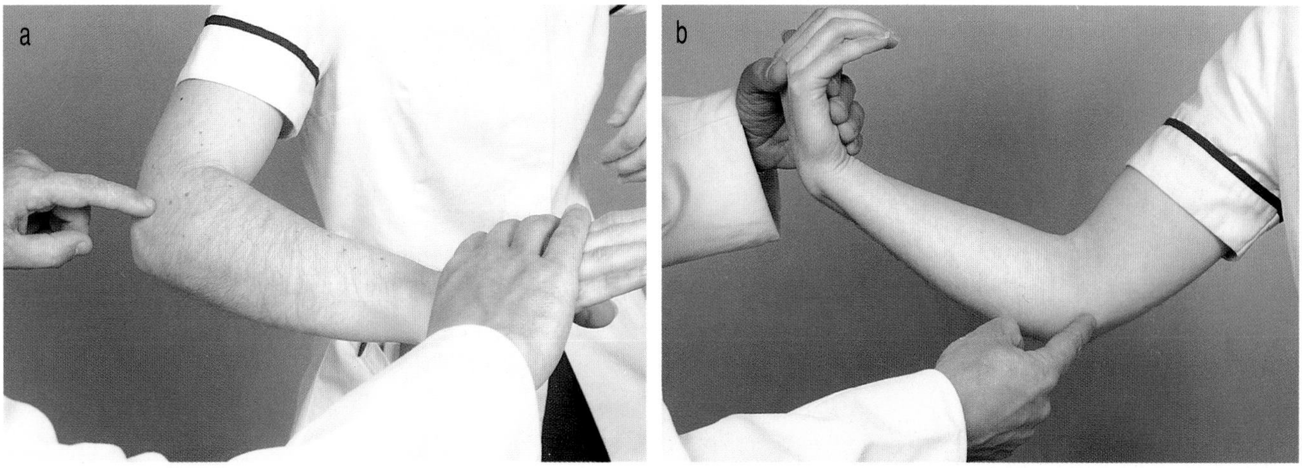

Fig. 11.53 Eliciting tenderness in a case of lateral (left) and (b) medial epicondylitis.

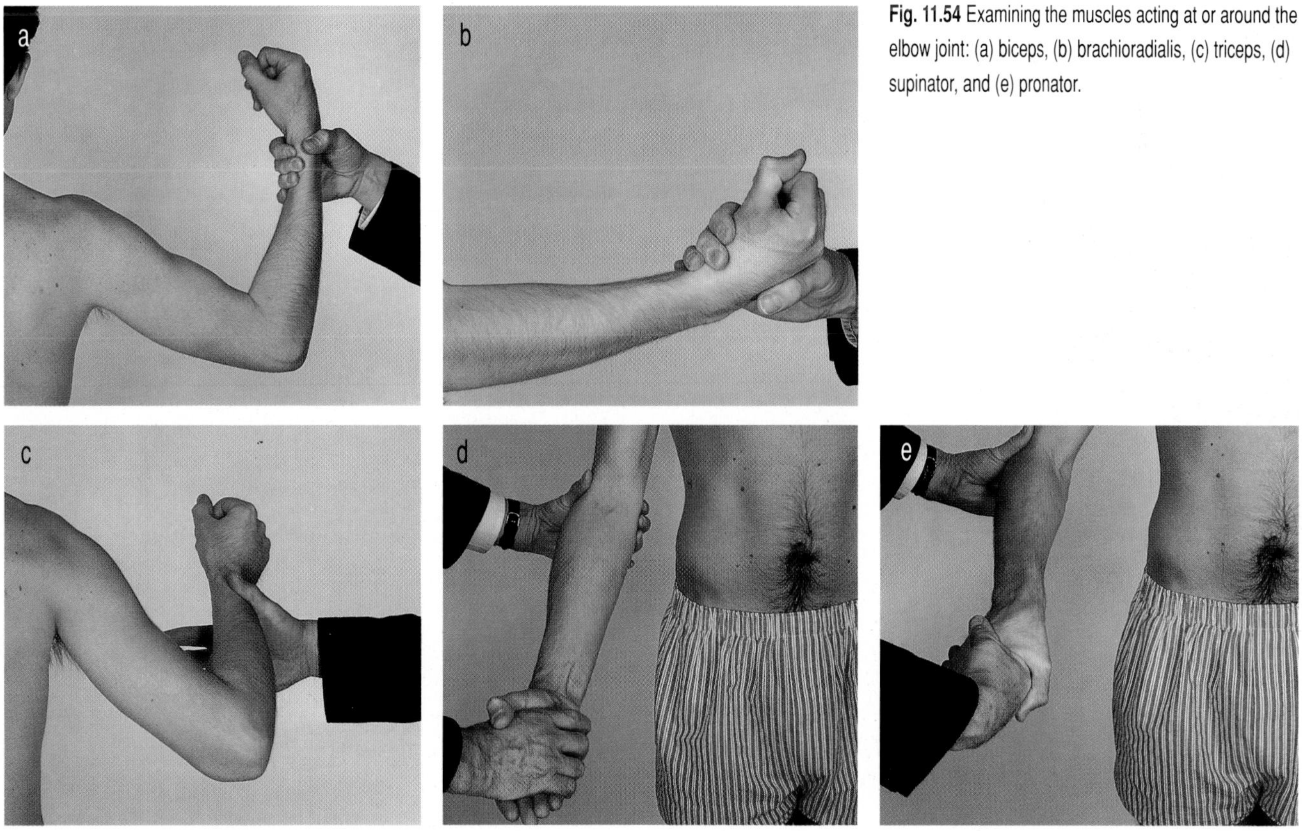

Fig. 11.54 Examining the muscles acting at or around the elbow joint: (a) biceps, (b) brachioradialis, (c) triceps, (d) supinator, and (e) pronator.

C6 root		
Muscles affected	**Dermatomal changes**	**Reflex changes**
Biceps	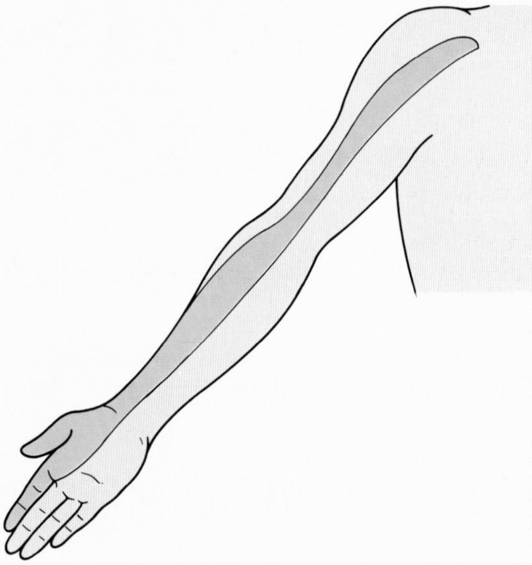	(Biceps)
Brachioradialis		Triceps
Supinator		
Triceps		

Fig. 11.55 C6 root syndrome.

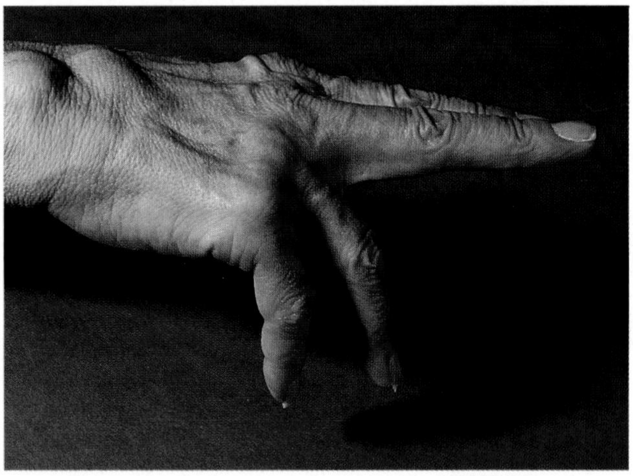

Fig. 11.56 Elevation of the ulnar head in rheumatoid arthritis. The flexion deformity of the 4th and 5th digits is due to rupture of their extensor tendons.

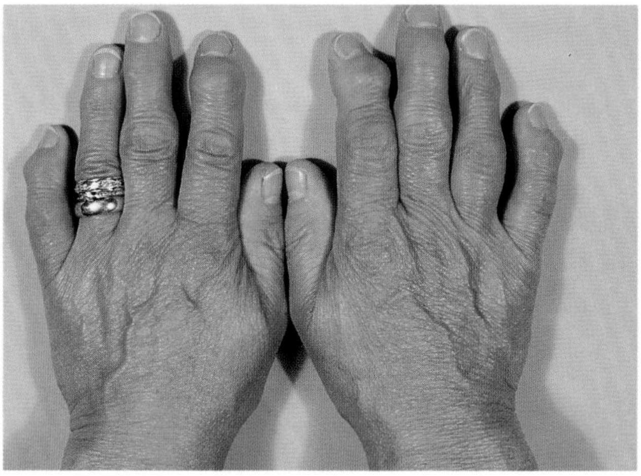

Fig. 11.57 The square hand of osteoarthritis.

press the palms together while elevating the elbows so that the forearms are in a straight line. The range of palmar flexion can be similarly compared with the backs of the hands pressed together. Now assess radial and ulnar deviation of the wrist. Wrist involvement is common in rheumatoid arthritis. Besides pain and limitation of movement, stretching of the ulnar collateral ligament allows the head of the ulna to subluxate upwards (Fig. 11.56). Osteoarthritis commonly affects the carpometacarpal joint of the thumb. In combination with changes in the distal interphalangeal joints, the appearance of a square hand results (Fig. 11.57).

Muscle function

Now test the muscles acting at the wrist (Fig. 11.58) and the long flexors and extensors of the fingers (Fig. 11.59).

A *C7 root lesion* affects triceps together with wrist and finger extension. The triceps jerk may be depressed and sensory loss, if present, occurs over the middle finger.

A *radial palsy* most commonly results from damage to the nerve in the spiral groove. There is weakness of supinator, brachioradialis, and wrist and finger extension (Fig. 11.60). The brachioradialis component of the supinator reflex is depressed.

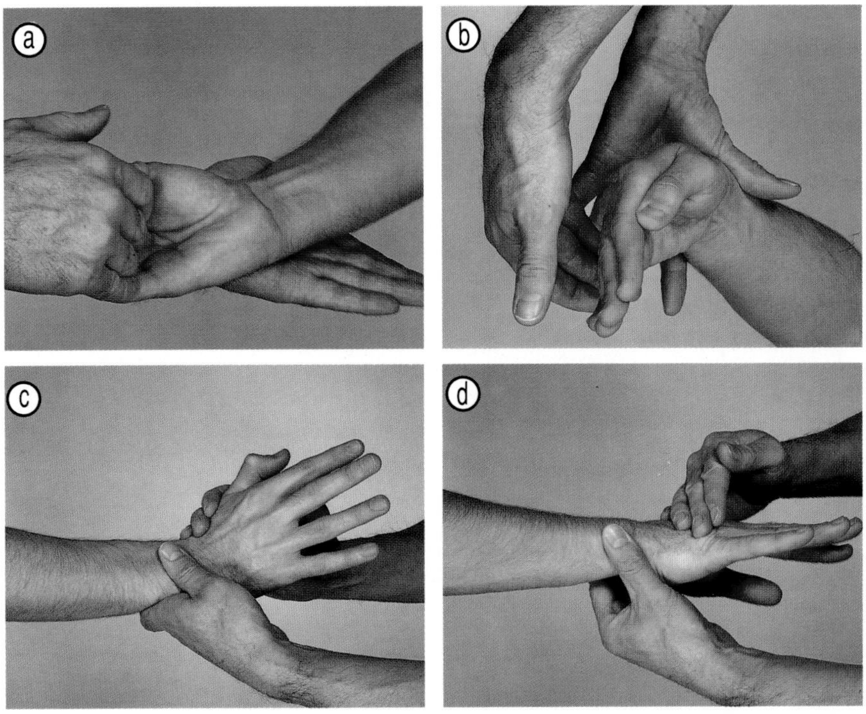

Fig. 11.58 Examining some of the muscles of the forearm: (a) flexor carpi radialis, (b) flexor carpi ulnaris, (c) extensor carpi radialis longus, (d) extensor carpi ulnaris.

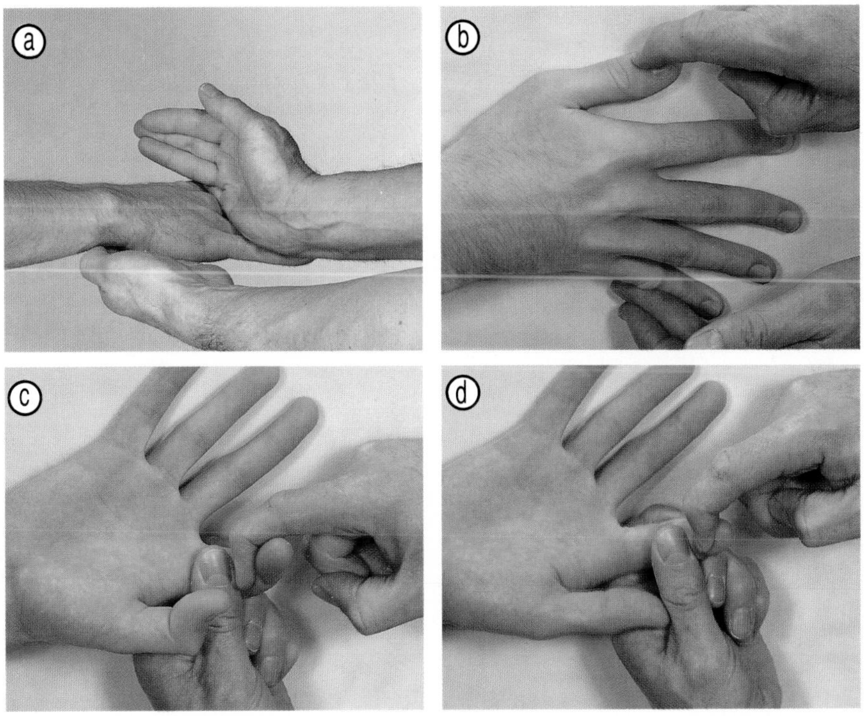

Fig. 11.59 Examining the long finger flexors and extensors: (a) extensor digitorum, (b) extensor pollicis longus, (c) flexor digitorum sublimis, (d) flexor digitorum profundus.

Sensory loss is often slight, mainly involving an area of skin in the region of the anatomical snuff box.

THE HAND

The joint and muscle function of the hand are best considered separately.

THE HAND JOINTS

Inspection and palpation

A good way to examine the hands both for joint and muscle function is to ask the patient to sit opposite you with his hands spread on a flat surface. You are looking for signs of joint deformity and whether any deformity is generalized or focal. If the latter, are particular joints affected? While inspecting the joints, remember to look at the state of the skin and whether the nails are deformed. Now turn the hands over to look at the palmar aspects. Is there evidence of tendon thickening?

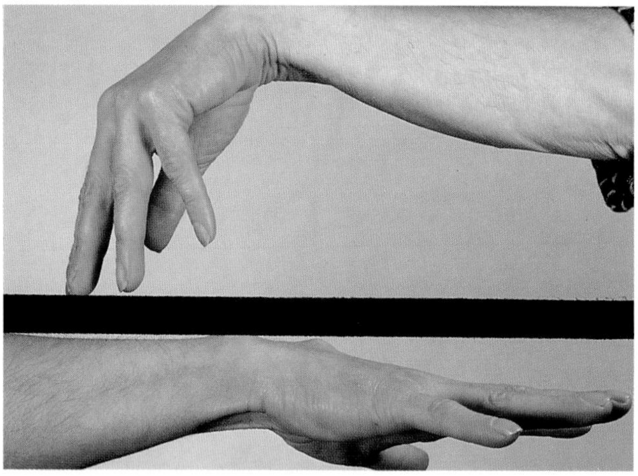

Next carefully palpate the joints. Is there joint tenderness? Assess the quality of any swelling (Fig. 11.61). Can you feel any nodules along the tendon sheaths?

In *early rheumatoid arthritis*, slight swelling of the proximal interphalangeal joints is accompanied by tenderness (Fig. 11.62). At a later stage of the condition, substantial deformities occur (see Fig. 11.24) accompanied by wasting of the small muscles. If the changes predominate in the distal interphalangeal joints, carefully inspect the nails for signs suggesting a diagnosis of *psoriasis* (Fig. 11.63). In *osteoarthritis*, nodules (Heberden's nodes) typically appear over the distal interphalangeal joints, but are also seen at the proximal interphalangeal joints (Bouchard's nodes) (Fig. 11.64). Nodule formation on the flexor tendon can lead to the tendon being caught in a localized narrowing of the sheath. The result, *trigger finger*, is a flexion deformity from which the finger can be extended only by force (Fig. 11.65).

Movement

Test the range of movement in the thumb and fingers. For abduction and adduction of the fingers, outlining the fingers on

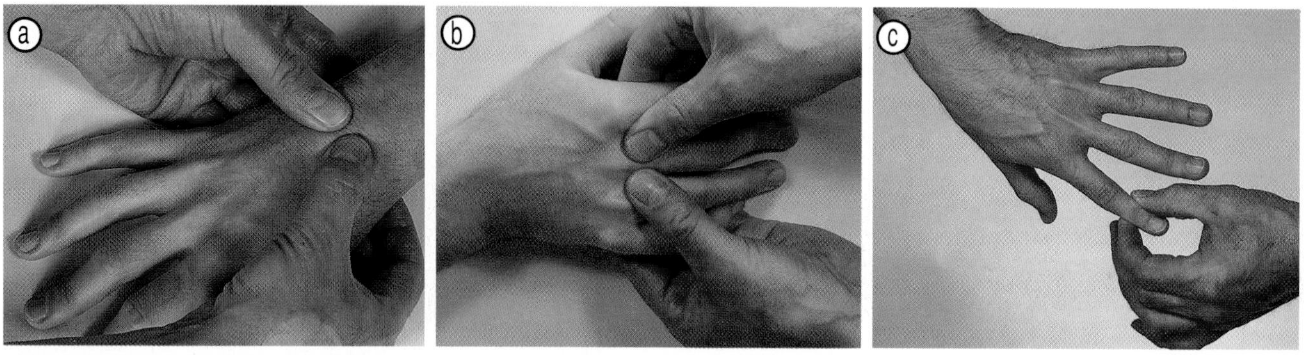

Fig. 11.61 Palpating the (a) wrist, (b) metacarpophalangeal, and (c) interphalangeal joints.

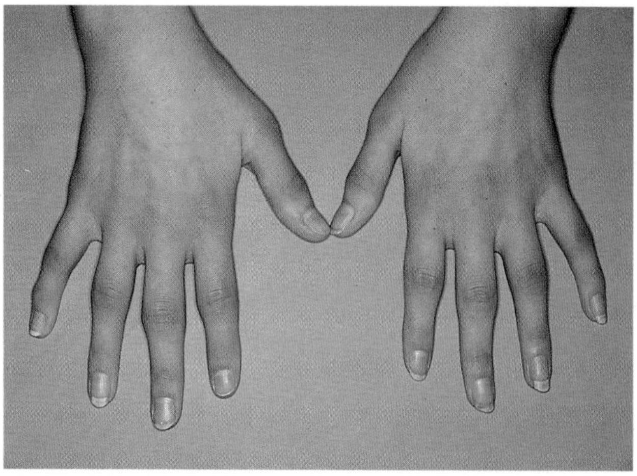

Fig. 11.62 Early rheumatoid arthritis. Slight spindling of the PIP joints.

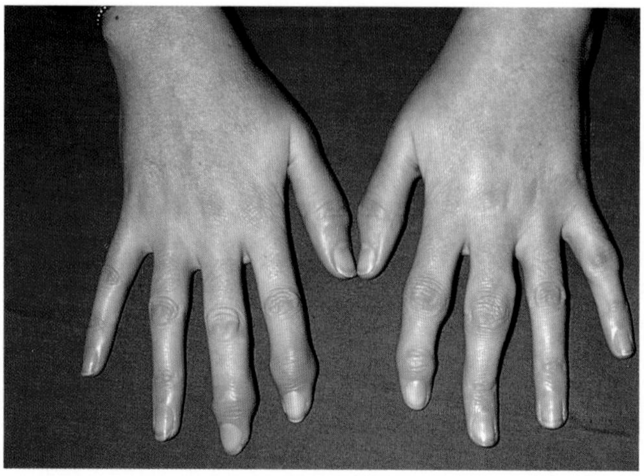

Fig. 11.63 Psoriatic arthropathy.

blank paper gives a quantitative assessment of the degree of their abduction from the neutral position.

THE HAND MUSCLES

Muscle and joint function cannot always be conveniently separated. A generalized joint disorder (e.g. rheumatoid arthritis) may well lead to wasting of the small hand muscles due to disuse, or may lead to focal wasting due to entrapment of a particular nerve (e.g. the median).

Inspection

First inspect the dorsum of the hands. In this position, all the muscles that are visible are supplied by the ulnar nerve. In the elderly, muscle bulk in the hand reduces, but without accompanying weakness. Wasting produces guttering between the extensor tendons, hollowing between the index finger and thumb, and loss of the convexity of the hypothenar eminence. Look for fasciculation. Now turn the hands over and inspect the palmar surfaces. For the first time, you have the opportunity to assess the bulk of muscles supplied by the median nerve by examining the thenar eminence. By now you have determined whether there is any small muscle wasting, whether it is bilateral or unilateral and, if unilateral, whether it is global or confined to the distribution of the median or ulnar nerve.

Testing power

Start with a muscle supplied by the ulnar nerve. A good choice is the first dorsal interosseous (Fig. 11.66). If the muscle is weak, test

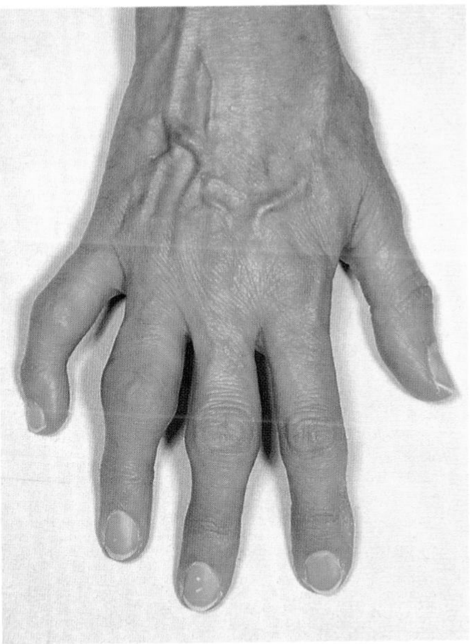

Fig. 11.64 Osteoarthritis at the PIP joints.

Trigger finger

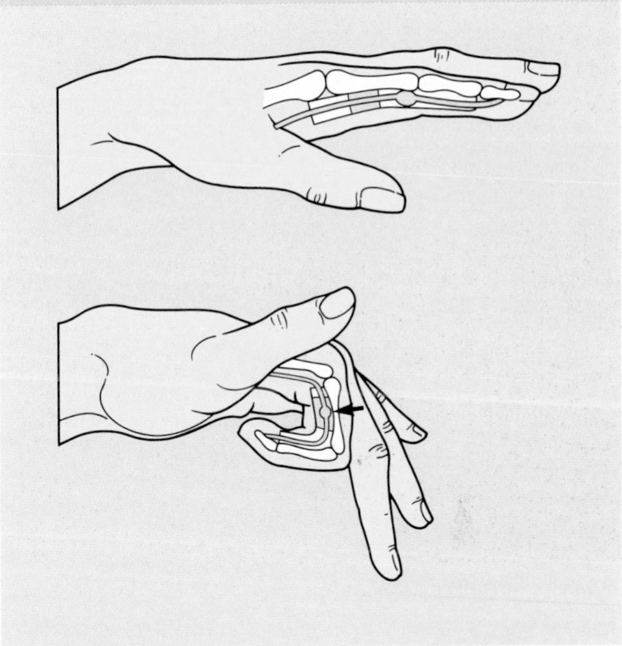

Fig. 11.65 Trigger finger. The thickened area becomes trapped in an area of narrowing of the tendon sheath (arrow).

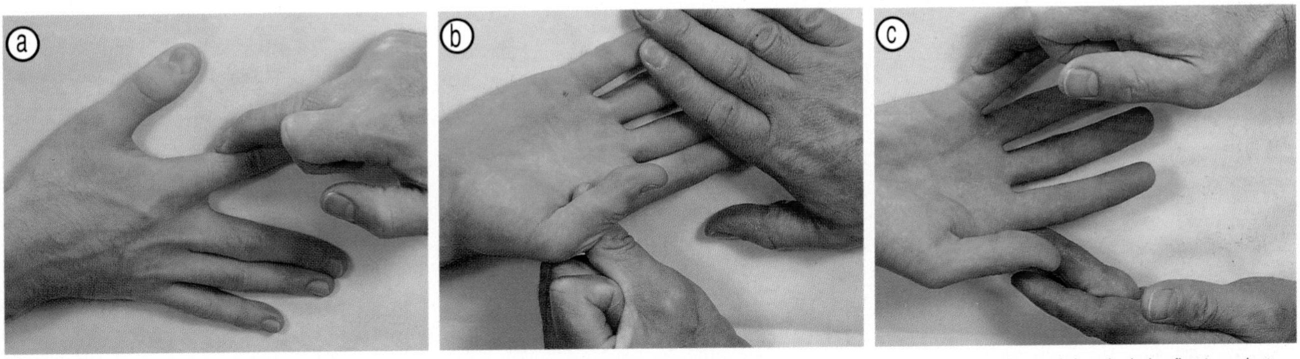

Fig. 11.66 Testing some of the small muscles supplied by the ulnar nerve. (a) First dorsal interosseous; with the fingers flat, the patient is trying to abduct the index finger against resistance. (b) Adductor pollicis; the patient is forcibly adducting the thumb towards the palmar surface of the index finger. (c) Abductor digiti minimi; the patient is abducting the little finger against resistance.

two other readily accessible muscles supplied by the nerve, adductor pollicis and abductor digiti minimi. Now move on to muscles supplied by the median nerve. Start with abductor pollicis brevis then proceed to test opponens pollicis (Fig. 11.67).

Clinical application

If the weakness is confined to the muscles of the thenar eminence, you are dealing with a distal *median nerve lesion* – most likely within the carpal tunnel. Weakness with or without wasting of the muscles of the thenar eminence is accompanied by a characteristic failure of the thumb to rotate during attempted opposition (Fig. 11.68). The *carpal tunnel syndrome* predominates in women, often triggered by pregnancy. Though usually idiopathic it can be triggered by other conditions, including rheumatoid arthritis, acromegaly, myxoedema, and previous wrist fracture. Typically the patient complains of nocturnal pain and paraesthesiae. The symptoms are often felt diffusely in the hand and forearm rather than being confined to the digits supplied by the nerve. Sensory loss is often not conspicuous. Ask the patient to compare touch sensation on the two sides of the ring finger. If percussion of the median nerve at the wrist produces tingling in the digits (Tinel's

Weakness of the hand

Is the weakness associated with joint pain?

Is the weakness confined to the muscles supplied by the median or ulnar nerve?

If the weakness is global, are both hands or just one hand affected?

Is there accompanying sensory loss?

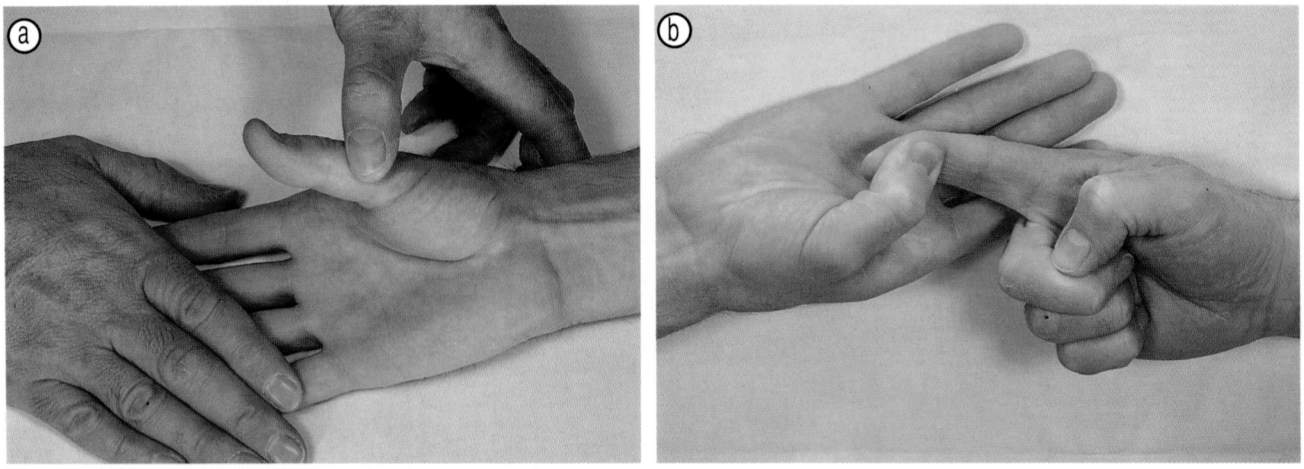

Fig. 11.67 Testing the muscles of the thenar eminence. Abductor pollicis brevis (left); the patient is lifting the thumb vertically from the plane of the palm of the hand. Opponens pollicis (right); against resistance, the patient is trying to touch the base of the little finger with the tip of the thumb.

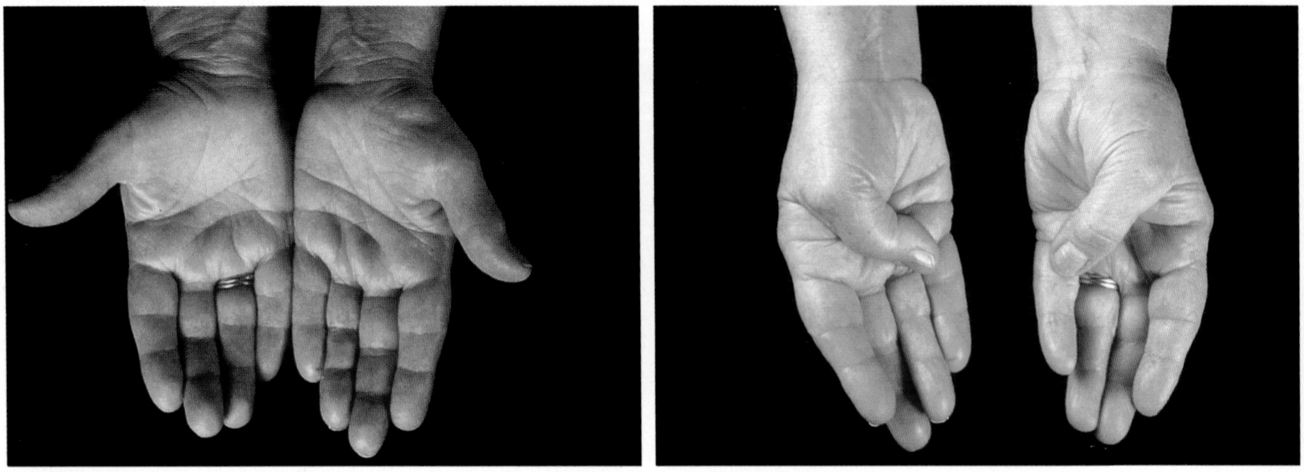

Fig. 11.68 Carpal tunnel syndrome. Wasting of the left thenar eminence (left). Failure of opposition of the left thumb (right).

sign) compression at the site of percussion is likely; the test, however, is frequently negative even in proven cases.

If the weakness is confined to the muscles supplied by the *ulnar nerve*, you next need to determine the site of the lesion. The commonest site is in the region of the ulnar groove at the elbow, usually the consequence of recurrent trauma and angulation. The hand muscles affected include the interossei, the hypothenar muscles, and the third and fourth lumbricals. A characteristic deformity affects the fourth and fifth digits (Fig. 11.69). In addition, there should theoretically be weakness of flexor carpi ulnaris, and of flexor digitorum profundus to the fourth and fifth digits. In practice, these long muscles may be spared, even though the lesion is proximal. Distal ulnar lesions occur. According to the site, there may be sparing of the muscles of the hypothenar eminence and absence of sensory change.

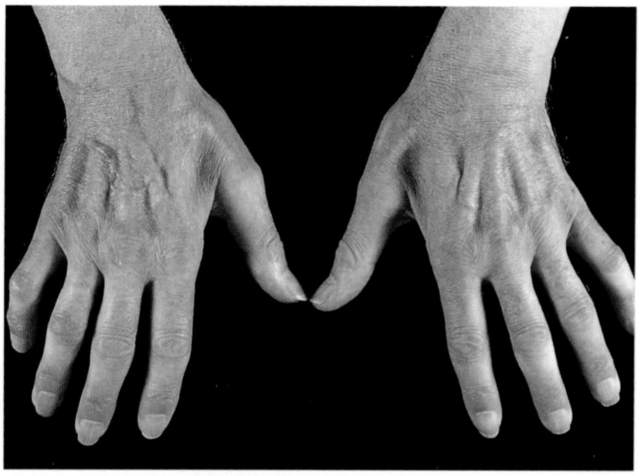

Fig. 11.69 Bilateral ulnar nerve lesions.

If there is weakness of all the small hand muscles, you are probably dealing with a proximal lesion – combined median and ulnar lesions are uncommon. If the other hand is normal, suspect a problem at the level of the brachial plexus or of the T1 root. The *brachial plexus* can be damaged by trauma or invaded by tumor. Damage to the upper trunk affects the fifth and sixth cervical segments, to the middle trunk predominantly affects fibres supplying the radial nerve, and to the lower trunk produces a global weakness of the hand. If the sympathetic fibres in the T1 root are involved, there will be an accompanying Horner's syndrome (Fig. 11.70).

The *cervical rib (thoracic outlet) syndrome* results from compression of the C8 and T1 roots, or the lower trunk of the plexus, by a fibrous band passing from the transverse process of the seventh cervical vertebra to the first rib. Curiously the hand weakness affects the muscles of the thenar eminence much more than those supplied by the ulnar nerve. A typical radiological feature is beaking of the C7 transverse process (Fig. 11.71). If you find bilateral weakness, with or without wasting, of the small hand muscles, you are dealing with a more diffuse process. (Bilateral brachial plexus lesions are rare.) You have to consider a peripheral neuropathy, or a lesion of the anterior horn cell (e.g. syringomyelia or motor neurone disease) (Fig. 11.72).

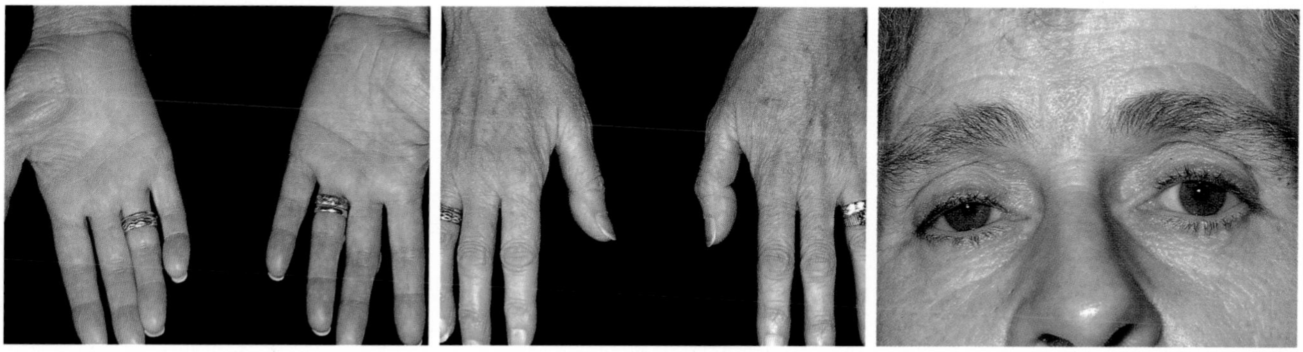

Fig. 11.70 Global wasting of the right hand (left and middle), together with a Horner's syndrome (right). Malignant invasion of the lower trunk of the brachial plexus and the T1 root.

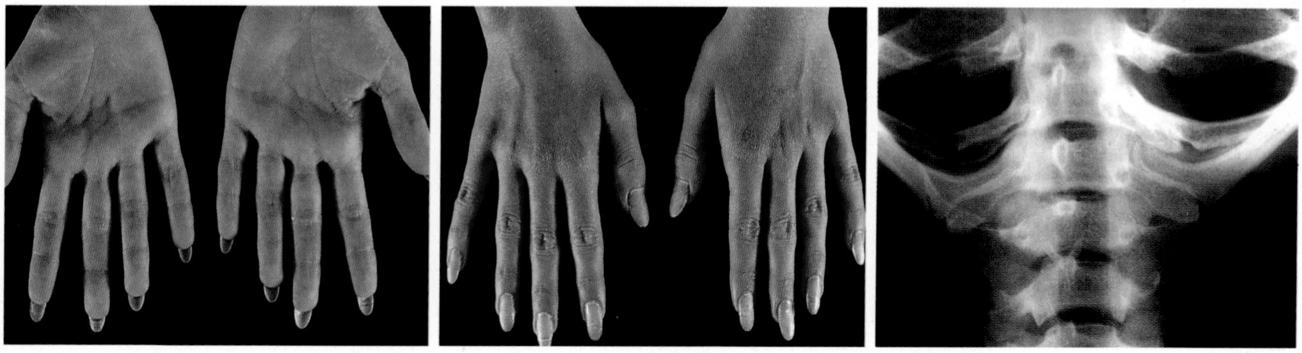

Fig. 11.71 Wasting of the small muscles of the right hand (left and middle) associated with breaking of the C7 transverse process (right).

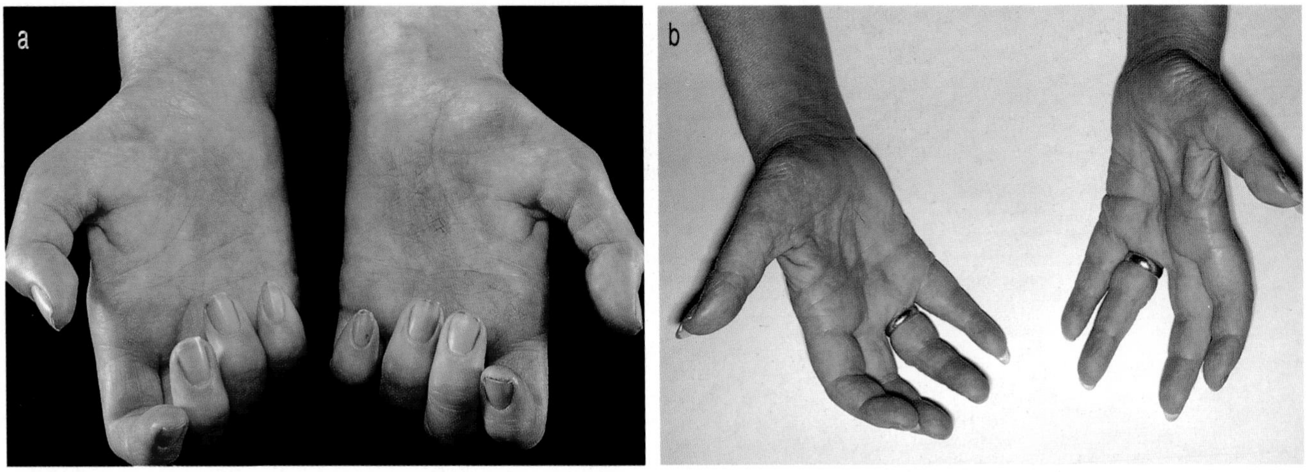

Fig. 11.72 Bilateral wasting of the small hand muscles in (a) hereditary sensori-motor neuropathy and in (b) motor neurone disease.

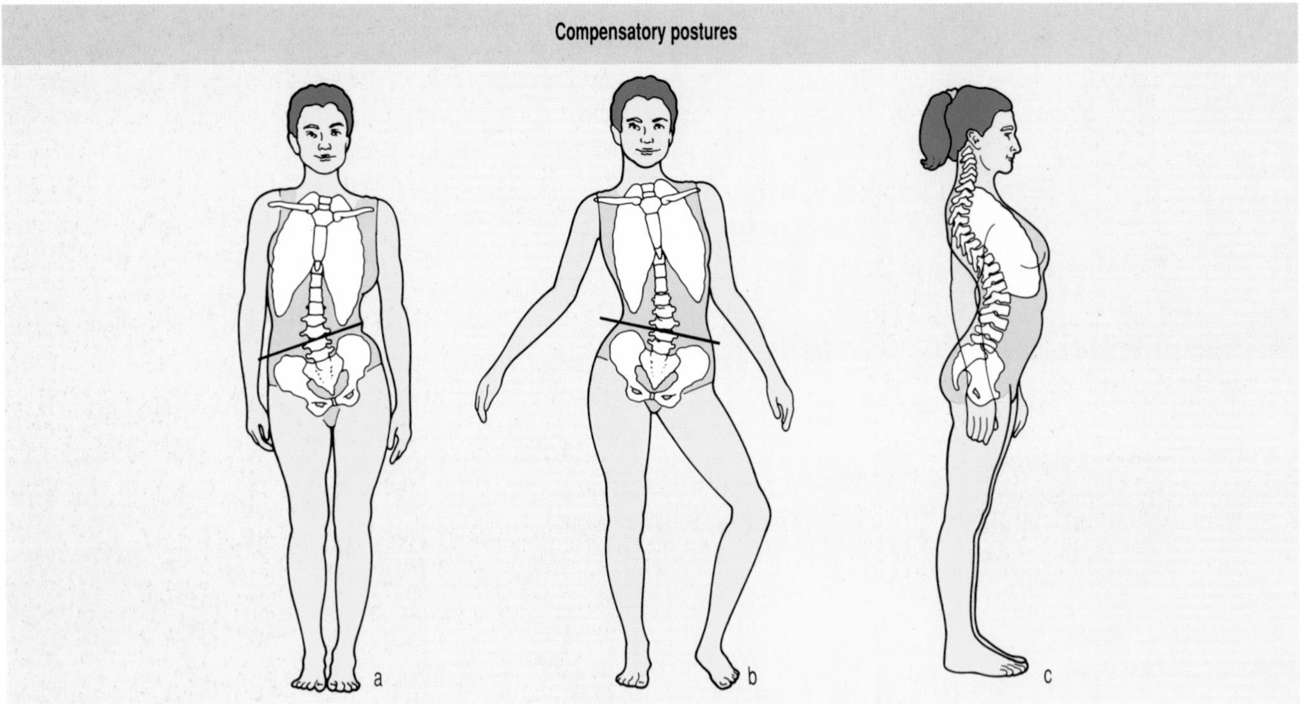

Fig. 11.73 Compensatory postures associated with (a) shortening of one leg, (b) adduction deformity of right leg, and (c) flexed deformity of the hips.

THE HIP

Inspection and palpation

The patient should be wearing only underpants if you are to examine the hip joints satisfactorily. Begin with the patient standing. Look for evidence of shortening of one of the legs. Compensation for this is achieved by a scoliotic posture or by flexion of the longer leg. An abduction deformity is compensated by flexion of the ipsilateral knee, and an adduction deformity by flexing the contralateral knee (Fig. 11.73). A flexion deformity is compensated by an exaggerated lordosis.

With the patient still standing, assess the integrity of each hip joint, and its surrounding muscles, by asking the patient to stand first on one leg then the other (Trendelenberg test). Normally as the foot is lifted the pelvis tilts upwards on the same side. If there is an abnormality in the hip joint or weakness of the muscle activity across it, the pelvis sinks downwards (Fig. 11.74).

Now lie the patient flat. First determine whether the iliac crests can be positioned in the same horizontal plane at right angles to the spine (Fig. 11.75). If this is not possible, there is an abduction or adduction deformity of one or other hip. Beware of the fact that a flexion deformity of the hip can be concealed as the patient lies flat by a compensatory lumbar lordosis. To check for this, flex the

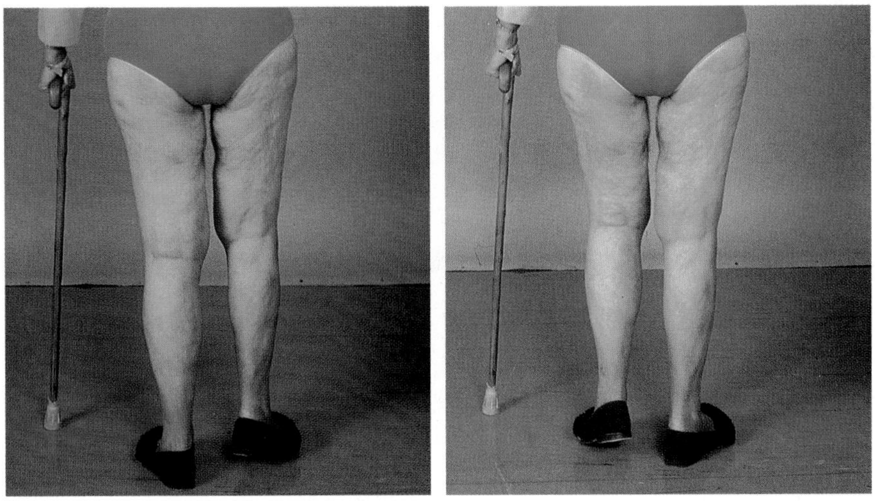

Fig. 11.74 Trendelenberg's sign. When the patient stands on the normal left leg the pelvis tilts to the left (left). (right) When she stands on the right leg (where there was osteoarthritis at the hip) the pelvis fails to tilt to the right.

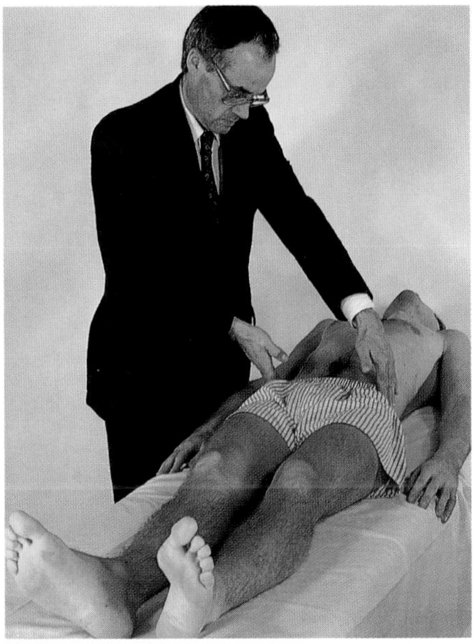

Fig. 11.75 Positioning the pelvis.

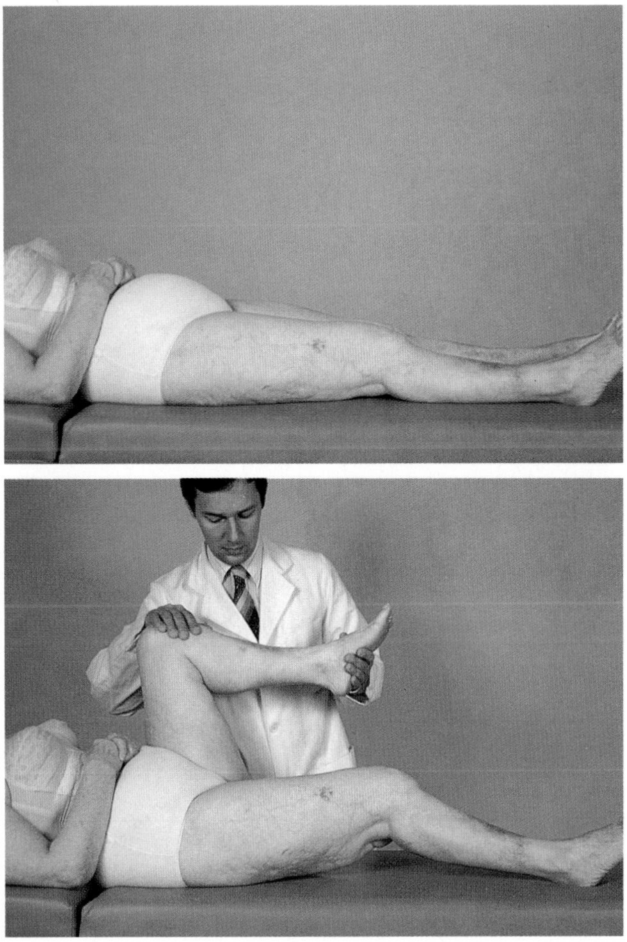

Fig. 11.76 Thomas' test. The fixed flexion deformity of the right hip can be obscured by a compensatory lumbar lordosis (above). When the lordosis is overcome by flexing the left hip, the right leg then lifts (below).

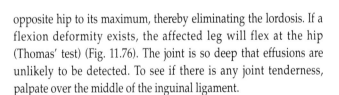

opposite hip to its maximum, thereby eliminating the lordosis. If a flexion deformity exists, the affected leg will flex at the hip (Thomas' test) (Fig. 11.76). The joint is so deep that effusions are unlikely to be detected. To see if there is any joint tenderness, palpate over the middle of the inguinal ligament.

Measurement of limb length

When measuring limb length, you need to distinguish between true and apparent shortening. When measuring, make sure that the position of the two hip joints is comparable. The true length is measured from the anterior superior iliac spine to the medial malleolus (Fig. 11.77). If one leg is shorter, suspect pathology in or around the hip joint of that side. Apparent length is measured from the umbilicus to the medial malleolus. A difference here, without a difference in true lengths, indicates a lateral tilt of the pelvis, most often due to an adduction deformity of the hip.

Joint movement

When measuring the range of hip movement, you need to ensure that the pelvis remains stationary. To do this, keep your free hand on the anterior superior iliac spine to detect any movement.

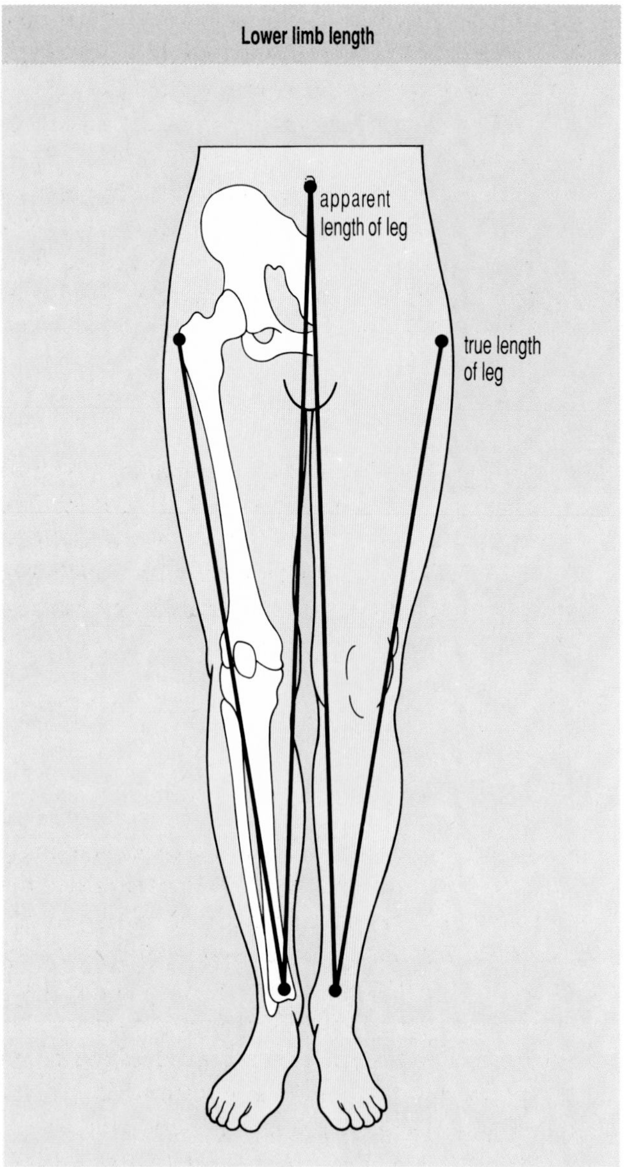

Fig. 11.77 True and apparent lengths of the lower limbs.

Causes of hip pain	
Trauma	Fracture Dislocation
Arthritis	Osteo- Rheumatoid
Slipped femoral epiphysis	
Osteochondritis (Perthe's disease)	
Infection	e.g. osteomyelitis

Fig. 11.79 Causes of hip pain.

To test flexion, bend the leg, with the knee flexed, into th abdomen. Extension is best assessed by standing behind the patien and drawing the leg backwards until the point at which the pelvi starts to rotate. Abduction is measured by taking the leg outwards again to the point where, by using the opposite hand, the pelvis i felt to move. Internal and external rotation are tested with the hi and knee flexed to 90° (Fig. 11.78).

Causes of hip pain vary, in terms of frequency, according to th age of the patient (Fig. 11.79).

Fractures of the neck of the femur are common in the elderly. Th leg becomes externally rotated, adducted and shortened.

Dislocations of the joint are rare, require considerable force, an are usually posterior. *Slippage of the femoral epiphysis* i

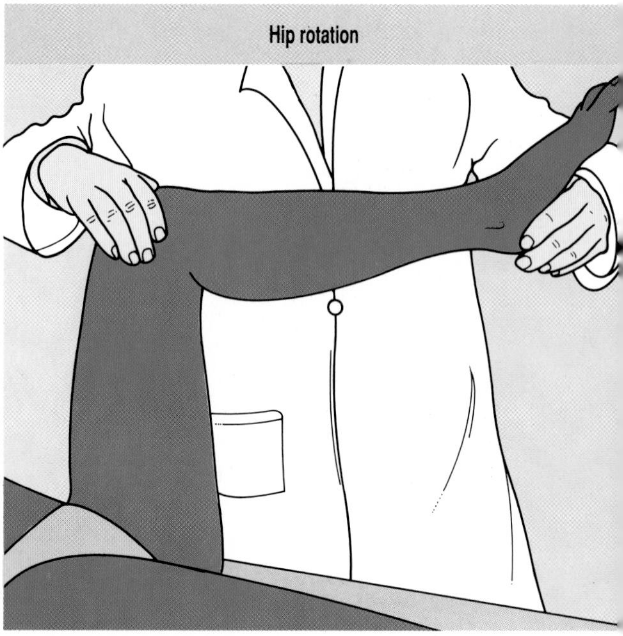

Fig. 11.78 Measuring the extent of hip rotation.

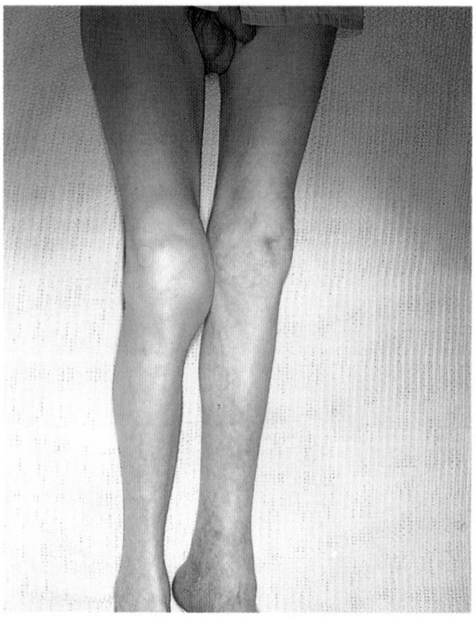

Fig. 11.80 Advanced osteoarthritis of the left hip. The leg is shortened and externally rotated.

predominantly seen in the second decade of life. It leads to pain and a limp. The pain can be referred to the knee (see Fig. 11.20). Typically there is limitation of flexion, abduction and medial rotation. *Osteoarthritis* frequently involves the hip joint. Pain is either local or referred. Movements of the joint are both restricted and painful. In advanced cases shortening of the limb occurs with external rotation (Fig. 11.80). *Groin strains* are common in those involved in sporting activities. The pain is usually a dull one exacerbated by hip movement and is most commonly the result of tears in the fibres of the hip flexors.

Muscle function

Test the power of hip flexion, extension, abduction, and adduction (Fig. 11.81). *Sciatic palsies* are associated with pelvic trauma, injuries to the buttock or thigh, and infiltration by tumor. The muscles supplied by the lateral popliteal component of the nerve tend to be more affected than those supplied by the medial popliteal branch (Fig. 11.82).

THE KNEE

Inspection and palpation

With the patient standing, look for a knee deformity, either *genu valgum* (knock-knee) or *genu varum* (bow leg). Now continue your inspection with the patient lying supine. The bulk of the quadriceps muscle is a sensitive guide to the presence of knee-joint pathology. If necessary measure the thigh of each leg at a comparable distance from the joint margin. Next look for an effusion. If this is large, the swelling will extend from the suprapatellar region down either side of the patella (Fig. 11.83). Smaller effusions are only detectable by palpation. First try ballottement – *the patella tap test.* Use your left hand to force any fluid out of the suprapatellar pouch then gently press the patella into the femur with the second and third fingers of your right hand. If there is a substantial effusion the patella will spring back

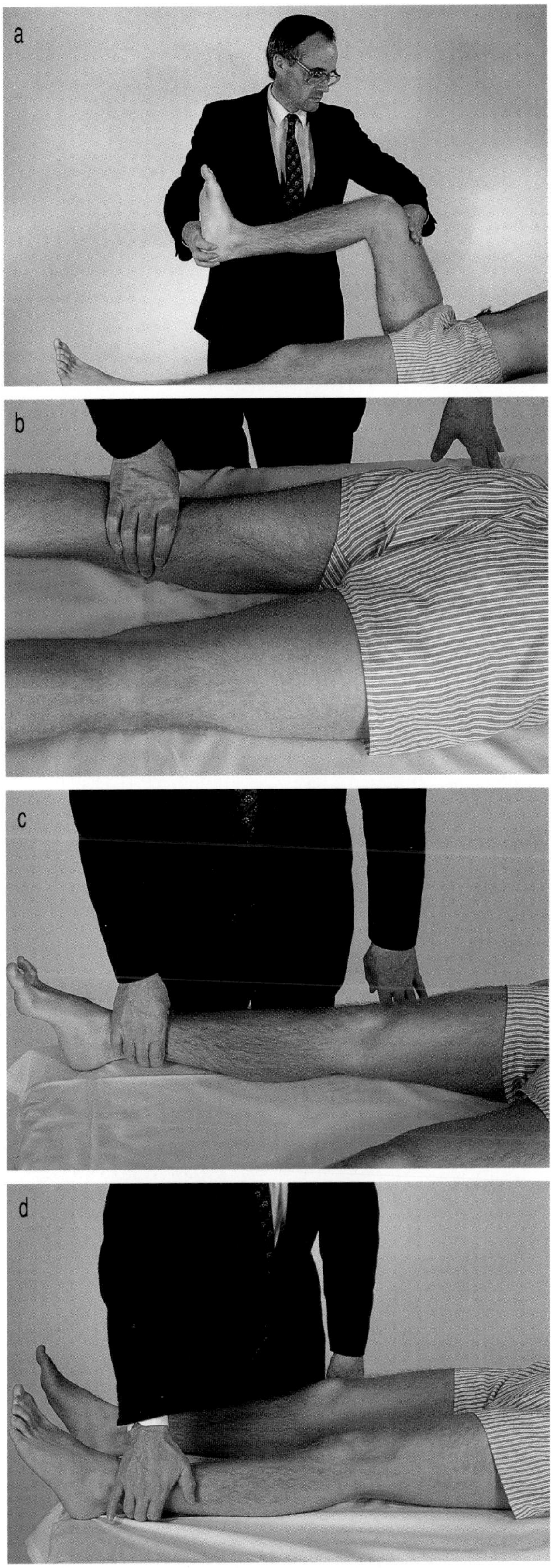

Fig. 11.81 Testing the muscles acting at the hip joint.

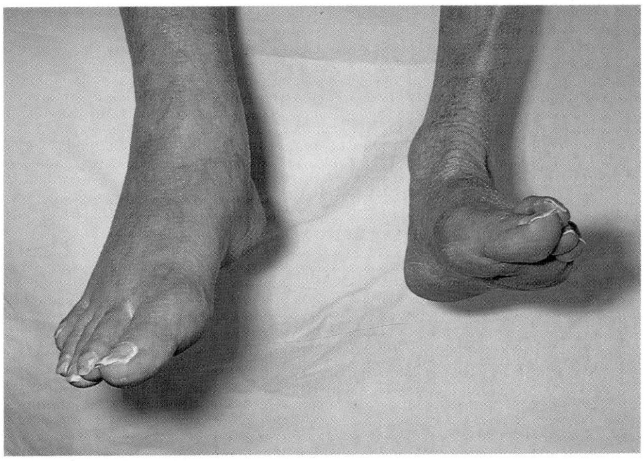

Fig. 11.82 Right sciatic palsy.

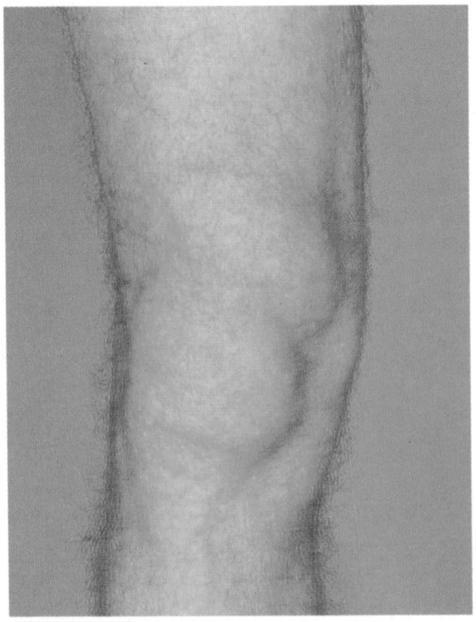

Fig. 11.83 Effusion in the suprapatellar pouch in a patient with rheumatoid arthritis.

against your fingers (Fig. 11.84a). For smaller effusions, look for the *bulge sign*. Again force any fluid out of the suprapatellar pouch but at the same time anchor the patella with the index finger of the same hand. Next, gently stroke down between the patella and the femoral condyles, first on one side then the other. If an effusion is present, a bulge appears on the other side of the knee during the manoeuvre (Fig. 11.84b).

Palpate the joint and surrounding structures, looking for any tenderness and also to assess the 'feel' of any swelling (Fig. 11.85). In *osteoarthritis*, periarticular tenderness, particularly at the insertion of the capsule and collateral ligaments, is an important diagnostic clue. Later bony swellings around the joint and secondary quadriceps wasting are common (Fig. 11.86). Remember to look at the back of the joint, i.e. the popliteal fossa. Posterior synovial protrusions (Baker's cysts) are visible here. They can complicate *rheumatoid arthritis*, in which additional features include effusions, synovial swelling and deformity (Fig. 11.87).

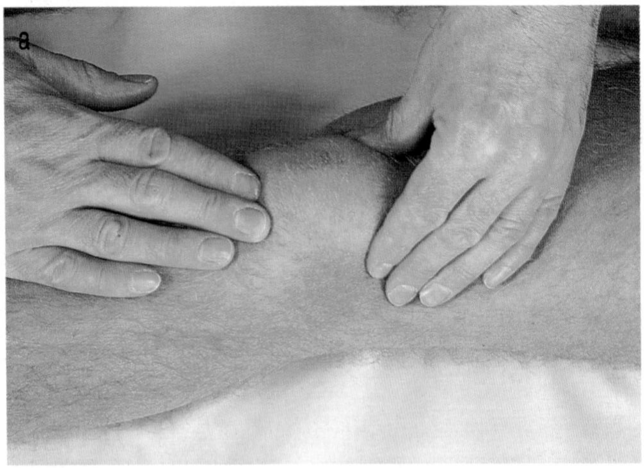

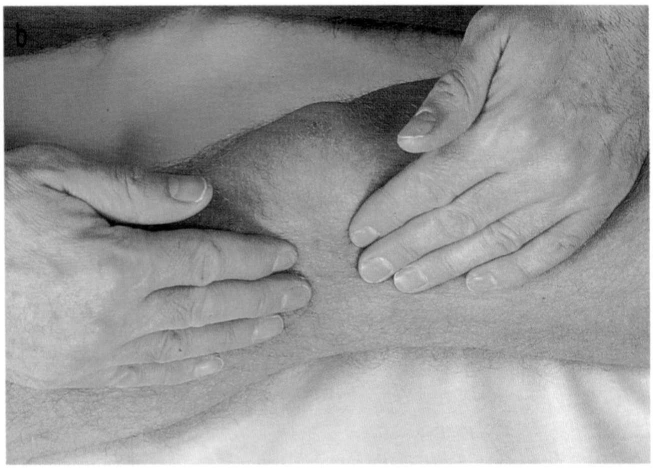

Fig. 11.84 Detection of an effusion: (a) patella tap, (b) bulge sign.

Causes of knee pain	
Trauma	Fracture Dislocation Ligament damage cartilage damage
Arthritis	Osteo- Rheumatoid
Osteochondritis dissecans	
Infection	e.g. osteomyelitis
Bone tumors	
Referred	e.g. from the hip-

Fig. 11.85 Causes of knee pain.

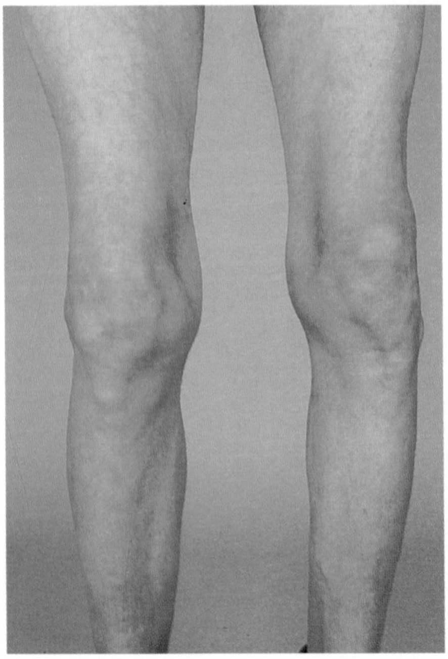

Fig. 11.86 Osteoarthritis of the knee. Bony swellings associated with quadriceps wasting.

Joint movement

Test the range of movement with the patient lying supine. Flexion occurs to about 135°. A small degree of extension (10°) can occur in

> **Knee pain**
>
> Is the pain unilateral or bilateral?
>
> Has the patient noticed swelling of the joint?
>
> Does the knee lock in certain positions?

some normal individuals. As you record the movement, palpate the joint for any crepitus. In addition, move the patella laterally and medially across the femoral condyles. Is the movement painful or does it elicit crepitus?

Stability

There are several important procedures which allow you to determine the integrity of the collateral and cruciate ligaments.

To test the *collateral ligaments*, attempt to abduct and adduct the lower leg. If there is lateral instability, record its degree (Fig. 11.88). For the assessment of the *cruciate ligaments*, bend the knee to a slight angle, sit on the patient's foot (better to ask permission first!) then tense the lower leg first forwards then backwards. If either ligament is lax excessive movement will occur (Fig. 11.89). Damage to these ligaments is almost always the consequence of trauma. If the ligaments rupture, a bloodstained effusion results. Damage to the synovial lining will allow the blood to track outside the joint margin.

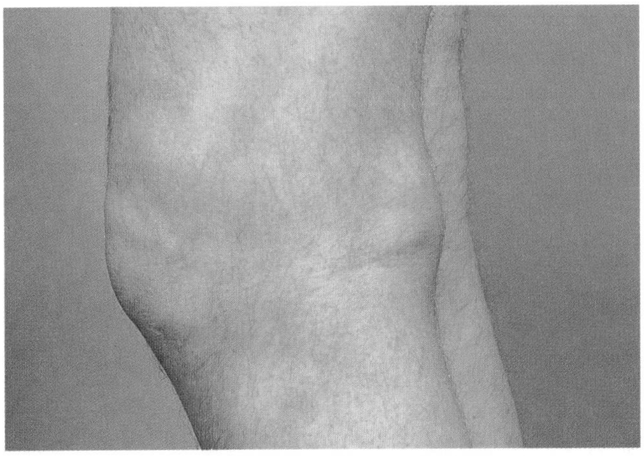

Fig. 11.87 A Baker's cyst which has partially ruptured into the calf.

Assessment of the semilunar cartilages

Damage to the cartilages is common. In order to test their integrity, bend the hip and knee to 90° and grip the heel with your right hand whilst pressing on the medial then lateral cartilage with your left (Fig. 11.90). Now internally and externally rotate the tibia while extending the knee. If there is a cartilage tear, its engagement between the tibia and femur during the manoeuvre leads to severe pain, a clunking noise, and, sometimes, actual locking of the joint (McMurray's test).

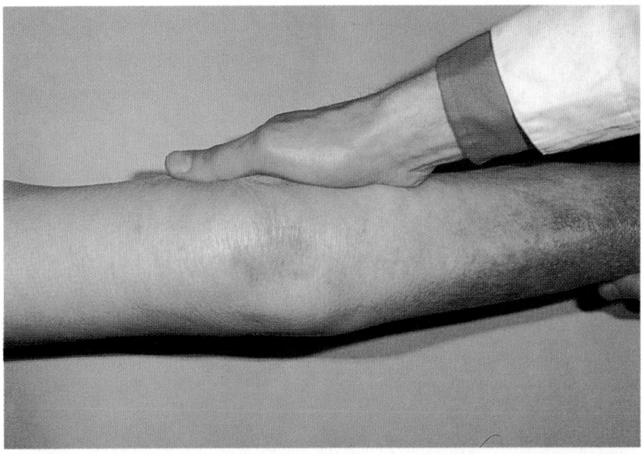

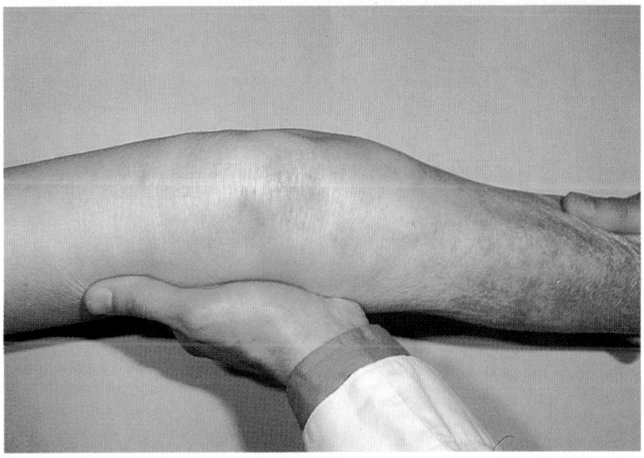

Fig. 11.88 Testing the collateral ligaments of the knee.

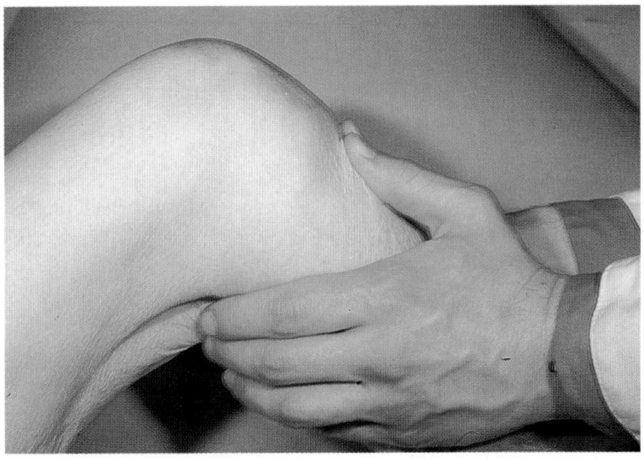

Fig. 11.89 Testing the cruciate ligaments.

Muscle function

Test the muscles responsible for knee extension and flexion: quadriceps and the hamstrings, respectively (Fig. 11.91). Both quadriceps weakness and wasting can accompany joint disease. If the knee joint is normal, unilateral quadriceps weakness suggests either a *femoral neuropathy* or an *L3 root syndrome*. In the latter, there is weakness of both quadriceps and the hip adductors associated with a depressed knee jerk and sensory change over the medial aspect of the thigh and knee (Fig. 11.92). A femoral neuropathy can result from thigh trauma or haemorrhage into the psoas sheath. In

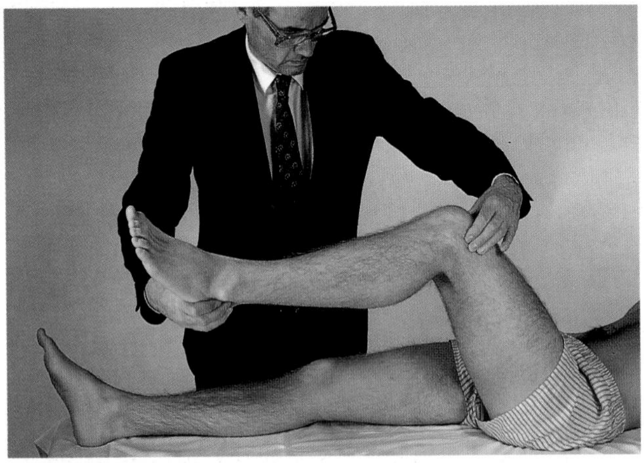

Fig. 11.90 McMurray's test.

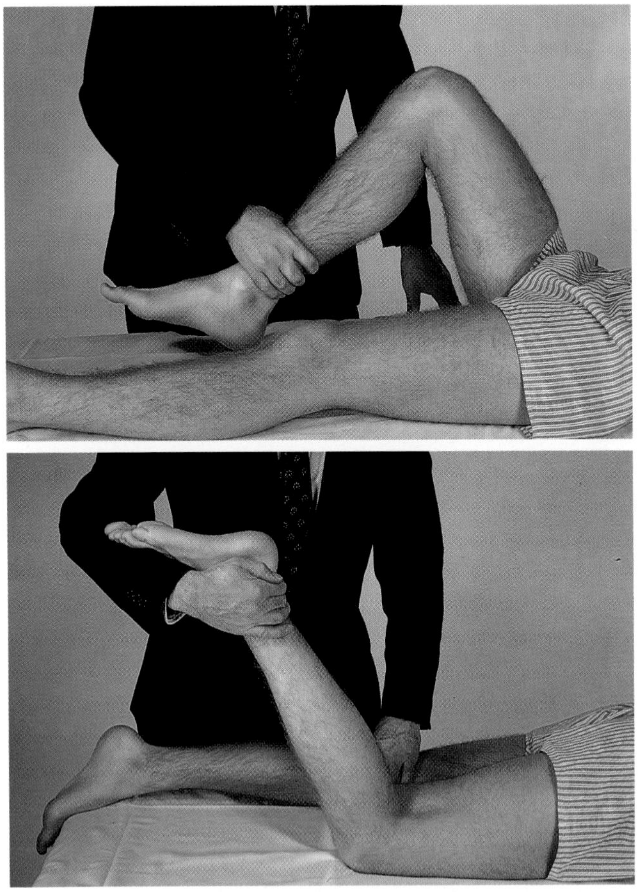

Fig. 11.91 Testing knee extension (above) and flexion (below).

L3 syndrome		
Muscle weakness	**Segmentary sensory change**	**Reflex depression**
Quadriceps Hip adductors	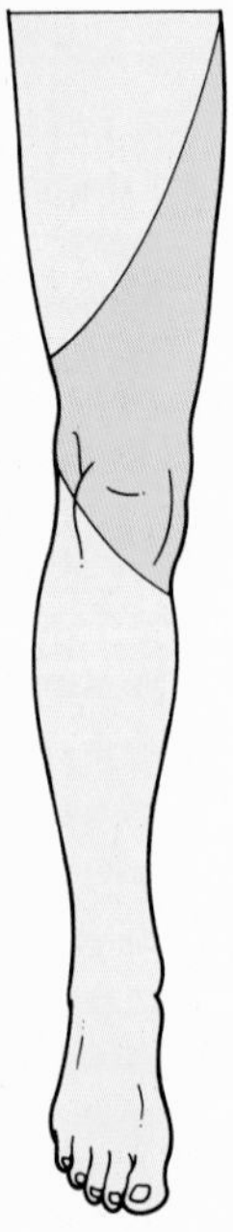	Knee

Fig. 11.92 L3 root syndrome. Motor, sensory, and reflex abnormalities.

diabetes mellitus, wasting of the thigh is more often the result of ischaemia of the lumbar roots rather than being due to a femoral neuropathy. Consequently, the thigh adductors are also affected. *Femoral neuropathy* leads to weakness and wasting of the quadriceps, loss of the knee jerk, and sensory change over the anterior thigh and the medial aspect of the lower leg (Fig. 11.93). If the nerve is damaged at the level of the psoas sheath, hip flexion is also affected. An *obturator palsy* can follow surgery or pelvic fracture, or be secondary to an obturator hernia. Weakness is confined to the thigh adductors with altered sensation over the thigh's inner aspect.

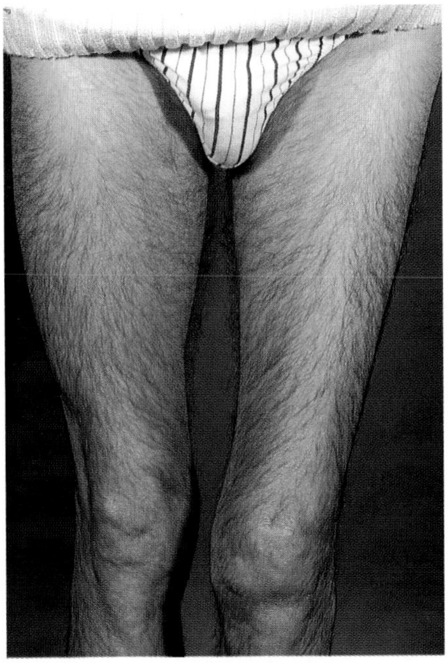

Fig. 11.93 Left femoral neuropathy following profundoplasty.

It is worth mentioning the condition of *meralgia paraesthetica*. The patient complains of pain, tingling and numbness over the anterolateral aspect of the thigh. There are no motor changes. The condition is due to compression of the lateral cutaneous nerve of thigh at the level of the groin.

THE ANKLE AND FOOT

Inspection and palpation

To assess the alignment of the feet at the subtalar joints, look at the ankles from behind with the patient standing. In a varus deformity the foot will be deviated towards the midline, in a valgus deformity away from it. With the patient still standing, look for any foot deformity. Is the arch of the foot exaggerated or absent? Is there deformity or swelling of the toe joints? Remember to inspect the sole of the foot as well as its dorsal aspect. Now palpate the margins of the ankle joint. In an inflammatory arthropathy the whole joint is likely to be tender, with corresponding pain on all movement. In ankle strain, the tenderness is likely to be confined to one site with pain predominantly occurring when the joint is moved in one direction. Next palpate the heel and Achilles tendon. The latter is a fairly common site for rheumatoid nodules. To detect tenderness in the metatarsophalangeal joints, compress each one between your thumb and finger (Fig. 11.94). To test the integrity of the Achilles tendon, squeeze the calf just below its maximal circumference. If the tendon is intact, the foot plantar flexes, if ruptured, no movement occurs.

Deformity of the foot is common. In *flat foot* the longitudinal arch is lost with the consequence that most or the whole of the sole comes into contact with the ground (Fig. 11.95a). In *pes cavus* the

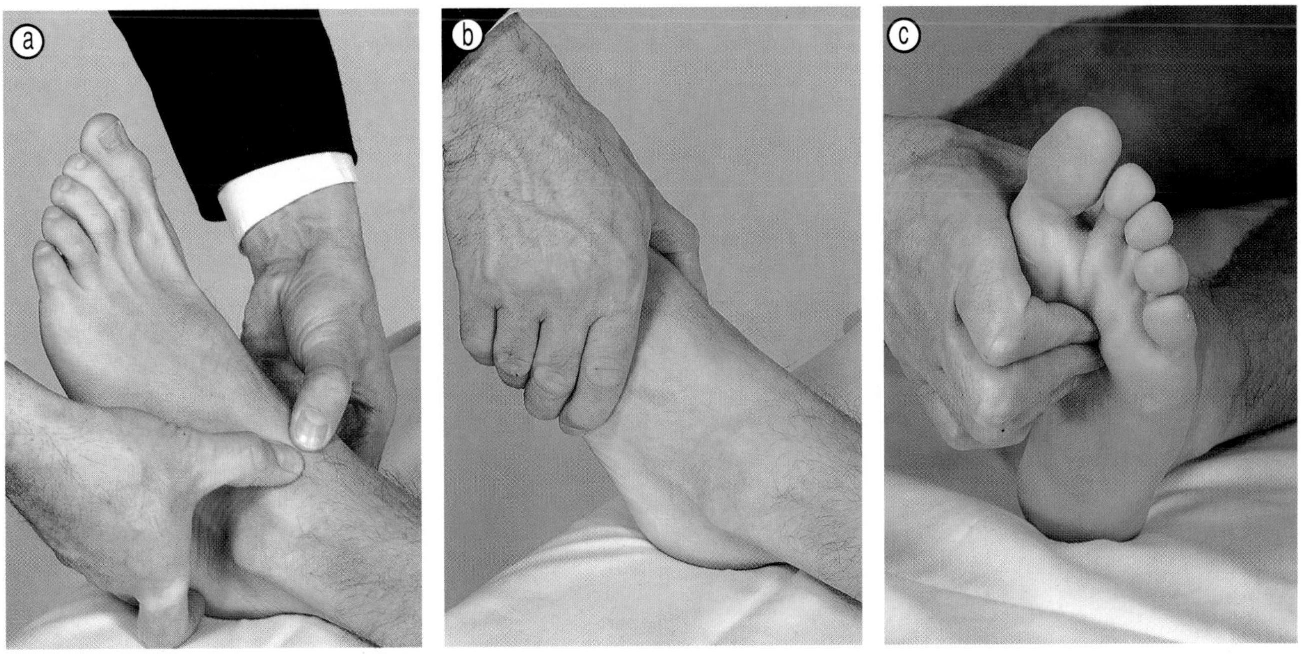

Fig. 11.94 Palpating (a) the anterior aspect of the ankle joint, and (b and c) testing for tenderness of the metatarsophalangeal joints.

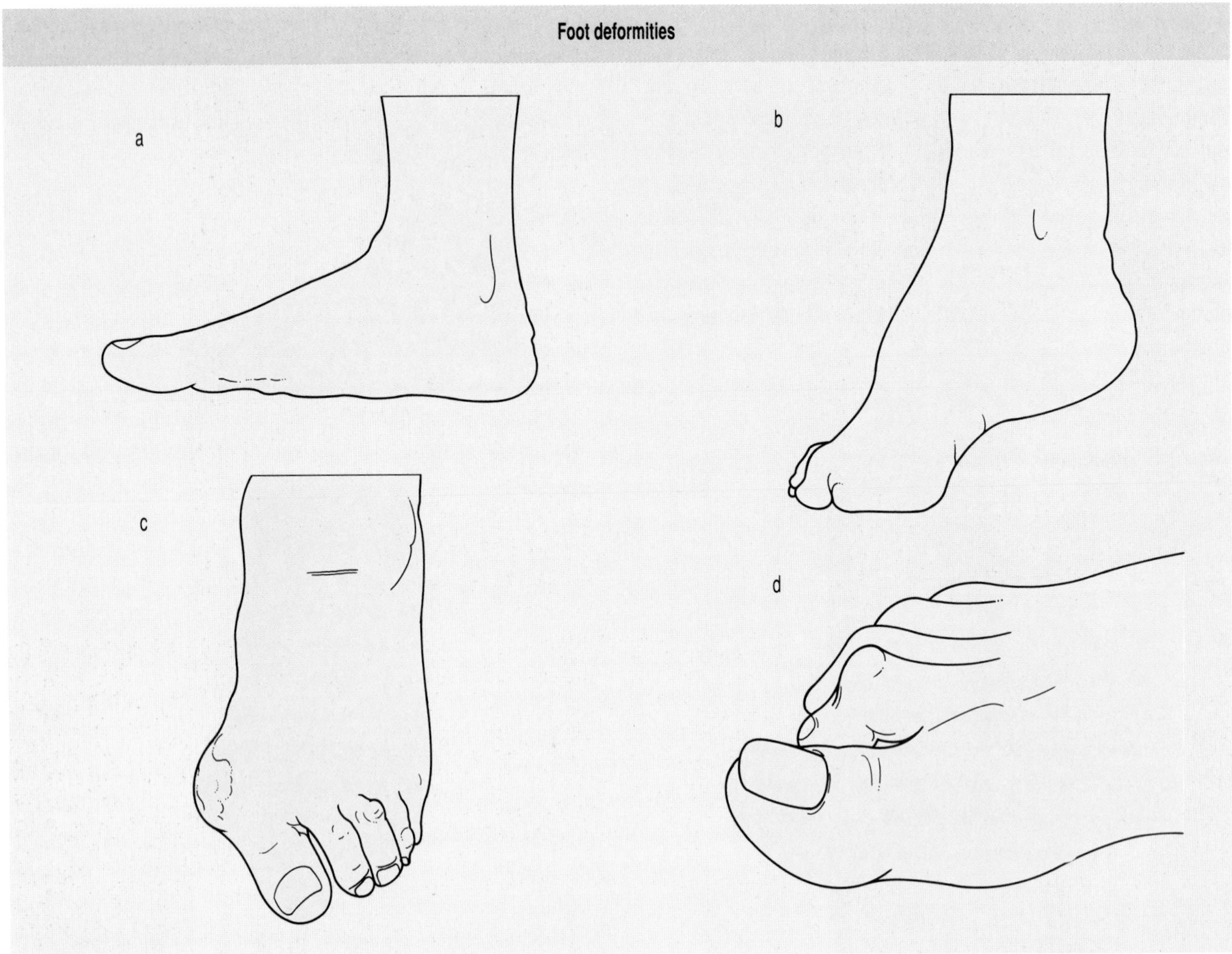

Fig. 11.95 Foot deformities. (a) pes planus, (b) pes cavus, (c) hallux valgus, (d) hammer toe.

Foot deformities

Has the deformity been present from birth?

Does it affect both feet?

Is it associated with joint pain or tenderness?

arch of the foot is exaggerated with accompanying hyperextension of the toes (Fig. 11.95b). *Hallux valgus* predominates in women. It consists of abnormal adduction of the big toe at the metatarsophalangeal joint, with a bursa at the pressure point over the head of the first metatarsal (Fig. 11.95c). A *hammer toe* is characterized by hyperextension at the metatarsophalangeal joint with flexion at the interphalangeal joint. Painful thickenings of the skin (corns) are liable to develop at the pressure points (e.g. over the proximal interphalangeal joints) (Fig. 11.95d).

Joint movement

The ankle joint proper is concerned with plantar and dorsiflexion. Inversion and eversion of the foot occur both at the subtalar and midtarsal joints. To test this movement, hold the heel firmly with one hand while inverting and everting the foot with the other hand. You have already looked for tenderness in the metatarsophalangeal joints. Now test the range of flexion and extension.

Osteoarthritis can affect both the ankle and the foot. In the foot, involvement of the first metatarsophalangeal joint leads either to deformity (hallux valgus) or fixation (hallux rigidus). *Gout* typically affects the same joint. In an acute attack there is intense pain associated with swelling and erythema of the overlying skin (see Fig. 11.95). The reaction is secondary to deposition of urate

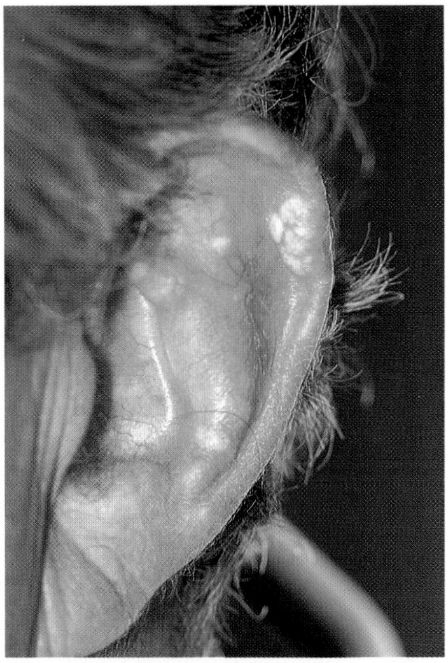

Fig. 11.96 Tophi on the helix of the ear.

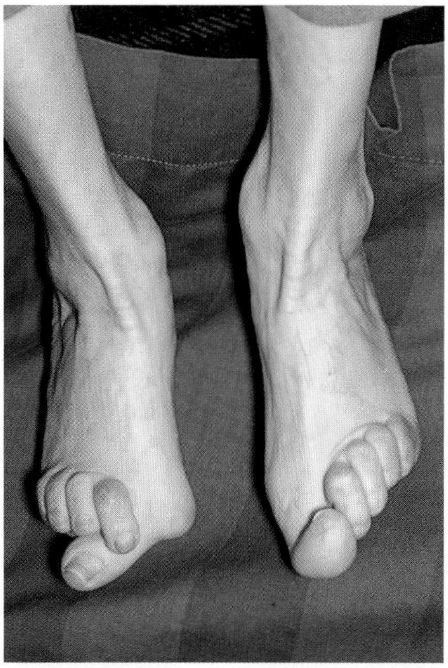

Fig. 11.97 Rheumatoid arthritis of the feet.

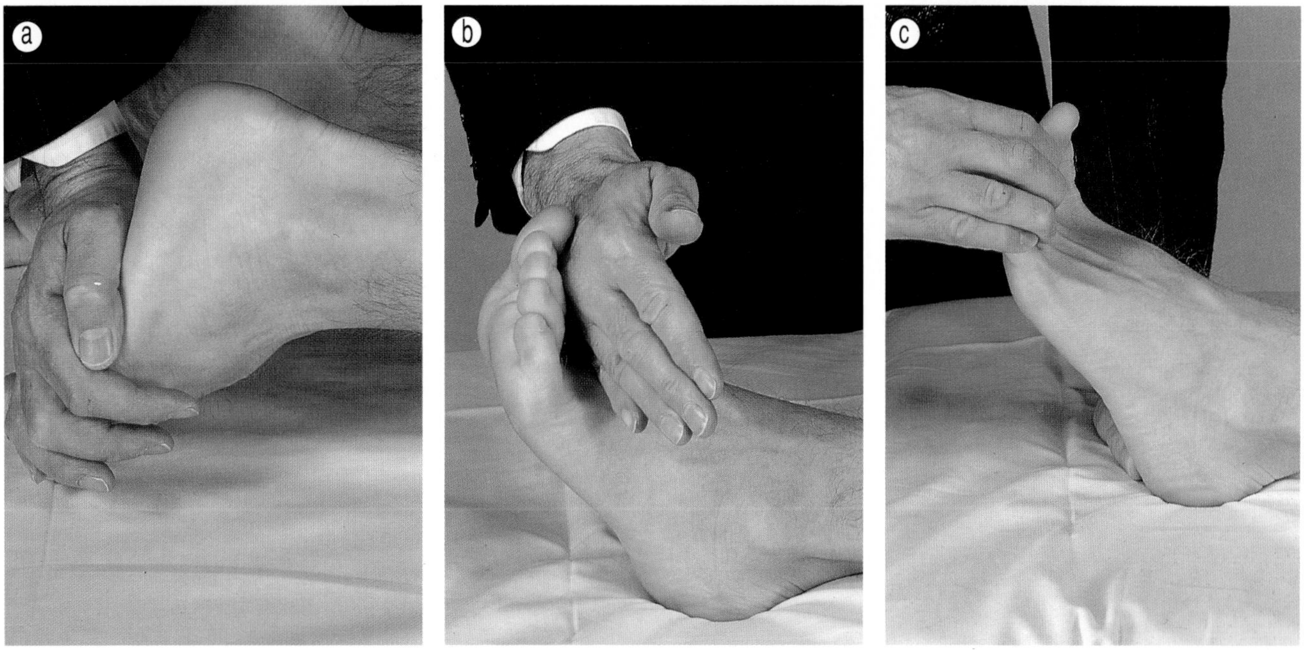

Fig. 11.98 Testing (a) plantar-flexion and dorsi-flexion of (b) the ankle and (c) toes.

salts within the connective tissues. If the hyperuricaemia is inadequately treated, urate deposits appear in periarticular and subcutaneous tissues. Typical sites include the first metatarsophalangeal joint, the elbow, the Achilles tendon and the ear (Fig. 11.96).

Rheumatoid arthritis involves both the ankle and the foot. When the disease is established, subluxation of the metatarsophalangeal joint is associated with flexion deformity at the proximal interphalangeal joints (Fig. 11.97). A variety of other inflammatory reactions can affect the ligamentous and tendon insertions around the heel. Causative agents include trauma and the seronegative arthritides.

Muscle function

Test the individual muscles concerned with movement at the ankle and foot. Start with the plantar and dorsiflexors of the ankle, then of the toes. Specifically test the extensor of the big toe, extensor hallucis longus (Figs 11.98 and 11.99). Finally test the evertors and invertors of the foot.

Lumbar spondylosis commonly affects the L5 and S1 roots. The motor deficit with the former is often confined to extensor hallucis longus. There is no reflex change, but there may be sensory change over the medial aspect of the foot. In an S1 root syndrome, there is weakness of plantar flexion of the foot (and potentially also of the calf and buttock muscles) together with a depressed or absent ankle jerk and sensory loss over the lateral border of the dorsal and plantar aspects of the foot (Fig. 11.100).

In *lateral popliteal palsy* there is weakness of dorsiflexion of the foot and toes and of the foot everters. The sensory change is often relatively inconspicuous, sometimes being confined to a small area of loss over the dorsum of the foot around the base of the first and second toes. There are no reflex changes.

PATTERNS OF WEAKNESS IN MUSCLE DISEASE

The pattern of weakness found in primary muscle disease differs from that seen in nerve root or peripheral nerve disorders. Conditions primarily affecting muscle include a group of genetically-determined disorders (the muscular dystrophies), a group of inflammatory disorders (e.g. polymyositis), various biochemical and endocrinological dysfunctions, and, finally, a further genetically-determined group associated with myotonia.

Certain characteristics support a clinical diagnosis of primary muscle disease. The weakness, which is usually symmetrical, tends to predominate proximally. In the upper limbs, the periscapular muscles and deltoid are weak, but the hand muscles are spared. In the lower limbs, weakness of hip flexion and extension is often conspicuous. The patient adopts a lordotic posture and has a waddling gait.

Patterns of weakness

Is the weakness associated with sensory symptoms or signs?

Is there a family history of muscle disease?

Is the weakness symmetrical?

Is the weakness predominantly proximal or distal?

Trendelenberg's sign is likely to be positive bilaterally (see Fig. 11.74). There is particular difficulty getting upright from a lying position. Typically the patient turns into the prone position, kneels then climbs up his legs using the upper limbs in order to extend the trunk (Gowers' manoeuvre) (Fig. 11.101). Muscle wasting and loss of tendon reflexes are late features in the myopathies. In some of the muscular dystrophies pseudohypertrophy of muscle occurs due to infiltration by fat and

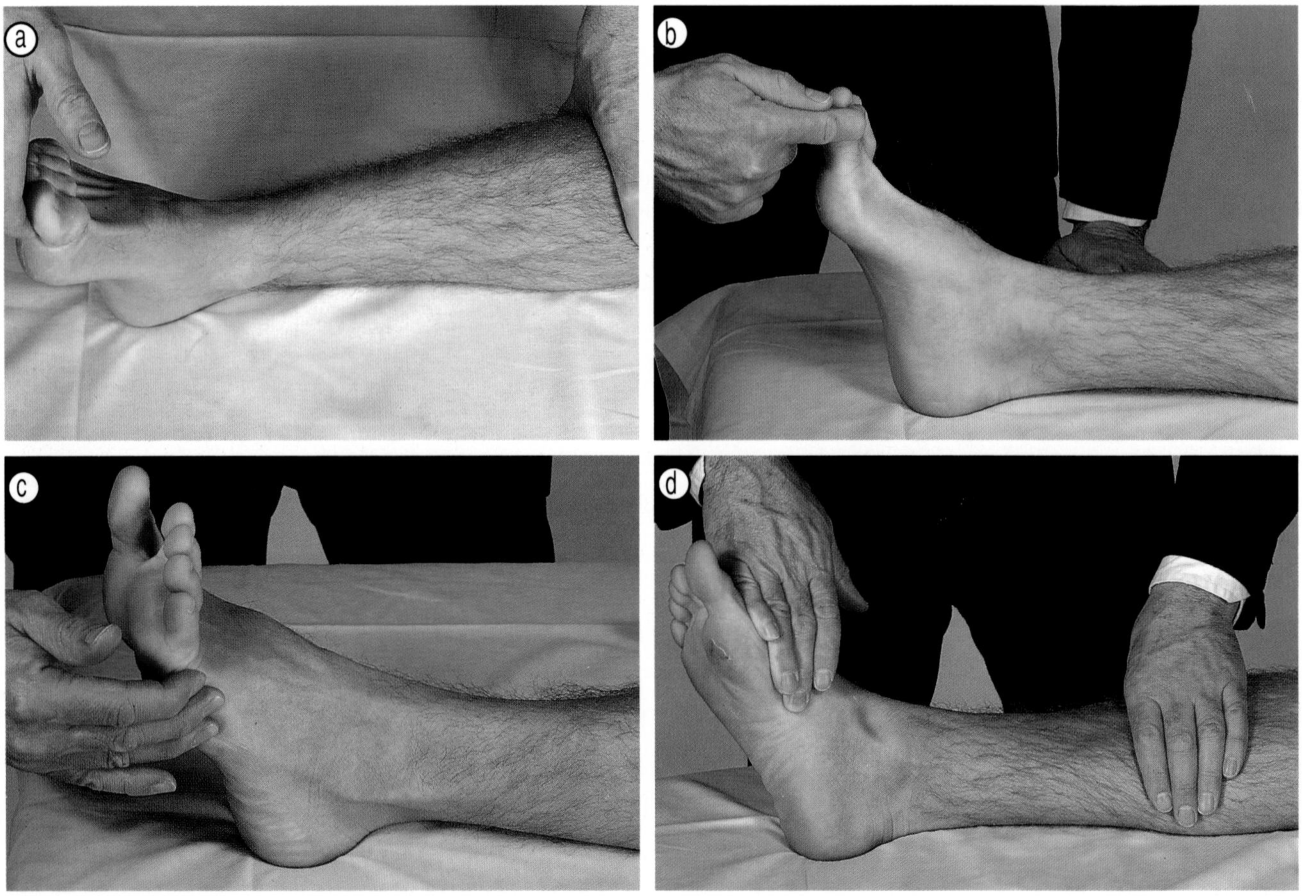

Fig. 11.99 Testing the (a) long toe flexors, (b) extensor hallucis longus, (c) peroneus longus and brevis and (d) tibialis posterior.

L5 and S1 syndromes			
	Muscle weakness	Sensory change	Reflex depression
L5	Extensor hallucis longus Eversion Hip extension	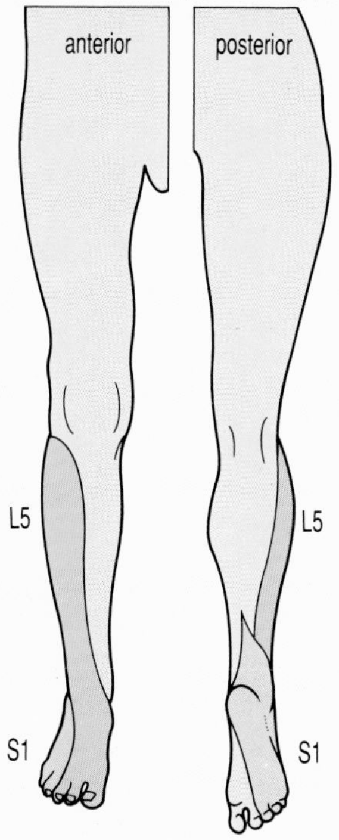	Nil
S1	Plantar flexion Knee flexion Hip extension and abduction		Ankle

Fig. 11.100 L5 and S1 root syndromes.

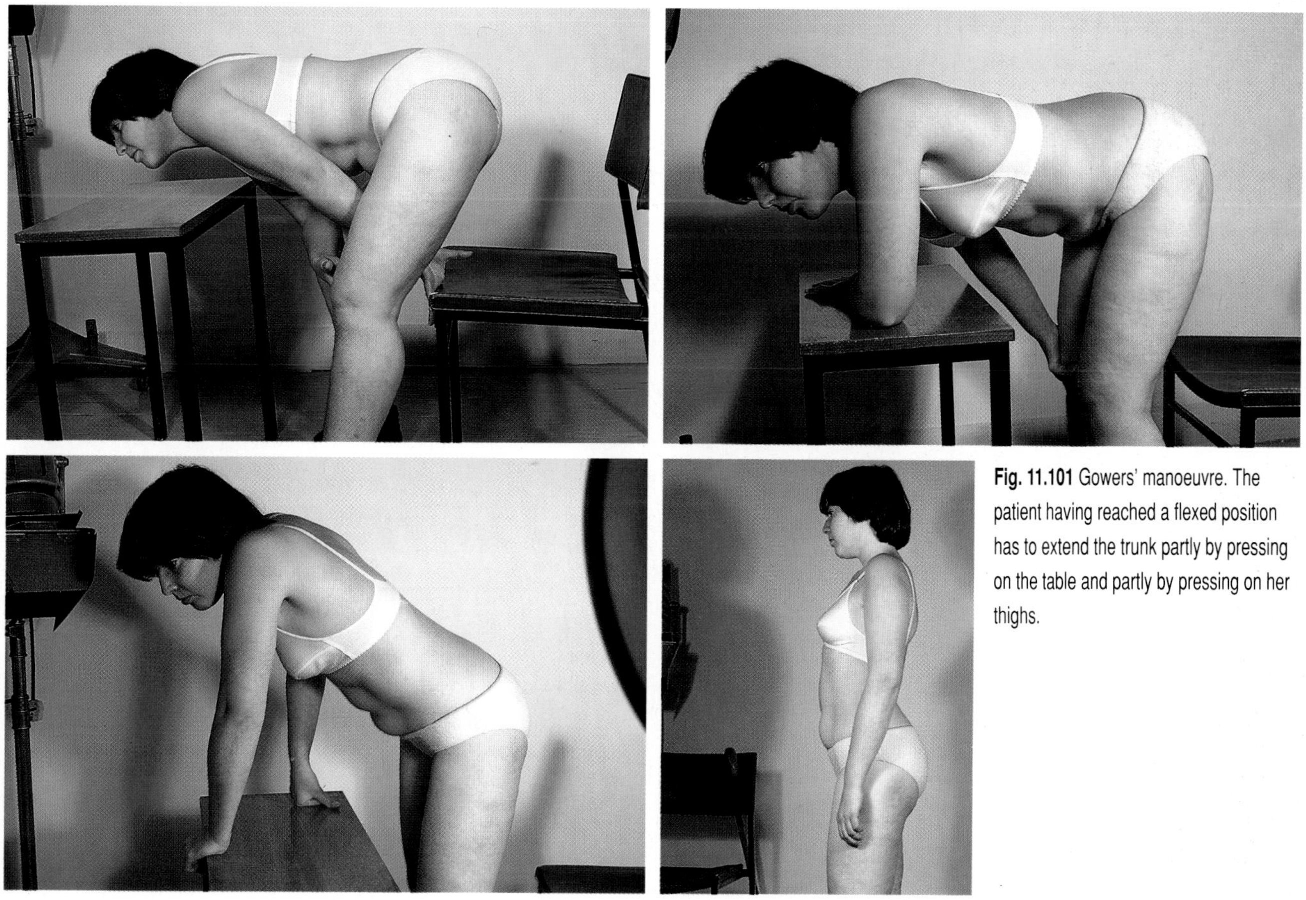

Fig. 11.101 Gowers' manoeuvre. The patient having reached a flexed position has to extend the trunk partly by pressing on the table and partly by pressing on her thighs.

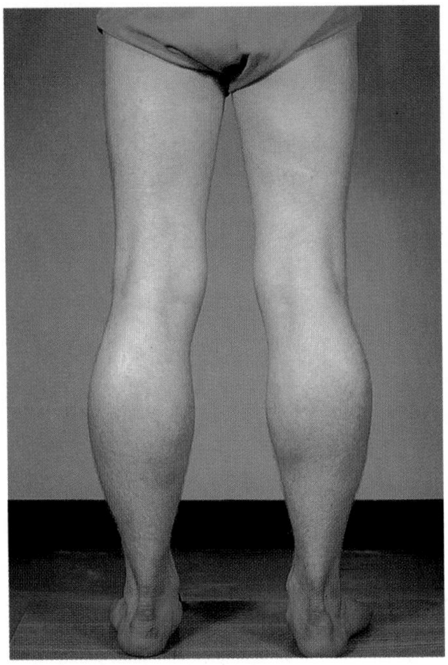

Fig. 11.102 Pseudohypertrophy of the calves.

connective tissue (Fig. 11.102). Distal weakness sometimes occurs in primary muscle disease, often then showing a characteristic distribution. Weakness of the hands is a prominent feature of dystrophia myotonica, in which muscle weakness is accompanied by myotonia, particularly of grip.

GAIT

You will have noticed how the patient walks when he enters the consulting room. Having completed your limb assessment of joint and muscle you can now examine the gait formally. Remember that disease of the joints of the lower limb can affect walking. The possibility will have been raised by the history and suggested by the joint examination. If the patient has described a substantial problem with gait, be ready to provide support when the patient starts to walk. Ask the patient to walk in their usual fashion for a few metres, then turn and walk back towards you. You should observe both the pattern of leg movement and the posture of the arms together with control of the trunk. If gait appears normal, ask the patient to walk heel-toe, i.e. 'as if on a tightrope'. If the patient appears nervous, walk alongside them.

Gait

Does the patient trip?

Is one shoe worn out more readily than the other?

Does the patient stagger to one particular side?

Does the patient, despite apparently severe ataxia, seldom sustain injury?

Spastic gait (Fig. 11.103a)

In a hemiplegia the arm is held flexed and adducted while the leg is extended. In order to move the leg, the patient tilts the pelvis which produces an outward and forward loop of the leg (circumduction). Failure to dorsiflex the foot leads to it scraping along the ground. If both legs are spastic, for example due to spinal cord disease, the whole movement is stiff, with thrusts of the trunk being used to assist locomotion.

Foot-drop gait (Fig. 11.103b)

Foot drop can be either unilateral or bilateral. The former is usually the result of a lateral popliteal palsy, the latter the consequence of a peripheral neuropathy. Increased flexion at the hip and knee allows the plantar flexed foot to clear the ground.

Ataxic gait (Figs 11.103c and d)

An ataxic gait can reflect either loss of sensory information from the feet or a disorder of cerebellar function. In the former case the patient stamps the feet down in order to overcome the instability; consequently, patients with this problem are much more unstable in the dark, or with their eyes closed (positive Romberg's test).

Cerebellar disease leads to a broad-based gait which is unaffected by the presence or absence of visual information. Loss of truncal control produces erratic body movement. With unilateral cerebellar disease the patient staggers to the affected side.

Waddling gait

Patients with substantial proximal lower limb weakness waddle from side-to-side as they walk from a failure to tilt the pelvis when one leg is raised from the ground. There is usually an exaggerated lumbar lordosis. The findings suggest a proximal myopathy.

Parkinsonian gait (Fig. 11.103e)

Patients with Parkinson's disease develop an increasingly flexed posture. Stride length diminishes and one or both arms fail to swing. There may be a problem initiating or arresting gait. Turning is difficult and requires an exaggerated number of steps.

Apraxic gait

In certain conditions (e.g. normal pressure hydrocephalus) there is a particular problem with the organization of gait even though other skilled lower limb movements are spared. The patient is liable to freeze to the ground, unable to initiate movement.

Hysterical gait

Here walking is erratic and unpredictable. The patient staggers wildly, often with an exaggerated movement of the arms. Falls and injuries do not exclude the possibility of a hysterical conversion reaction. There is often a violently positive Romberg's test which the patient self-corrects.

Gait disorders

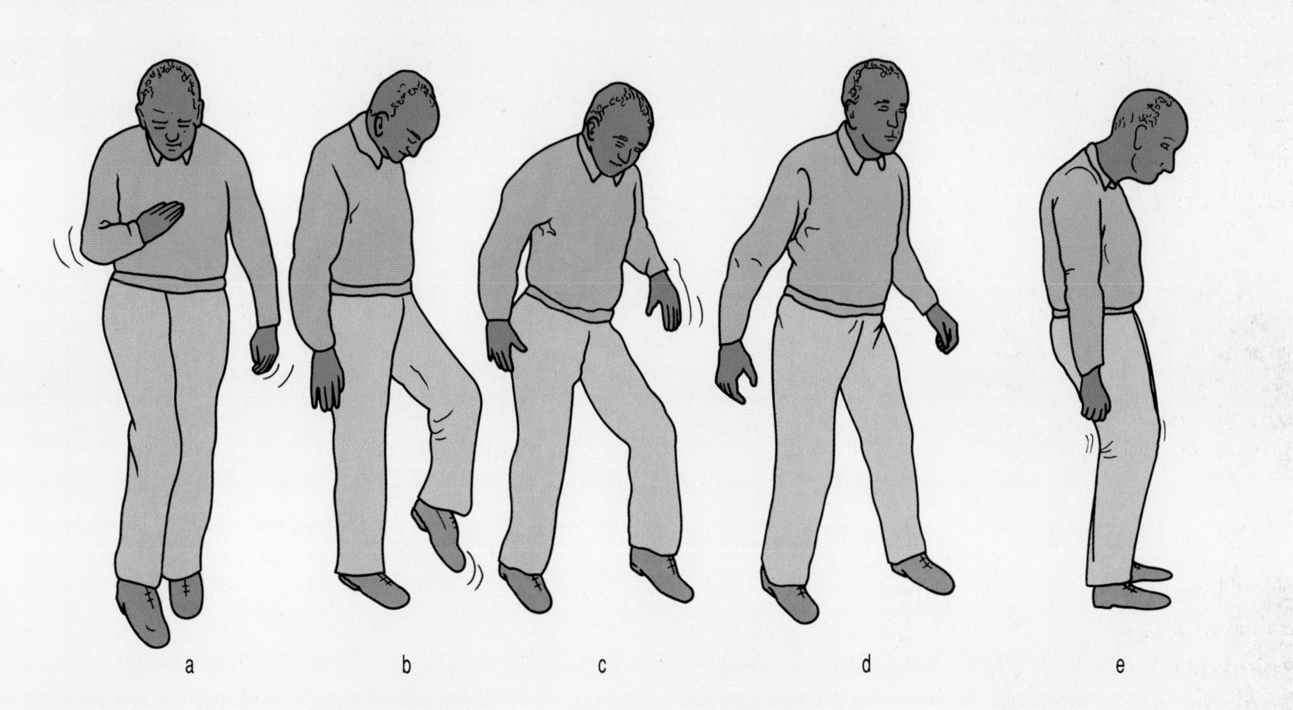

Fig. 11.103 Gait disorders. (a) Hemiplegic, (b) unilateral foot drop, (c) sensory ataxia, (d) cerebellar ataxia, and (e) Parkinsonian.

Medical students often approach the neurological examination with trepidation, and indeed there is no denying the complexities of the nervous system, or the difficulties sometimes experienced in attempting anatomical localization on the basis of abnormal physical signs. The problem for the student, however, often begins with a failure to acquire the skills necessary to elicit these signs. If these are not identified correctly, mistakes in interpretation and diagnosis inevitably follow.

This chapter summarizes the examination of the central and peripheral nervous systems, though it will seldom be necessary to examine all the areas covered. Selection is influenced partly by the patient's history, but also by their cooperation, their conscious state, and the level of fatigue. Certain examination techniques demand a good deal of both patient and examiner, and if responses become erratic it is better to return to the examination later. Students, and sometimes doctors, are prone to examine only those areas immediately accessible with the patient supine. Remember to turn the patient over in order to assess the spine and the muscles of the shoulder and pelvic girdles. Always record your findings in full, avoiding irritating acronyms (e.g. PERLA for pupils equal, reacting to light and accommodation) and, if your examination has been limited, state exactly what you have done (rather than just 'CNS' followed by a tick). Remember that physical signs can alter, sometimes rapidly, and repeating your examination can give you useful insight into the mechanisms of certain disorders.

THE CORTEX

STRUCTURE AND FUNCTION

On the basis of differences in histological structure, distinct areas can be identified within the cerebral cortex (Fig. 12.1). Tracts within the cortex comprise efferent pathways such as the pyramidal system, afferent pathways such as the thalamo-cortical projections, association fibres passing from regions within the hemisphere, and commissural fibres connecting regions contralateral to one another. Surrounding the classical primary cortical areas for movement, sensation and vision are the cortical association areas. For example, the lateral geniculate body projects not just to the visual cortex (area 17) but also to areas 18 and 19 – parts of the visual association cortex (Fig. 12.1).

Brodmann's cortical areas

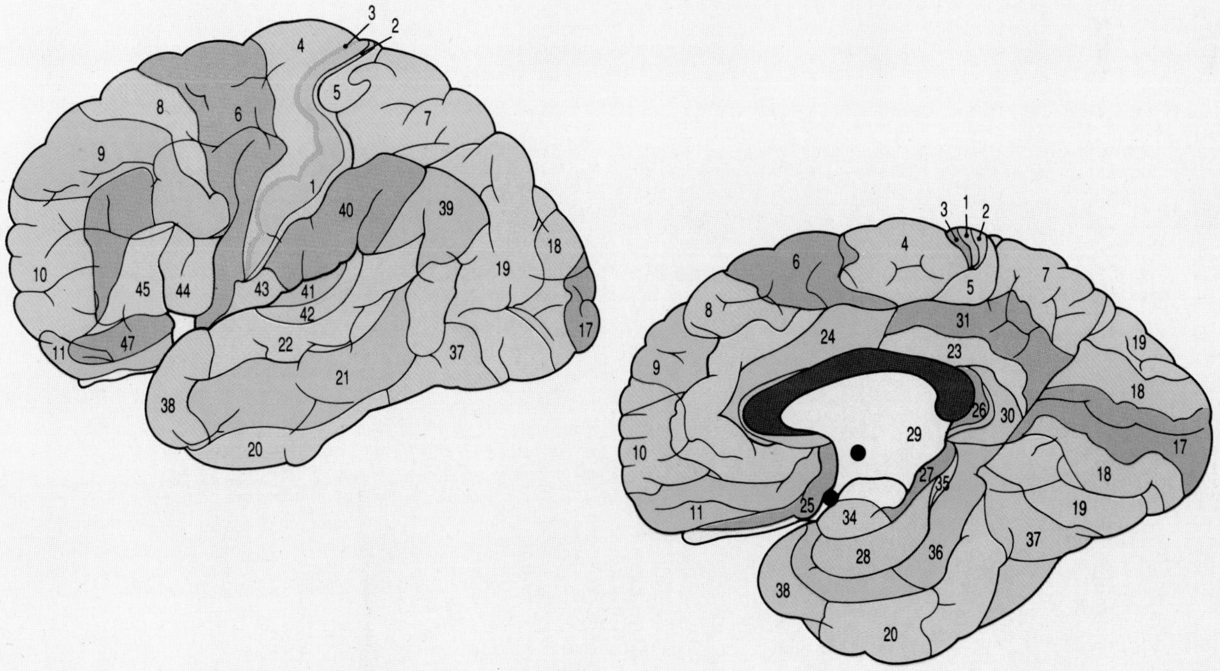

Fig. 12.1 Lateral and medial aspects of the cerebral hemisphere showing Brodmann's cortical areas.

The frontal lobe is separated from the parietal lobe posteriorly by the central (Rolandic) sulcus, while the temporal lobe lies below the lateral (Sylvian) sulcus. The boundaries of the parietal, temporal, and occipital lobes are not defined by a specific sulcus (Fig. 12.2).

The brain is supplied by four arteries, the paired vertebral and paired internal carotid vessels. The former terminate in the anterior and middle cerebral arteries, and the anterior cerebral arteries are connected by an anterior communicating artery. The vertebral arteries unite to form the basilar artery which ends by forming the posterior cerebral arteries (Fig. 12.3). An anastomotic system at the base of the brain (the circle of Willis) provides connections between these various components. The lateral surface of the cortex is supplied predominantly by the middle cerebral artery. The anterior cerebral artery supplies a strip of cortex spanning its superior margin, while the posterior cerebral artery supplies the occipital lobe and the

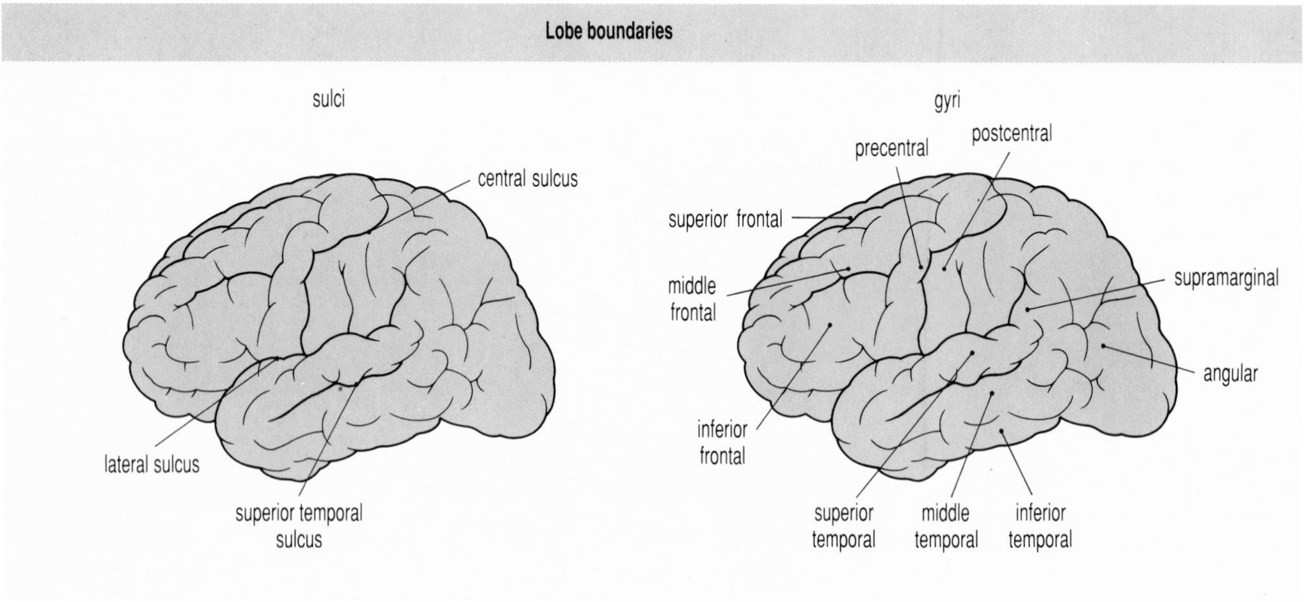

Fig. 12.2 Lateral surface of the cerebral hemisphere.

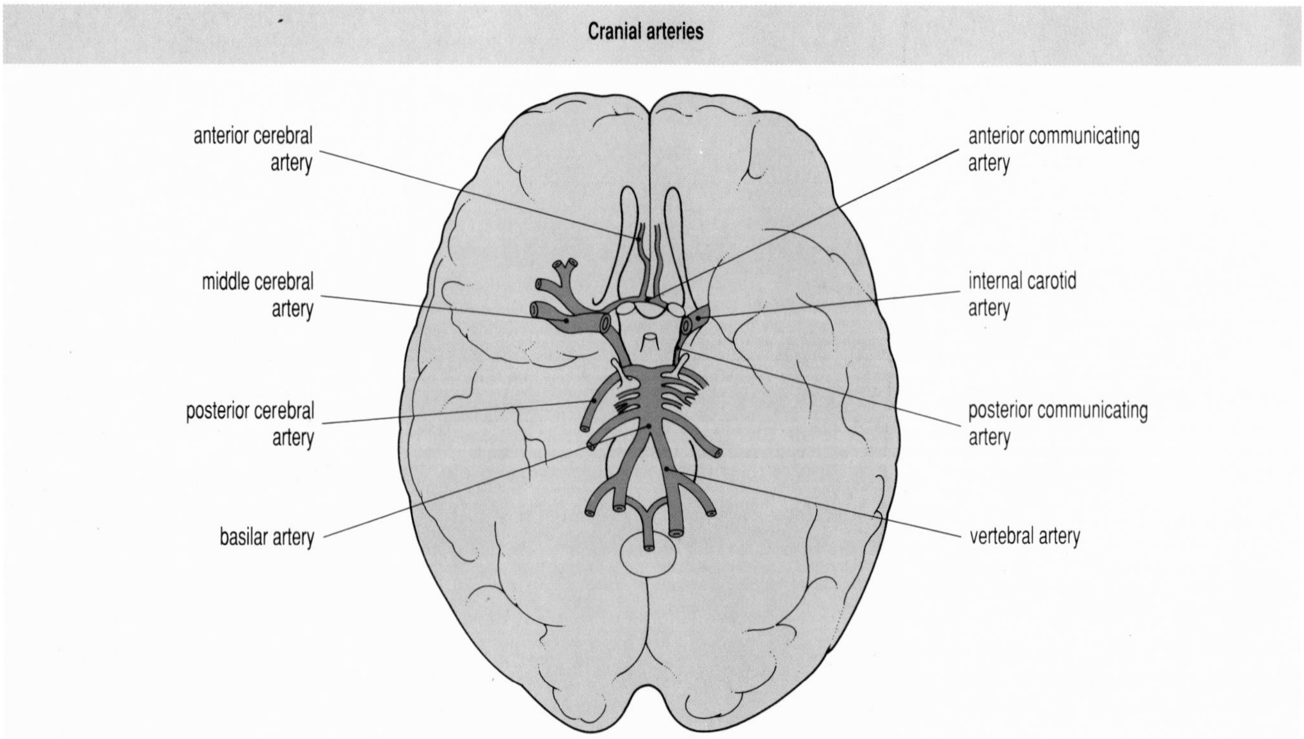

Fig. 12.3 Arteries at the base of the brain.

inferior aspect of the temporal lobe (Fig. 12.4) Normal cerebral blood flow, at around 55ml/100g/minute, represents about 15 per cent of cardiac output. The level of blood flow is largely dependent on the $PC0_2$ of arterial blood. Vasodilatation and increased flow occur as $PC0_2$ rises. During a specific task orientated to speech, vision, hearing, or motor activity, a focal increase in flow occurs in the appropriate part of the cortex.

The ventricular system contains cerebrospinal fluid (CSF) which originates predominantly in the choroid plexuses of the lateral ventricles then circulates through the third ventricle and aqueduct before reaching the fourth ventricle. The CSF exits through the foramina of the fourth ventricle and is eventually reabsorbed through the arachnoid villae. The rate of CSF production is approximately 120ml/24 hours.

Though certain functions (e.g. language and visuo-spatial ability) can be localized to specific cortical areas, other aspects of higher cortical function are represented more diffusely. Abstract thinking is probably located predominantly posteriorly. Calculation ability is more affected by lesions of the dominant rather than the non-dominant hemisphere.

Acquisition of memory requires a number of stages. All data, whether visual or verbal, is recorded temporarily in a short-term pool. A selective and active process then passes some of the data into a long-term memory store. Finally, an active process of retrieval restores the memory to consciousness. Conventionally, the memory is divided into the immediate, recent, and remote components, though these divisions are not absolute. Immediate, or short-term, memory lasts a few seconds; recent memory relates to activities or events occurring within a few hours or days; and remote memory refers to events of the past, for example the individual's youth. Structures particularly associated with learning storage include the hippocampi, the mamillary bodies and the dorsomedial nuclei of the thalami – the limbic system. Remote memory, however, can be retrieved even if these structures are damaged, suggesting that it is stored predominantly in the association cortex appropriate to the memory modality.

Visuo-spatial ability is dependent mainly upon parietal lobe function. Though damage to the non-dominant hemisphere produces a greater degree of constructional apraxia, the disorder occurs with lesions of either parietal lobe.

Language function is located in the left hemisphere in over 99 per cent of right-handed individuals. For left-handed individuals, some 60 per cent have language dominance in the left hemisphere, with 40 per cent in the right hemisphere. Something like 80 per cent of all left-handed individuals have mixed dominance – in other words, language is represented in both hemispheres. Within the hemisphere, a posteriorly placed area (Wernicke) is concerned with the comprehension of spoken language and an anterior area (Broca) with language output. The two are connected by the arcuate fasciculus (Fig. 12.5). The integration of the auditory and visual data required for reading and writing is achieved by the angular gyrus (area 39) (Fig 12.1).

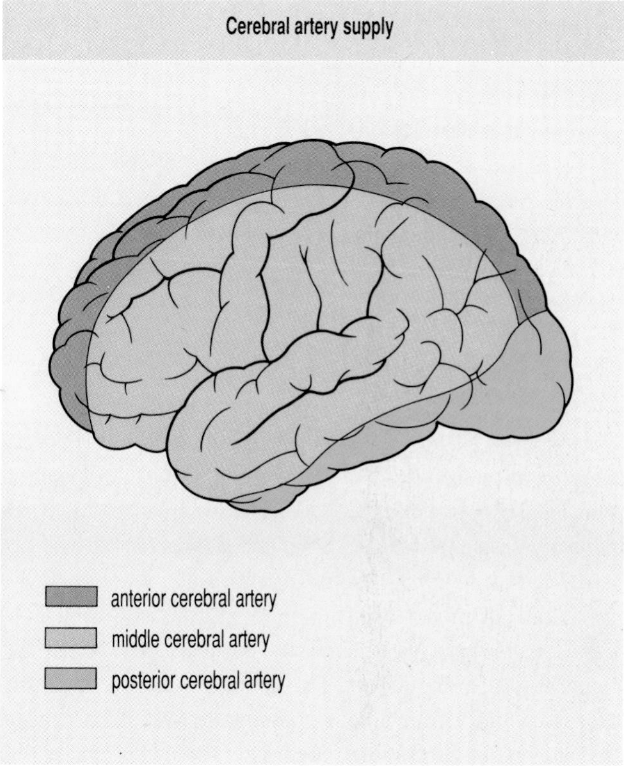

Fig. 12.4 The arterial supply of the lateral surface of the cerebral hemisphere.

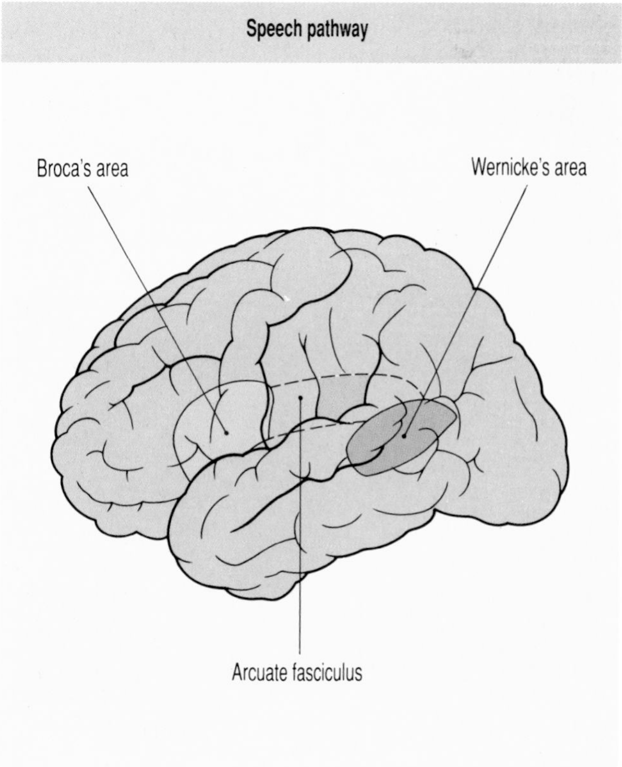

Fig. 12.5 Broca's and Wernicke's areas and their connecting arcuate fasciculus.

SYMPTOMS

Many of the symptoms arising from a disorder of higher cortical function will be more evident to a close friend or relative than to the patient. Areas to cover, though some will be more evident during formal examination, include:

Higher cortical function

Has there been a change in your mood?

Has your memory deteriorated?

Do you have difficult finding the right word in conversation?

Have your ever become lost while travelling a familar route?

Do you have difficulty dressing?

Mood

This can be assessed by direct questioning but also by observation of the patient's behaviour. Is the mood appropriate to the setting of the interview? Is the patient passive, apparently disinterested, or even denying disability? Is there evident anxiety or a heightened state of arousal, accompanied by restlessness and pressure of talk? Does the history suggest delusions or hallucinations?

Memory

Often the demented patient denies loss of memory, particularly once the condition is established. In the early stages, however, patients can retain awareness of their difficulty, and sometimes they volunteer that remote memory is partly spared, though it never escapes the effects of the disease.

Aphasia

Aphasic patients have word-finding difficulty into which they usually retain insight. At times the defect is so substantial that history taking from the patient becomes impossible. Listening to the history allows estimation of the degree of fluency in speech production, an assessment which will continue during the course of the examination. Patients are likely to volunteer any associated difficulty with reading (dyslexia) or writing (dysgraphia).

Geographical disorientation

The first sign of this problem may be the inability to follow a familiar route. If the impairment is severe patients can become lost in their own home, but at this level of disability the problem will be volunteered by relatives rather than the patient.

Dressing

Ask the patient if they have encountered any problems while dressing. Mistakes will usually have been rectified by a relative, but sometimes it is evident that the patient has lost the concept of the order and appropriate arrangement for items of dress.

EXAMINATION

Assessment of the mental state begins as soon as the patient enters the consulting room. During the history-taking it will become apparent if there is an alteration of mood, whether there is any disturbance in the comprehension or production of speech, and whether the patient has retained insight. The physical appearance can be helpful. Demented patients often have a bemused look, wondering quite what they are doing in this particular situation. Evidence of self-neglect is usually concealed by the attentions of friends or relatives. The way in which the patient responds to questioning is of value in diagnosis. Demented patients tend to be inert and apathetic, but a similar impression can be given by depressed individuals.

Orientation

Begin by assessing the patient's orientation in time and space. Establish the patient's age, and ask the time, date, and the name of the hospital in which the interview is taking place. Ask either how long the patient has been in hospital, or the duration of the interview. Normal individuals readily answer these questions.

Memory

Immediate recall

For testing recall, you can use digit repetition, though a normal response also requires intact attention and adequate comprehension. Start with two or three figures, at 1 second intervals, avoiding recognizable sequences. Normal individuals can repeat a five to seven digit sequence. Reverse repetition of a set of digits is a more difficult process which requires psychological functions other than memory. Normal individuals can achieve a four to five figure sequence. The performance of serial 7's (subtracting 7 serially from 100) is dependent on many factors. An abnormal response to this test does not specifically identify the patient with dementia.

Recent memory (new learning ability)

Your examination begins by asking the patient about recent events, though interpretation of the responses must take account of the patient's premorbid intelligence and level of culture. Next ask the patient to memorize four words, or alternatively a name, an address, and a flower. Repeat the words immediately, and ask the patient to repeat them, so that they have clearly been registered. Over the next 10 minutes distract the patient so that there is no opportunity for mental rehearsal, then ask the patient to repeat the data. Most normal individuals can recall all the data at 10 minutes, and 75 per cent at 30 minutes. For further testing of verbal recall, give the patient a short story containing a standard number of items and as soon as the story has been told, ask the patient to recount it.

Visual memory can be tested by displaying drawings for a 5-second period then asking the patient to reproduce the design 10 seconds later. Patients with visuo-spatial disorders will have problems with the task even if their visual memory is intact. The copies can be graded on a four point scale, with a score of two, for example, indicating a recognizable design containing minor flaws, and three a near-perfect or perfect reproduction. Average individuals score two or three on each test item (Fig. 12.6).

Visual memory test

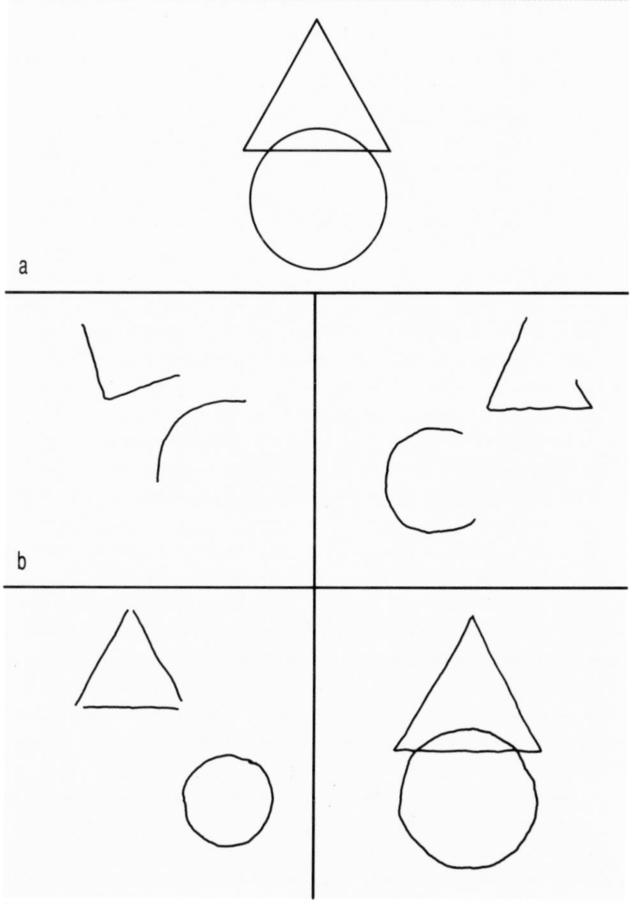

Fig. 12.6 (a) Standard design and (b) reproductions scored from 0–3.

Remote memory

Ask the patient about schooling, childhood, work history, marriage, and, if relevant, the ages of any children. The accuracy of the responses will need verification by a relative. Remote memory is spared in individuals with minor degrees of brain damage but will inevitably be eroded in those suffering from dementia.

Intelligence

Testing a patient's knowledge and abstract thinking must be performed in the light of the social background to which the patient has been exposed. Inherent in all assessments of intelligence is an estimate of the patient's premorbid ability.

Level of information

An example of test questions is shown in Fig. 12.7. Certain elements need to be amended according to the patient's country of residence. An average individual will correctly answer at least six items.

Items for testing patient information level

Questions	Acceptable responses
1. How many weeks are there in a year?	52.
2. Why do people have lungs?	To transfer oxygen from air to blood; to breathe.
3. Name four people who have been prime minister of Great Britain since 1945.	Atlee, Churchill, Eden, Macmillan, Home, Wilson, Heath, Callaghan, Thatcher, Major.
4. Where is Denmark?	Scandinavia.
5. How far is it from London to Edinburgh?	Any answer between 200 and 300 miles.
6. Why are light coloured clothes cooler in the summer than dark coloured clothes?	Light coloured clothes reflect heat from the sun, whereas dark colours absorb heat.
7. What is the capital of Spain?	Madrid.
8. What causes rust?	Oxidation: a chemical reaction of metal, oxygen, and moisture.
9. Who wrote the Odyssey?	Homer.
10. What is the Acropolis?	Site of the Parthenon in Athens.

Fig. 12.7 Items used for testing patient's information level.

Construction test

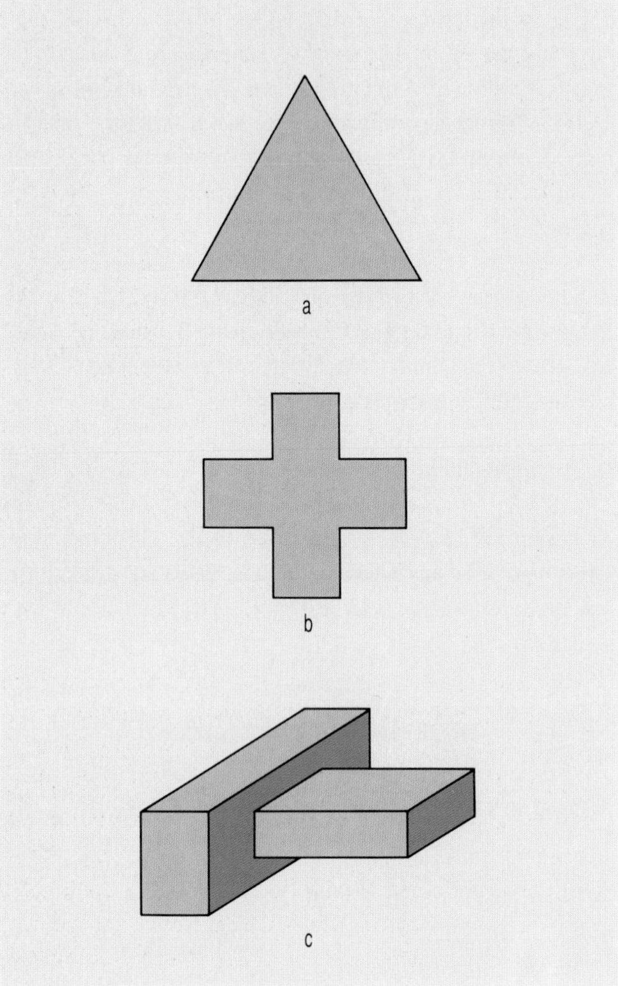

Fig. 12.8 Drawings of increasing complexity to be reproduced by the patient.

Defect of geographical localization

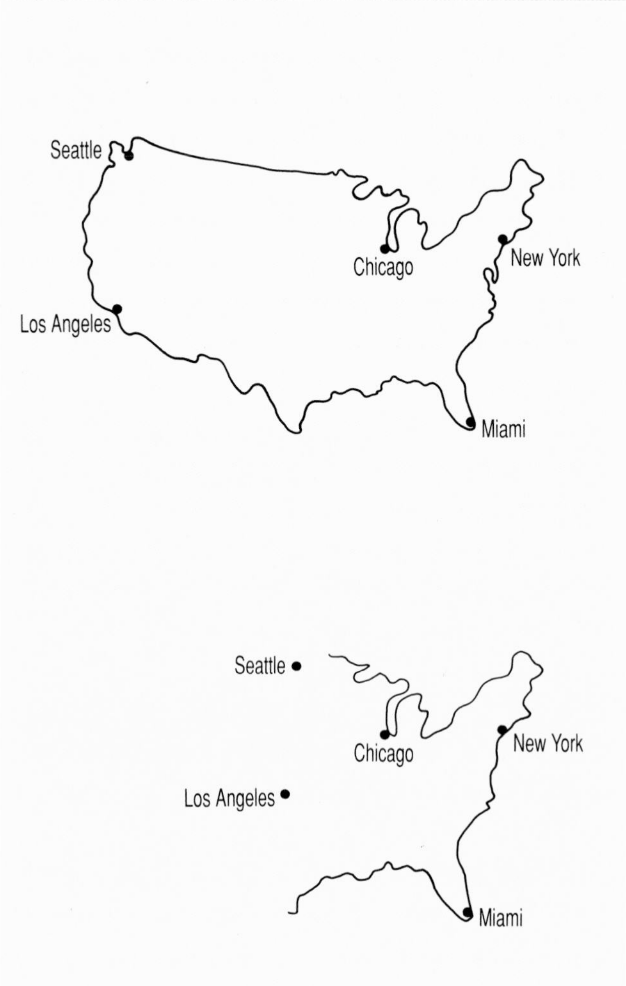

Fig. 12.9 Map. Control (above), patient with left-sided neglect (below).

Calculation

Give the patient simple addition, subtraction, multiplication, and division sums. These can be followed by written tests. At times there may be a calculation difficulty specific to a particular function. Assessment of the results must take account of the patient's education.

Proverb interpretation

Interpretation of proverbs tests both general knowledge and capacity for abstract thinking. Proverbs of increasing complexity are read out to the patient, and their interpretation recorded. A simple proverb to interpret would be 'A bird in the hand is worth two in the bush'; more difficult would be 'People in glass houses should not throw stones'. Concrete responses are made by patients who fail to see beyond the immediate implications of the proverb – for example, a concrete response to the second example would be that the glass would get broken.

Further tests of abstract thinking include the capacity to identify similarities between two objects or situations, and the ability to complete letter or number sequences.

Constructional ability

Constructional capacity can be tested by asking the patient to copy designs of increasing complexity (Fig. 12.8). A scoring system can be devised, low values for which correlate well with the presence of brain damage. When assessing the patient's drawing, look for evidence of unilateral neglect, suggesting the probability of a contralateral parietal lobe syndrome.

Geographical orientation

Evidence concerning this may have been forthcoming during history-taking, but to test it specifically ask the patient to draw an outline of their native country and to place within it a few of the principal cities. From the figure it should be apparent whether or not the patient has an overall defect of geographical localization, or one based on neglect of one half of the visual field (Fig. 12.9).

Speech and speech defects

Elicit the patient's handedness. Asking which hand is used for writing is insufficient since some left-handed individuals have been taugnt to write with their right hand. Ask which hand is used for holding a knife, using a hair brush, using a screwdriver or for playing racket sports. Check on the family history of handedness.

Dysarthria

This is a defect of articulation without any disturbance of language function. Dysarthric patients have a normal speech content, and if they are able to write, their script will be free of dysphasic errors. Production of certain consonants depends on specific parts of the vocal apparatus; P and B are labial sounds, D and T are lingual. Ask the patient to produce particular sounds.As a measure of phonation, ask the patient to hum with the mouth open. As a measure of articulation, ask them to whisper.

In a bulbar palsy, lips, tongue and palate are all likely to be affected. If the palate is principally involved, speech becomes nasal. The sound quality produced by a patient with a palatal palsy is similar to that produced by speaking with your nose occluded. In a pseudobulbar palsy, there may be a gross impairment of diction (anarthria). When the disorder is less severe, the speech is hesitant, with an explosive, strangulated quality. Speech is hoarse and of reduced volume in the presence of a unilateral vocal cord paralysis and virtually lost in bilateral vocal cord paresis. If the cords are adducted, you will hear an inspiratory stridor. The sound is easily mimicked. Patients with cerebellar dysarthria are unable to achieve a normal speech rhythm, and speech volume and inflexion fluctuate wildly. A staccato quality emerges when the problem is severe.

Dysphonia

Dysphonia is a defect of speech volume and is usually the result of a disorder limiting the excursion either of the muscles of respiration or the vocal cords. Spastic dysphonia is a form of focal dystonia in which inappropriate muscle contraction produces speech which is strained and strangulated.

Dysphasia

This is a defect of language function in which there is either abnormal comprehension or production of speech, or both. Much of the patient's language function will have been tested, though not deliberately, while taking the history. Seldom is there no spontaneous speech, though in certain types of dysphasia, the patient may be reduced to uttering short, meaningless phrases. Aphasic speech lacks grammatical content, displays word-finding difficulty, and contains word substitutions (paraphasias). Paraphasias are either whole word substitutions (verbal) (e.g. bread for table), syllable substitutions (literal) (e.g. speed for feed), or complete nonsense words (neologisms) (e.g. tersh).

Assessment of dysphasia

What is the patient's handedness?

Is the speech fluent or non-fluent?

What is the level of comprehension?

Can the patient repeat words or phrases?

Can the patient name objects?

Fluency

Fluency may be defined as the amount of speech produced in a given period of time. Non-fluent speech, therefore, contains a limited number of words. Typically the patient displays greater effort in speech production, the output is often dysarthric, and the phrase length limited. The overall result is a loss of rhythm and melody (dysprosody). Fluent dysphasia is near or even above normal in terms of output. Melody tends to be retained and phrase length is normal. Despite this the patient fails to produce critical, meaningful words, and output is incoherent. Many fluent dysphasics are labelled as confused. Paraphasias are particularly prominent. Non-fluent speech is associated with anterior, and fluent speech with posterior hemisphere lesions.Verbal fluency can be formally tested by asking the patient to name as many objects as possible in a particular category (e.g. fruits and vegetables) in a set length of time.

Comprehension

In testing comprehension, increasingly complex questions can be asked, but all should be answerable by a simple yes or no response. A substantial number of questions requiring randomly distributed yes/no responses are needed to avoid errors in interpretation. Avoid asking the patient to perform a skilled task – those with apraxia will fail even if their comprehension is intact.

Repetition

Repetition can be selectively spared or involved in a dysphasic process and should be tested separately. Start by asking the patient to repeat simple words, then give sentences of increasing complexity. Patients with repetition difficulty often have a particular problem repeating 'no, ifs, ands, or buts'. Normal individuals can repeat sentences of 19 syllables.

Naming

A naming defect is common to virtually all dysphasic problems. Point to a succession of items, and ask the patient to name each one. Use objects commonly and less commonly encountered, and mix the categories rather than restrict the test to, say, parts of the body.

Reading

Reading assessment must take account of the patient's educational background. Ask the patient to read aloud, then test comprehension by asking questions requiring simple yes/no responses.

Writing

Agraphia is an inevitable accompaniment of aphasia. Begin testing writing ability by asking the patient first to write single words, then sentences, initially writing them spontaneously and then in response to dictation. After checking word content, note whether the writing is crammed into one side of the page, suggesting the possibility of unilateral neglect.

Praxis

Apraxia is a disorder of skilled movement not attributable to weakness, incoordination, sensory loss, or failure to comprehend what is required. The problem in movement may be confined to the limbs, to the trunk, or even to the buccofacial musculature. A defect for a single skilled task is termed ideomotor apraxia. Ideational apraxia is a failure to perform a more complex sequence of skilled activity.

Start by asking the patient to carry out a particular task (e.g. 'pretend to use a screwdriver'). If the patient is unable to perform the task, do it yourself and then ask the patient to copy your movement. If a response is still not forthcoming, provide the object in question and ask the patient to demonstrate its use. These three tiers of command are in descending order of difficulty for the apraxic patient. Instructions that will test relevant movements include, 'put out your tongue', 'pretend to whistle', 'salute', 'show how you would use a toothbrush, or a hair brush'. For whole body movements, ask the patient to stand to attention, or to stand as if about to start dancing. A more complex motor sequence is tested by asking the patient to go through a series of related movements. For example, taking the cap off a toothpaste tube, squeezing the toothpaste onto a brush, then replacing the cap.

Right-left orientation

A proportion of normal individuals have some problem with right-left orientation. Patients who are dysphasic can have problems understanding your commands. Start testing with simple tasks (e.g. 'show me your right hand') then gradually increase their complexity (e.g. 'put your left hand on your right ear').

Agnosia

Patients with visual agnosia are unable to recognize objects they see, despite intact visual pathways and speech capacity. Show objects to the patient, asking them to name each one, and then allow the patient to manipulate the object to see if this improves recognition. Other forms of agnosia which can be tested include the ability to name and recognize individual fingers (finger agnosia) and colours (colour agnosia).

Conclusion

It is clearly not appropriate to go through such an extensive testing of higher cortical function in every patient. Screening tests have been devised which allow a rapid assessment of function. Such tests – for example the mini-mental state test (Fig. 12.10) — are useful, though their limitations need to be remembered when using them for screening purposes. A score of 20 or less suggests the possibility of a cognitive disorder, particularly dementia.

Mini-mental state examination

Orientation

1. What is the year, season, date, month, day? (One point for each correct answer.)
2. Where are we? Country, county, town, hospital, floor? (One point for each correct answer.)

Registration

3. Name three objects taking one second to say each. Then ask the patient all three once you have said them. One point for each correct answer. Repeat the questions until the patient learns all three.

Attention & Calculation

4. Serial sevens. One point for each correct answer. Stop after five answers. Alternative: spell WORLD backwards.

Recall

5. Ask for names of three objects asked in Question 3. One point for each correct answer.

Language

6. Point to a pencil and a watch. Have the patient name them for you.One point for each correct answer
7. Have the patient repeat "No ifs, ands, or buts. One point.
8. Have the patient follow a 3-stage command: "Take the paper in your right hand; fold the paper in half; put the paper on the floor." Three points.
9. Have the patient read and obey the following: CLOSE YOUR EYES. (Write this in large letters) One point.
10. Have the patient write a sentence of his/her own choice. (The sentence must contain a subject and an object and make some sense). Ignore spelling errors when scoring. One point.
11. Have the patient draw two intersecting pentagons with equal sides. Give one point if all the sides and angles are preserved, and if the intersecting sides form a quadrangle.

Maximum score = 30 points

Fig. 12.10 The mini-mental state test.

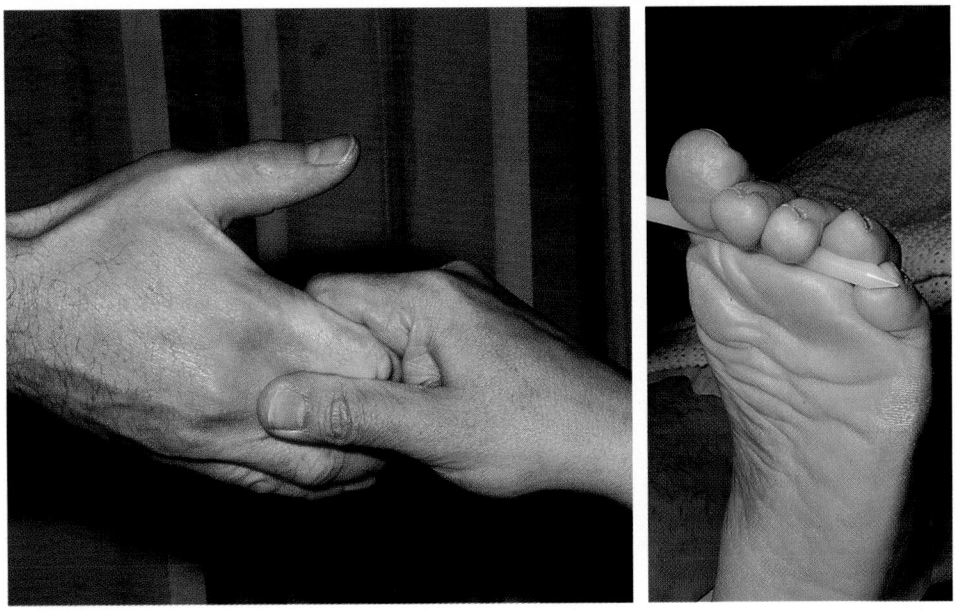

Fig. 12.11 Primitive reflexes.

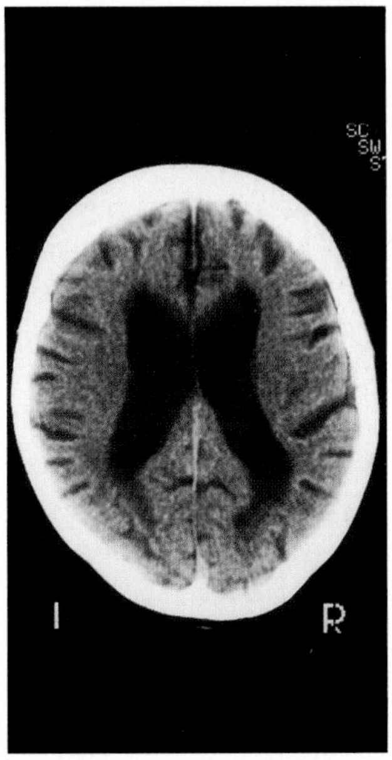

Fig. 12.12 CT scan of a patient with dementia.

PRIMITIVE REFLEXES

At this stage it is worth testing a number of primitive reflexes (Fig. 12.11) before passing on to the cranial nerve examination.

The glabellar tap

Tap repetitively with the tip of your index finger on the glabella. The blinking response should inhibit after 3 – 4 taps. In certain disorders, particularly the dementias and Parkinson's disease, the response persists.

The palmo-mental reflex

Apply firm and fairly sharp pressure to the palm of the hand alongside the thenar eminence. If the response is positive, contraction of the ipsilateral mentalis causes a puckering of the chin.

Pout and suckling reflexes

A positive pout response results in protrusion of the lips when they are lightly tapped by the index finger. A positive suckling reflex consists of a suckling movement of the lips when the angle of the mouth is stimulated.

Grasp reflex

Stroke firmly across the palmar surface of the hand from the radial to the ulnar aspect. In a positive response the examiner's hand is gripped by the patient's fingers with such force that release is difficult. A foot grasp reflex is elicited by stroking the sole of the foot towards the toes with the handle of the patella hammer. A positive response leads to plantar flexion of the toes.

CLINICAL APPLICATION

Dementia

The majority of patients with dementia have Alzheimer's disease, or senile dementia of Alzheimer-type. Most of the remainder have either cerebrovascular disease or a mixed pathology. In the early stages of dementia the most prominent symptoms are apathy and lack of concentration, together with defects in memory and performance. Later, word-finding difficulty appears with impaired comprehension and paraphasic substitutions. The patient becomes apraxic. There is a surprisingly poor correlation between the presence of dementia and the size of the cortical sulci as demonstrated on computerized tomography. Ventricular size provides a better correlate (Fig. 12.12).

Memory

Damage to the limbic system results in a failure to learn new memories (antegrade amnesia) associated with a defect of memory for the more recent past (retrograde amnesia). In some instances the patient confabulates responses, particularly soon after the onset. Immediate memory remains intact. Conditions causing this picture include herpes simplex encephalitis, and alcoholism. Unilateral temporal lobe lesions can have a selective effect on verbal or visual memory according to whether the dominant or non-dominant hemisphere is affected.

Dyscalculia

Dyscalculia can occur with bilateral or unilateral lesions. Generally the dyscalculia is greater when the dominant hemisphere is affected.

Constructional ability and geographical orientation

Constructional difficulty is particularly associated with parietal lobe lesions of the non-dominant hemisphere. It appears relatively early in the course of Alzheimer's disease. Geographical disorientation has a similar topographical significance.

Aphasia

A number of aphasic syndromes have been described on the basis of the findings from testing of fluency, comprehension, repetition and naming (Fig. 12.13).

Broca's aphasia

In this aphasia the output is non-fluent and usually dysarthric, comprehension is intact except for complex phrases, and there are naming errors. The lesion lies in and around area 44 (Fig. 12.1) of the frontal lobe and may be vascular or neoplastic.

Transcortical motor aphasia

This is similar to Broca's aphasia except that the patient's powers of repetition are retained. The pathological process (again usually vascular or neoplastic) is located above or anterior to Broca's area.

Wernicke's aphasia

Here the patient has fluent, easily articulated speech, but there are frequent paraphasias and meaning is largely absent. Comprehension and repetition are severely impaired, and attempts at naming produce paraphasic errors. If the lesion is confined to Wernicke's area, auditory comprehension is severely affected; if it is in the parietal lobe, comprehension of single words is retained.

Conduction aphasia

Conduction aphasia is fluent but not to the degree seen in Wernicke's aphasia. Interruptions to the speech rhythm are frequent, but there is no dysarthria. Naming is imperfect but comprehension good. Despite this, repetition is severely abnormal. Reading, at least out loud, and writing are impaired. Cerebrovascular disease is the commonest cause of conduction aphasia. The condition occurs with disruption of the arcuate fasciculus connecting the posterior temporal lobe to the motor association cortex (Fig. 12.13), and is also seen with lesions in the region of Wernicke's area.

Transcortical sensory aphasia

Transcortical sensory aphasia is fluent but frequently interrupted by repetition of words or phrases initiated by the examiner (echolalia). Despite the readiness and accuracy of the patient's repetition, comprehension is severely impaired. Naming is poor and reading comprehension defective. The anatomical site responsible for this form of aphasia is less well localized than for some of the others, but lies in the borderlands of the temporal and parietal lobes of the dominant hemisphere.

Anomic aphasia

Anomic aphasia is fluent and interrupted more by pauses than by paraphasic substitutions. Comprehension is relatively preserved, repetition is good and naming is affected but to a varying degree. There is no specific anatomical location. Anomic aphasia can be the final stage of recovery from other forms of aphasia and is seen with both structural and metabolic disease of the brain.

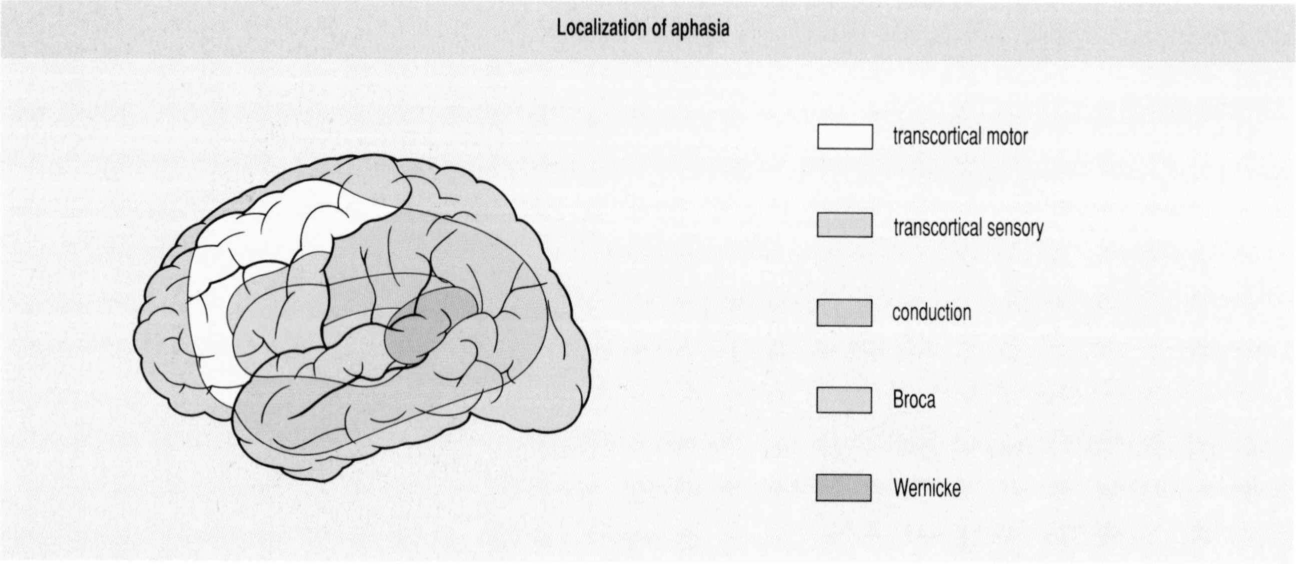

Fig. 12.13 Anatomical sites associated with the various aphasic syndromes.

Global aphasia

As the title implies, global aphasia affects all aspects of speech function. Output is non-fluent and comprehension, repetition, naming, reading, and writing are all affected, often to a severe degree. The causative pathology occupies a substantial part of the language area of the dominant hemisphere and is most commonly the consequence of an extensive infarct in middle cerebral artery territory.

Dyslexia and alexia

The term dyslexia is generally restricted to developmental disorders of reading, and alexia to disorders secondary to acquired brain damage. Alexia with agraphia is found with lesions of the angular gyrus of the dominant hemisphere. Alexia without agraphia is associated with lesions affecting both the left occipital cortex and the splenium of the corpus callosum. Most commonly it is the result of an occlusion of the posterior cerebral artery to the dominant hemisphere.

Agraphia

While it is true to say that virtually all aphasic patients have agraphia, many patients with agraphia are not aphasic. Writing skill is affected by motor disability, involuntary movements, and visuo-spatial disorders.

Apraxia

The pathway involved in performing a skilled task to command begins in the auditory association cortex of the dominant hemisphere then passes to the parietal association cortex, subsequently travelling forwards to the premotor cortex and finally the motor cortex itself. Interruption of this pathway at any point results in an ideomotor apraxia affecting both the dominant and non-dominant hands (Fig. 12.14). The pathway from the dominant to the non-dominant premotor cortex (D – D) passes through the anterior corpus callosum. A lesion at that site will produce an apraxia confined to the left hand. Whole body movements tend to be relatively spared even when limb ideomotor apraxia is substantial. Ideational apraxia is usually the consequence of bilateral hemisphere lesions.

Right-left disorientation

Right-left disorientation is most likely to result from posteriorly placed dominant hemisphere lesions. Gerstmann's syndrome comprises right-left disorientation, finger agnosia, dysgraphia, and dyscalculia. If all four components are present, the causative pathology is likely to lie in the dominant parietal lobe.

Visual agnosia

One form of visual agnosia is due to a disconnection between the visual cortex and the speech area. Patients can recognize objects, and demonstrate their use, but are unable to name them. Bilateral temporo-occipital lesions are the usual cause. In the other form of visual agnosia, recognition of objects fails, but their use can be demonstrated if the object is placed in the hand. In other words, sensory information can bypass the defect of visual recognition, which is a consequence of damage to the visual association cortex in both hemispheres.

Primitive reflexes

The palmo-mental reflex is found bilaterally in some normal individuals, but a unilateral palmo-mental reflex suggests a contralateral frontal lobe lesion. Snout and suckling reflexes are elicited in

Skilled motor task pathways

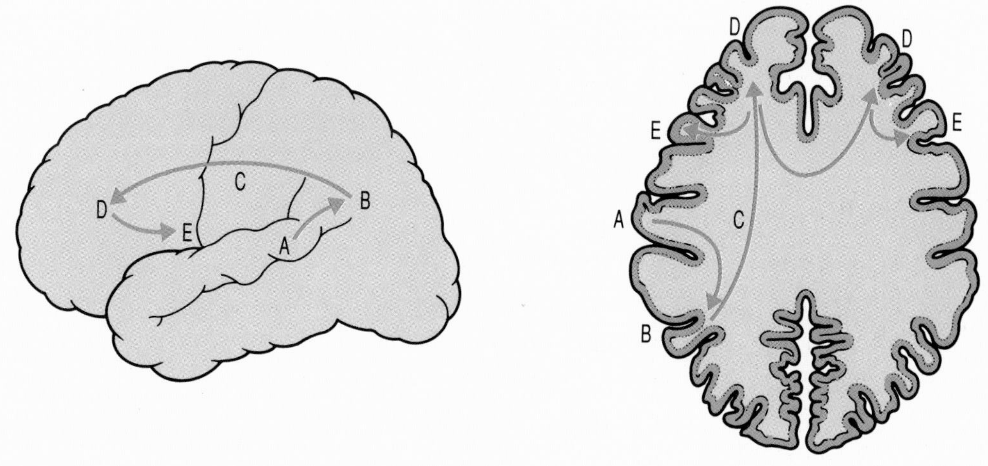

Fig. 12.14 Pathways involved in the formulation and performance of a skilled motor task.

patients with diffuse bilateral hemisphere disease. Bilateral grasp reflexes are of limited localizing value, but a unilateral response is associated with pathology in the contralateral frontal lobe. A foot grasp, or tonic plantar reflex, can be one of the earliest signs of a frontal lobe lesion.

THE PSYCHIATRIC ASSESSMENT

SYMPTOMS

The most important part of the psychiatric assessment is the interview, in which the patient's mood and personality can be gauged while the history unfolds. Many symptoms are common to both physical and psychiatric disease but others are more specifically the territory of psychiatry.

Psychiatric assessment

Do you feel unduly anxious or depressed?

Do you repeat certain tasks over and over again?

Do you feel people are against you?

Have you heard or seen things which are not there?

Do you ever lose the sense of yourself or your environment?

Somatic and psychic symptoms of anxiety and depression

	Anxiety	Depression
Somatic	palpitations tremor breathlessness dizziness fatigue diarrhoea sweating	altered appetite constipation headache bodily fatigue tiredness
Psychic	feelings of tension Irritability difficulty getting to sleep fear depersonalization	apathy poor concentration early morning waking diurnal mood change retardation feelings of guilt

Fig. 12.15 Somatic and psychic symptoms of anxiety and depression.

Anxiety

Patients will usually complain specifically of anxiety, but sometimes its somatic manifestations, for example palpitations, sweating and tremulousness predominate (Fig. 12.15). The anxiety may be chronic and spontaneous or triggered acutely by a specific stimulus – phobic anxiety.

Depression

The somatic manifestations of depression are often as conspicuous as the mood change itself. The patient will have noticed a flattening of mood, with loss of interest and difficulty in concentration. The mood may fluctuate during the course of the day, but patients describe an overall sadness, with a grey dreary aspect to their lives. Suicidal thoughts are sometimes expressed spontaneously. If not, they should be sought for specifically.

Euphoria

The patient is hardly likely to complain of euphoria, a feeling of boundless physical and mental energy. There is likely to be a pressurized, manic quality to the patient's conversation accompanied by physical restlessness.

Obsessiveness

The obsessional patient has become a victim to ritualistic thoughts or actions. When translated into physical activity, these rituals (e.g. washing of the body) are repeated with monotonous regularity and in a set order. Examples of obsessional thought include convictions that a particular individual is antagonistic, or that a spouse is unfaithful.

Delusions

Delusions are ideas which cannot be dismissed by the patient despite evidence indicating their falsity. Often there is an element of reference – in other words, that actions or words are directed specifically at that individual even if they appear on a global platform, for example the radio. Paranoid delusions contain a persecutory element. Delusions of worthlessness are particularly associated with depressive illness.

Abnormal perceptions

Illusions are misinterpretations of an external reality. They are usually visual and affect normal individuals as well as patients with psychiatric disorders. Hallucinations are experiences which have no objective equivalent to explain them. They are predominantly either visual or auditory, although other forms of hallucination occur, for example of smell or taste. These are particularly associated with complex partial seizures.

Visual hallucinations

These may be unformed, for example an ill-defined pattern of lights, or formed, the patient then describing individuals or animals, often of a frightening aspect. Visual hallucinations are more usually a feature of an organic brain syndrome (e.g. delirium tremens) rather than the functional psychoses (e.g. schizophrenia).

Auditory hallucinations

Auditory hallucinations are also either unformed or formed. The patient is sometimes able to identify the voice if the hallucination is formed. Auditory hallucinations are found more often in the functional psychoses than in organic brain disease. The voices can take on a persecutory quality in schizophrenia, and an accusatory element in depression.

Déja and jamais vu

Déja and jamais vu refer, respectively, to an intense feeling of a relived experience, and a sensation of strangeness in familiar surroundings. Both are sometimes an experience of everyday life, but when pathological they are usually epileptic in origin.

Depersonalization and derealization

In depersonalization the patient feels a sense of bodily strangeness, amounting at times to a sense of being outside the body, watching its actions as an external witness. Derealization results in a sense of loss of reality of the environment. Both are experienced in depressive and anxiety states.

EXAMINATION

The concept of the psychiatric examination needs to be interpreted in a broad sense. A physical examination is necessary but the most telling diagnostic details will be revealed by an exploration of the patient's mental state, emerging as much from the history as from the answers to specific questions. History taking from the psychiatric patient follows that used in other settings (see Chapter 1) but certain areas should be covered in greater detail.

Family history

Genetic factors are particularly strong in schizophrenia and manic depressive psychosis. In addition, the family environment is likely to be a factor in many psychiatric disorders. Enquiry should include the parental background; establish whether they are still alive, or, if dead, the patient's age when this occurred. The quality of the parents' marriage is relevant to the patient's development.

Personal history

A detailed personal history is time-consuming. It must embrace the patient's childhood, adolescence and schooling, sexual development, and present occupation or training. Relevant details include neurotic traits in childhood, for example bed-wetting, failure to achieve close relationships in childhood, frequent truanting, frequent job changes, and problems achieving close adult relationships including marriage. It can take several interviews before sensitive issues emerge.

Past history

The past history should not simply cover previous psychiatric illness, which can be relevant whether or not it led to specialist referral, but also episodes of physical illness with their potential for acting as a catalyst for subsequent mental disorder.

Drug history

Try to determine the degree of alcohol consumption, though few alcoholics will answer accurately. Features suggestive of alcohol dependency include early morning drinking, morning vomiting, taking a drink prior to the interview, erratic work attendance, and drinking in isolation. Ask about narcotic exposure, the use of softer drugs such as cannabis, and exposure to tranquillizers. If the patient is using codeine derivatives, ascertain for what purpose and the dosage.

Personality profile

Evidence suggesting changing personality and mood is often better provided by colleagues, relatives, or friends than by the patient. Questionnaires have been devised for the assessment of personality, but without using a formal questionaire, the patient's attitudes and behaviour, in terms of work and social relationships, personal ambitions, drive, level of independence and authority, and response to stress will indicate the nature of the personality.

CLINICAL APPLICATION

Organic mental states

In organic mental states a specific pathological basis for the mental disorder has been established. Acute forms include the toxic confusional states, characterized by alteration of the conscious level, disordered perceptions (e.g. visual hallucinations), restlessness, and thought disorder. Almost any structural or metabolic disorder can trigger the reaction. Examples include encephalitis, head injury, and alcohol withdrawal. The principal chronic organic mental state is dementia.

Functional mental states

In functional mental states a specific underlying pathological or metabolic cause has not been identified. Psychotic states are those in which the individual has lost insight, and neurotic states those in which insight is preserved. The distinction is not absolute, however, and the terms are best avoided. In affective disorders an alteration of mood is a major feature of the illness. Such disorders include anxiety, depression, and mania.

Phobias

Phobias are a particular form of anxiety triggered by a specific environment or circumstance. Agoraphobia, for example, results in a fear of leaving the home, particularly if this involves entering crowded places.

Depressive illness

Depressive illnesses include those triggered primarily by genetic or constitutional factors (endogenous), and those precipitated by adverse external events (reactive).

Mania and hypomania

Mania and hypomania (its lesser form) represent the opposite end of the mood spectrum. There is pressure of talk and physical activity. Patients lack insight and react adversely if their grandiose schemes are questioned. In manic-depressive illness, the mood fluctuates between two extremes.

Schizophrenia

Schizophrenia has been classified into a number of different types, though the entities so defined are not absolutely distinct. The condition is characterized by the presence of thought disorder, blunting of emotional responses, paranoid tendencies, and perceptual disorders. Thought disorder leads to irrational conversation, in which the development of ideas either is blocked, or moves suddenly into unconnected channels. The emotions are blunted and the patient becomes increasingly withdrawn. Delusions are prominent and frequently contain paranoid elements. Auditory hallucinations are particularly characteristic of schizophrenia.

Obsessional states

In obsessional states, preoccupation with mental or physical acts predominates. An obsessional personality displays these characteristics but not to the point where they interfere with the normal activities of life. In obsessional states, however, the relevant thought or action takes on a compulsive quality, ineffectively countered by resistance on the part of the patient. Obsessional symptoms can feature in other psychiatric illnesses.

Hysteria (conversion hysteria)

Hysteria is a disorder in which physical symptoms or signs exist for which there is no objective counterpart, and which require, in the case of signs, an elaboration on the part of the patient of which he or she is unaware. Many of the symptoms are referred to the nervous system – for example memory loss, paralysis, unsteadiness and visual impairment. Malingerers, on the other hand, consciously elaborate their disability.

For anxiety

Are the symptoms provoked by particular environments?

For depression

Are there suicidal thoughts?

For schizophrenia

Has the patient had auditory hallucinations?
Does the patient believe his thoughts are controlled by others?

Hysterical personality

Hysterical personality is distinct from hysteria, though those with this personality trait may develop conversion reactions. The hysterical personality state is characterized by superficiality and shallow emotional responsiveness combined with a histrionic overwrought reaction to events.

THE CRANIAL NERVES

THE OLFACTORY (1ST) NERVE

STRUCTURE AND FUNCTION

The olfactory epithelium contains specialized receptor cells and free nerve endings, the latter derived from the first and second divisions of the trigeminal nerve. Unmyelinated axons from the receptor cells traverse the cribriform plate before synapsing in the olfactory bulb. From here, the olfactory tract passes backwards, dividing into lateral and medial roots in the region of the anterior perforated substance. The more important lateral root projects predominantly to the uncus of the ipsilateral temporal lobe.

Molecules derived from particular odours are absorbed into the mucus covering the olfactory epithelium. From here they diffuse via ciliary processes to the terminal processes of the receptor cells where they bind reversibly to receptor sites. This initiates an action potential in the olfactory nerve with a firing frequency related to the intensity of the stimulus.

Women have a more sensitive sense of smell than men. In both sexes, smell sensitivity declines after the fifth decade of life. Many healthy individuals have difficulty naming or describing the quality of a particular odour even though they can distinguish it from others. The value of a particular odour for the testing of olfactory nerve function is determined principally by how selectively it stimulates the specialized receptor cells rather than the free trigeminal endings. Odours stimulating the trigeminal nerve include peppermint, camphor, ammonia, menthol, and anisol. Highly selective stimulants of olfactory nerve endings include ß-phenyl ethyl alcohol, methyl cyclopentenolone and isovaleric acid. Coffee, cinnamon, and chocolate are useful everyday odours for the bedside testing of smell.

EXAMINATION

The most convenient method for testing smell utilizes squeeze bottles bearing a nozzle which can be inserted into each nostril in turn. The patient is asked either to identify the smell or describe its quality. Quantitative measurement is unnecessary for routine clinical evaluation, but can be achieved by using serial dilutions of a particular odour presented on a strip of filter paper, or by dispersing the odour in a varying volume of air.

CLINICAL APPLICATION

Olfaction is commonly disturbed by upper respiratory tract infection or local nasal pathology (Fig. 12.16). Hyposmia can persist after an apparently banal viral illness, and following head injury. Smell sensitivity is diminished in dementia. Unilateral hyposmia is rarely the presenting symptom of a subfrontal meningioma. Olfactory hallucinations occur in complex partial seizures (temporal lobe epilepsy).

THE OPTIC (2ND) NERVE

STRUCTURE AND FUNCTION

Two types of photoreceptor, rods and cones, have been identified in man. At the fovea only cones are found, with rods predominating in the periphery of the retina. Fibres from the nasal aspect of the fovea pass directly to the optic disc. Those from above and below the fovea pass almost directly, but fibres from the temporal border pass almost vertically, both superiorly and inferiorly, before arching around the other foveal fibres on their way to the optic disc (Fig. 12.17). Axons from the papillomacular bundle originate in the cones of the fovea and occupy a substantial proportion of the temporal aspect of the optic disc. Fibres from the superior and inferior parts of the periphery of the retina occupy corresponding areas in the optic nerve. As the papillomacular bundle approaches the chiasm it moves centrally. The crossing, nasal, macular fibres occupy the central and posterior part of the chiasm. The superior peripheral nasal

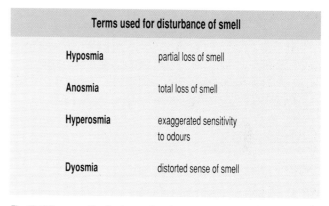

Terms used for disturbance of smell	
Hyposmia	partial loss of smell
Anosmia	total loss of smell
Hyperosmia	exaggerated sensitivity to odours
Dyosmia	distorted sense of smell

Fig. 12.16 Terms used for disturbance of smell.

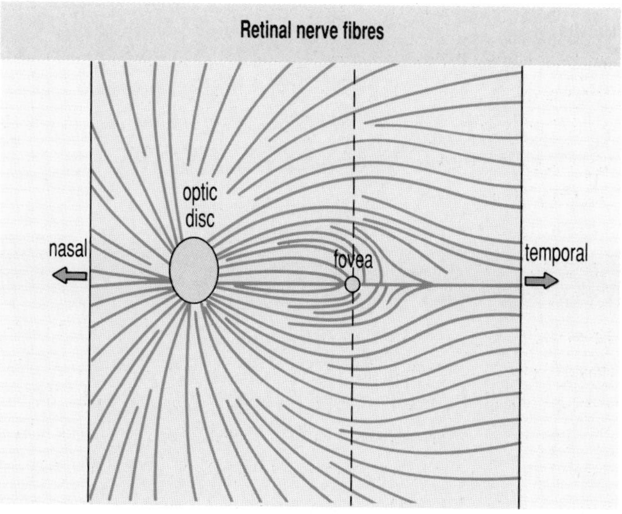

Fig. 12.17 Representation of the course of the retinal nerve fibres.

fibres cross more posteriorly than the ventral fibres, which loop slightly into the terminal part of the opposite optic nerve (Fig. 12.18). In the optic tract the macular fibres are dorsolateral, the upper retinal fibres dorsomedial, and the lower retinal fibres ventrolateral. Crossed and uncrossed fibres are arranged in alternate layers in the lateral geniculate body. The optic radiation extends from the lateral geniculate body to the visual (striate) cortex, area 17 (Fig. 12.1). The ventral fibres of the radiation loop forward towards the tip of the temporal lobe. The visual cortex is situated along the superior and inferior margins of the calcarine fissure, extending about 1.5cm around the posterior pole. The macular representation lies posteriorly, with dorsal and ventral retina above and below the fissure, respectively. The unpaired outer 30° of the temporal field is represented in the contralateral hemisphere at the anterior limit of the striate cortex (Fig. 12.19).

Conditions of high (photopic) illumination activate cone photoreceptors, providing high spatial resolution and colour vision sense. Low-illumination (scotopic) responses are mediated by rods. The receptive field of a ganglion cell is defined as the retinal area which, when stimulated, results in a response from that cell. Each retinal area projects to a specific site in the primary visual cortex. Fibres originating from retina nasal to the fovea are predominantly crossed, while those originating from retina temporal to the vertical meridian are predominantly uncrossed. Within a narrow strip centred on the vertical meridian, cells projecting either ipsilaterally or contralaterally intermingle.

Crossed and uncrossed fibres

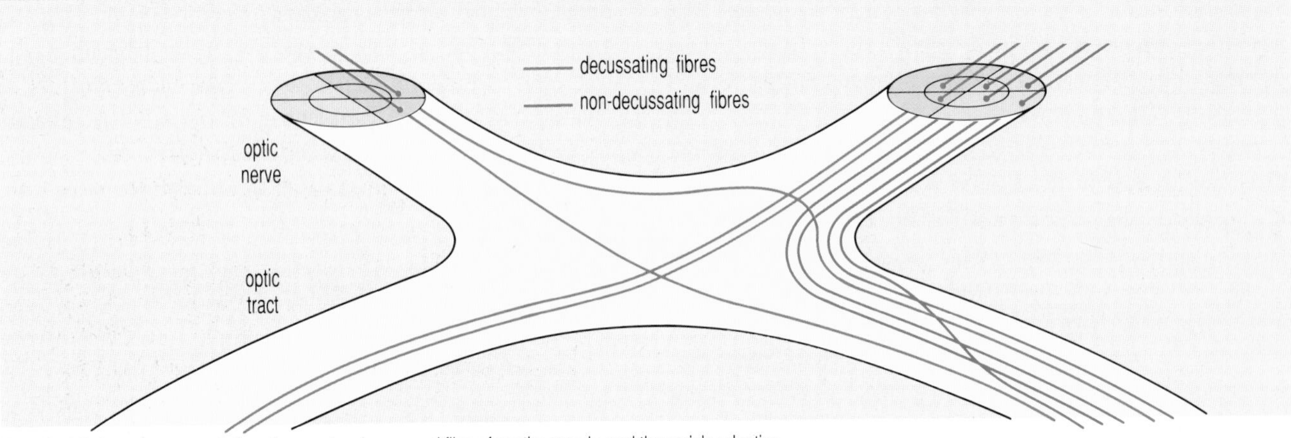

Fig. 12.18 Schematic representation of crossed and uncrossed fibres from the macula, and the peripheral retina.

Representation of right visual field

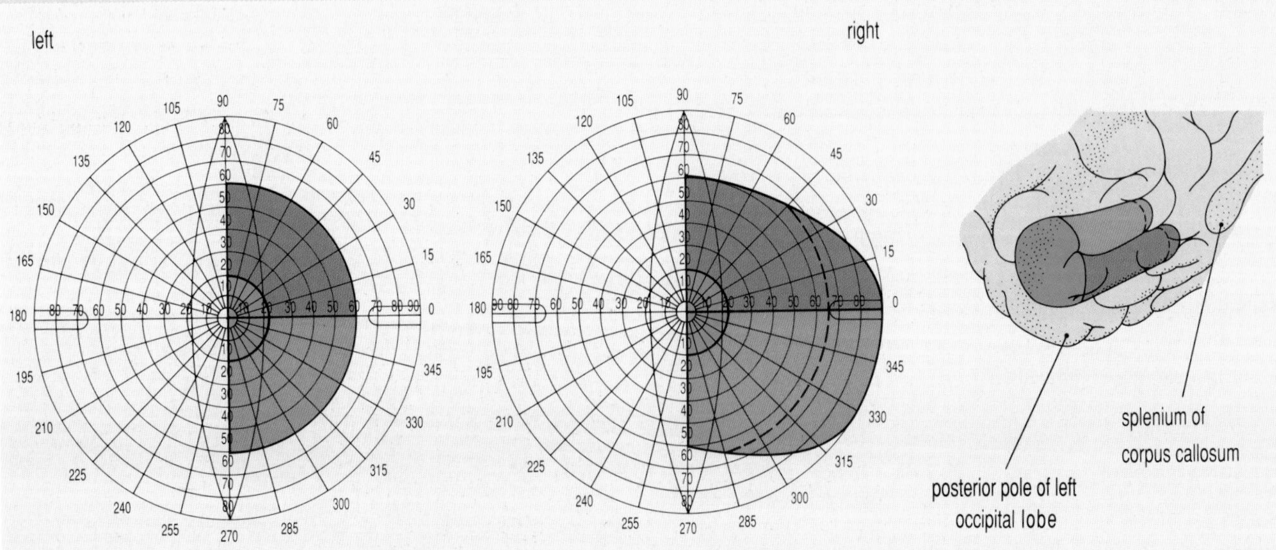

Fig. 12.19 Representation of the right visual field in the left occipital cortex.

EXAMINATION

Visual acuity

Visual acuity is tested in conditions of high illumination, producing a measure of cone function. The Snellen chart is used for testing distance vision. Any object in the visual field subtends an angle at the eye, the visual angle. With the patient at the distance shown above a particular line, the visual angle subtended by a letter in that line would be 5′ and by individual components of the letter, 1′ (Fig. 12.20).

Seat or stand the patient 6m from the card. Ask the patient to cover each eye in turn (with the palm rather than the potentially separating fingers) and find which is the smallest line of print that can be read comfortably. The visual acuity is then expressed as the ratio of the distance between the patient and the card (usually 6m), to the figure on the chart immediately above the smallest visible line. An acuity of 6/18, therefore, indicates that, when positioned 6m from the chart, the patient is able to read down only to the 18m line. Make sure the patient wears glasses if they contain a distance correction. If the patient's glasses are not available, reading through a pinhole will partly correct for any myopia. Illiterate patients can be asked to indicate the orientation of a single letter (Fig. 12.21). If a patient is unable to read the 60m line at 6m they can move nearer the test type, say to 3m. If the patient can then just read the 60m line, the visual acuity, for that particular eye, would be 3/60. A visual acuity of less than 1/60 can be recorded as counting fingers (CF), hand movements (HM), perception of light (PL), or no perception of light (N PL). Near vision is tested by using reading test types, such asthat produced by the Faculty of Ophthalmologists (Fig. 12.22). Near visual acuity does not necessarily correlate well with distance acuity.

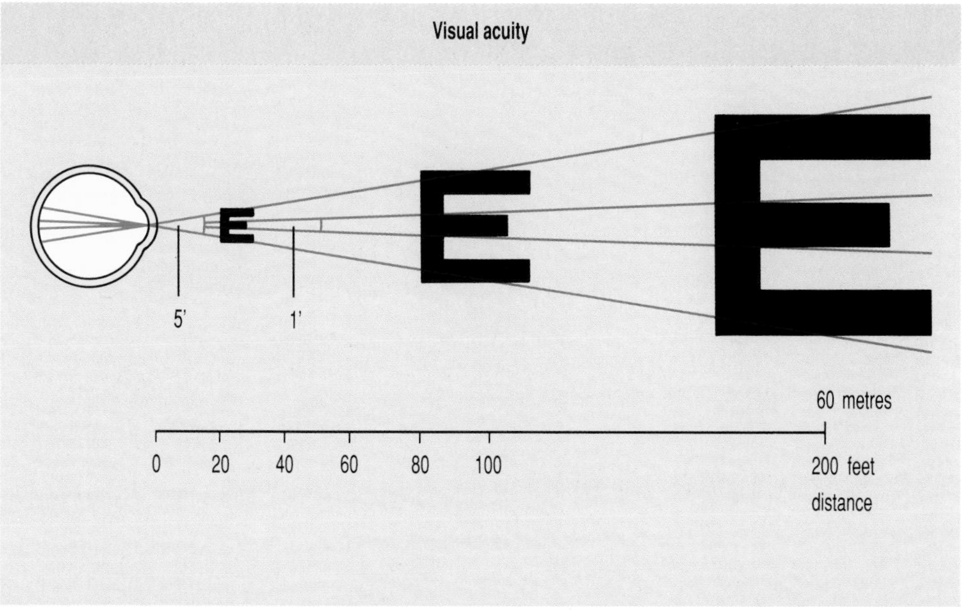

Fig. 12.20 The angles subtended by standard Snellen type.

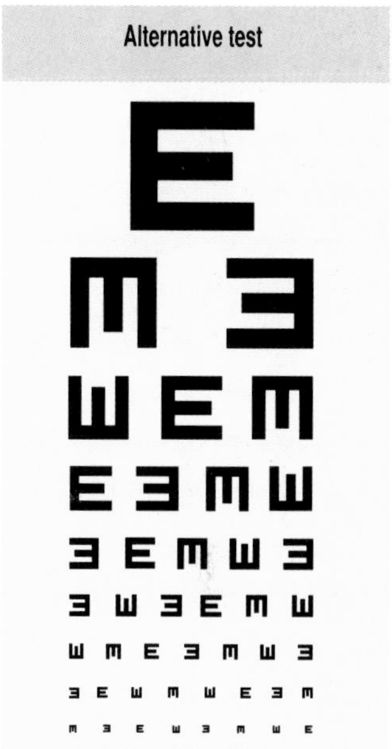

Fig. 12.21 Alternative test types for illiterate patients.

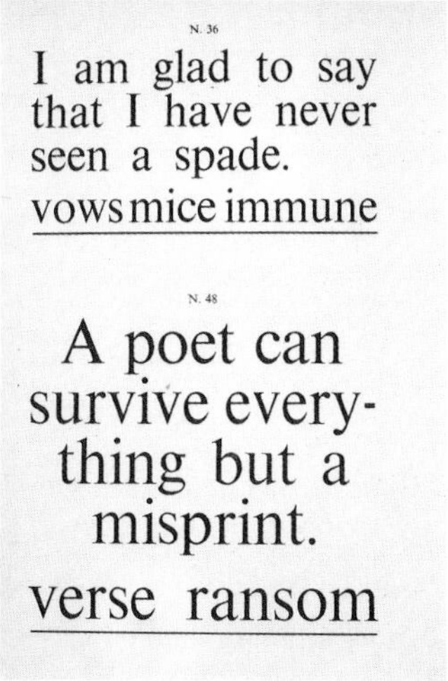
N. 36

I am glad to say that I have never seen a spade.

vows mice immune

N. 48

A poet can survive everything but a misprint.

verse ransom

Fig. 12.22 Page from standard reading type.

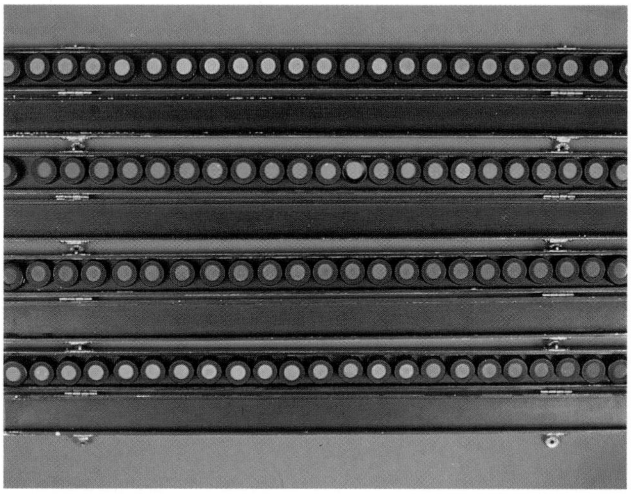

Fig. 12.23 Farnsworth Munsell coloured tiles.

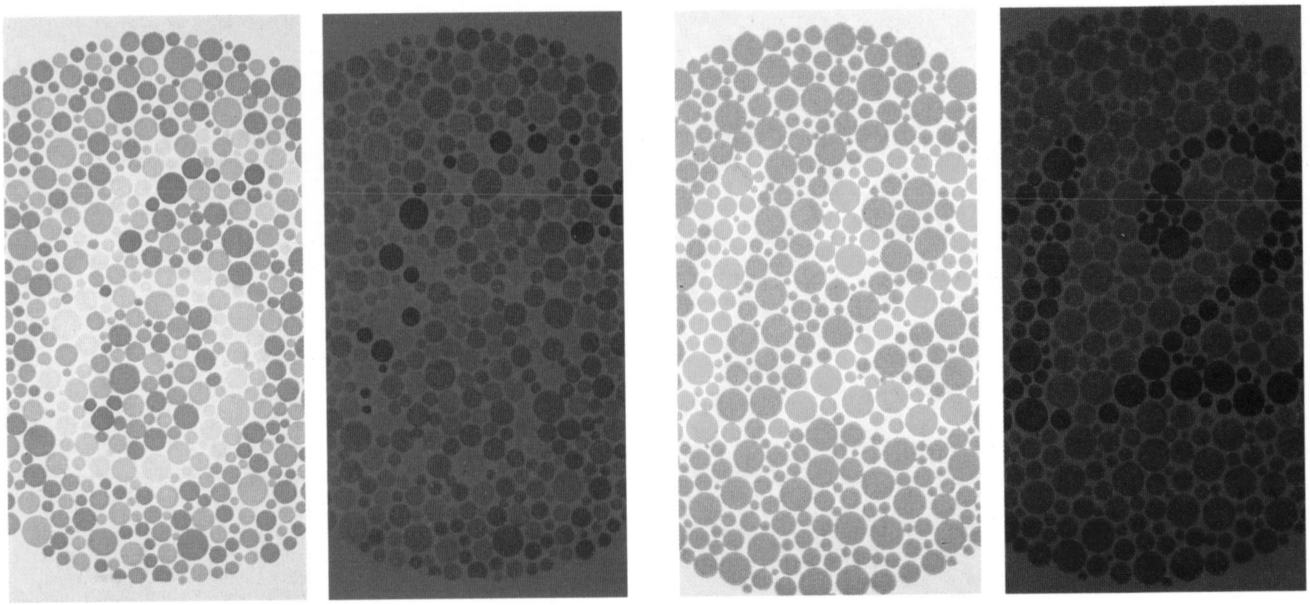

Fig. 12.24 Two plates from the Ishihara series. A patient with normal vision reads both (a) and (c) without difficulty; however, a patient with red-green deficiency is unable to read the figure 6 (b) but is able to read the figure 12 (d) correctly.

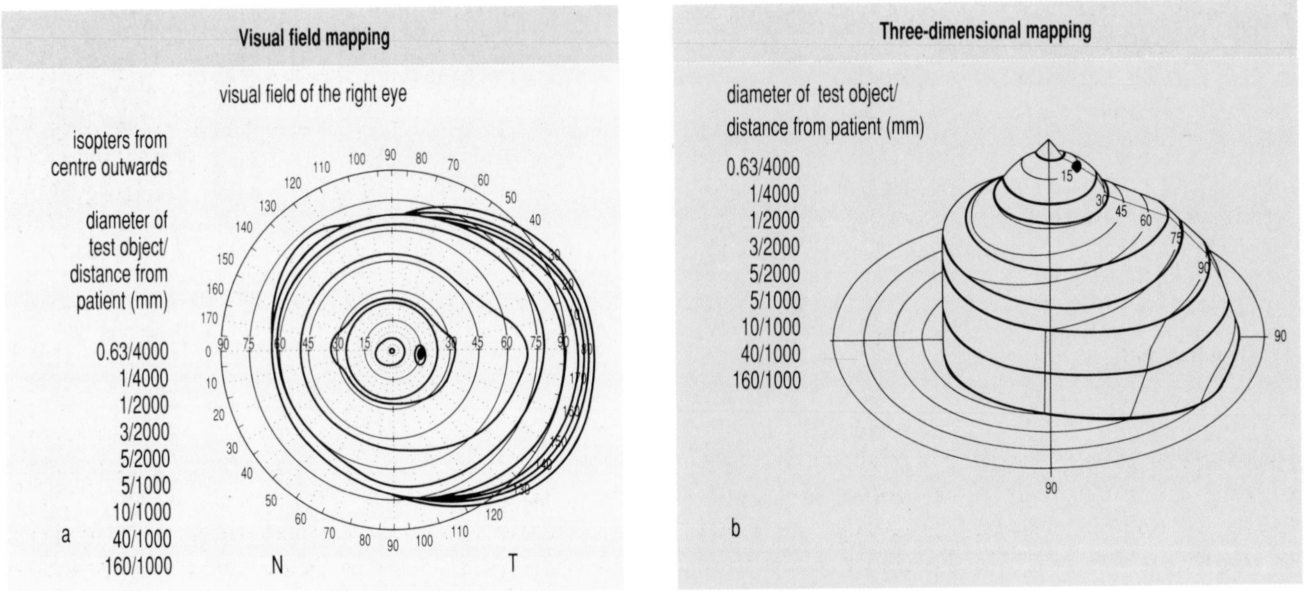

Fig. 12.25 (a) Visual field on a Bjerrum screen to targets of different size. (b) The same field plotted in three-dimensional form.

Colour vision

Colour appreciation depends on the possession of three types of cone with spectral sensitivities spanning the range of colour vision. Bedside tests of colour vision are designed principally to detect congenital defects. In the Farnsworth Munsell test (Fig. 12.23) the patient grades the shading of 84 coloured tiles. Red-green deficiency can be assessed more rapidly using the Ishihara test plates (Fig. 12.24). These are designed to be used in a room lit by daylight, and artificial lighting can slightly distort the shades of the colours. With the plates at about 75cm from the eyes, which are covered in turn, ask the patient to read plates 1 to 15. If 13 or more plates are read correctly, colour vision can be regarded as normal.

Visual fields

Retinal sensitivity diminishes with increasing distance from the fovea. Visual field mapping defines points in the visual field at which an object of a particular size or illumination is detected. An isopter is the outline obtained by joining these points together. Usually a visual field is plotted for one or two targets, but if multiple targets are used, a picture resembling a contour map emerges

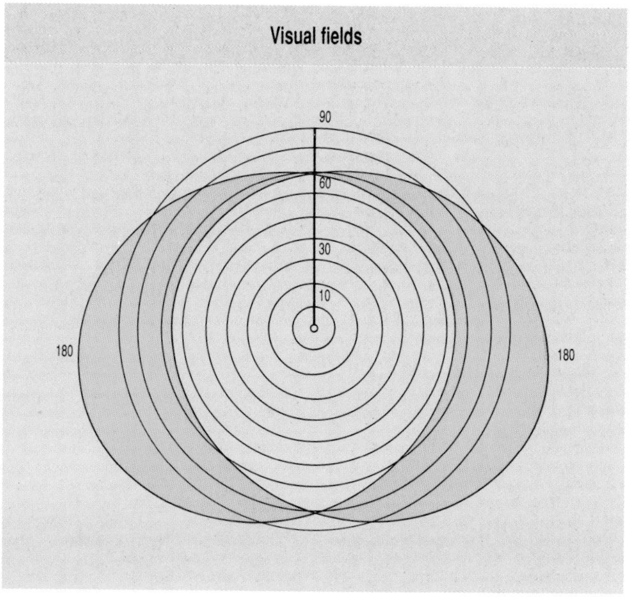

Fig. 12.26 Superimposed fields indicating binocular and monocular components.

(Fig. 12.25). Note that the visual field is not symmetrical. It extends superiorly and medially for about 60° , temporally for about 100°, and inferiorly for about 75°. The blind spot, situated approximately 15° from fixation in the temporal field, marks the position of the optic disc. The field of vision to a coloured object, reflecting cone function, is more restricted than the field of a white object of the same size. Only the central portions of the two visual fields are binocular, the temporal margins being monocular (Fig. 12.26). Static perimetry involves the detection of a stationary target of varying brightness, while kinetic perimetry involves the detection of a moving target.

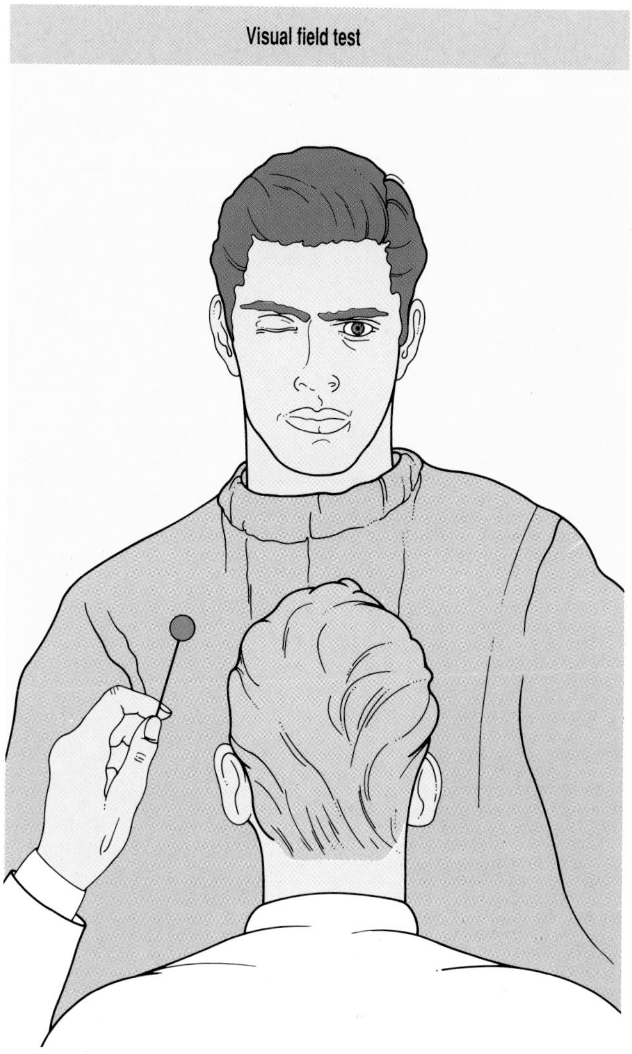

Fig. 12.27 Testing visual fields by confrontation.

Visual assessment

For bedside testing of the visual field sit about 1m from the patient. The choice of target is determined partly by the patient's age and cooperation, and partly by the type of field defect being looked for. In infants or poorly cooperating adults, a meaningful response may be impossible to elicit, or may be obtained only by using visual threat – in other words a sudden, unexpected hand movement. For cooperative adults, and older children, either finger movements or coloured objects can be used. For testing the right visual field, ask the patient to cover the left eye with the left hand, and cover your own right eye (Fig. 12.27). Ensure that the patient's right eye remains fixed on your left eye throughout the examination. The limits of the peripheral field can be determined by bringing the moving fingers of your left hand into the four quadrants of the patient's field.

Hand or finger movements are too crude a stimulus for assessing central field defects, and here a small coloured object is used. It is useful to outline the blind spot first, partly because its successful identification increases confidence in one's own technique and partly because it indicates good fixation on the part of the patient. Move a red pin of some 10mm in diameter into the temporal field along the horizontal meridian. First explain to the patient that the object will disappear briefly then reappear, and that they should indicate when this happens. Once you have found the position of the blind spot its shape can be mapped. Remember that the patient's blind spot will coincide with your own only if your head positions are exactly comparable. This is seldom the case, so that you will find you map the position of your own and the patient's blind spot independently. Having identified the blind spot, assess the central visual field.

Visual field abnormalities

Scotoma

A scotoma is an area of diminished vision surrounded by an area of more normal, or normal, vision. An absolute central scotoma is an area around fixation in which there is no appreciation of the visual stimulus. A relative central scotoma is an area in which the object is still detected but where its colour appears diminished, or desaturated, compared to surrounding areas (Fig. 12.28). A centrocaecal scotoma extends temporally from fixation towards the blind spot.

Bitemporal hemianopia

A bitemporal hemianopia, in which the temporal halves of the fields are lost, is due to a lesion of the optic chiasm. In its earliest stages the field defect can be detected only by moving a coloured target across the vertical meridian. As the target moves from the intact nasal field into the impaired temporal field its colour becomes less intense (Fig. 12.29).

Homonymous hemianopia

A homonymous hemianopia is a field defect in which the left or right half field is affected. In a complete right homonymous hemianopia, therefore, the temporal field of the right eye and the nasal field of the left eye are lost. Homonymous hemianopias are detectable, according to their size, by using finger movements or coloured targets. If individual half fields are full, then the target object, usually your moving fingers, should be presented in both peripheral fields simultaneously. In parietal lobe lesions, particularly of the non-dominant hemisphere, a visual target presented in isolation in the contralateral field is perceived, but it is missed (visual suppression or inattention) when a comparable target is presented simultaneously in the ipsilateral half field (Fig. 12.30).

Fundoscopy

Normally it is not necessary to dilate the pupils in order to examine the central fundus, but if the patient has small pupils, or the background illumination is high, take the patient into a darkened room for the examination. If this fails to dilate the pupils sufficiently, then a mydriatic, for example Mydrilate (1 per cent cyclopentolate), can be instilled. This should never be done in the unconscious patient and must always be recorded in the patient's notes. Do not use mydriatics in a patient with glaucoma. Remember to reverse the effects of the mydriatic at the end of the examination by instilling 2 per cent pilocarpine.

The direct ophthalmoscope incorporates a light source, which is directed on to the retina via a mirror, together with a series of lenses of varying strength which allow the reflected light to be focused on to the examiner's own retina. The field of view extends over about 6.5° and the image is upright. If the patient wears glasses with a substantial correction, it sometimes facilitates the examination to perform it with the patient's glasses in place. Ask the patient to fixate on a distant target (Fig. 12.31).

The optic disc is examined first to assess its shape, colour and clarity. The temporal margin of the disc is slightly paler than the nasal margin. The physiological cup varies in size but seldom extends to the temporal, and never to the nasal margins of the disc. The blood vessels are not obscured as they cross the disc margin, nor are they elevated (Fig. 12.32).

The vessels are examined next. The arteries are narrower than the veins and a brighter colour. They possess a longitudinal pale streak as a consequence of light reflecting from their walls. The retinal veins should be closely inspected where they enter the optic disc. In around 80 per cent of normal individuals the veins pulsate, their walls alternately expanding and collapsing. This pulsation ceases when CSF pressure exceeds 200mm of water. Therefore the presence of retinal venous pulsation in these individuals is a very sensitive index of normal intracranial pressure. Learn to identify this physical sign. It will save countless references to 'swollen optic discs?' The fundus is examined for the presence of haemorrhages and exudates, the positions of which are best shown by a small diagram in the patient's notes, or by a description which uses the optic disc as a clock face for localization purposes; for example, 'one large haemorrhage at 6 o'clock, one disc diameter from the disc.' Finally, the pattern of the retinal nerve fibres can be assessed using a red-free light.

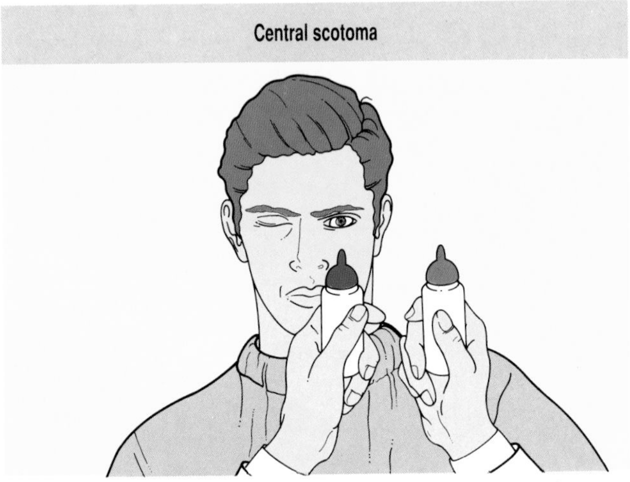

Fig. 12.28 Comparison of colour sensitivity between central and peripheral field. In this patient with a central scotoma the red object appears brown in the central field.

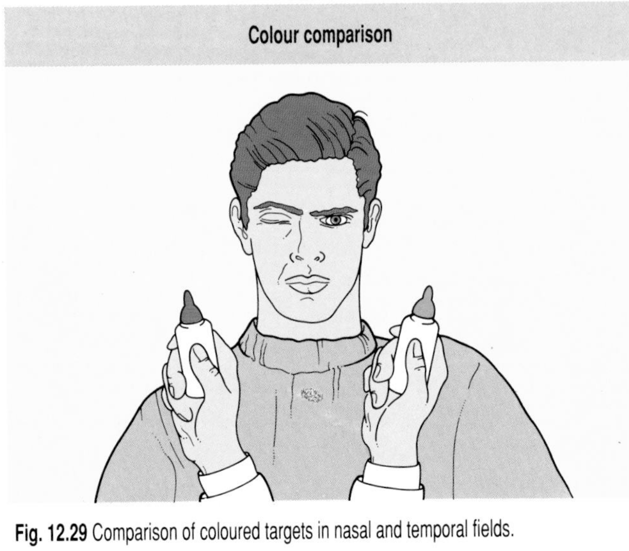

Fig. 12.29 Comparison of coloured targets in nasal and temporal fields.

CLINICAL APPLICATION

Optic atrophy

Optic atrophy follows any process which damages the ganglion cells or the axons between the retinal nerve fibre layer and the lateral geniculate body. It is associated with loss of bulk of the nerve. In the past the terms primary, secondary, and consecutive optic atrophy have been used, but these definitions have not been consistent and should be avoided.

Optic atrophy results in pallor of the disc (Fig. 12.33). This is probably partly due to a reduction of blood supply, and partly the consequence of glial tissue formation with a contribution from changes in the structure of the nerve fibre bundles at the optic disc head. The pallor may be diffuse or segmental. Temporal pallor is the most common form of segmental atrophy, attributable to the susceptibility of the papillomacular bundle to degenerate following optic nerve damage by compression or metabolic disturbance. Atrophy of the retinal nerve fibre layer in the region of the optic disc produces dark slits or wedges within which there is a loss of normal retinal striation (Fig. 12.34).

Visual inattention

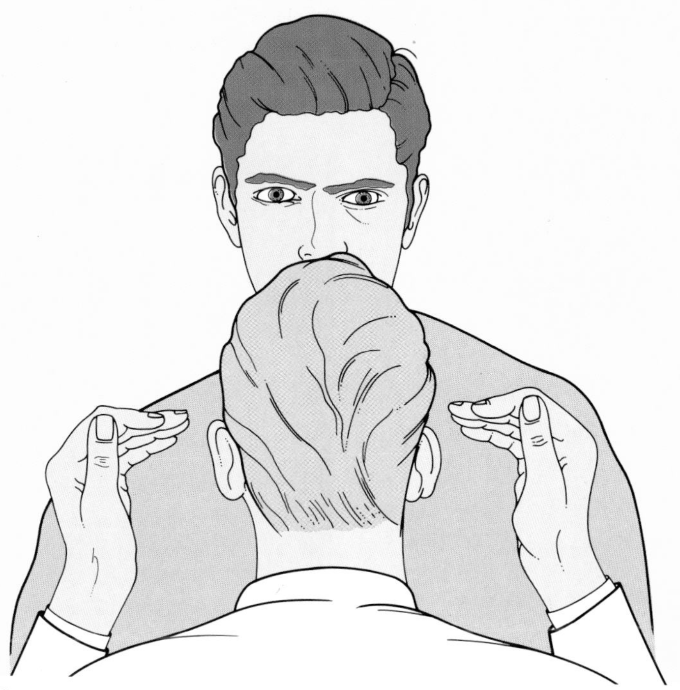

Fig. 12.30 Simultaneous presentation of finger movements in the two half fields.

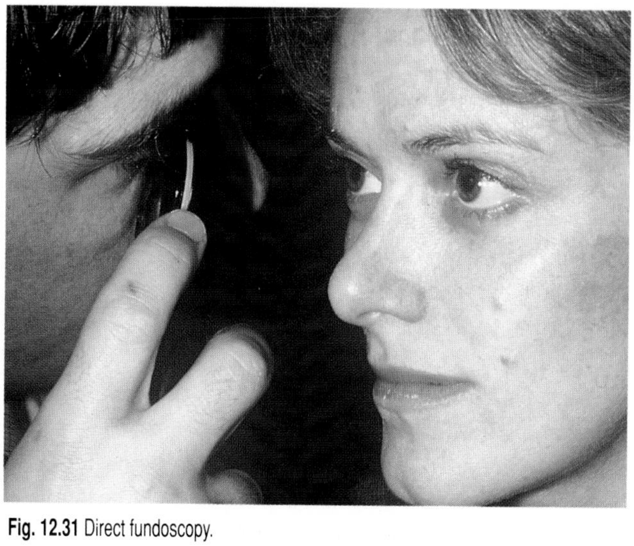

Fig. 12.31 Direct fundoscopy.

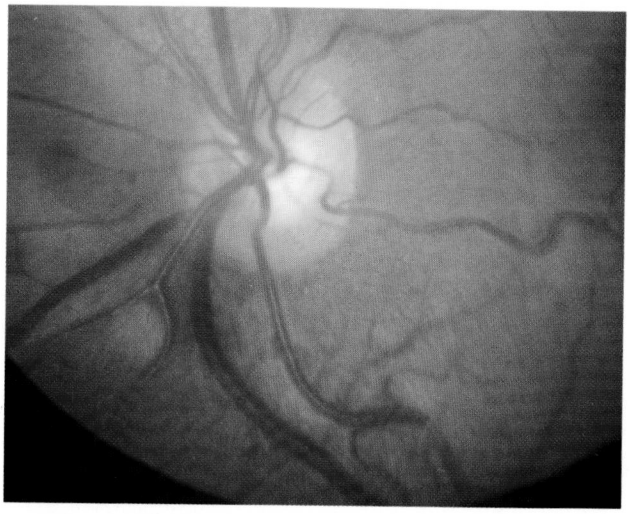

Fig. 12.32 The normal fundus..

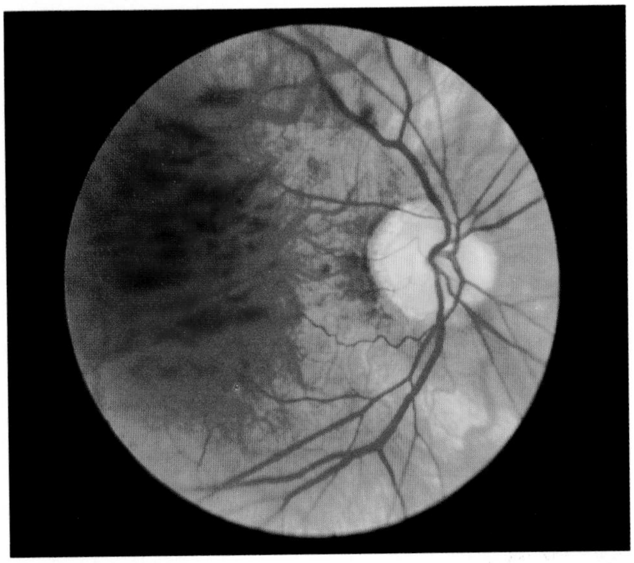

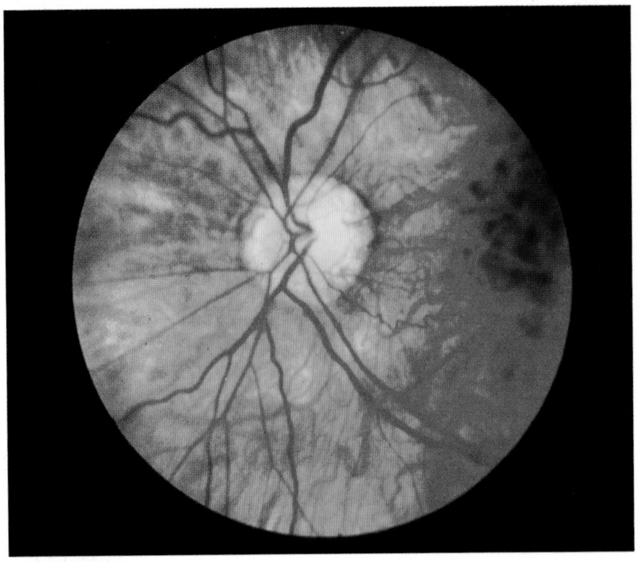

Fig. 12.33 Optic atrophy.

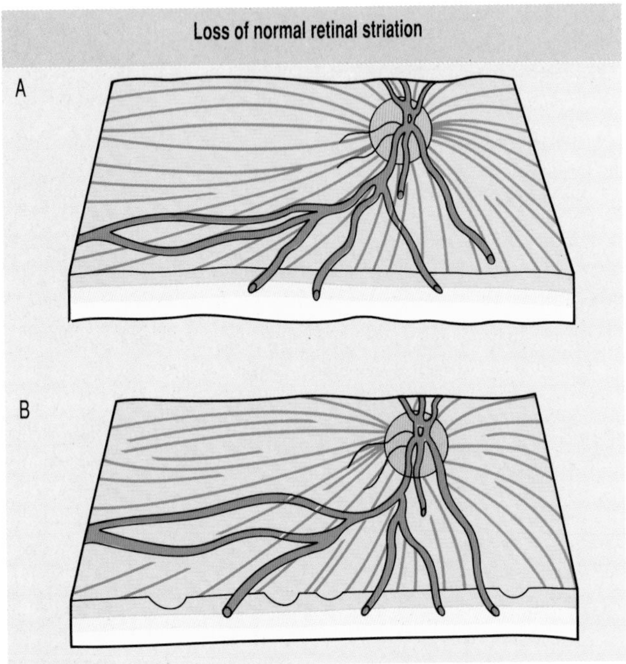

Fig. 12.34 Schematic representation of normal (above) and atrophic retinal nerve fibres (below).

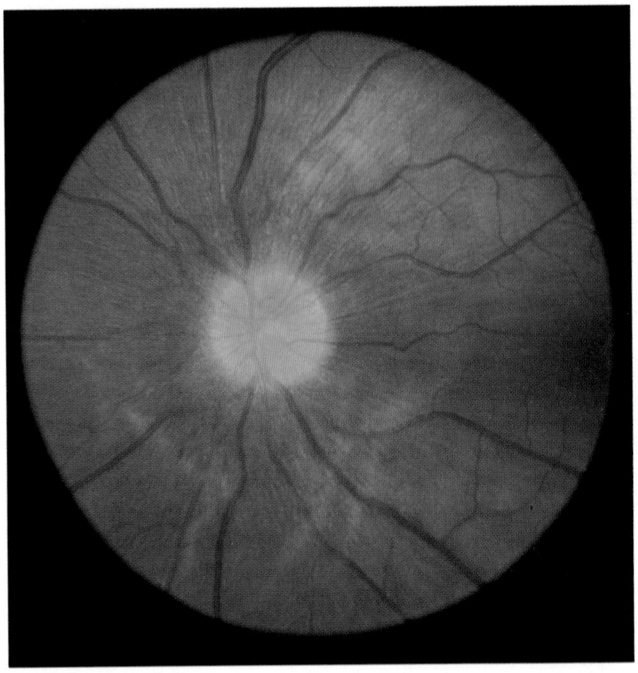

Fig. 12.35 Early papilloedema. Dilated nerve-fibres bundles, superficial haemorrhages and disc hyperaemia.

The colour of the normal optic disc is variable, and the ophthalmoscopic diagnosis of optic atrophy notoriously subjective. It is unwise to make a confident diagnosis of optic atrophy if there are no other criteria suggesting optic nerve damage (see below). Additional features which may help the diagnosis have been suggested, including a count of the number of capillaries visible on the optic disc, and the presence of retinal nerve fibre atrophy. The former criterion has not been substantiated and detection of the latter requires considerable experience. Inspection of the retinal vessels is worthwhile. The presence of sheathing or attenuation of the retinal arterioles suggests that the optic atrophy is secondary to ischaemic optic neuropathy or central retinal artery occlusion.

Papilloedema

Patients with papilloedema often have no visual complaints, though some describe transient obscurations of vision either occurring spontaneously or being triggered by postural change. Papilloedema is usually bilateral, though sometimes asymmetrical. Its pathogenesis remains unsettled. The term papilloedema is best reserved for cases where the disc swelling is secondary to raised intracranial pressure. Transmission of the raised intracranial pressure, via the sub-arachnoid space of the optic nerve, results in venous stasis and also interrupts both fast and slow axoplasmic flow in the optic nerve.

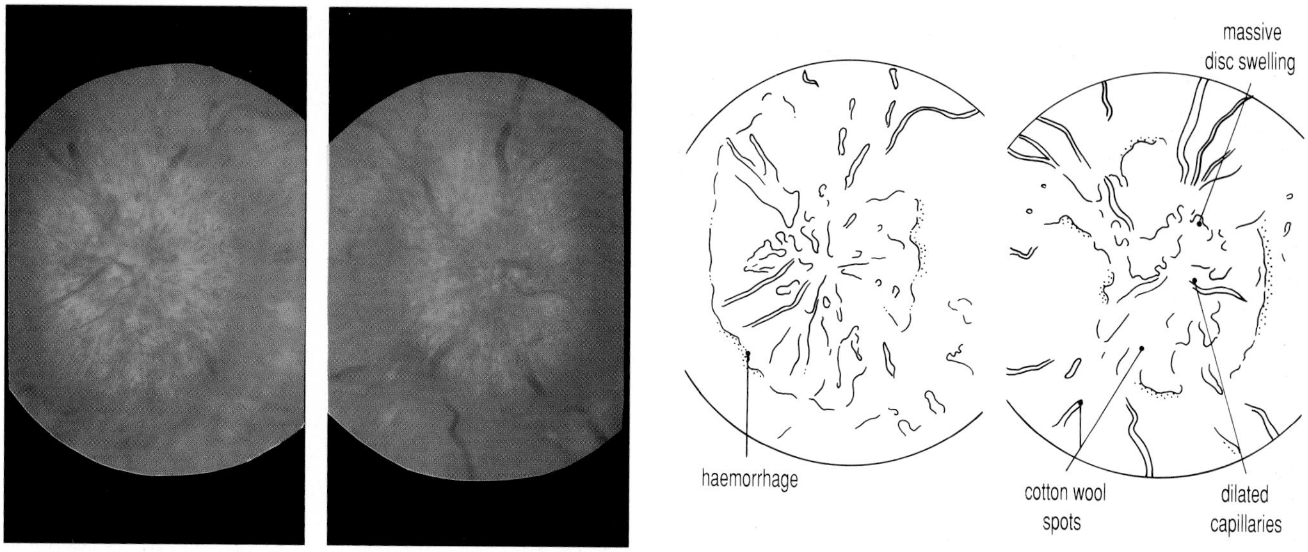

Fig. 12.36 Chronic papilloedema. Swollen optic discs, dilated capillaries, haemorrhages and cotton-wool spots.

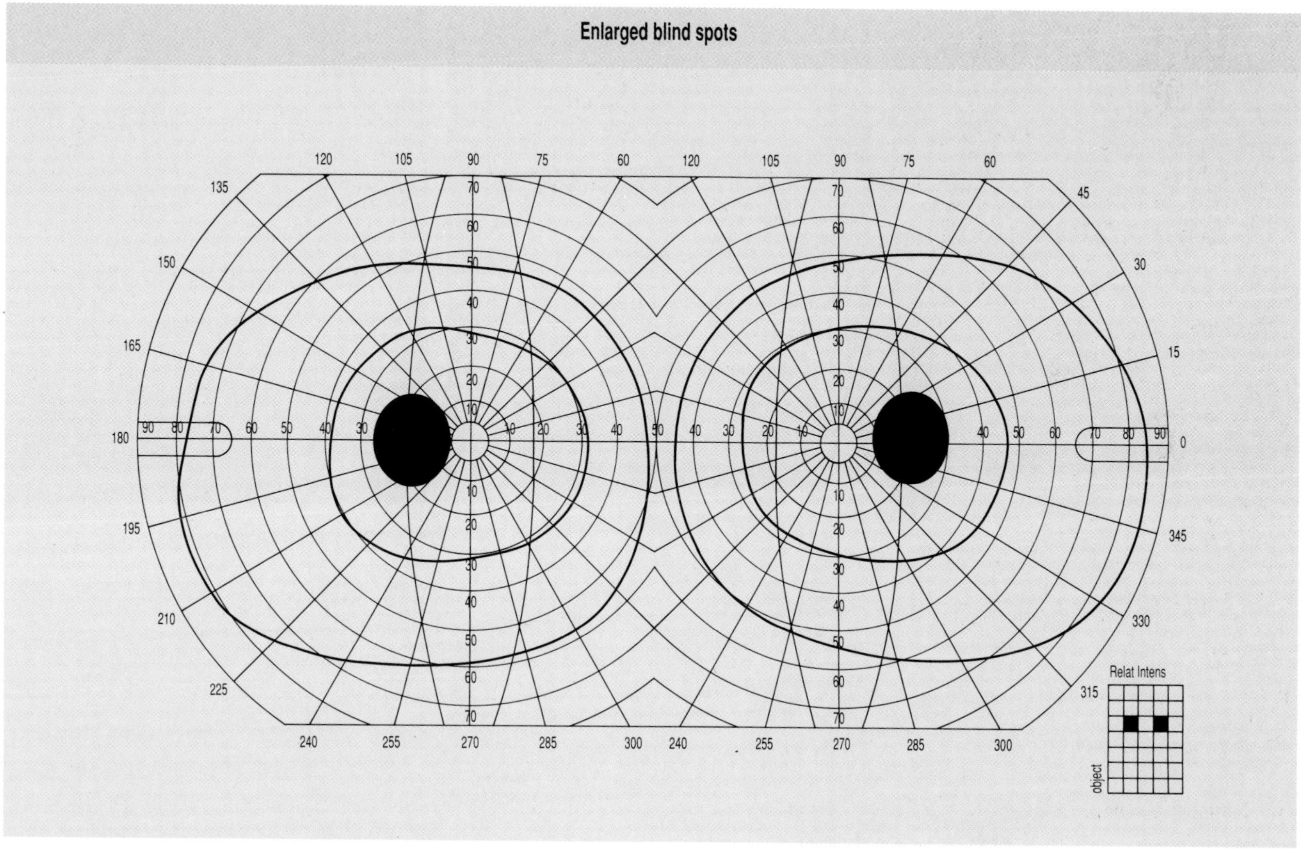

Fig. 12.37 Papilloedema. Visual fields showing bilaterally enlarged blind spots.

As papilloedema develops, swelling of the nerve fibre layer appears (best seen with a red-free light) within which haemorrhages are visible. The disc becomes hyperaemic (due to capillary dilatation) with a loss of definition of its margins, and retinal venous pulsation disappears (Fig. 12.35). In fully developed papilloedema there is engorgement of retinal veins, obscuration of the disc margins, flame haemorrhages, and cotton-wool spots (the consequence of retinal infarction). The vessels are tortuous (Fig. 12.36). Often the only visual field change at this stage is an enlargement of the blind spot (Fig. 12.37). In the later stages of papilloedema hard exudates appear on the disc, which becomes atrophic, and other visual field abnormalities appear, including arcuate fibre defects and peripheral constriction.

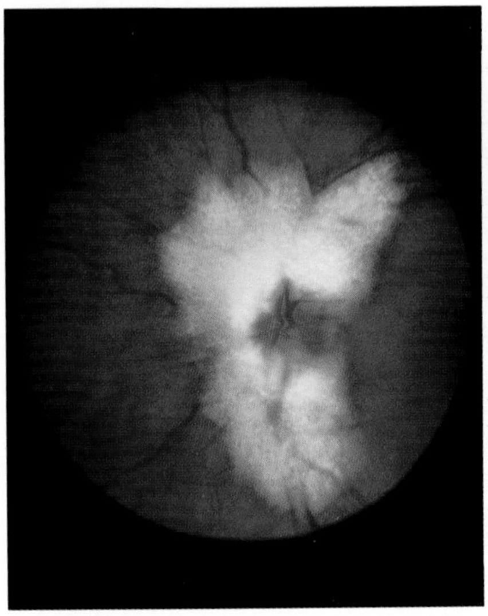

Fig. 12.38 Myelinated nerve fibres.

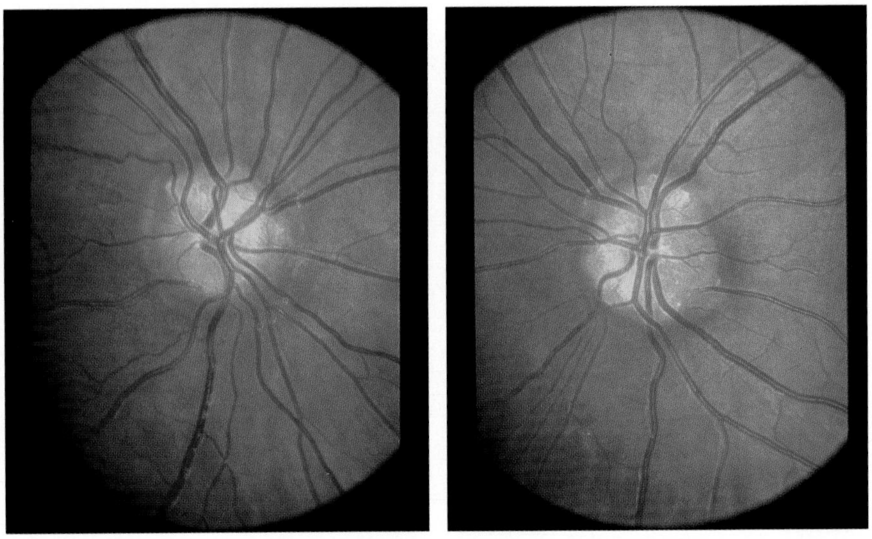

Fig. 12.39 Bilateral drusen (associated with peripapillary haemorrhage on right).

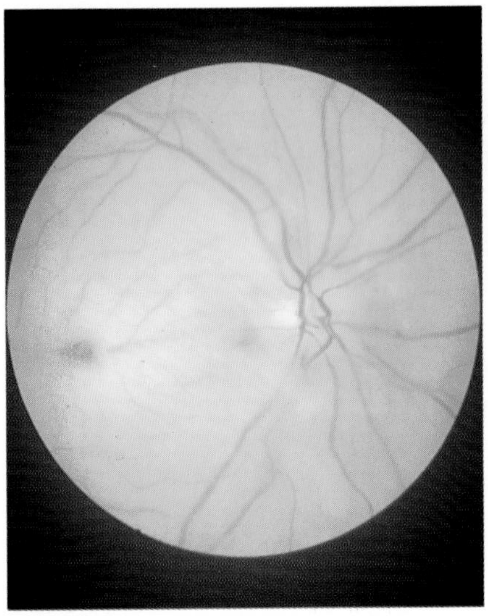

Fig. 12.40 Central retinal artery occlusion.

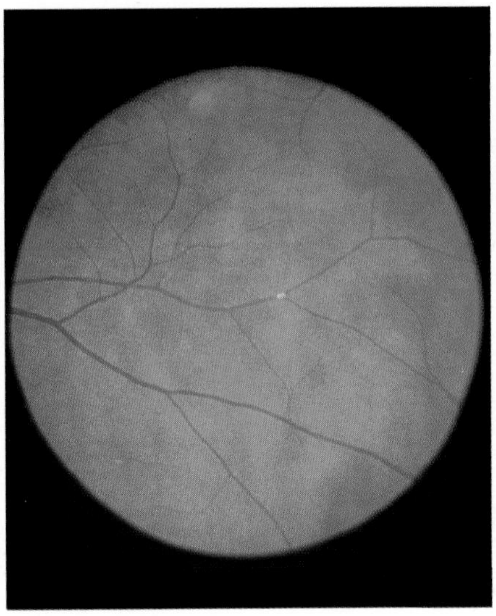

Fig. 12.41 Cholesterol embolus.

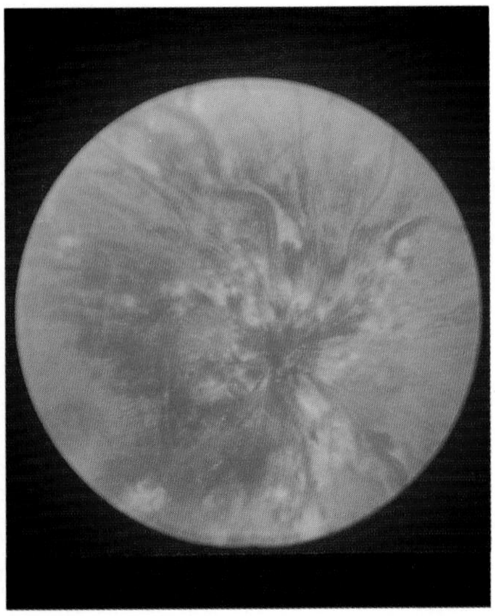

Fig. 12.42 Central retinal vein occlusion.

Papilloedema can probably appear within 4–5 hours of the development of intracranial hypertension, and may not resolve for some weeks after its reduction.

Other fundus abnormalities

Myelinated nerve fibres

A congenital anomaly affecting the retina is the presence of myelinated, and therefore visible, nerve fibres at, or adjacent to, the disc margin (Fig. 12.38).

Drusen (hyaline bodies)

Drusen are thought to be derived from axonal debris, and are situated in the disc anterior to the lamina cribrosa, where they appear as yellow excrescences, often distorting the disc margin. They do not usually produce visual symptoms (Fig. 12.39).

RETINAL VASCULAR DISEASE

Retinal artery and vein occlusion

Following occlusion of the central retinal artery the retina becomes pale and opaque with a cherry red spot at the macula. The optic disc, initially swollen, becomes atrophic (Fig. 12.40). The presence of micro-emboli, containing either cholesterol or a fibrin-platelet mixture, establishes that the occlusion is embolic (Fig. 12.41). A branch occlusion produces a corresponding sector-shaped visual defect. In central retinal vein occlusion there is swelling of the optic disc, dilatation of the retinal veins, and fundal haemorrhages (Fig. 12.42).

Hypertensive retinopathy

In hypertensive retinopathy, the light reflex from the arteriolar wall is abnormal, and constriction of the venous wall appears at sites of

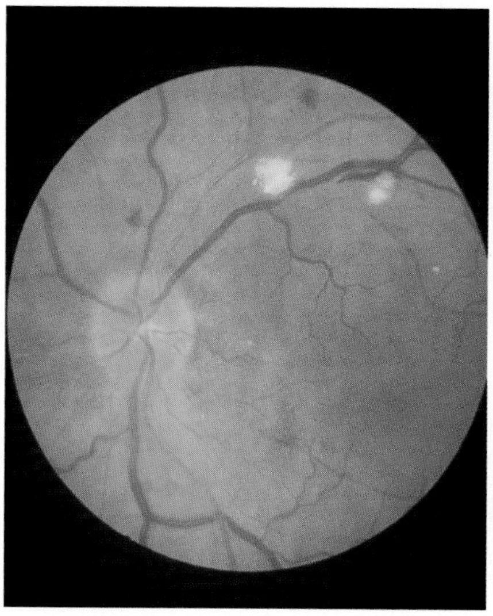

Fig. 12.43 Hypertensive retinopathy with haemorrhages, cotton-wool spots and variation in arteriolar calibre.

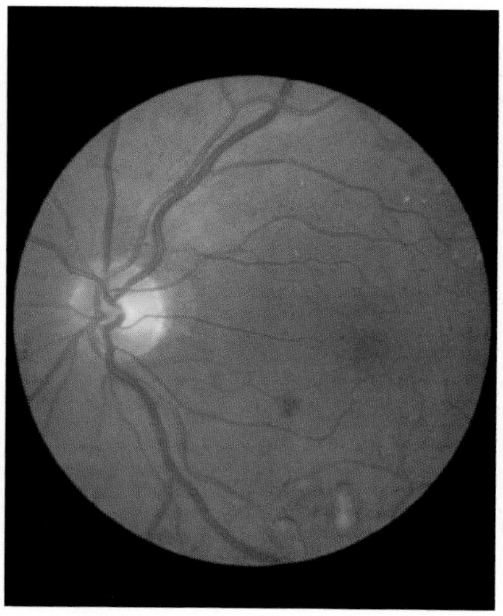

Fig. 12.44 Diabetic retinopathy. Microaneurysms, haemorrhages, exudates and cotton-wool spots.

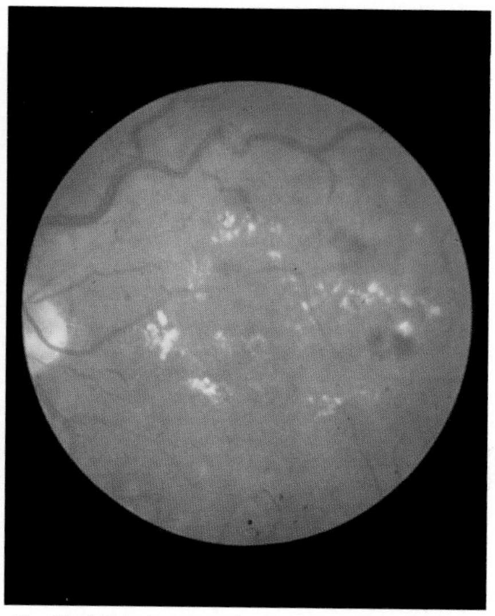

Fig. 12.45 Diabetic retinopathy. Hard exudates at macula.

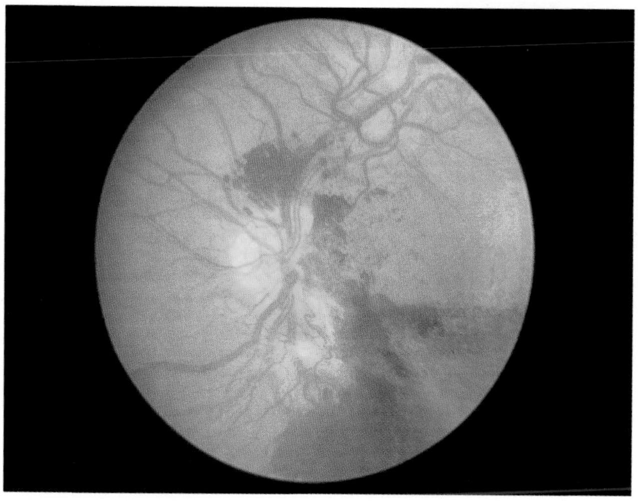

Fig. 12.46 Vitreous haemorrhage with evidence of new vessel formation at the disc margin.

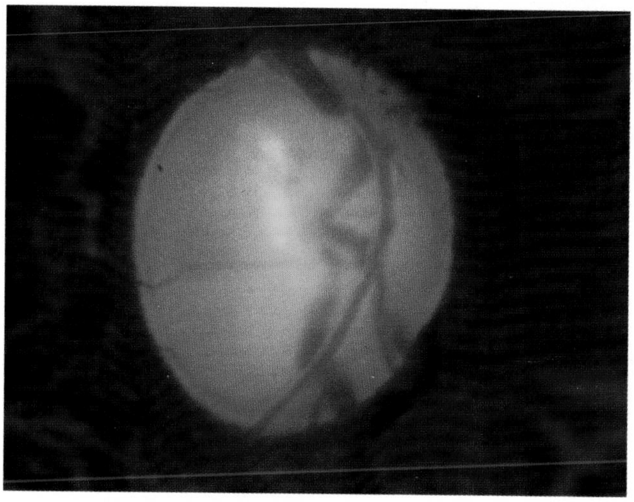

Fig. 12.47 Advanced chronic simple glaucoma.

arteriovenous crossing. Both changes, the former described as silver or copper-wiring and the latter as A–V nipping, are encountered as an age-related phenomenon in normal individuals. In other words, they have a low specificity, particularly in older patients. A more reliable sign of hypertensive retinopathy is variation in the calibre of the retinal arterioles. As the retinopathy advances haemorrhages and cotton wool spots appear (Fig. 12.43) and, in malignant or accelerated hypertension, disc swelling occurs.

Diabetic retinopathy

Diabetic retinopathy in its early stages principally affects the retinal microcirculation producing the characteristic, though not pathognomonic, micro-aneurysm (Fig. 12.44). Subsequently small haemorrhages, exudates, and cotton wool spots appear. Visual failure is usually due either to macular disease, in the form of oedema, infarction or lipid deposition (Fig. 12.45), or to the appearance of new vessel formation (proliferative diabetic retinopathy), leading to vitreous haemorrhage and retinal detachment due to traction by fibrous tissue (Fig. 12.46).

Glaucoma

Glaucoma, characterized by raised intra-ocular pressure, can occur either secondarily to various ocular pathologies (e.g. uveitis) or in a primary form. The latter is far more common. Primary glaucoma can be classified into three types: open angle, closed angle and congenital. The first of these is responsible for some 66 per cent of all cases. Resulting changes in the optic disc include enlargement of the physiological cup (particularly significant if in the vertical axis), an increase in the ratio of cup size to vertical disc diameter beyond 0.6, and retinal nerve fibre atrophy. Arcuate field defects accompany these changes. With advanced glaucoma there is marked undermining of the disc margins and bowing of the blood vessels (Fig. 12.47).

OPTIC NERVE DISEASE

In lesions of the optic nerve the visual defect is monocular. Visual acuity is usually reduced, and colour perception is disturbed (particularly for red-green). There is an afferent pupillary defect (see page 2.33). The most likely visual field defect is a central scotoma (Fig. 12.48). Optic atrophy is a relatively late development in cases of optic nerve compression. Proptosis is likely if the lesion is within the orbit.

CHIASMATIC LESIONS

Most chiasmatic syndromes are the result of compression by pituitary tumour, meningioma, or craniopharyngioma. The result is a bitemporal hemianopia, though the type of defect relates to the position of the growth and its relation to the chiasm. Typically, the visual defect is asymmetrical (Fig. 12.49). Patients frequently complain of blurred or double vision, a consequence of lost integration between independent nasal fields. The development of optic

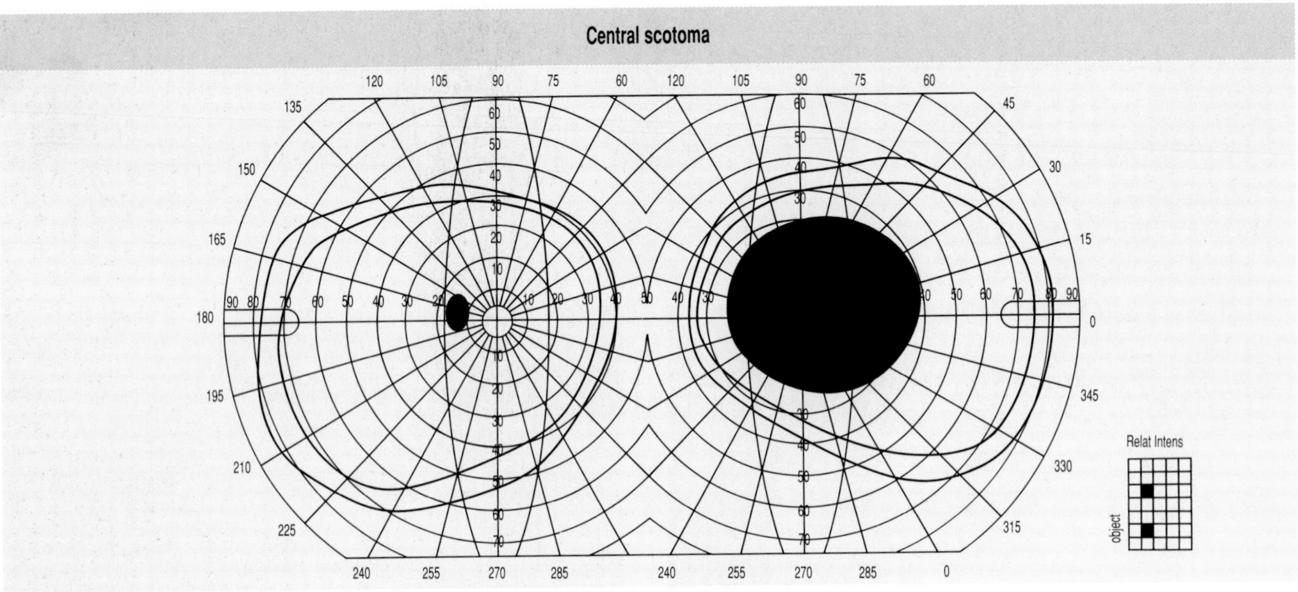

Fig. 12.48 Large right central scotoma.

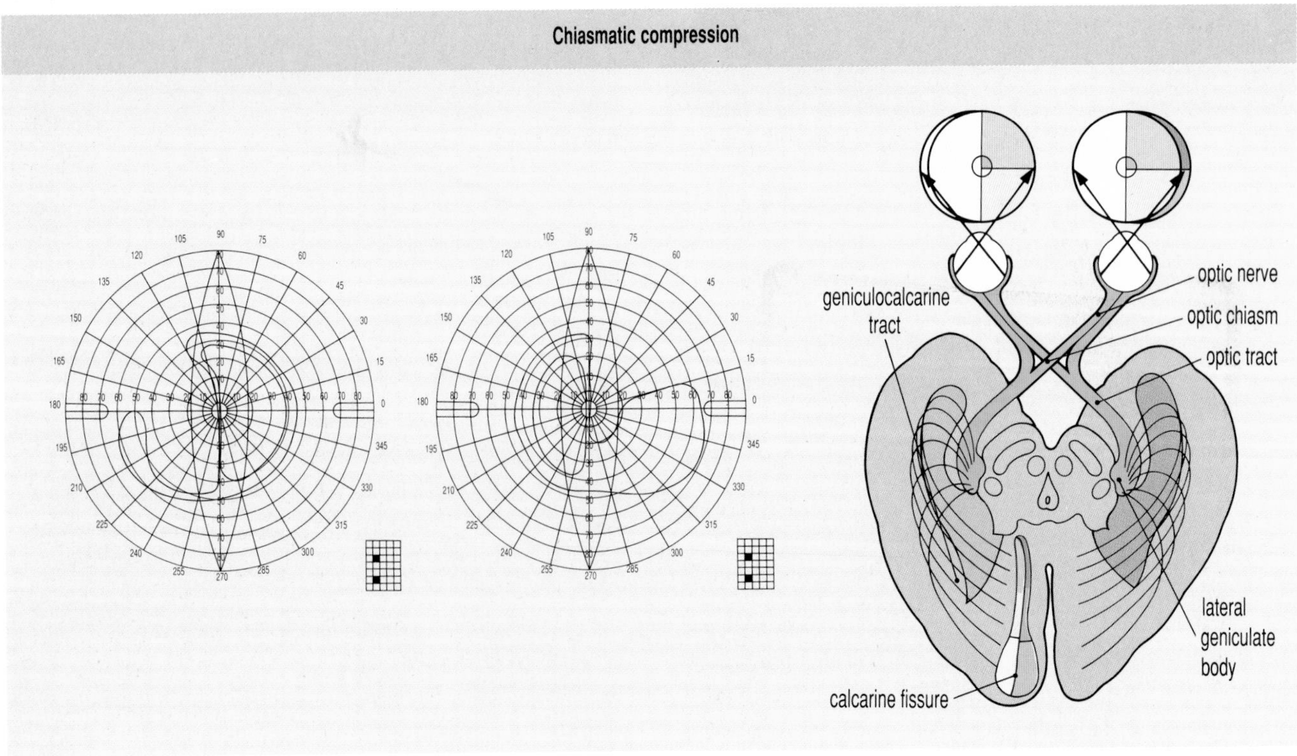

Fig. 12.49 Visual pathways (left) with field defect produced by chiasmatic compression (right).

atrophy may be delayed for some years. Since the nasal retinal fibres (subserving the temporal field) enter the disc horizontally on both sides, the atrophy predominantly occupies a sector around the horizontal meridian on both sides of the disc (Fig. 12.50).

Optic tract and lateral geniculate body lesions

These are uncommon. A lesion in the anterior part of the optic tract, before the homonymous fibres have joined, produces an incongruous homonymous hemianopia, that is, one in which the two half field losses are not equal (Fig. 12.51). The optic atrophy that appears with damage to the optic tract will affect the nasal aspect of the contralateral eye, but the temporal aspect of the ipsilateral eye.

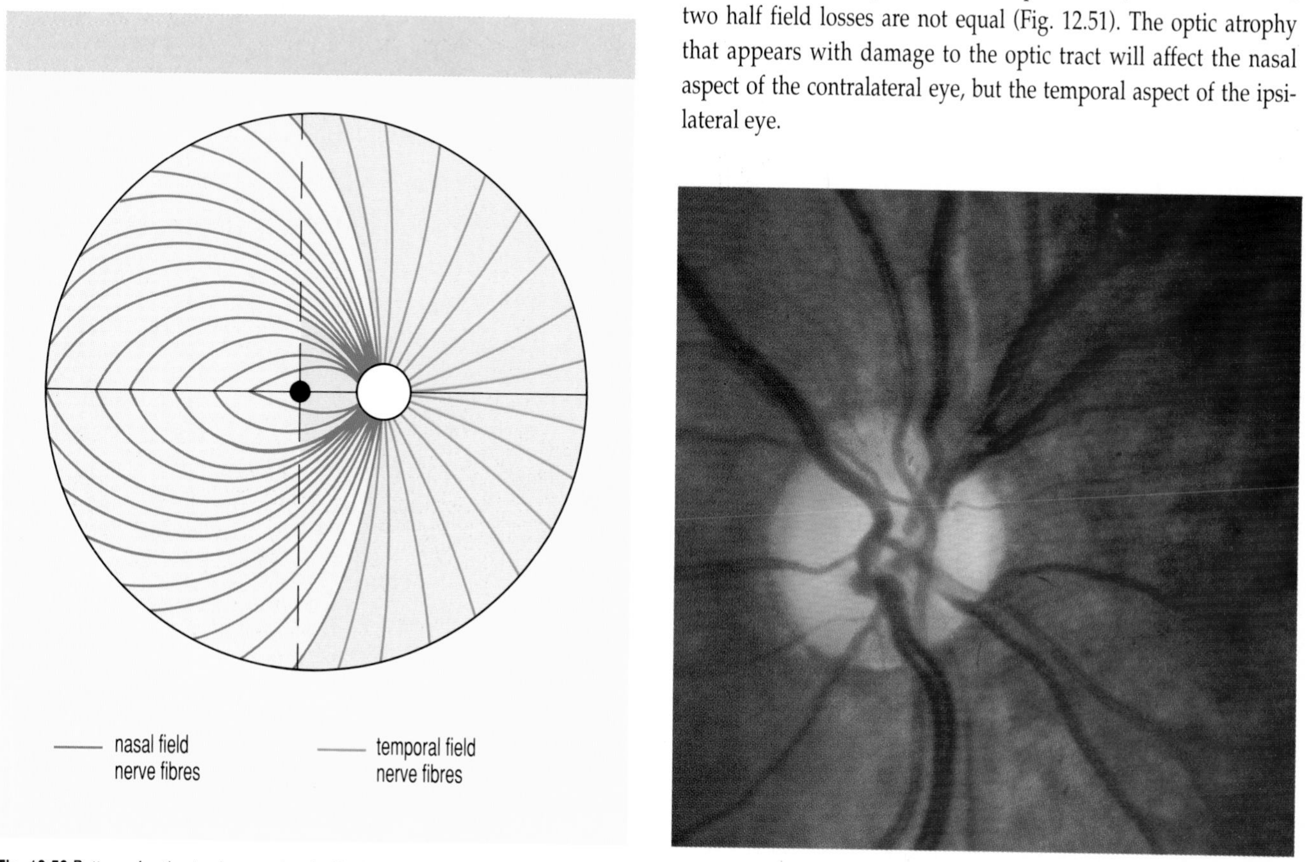

Fig. 12.50 Pattern of optic atrophy associated with chiasmatic compression. Initially, temporal and nasal horizontal sectors are affected.

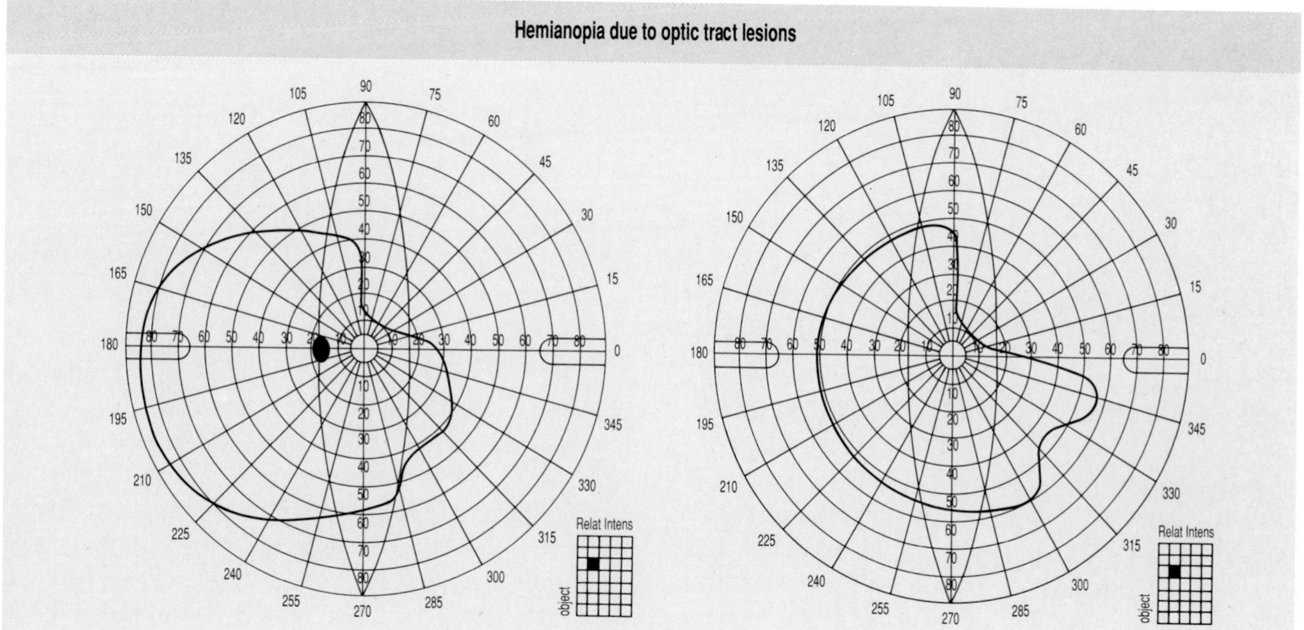

Fig. 12.51 Incongruous right homonymous hemianopia associated with a left optic tract lesion.

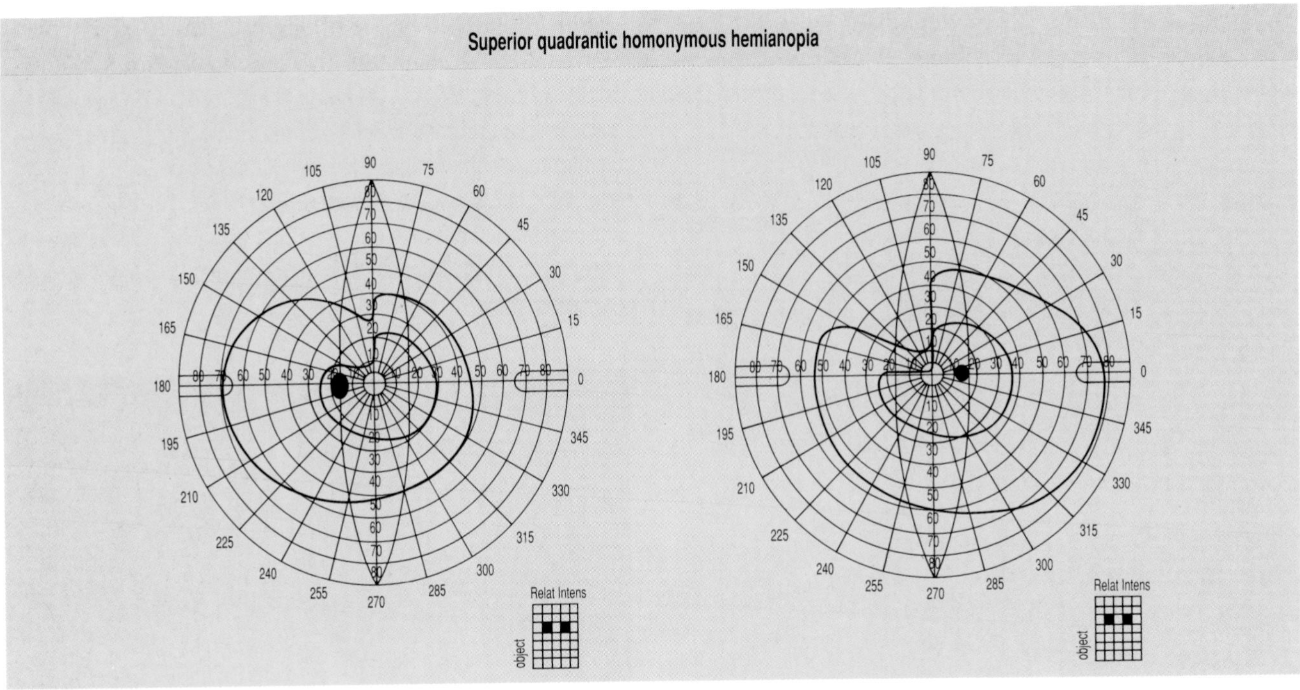

Fig. 12.52 Incongruous left superior quadrantic homonymous hemianopia associated with a lesion of the temporal part of the right optic radiation.

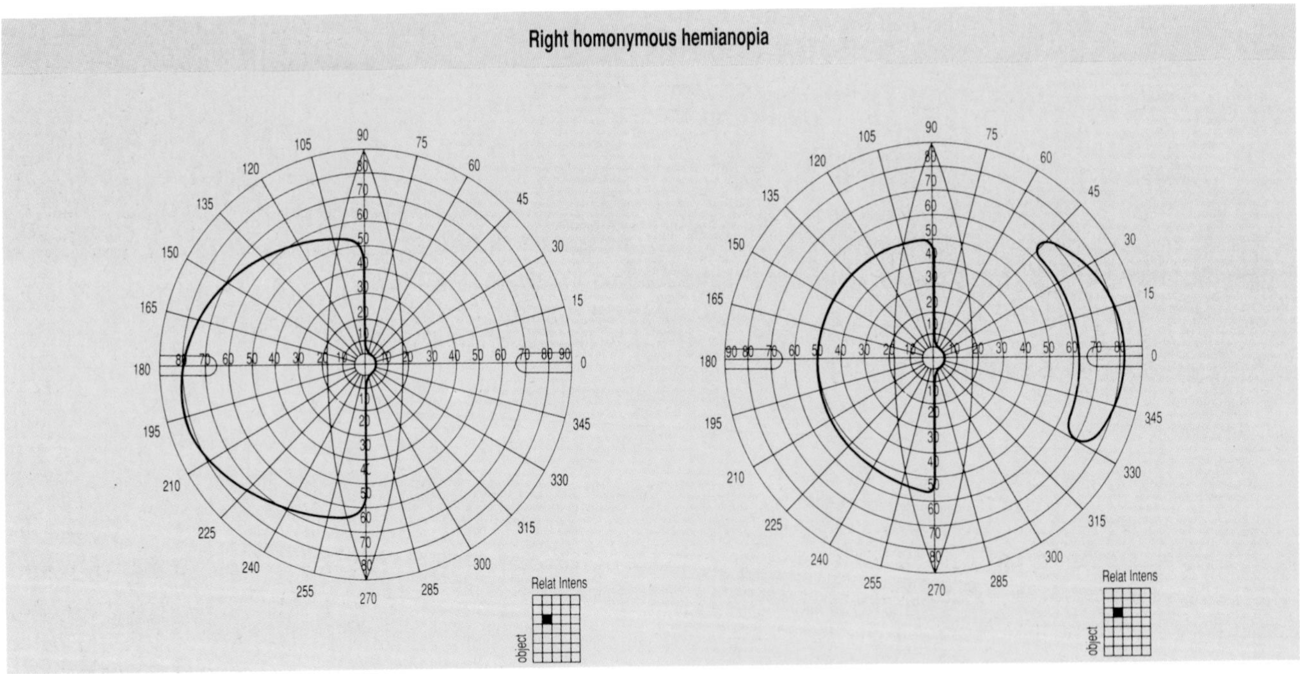

Fig. 12.53 A right homonymous hemianopia, sparing the macula and the peripheral temporal crescent of the right eye.

OPTIC RADIATION AND OCCIPITAL CORTEX LESIONS

The type of visual field loss from lesions of the optic radiation depends on their localization. All the defects are homonymous but not necessarily congruous. In lesions affecting the temporal radiation, the superior quadrantic field is more affected than the inferior. If the defect is incongruous the nasal loss in the ipsilateral eye is more extensive than the temporal loss in the contralateral eye (Fig. 12.52).

With parietal lobe lesions the defect is often complete, but rarely principally affects the inferior quadrants. Occipital lobe pathology produces congruous defects which can be total, quadrantic, or scotomatous. In some instances there is macular sparing, probably due to a dual vascular supply to the macular area of the occipital cortex (Fig. 12.53). An isolated homonymous hemianopia is usually occipital in origin, and almost always due to vascular disease. Temporal or parietal lobe pathology associated with visual field defects will usually produce additional symptoms and signs. Furthermore, the pathology is often neoplastic rather than vascular.

Pupillary light pathway

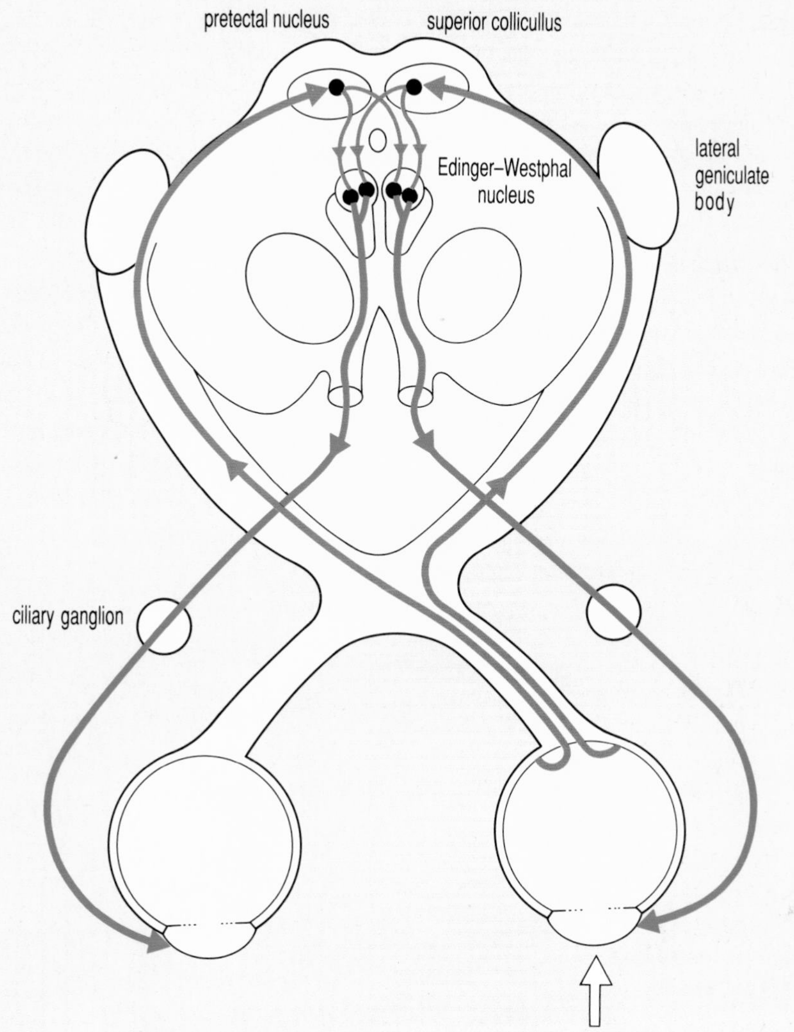

Fig. 12.54 Pupillary light pathway. The input from the left eye decussates at the chiasm and reaches both third nerve nuclei.

Bilateral occipital infarction results in cortical blindness. The pupillary responses are normal. In some instances there is denial of visual disability and confabulation of visual detail (Anton's syndrome).

THE OCULOMOTOR, TROCHLEAR, AND ABDUCENS (3RD, 4TH, & 6TH) NERVES

STRUCTURE AND FUNCTION

Pupillary light response pathway

The pupillary light response pathway originates in the same rods and cones that register visual stimuli. Fibres from the receptors partly decussate in the chiasm, then leave the optic tract before the lateral geniculate body on their way to the brachium of the superior colliculus, and hence the Edinger–Westphal nucleus, via the pretectal nuclear complex (Fig. 12.54). A light stimulus to one eye triggers a bilateral, symmetric, pupillary response. The pupillomotor fibres lie superficially in the oculomotor nerve before joining the inferior division of the nerve on their way to the ciliary ganglion. After synapsing, the fibres enter the short ciliary nerve.

Near reaction

The near reaction comprises pupillary constriction, ocular convergence and increased accommodation of the lens. The accommodation reaction is controlled by the rostral and mid-portion of the Edinger-Westphal nucleus. The efferent pathway passes through the oculomotor nerve, ciliary ganglion, and short ciliary nerve.

Ocular sympathetic fibres

The ocular sympathetic fibres originate in the hypothalamus and remain uncrossed. The first order neurones terminate in the spinal cord in the intermediolateral cell column between the spinal segments of C8 and T2. Second order neurones exit from the cord, principally in the first ventral thoracic root, and pass through the inferior and middle cervical ganglia before terminating in the superior cervical ganglion (Fig. 12.55). Sudomotor and vasoconstrictor fibres to the face, except for those to a small area on the forehead, run with branches of the external carotid artery. Fibres accompanying the internal carotid artery reach the pupil via branches of the ophthalmic division of the trigeminal nerve, and the eyelids via branches of the ophthalmic artery. The fibres supply the dilator muscle of the iris, and smooth muscle in the upper and lower lids.

Horizontal and vertical saccades

There are supranuclear, internuclear, and infranuclear components in the anatomical pathways for eye movements, with different supranuclear pathways for saccadic (refixation) movements and pursuit (following) movements. Horizontal saccades originate in both the frontal and parietal lobes. From the former the principal descending pathway passes through the anterior limb of the internal capsule, continues along the ventrolateral aspect of the thalamus, decussates in the lower midbrain, then passes in the paramedian pontine reticular formation to end at the excitatory burst neurones in the pontine gaze centre (Fig. 12.56). From here neurones project to the ipsilateral abducens nucleus and through it, via the medial longitudinal fasciculus, to the medial rectus component of the contralateral third nerve nucleus. The pathway for vertical saccades has been less clearly defined, but it projects eventually to the rostral interstitial nucleus of the medial longitudinal fasciculus (Fig. 12.57), which is located at the junction of midbrain and thalamus. The nucleus receives additional ascending inputs through the medial longitudinal fasciculus and, directly, from the paramedian pontine reticular formation. From this nucleus, the pathway for downward saccades passes caudally to the third and fourth cranial nerve nuclei; that for upward saccades traverses the posterior commissure.

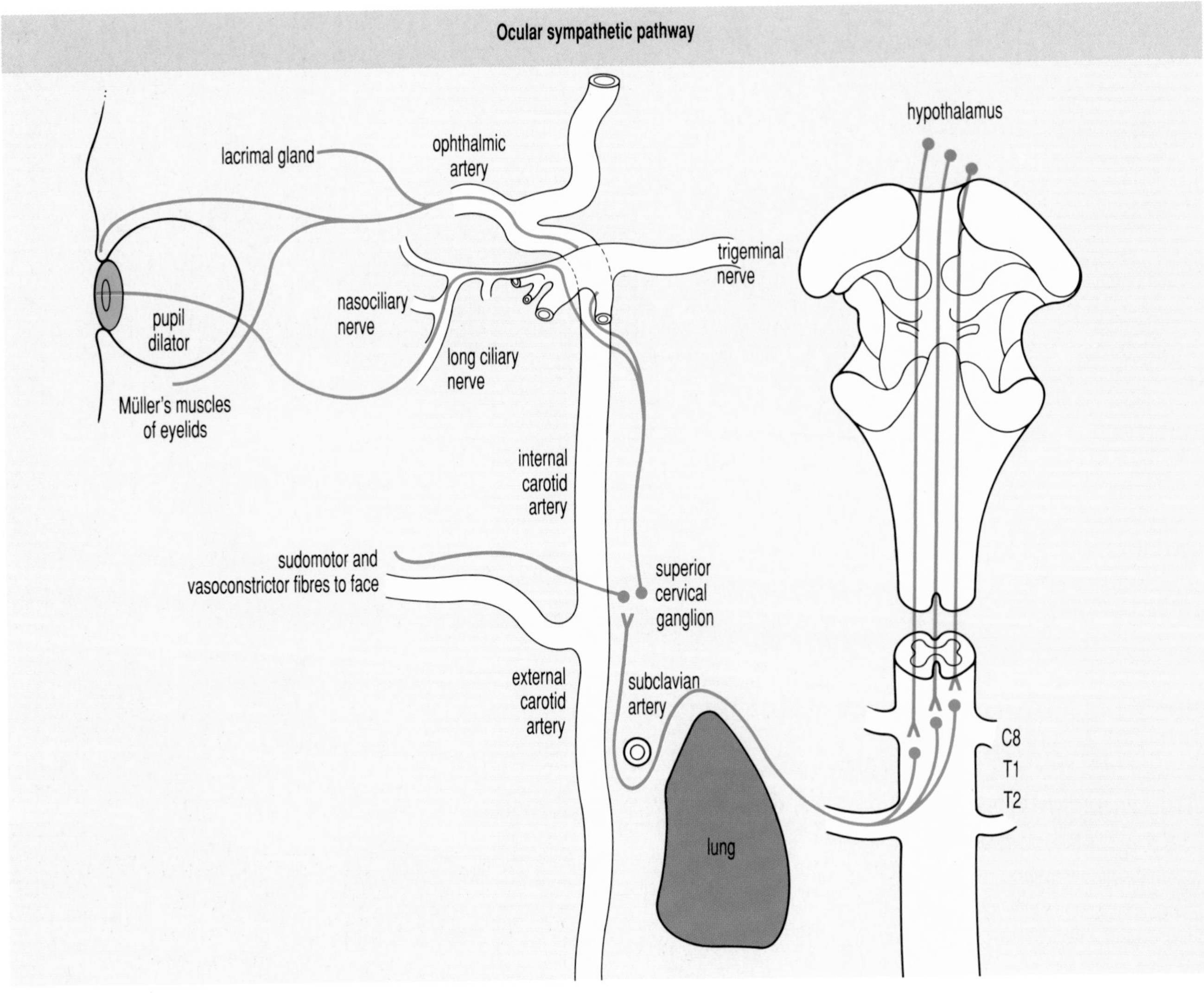

Fig. 12.55 The ocular sympathetic pathway.

Pursuit movements in both the horizontal and vertical planes originate in the parieto-occipital cortex, then descend in an uncrossed pathway whose exact location remains undetermined. That for horizontal pursuit is known to pass through the paramedian pontine reticular formation and that for vertical pursuit is controlled, at least in part, by fibres passing rostrally through the medial longitudinal fasciculus.

The globe has an innate tendency to return to the primary position of gaze following ocular de¡viation, so the stimulus for a sudden horizontal or vertical movement needs to be followed by a sustained neuronal discharge to the relevant muscles if ocular deviation is to be sustained. Burst neurones trigger the initial saccade; at other times their output is suppressed by pause neurones. Simultaneously there is inhibition of the nucleus supplying the contralateral antagonist muscle. For sustained deviation, a tonic neuronal discharge occurs that utilizes the same final common pathway as the burst neurones but which is influenced by other structures including the cerebellum and the medial vestibular nucleus. A similar tonic mechanism exists for other forms of eye movement.

Saccadic movements with a velocity of up to 700°/s permit a rapid refixation of gaze from one object to another, whereas pursuit movements allow tracking of a slowly moving target at velocities up to 50°/s. Vestibular movements are initiated in the semicircular canals by head movement or, reflexly, by caloric stimulation. These movements maintain a stable perception of the environment during bodily movement.

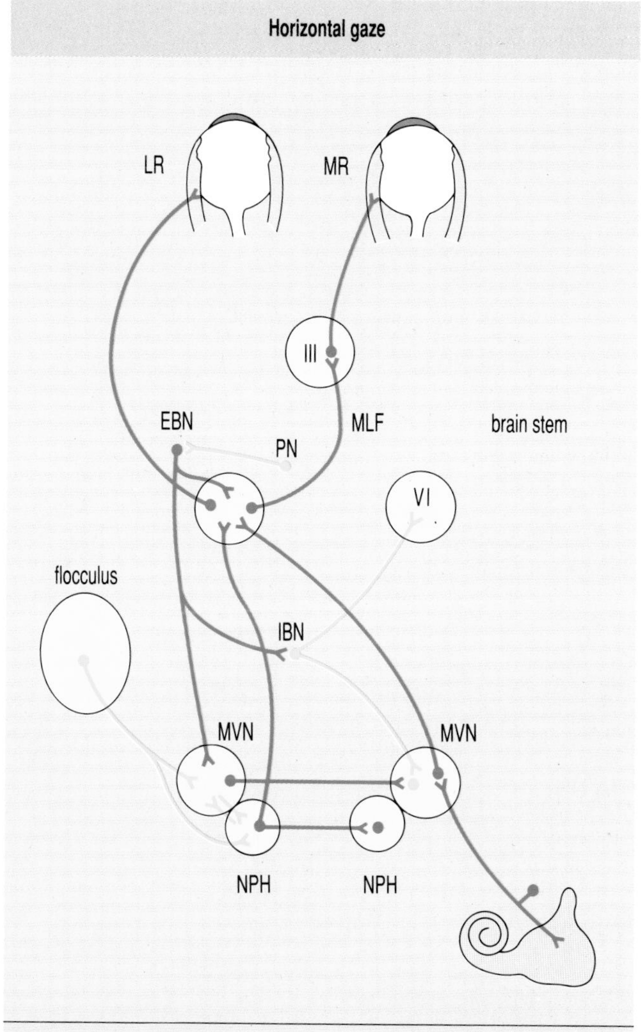

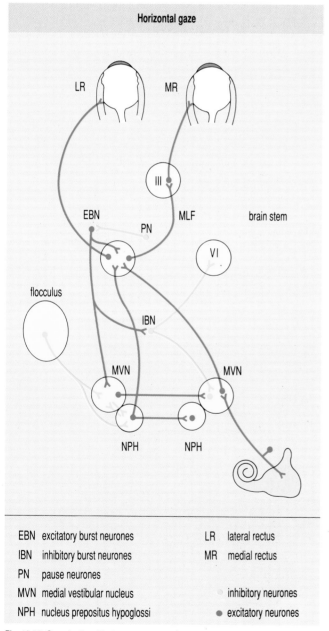

EBN excitatory burst neurones
IBN inhibitory burst neurones
PN pause neurones
MVN medial vestibular nucleus
NPH nucleus prepositus hypoglossi
LR lateral rectus
MR medial rectus
inhibitory neurones
excitatory neurones

Fig. 12.56 Organization of horizontal gaze.

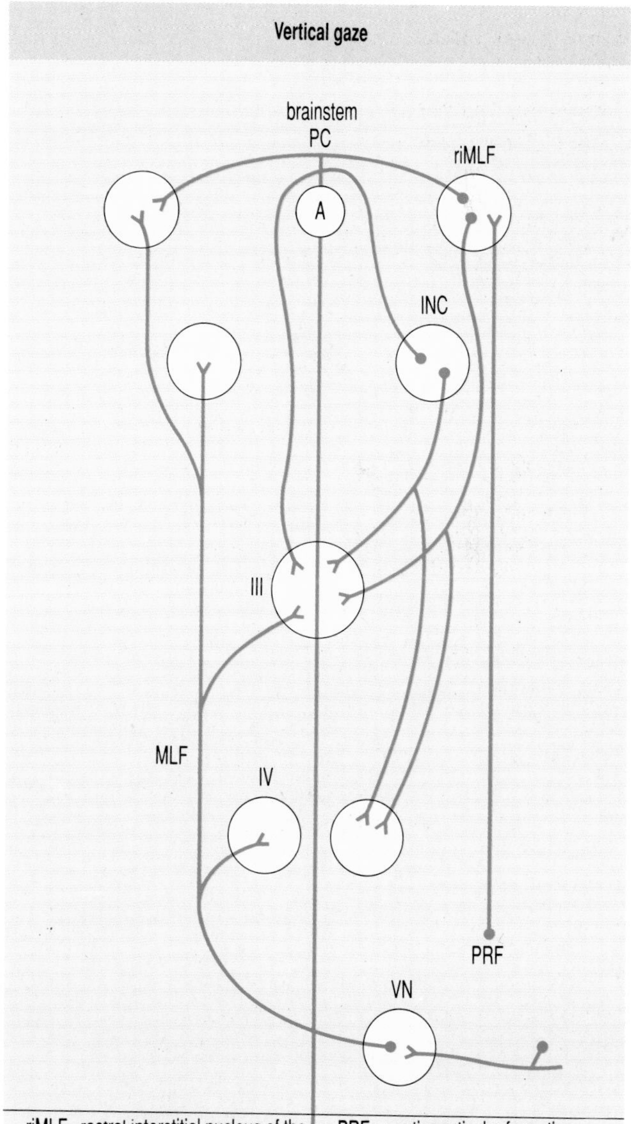

riMLF rostral interstitial nucleus of the medial longitudinal bundle
INC interstitial nucleus of Cahal
PRF pontine reticular formation
A aqueduct
PC posterior commisure
VN vestibular nucleus

Fig. 12.57 Organization of vertical gaze.

Third nerve

The third nerve nucleus is located in the midbrain at the level of the superior colliculus. All its neurones project ipsilaterally apart from those passing to the contralateral superior rectus muscle (Fig. 12.58). The levators of the upper lids are supplied by a single midline nucleus. The third nerve emerges from the anterior aspect of the midbrain and lies close to the posterior communicating artery before entering the cavernous sinus in which it runs superiorly (Fig. 12.59). It terminates in superior and inferior divisions, the latter containing pupillomotor fibres.

Fourth nerve

The fourth nerve decussates before exiting from the dorsal aspect of the midbrain, eventually innervating the contralateral superior oblique muscle. It lies immediately below the third nerve in the cavernous sinus and enters the orbit through the superior orbital fissure, along with the other nerves supplying the eye muscles.

Sixth nerve

The sixth nerve emerges from the lower border of the pons, runs beneath the petroclinoid ligament then lies close to the internal carotid artery in the medial aspect of the cavernous sinus. It supplies the lateral rectus muscle.

Nystagmus

Nystagmus is a repetitive to-and-fro movement of the eyes. In pendular nystagmus the phases are of equal velocity, in phasic (jerk) nystagmus they differ. The slow phase of jerk nystagmus may show a linear or non-linear time course. Vestibular dysfunction, either centrally or peripherally, is the usual cause of a jerk nystagmus in which the slow-phase is linear. In gaze-evoked nystagmus the eyes drift back from an eccentric position with a non-linear velocity, followed by a saccadic correction. This type of nystagmus is thought to result from dysfunction of the neural integrater, the mechanism which sustains a tonic discharge of neuronal activity during eccentric gaze (Fig. 12.60).

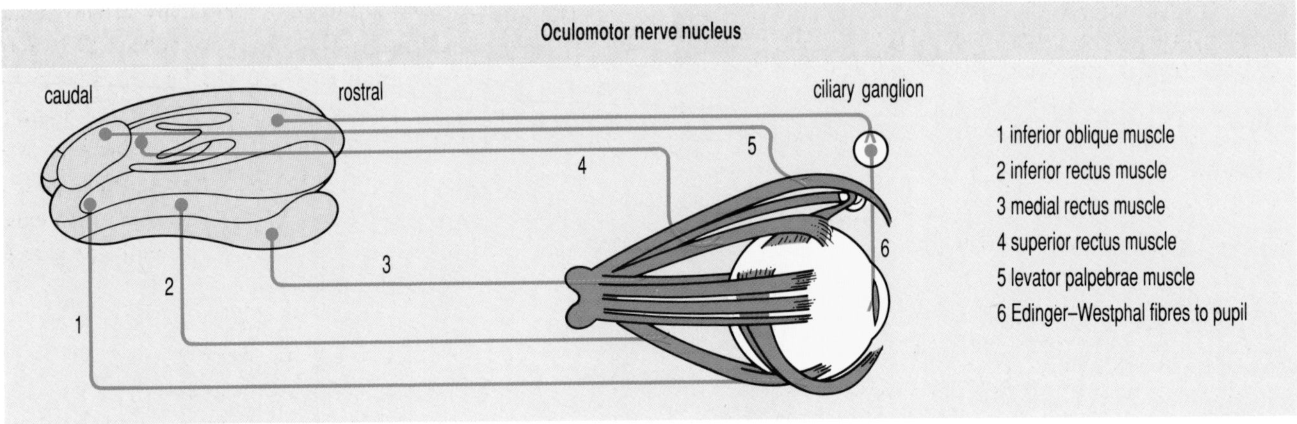

Fig. 12.58 Organization of the oculomotor nerve nucleus.

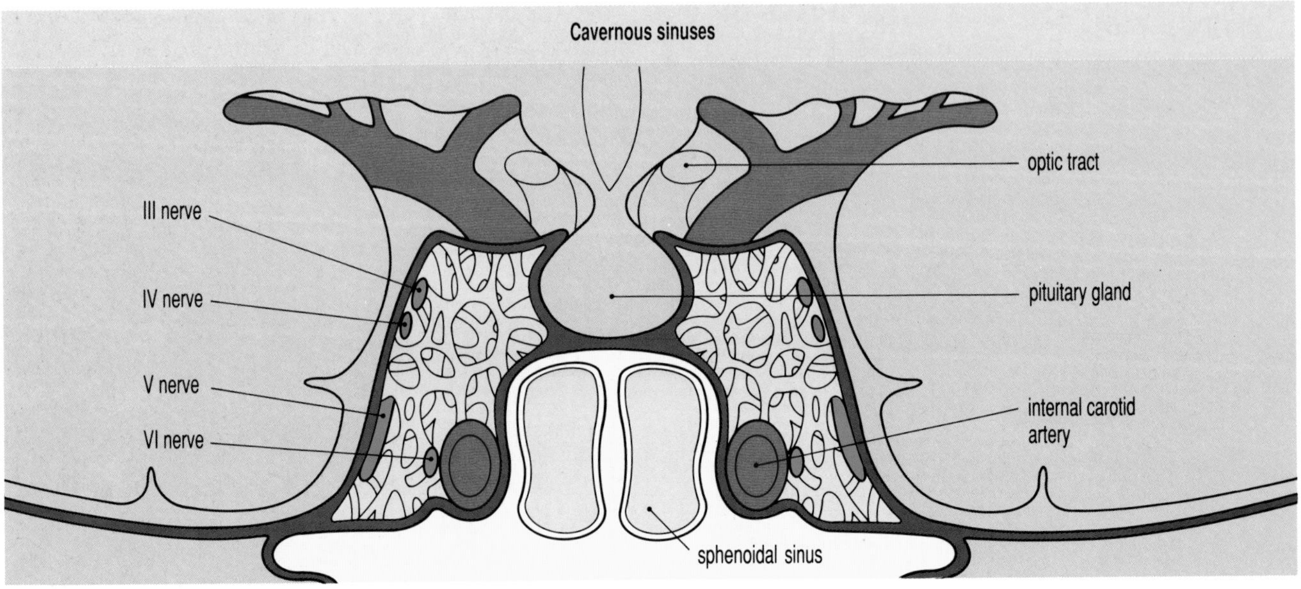

Fig. 12.59 Transverse section of cavernous sinuses.

covered, increased innervation attempts are made in order to achieve fixation with the paretic eye. This abnormal stimulus spills over to the yoke muscle, the medial rectus of the left eye, which accordingly over-adducts that eye (secondary deviation). In a paralytic strabismus, secondary deviation is greater than primary (Fig. 12.63).

If a muscle paresis is suspected, further questioning can help identify the likely culprit. A horizontal diplopia is due to paresis either of the lateral or medial rectus. Paresis of the other eye muscles produces an oblique or vertical diplopia. Having confirmed that the diplopia is binocular (in other words, that it disappears when one or the other eye is covered) ask the patient to look in the six directions illustrated in Fig. 12.64. Paresis of an eye muscle produces a diplopia which increases as the eye moves in the direction of action of that muscle. The false image (which often appears indistinct or blurred) is peripheral to the true image and belongs to the affected eye (Fig. 12.65). Having elicited the diplopia, cover first one eye, then the other, to establish to which eye the

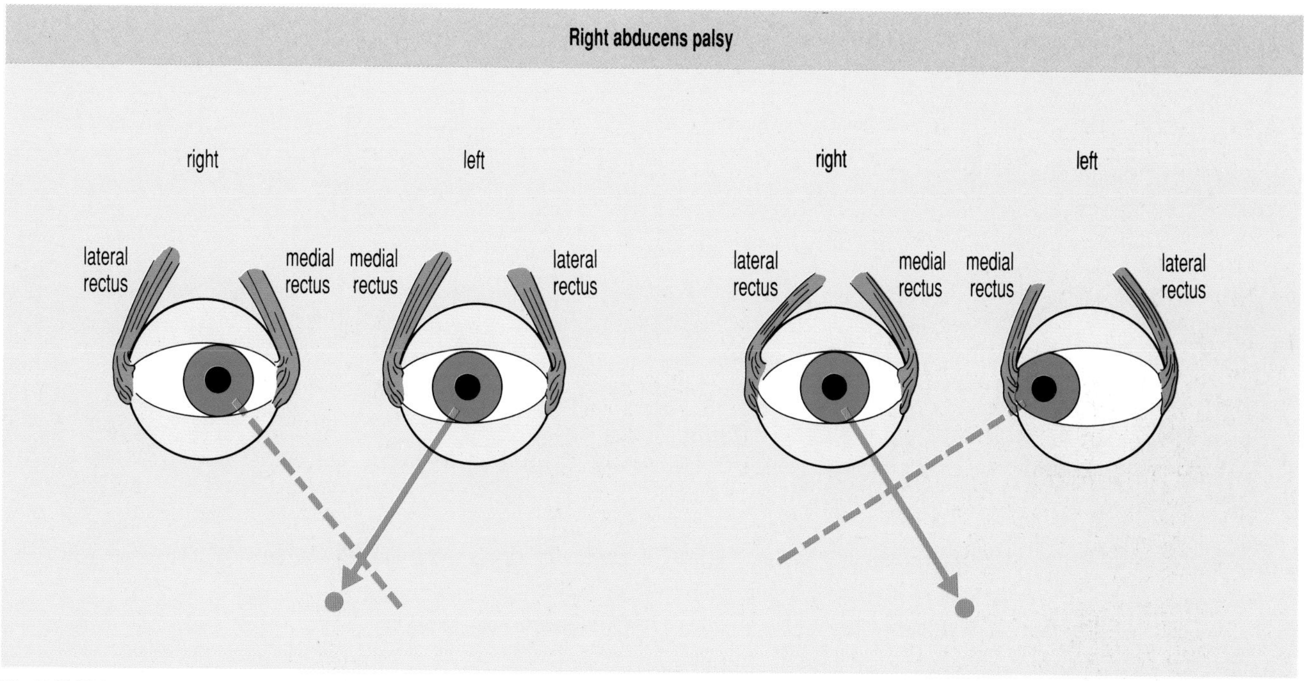

Fig. 12.63 Right abducens palsy. The right eye tends to converge, particularly when the left eye is used for fixation. When the right eye tries to fixate, overaction of the left medial rectus occurs.

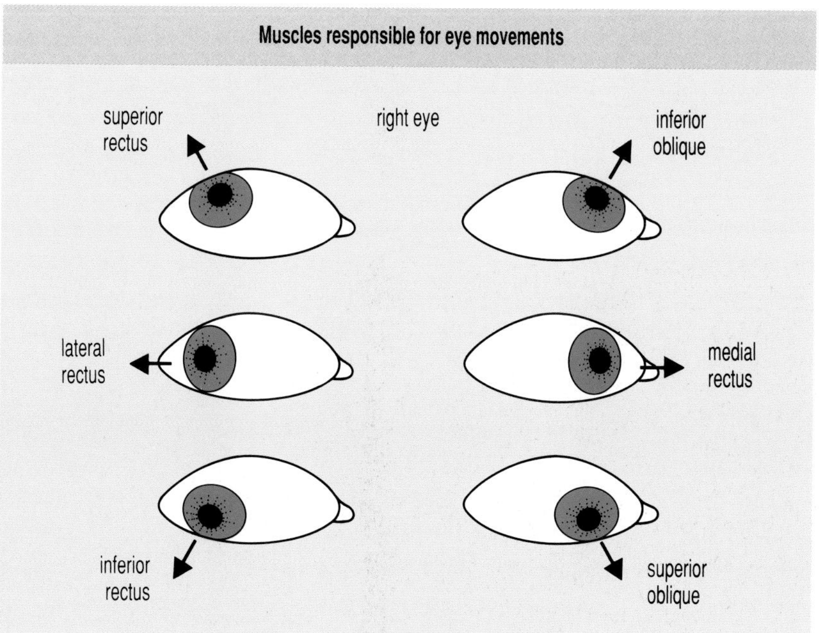

Fig. 12.64 The muscles responsible for eye movements in particular directions.

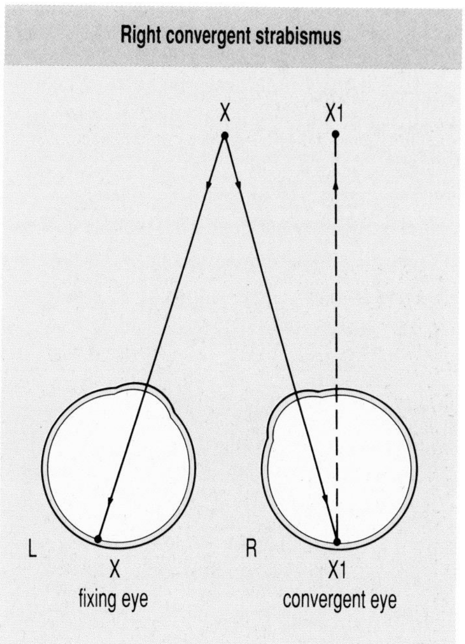

Fig. 12.65 Right convergent strabismus. The right eye falsely projects the object X to position X1.

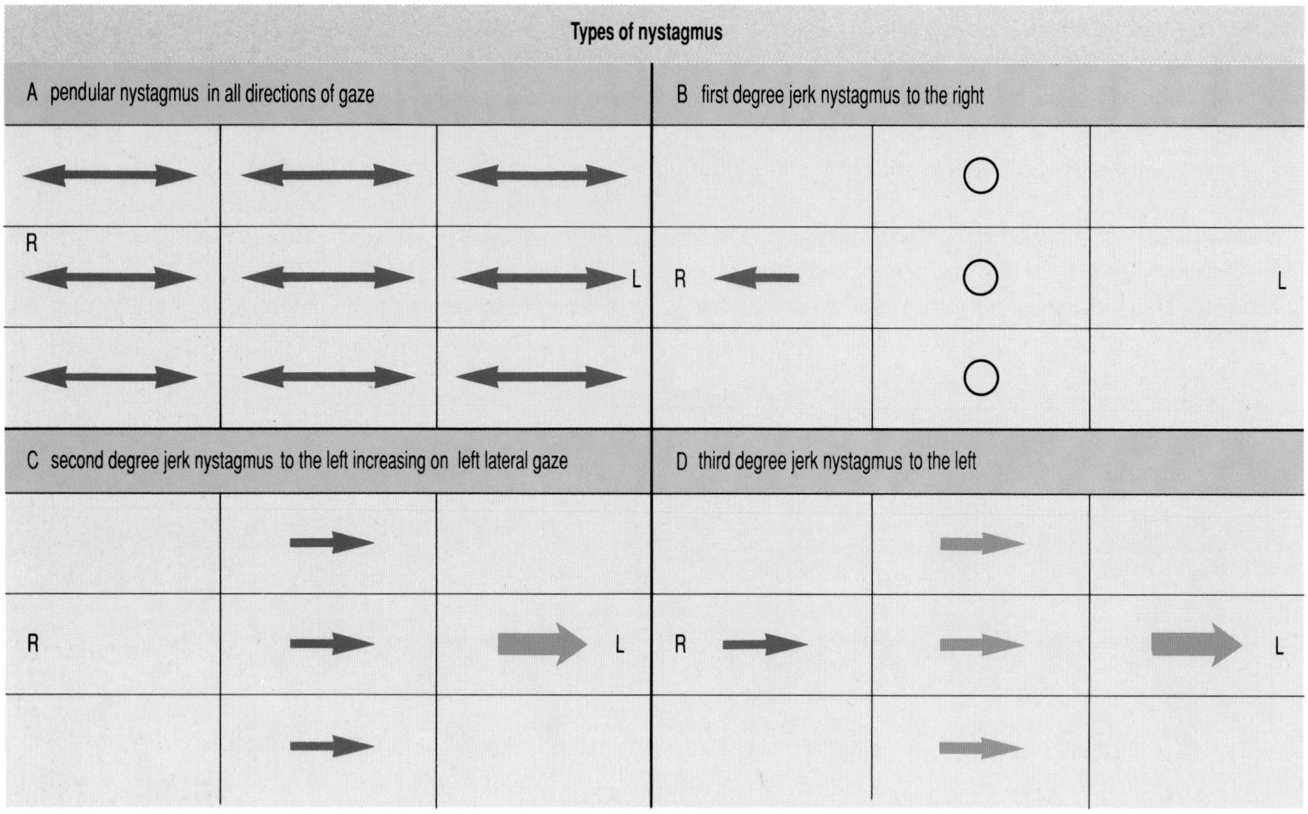

Fig. 12.66 Diagrammatic representation of pendular nystagmus in all directions of gaze, first degree jerk nystagmus to the right, second degree nystagmus to the left, and third degree jerk nystagmus to the left.

false image belongs. Observe if the patient has an abnormal head tilt as a compensation for the diplopia. To establish whether the head tilt is of long standing, examine old photographs. Finally, remember that a pattern of diplopia which is variable and difficult to interpret suggests the possibility of myasthenia gravis.

Nystagmus

Note the presence of nystagmus, and whether it is pendular or jerk. Record the amplitude (fine, medium, or coarse), persistence, and the direction of gaze in which it occurs. Additionally, indicate whether the movement is horizontal, vertical, rotary, or a mixture of several types. The nystagmus can be represented diagrammatically (Fig. 12.66). First degree nystagmus to the left is a fast beating nystagmus to the left on left lateral gaze. In second and third degree nystagmus to the left the same nystagmus is present on forward and right lateral gaze, respectively.

Barany or Hallpike manoeuvre

If the patient has described attacks of intense vertigo triggered by particular positions, assess whether certain postures can elicit nystagmus. With the patient sitting on the edge of the couch, turn the head to one side then rapidly depress the head and upper trunk so that they are slightly below the horizontal (Barany or Hallpike manoeuvre). A positive result is a rotary nystagmus towards the dependent ear. Observe whether the nystagmus is sustained or fatigues, and if it reappears on returning to the sitting position. Repeat the manoeuvre with the head rotated to the other side.

Optokinetic nystagmus

Optokinetic responses are assessed using a drum painted with vertical lines, which is rotated first in the horizontal and then in the vertical plane. As the patient looks at the drum a pursuit movement is seen in the direction of its rotation, followed by a saccade returning the eyes to the mid-position (Fig. 12.67). Both movements are generated by the hemisphere towards which the drum is rotating. Thus, with the drum rotating to the right, pursuit is controlled by the right parieto-occipital cortex, and the correcting saccade by the right frontal cortex.

CLINICAL APPLICATION

THE PUPIL

Horner's syndrome

Horner's syndrome results from interruption of the sympathetic fibres to the eye. The pupil is miosed, and the palpebral fissure is narrowed due to mild ptosis of the upper lid and elevation of the lower lid. The pupillary asymmetry is often slight but can be accentuated by taking the patient into a darkened room. Though enophthalmos is suggested by the appearance of the eye, this is not con-

Fig. 12.67 Optokinetic nystagmus. As the drum rotates to the right, pursuit movements to the right are interrupted by correcting saccades to the left.

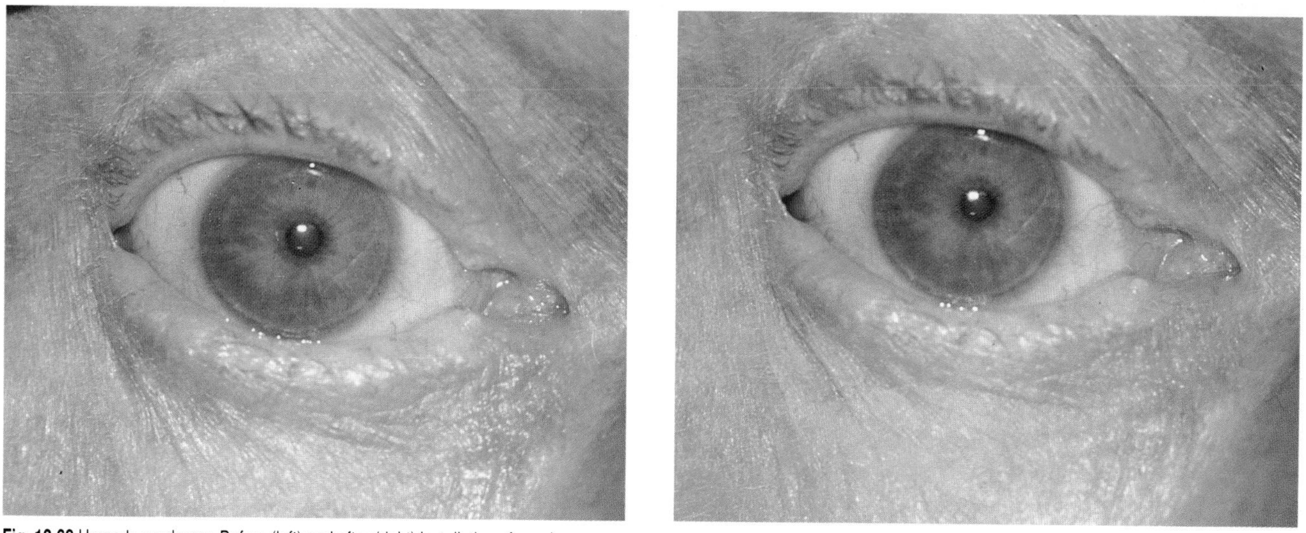

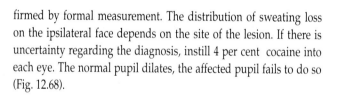

Fig. 12.68 Horner's syndrome. Before (left) and after (right) installation of cocaine.

firmed by formal measurement. The distribution of sweating loss on the ipsilateral face depends on the site of the lesion. If there is uncertainty regarding the diagnosis, instill 4 per cent cocaine into each eye. The normal pupil dilates, the affected pupil fails to do so (Fig. 12.68).

Tonic pupil syndrome

The tonic pupil syndrome is usually unilateral. The affected pupil is dilated, though in long-standing cases it tends to become progressively smaller. The light response is absent or markedly depressed and consequently, in a darkened room, the affected pupil becomes smaller than its fellow due to a failure of reflex dilatation. The near reaction is delayed but sometimes more marked than that of the normal pupil. On relaxing the near effort, dilatation is delayed so that for a period the previously larger pupil is the smaller one (Fig. 12.69). The accommodation reaction is often sustained, resulting in blurred vision when switching from a distant to a near target or vice versa. The iris contains areas of focal atrophy, and characteristically the pupils are hypersensive to dilute parasympathomimetic agents (e.g. 0.125 per cent pilocarpine). Tonic pupil syndrome is sometimes associated with depression of the deep tendon reflexes – the Holmes – Adie syndrome.

Argyll Robertson pupil

The Argyll Robertson pupil is miosed, with a light response which is diminished compared to the near reaction (light-near dissociation). When the defect is fully developed , the pupil is fixed to light and fails to dilate in the dark. The pupil is often irregular with evidence of iris atrophy (Fig. 12.70). When complete the syndrome is pathognomonic of neurosyphilis. The lesion responsible is thought to lie in the midbrain immediately above the Edinger – Westphal nucleus. A pupil of normal size with light-near dissociation can occur in other circumstances (e.g. in a blind eye).

Relative afferent pupillary defect

This results from a lesion of the afferent light reflex pathway between the retina and the optic tract. It is not found with disease of the lens or vitreous. The conducting systems of the two optic nerves are best compared by performing the swinging light test. In the presence of a unilateral optic nerve lesion, for example due to optic neuritis, the affected pupil dilates as the torch is swung on to it from the sound eye (Fig. 12.71).

Hippus

Hippus is a rhythmic alteration in pupil size found in many individuals and is of no significance.

DISORDERS OF EYE MOVEMENTS

Gaze paresis

In an acute frontal lobe lesion, contralateral saccadic eye movements in the horizontal plane are depressed or absent, and there is limb paresis ipsilateral to the gaze palsy (Fig. 12.72). Both pursuit movements and the oculocephalic responses are spared. Saccades return later, but now initiated by the contralateral frontal lobe. Damage to that frontal lobe will result in a complete horizontal saccadic palsy. A lesion at the level of the paramedian pontine reticular formation produces an ipsilateral gaze paresis for both saccadic and pursuit movement (Fig. 12.73). The limb paresis is contralateral. An ipsilateral pursuit paresis occurs with posterior hemisphere disease and is associated with a contralateral homonymous field defect.

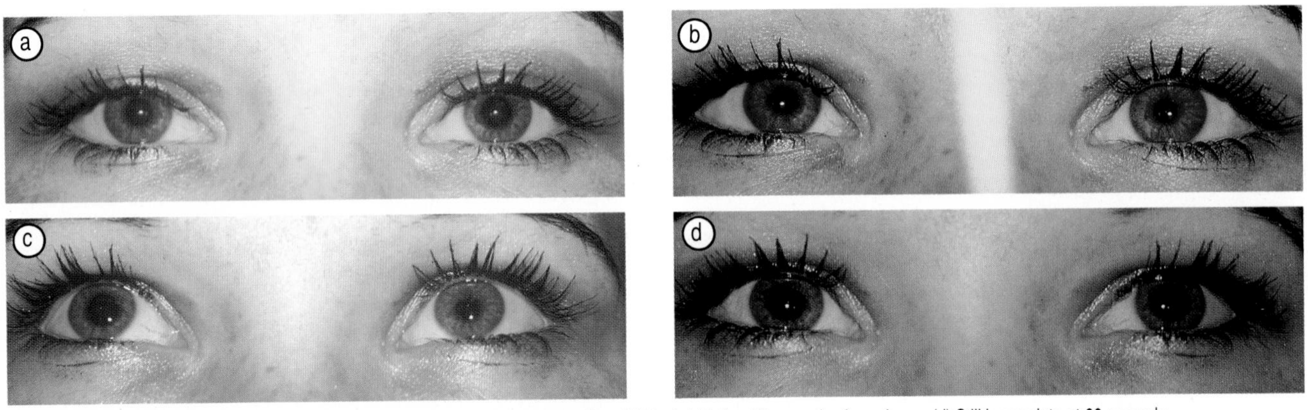

Fig. 12.69 Tonic pupil syndrome. (a) Left pupil is dilated. (b) After a minute's near-effort. (c) Partial dilation 15 seconds after release. (d) Still incomplete at 60 seconds.

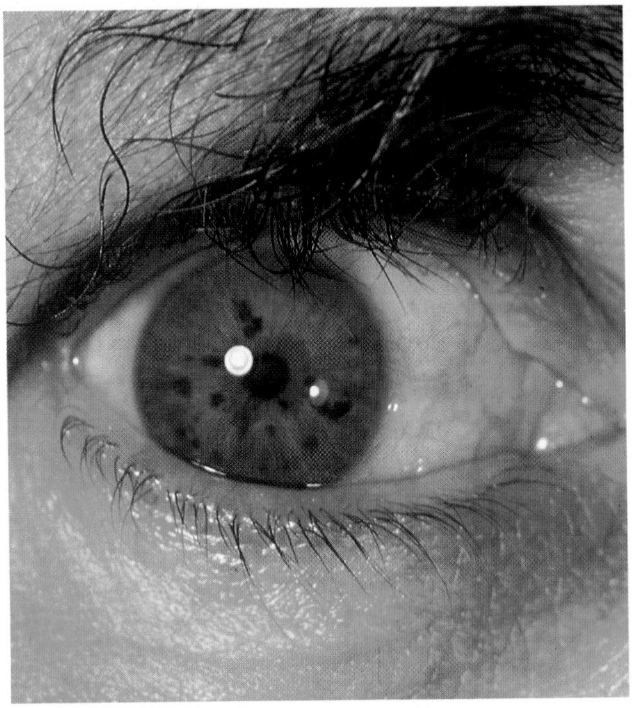

Fig. 12.70 Argyll Robertson pupil.

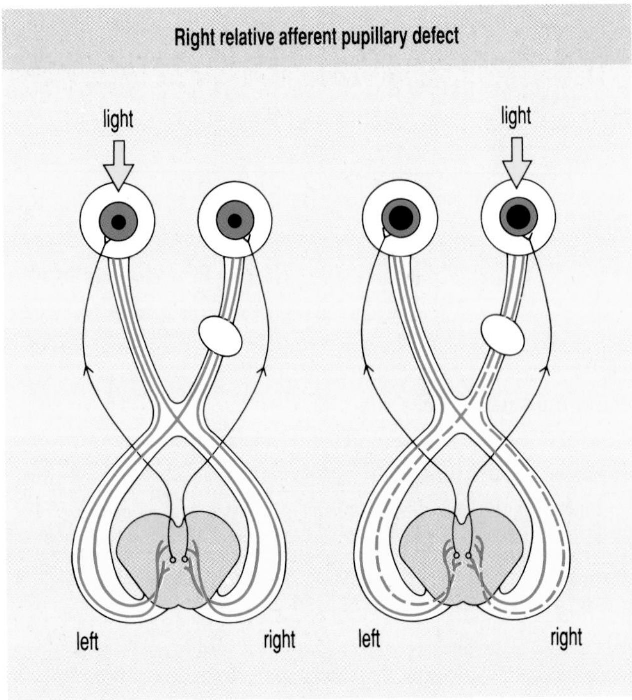

Fig. 12.71 Right relative afferent pupillary defect. Constriction of both pupils occurs when the light is shone in the left eye. As the torch is swung to the right eye, its pupil dilates due to loss of the consensual response.

A paresis of upward saccades, initially with relative preservation of pursuit, is a feature of the dorsal midbrain (Parinaud's) syndrome (Fig. 12.74). Other findings include impaired convergence and dilated, light-near dissociated pupils. At a later stage upward pursuit and down gaze become affected. Causes include vascular disease and pinealoma.

Other saccadic and pursuit movement disorders

Saccadic slowing, accompanied by disorganized pursuit movements, is found in both Huntington's and Parkinson's disease. In progressive supranuclear palsy, downward saccades and pursuit fail first, followed by involvement of upward and, finally horizontal

Eye movements in frontal, pontine, and dorsal–midbrain lesions

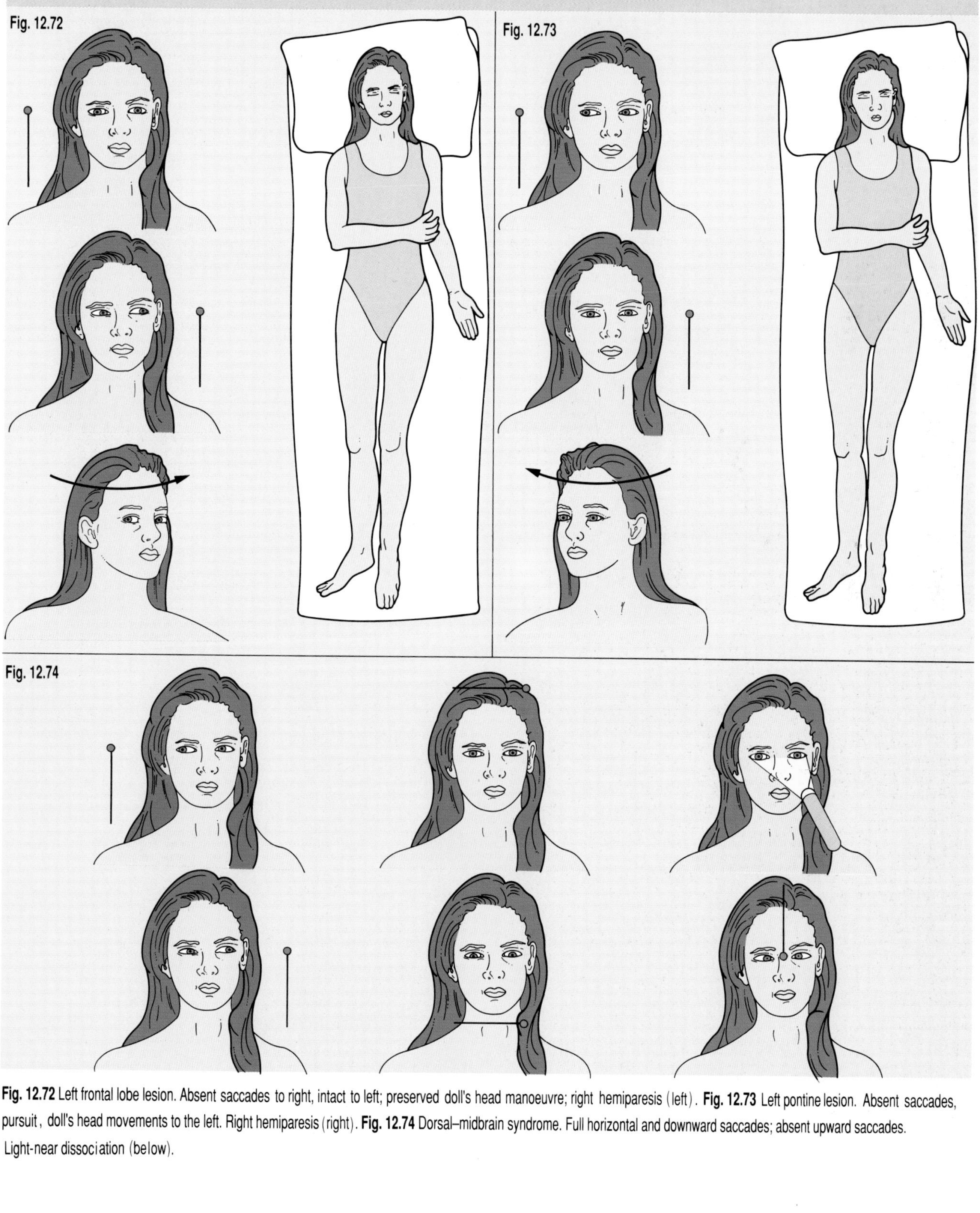

Fig. 12.72 Left frontal lobe lesion. Absent saccades to right, intact to left; preserved doll's head manoeuvre; right hemiparesis (left). **Fig. 12.73** Left pontine lesion. Absent saccades, pursuit, doll's head movements to the left. Right hemiparesis (right). **Fig. 12.74** Dorsal–midbrain syndrome. Full horizontal and downward saccades; absent upward saccades. Light-near dissociation (below).

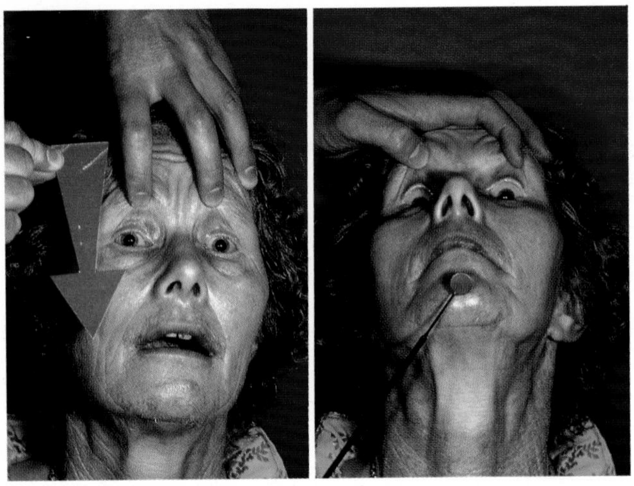

Fig. 12.75 Progressive supranuclear palsy. Failure of down gaze (left) is improved by the doll's head manoeuvre (right).

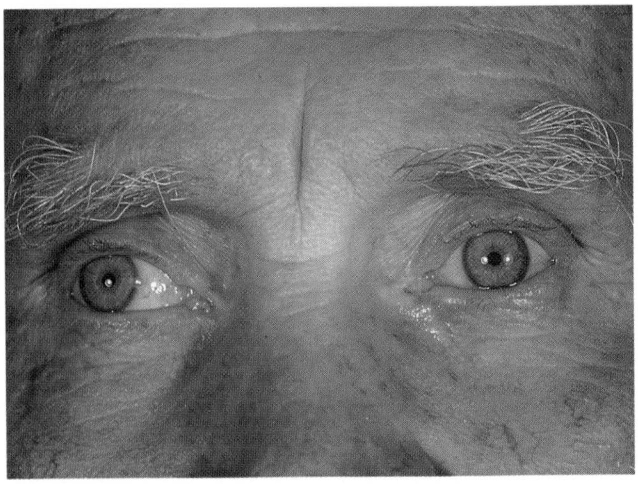

Fig. 12.76 Left internuclear ophthalmoplegia. Failure of adduction of the left eye on right lateral gaze.

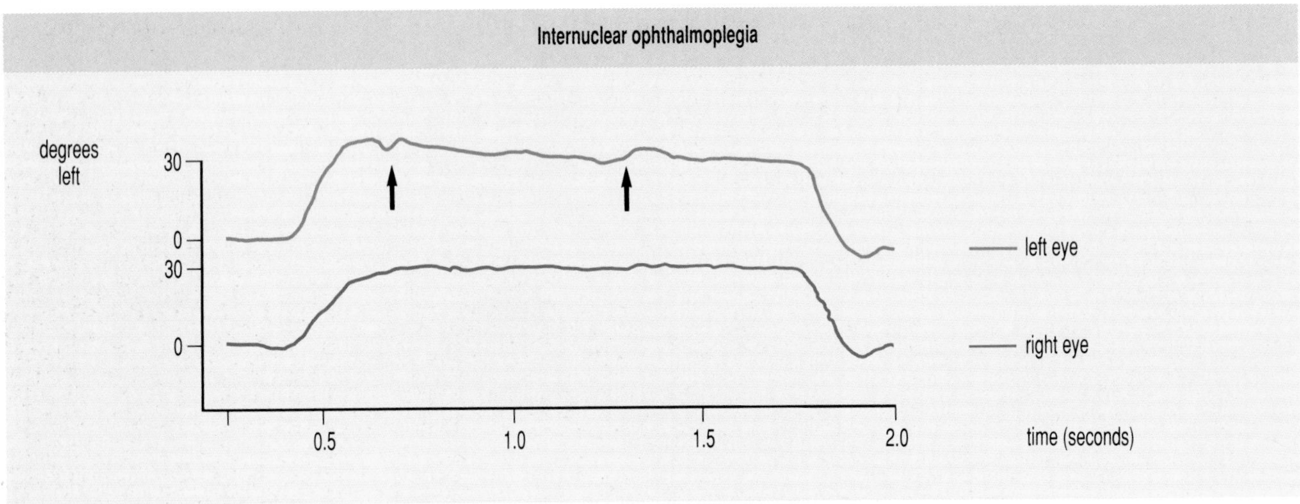

Fig. 12.77 Right internuclear ophthalmoplegia. Adduction of the right eye is slower than abduction of the left. The abduction is interrupted by nystagmus (arrows).

movements. Doll's head movements are spared (Fig. 12.75). A delay in the initiation of saccades occurs in many extrapyramidal disorders. Overshooting or undershooting saccades (hypermetria and hypometria, respectively) occur with cerebellar disease. Large or small inappropriate saccades can interrupt fixation. Causes include multiple sclerosis and cerebellar disease. Slowing of pursuit movement is most commonly due to sedative medication.

Internuclear ophthalmoplegia

A lesion of the medial longitudinal fasciculus leads to slowing, or total failure, of medial rectus contraction during lateral gaze (Fig. 12.76). The slowing affects all movement, whether saccadic, pursuit, or reflex. To assess subtle slowing, observe the relative velocity of the two eyes while the patient rapidly fixates between two targets. There is usually an accompanying nystagmus in the abducting eye (Fig. 12.77). Bilateral internuclear ophthalmoplegia is accompanied by upbeat vertical nystagmus. Multiple sclerosis is the commonest cause in younger subjects, vascular disease in the elderly.

The 'one-and-a-half'syndrome

If the lesion responsible for a unilateral internuclear ophthalmoplegia spreads into the pontine gaze centre a more profound loss of ocular motility results (Fig. 12.78). The only normal horizontal movement possible is abduction of the opposite eye (Fig. 12.79). The finding is usually the consequence of vascular disease.

Abducens palsy

Ironically, a lesion of the sixth nerve nucleus produces a gaze paresis rather than an isolated lateral rectus weakness. The latter is usually due to a lesion of the central or peripheral course of the sixth nerve, but it can be caused by myasthenia or orbital disease. The eye fails to abduct. When the defect is complete, there may be a convergent strabismus due to unopposed action of the ipsilateral medial rectus (Fig. 12.80). Unilateral or bilateral sixth nerve palsies sometimes result from the effects of raised intracranial pressure (Fig. 12.81).

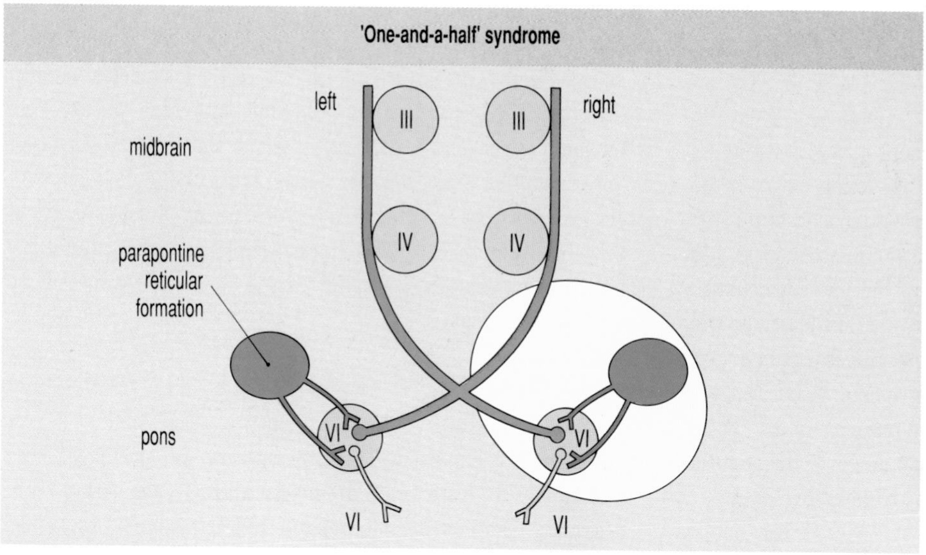

Fig. 12.78 Diagram of lesion causing the 'one-and-a-half' syndrome. There is involvement of the right pontine gaze centre and the medial longitudinal fasciculus destined for the medial rectus component of the right third nerve nucleus.

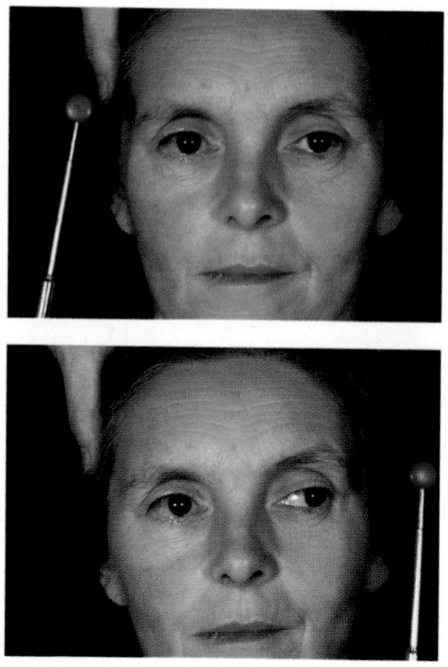

Fig. 12.79 'One-and-a-half' syndrome. Right gaze paresis plus right internuclear ophthalmoplegia.

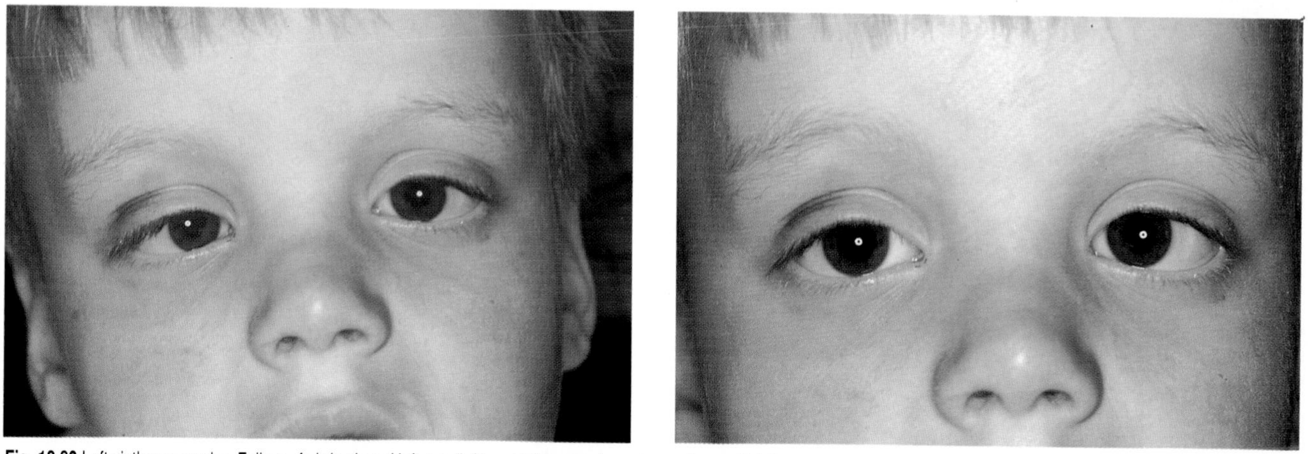

Fig. 12.80 Left sixth nerve palsy. Failure of abduction of left eye (left) and left esotropia on forward gaze (right).

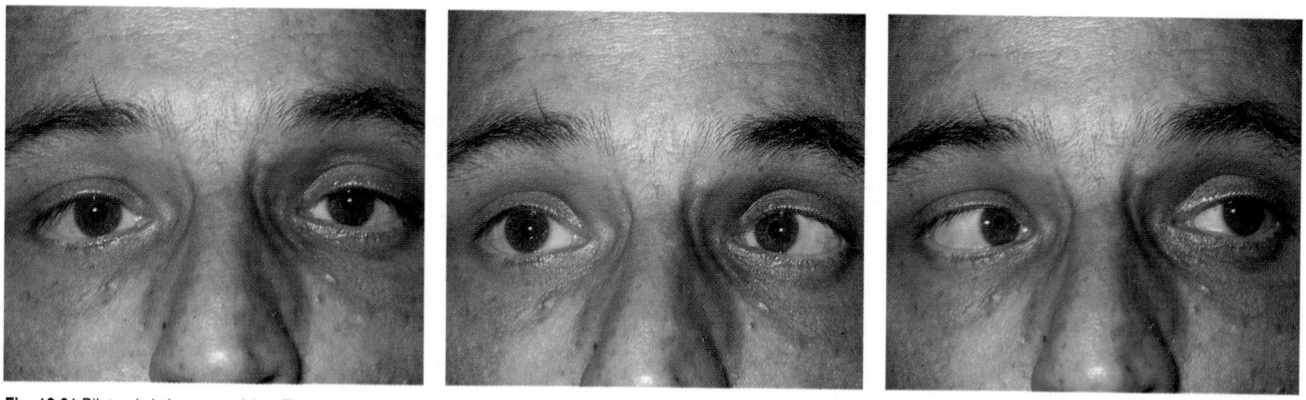

Fig. 12.81 Bilateral sixth nerve palsies. There is a tendency for the eyes to converge on forward gaze (left), with partial failure of abduction to right (middle), and to left (right).

Trochlear palsy

Though normally a result of trochlear nerve palsy, weakness of the superior oblique muscle can occur with myasthenia or dysthyroid eye disease. An isolated trochlear nerve palsy sometimes follows a closed head injury. The head tilts to the side opposite the affected eye, and the patient complains of diplopia, particularly on downward gaze. There is defective depression of the adducted eye (Fig. 12.82).

Oculomotor palsy

Nuclear oculomotor palsies tend to be either incomplete or complete but with pupillary sparing. A complete third nerve palsy cannot be nuclear unless there is involvement of the contralateral superior rectus muscle. Peripheral third nerve lesions are commonly due to diabetes. The paresis is typically painful, and pupil-sparing in about 50 per cent of cases (Fig. 12.83). In a complete third nerve palsy there is a substantial ptosis, and the eye is deviated laterally and slightly downwards. Compression of the oculomotor nerve, for example by a posterior communicating aneurysm, almost always results in pupillary dilatation (Fig. 12.84). To assess whether the fourth nerve is intact in the presence of a complete third nerve palsy, ask the patient to look down. If the superior oblique muscle is still functioning, the abducted eye shows an inwardly rotating twitch.

Combined palsies

A lesion within the cavernous sinus is particularly liable to affect the eye nerves in combination rather than individually. At risk are the third, fourth, and sixth nerves, the first and second divisions of the trigeminal nerve, and the ocular sympathetic fibres. A cavernous aneurysm is commonly responsible for pressure effects at this site. A complex, mixed ophthalmoplegia without pupillary involvement raises the possibility of myasthenia or dysthyroid eye disease (Fig. 12.85).

Nystagmus

Pendular nystagmus is usually congenital but is sometimes found in association with brain stem vascular disease or multiple sclerosis. Vestibular nystagmus due to labyrinthine disease has

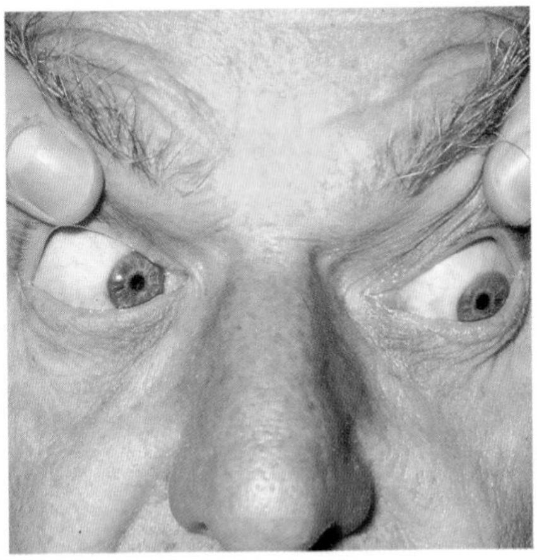

Fig. 12.82 Right superior oblique palsy.

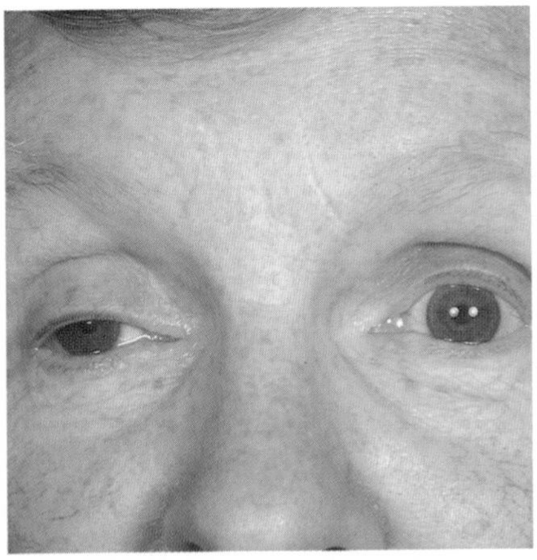

Fig. 12.83 Pupil-sparing right oculomotor palsy due to diabetes.

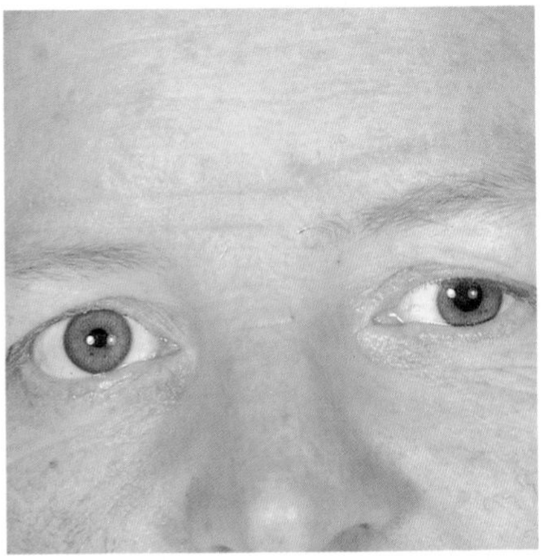

Fig. 12.84 Left third nerve paresis. The pupil is dilated.

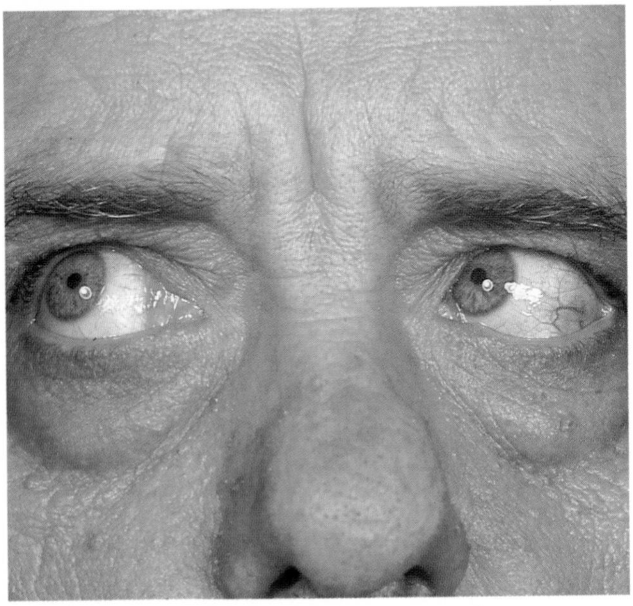

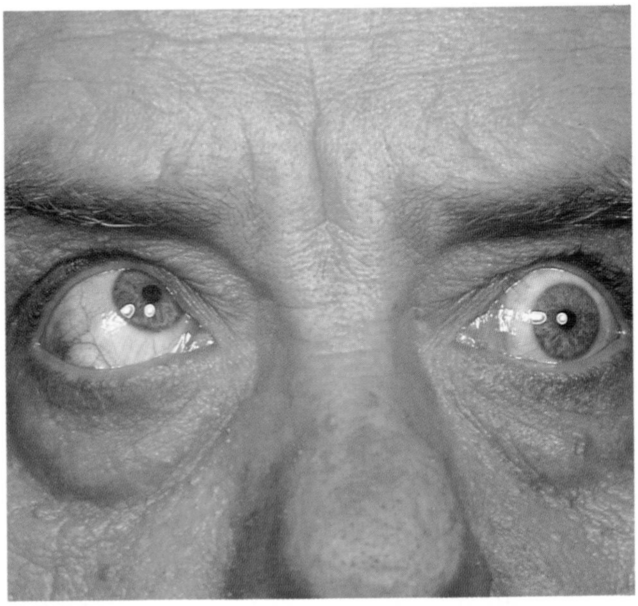

Fig. 12.85 Dysthyroid eye disease. Failure of laevo-elevation of the left eye.

both horizontal and rotary components, and is suppressed by visual fixation. The slow phase is directed to the side of the lesion. The nystagmus resulting from disease of the central vestibular pathways is more variable and may be rotary, horizontal, vertical, or a mixture of several types. Fixation does not affect it.

Nystagmus triggered by a change in head posture commonly results from labyrinthine disease. In benign positional vertigo, the patient complains of vertigo triggered by a particular head posture (e.g. lying down in bed on one or other side). Head positioning produces a nystagmus, with both horizontal and rotary components, which appears after a delay and then fatigues rapidly. As the patient returns to the sitting position, the nystagmus is liable to recur. The positional nystagmus of central vestibular disease is less likely to fatigue and is more variable in its direction.

Gaze-evoked nystagmus is often drug-induced but is also seen with disease of the cerebellum or brain stem. The presence of vertical nystagmus implies either brain stem or cerebellar disease. A vertical or oblique nystagmus on down and out gaze is particularly associated with lesions at the foramen magnum, for instance the Chiari malformation. In convergence-retractory nystagmus, a feature of the dorsal midbrain syndrome, attempts at upward saccades produce retractory movements of the globes. The movement is best elicited by asking the patient to look at the optokinetic drum as it rotates downwards (Fig. 12.86). End-point nystagmus is a physiological phenomenon. It occurs at extremes of lateral gaze, is variable and tends to affect one eye more than the other

THE TRIGEMINAL (5TH) NERVE

STRUCTURE AND FUNCTION

The motor nucleus of the nerve lies in the floor of the upper part of the fourth ventricle and receives fibres from both hemispheres, but principally the contralateral one. Initially the motor root remains separate, running below the Gasserian ganglion before joining the mandibular divison of the nerve to emerge through the foramen ovale. The principal muscles supplied by the nerve are the medial and lateral pterygoids, temporalis and masseter. Smaller muscles supplied include tensor tympani and tensor palati. Jaw closure is achieved by contraction of temporalis, and masseter. Jaw opening, and lateral movements, are performed by the pterygoids.

There are three sensory nuclei: the main (principal) nucleus, the mesencephalic nucleus, and the nucleus of the spinal tract (Fig. 12.87). Tactile stimuli are relayed through the main nucleus. From here ascending fibres, most of which decussate, terminate in the thalamus. The spinal nucleus, continuous above with the main nucleus, extends caudally to the second cervical segment where it lies in the posterior horn continuous with the substantia gelatinosa. A rostrocaudal organization of fibres from concentric segments over the face and head has been suggested, based on the pattern of facial sensory loss sometimes seen with lesions of the spinal tract (Fig. 12.88). Terminating in close proximity to the nucleus of the spinal tract are fibres from the seventh, ninth, and tenth cranial

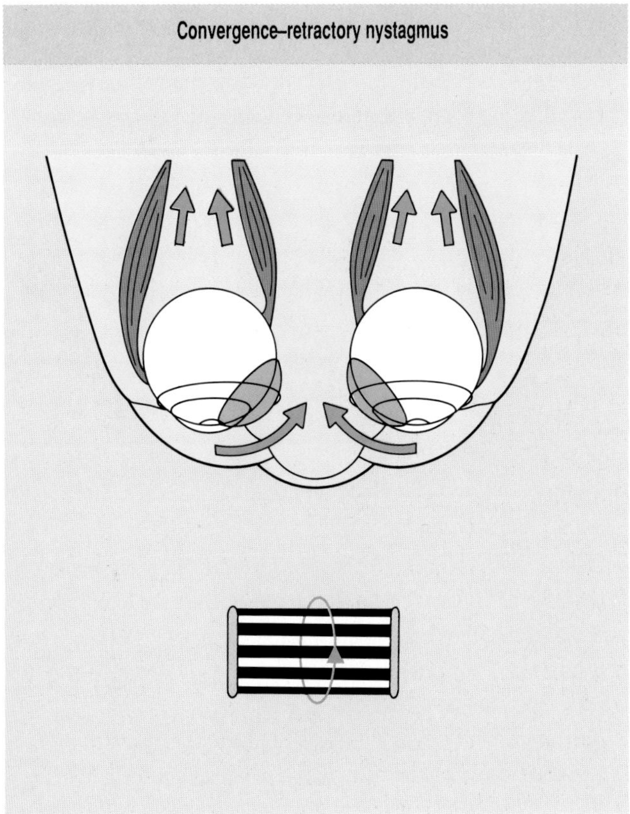

Fig. 12.86 Convergence-retractory nystagmus.

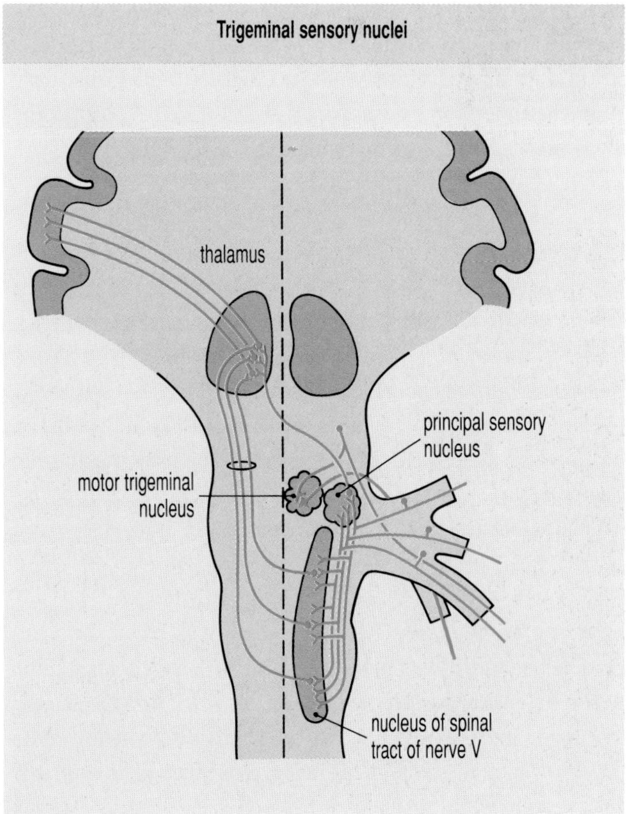

Fig. 12.87 Organization of trigeminal sensory nuclei within the brain stem.

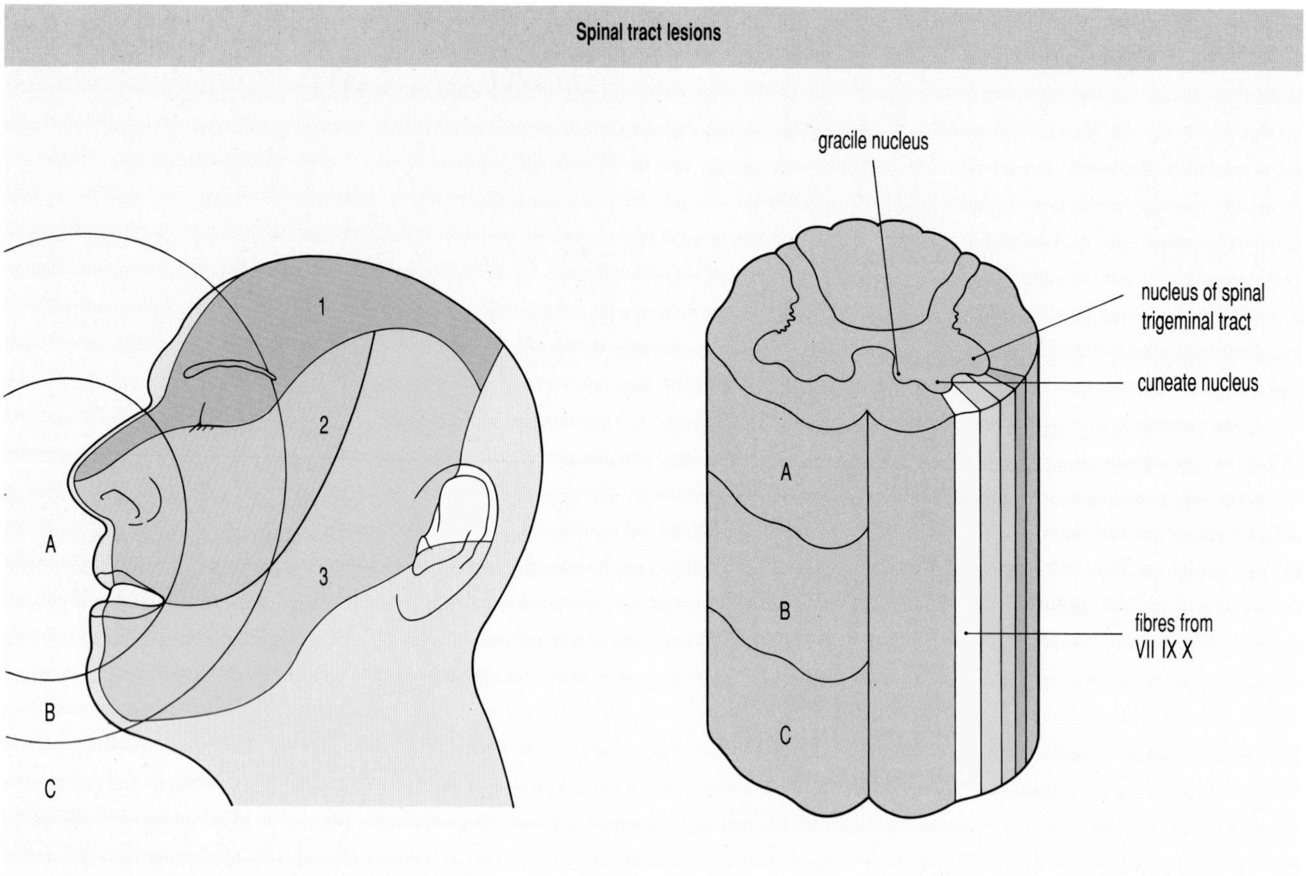

Fig. 12.88 Suggested organization of concentric segments of facial cutaneous innervation within the spinal tract.

nerves which supply cutaneous fibres to the region of the ear. The nucleus contains fibres concerned principally with pain and temperature sensation. Fibres from the nucleus decussate then ascend to the thalamus. The mesencephalic nucleus receives proprioceptive fibres from the muscles of mastication. Collaterals from the afferent fibres synapse on cells in the motor nucleus.

The sensory root accompanies the motor root through the pontine cistern before entering the Gasserian ganglion, which is situated in a depression in the petrous temporal bone (Fig. 12.89). From here the ophthalmic division enters the orbit through the superior orbital fissure, and the maxillary and mandibular divisions leave the skull through the foramina rotundum and ovale, respectively. The facial and scalp innervation of the three divisions is depicted in Fig. 12.90. In addition the trigeminal nerve innervates the mucous membranes of the nose and mouth, certain sinuses, part of the external auditory meatus, and most of the dura.

The jaw jerk

The afferent part of this reflex is formed by large afferents from muscle spindles in masseter and temporalis, which pass to the mesencephalic nucleus in the motor rather than the sensory root. Collaterals from the axons of the unipolar mesencephalic neurones synapse with cells in the motor nucleus, producing a monosynaptic reflex arc, the efferent pathway being within the motor root.

The corneal reflex

The afferent limb of the corneal reflex is contained in the ophthalmic division of the trigeminal. The efferent pathway is within the seventh nerve. Stimulation of the cornea produces both an ipsilateral and a contralateral blink response, the latter being about 5ms slower than the former. The central conduction time for the reflex, approximately 40ms, indicates it is polysynaptic. Scleral, rather than corneal, stimulation results in a reflex with a considerably longer latency.

EXAMINATION

SENSORY

Details of the techniques for sensory examination are given on pages 12.81–12.85 Convenient sites for testing are the forehead, the medial aspect of the cheek, and the chin. Normally it suffices to test light touch and pin prick alone, but occasionally it is necessary to assess temperature appreciation.

With the patient's eyes closed test light touch by touching the appropriate areas of the face with a wisp of cotton wool (Fig. 12.91). Wait for a response after each contact and do not prompt the patient. Avoid dragging the stimulus across the skin. A partial loss

Course of the trigeminal nerve

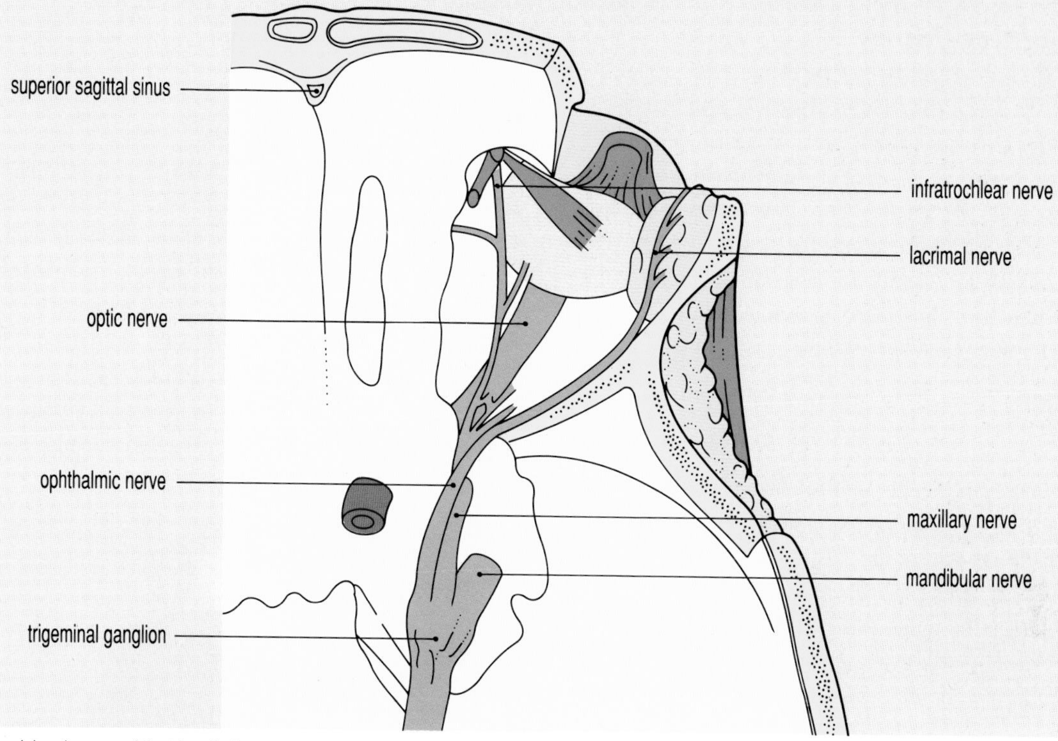

Fig. 12.89 The peripheral course of the trigeminal nerve.

Divisions of the trigeminal nerve

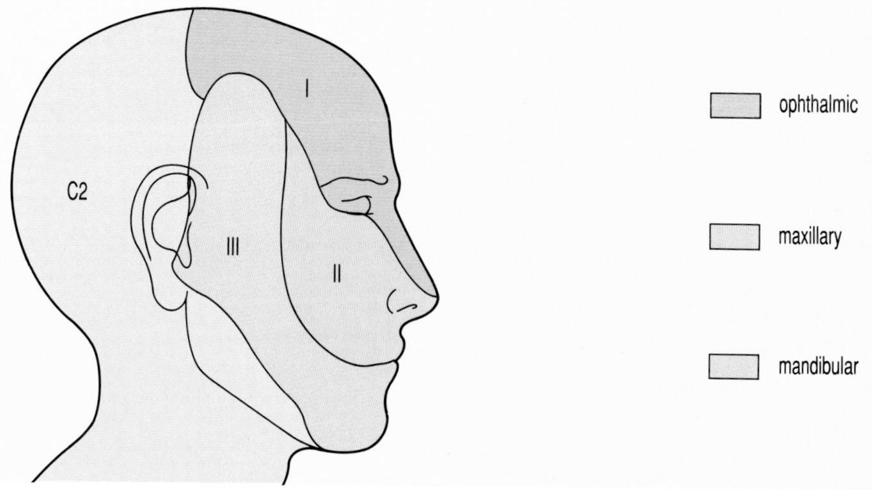

Fig. 12.90 Cutaneous distribution of the three divisions of the trigeminal nerve.

of sensation is more likely than total anaesthesia, so ask the patient to compare the stimulus with sites in other divisions of the nerve on that side, then with comparable areas on the other side of the face. Now test pin prick sensation at the same sites. In addition, the pin can be moved backwards across the scalp and the patient's responses noted. If there is a sensory loss confined to the trigeminal nerve distribution, the response to this stimulus becomes normal at the level of the vertex. Remember that the border between the territory of the mandibular division and the second cervical segment does not correspond to the jaw line, but extends well above it on to the cheek (Fig. 12.90). Again, variations in the response at different sites should be noted. Since it is difficult to repeat the stimulus with equal force, minor differences of sensitivity should be ignored unless they are consistent.

Malignant invasion of the nerve, or its ganglion, produces both pain and functional disturbance. In isolated trigeminal neuropathy, motor function is spared, but there is progressive loss of facial sensation. When the sensory loss is profound, inadvertent self-injury can result in tissue necrosis (Fig. 12.92).

Disorders of the central sensory pathways can result in selective loss of function. In spinal cord lesions above C2, selective loss of facial pain and temperature sense is possible, sometimes with an 'onion ring' distribution which crosses dermatomal boundaries (Fig. 12.88). Loss of facial pain and temperature sense occurs ipsilateral to an infarct in the distribution of the posterior inferior cerebellar artery. Depression of light touch alone results from pontine damage confined to the main sensory nucleus. A hemisensory loss which includes the face can follow thalamic infarction.

The corneal response

The corneal response is elicited by lightly touching the cornea with cotton wool. Carefully explain the procedure to the patient before proceeding. The lower part of the cornea can be tested without depressing the lid, by asking the patient to look slightly upwards. In order to stimulate the upper cornea, the upper lid should be retracted. The patient's subjective reaction is assessed and the ipsilateral and contralateral blink reaction noted. Corneal sensitivity varies considerably. Patients who wear contact lenses will need to remove them first; even then dulling of the response is likely, but it will be symmetrical. If the response is substantially depressed, the cotton wool can be held against the cornea without provoking a reaction (Fig. 12.93). Testing the response in an unconscious patient must be done with great care. Repeated stimulation can easily traumatize the cornea. The response will be depressed or absent ipsilateral to a facial palsy affecting orbicularis oculi; the contralateral reaction remains intact.

Loss of the corneal response is sometimes the first or an early sign of the effect of nerve compression, and should be looked for in all patients complaining of facial pain. A depressed response ipsilateral to a deaf ear is a valuable clue to the presence of a cerebellopontine angle tumour.

MOTOR

Look for muscle wasting before testing the muscles of mastication. Wasting of temporalis produces hollowing above the zygoma (Fig. 12.94). Wasting of the masseter is more difficult to detect, but both masseter and temporalis can be palpated while the teeth are clenched (Fig. 12.95). The power of pterygoids and of masseter and temporalis can be assessed by resisting the patient's attempts at opening and closing the jaw respectively. Ask the patient to open the jaw first without, then with, resistance. In a unilateral trigeminal lesion the jaw deviates to the paralysed side (Fig. 12.96).

Light touch

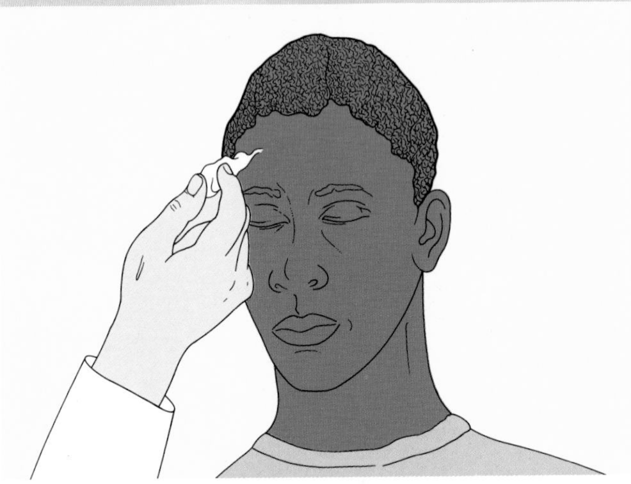

Fig. 12.91 Testing light touch sensation.

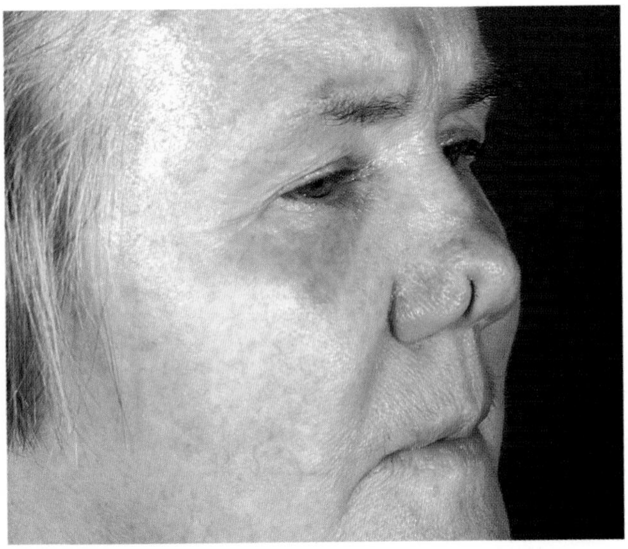

Fig. 12.92 Tissue necrosis consequent to loss of nasal sensation.

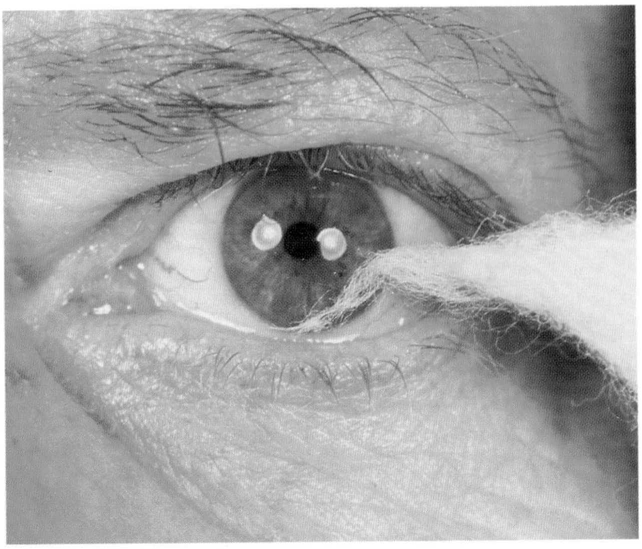

Fig. 12.93 A depressed left corneal response.

The jaw jerk

Ask the patient to open the mouth slightly. Rest your index finger on the apex of the jaw and tap it with the patella hammer (Fig. 12.97). The response, a contraction of the pterygoid muscles, varies widely in normal individuals. In many it is imperceptible, in others surprisingly brisk.

THE FACIAL (7TH) NERVE

STRUCTURE AND FUNCTION

Fibres from the seventh nerve nucleus loop around the lower end of the abducens nucleus before leaving the pons in close proximity to the acoustic nerve. Having crossed the cerebellopontine angle, the nerve enters the internal auditory meatus along with the

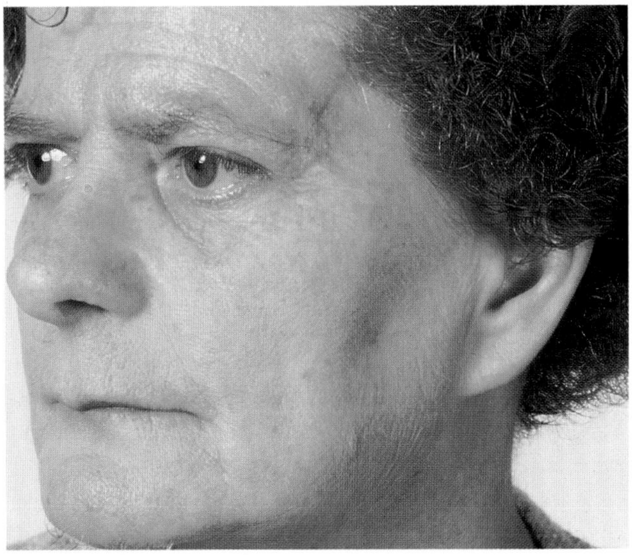

Fig. 12.94 Wasting of the temporalis producing hollowing above the zygoma.

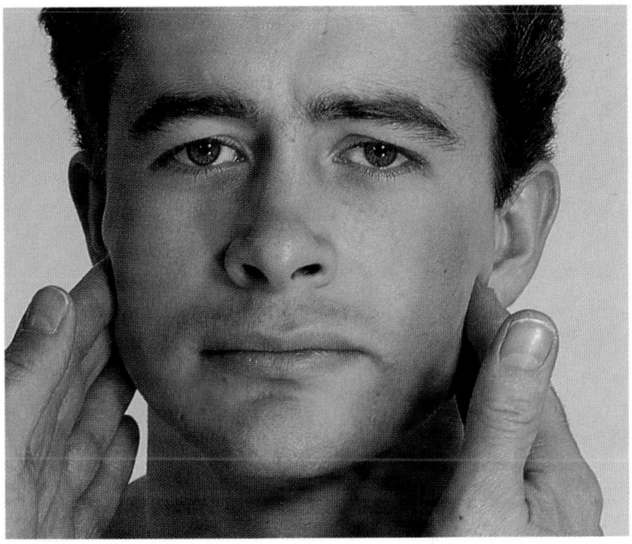

Fig. 12.95 Palpating the masseter muscles.

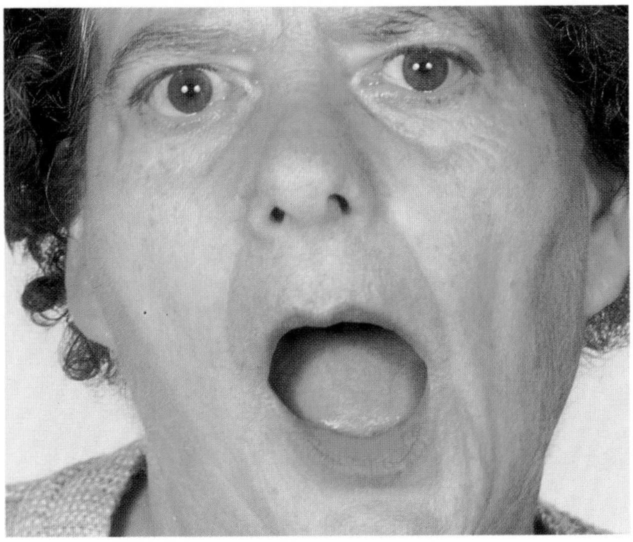

Fig. 12.96 Left trigeminal nerve lesion. Jaw deviation to the left.

The jaw jerk

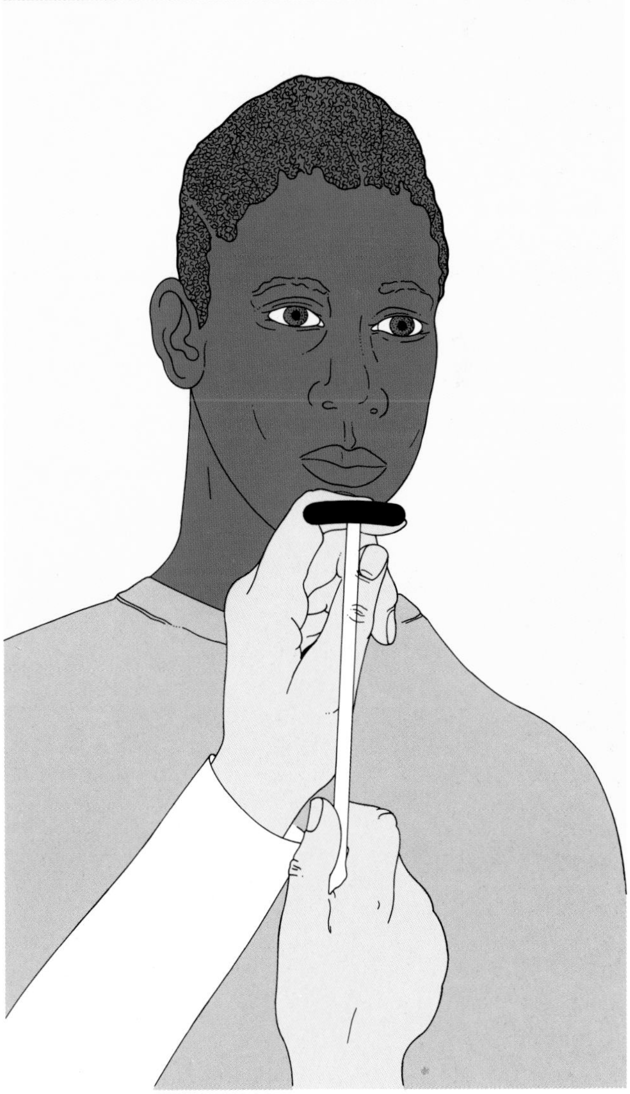

Fig. 12.97 Testing the jaw jerk.

acoustic nerve and the internal auditory artery and vein. Shortly afterwards the facial nerve enters its own canal, passing forwards above the cochlea before bending sharply backwards, at which point the nerve expands to form the geniculate ganglion. Here the greater superficial petrosal nerve leaves, its fibres eventually reaching the lacrimal gland via the sphenopalatine ganglion (Fig. 12.98). The nerve to stapedius and the chorda tympani leave the facial nerve before its exit from the stylomastoid foramen. Parasympathetic fibres in the chorda tympani supply the submandibular and sublingual glands. Special afferent fibres in the nerve supply taste sensation to the anterior two-thirds of the tongue. After leaving the stylomastoid foramen the nerve courses through the parotid gland on its way to the muscles of facial expression. Of these, frontalis elevates the eyebrow, orbicularis oculi closes the eye and orbicularis oris the mouth, while platysma depresses the angle of the mouth. The buccinator muscle, also supplied by the facial nerve, assists in mastication.

Frontalis receives an innervation from both cortices, but the muscles of the lower face are innervated solely by the contralateral hemisphere (Fig. 12.99). Emotional movements receive an additional supply from other sources,including the thalamus and globus pallidus.

The sensory component of the nerve innervates the external auditory meatus, the tympanic membrane and a small area of skin behind the ear. The taste fibres, having entered the pons, terminate in the nucleus of the tractus solitarius. From here, fibres project to the thalamus and hence the cortical gustatory area.

The intensity of a taste experience is determined by the size of the neural response. Taste buds are found in the tongue, soft palate, pharynx, larynx, and oesophagus. A particular taste represents an amalgam of four primary taste functions, sweet, sour, bitter, and salt, combined with any olfactory stimulating effect that the food or beverage possesses. There is some decline in taste acuity with age, but to a lesser extent than occurs with olfaction.

EXAMINATION

Facial asymmetry is common, as is an asymmetry of movement of the lower face during conversation. Carefully observe the movements of the patient's face while you are taking the history. An asymmetry of blinking is a useful indicator of mild weakness of orbicularis oculi. Decide whether the nasolabial folds are equally well – defined. Note any difference in the position of the two angles of the mouth, but remember that in a long-standing facial weakness fibrotic contracture of the muscles can elevate the angle of the mouth, suggesting that the facial weakness is on the other side. Bilateral facial weakness is easily overlooked. The face lacks expression and appears to sag (Fig. 12.100).

Ask the patient to elevate the eyebrows (Fig. 12.101) then close the eyes tightly. Normally, the eyelashes virtually disappear. A useful sign of a mild weakness is a more marked protrusion of the eyelashes on the affected side (Fig. 12.102). Try to open the eyes by pressing the eyelids apart with your thumbs. If there is no weakness, the patient can prevent the eyelids separating. Now ask the patient to blow out the cheeks, then purse the lips tightly together (Fig. 12.103). At times you will notice a discrepancy between the degree of weakness around the mouth when smiling compared to

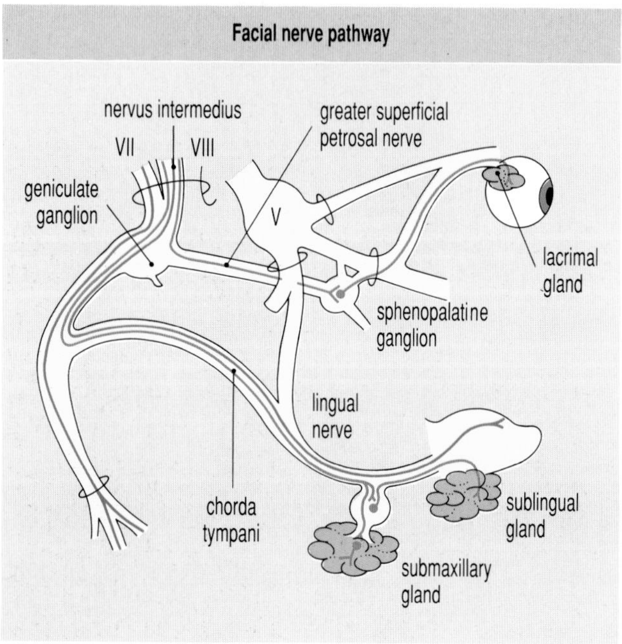

Fig. 12.98 Pathway of the facial nerve.

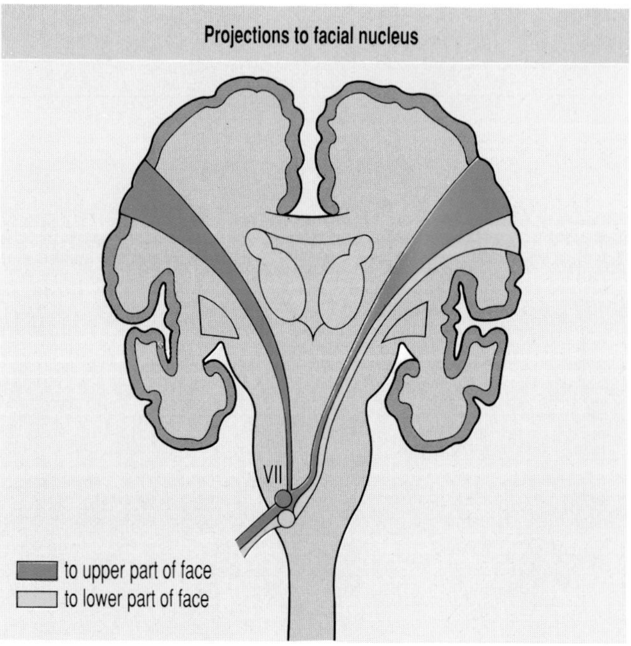

Fig. 12.99 Cortical projections to the facial nerve nucleus.

when making voluntary movements. Finally ask the patient to tighten the neck muscles in order to assess platysma. Weakness of stapedius is suggested if the patient complains of an undue sensitivity (hyperacusis) to noise in the affected ear.

Many patients who complain of an altered sensation of taste are found to have a disturbance of olfaction. Taste is difficult to test. Simply applying drops of a test solution on the protruded tongue seldom produces a consistent response. For assessing seventh nerve function, the stimulus should be confined to the anterior two-thirds of the tongue, each side of which is tested separately. Sweet (sugar), salt, bitter (quinine), and sour (vinegar) solutions are applied in turn, the mouth being washed out with distilled water between testing. The difficulties of testing and the problems in interpretation are such that taste assessment is seldom justified for routine diagnostic purposes. Electrical stimulation of the tongue allows a more objective and accurate measure of taste, although, using a direct current, anodal stimulation produces a sour taste and cathodal stimulation a less clearly definable sensation.The procedure is not used routinely.

The area of skin around the ear which is supplied by the seventh nerve receives overlapping innervation from the fifth and ninth nerves. Nothing is gained, therefore, by testing sensation in this area. The patient can be asked if there has been loss of lacrimation from the eye. Finally look for evidence of abnormal facial movement.

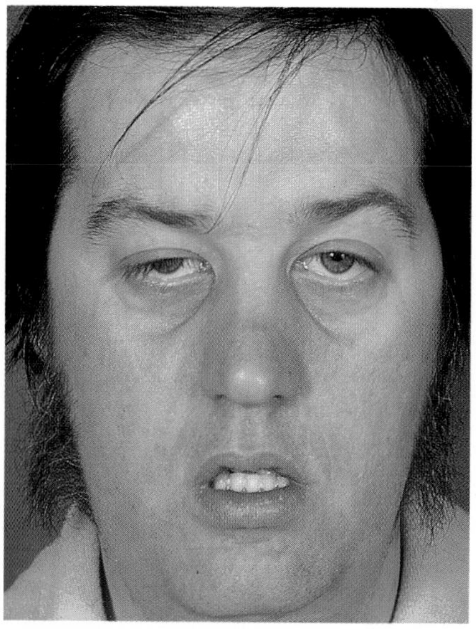

Fig. 12.100 Bilateral facial weakness.

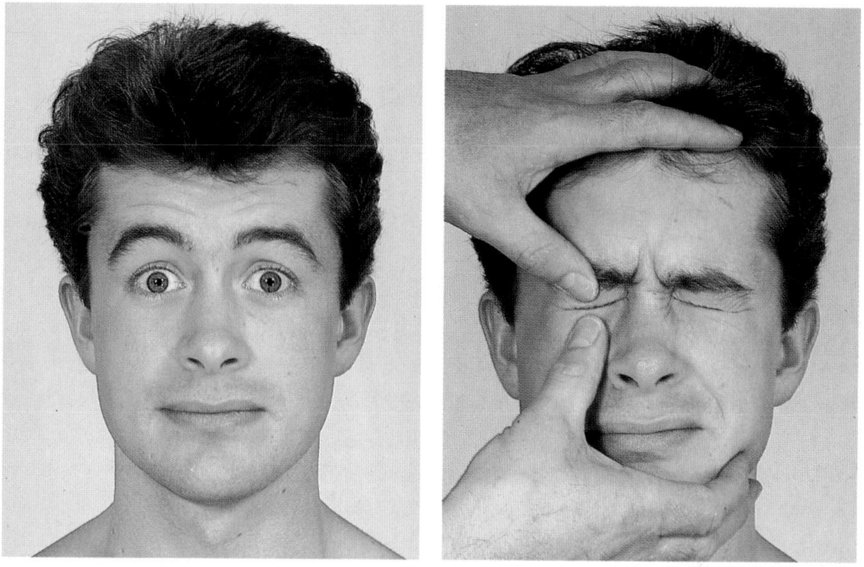

Fig. 12.101 The patient has been asked to elevate the eyebrows, then to close the eyebrows tightly.

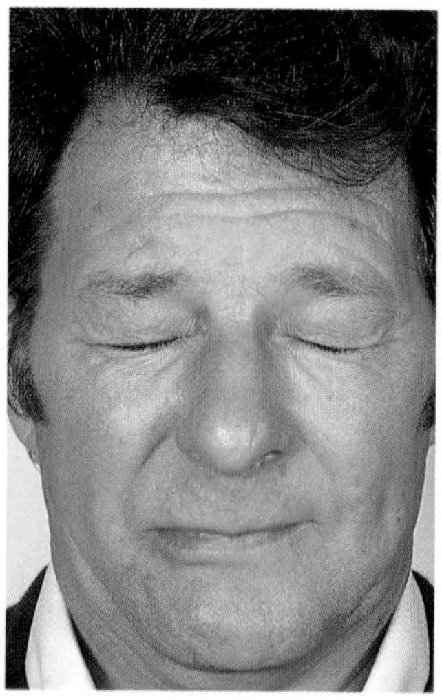

Fig. 12.102 The patient has been asked to close his eyes tightly. The eyelashes on the right are slightly more prominent than those on the left.

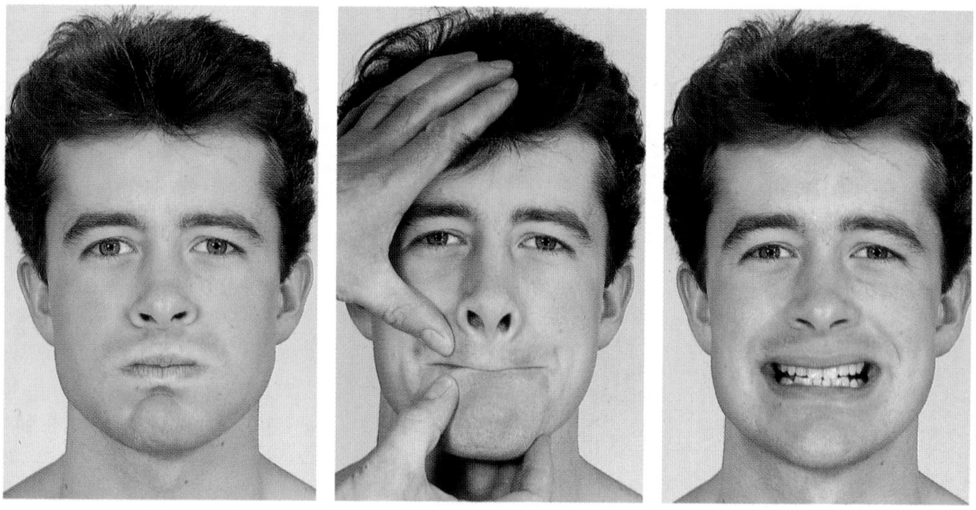

Fig. 12.103 The patient is blowing out the cheeks, pursing his lips and baring his teeth.

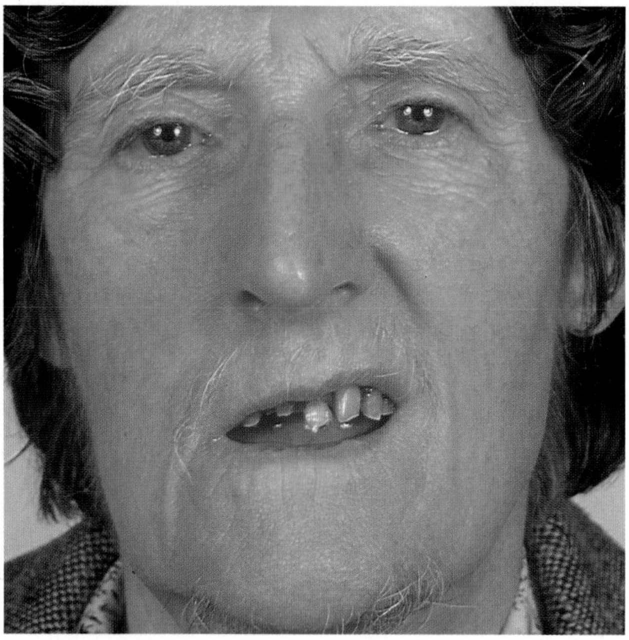

Fig. 12.104 Upper motor neurone facial weakness. The patient has been asked to bare her teeth.

Causes of lower motor neurone facial weakness
Bell's palsy
Ramsay Hunt syndrome
Trauma
Parotid carcinoma
Sarcoidosis
Multiple sclerosis

Fig. 12.105 Causes of lower motor neurone weakness.

Upper motor neurone facial weakness

An upper motor neurone facial weakness results from interruption of descending fibres passing from the contralateral motor cortex to the ipsilateral facial nerve nucleus. There is minimal asymmetry of frontalis contraction on the two sides, but substantial asymmetry of the lower face (Fig. 12.104).

In a lower motor neurone facial weakness, all the facial muscles are equally affected unless the lesion lies so distally that it involves individual branches of the nerve (Fig. 12.105). The site of the lesion can be deduced from the presence or absence of certain symptoms and signs. If it lies at or beyond the stylomastoid foramen,there will be no disturbance of taste, hearing, or lacrimation. Involvement of the nerve immediately proximal to the origin of chorda tympani will result in loss of taste over the anterior two-thirds of the tongue, and still more proximal interruption of stapedius fibres will result in hyperacusis. Loss of lacrimation is added to these other symptoms if the nerve is damaged at, or proximal to, the Gasserian ganglion.

Facial weakness of lower motor neurone type

Q

Have you noticed any loss of taste on the front part of the tongue?

Have you noticed that noises appear excessively loud in the ear on the same side?

Does the eye on that side still water?

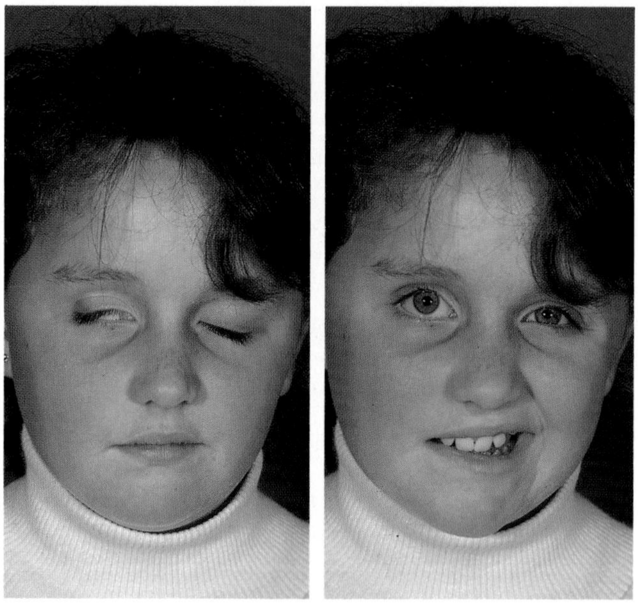

Fig. 12.106 A right Bell's palsy in a girl of 11.

Bell's palsy

Bell's palsy is an idiopathic paralysis of the facial nerve. When the resulting facial weakness is substantial, there is loss of forehead furrowing, eye closure, and mouth elevation (Fig. 12.106). If denervation occurs, regrowth of fibres may extend to muscles not originally part of their innervation (aberrant re-innervation). In such cases blinking can result in synkinetic contraction of muscles in the lower face (Fig. 12.107), and misdirection to the lacrimal gland of fibres originally destined for the salivary glands results in eye watering when a food stimulus appears (crocodile tears).

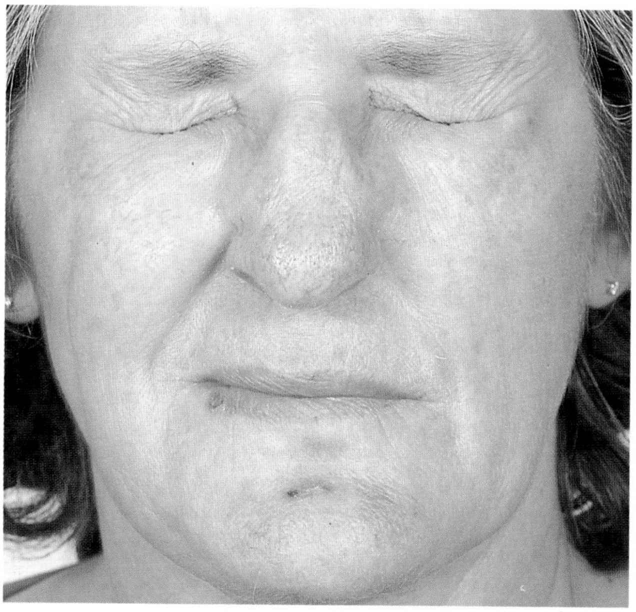

Fig. 12. 107 Aberrant re-innervation. The right angle of the mouth elevates during eye closure. Previous right Bell's palsy.

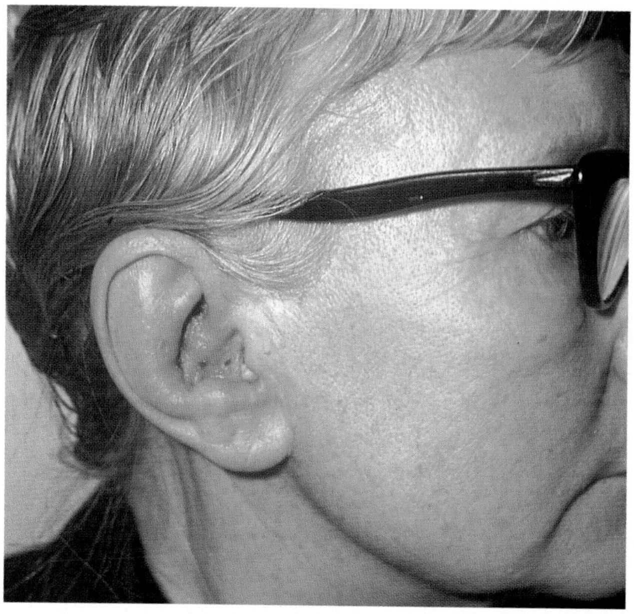

Fig. 12.108 Vesicular eruption in a case of the Ramsay Hunt syndrome.

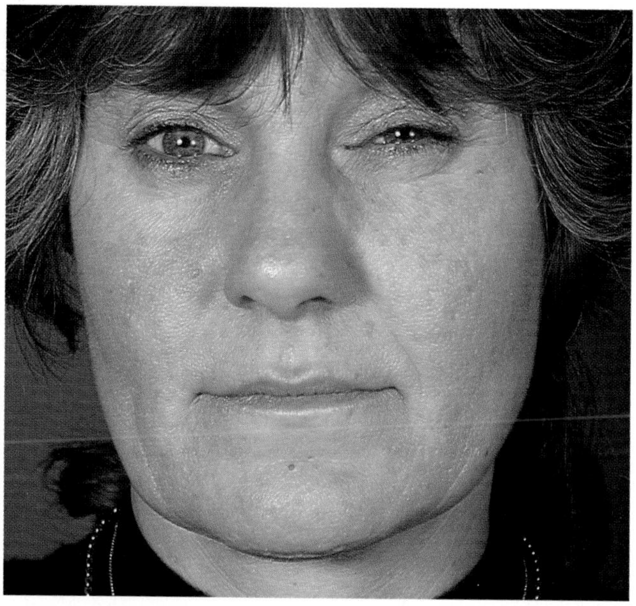

Fig. 12.109 Left hemifacial spasm. The left palpbebral fissure has narrowed during the contraction.

Ramsay Hunt syndrome

The Ramsay Hunt syndrome is the consequence of herpetic involvement of the geniculate ganglion. A vesicular eruption can occur at a number of sites, including the pinna (Fig. 12.108).

Facial movement disorders

Facial fasciculation is virtually confined to patients with motor neurone disease. Facial myokymia is a subtle movement disorder in which a fine, more or less continuous, shimmering contraction of muscles occurs in part or all of the facial nerve distribution. Multiple sclerosis is the commonest cause. In hemifacial spasm, involuntary contraction of facial muscle, often initially confined to orbicularis oculi, occurs in a haphazard fashion (Fig. 12.109). Eventually a mild facial weakness develops. Blepharospasm produces forced repetitive blinking over which the patient has no control. This condition is discussed, along with the other focal dystonias, on page 12.71. Facial tics are repetitive stereotyped movements, partly under voluntary control. Orofacial dyskinesia is an involuntary, semi-repetitive contraction of muscles around the mouth, usually accompanied by abnormal movements of the tongue. It can occur spontaneously, or secondary to phenothiazine therapy. Loss of taste (ageusia) can accompany a facial palsy. It rarely occurs in isolation, the commonest cause being major head injury. A distortion of taste can result from the use of drugs, including captopril.

THE ACOUSTIC (8TH) NERVE

STRUCTURE AND FUNCTION

The eighth nerve comprises vestibular and cochlear divisions which unite within the internal auditory canal. The nerve then crosses the subarachnoid space and enters the brain stem at the junction of pons and medulla, lateral to the facial nerve. In the brain stem the acoustic nerve projects predominantly to the contralateral inferior colliculus. From here fibres pass to the medial geniculate body and then in the auditory radiation to the auditory cortex in the upper aspect of the temporal lobe (Heschl's gyrus). The fibres of the vestibular nerve terminate in four separate nuclei. A projection from the lateral vestibular nucleus forms the vestibulospinal tract, which descends, mainly ipsilaterally, to the cervical and lumbar motor neurones. The medial vestibular nucleus has connections to the contralateral abducens nucleus and the cerebellum. These pathways are important in gaze-holding and for the control of smooth pursuit eye movements (see page 12.31).

Vibration of the tympanic membrane, triggered by a sound stimulus, is transmitted through a chain of three ossicles (the malleus, incus, and stapes) situated in the middle ear (Fig. 12.110). The movements of the ossicles are also influenced by the tensor tympani and stapedius muscles. The base of the stapes is attached to the oval window. Vibration of the oval window sets up movement in the perilymph which occupies the bony labyrinth, comprising the cochlea, the vestibule, and the semicircular canals. Lying within the bony labyrinth, and containing endolymph, is the membranous labyrinth comprising the cochlear duct, the saccule, the utricle, and three semicircular ducts. The semicircular canals, each surrounding a semicircular duct, are arranged in planes roughly at right angles to each other. The canals open into the vestibule which contains the saccule and utricle. Specialized receptor areas (maculae) are found in the saccule and utricle. At one end of each semicircular canal is a receptor organ (crista ampullaris).

The inferior part of the bony labyrinth contains the osseous canal of the cochlea. A bony spur, the osseous spiral lamina projects into the canal dividing it into two corridors: the scala vestibuli and the scala tympani (Fig. 12.111). In the wall of the cochlear duct, resting on the basilar membrane, is the spiral organ of Corti which is innervated by the cochlear component of the auditory nerve. The vestibular component innervates the specialized receptor areas of the utricle and the semicircular canals. The saccule, and part of the posterior semicircular canal, receives fibres from the cochlear division (Fig. 12.112).

Sound waves, transmitted through the perilymph, reach the organ of Corti via the ossicular chain, by vibration of the round window or by bony transmission. High-frequency waves produce a maximal response in the basal part of the cochlea, and low-frequency waves at its apex. Activity in the components of the auditory brain stem pathway is reflected in a succession of negative potentials recorded from mastoid and scalp electrodes following a click stimulus. Seven potentials occurring within the first 10 ms of the stimulus are thought to relate to specific anatomical sites (Fig. 12.113).

Middle and inner ear

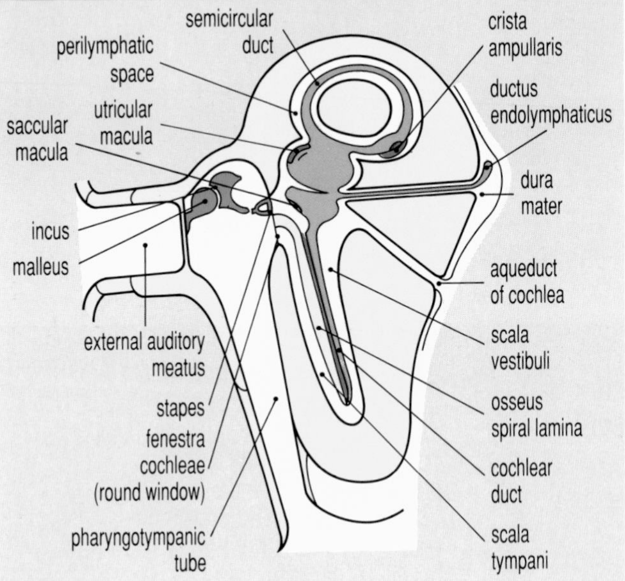

Fig. 12.110 Organization of the middle and inner ear. The endolymphatic system is coloured.

Acoustic nerve

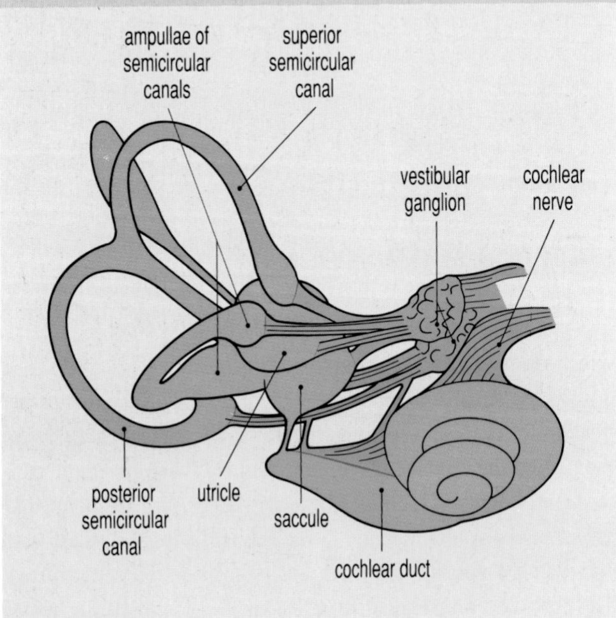

Fig. 12.111 Distribution of the vestibular and cochlear compartments of the acoustic nerve.

Cochlea

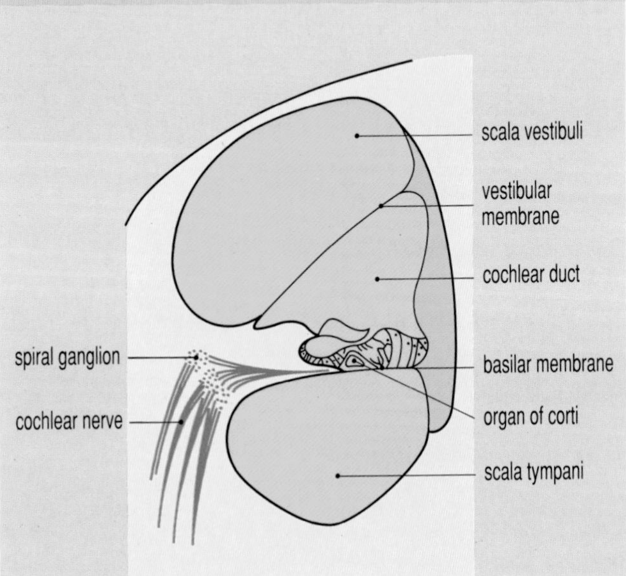

Fig. 12.112 The cochlea.

The nerve endings in the cristae and maculae are triggered by movements of the endolymph either from stimulation of the hair processes of the cristae or by movements of small calcific particles (the otoliths) embedded in a membrane of the maculae of the utricle and saccule. Head position is coded by the receptors of the utricle and saccule. Head tilt shifts the otoliths, displaces the hair cells and initiates an action potential in the fibres of the vestibular nerve. The semicircular canals are responsible for the detection of rotational head movements, via patterns of flow produced in the endolymphatic system.

Overall the vestibular system provides information on head posture and movement, integrated with visual data and proprioceptive information arising from neck muscle receptors.

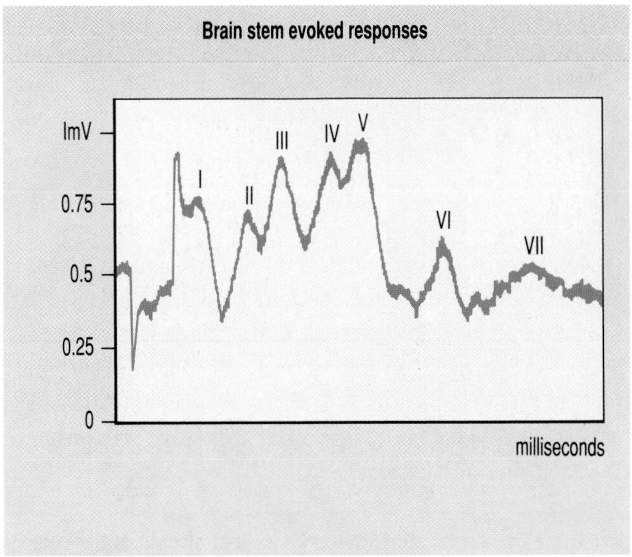

Fig. 12.113 Normal brain stem auditory evoked responses.

EXAMINATION

AUDITORY FUNCTION

Each ear is tested separately. Ask the patient to occlude the ear not being tested by pressing on the tragus. Hearing sensitivity can be assessed by the capacity to hear a whispered sound (normally possible at least 0.8m away), a wristwatch (possible at about 0.75m) or the sound of the fingers being rubbed together. Further tests are required to determine whether any loss of hearing is the result of damage to the cochlea or cochlear nerve (perceptive or nerve deafness) or the conducting system leading to the cochlea (conductive deafness).

Rinne test

Place a 512Hz tuning fork on the mastoid process then hold it adjacent to the pinna (Fig. 12.114a and b). Ask the patient which sound appears louder. Normally, air conduction is better perceived than bone conduction (Rinne positive). In perceptive deafness this discrepancy remains, but in conductive deafness it is reversed (Fig. 114c and d).

Weber's test

Place a 512Hz tuning fork at the midline over the vertex or on the forehead and ask the patient whether the sound appears equally loud in each ear, or more so in one than the other. Normally, the sound is perceived equally by the two ears, but it is heard better by the intact ear in perceptive deafness, and by the affected ear in conductive deafness (Fig. 12.115).

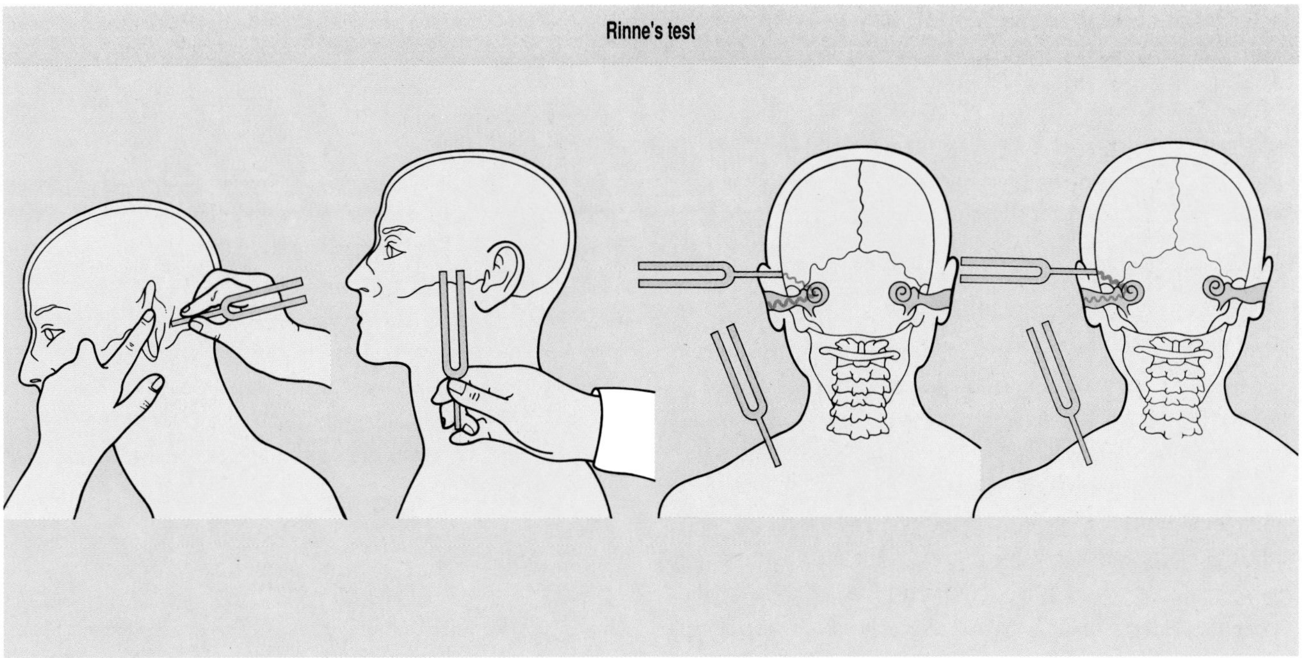

Fig. 12.114 Rinne's test. Comparison of (a) bone conduction and (b) air conduction. (c) Perceptive deafness (d) conductive deafness

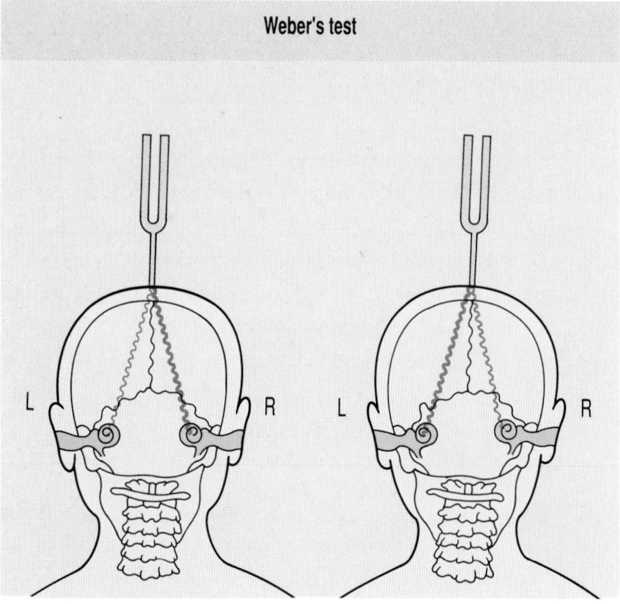

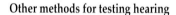

Fig. 12.115 Weber's test. Left sided perceptive deafness (left) and left sided conductive deafness (right).

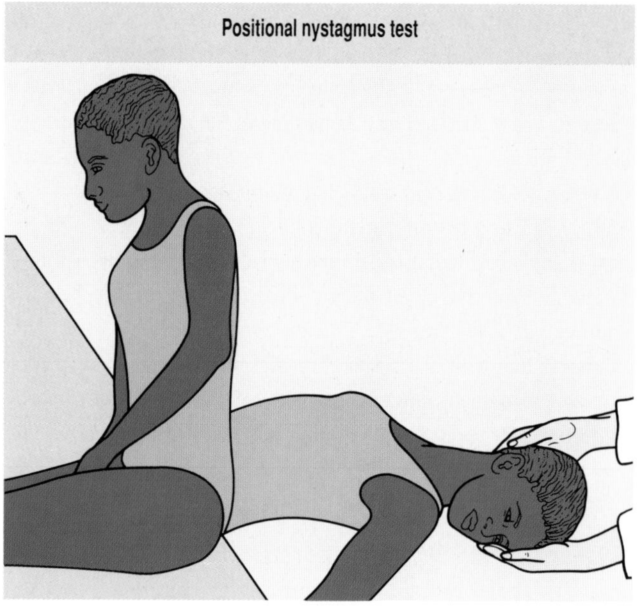

Fig. 12.116 Testing for positional nystagmus.

Other methods for testing hearing

More accurate measurement of hearing requires specialized techniques. Pure tone audiometry delivers tones between 250 and 8000Hz either to the ear or the mastoid process. Perceptive deafness principally affects the higher frequencies. Speech audiometry measures the threshold for speech sounds of differing intensity. When a cochlear lesion causes nerve deafness, speech recognition initially improves but later deteriorates as the sound intensity increases. In conductive deafness, discrimination tends to be preserved if a sufficiently loud stimulus is used. Loudness recruitment is tested by presenting sounds of gradually increasing intensity to each ear separately. Recruitment is present when loud sounds are heard equally well in the two ears but quiet sounds less well in the deaf ear. Recruitment is a feature of cochlear deafness. Tone decay assesses to what degree and how quickly a sound of fixed intensity appears to diminish. Abnormal tone decay is more marked in nerve, rather than conductive, deafness.

VESTIBULAR FUNCTION

There are no direct bedside methods for assessing vestibular function. An acute peripheral vestibular disturbance is suggested by a combination of physical findings. A unidirectional jerk/rotatory nystagmus occurs, with the slow component to the side of the affected ear. With the eyes closed the patient tends to fall to the side of the slow phase of the nystagmus and will point to that side of a stationary target. A sense of rotation of the environment is experienced in the direction of the fast phase of the nystagmus. If these findings are less clear-cut, then a disorder of the central vestibular pathways is likely. If a patient complains of positional vertigo, then the effect of posture should be included in the examination (see also page 12.36). Position the patient at the edge of the examination couch, facing away from the edge, then depress the head and trunk so that the head is almost 30° below the horizontal but turned first to one side then the other (Fig. 12.116). Do make sure that you are able to support the patient's weight before attempting the manoeuvre. If nystagmus appears, record whether it begins immediately or after an interval, whether it persists or fatigues and if it then reappears when the patient returns to the sitting position. Warn the patient that vertigo may be experienced, and explain that the eyes should be kept open during the manoeuvre. If the test proves positive, ask the patient whether the symptoms resembled those of the presenting disorder.

Caloric testing

Caloric testing is used to assess vestibular function. The patient lies supine with the head at 30° above the horizontal. In this position, the lateral semicircular canal lies in the vertical plane. Water at 7°C above and below body temperature is instilled into the external auditory meatus. Around 250 ml of water is instilled over 40s. With cold water the normal response is a second degree jerk nystagmus beating away from the irrigated ear. The time is recorded from the beginning of irrigation to the cessation of nystagmus. The nystagmus is enhanced if ocular fixation is abolished.

Canal paresis

In the presence of labyrinthine disease, responses from one ear, whether to hot or cold water, may be diminished or absent – canal paresis (Fig. 12.117).

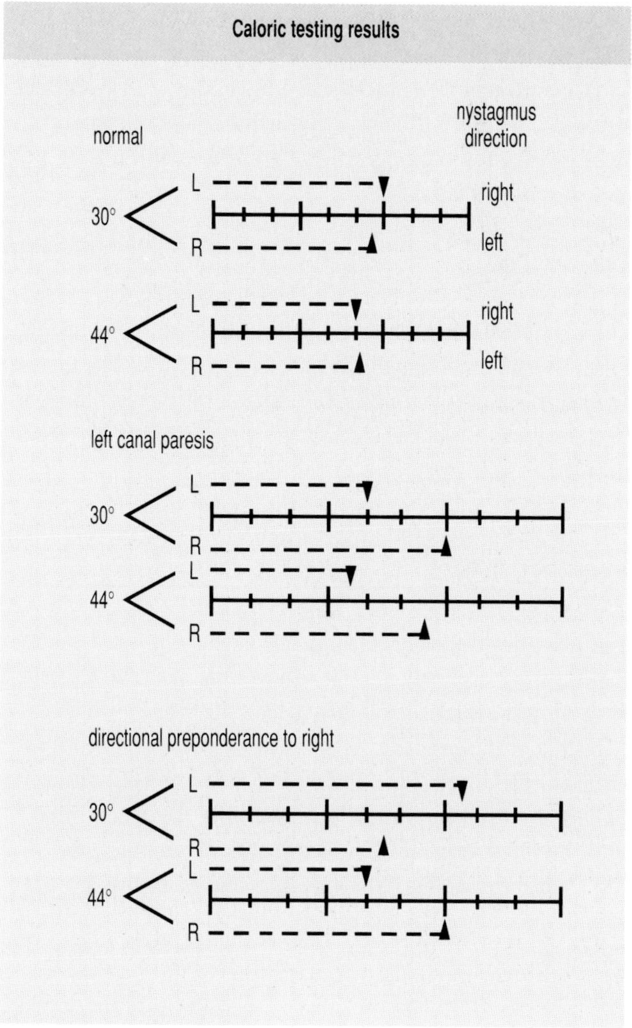

Fig. 12.117 Results of caloric testing.

Directional preponderance

Directional preponderance exists if the duration of nystagmus in one direction, whether triggered by hot or cold water, exceeds that in the other. Directional preponderance is found with both temporal lobe and brain stem lesions.

CLINICAL APPLICATION

Deafness

Conductive deafness is usually due to either debris or wax in the external auditory meatus, loss of elasticity of the ossicular chain (otosclerosis), or disease of the middle ear. Nerve deafness occurs with end-organ change (e.g. in Menière's disease) or consequent to a disturbance of the auditory nerve itself (e.g. following occlusion of the internal auditory artery). Lesions of the central nervous system rarely cause deafness because of the bilateral projections of the central auditory pathways at multiple levels.

Dizziness

Does the patient describe dizziness or giddiness or is there an experience of rotation, either of the patient or of the environment (vertigo)?

Is the dizziness accompained by an unsteadiness when walking?

Is any vertigo triggered only by a certain movement or head posture?

Tinnitus

Patients with tinnitus complain of noise in one or both ears. The noise may be continuous or intermittent and of varying pitch. The symptom occurs with cochlear disease or damage, or with compression of the auditory nerve. Some patients with abnormal intracranial blood flow, for example through an arteriovenous malformation, are able to hear the flow and describe it as a form of pulsatile tinnitus. In these patients a bruit is usually audible over the skull.

Vertigo

Vertigo is a sense of rotation either of the individual or of the environment. Patients rarely complain of persistent vertigo though many describe a persistent dizziness or giddiness, much less clear-cut symptoms which commonly elude diagnosis. Vertigo is usually a result of disruption of either the labyrinthine system (peripheral vertigo) or the central connections of the vestibular nerve (central vertigo).

Epidemic labyrinthitis and acute vestibular neuronitis

These diagnoses have been applied to patients who give a history of acute vertigo, often with vomiting, together with ataxia and malaise on the assumption that an acute disruption of the labyrinth or the vestibular nerve has occurred.

Benign positional vertigo

Benign positional vertigo is a more specific, peripheral, vestibular dysfunction. Patients complain of attacks of vertigo, typically triggered by lying down in bed on one particular side. Tests for positional nystagmus are positive. The condition, sometimes triggered by head injury but often spontaneous, remits within a few weeks but is liable to briefly relapse over subsequent years. Patients with peripheral vestibular disorders are ataxic while the vertigo persists, but not at other times.

Meniére's disease

In Meniére's disease, thought to be the consequence of a distention of the endolymphatic space, paroxysms of vertigo occur together with a persistent unilateral tinnitus and progressive sensorineural deafness.

Central vertigo

Central vertigo is likely to persist longer than peripheral vertigo; and if posture related, is less likely to be delayed in onset, or to fatigue, after posture change than benign positional vertigo. Both cerebrovascular disease and multiple sclerosis are common causes of a central vestibular disturbance. Usually other signs of brain stem disease are evident.

THE GLOSSOPHARYNGEAL (9TH) NERVE

STRUCTURE AND FUNCTION

The ninth, tenth, and eleventh cranial nerves share a motor nucleus (nucleus ambiguus) which innervates the striated muscle of the pharynx, larynx, and upper oesophagus (Fig. 12.118). Corticobulbar fibres destined for each nucleus ambiguus originate in both cerebral hemispheres. The glossopharyngeal nerve emerges from the upper part of the medulla bounded above and below by the facial nerve and the vagus. It leaves the skull through the jugular foramen in company with the vagus and the accessory nerves. The general visceral efferent and special visceral afferent fibres are not readily testable. Somatic afferent components in the glossopharyngeal nerve supply a number of structures including the tonsillar fossa and parts of the pharynx. For a discussion of taste function, see page 12.49. Arterial baroreceptors in the carotid sinus are innervated by the glossopharyngeal nerve, while those in the aortic arch are innervated by the vagus.

The gag reflex

The gag reflex is triggered by applying a stimulus to the tonsillar fossa. The end result is midline elevation of the palate. The afferent arc probably travels in the glossopharyngeal nerve only if the stimulus is painful. The efferent arc, supplying levator palati, passes in the vagus.

EXAMINATION

The motor innervation of the ninth nerve cannot be tested, nor can the cutaneous distribution in the region of the pinna be separated from the overlapping contribution of the seventh and tenth nerves.

Testing of the gag reflex is an uncomfortable experience and should be performed only if there is a suspicion of a disturbance of the lower cranial nerves. Clearly indicate to the patient what is involved. Press the end of an orange stick first into one tonsillar fossa then the other (Fig. 12.119). Besides confirming that the palate rises in the midline, ask the patient if the sensation is comparable on the two sides. In the presence of a glossopharyngeal lesion, the gag reflex is depressed or absent on that side.

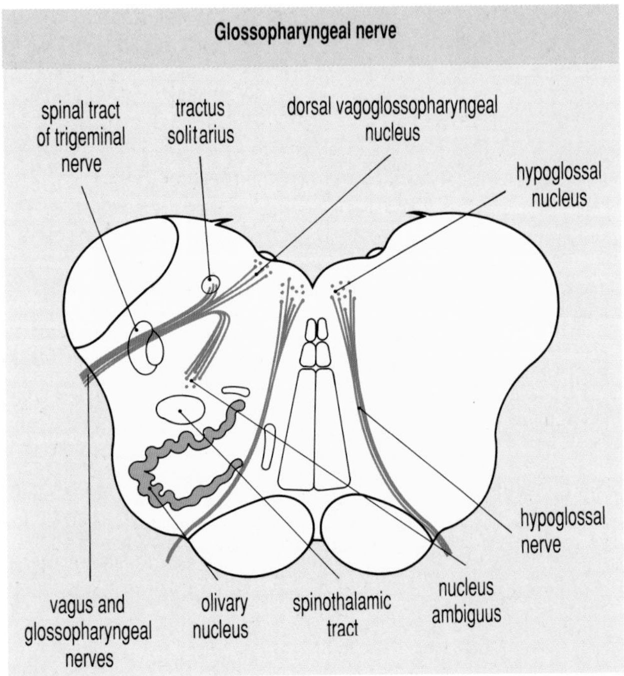

Fig. 12.118 Relationship of the central components of the glossopharyngeal nerve.

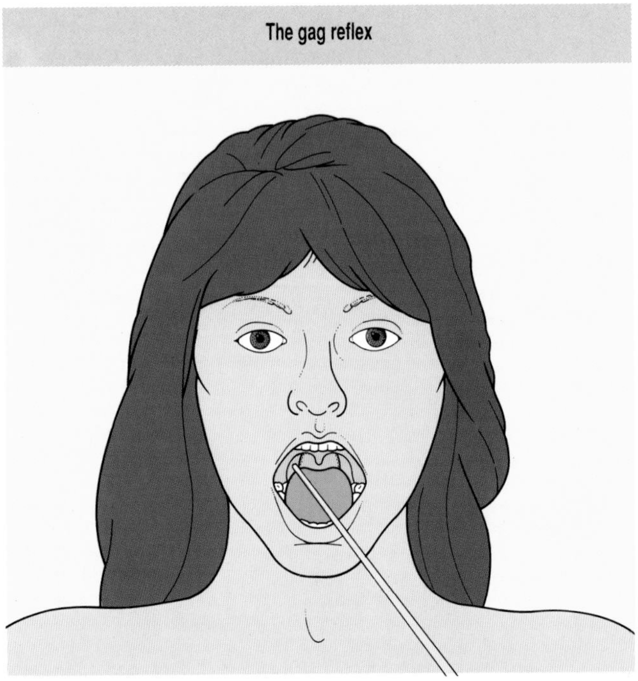

Fig. 12.119 The gag reflex. The orange stick is pressed into the base of the tonsillar fossa.

CLINICAL APPLICATION

Isolated lesions of the ninth nerve are almost unknown. A destructive process in the region of the jugular foramen, most commonly a nasopharyngeal carcinoma, disrupts the ninth, tenth, and eleventh cranial nerves. In the Chiari malformation, stretching of the ninth nerve can lead to depression of the gag reflex on one or both sides. Glossopharyngeal neuralgia usually results from distortion of the nerve by a tumour or a vascular anomaly. Paroxysms of pain in the tongue, soft palate, or tonsil are triggered by swallowing, chewing, or protruding the tongue. Involvement of fibres from the carotid sinus can result in syncopal attacks occurring at the time of the painful paroxysms, or triggered independently by swallowing.

THE VAGUS (10TH) NERVE

STRUCTURE AND FUNCTION

The roots of the vagus leave the medulla immediately below the glossopharyngeal nerve. Both nerves pass through the jugular foramen alongside the accessory nerve. The components of the vagus mirror those of the glossopharyngeal nerve. The special efferent fibres innervate the striated muscle of the pharynx, larynx, and upper oesophagus. The recurrent laryngeal branch of the vagus supplies all the intrinsic muscles of the larynx except for cricothyroid, which is supplied by the external branch of the nerve.

In the heart, fibres from the right vagus end principally around the sinoatrial node, while those from the left end principally around the atrio-ventricular node. Vagal fibres innervating the aortic arch are concerned with the baroreceptor reflex.

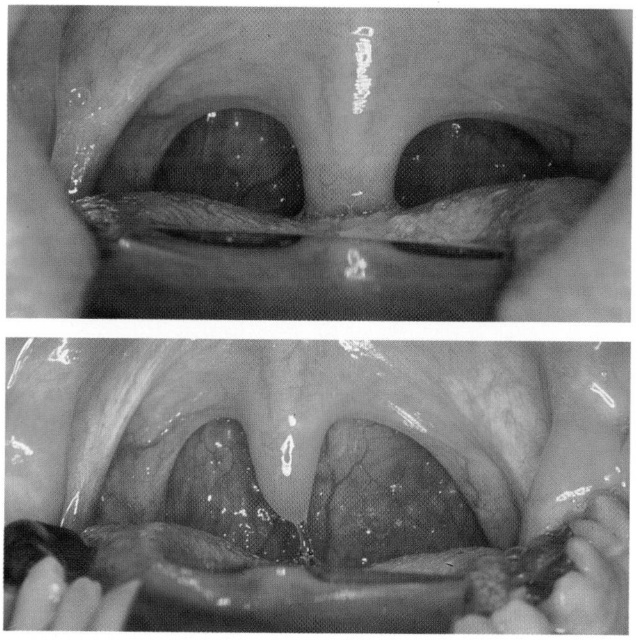

Fig. 12.120 Palsy of the left vagus. The palate deviates to the right on phonation (below).

EXAMINATION

Bedside evaluation is confined to assessment of spontaneous and reflex movements of the uvula and posterior pharyngeal wall. A unilateral lesion of the vagus produces paralysis of the ipsilateral soft palate. At rest, the palate lies slightly lower on the affected side then deviates to the intact side during phonation or on testing the gag reflex (Fig. 12.120). An accompanying deviation of the median raphe of the posterior pharyngeal wall is more characteristic of a glossopharyngeal, rather than a vagal, lesion. Minor deviations of the uvula, particularly if not consistent, should be ignored.

Indirect laryngoscopy is not considered part of the clinical examination, but it is worth summarizing the findings of this technique in unilateral or bilateral vagal lesions. In a unilateral lesion of the vagus there is ipsilateral paralysis of the vocal cord. An initial hoarseness tends to lessen. When the lesion is of the recurrent laryngeal nerve, the abductors tend to be paralysed before the adductors (Fig. 12.121), so that the affected cord lies close to the midline. When the lesion is more complete, the cord comes to lie in a position between adduction and abduction. Bilateral palsies of the vagus produce severe palatal palsy, with nasal regurgitation and aphonia. If there are bilateral palsies of the recurrent laryngeal nerves, and adduction is relatively spared, the cords lie close to the midline and severe restriction of the airway results in stridor. Unilateral loss of the parasympathetic component of the vagus is not detectable clinically. Bilateral loss can lead to a short-lived tachycardia.

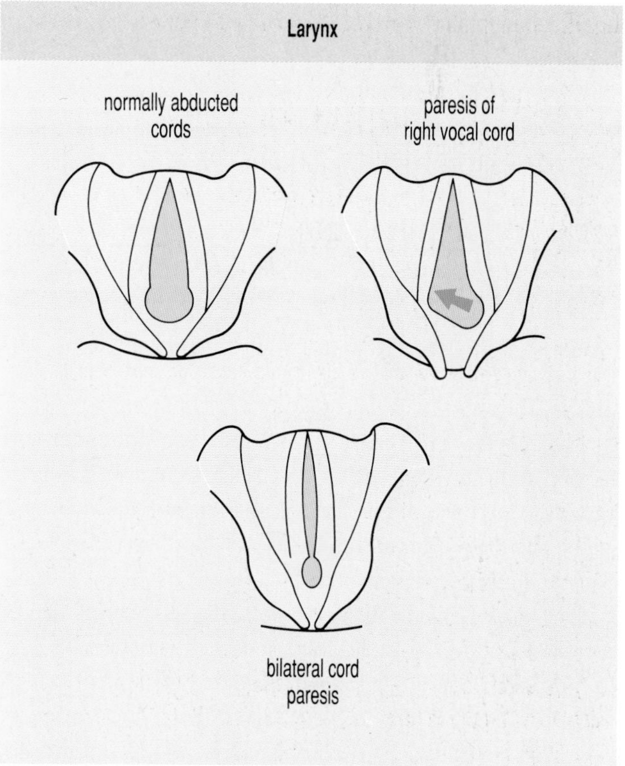

Fig. 12.121 View of the larynx by indirect laryngoscopy. Normally abducted cords (top), paresis of the right vocal cord (centre) and bilateral cord paresis (bottom).

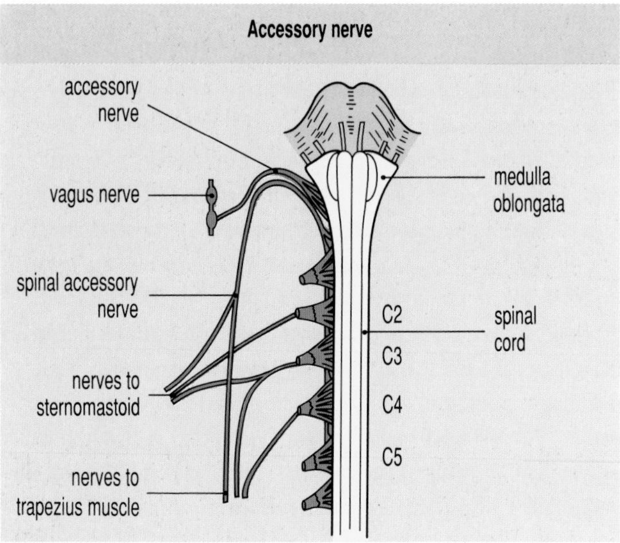

Fig. 12.122 Distribution of the components of the accessory nerve.

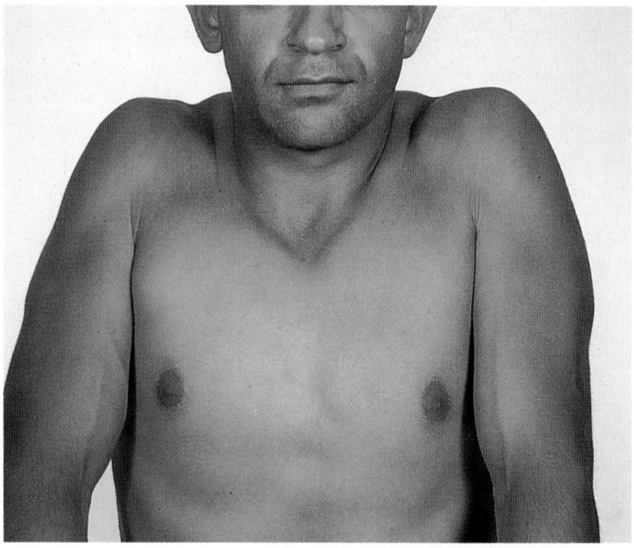

Fig. 12.123 Testing the trapezius muscles. The shoulders are elevated first without, then with resistance.

CLINICAL APPLICATION

A unilateral disturbance of the corticobulbar projection to the nucleus ambiguus is usually without consequence. However, bilateral supranuclear lesions, for example due to cerebrovascular disease, are symptomatic (see page 12.60). Nuclear vagal lesions occur in polio and following lateral medullary infarction. The main branch of the vagus is seldom affected in isolation. Recurrent laryngeal palsies are more common, and are usually left-sided because of the longer course of the nerve on that side. Causes include aortic aneurysm, thyroid surgery, and malignant invasion of the mediastinum. Isolated laryngeal palsies are often of unknown etiology.

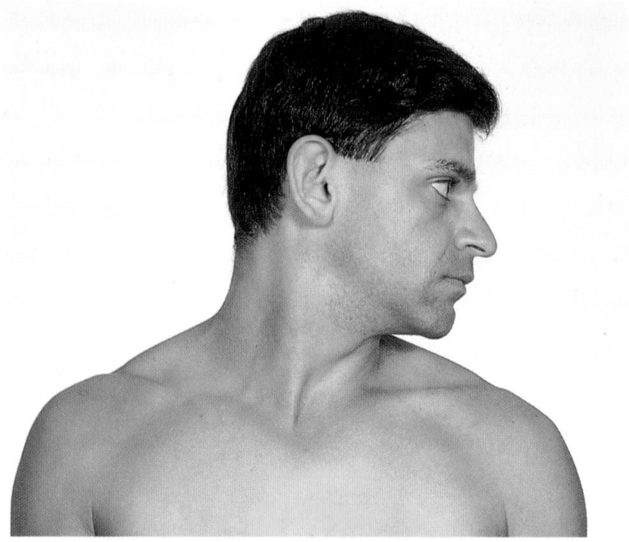

Fig. 12.124 Testing head rotation.

THE ACCESSORY (11TH) NERVE

STRUCTURE AND FUNCTION

The accessory nerve has both cranial and spinal components. The cranial part originates from the nucleus ambiguus and exits from the medulla in line with the ninth and tenth cranial nerves (Fig. 12.122). The spinal part is formed by a series of rootlets which emerge from the lateral aspect of the cervical spinal cord down to the fifth segment. The rootlets form a single trunk which ascends alongside the cord, passes through the foramen magnum and unites with the cranial component. The combined nerve leaves the skull through the jugular foramen.

The cranial root joins the vagus while the spinal root receives contributions from the second, third, and fourth cervical roots (Fig. 12.122) before innervating sternomastoid and the upper fibres of trapezius. The fibres from the second and third cervical roots passing to the sternomastoid are probably proprioceptive, whereas the fibres from the third and fourth roots to the lower part of trapezius are purely motor.

The spinal accessory nucleus receives innervation from both cerebral hemispheres. Those fibres concerned with the innervation of sternomastoid possibly undergo a double decussation within the brain stem.

EXAMINATION

There is no way of assessing the innervation of the cranial component of the accessory nerve, but that of the spinal component can be assessed by examining trapezius and sternomastoid. The function of trapezius is assessed by asking the patient to elevate the shoulder, first without, then with, resistance (Fig. 12.123). The strength of contraction of sternomastoid can be gauged by asking the patient to rotate the head to the relevant side against resistance (Fig. 12.124).

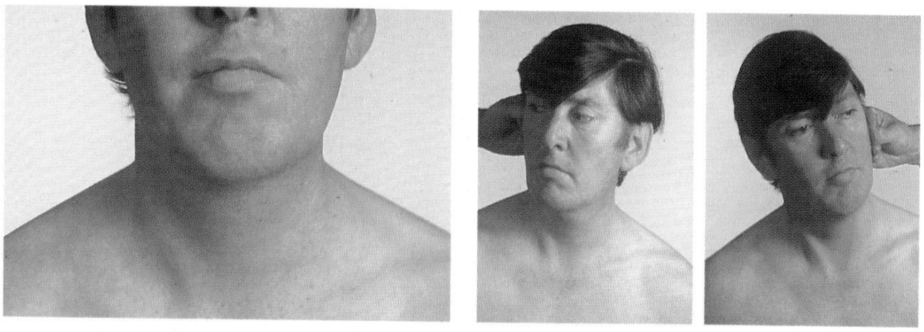

Fig. 12.125 Left accessory nerve lesion. The left sternomastoid is less conspicuous (left) and fails to stand out during neck rotation (right).

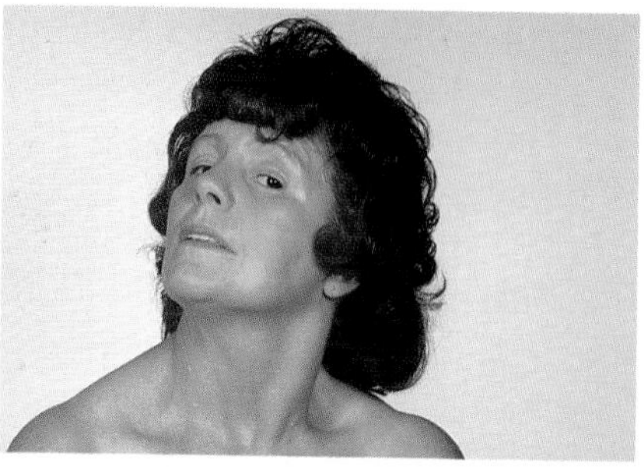

Fig. 12.126 Spasmodic torticollis associated with contraction of the left sternomastoid.

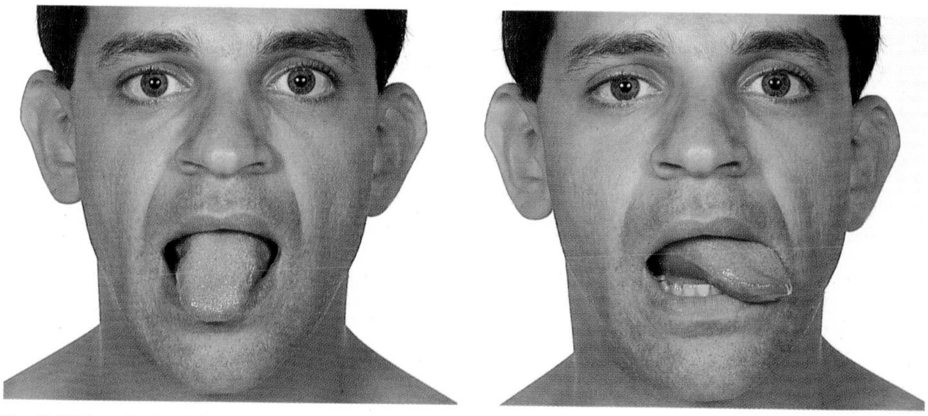

Fig. 12.127 Examination of the tongue. Protusion (left) and lateral movements (right).

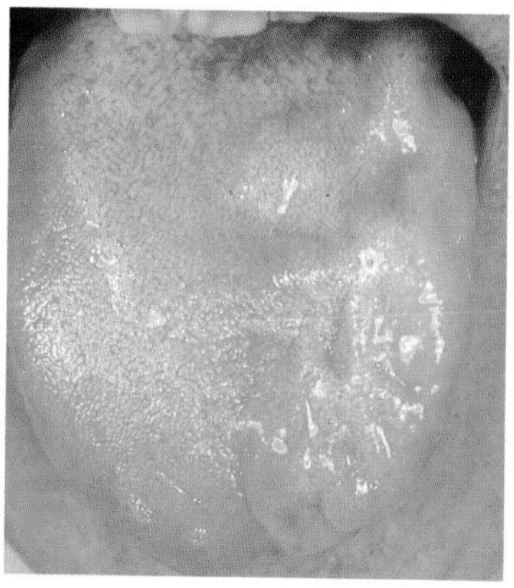

Fig. 12.128 Left hypoglossal nerve lesion.

CLINICAL APPLICATION

Isolated lesions of the eleventh cranial nerve are rare. Tumours in the region of the jugular foramen are likely to produce a combined palsy of the ninth, tenth and eleventh nerves (Fig. 12.125). In the presence of a hemiplegia, the trapezius muscle on the hemiplegic side is affected. A delay in shoulder shrug may be an early sign. The same hemiplegia, however, will affect the contralateral sternomastoid, that is the muscle rotating the neck towards the hemiplegic limbs. The weakness in such cases is incomplete. Spasmodic torticollis is a focal dystonia particularly affecting the sternomastoid muscle. Typically there are repetitive rotatory movements of the head and neck, which lead to hypertrophy of the relevant muscles in long-standing cases (Fig. 12.126).

THE HYPOGLOSSAL (12TH) NERVE

STRUCTURE AND FUNCTION

The hypoglossal nucleus lies close to the midline in the floor of the fourth ventricle and receives supranuclear fibres from both cerebral hemispheres, but principally the contralateral one. The hypoglossal nerve leaves the skull through the anterior condylar canal and supplies all the intrinsic muscles of the tongue, and all its extrinsic muscles except palatoglossus.

EXAMINATION

First inspect the tongue as it lies in the base of the oral cavity. In many patients there are tremulous movements which are often hard to distinguish from fasciculation or true involuntary movements. Fasciculation imparts a shimmering motion to the surface of the tongue. Involuntary movements include a coarse tremor, for example in Parkinson's disease, and complex, unpredictable movements found in such conditions as Huntington's disease and orofacial dyskinesia. While assessing the tongue for spontaneous contractions, observe its bulk. As the tongue wastes it becomes thinner and more wrinkled. Now ask the patient to protrude the tongue. Minor deviations from the midline are sometimes seen in normal individuals. Finally ask the patient to move the tongue rapidly from side to side, and assess its power by instructing the patient to push the tongue against the side of the cheek (Fig. 12.127). A disturbance of the speed of tongue movement occurs in extrapyramidal diseases, including Parkinson's disease.

Unilateral and bilateral lower motor neurone lesions

In a unilateral hypoglossal nerve lesion, there is focal atrophy, fasciculation and deviation to the paralyzed side (Fig. 12.128). Such a lesion can occur in isolation, or as the consequence of malignant invasion of the skull base. Bilateral involvement of the lower motor neurone projections to the tongue is usually part of a bulbar palsy.

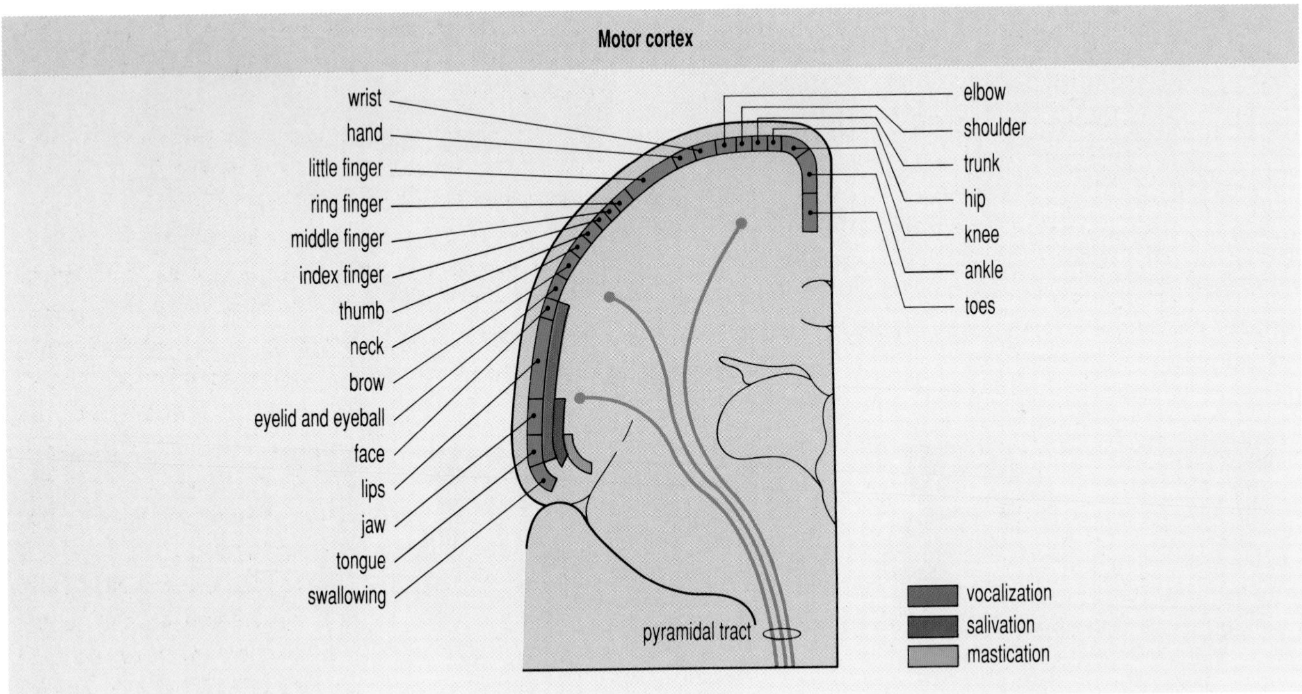

Fig. 12.129 Organization of the motor cortex.

There is additional involvement of the other lower brain stem motor nuclei, resulting in dysphagia and dysarthria. The tongue is wasted and immobile.

Unilateral upper motor neurone lesion

A unilateral upper motor neurone lesion has little effect on tongue function, though it may protrude slightly to the side of the hemiparesis.

Bilateral upper motor neurone lesion

Bilateral involvement of the pyramidal projections to the brain stem nuclei, usually the consequence of cerebrovascular disease, results in a pseudobulbar palsy. There is dysphagia, dysarthria and emotional lability. The tongue is stiff and immobile, and there is weakness of palatal elevation combined with a brisk gag reflex and jaw jerk.

THE MOTOR SYSTEM

STRUCTURE AND FUNCTION

The major supraspinal influences on motor activity are the sensorimotor cortex (exerting its role primarily through the pyramidal system), the basal ganglia, a number of tracts descending from the brain stem, and the cerebellum. The upper motor neurone defines that part of the motor pathway between the cerebral cortex and the anterior horn cell. The lower motor neurone consists of the anterior horn cell and its motor axon.

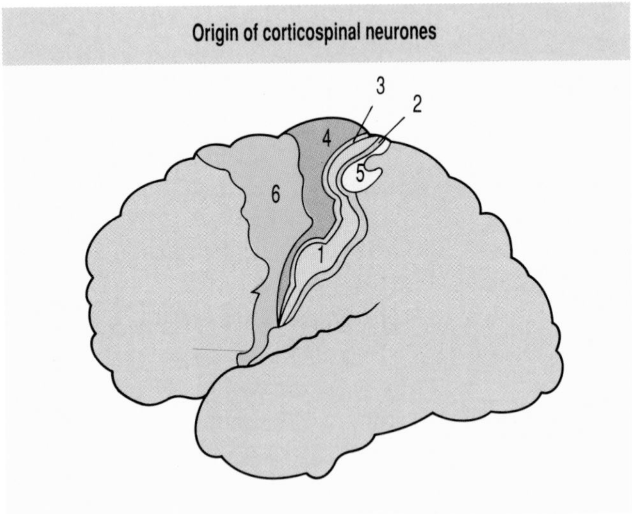

Fig. 12.130 Location of the areas contributing to corticospinal neurones.

The pyramidal tract

The motor cortex is situated in the precentral convolution, anterior to the rolandic fissure (area 4). Movements of the contralateral half of the body are represented inversely, with a large area responsible for the hand, thumb, and fingers, and a much smaller area, on the medial aspect of the hemisphere responsible for the lower limb (Fig. 12.129). Corticospinal neurones originate in the premotor association area (6), the motor area (4), the sensory area, and part of the sensory association area. The medial aspect of area 6 is called the supplementary motor area (Fig. 12.130). Both the motor and sensory cortices are arranged in radial and horizontal layers. The afferent inflow to the radial columns of the corticospinal neurones

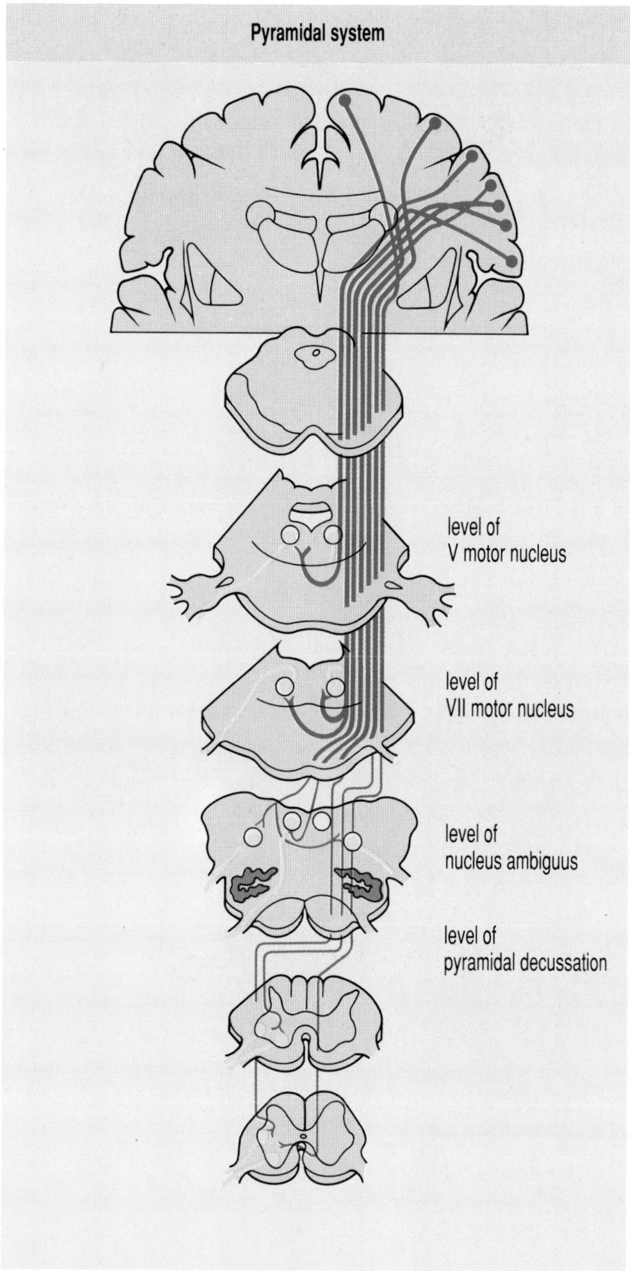

Fig. 12.131 Pathway of the pyramidal system

comes from those parts of the body receiving the motor outflow from that area. About 66 per cent of the neurones in the columns of the motor cortex are outflow. Afferent inputs include those from the cerebellum, the spinothalamic tracts, and the lemniscal system.

The motor cortex sends about a million pyramidal tract axons to the medulla. Less than 50 per cent of the neurones providing the fibres traversing the medullary pyramids are located in the precentral primary and supplementary motor areas, with the rest coming from the post-central cortex. The fibres from the cortex pass through the corona radiata and internal capsule before traversing the midbrain and pons on their way to the medulla (Fig. 12.131). About 75 per cent of the fibres reaching the medulla continue into the spinal cord, forming the lateral and ventral corticospinal tracts. About three-quarters of the fibres decussate. Some pyramidal fibres terminate directly on anterior horn cells but most synapse with internuncial neurones in the spinal grey matter, which in turn transmit to the anterior horn cells.

The motor cortex is particularly concerned with skilled activities requiring finely tuned movements of the hand and fingers. The corticospinal neurones innervate anterior horn cells related to a particular movement, even if those cells are located in separate spinal segments. Consequently, some muscles can be activated from cortical areas several millimetres apart, while several muscles may be activated by minimal stimulation confined to a single area of the cortex. Distinct populations of neurones within the sensorimotor cortex are concerned with the initiation of movement, its maintenance and control, and its termination. Different parts of area 4, projecting to specific populations of corticospinal neurones, respond to proprioceptive and cutaneous stimulation, allowing movement to be modified according to positional or tactile information.

Less than 25 per cent of the corticospinal neurones conduct at a velocity exceeding 25 m/s. The majority are small and slowly conducting, influencing fine gradations of force by being recruited early in the performance of a motor task. The larger, more rapidly conducting neurones are recruited late when larger movements are required. Discharge rates in the neurones relate to the force being exerted and its rate of change.

Activity within the corticospinal system also releases limbs from the postures imposed by gravity. In the upper limbs, this results in inhibition of flexors and facilitation of extensors, with the reverse effects in the lower limbs.

The extrapyramidal system

The basal ganglia are located in the basal forebrain and the midbrain. They include the nucleus accumbens, the putamen, globus pallidus, and caudate nucleus, the substantia nigra, and the subthalamic nucleus. Major inputs to the basal ganglia come from the cortex, the thalamus, and the reticular formation. Major outputs pass from the globus pallidus to the thalamus and pons, and from the substantia nigra to the thalamus, superior colliculus, and reticular formation. Finally, there are multiple interconnections between the various components of the system. The pigmented structures of the basal ganglia give rise to dopaminergic driven pathways passing from the pars compacta of the substantia nigra to the striatum (caudate nucleus and putamen) and from the ventral tegmentum to the nucleus accumbens and the frontal cortex.

The basal ganglia modify the programme of muscular action. Striatal neurones discharge after the neurones in the cortex from which they receive their connections. Efferent neurones in the globus pallidus and substantia nigra discharge still later. The basal ganglia integrate the individual components of skilled motor tasks and are important in the control of heavily learned motor activity. Lesions of the globus pallidus lead to increased duration of movement in the contralateral limbs. Output from the globus pallidus, if disinhibited by lesions of the subthalamic nucleus, leads to involuntary movement of the contralateral limbs.

The tracts descending from the brain stem

Vestibulospinal tract

The vestibulospinal tract descends uncrossed from the lateral vestibular nucleus. Its principal projection is to the cervical cord.

Reticulospinal tracts

Inhibitory and facilitatory reticulospinal tracts descend from the region of the midbrain and pons (Fig. 12.132).There are four inhibitory pathways, two of which are monoaminergic. A dorsal reticulospinal system passes from the pontomedullary reticular formation to the dorsolateral column of the spinal cord. The final inhibitory pathway originates in the medulla and descends ventral to the lateral corticospinal tract. The facilitatory reticulospinal tract passes from the pons and runs in the anterior column of the cord close to the ventral sulcus.

The initiating signals for locomotion are largely the responsibility of the reticulospinal and vestibulospinal tracts. The two monoaminergic inhibitory reticulospinal pathways alter the effects of the flexor reflex afferents. The dorsal reticulospinal tract inhibits segmentally active flexor reflex afferents and Ib polysynaptic paths. By doing so, it allows the activation of coordinated stepping movements. The ventral reticulospinal pathway inhibits the monosynaptic reflex arc, particularly of extensors, again in preparation for the release of spinal cord structures from their anti-gravity function. Interruption of this pathway results in hypertonicity and increased reflexes.The anti-gravity reflexes for standing are promoted by the facilitatory reticulospinal tract. Stimulation of this pathway tonically augments flexors in the upper limbs and extensors in the lower limbs. The vestibulospinal pathway has similar properties. The cerebellum has major inputs to the lateral vestibular nucleus and hence its descending pathway.

The spinal cord and lower motor neurone

The anterior horn cell contains alpha, beta and gamma motor neurones. The alpha axons are of large diameter conducting at around 45 m/s in the lower limb and 55 m/s in the upper limb. A motor unit comprises the anterior horn cell, its axon, and the muscle fibres it innervates, which may range from ten to several hundred.

The stretch reflex

The afferent limb of the stretch reflex arc is contained in Ia fibres innervating the muscle spindle. The fibres synapse with anterior horn cells which supply alpha motor neurones to the skeletal muscle containing that spindle. The muscle spindle is innervated by gamma fibres. Ib afferent fibres, originating from the Golgi tendon organ have an inhibiting effect on the stretch reflex via interneurones (Fig. 12.133).

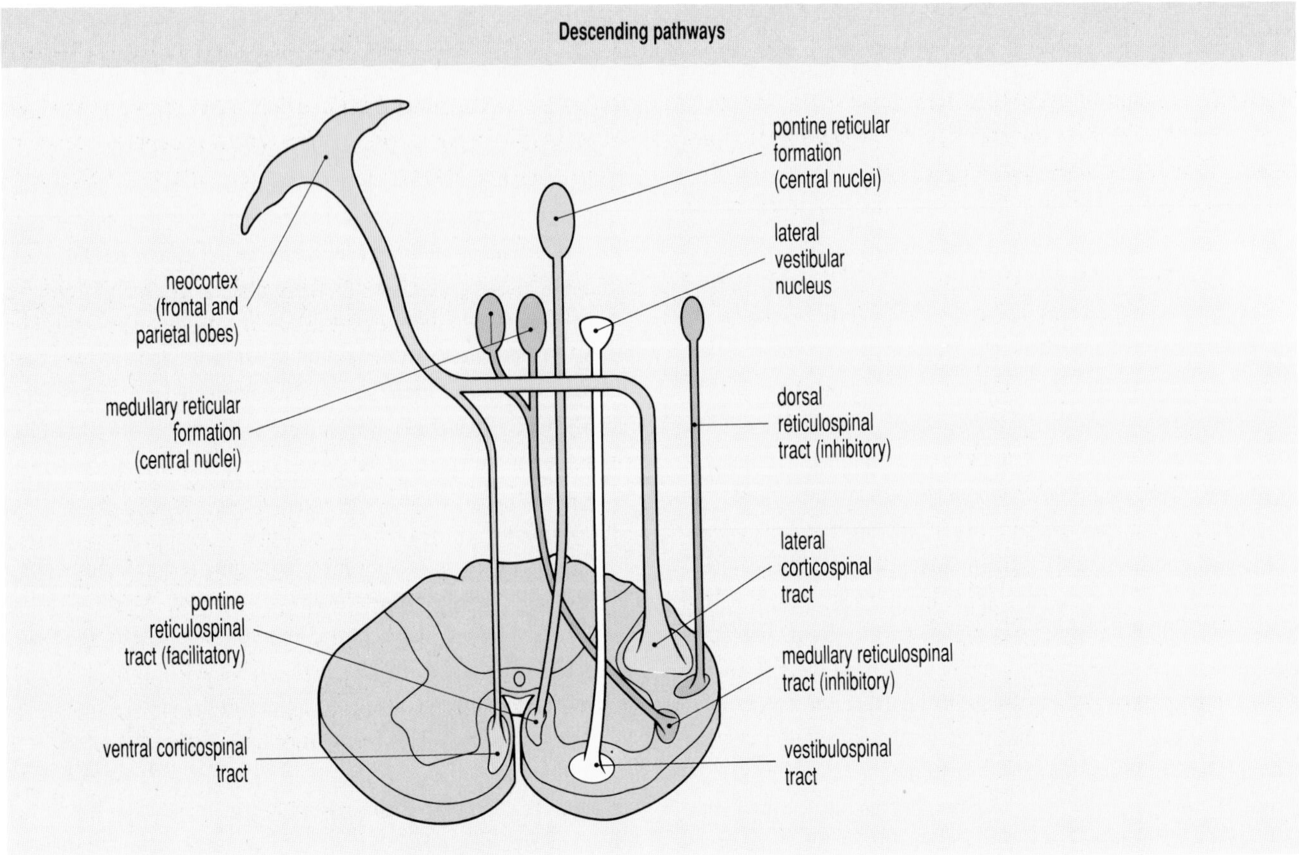

Fig. 12.132 Descending pathways from brain stem concerned with movement.

Other reflexes

Flexor reflex afferents (FRA), contained in small fibres, are excited by painful stimulation of the skin and deeper structures. They reach the motor neurones by polysynaptic pathways through interneurones within the spinal cord. For the lower limb these polysynaptic pathways innervate those segments needed to evoke a flexor withdrawal reaction to a painful stimulus. Connections to the other side of the cord facilitate extensor tone there.

Muscle

The fibres of skeletal muscle consist of myofibrils bounded by a sarcolemmal membrane. There are at least two types of muscle fibre with differing histochemical characteristics. Type 1 fibres are slow contracting, type 2 fast contracting.

The reflexes and abnormal muscle tone

The stretch reflex has phasic and tonic components. The tendon reflexes are phasic. Tonic stretch reflexes result in a sustained muscle contraction which has both dynamic (velocity-dependent) and static (length-dependent) components. Patients who relax poorly are activating tonic stretch reflexes which then hinder displacement of the limb. The tonic reflexes probably provide a means for damping the frequent motor responses which would otherwise occur if the phasic reflexes were unopposed.

Spasticity

Spasticity is a feature of an upper motor neurone lesion, though its appearance owes more to disruption of the ventral reticulospinal pathway than to altered pyramidal tract function. Indeed, selective damage of the latter results in hypotonia rather than spasticity. In spasticity the increase in muscle tone is velocity-dependent, probably the consequence of the dynamic sensitivity of the primary spindle ending. As the speed of displacement is increased, a critical velocity is reached at which muscle tone suddenly increases and resistance appears. Following a pyramidal tract lesion, the development of increased tone in anti-gravity muscles results in extension of the lower limbs. At a certain point of flexion of the extended limb the hypertonicity suddenly resolves because of a length-dependent inhibition of the quadriceps stretch reflex: the clasp-knife effect. The phenomenon is less evident in the upper limbs, and is particularly evident in spinal lesions. The inhibition of lower limb extensors at a critical level of stretch results from interruption of the inhibitory effect of the dorsal reticulospinal system on the flexor reflex afferent system. The degree of loss of flexor inhibition determines the likelihood of flexor spasms emerging.

Rigidity

The rigidity of Parkinson's disease and other extrapyramidal disorders is fundamentally different to spasticity. The increased tone is more uniformly distributed between flexors and extensors and is not velocity-dependent. Furthermore, a clasp-knife effect does not occur. In some cases, the rigidity is fluctuant, producing a cogwheel effect. The frequency of the cogwheeling is more closely linked to the frequency of the action than to the resting tremor found in Parkinsonian patients.

EXAMINATION

A detailed outline of the limb muscles, and their examination, is contained in Chapter 11. This section concentrates on an overview of patterns of weakness and how that pattern is helpful in diagnosis.

Stretch reflex arc

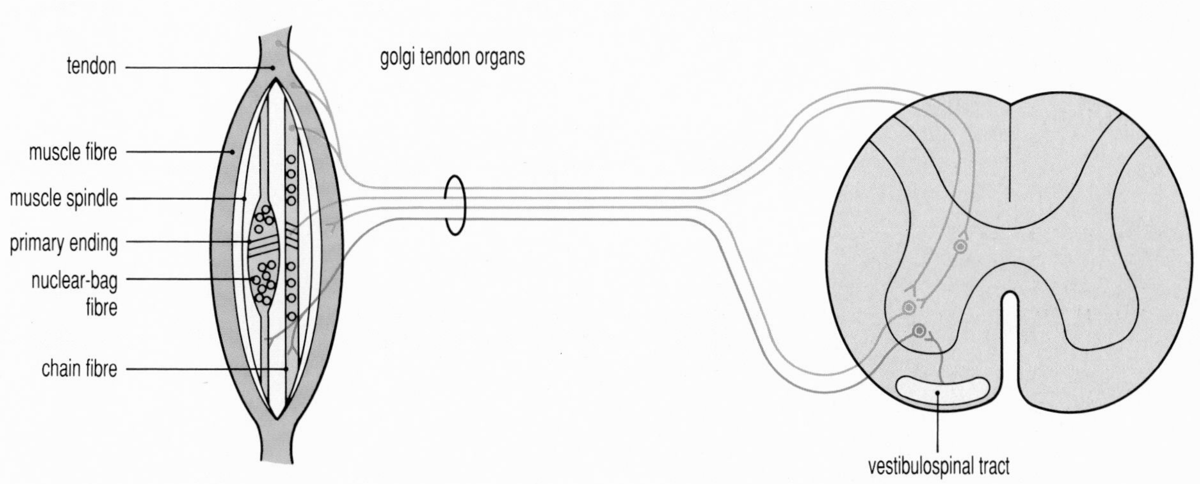

Fig. 12.133 The stretch reflex arc.

Appearance

Some thinning of the small hand muscles is common in the elderly but is not associated with weakness. When assessing muscle wasting, do not neglect areas hidden when the patient lies in the supine position. Sit the patient forward to look at the periscapular muscles, and turn the patient over to assess the bulk of the glutei, hamstrings, and calves. A global loss of muscle bulk is more likely to be the result of either impaired nutrition or malignancy rather than neurological disease. Focal muscle wasting can rapidly appear following injury of a joint with consequent immobilization. If you suspect a discrepancy in size between two limbs, use a tape measure to record the limb cirumference. Choose a suitable landmark, for instance the joint margin of the knee, then measure the circumference of the limb at a specified distance from the landmark. Remember that the circumference of the dominant limb is likely to be slightly greater. The pattern of wasting often suggests a particular peripheral nerve or root disorder (Fig. 12.134).

While inspecting the muscle, look for spontaneous contractions. Many patients, whether through nervousness or cold, display tremulous movements of the limbs, and these relatively coarse movements need to be distinguished from fasciculation. Fasciculation is due to spontaneous contraction of the fibres belonging to a single motor unit. Depending on the size of the motor unit, the fasciculation appears either as a fine flicker (e.g. in a hand muscle) or as a coarse twitch (e.g. in the thigh). Fasciculation often appears in short bursts before disappearing for several minutes. Muscles may hypertrophy as well as atrophy. Pseudohypertrophic muscles are infiltrated by fat and connective tissue and are weak on formal testing (Fig. 12.135). Muscle palpation provides little information, though ischaemic, fibrotic muscle feels harder than normal. Acutely inflamed muscle is tender but, a similar sensitivity can be found in subjects without evidence of organic disease.

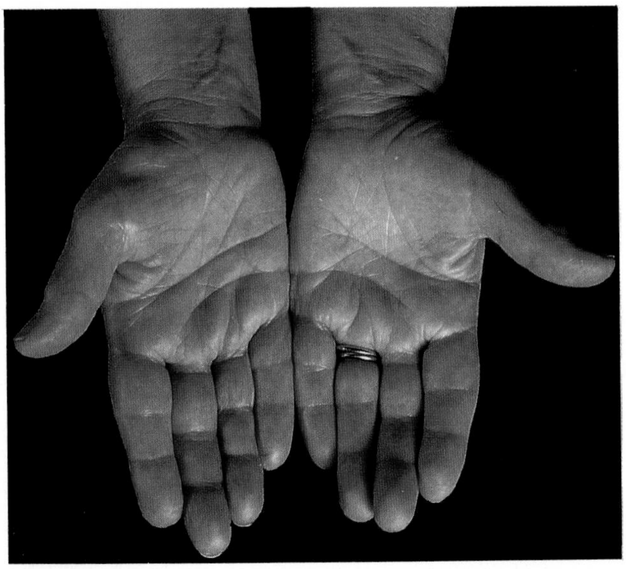

Fig. 12.134 Focal wasting of the thenar eminence secondary to median nerve compression.

Tone

Assessment of muscle tone is one of the most difficult parts of the neurological examination. It requires both skill on the part of the examiner, and relaxation on the part of the patient. Ensure that the patient is comfortable and warm. First observe the limb posture; this may indicate the distribution of altered tone between the flexors and extensors of the limb. You do not need to examine movement at all joints to assess tone. For screening purposes, assess flexion-extension at the elbow, pronation and supination of the forearm, and flexion-extension at the knee, using a range of speeds rather than a fixed velocity. Remember to take account of any painful limb or joint.

Spastic limbs

In spastic limbs at a critical velocity a catch appears which is absent during slower displacements. Subsequently the hypertonus fades away as stretch continues. Spasticity is selectively distributed. In the upper limbs it predominates in flexors, and it is more evident when the forearm is supinated than when it is pronated. In the lower limb it is greater in quadriceps than in the hamstrings. This selectivity may vary, particularly in spinal cord disease, but the finding is highly suggestive of a disorder affecting the upper motor neurone. In spinal cord disease, release of flexor reflex afferents may be so prominent that mild stimulation of the lower limb produces a flexor reaction at the hip and knee. In long-standing spasticity you may find that the limb can no longer be fully displaced at the affected joint. For example, in the leg persistent hypertonia in the plantar flexors can lead to shortening of the tendo Achilles.

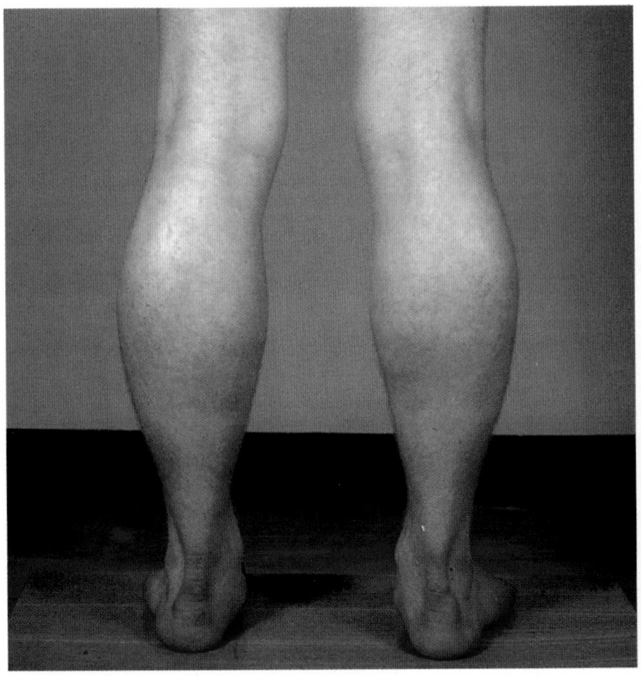

Fig. 12.135 Pseudohypertrophy of the calf muscles.

Rigidity

Rigidity is more uniformly distributed in the limb. It may begin unilaterally and is sometimes easier to detect in one joint rather than another. The resistance is felt at low speeds of displacement and does not 'melt away'. Rigidity is activated by contraction of muscle in an unaffected limb. If you have doubts regarding an increase in tone, ask the patient either to clench their teeth or grip the hand not being tested. In patients with rigidity the increased tone becomes more evident during this procedure. At times rigidity is not uniform but fluctuates in a phasic manner, aptly described as cogwheeling.

Many tense, nervous patients will appear to have a fluctuant increase in tone, but the variability should suggest there is no significant pathology.

Gegenhalten

A more diffuse increase in tone, Gegenhalten, can be found in patients with an altered level of consciousness, and in those with frontal lobe lesions.

Hypotonia

Reduced tone is more difficult to detect. The limb is floppy and is liable to show abnormal excursions when moved passively. Hypotonia occurs in the presence of a lower motor neurone lesion and in cerebellar disease.

MUSCLE POWER

Muscle weakness is often suggested by lack of spontaneous movement in the affected part during conversation or when the patient walks. In Parkinson's disease, however, certain automatic movements can disappear even in the absence of weakness.

Grade	Definition
0	Total paralysis
1	Flicker of contraction
2	Movement with gravity eliminated
3	Movement against gravity
4	Movement against resistance but incomplete
5	Normal power

Fig. 12.136 MRC classification of muscle power.

It is helpful to use an accepted numerical system for grading muscle power rather than resorting to descriptive terms; 'rather weak' covers a broad spectrum of disability. The MRC system of classification is recommended (Fig. 12.136).

To apply this system to a muscle test its strength as shown for biceps in Fig. 12.137. Remember to take account of the patient's age, occupation, and your own physical development. In practice grades 4 and 5 are separated by a wide range of strength, but as you gain experience you can overcome this problem by using the grades 4+, 4++, and 5-.

Testing biceps

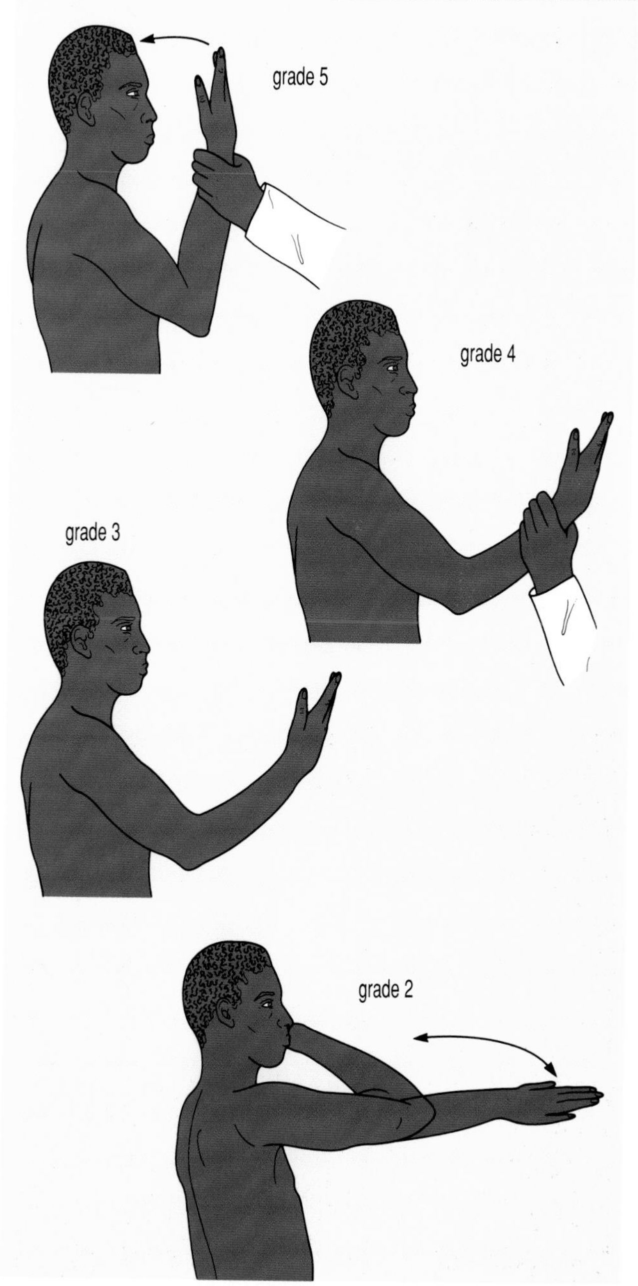

Fig. 12.137 The application of the MRC system of grading muscle power to the examination of biceps.

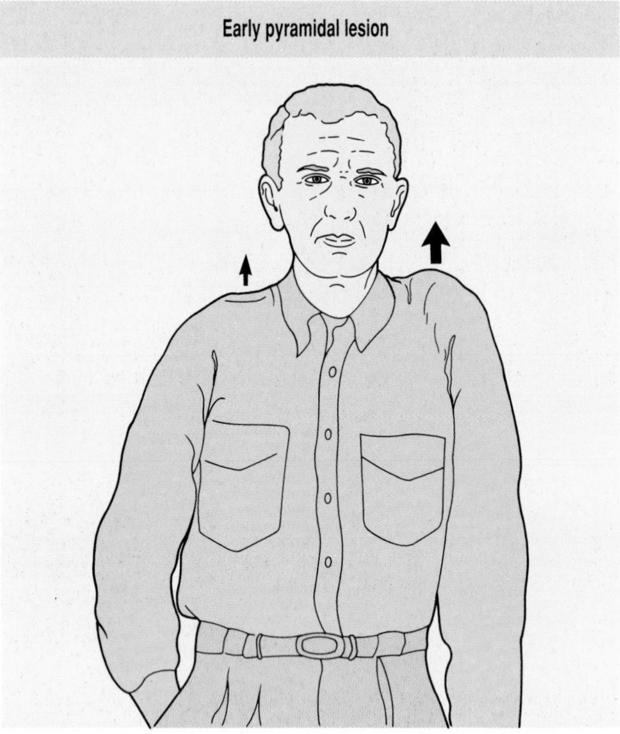

Fig. 12.138 Delayed right shoulder shrug in a patient with an early pyramidal lesion.

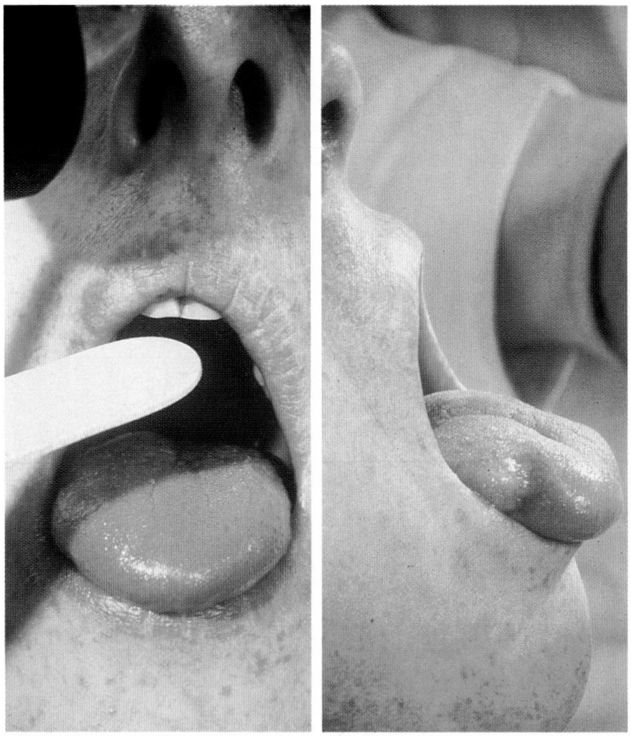

Fig. 12.139 Percussion myotonia of the tongue.

A description of the methods of assessing individual muscles is given In Chapter 4. Looking at a limited number can screen for many neurological disorders. In the upper limbs, first ask the patient to shrug his shoulder. In an early pyramidal lesion above the level of C2 (but also in unilateral Parkinson's disease) the affected shoulder lags behind its fellow (Fig. 12.138). Next, test deltoid, biceps, triceps, then the first dorsal interosseous, and abductor pollicis brevis. Score each muscle on the MRC scale. Test one arm at a time rather than trying to test both arms together. In the lower limb, look at hip flexion and extension, knee flexion and extension, and dorsi- and plantar flexion of the feet.

Muscle weakness

Is the weakness confined to one limb, or to one side of the body?

Is the weakness static, progressive, or does it fluctuate in degree?

Is the weakness accompanied by a feeling of stiffness, or is the affected limb 'floppy'.

Patterns of weakness

Strictly speaking paresis and plegia indicate incomplete and complete paralysis, respectively. However, these terms tend to be used interchangeably. The distribution of muscle weakness is described as monoplegia if the paralysis is confined to a single limb, hemiplegia if there is paralysis of one half of the body (with or without facial involvement), paraplegia if there is paralysis of the legs, and tetraplegia, or a quadriplegia, if there is weakness of all four limbs.

If the degree of muscle weakness fluctuates during the course of the examination, test for fatiguability. In the upper limb, shoulder abduction is a convenient movement for this purpose. First attempt to overcome the arms when abducted to 90°. Then ask the patient to maintain this posture for a minute and retest. In the lower limb hip flexion can be tested in a similar fashion. Remember that a fluctuating performance is also often prominent in non-organic weakness.

Myotonia results in impaired relaxation of skeletal muscle following contraction. Ask the patient to clench the fists tightly then release them; if the patient has myotonia there is a significant delay before the fingers can be fully extended. There is likely to be abnormal dimpling of muscle following percussion. Tap the thenar eminence with the patella hammer. In the presence of myotonia, the muscle dimples, and stays dimpled, for several seconds. The same sign can be elicited in the tongue (Fig. 12.139).

Deep tendon reflexes

Because the clinical examination is performed standing on the patient's right, left-handed individuals are at a considerable disadvantage when testing the reflexes. However, it is better to learn to hold the patella hammer in the right hand rather than examining the patient on their left. Some patients tend to assist the reflex response by a reflex contraction, but this is usually readily distinguished from a true reflex contraction.

Grade	Definition
0	Absent
±	Present only with reinforcement
+	Just present
++	Brisk normal
+++	Exaggerated response

Fig. 12.140 Grading reflexes.

Testing the reflexes assesses the reflex arc and the supraspinal influences which operate upon it. Each reflex is graded according to strength of response as shown in Fig. 12.140.

Reflexes are remarkably variable in normal individuals. Some patients have very brisk reflexes, though unaccompanied by clonus. Others have very depressed responses which often appear better preserved at the ankle than elsewhere, the opposite of what one would find if a neuropathy was the cause of the hyporeflexia.

The upper limb

The reflexes of the upper limb routinely tested are the biceps, triceps, and supinator (the roots subserving each reflex are shown in brackets below). The biceps and supinator reflexes are tested first, with the patient in the posture shown in Fig. 12.141.

Biceps (C5/6)

The whole arm must be exposed when testing this reflex. Place the thumb or index finger of your left hand on the biceps tendon then strike it with the patella hammer using a pendular motion by extending then flexing your wrist. Grasp the hammer at the end rather than halfway down the shaft (Fig. 12.142). The response consists of contraction of the biceps muscle. If there is no response, ask the patient to clench their teeth, or grip the fingers of the other hand shortly before testing (Jendrassik manoeuvre). Now examine the reflex in the left arm. Lean over and use your inverted thumb to mark the position of the tendon. It is tempting, particularly for the left handed, to walk round the couch and examine from the other side. Avoid the temptation. It is time-consuming and unnecessary.

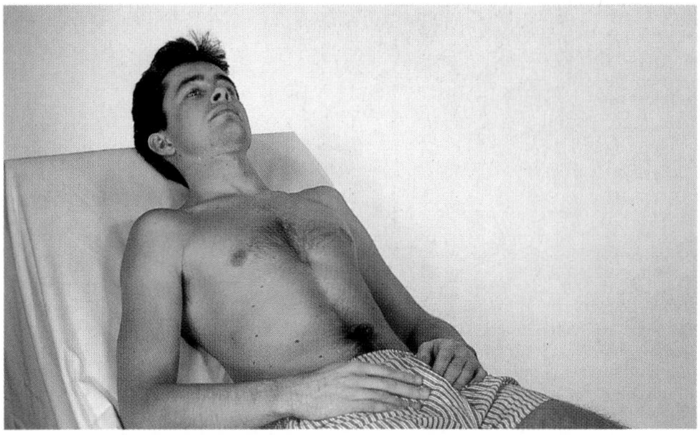

Fig. 12.141 Posture of the upper limbs for testing the biceps and supinator reflexes.

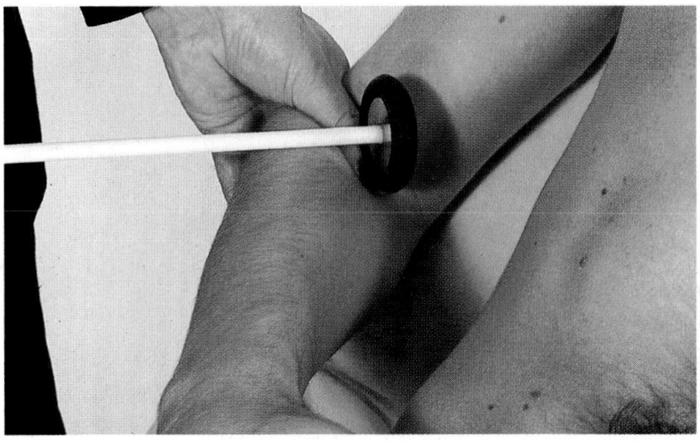

Fig. 12.142 Testing the right biceps reflex.

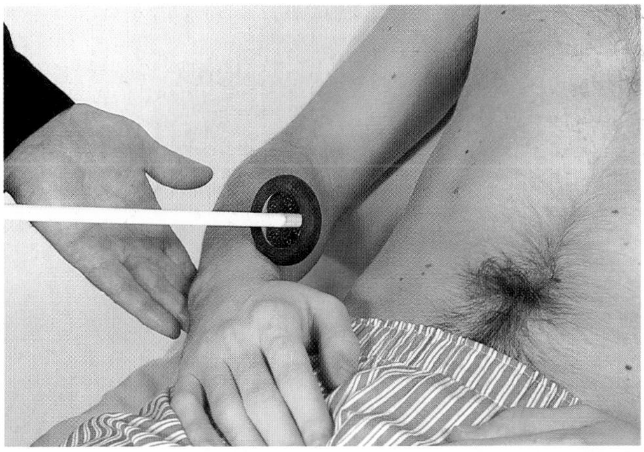

Fig. 12.143 Testing the right supinator reflex.

Supinator (C5/6)

With the patient's arm in the semi-pronated position, strike the radial margin of the forearm about 5cm above the wrist (Fig. 12.143). You do not need to interpose your finger. The response is a contraction of brachioradialis and biceps. When measuring the biceps and supinator reflexes, observe also the fingers of the hand. A brisk reflex is accompanied by finger flexion. In certain instances, despite a depression of the direct reflex, flexion of the fingers still occurs (inversion). This physical finding, usually due to cervical spondylosis, suggests the combination of a depression of the reflex arc at the C5/C6 level, together with an exaggeration of reflexes at a lower level due to a co-existent pyramidal tract disorder.

Triceps (C6/7)

To test the right triceps jerk, bring the patient's right arm well across the body, with the elbow flexed at about 90° so that the triceps tendon is adequately exposed (Fig. 12.144). Strike the tendon with the patella hammer. A normal response is contraction of the triceps. Having tested the reflex on the right, bring the left arm over and test the reflex on that side.

Finger (C/8)

The finger jerk is usually present only when there is a pathological exaggeration of the reflexes. With the patient's arm pronated exert slight pressure on the flexed fingers with the fingers of your left hand. Now strike the back of your own fingers with the hammer. A positive response leads to a brief flexion of the fingertips (Fig. 12.145).

Lower limb

Knee (L2/3/4)

To test the knee jerks insert your left arm underneath the patient's knees and flex them to about 60° (Fig. 12.146). If the patient is properly relaxed the legs will sag when you remove their support. Tap first the right patella tendon and then the left. If one or both reflexes is particularly brisk, test for knee clonus by fitting your thumb and index finger along the upper border of the patella with the knee extended (Fig. 12.147). Exert a sudden, downward (but not violent) stretch and maintain it. Any repetitive contraction of the quadriceps (i.e. clonus) even if only two or three beats, is strongly suggestive of a pyramidal tract disorder affecting the relevant segment of that limb.

Ankle (S1)

Positioning is important when eliciting the ankle jerk. The patient's leg is abducted and externally rotated at the hip, flexed at the knee and flexed at the ankle. If hip abduction is limited, rest the leg on its fellow to allow adequate access to the Achilles tendon (Fig. 12.148). If the reflex is brisk, look for clonus. With the limb in the same position, forcibly dorsiflex the ankle and maintain that position (Fig. 12.149). Three to four beats of symmetrical ankle clonus is acceptable in normal individuals, but asymmetric or more sustained clonus is pathological.

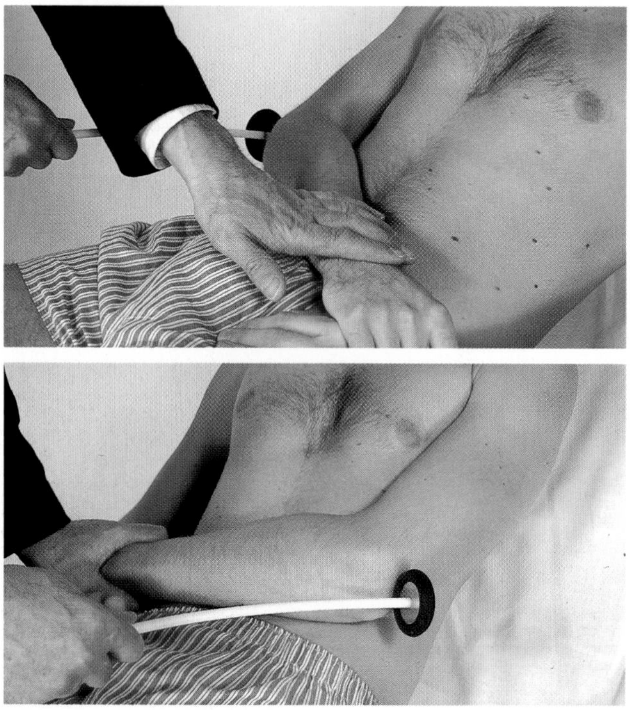

Fig. 12.144 Testing the right and left triceps reflexes.

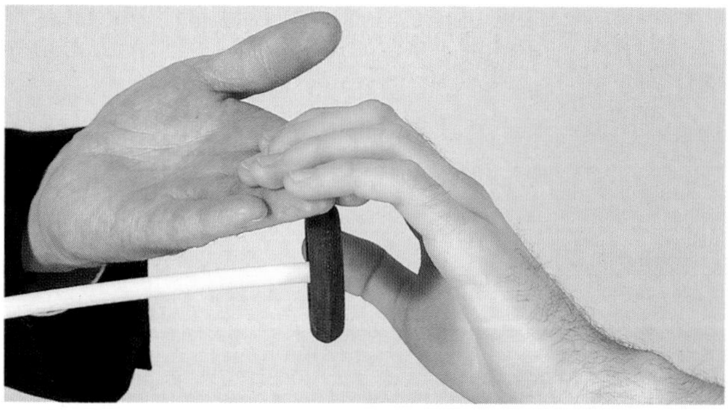

Fig. 12.145 Eliciting a finger jerk.

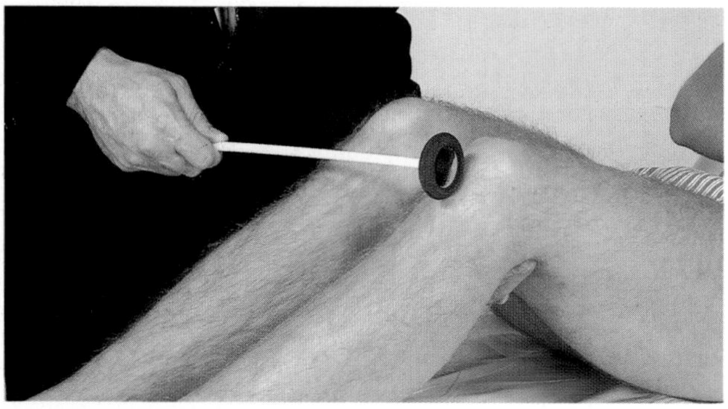

Fig. 12.146 Eliciting the knee reflexes.

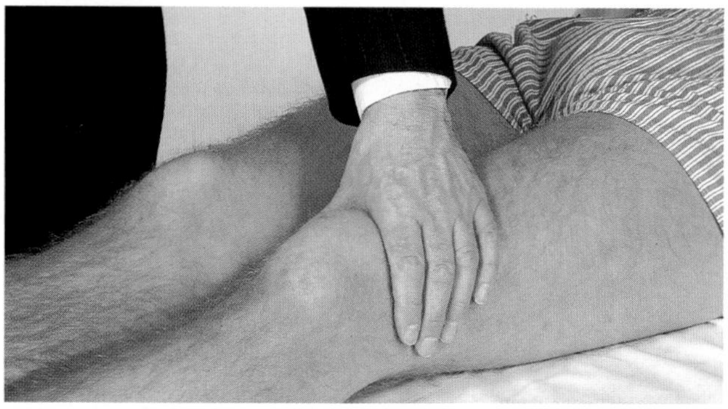

Fig. 12.147 Testing for knee clonus.

Other reflexes

Abdominal responses

The abdominal responses are notoriously variable. They diminish with age and are more difficult to elicit in the obese or in women who have had children. They are cutaneous reflexes whose latency suggests mediation through a spinal reflex arc. Before you can assess the abdominal reflexes the patient must be relaxed and lying flat. Lightly draw the end of an orange stick across the four segments of the abdomen around the umbilicus (Fig. 12.150). Normally there is a reflex contraction in each segment. To summarize the findings in your notes draw a cross with a 0, ± or + in each segment according to response.

Cremasteric reflex

The cremasteric reflex is elicited by stroking the upper inner aspect of the thigh. It is mediated through segments Ll and L2 and leads to retraction of the ipsilateral testicle.

Plantar response

The plantar response is elicited by applying firm pressure (use an orange stick) to the lateral aspect of the sole of the foot, moving from the heel to the base of the fifth toe, then, if necessary, across the base of the toes (Fig. 12.151). While you do this observe the metatarsophalangeal joint of the big toe. In the normal adult, the toe plantar flexes. In the presence of a pyramidal tract lesion, the toe dorsiflexes. The same dorsiflexion appears in normal individuals if a sharp stimulus is applied to the big toe and in infants if the stimulus is applied over a wider area. The reflex is considered to be part of a flexor withdrawal response to a noxious stimulus. With the development of the upright posture, descending pathways, one of which is the pyramidal tract, inhibit the reaction except when stimulation is applied directly to the big toe. Damage to descending pathways, particularly the corticospinal system, releases the inhibition and allows the appearance of the pathological response. In certain spinal cord disorders, where the flexor withdrawal response is totally disinhibited, minor stimulation of the foot or other part of the leg results in flexion at hip, knee, ankle, and toe. There is no point in testing the plantar response if the big toe is immobile, or if there is severe loss of S1 cutaneous innervation. Other toe movements accompany the flexor and extensor response, and other ways of eliciting the reflex are described, but neither add any useful information to the interpretation of the response. Summarize your findings with arrows: for flexor ↓, for extensor ↑ and for equivocal ↑↓.

Anal reflex

The anal reflex is assessed by pricking the skin at the anal margin. In normal subjects there is a brisk contraction of the anal sphincter. The tone of the anal sphincter can be assessed by inserting a finger into the anus and asking the patient to bear down on it.

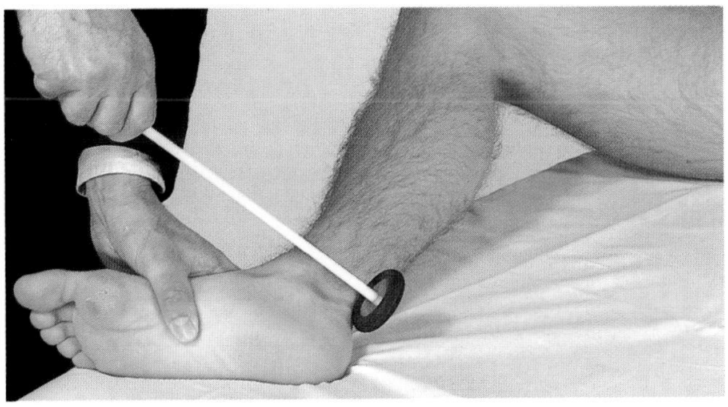

Fig. 12.148 Eliciting the ankle reflex.

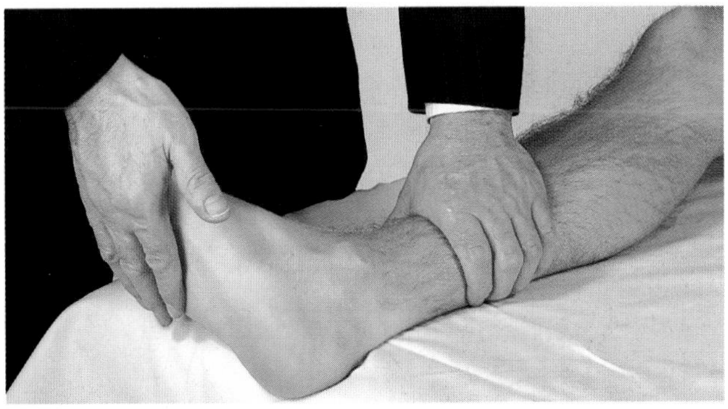

Fig. 12.149 Testing for ankle clonus.

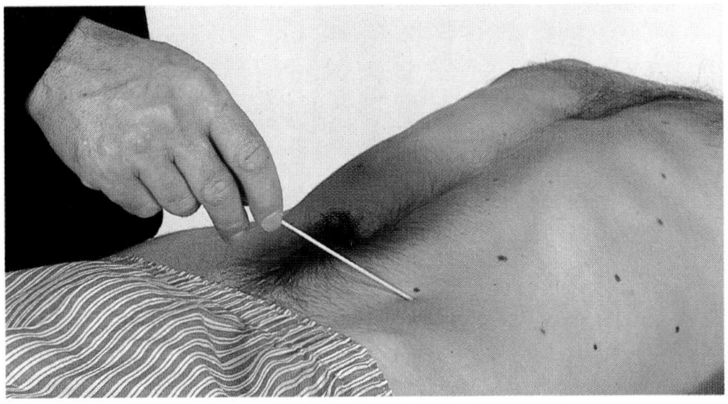

Fig. 12.150 Testing the abdominal responses.

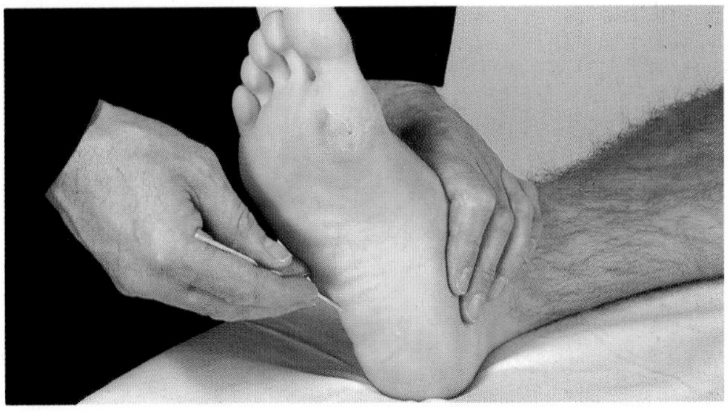

Fig. 12.151 Testing the plantar response.

The extrapyramidal system

Examination of tone has already been considered, and the interpretation of abnormal movements including tremor will be considered later.

Bradykinesia

Bradykinesia is particularly associated with Parkinson's disease. The problem may be confined to one limb, at least initially, or it may be generalized. Initiation of movement is delayed, the actual movement slowed and its adjustment insensitive. To look for bradykinesia in the upper limbs, ask the patient to tap repetitively the back of one hand with the other. In a patient with Parkinson's disease the movement tails off. Ask the patient to use such force that the tapping is audible. Typically, if the movement is bradykinetic its sound diminishes and falters. Now ask the patient to 'polish' the back of one hand with the other. Parkinsonian patients display a movement of reduced amplitude which eventually may cease completely. To assess bradykinesia in the lower limbs, ask the patient to tap your hand repetitively, first with one foot, then the other. Many individuals find it difficult to sustain a rhythm but in Parkinsonian patients the movement will again fade away. There are many ways of assessing bradykinesia without recourse to formal examination. Watch the patient dressing, or using a knife and fork. Ask them to write and examine the size of the script and its legibility. See how easily they stand from a sitting posture and time how long they take to walk a set distance.

Involuntary movement

You may reasonably be dismayed when trying to describe a movement disorder. Begin by detailing the characteristics of the movement. Is it present at rest, with the limb completely supported, or when the limb takes up a particular posture, or only when the patient carries out a skilled activity? Ascertain the frequency of the movement, and its distribution. Is the problem mainly proximal or distal? Are the movements brief, or sufficiently prolonged to cause an abnormal posture?

Tremor

Is your tremor mainly present at rest,

When you hold the hands out, or when you use your hands?

Is the tremor relieved by alcohol?

Does anybody in your family have a tremor?

Tremor

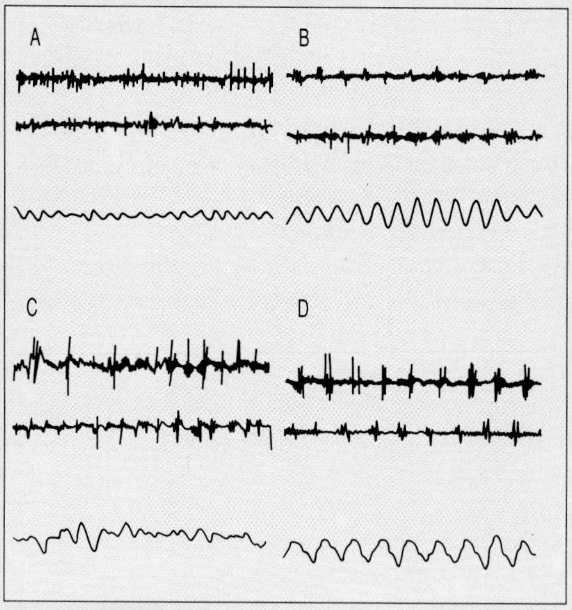

A physiological tremor

B essential tremor (EMG bursts in flexors and extensors are synchronized)

C tremor due to deafferentation

D Parkinsonian tremor (EMG bursts in flexors and extensors alternate)

Fig. 12.152 EMG traces from wrist extensors (top) and flexors (middle) with tremor recording from hand (bottom).

Tremor

Tremor is a rhythmic movement which, at a particular joint, is usually confined to a single plane (Fig. 12.152). Physiological tremor is a normal finding, usually detectable only with EMG recording. Enhanced physiological tremor is triggered by agitation, the use of sympathomimetic agents and thyrotoxicosis. Its frequency is around 9Hz in younger subjects. Stimulation of β2-adrenergic receptors in muscle accounts for enhanced physiological tremor.

Essential (familial) tremor is absent at rest. Besides the upper limbs, it can affect the head and neck, and the voice. It is not dependent on the integrity of the reflex arc and appears to be sustained by central mechanisms. The amplitude of the tremor tends to increase towards the end of a skilled movement, but not to the degree found with cerebellar disease. The same factors which trigger enhanced physiological tremor can exacerbate essential tremor. It is often diminished by alcohol.

Several types of tremor occur in Parkinsonian patients. Classically there is a resting tremor, firing at about 4–5Hz. EMG shows alternate contraction of antagonist muscle groups. Typical movements include flexion/extension at the wrist and fingers, pronator-supinator movements of the forearm, and complex com-

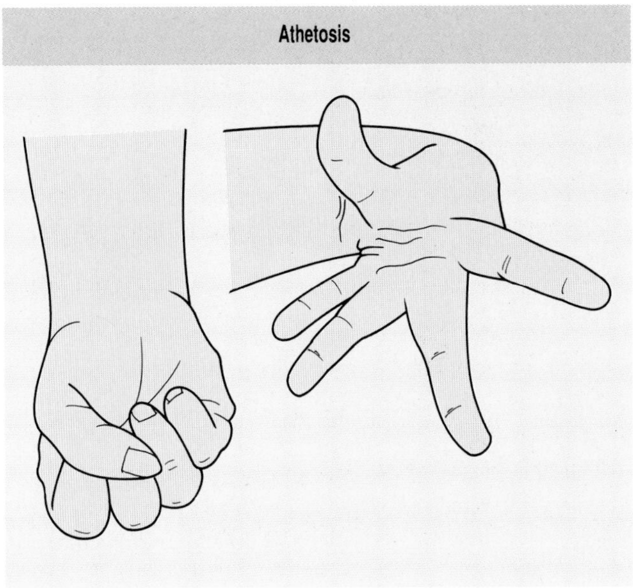

Fig. 12.153 Athetoid hand postures.

binations. A similar tremor can be seen in the head, neck, or lower limb. Typically, it is inhibited for a few seconds by skilled activity. If you find the combination of a resting tremor which briefly remits during activity, then you can be confident of making a diagnosis of Parkinson's disease. In addition to the resting tremor, many Parkinsonian patients have an action tremor which has the characteristics of exaggerated physiological tremor.

Myoclonus

Myoclonus is characterized by rapid, recurring muscle jerks. The movement is similar to the startle reaction described as 'jumping out of one's skin'. The movements are either generalized or confined to one part of the body. In some cases they appear only when the limb is activated. One form of focal myoclonus principally affects the palate. Following damage to the brain stem, usually from cerebrovascular disease, myoclonus appears in the palate and also the larynx and face. Other structures can be affected. The movement frequency is around 2–3Hz. The patient may have noticed an inability to sustain an even pitch when speaking or singing. If you detect rhythmic contractions in the facial muscles, look at the palate, where myoclonus produces a rhythmic oscillation, the movement showing little tendency to alter in frequency or amplitude.

Causes of generalized myoclonus include subacute sclerosing panencephalitis and Creutzfeldt–Jakob disease. Familial generalized myoclonus occurs either in isolation or with epilepsy. Segmental myocolonus can occur with spinal cord disease.

Chorea

Patients with chorea appear to fidget. They show brief, random movements which do not have the shock-like quality of myoclonus. Typical movements include furrowing of the eyebrows, pursing of the lips, elevation of a shoulder, and random contraction of the fingers. Both proximal and distal limb muscles can be affected. Because the movements are short-lived, sustained postures do not occur. Ask the patient to grip your hand – you will find that the grip waxes and wanes with the fluctuations of the chorea. The tendon reflexes may be prolonged due to the superimposition of a late, sustained contraction on the phasic reflex. The choreiform movements tend to be accentuated by a skilled action. Chorea associated with rheumatic fever (Sydenhams's chorea) is rare but is usually a prominent feature of Huntington's disease. Chorea can occur with dopa therapy and is sometimes associated with the use of the oral contraceptive. It is sometimes seen in thyrotoxicosis and systemic lupus erythematosus.

Athetosis

Athetoid movements are slower still than chorea and become prominent during the performance of voluntary activity. The distal parts of the limbs are predominantly affected. In the hand the posture oscillates between hyperextension of the fingers and thumb, usually with pronation of the forearm, and flexion of the digits associated with supination (Fig. 12.153). In some cases the movements are superimposed on more sustained postures. In the hand this combines flexion of the wrist with extension of the fingers, and in the foot flexion of the toes associated with inversion at the ankle. In progressive disease states the abnormal sustained postures become dominant. Assessment of the plantar response is difficult if athetosis is affecting the foot. Stimulation of the sole is liable to produce extension of the toes whether or not there is a pyramidal tract disorder. A combination of choreiform and athetoid movements is called choreo-athetosis.

Hemiballismus

Hemiballismus results in violent swinging movements of the contralateral arm and leg. The movements, in which rotation is prominent, are of maximal amplitude at the shoulder and hip. The affected limbs are relatively flaccid. The condition is usually the consequence of a vascular lesion in the contralateral subthalamic nucleus. If the lesion extends into the ipsilateral globus pallidus, the movement resolves.

Dystonia

In dystonia abnormal postures result from the contraction of antagonistic muscle groups. It is exacerbated by attempts at voluntary movement. The dystonia may be generalized or localized to one area. Torsion dystonia (dystonia musculorum deformans) is a familial generalized dystonia which predominates in either axial or limb musculature. In adults, dystonia is often drug-induced. Examples of focal dystonia include blepharospasm, spasmodic torticollis, and writer's cramp. The movements are not under voluntary control and the patient is unable to restrain them. They cease in sleep, as do all the other involuntary movements apart from hemiballismus and palatal myoclonus. In certain, long-standing extrapyramidal disorders, the body assumes either an overall flexed posture (generalized flexion dystonia) or one in which flexion of the upper limbs is associated with extension of the lower limbs (hemiplegic dystonia).

Tics

Tics are repetitive movements which appear, at least briefly, to be under voluntary control. They predominate in younger people. Typical examples are head nodding and jerking. The movement is easily mimicked. There will be no abnormal signs on examination.

Dyskinesia

Brief, involuntary movements around the mouth and face are relatively common in the elderly (orofacial dyskinesia). Similar movements can be induced by long-term phenothiazine therapy and in patients on L-dopa. The former problem tends to persist whatever adjustment is made to the medication, but the latter is dose-dependent.

Myokymia

Myokymia confined to the eyelid is a common experience in normal individuals and is felt as a fine twitching. In pathological myokymia this fine movement extends to other parts of the facial musculature. The movements are easily missed, but on examination a continuous, fine flickering motion can be seen. If the movements are extensive, the eye may close slightly and the mouth retract (Fig. 12.154). Causes include multiple sclerosis and brain stem tumour.

Asterixis

In certain metabolic disorders, particularly hepatic and renal failure, there is a defect of limb posture control. If the patient is asked to extend his arms and hold the fingers in the horizontal plane, a downward drift of the fingers and hands is interrupted by a sudden, upward, corrective jerk.

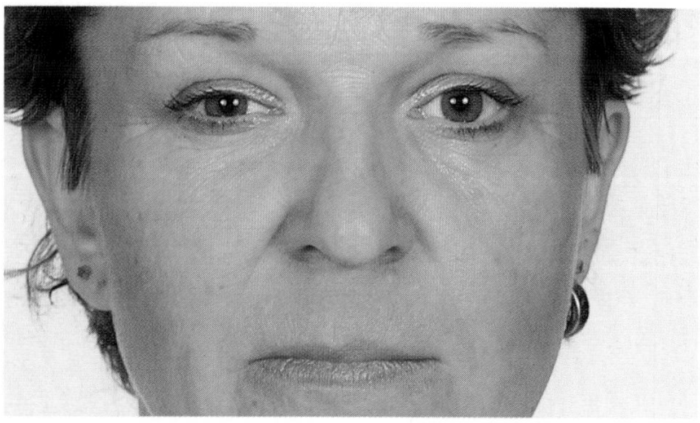

Fig. 12.154 Facial myokyia.

CLINICAL APPLICATION

Upper motor neurone lesion

An upper motor neurone lesion results from disruption of the pyramidal pathway at any point between the motor cortex and the anterior horn cell. Its characteristic features are shown in Fig. 12.155.

The pattern of weakness is influenced by the site of the lesion, but generally it predominates in the upper limb extensors and the lower limb flexors. With cortical lesions, for instance one affecting the hand, a more global loss of function results. If the pathway is disturbed above the brain stem, then certain cranial nerve signs are likely to accompany the limb weakness. The most common cause of a hemiplegia is cerebrovascular disease. The distribution of the weakness, and certain accompanying physical signs due to disruption of other pathways, often allows an accurate anatomical localization of the lesion.

Lower motor neurone lesion

The characteristic findings in a lower motor neurone lesion secondary to disruption of the pathway between the motor nucleus and the neuromuscular junction are shown in Fig. 12.156.

The weakness is found in all the muscles supplied by the affected motor neurone. Wasting results from interruption of the nerve axon, or its parent cell, but can take several weeks to emerge. Fasciculation is particularly prominent when the anterior horn cells or cranial nerve motor nuclei are disrupted. Fibrillation, a sign of denervation, can be detected only by sampling the muscle with a

Features of an upper motor neurone lesion

- Muscle weakness
- Increased deep tendon reflexes
- Depressed abdominal responses
- An extensor plantar response
- Spasticity

Fig. 12.155 Features of an upper motor neurone lesion.

Features of a lower motor neurone lesion

- Muscle weakness
- Depressed deep tendon reflexes
- Fasciculation
- Wasting
- Flaccidity

Fig. 12.156 Features of a lower motor neurone lesion.

needle electrode. If the lesion is at the anterior horn cell level, for example in motor neurone disease, there will be no sensory signs. If the lesion affects the combined nerve root, or the peripheral nerve, sensory signs will almost certainly accompany the motor deficit.

Nerve root disorders are commonly the result of degenerative disease of the spine. Lesions of a single peripheral nerve are usually the consequence of abnormal angulation, stretch, or compression. A diffuse disorder of peripheral nerves (though the pattern of distribution can vary) is called a peripheral neuropathy. In most instances, both sensory and motor components of the nerves are affected, resulting in weakness, distal sensory loss, and reflex depression.

Myasthenia gravis

In myasthenia gravis, deposition of antibody on the postsynaptic acetylcholine receptor site interrupts the function of the neuromuscular junction. Fatiguable weakness can affect any skeletal muscle. Diplopia and ptosis are particularly common (Fig. 12.157). Muscle wasting is a late, and inconsistent feature. The tendon reflexes are preserved.

Extrapyramidal disorders

The disorder most frequently affecting the extrapyramidal system is Parkinson's disease. A combination of tremor, rigidity, and bradykinesia is the hallmark of the condition. The distribution can sometimes be disconcertingly focal, and often a patient with unilateral Parkinsonism is believed to have a hemiplegia. Postural problems are common; the neck and trunk become flexed. When walking, arm swing is reduced on one or both sides and turning is difficult, the patient taking more steps than usual. Eye movements are slowed, and convergence and upward gaze tend to be diminished in range. Some patients have an associated dementia. An identical clinical (and pathological) pattern can coexist with degeneration of the intermediolateral columns of the spinal cord, producing profound autonomic failure. The Shy–Drager syndrome is a somewhat different degenerative process (though again causing extrapyramidal features) which also affects pyramidal, cerebellar, and autonomic pathways. Many patients with rigidity and bradykinesia have had their symptoms induced by drugs affecting the release of dopamine or its receptor sites. Most commonly one of the phenothiazines is responsible. Another diffuse process affecting the extrapyramidal pathways also disrupts first the supranuclear, then the nuclear, gaze pathways: the Steele–Richardson–Olsczewski syndrome (progressive supranuclear palsy).

THE CEREBELLAR SYSTEM

STRUCTURE AND FUNCTION

The cerebellum comprises two hemispheres and a midline structure, the vermis. Between the vermis and each hemisphere lies the paravermis (intermediate zone). From above down, the cerebellar cortex is divided into the anterior and posterior lobes, and the flocculonodular lobe (Fig. 12.158). Phylogenetically, there are three components; the archi-, palaeo-: and neocerebellum. The archicerebellum (principally the flocculonodular lobe) receives its major input from the vestibular nuclei. The palaeocerebellum (predominantly the vermis) receives projections from the spinal cord, while the neocerebellum, located mainly in the cerebellar hemispheres, lies on a circuit incorporating the cerebral cortex and the pons (Fig. 12.159). The fibres projecting in and out of the cerebellum pass through the superior, middle, or inferior cerebellar peduncles.

Embedded in the white matter of each cerebellar hemisphere is the dentate (lateral) nucleus. The fastigial nucleus lies medially, beneath the vermis. Lateral to the fastigial nucleus is the nucleus interpositus.

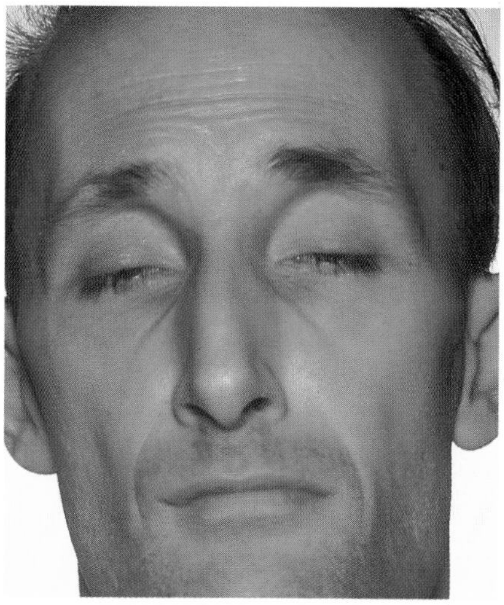

Fig. 12.157 Myasthenia gravis.

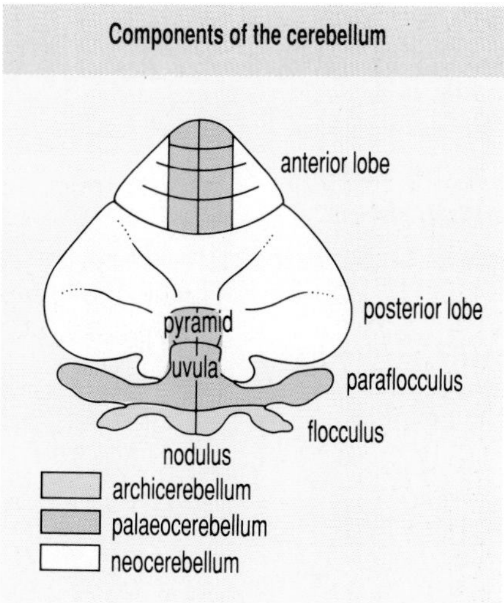

Fig. 12.158 Representation of the components of the cerebellum.

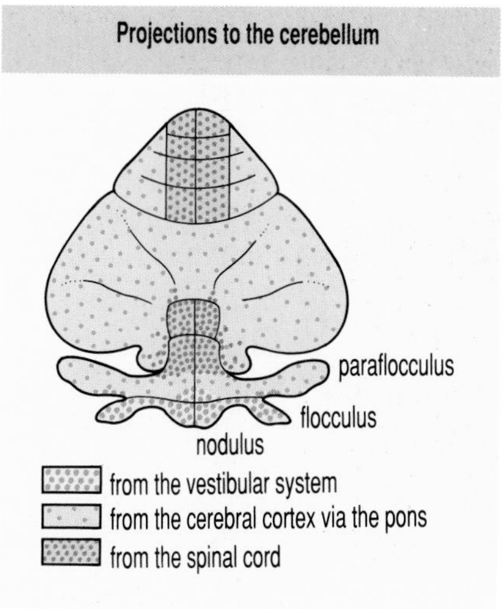

Fig. 12.159 Projections to cerebellum from vestibular system, spinal cord, and cerebral cortex via the pons.

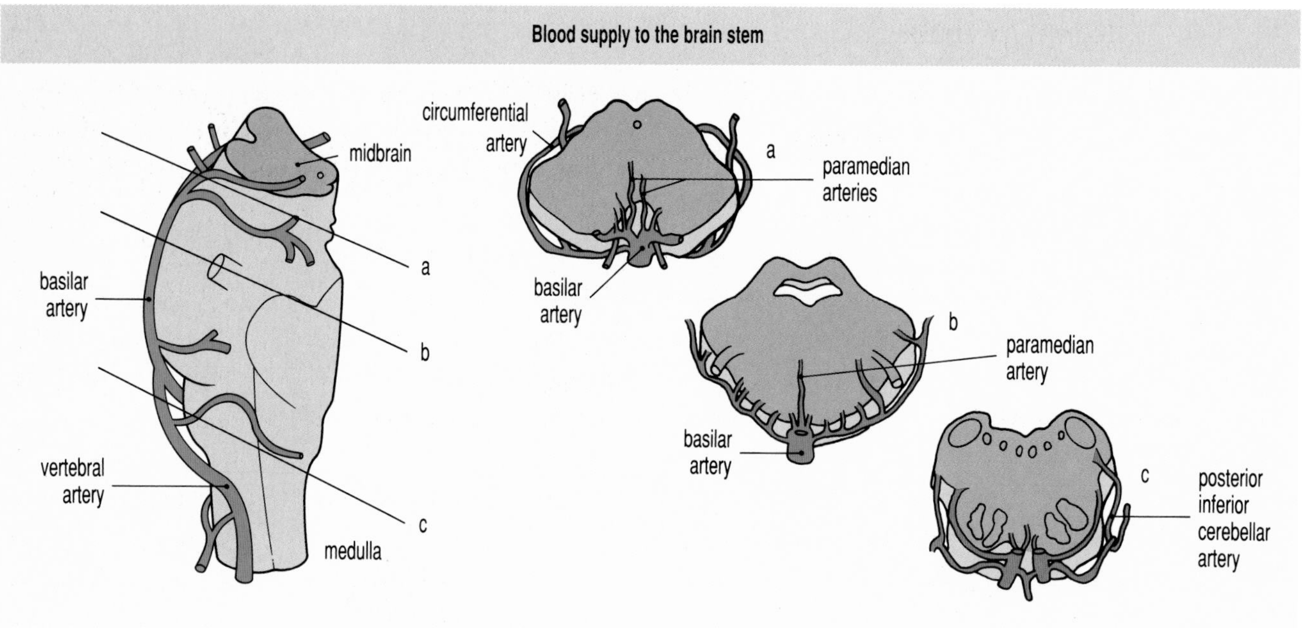

Fig. 12.160 Blood supply to the brain stem.

The cerebellar cortex is supplied by three vessels: the upper surface is supplied by the superior cerebellar arteries and the lower surface is supplied by the anterior inferior cerebellar arteries, with a contribution here from the posterior inferior cerebellar arteries. The first two pairs of vessels arise from the basilar artery, the last from the vertebral artery. The brain stem is supplied by penetrating branches arising directly from the basilar artery, from circumferential branches, and, at the level of the medulla, from the posterior inferior cerebellar artery (Fig. 12.160).

Dentate neurones discharge before the onset of motor activity, and even before the relevant motor cortical discharge. The nucleus interpositus is active during the control of movement, and at its termination. Both nuclei are concerned with posture control but activity in the interpositus nucleus appears more closely related to the force of muscle contraction and its velocity. Discharge in fastigial neurones relates partly to velocity and partly to force.

The cerebellum exerts an influence on muscle tone through an effect on motor neurone output to the muscle spindle. In the presence of a cerebellar lesion, the early phase of the stretch reflex is unaffected, but the later phases tend to be diminished. Efferents from the flocculus exert an inhibitory effect on the vestibulo-ocular reflex via the fastigial nucleus.

SYMPTOMS

The symptoms of a disruption of the cerebellar system include dysarthria, limb clumsiness and gait ataxia.

Dysarthria

Patients with dysarthria have a defect of pronunciation, though speech content remains normal.

Limb clumsiness

A unilateral cerebellar disorder results in an ipsilateral limb ataxia. If the dominant limb is affected, the patient may well have noticed an alteration in writing. Sometimes the patient may refer to an ataxic limb as being weak rather than clumsy.

Gait ataxia

If the cerebellar problem is confined to one hemisphere, the patient often complains of deviating to that side when walking. With disruption of midline cerebellar structures, however, unsteadiness when walking is the main complaint rather than a tendency to deviate to a particular side.

EXAMINATION

Speech

Dysarthria will be apparent while you take the history. Remember to take account of accent. There is no need to give the patient set phrases to pronounce; a brief conversation suffices. In cerebellar dysarthria speech volume and pitch are typically erratic, so that the rhythm of speech is lost, with pauses then accelerations. If the disorder is severe, speech is shot out in a staccato fashion.

Eye movements

In patients suspected of having cerebellar disease, you need to look for nystagmus, and for abnormalities of either saccadic or pursuit movements (Fig. 12.161). The assessment of eye movement has

Eye signs in cerebellar disease	
Location	**Sign**
flocculus	abnormal smooth pursuit gaze-evoked nystagmus
flocculus /nodulus	down-beat nystagmus
vermis/fastigial nucleus	ocular dysmetria
lateral zones	ocular dysmetria gaze-evoked nystagmus

Fig. 12.161 Eye signs in cerebellar disease.

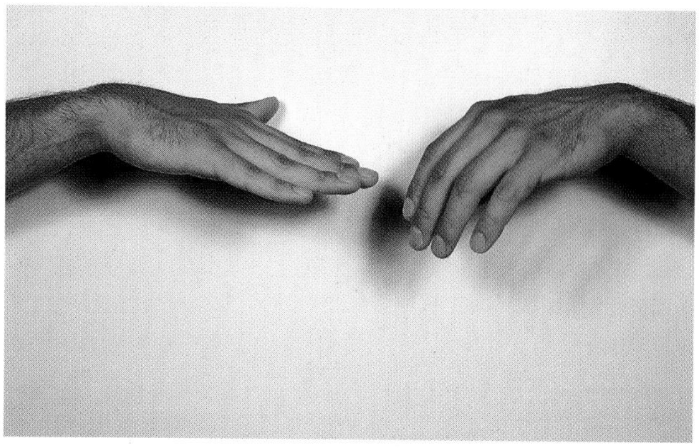

Fig. 12.162 Hypotonia of the left hand in a left cerebellar lesion.

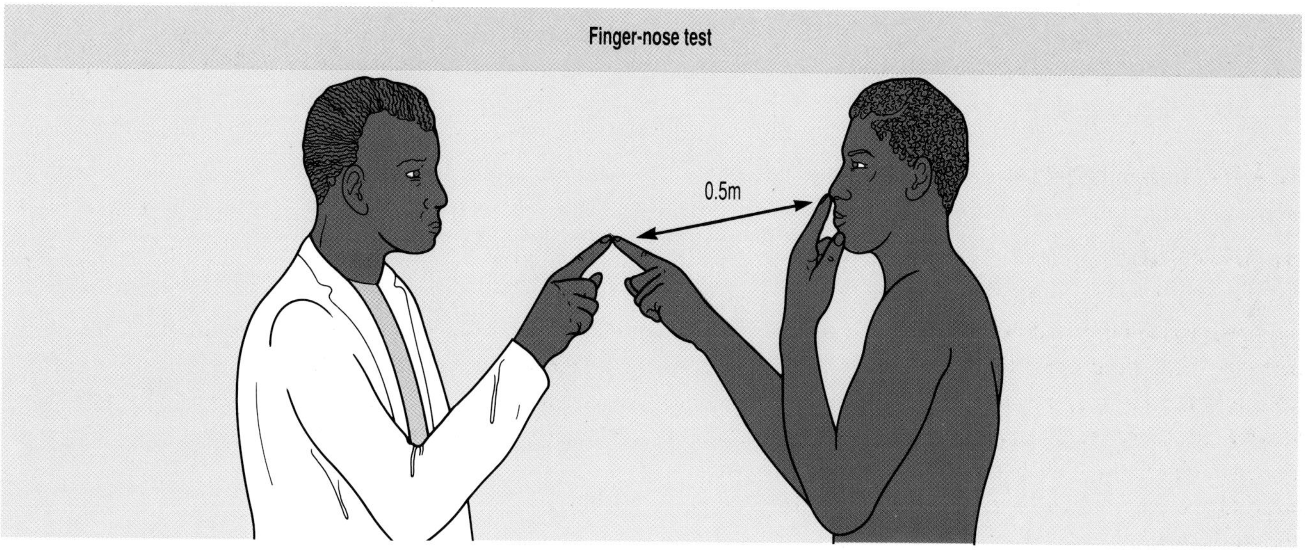

Fig. 12.163 The finger-nose test.

been discussed on pages 12.35–12.36. In archicerebellar lesions, particularly those of the flocculus, you will find a gaze-evoked nystagmus and a defect of smooth pursuit in which the movement is broken up by saccadic corrections. Downbeat nystagmus can occur in the presence of floccular or nodular lesions. Disruption of the vermis and the underlying fastigial nucleus causes ocular dysmetria, in which, during saccadic movement,the eyes over- or undershoot the target (hypermetria and hypometria, respectively). To elicit this physical sign ask the patient to rapidly fixate between two targets, one central and the other about 30° from fixation. Ocular dysmetria may also occur in hemisphere lesions, but it is uncertain whether a lesion confined to that site is associated with nystagmus.

Limb examination

The reduced limb tone associated with a cerebellar lesion is difficult to detect. If the problem is unilateral, ask the patient to hold the arms in the position shown in Fig. 12.162. If the limb is hypotonic, the hand tends to sag below the horizontal. If there is a severe cerebellar disturbance the outstretched hands may oscillate. More likely, however, is the presence of an intention tremor. To test this ask the patient to touch first his nose then your finger held about 0.5m in front of him (Fig. 12.163). In a cerebellar ataxia, a tremor emerges which becomes more apparent as the target is approached. If you are undecided, move your target finger in a random fashion while the patient tries to maintain a smooth pursuit. A mild ataxia may then become more evident.

Occasionally, in disease of the cerebellar pathway, a severe swinging tremor appears as a result of interruption of the cortico-cerebellar circuit at the level of the red nucleus (rubral tremor). While testing for intention tremor observe whether the patient's finger reaches the target accurately. It may reach beyond the target (hypermetria), fall short (hypometria), or even bounce against it in an uncontrolled fashion.

Now assess alternating movements in the upper limbs. Ask the patient to hold one hand steady, in the horizontal plane, with the fingers closed. Next ask the patient to tap first the dorsal then the palmar surface of one hand with the fingers of the other, pronating and supinating the forearm in the process. Test the movement in yourself, using the dominant and non-dominant movement in yourself, using the dominant and non-dominant hand to gauge the speed and accuracy in a normal individual. The patient with cerebellar ataxia is clumsy and there are fluctuations in both the speed and amplitude of the movement (dysdiadokokinesis). Listen to the sound of one hand slapping on another; normally it is easy to sustain a fairly even volume. The 'slaps' of a cerebellar hand lurch between a 'whisper' and a 'shout'.

Patients with cerebellar disease encounter difficulties in the initiation and termination of movement. Ask the patient to raise his arms rapidly from the sides but to stop them abruptly in the horizontal plane. In cerebellar disease the affected arm oscillates about its intended resting place due to a failure of the damping mechanism. You will already have examined the limb reflexes as part of the motor system examination. They may be unusually sustained in cerebellar disease ('hung up' reflex).

To assess lower limb coordination, ask the patient to slide the heel of one foot in a straight line down the shin of the other leg: the heel-knee-shin test (Fig. 12.164). In the presence of cerebellar ataxia the heel wavers around the intended pathway. When the heel has reached the bottom of the shin, ask the patient to flex the leg then bring the heel back down on to the shin just below the knee. If there is cerebellar incoordination, the heel may fall short of its target or thump into the shin rather than landing gently. Finally, ask the patient to tap your hand repetitively using first one foot then the other. Be aware, however, that the performance of this test is quite variable in normal individuals, and tends to be less smooth in the non-dominant limb.

Gait

Unless there is a substantial disturbance of midline cerebellar structures, patients do not display any instability of the trunk while sitting, but upon standing oscillations of the body may occur even before gait is initiated. When walking, the patient will use a wide-based gait and is likely to show caution when turning. Attempts to turn quickly will result in problems with posture control. Be prepared to support the ataxic patient when you ask them to walk independently. If the patient has a lesion of one cerebellar hemisphere, then deviation to that side occurs on walking. To detect a more subtle disturbance of cerebellar function, ask the patient to walk heel-toe (Fig. 12.165). Again you need to appreciate how variably normal individuals perform this test. Those lacking confidence in walking, for any reason, are likely to perform badly.

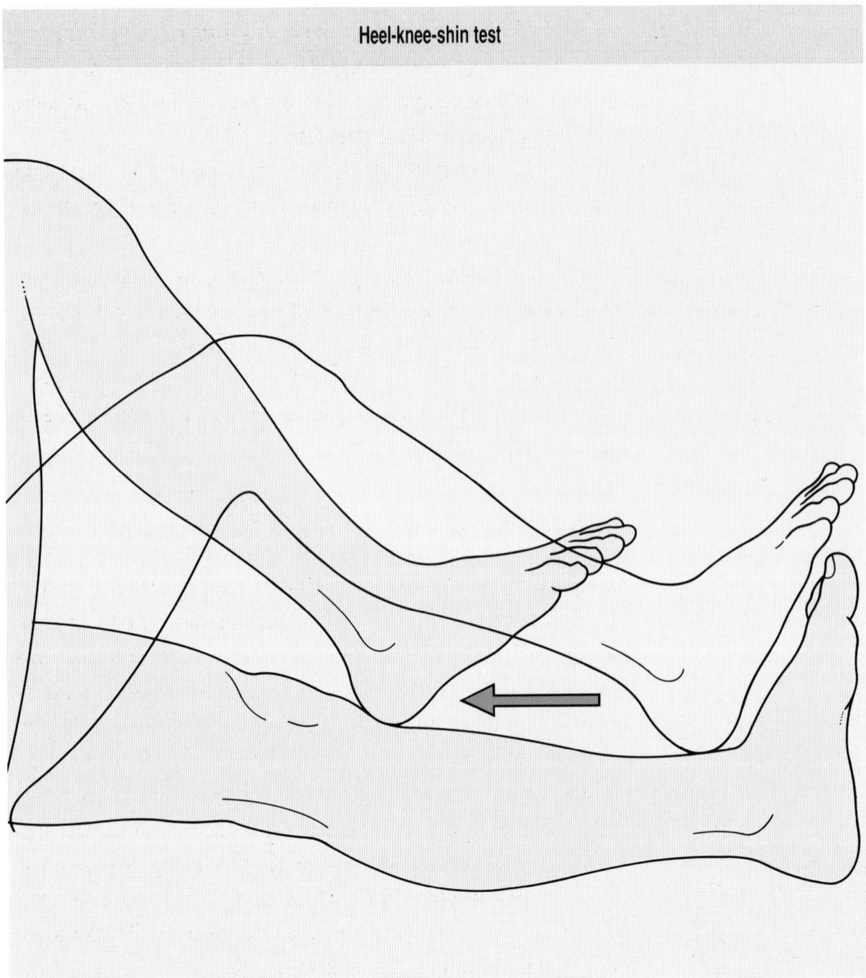

Fig. 12.164 Performing the heel-knee-shin test with the right leg.

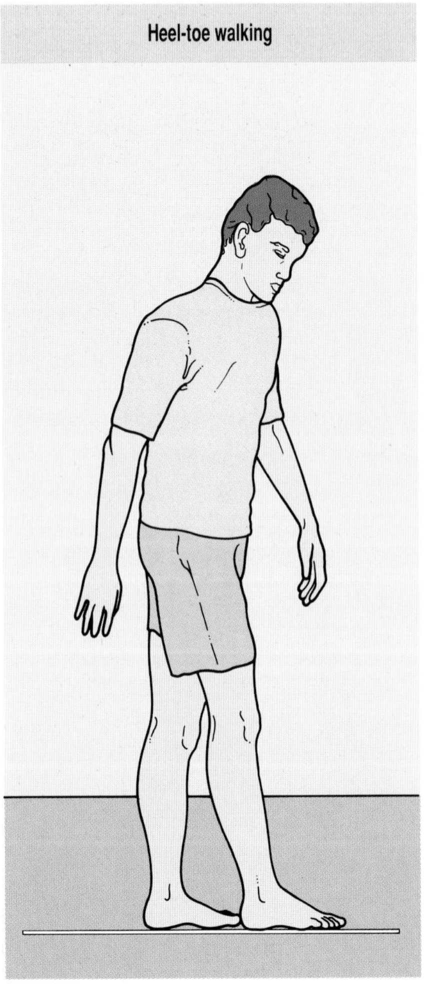

Fig. 12.165 Heel-toe walking.

CLINICAL APPLICATION

Lesions of the cerebellar hemisphere

The lesions most commonly affecting the cerebellar hemisphere are infarcts (Fig. 12.166), haemorrhage, and tumour. In adults a tumour involving the cerebellum is usually metastatic. Characteristic symptoms include an ipsilateral limb ataxia, a gait which tends to deviate to the affected side and an ocular dysmetria.

Midline cerebellar lesions

The predominant complaint in patients with lesions of the vermis or paravermis is a gait ataxia. Tumours are sometimes confined to this area but more often the syndrome is due to selective atrophy secondary, for example, to alcohol. The familial cerebellar atrophies tend to produce a more diffuse atrophy readily detectable by CT scanning (12.167).

Cerebellar signs are very common in patients with established multiple sclerosis, but the triad of tremor, dysarthria, and nystagmus, described by Charcot, is rare as an isolated clinical feature. More often it is accompanied by other features of the disease.

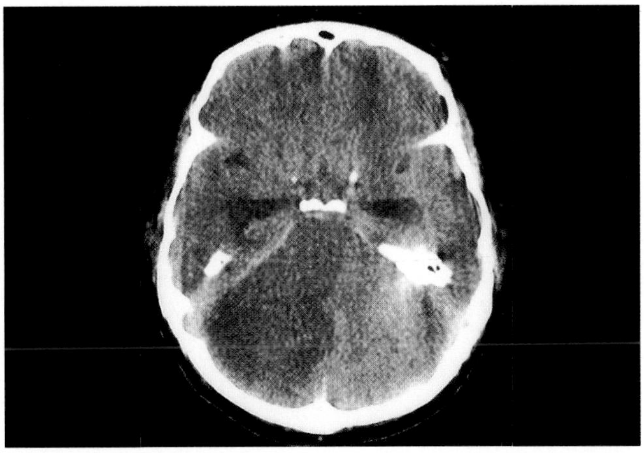

Fig. 12.166 CT scan showing a left cerebellar infarct.

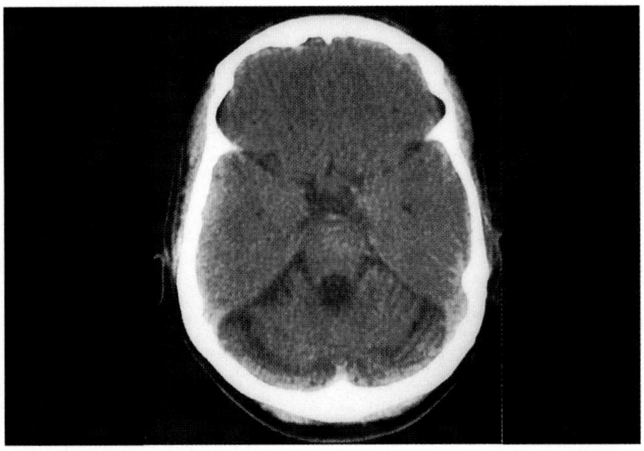

Fig. 12.167 CT scan showing diffuse cerebellar atrophy.

THE SENSORY SYSTEM

STRUCTURE AND FUNCTION

The sensory nerve endings

The majority of the sensory nerve endings in the skin are located in the epidermis. They are more common in the face, hands, and feet than in the trunk. The individual cutaneous receptors do not respond solely to a specific stimulus, but their sensitivity for one usually far exceeds that for the others. Cutaneous receptors include those responding to a deformity of the skin (mechanoreceptors), those responding to temperature (thermoreceptors), and those responding to pain (nociceptors). Information regarding the position and posture of the limbs (proprioception) is derived from end organs in muscle, the muscle spindle, and the Golgi tendon organ. The nerve fibres issuing from these various receptors are either myelinated or nonmyelinated.

Mechanoreceptors respond either to a change in skin position (rapidly adapting), or continue to discharge as long as the skin displacement persists. In general the mechanoreceptors are innervated by myelinated fibres.

The cutaneous thermoreceptors produce impulses in response to small changes in skin temperature. The thermoreceptors are innervated by thinly myelinated and nonmyelinated (C) fibres. The former conduct at around 15 m/s, the latter at around 1 m/s. The fibres conveying temperature sense travel in the spinothalamic tract closely associated with pain fibres.

Cutaneous nociceptors discharge almost specifically in relation to a potentially damaging thermal or mechanical stimulus to the skin.

Light touch responses are perceived principally by the Pacinian corpuscle and the hair follicle receptors. The information is transmitted predominantly by large myelinated fibres.

Pacinian corpuscles identify a vibrating stimulus when applied to the skin. The central pathway lies in the dorsal columns but also utilizes the spinothalamic system.

The spinal roots

The spinal cord has paired spinal roots at each segmental level. The dorsal roots (purely sensory) and the ventral roots (predominantly motor) join to form a mixed spinal nerve which then produces two branches: the posterior primary ramus and the anterior primary ramus. The brachial and lumbosacral plexuses, responsible for the nerve supply of the upper and lower limbs, are each supplied by the relevant anterior primary rami. In the trunk, the anterior and posterior primary rami are distributed to the hyaxial (ventral) and epaxial (dorsal) musculature respectively, and to the corresponding overlying skin (Figure 12.168). The areas of skin supplied by the branches of the dorsal roots are called dermatomes. The arrangement of dermatomes is straightforward in the trunk, but more complicated in the limbs (Fig. 12.169). The cutaneous distribution of the individual peripheral nerves is summarized in Figure 12.170. Considerable overlap of distribution exists both for adjacent dermatomes and peripheral nerves.

The posterior columns

All sensory fibres have their first cell station in the dorsal root ganglion. A proportion of fibres pass directly into the posterior columns, with about 25 per cent reaching the gracile and cuneate nuclei. Additional fibres in the posterior columns originate from cells in the ipsilateral posterior horn. Proprioceptive fibres tend to run the whole length of the cuneate fasciculus, but those in the gracile fasciculus leave in the upper lumbar segments of the cord, synapsing in Clarke's column before passing into the dorsal spinocerebellar tract. Above this level the fasciculus gracilis is occupied by fibres solely concerned with cutaneous sensation. Initially, as successive fibres enter the dorsal columns, distal segmental fibres are displaced medially, but in the neck area, the arrangement of fibres in the columns is related to their anatomical rather than their segmental source. In the nuclei, the lower limb is represented medially and the upper limb laterally. Immediately above the gracile nucleus is nucleus Z, believed to receive proprioceptive information from the ipsilateral lower limb. Second-order neurones from the gracile and cuneate nuclei, and from nucleus Z, decussate to form the medial lemniscus which in turn projects to the ventroposterior nucleus of the thalamus.

The spinothalamic tract

Another group of fibres enters the spinal cord and terminates in the posterior horn. The majority of the axons within the spinothalamic tract originate from layer V (Fig. 12.171). The fibres then pass ventral to the spinal canal before ascending in the anterolateral quadrant. Here the fibres from the sacral segments come to lie laterally, and superficially, as they are displaced by fibres from higher segmental levels. There is no firm evidence that the ascending spinothalamic tract is divided into discrete ventral and dorsal components.

Distribution of a spinal nerve

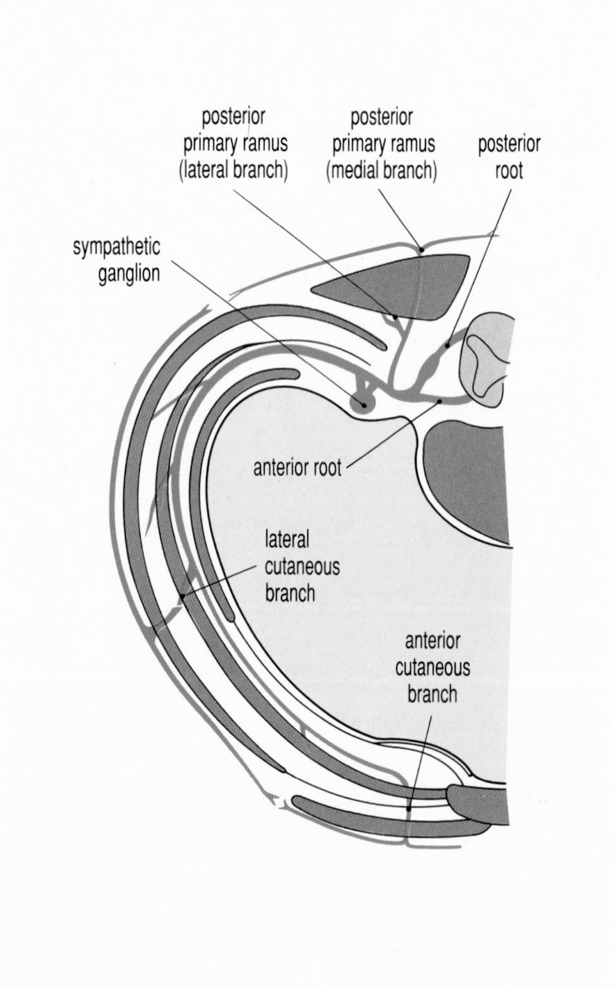

Fig. 12.168 Distribution of a spinal nerve.

Dermatome distribution

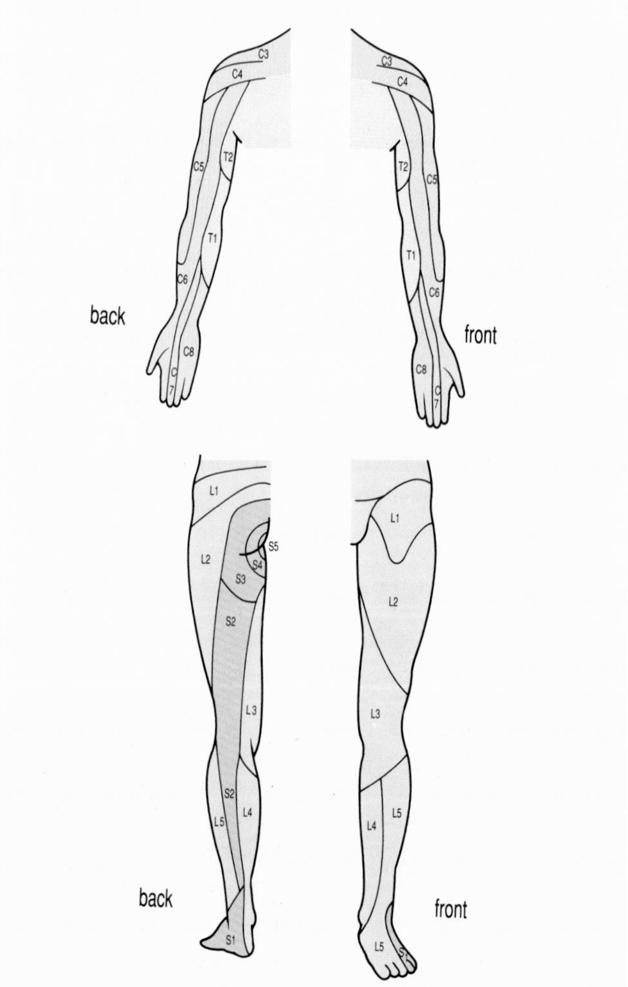

Fig. 12.169 Dermatomes of the upper and lower limbs.

The spinocervical tract

The third ascending pathway begins with cells from laminae IV and V of the dorsal horn which send fibres ipsilaterally in the spinocervical tract to the lateral cervical nucleus, which is situated lateral to the dorsal horn of the upper segments of the cervical cord (Fig. 12.171). From here fibres decussate and join the medial lemniscus. The spinocervical tract contains axons which respond

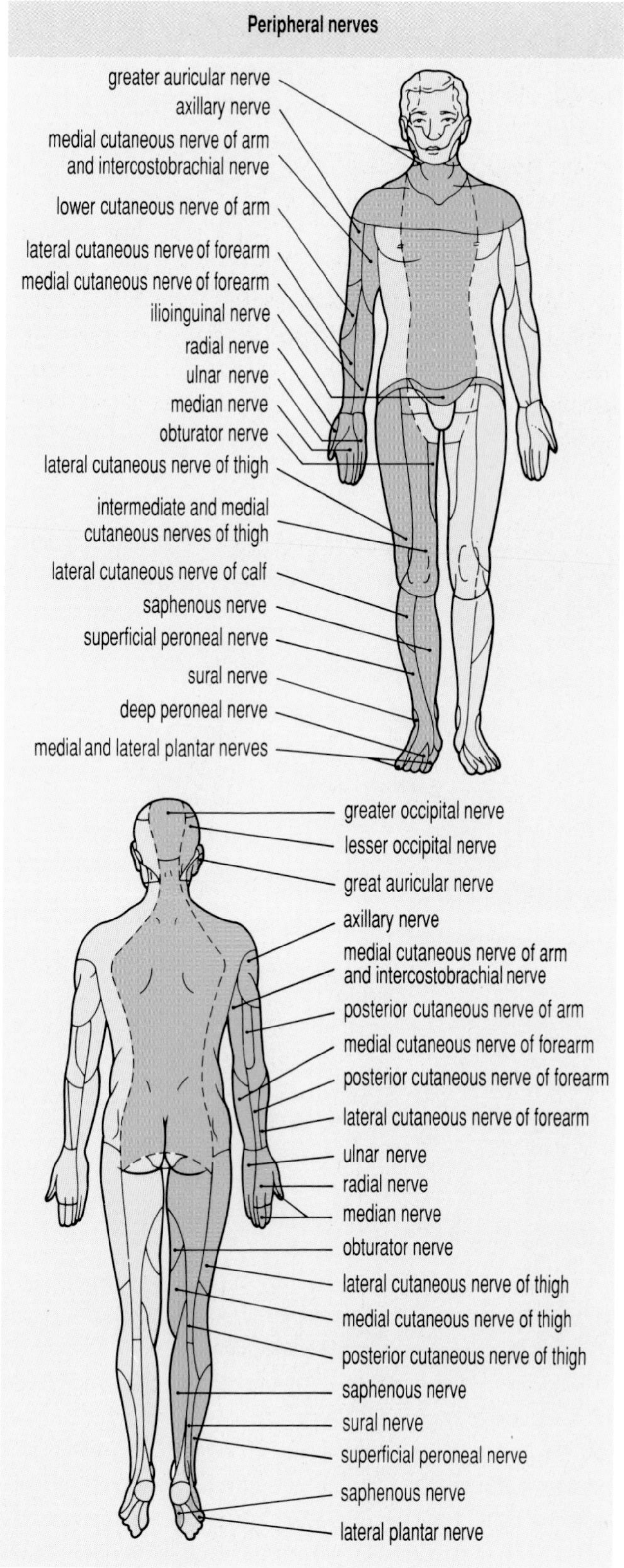

Fig. 12.170 Distribution of sensory components of the peripheral nerves.

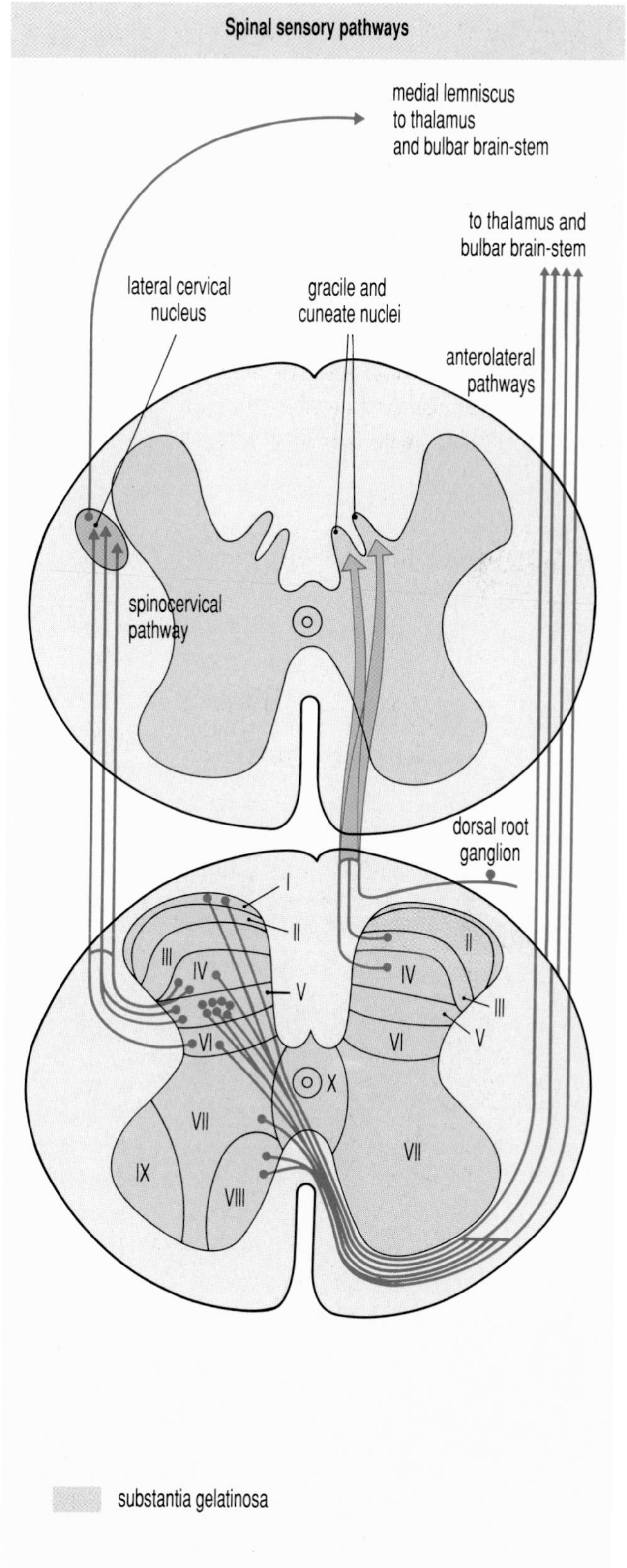

Fig. 12.171 Sensory pathways in the spinal cord.

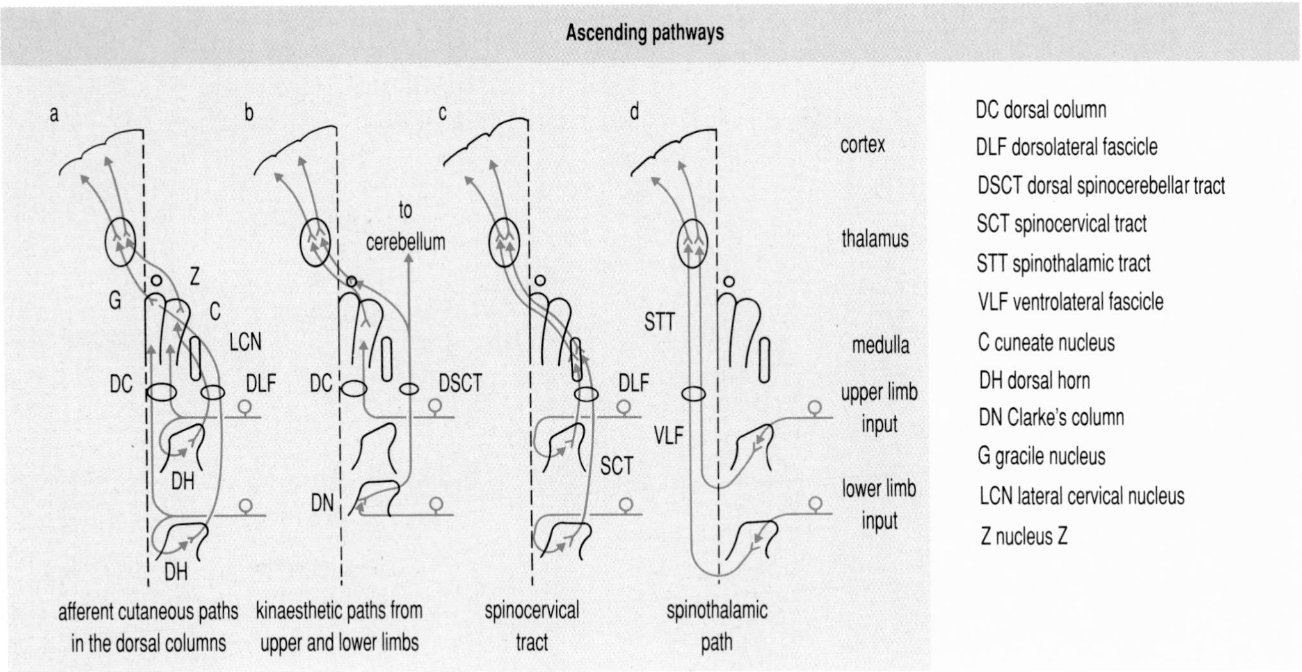

Fig. 12.172 Ascending pathways.

principally to light pressure but also contains fibres responding to noxious thermal and mechanical stimuli. A summary of the ascending pathways is shown in Fig. 12.172.

The thalamus

The medial part of the ventroposterior nucleus of the thalamus receives information from the face, and the lateral portion from the medial lemniscus and the spinothalamic tract. In practice, however, this neat parcelling of function is an over-simplification.

The cortex

Areas of the cortex concerned with the processing of ascending sensory information include the primary somatic area (SI), the secondary somatic area (SII) and the adjacent cortex (Fig. 12.173). Most of the afferent fibres to SI arise from the ventroposterior nucleus of the thalamus. Representation is parallel to that of the motor cortex (Fig. 12.174). The cells in the anterior part of the sensory cortex respond principally to cutaneous stimulation, and those in the posterior part to stimulation of deep tissues, including the joints. Group I muscle afferents project principally to the anterior part of SI. The cells in SII receive projections from both sides of the body. In its posterior part are cells which respond to a noxious stimulation of the limbs.

PAIN

According to the gate control theory of pain perception, the activity level of certain cells in the substantia gelatinosa (lamina II and III) can inhibit conduction of impulses in the central pain pathways.

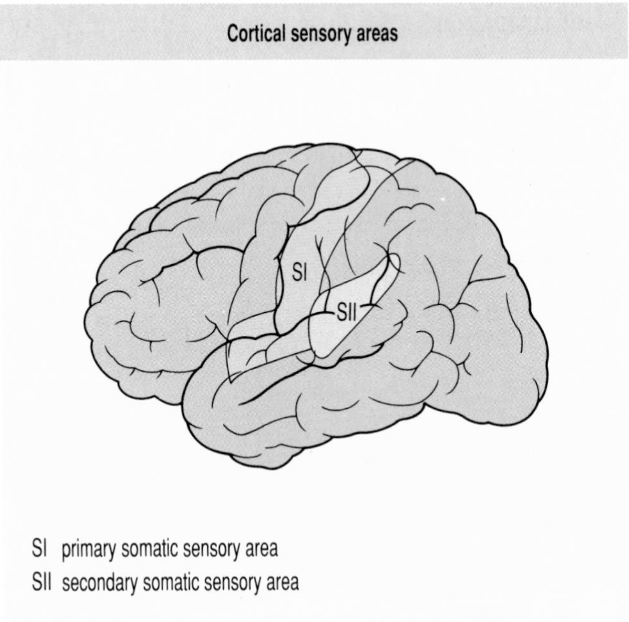

Fig. 12.173 Cortical sensory areas.

These inhibitory cells are activated by impulses in large diameter peripheral afferent fibres, and switched off by impulses in small diameter myelinated and unmyelinated fibres.

Visceral pain is transmitted by sympathetic or parasympathetic fibres. Impulses emanating from free nerve endings in the gut pass into the posterior root via the splanchnic nerves. Their central connections are similar to those of the spinothalamic fibres. In some instances pain from a viscus is interpreted as arising from a superficial body part possessing the same segmental innervation (referred pain).

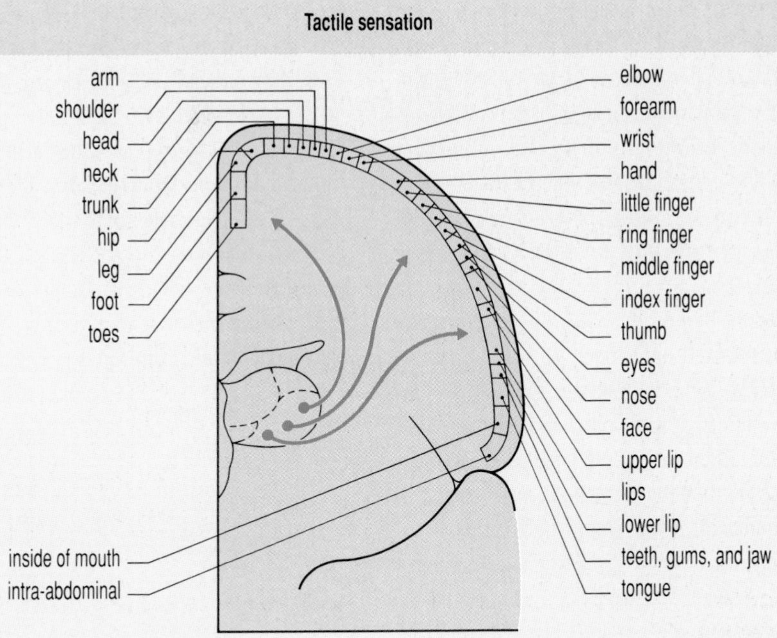

Fig. 12.174 Representation of tactile sensation in the left hemisphere.

SYMPTOMS

Sensory symptoms include pain, paraesthesiae, and numbness. Frequently the patient's understanding and use of these terms (though they are more likely to mention tingling, or pins and needles, than paraesthesiae) differ from that of the physician. Clearly establish what the patient means – many use numbness to describe a lack of use of a limb, rather than a defect of sensation.

Sensory disturbances

When the patient describes numbness, do they mean actual loss of cutaneous sensation?

Does the distribution of any numbness or tingling follow the distribution of a peripheral nerve or nerve root?

Does the patient describe loss or altered sensation ascending onto the abdomen or thorax?

Pain

Only rarely does the particular quality of a pain serve to identify its likely source. In peripheral nerve injury, signs of nerve damage may be accompanied by a distressing, persistent burning sensation known as causalgia. Pain related to peripheral nerve disease usually localizes to the distribution of the affected nerve. In nerve root disorders, the pain is not referred in a dermatomal distribution but follows a distribution corresponding to the muscles (myotome), or to other deep structures (sclerotome) supplied by that root. A particular type of pain can emerge after damage to the spinothalmic tract or the thalamus itself (thalamic pain). It is persistent, with a very unpleasant burning or scalding quality, and is exacerbated by painful or tactile contact.

Paraesthesiae and numbness

Patients often struggle when describing the nature of sensory disturbances. They tend to resort to a previous experience to assist their description (e.g. the recovery of sensation after a dental block). Few patients are able to provide a meticulous description of the distribution of their symptoms. Furthermore, the confined areas of sensory change from nerve or root damage, the consequence of the overlap of function between adjacent peripheral nerves or dermatomes, can hinder identification of the anatomical structures involved.

EXAMINATION

Sensory examination is difficult. There are few objective criteria, assessment being largely dependent on the patient's subjective responses. It is seldom necessary to test all sensory modalities, and even then certainly not in all parts of the body. The areas tested, and the modalities used, should be influenced by the type of sensory disturbance suggested by the patient's history. If the patient has an area of reduced cutaneous sensation, start testing within that area, moving out gradually to determine the zone of transition to normal sensation. When describing the patient's reaction to a stimulus, it is better to indicate the stimulus used, and the reaction observed, rather than relying on a term which may have an ambiguous meaning. Anaesthesia and hypaesthesia refer, respectively, to areas of lost and reduced light touch sense. For painful stimuli, the comparable terms are analgesia and hypalgesia. An exaggerated reaction to a painful stimulus at a normal threshold (hyperalgesia) is rare. More often, the exaggerated reaction coincides with an altered threshold (hyperpathia). Hyperaesthesia indicates an exaggerated reaction to, or perception of, light touch.

Try to avoid testing pin prick in younger children – an adverse response to the sight of the needle will interrupt the rest of the examination. Avoid being over persuasive when attempting to confirm a preconceived area of sensory deficit. The sensory examination is fatiguing for both patient and examiner, and it is better to return to complete the examination at another session rather than continuing an assessment which is yielding increasingly conflicting findings.

Light touch

Use a wisp of cotton wool to test light touch sensation (Fig. 12.175). Varying the size of the wisp, or the contact, alters the stimulus strength. A brush can be used as an alternative, but it may be more difficult to grade stimulus intensity by this method . Remember that different areas of the skin vary in sensitivity. The distal parts of the limb are more sensitive than the proximal and hair containing skin is more sensitive than smooth skin. Do not drag the cotton wool along the surface of the skin, but apply it at a single point then move on. Ask the patient to close his eyes and to respond when contact is made.

If the patient complains of unilateral sensory change, compare equivalent parts on the two sides of the body. Patients with cortical lesions tend to show an erratic response to cutaneous stimulation, which may even suggest non-organic disease. If the history suggests a cortical lesion, but cutaneous sensation appears intact, assess the effect of simultaneous stimulation of equivalent body parts. In parietal lesions, the half-body supplied by the damaged cortex may fail to register a stimulus when there is competition from the intact opposite side, even though a stimulus, applied in isolation, is appreciated (sensory suppression or extinction). In hemisensory loss, the change to normal appreciation will occur strictly at the midline.

Two-point discrimination

Two-point discrimination is tested with a pair of compasses specifically designed for this purpose, with gradations in centimetres indicating the separation of the tips, which are blunt rather than pointed. Apply the tips with equal, gentle pressure (Fig. 12.176) while the patient's eyes are closed, and establish the minimum separation at which two points are confidently identified. As an approximate guide, a young adult will detect a separation of around 3mm on the finger tips, 1cm on the palm of the hand, and 3cm on the sole of the foot.

The test findings do not necessarily mirror the responses to light touch and can provide useful information in peripheral nerve, cord and cortical sensory disturbances. Patients with cortical lesions have a fluctuating threshold.

Light touch test

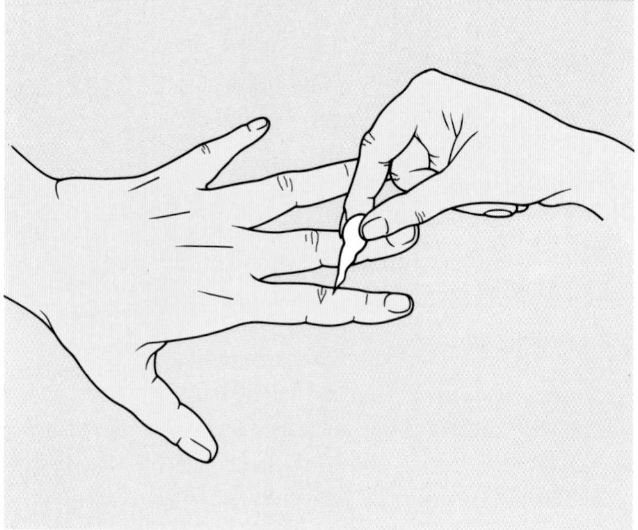

Fig. 12.175 Testing light touch with a wisp of cotton wool.

Two-point discrimination test

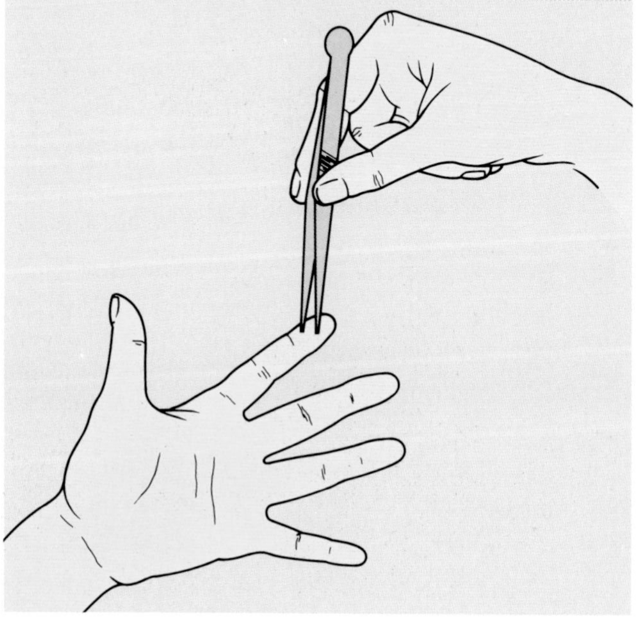

Fig. 12.176 Testing two-point discrimination.

Proprioception

While assessing joint position sense ensure that the patient's eyes remain closed throughout each test. Begin by testing the patient's ability to appreciate passive movements of the joints. It is rare to find a loss of proximal joint position sense; more often the problem is confined to the digits. During testing avoid pressing on the digit in such a way that the patient appreciates the direction of movement. To test the terminal interphalangeal joint of the index finger grip the sides of the phalanx with the thumb and forefinger of your right hand using your left to stabilize the proximal joints of the finger (Fig. 12.177). You will not at first realise how sensitive the responses to movement are. The movement appreciated will be barely perceptible to the naked eye. If the responses are inaccurate, move proximally until the movements are accurately perceived. Indicate your findings in the notes as 'JPS – intact to movement of the distal interphalangeal joint of 10°', or whatever range you have chosen. Remember that this amount would be above threshold for younger patients, but that proprioceptive sensitivity probably declines a little with age.

In addition to testing passive movement, you can test active proprioception by asking the patient with the eyes closed to locate a digit of one hand with the index finger of the other limb. Alternatively, move the limb with intact sensation into a certain posture and then ask the patient to mimic that position with the affected limb. Finally, ask the patient to hold the hands outstretched while the eyes are closed. With severe loss of distal proprioception, the fingers move in a curious, irregular, purposeless fashion, as if exploring their environment (pseudo-athetosis) (Fig. 12.178).

To test the quality of the proprioceptive information coming from the lower limbs, ask the patient to stand with their feet together and their eyes closed. Where there is loss of proprioception, the patient immediately loses stability (positive Romberg's test) (Fig. 12.179).

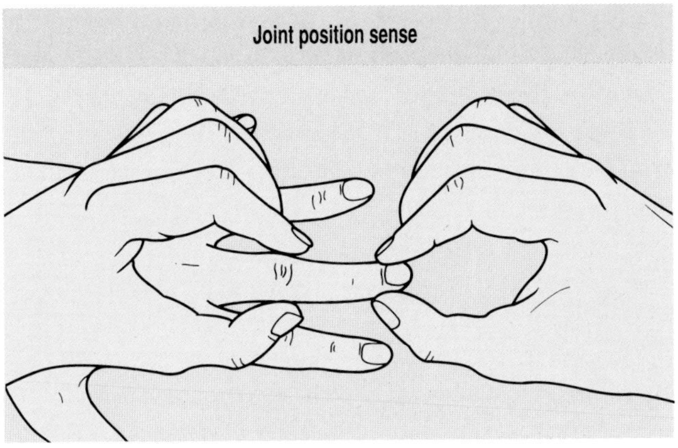

Fig. 12.177 Testing joint position sense.

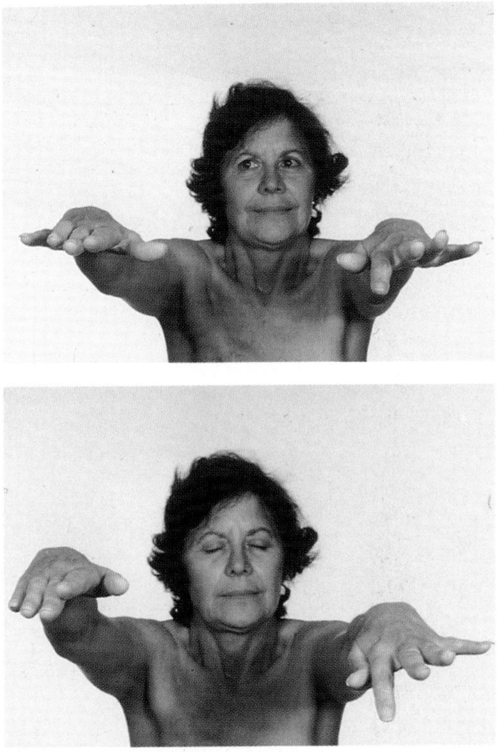

Fig. 12.178 Pseudo-athetoid posturing.

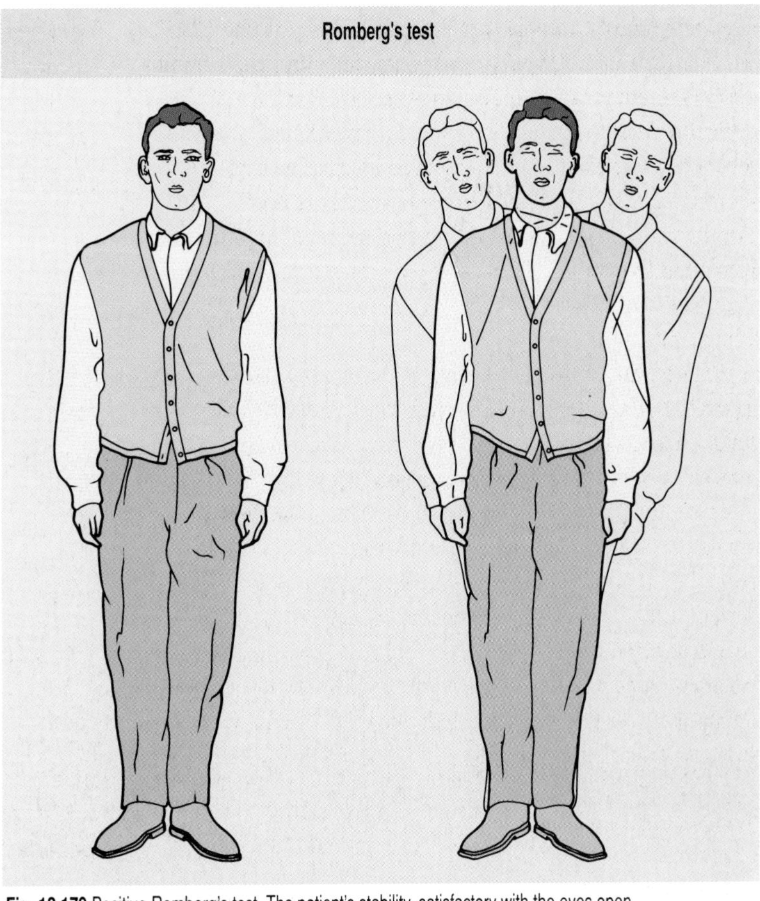

Fig. 12.179 Positive Romberg's test. The patient's stability, satisfactory with the eyes open, immediately deteriorates with the eyes closed.

Vibration sense

Testing the appreciation of vibration is of limited value in most patients, and it is not uncommon to find this sense reduced or absent in the toes of elderly people.

Vibration sense is tested using a 128Hz tuning fork. It is not necessary to have the tuning fork in close contiguity with underlying bone. To test sense in the finger, apply the gently vibrating base of the fork to the pulp of the finger, or the knuckle of the distal interphalangeal joint (Fig. 12.180). For the foot, start with the pad of the big toe or the dorsum of the interphalangeal joint. If vibration sense is absent there, test more proximally. In the upper limb, you can successively test a metacarpophalangeal joint, the wrist, and the elbow, and, in the lower limb, the ankle, knee, and anterior superior iliac spine, if necessary ending at the rib margin. The chest wall acts as a resonator, and a more accurate level of vibration loss on the trunk is obtained by applying the fork to a fold of skin pulled away from the underlying rib. In practice, this is seldom necessary. Semi-quantitative testing is achieved by waiting until the perception of vibration has ceased on one limb then transferring the tuning fork to the other limb.

Pain

Pain is best tested by using a sharp pin or needle (Fig. 12.181). Venepuncture needles are unsuitable because they are so sharp that the skin is readily punctured and bleeding results, particularly in the elderly. It is preferable, therefore, to use a dressmaker's pin which, though sharp, is unlikely to pierce the epidermis unless applied with excessive force. Standard 'sharps' safety procedures should be followed, discarding the pin immediately after use.

Remember that you are testing the painful quality of the stimulus, rather than merely an appreciation of contact. Either ask the patient to close their eyes and identify if the contact is painful, or present the sharp and blunt ends of the pin in a random fashion, asking the patient to distinguish one stimulus from another. Apply a series of three of four contacts to, say, the right thumb before testing a similar area on the left. Usually the patient accurately identifies the point of stimulation, but in some pathological states a more diffuse pain radiates out from the site of contact. Remember that certain areas, for instance callouses, are liable to show diminished sensitivity to pain. Deep pain sense can be tested by applying pressure to deeper structures, for example by pinching the tendo Achilles. Be aware, however, that the discomfort felt, and the corresponding reaction, are likely to exceed those triggered by pricking the skin.

The sense of tickle can be tested by drawing the finger along the skin. The peripheral and central pathways for this sense follow those for pain.

Temperature

Testing temperature sense is time-consuming and the findings are often difficult to interpret. There are, however, certain conditions where selective loss of thermal sensitivity occurs, and where temperature testing remains important.

A reduced or exaggerated response to a thermal stimulus can exist over a fairly narrow band of temperature, but to test temperature sense it generally suffices to use two metal tubes, one containing water mixed with ice chips, the other containing hot water. Do test skin sensitivity on yourself before testing the patient. Ask the patient to distinguish hot from cold on comparable parts of the two sides of the body. You will need to renew the tubes if the examination is protracted.

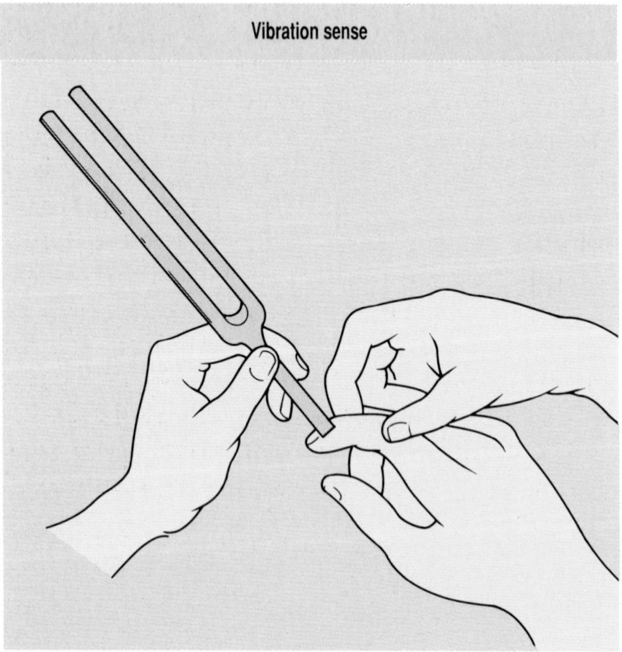

Fig. 12.180 Testing vibration sense in the left index finger.

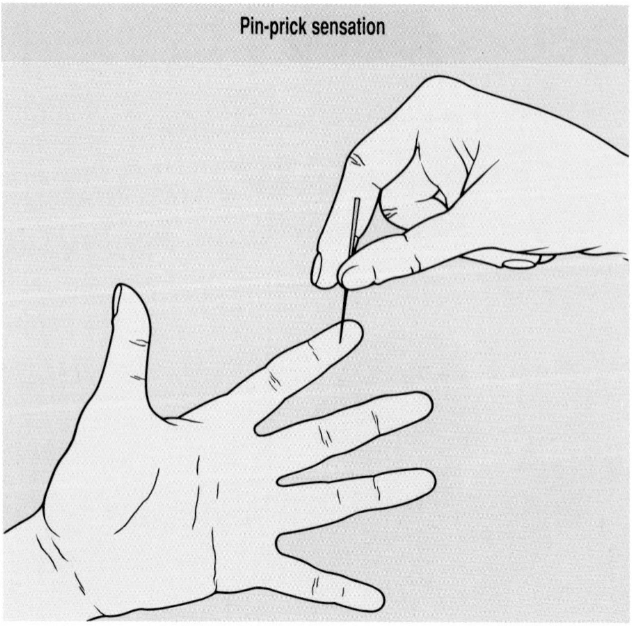

Fig. 12.181 Testing pin-prick sensation.

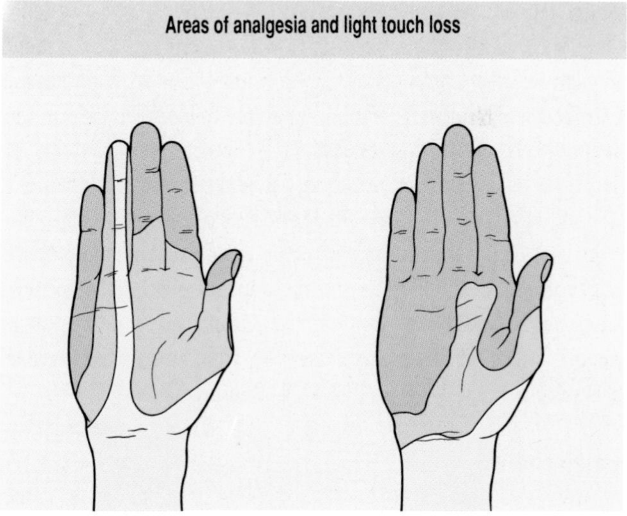

Fig. 12.182 Areas of analgesia and light touch loss with isolated median and ulnar nerve lesions (left) and combined lesions (right).

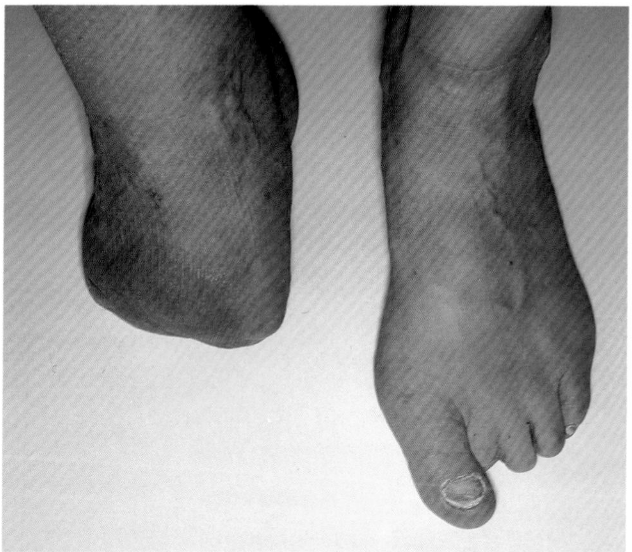

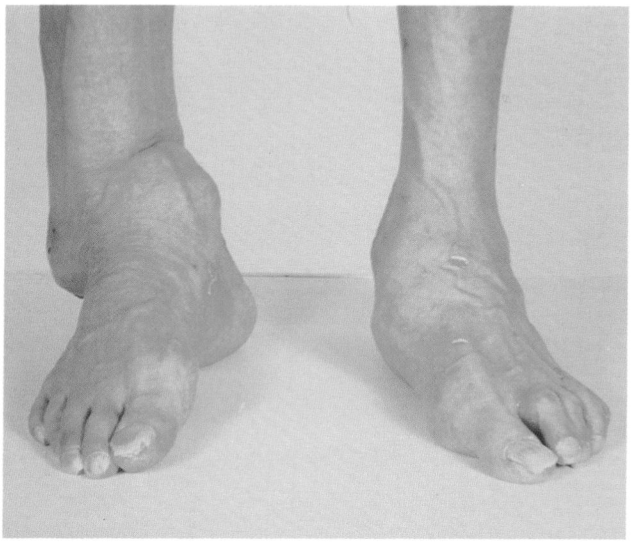

Fig. 12.183 Amputation of the right fore-foot and of several toes of the left foot in a patient with sensory neuropathy (upper). Charcot joint. Right ankle (lower).

Weight, shape, size, and texture

Certain sensory modalities are particularly worth testing if a disturbance of cortical function is suspected. To test weight appreciation put an object in the patient's palm, allowing the hand to move up and down so the patient appreciates both the pressure exerted by the weight and the resistance experienced when the hand is moved against gravity. Compare the effect of the same weight in the other hand, or alternate differing weights between the two hands and ask the patient to distinguish them.

Shape recognition is also heavily dependent on cortical function. Everyday objects, such as a series of coins of different values, can be used when testing this modality. Ask the patient to assess the shape of the coin, and also (though this involves other sensory modalities) whether it possesses a milled edge. If the hand is paretic the patient will experience great difficulty in manipulating the object, but in this case you can guide their finger over the surface and edge of the coin. In fact watching the patient manipulate the coin gives you valuable information about both the motor and sensory status of the digits. Another problem arises if the patient is aphasic or agnosic. Such patients will face difficulties in describing the object, even in the absence of any sensory loss (see pages 12.7–12.8). Coins can also be used for testing size recognition. You can use materials of different form (velvet, wool, linen, etc.) to test the patient's appreciation of texture.

CLINICAL APPLICATION

Nerve and root disorders

You may well suspect from the history that the patient has a neuropathic or radicular sensory loss. Besides the problem of overlap of contiguous nerves or dermatomes (Fig. 12.170), you need to appreciate that considerable anatomical variation exists in the classical cutaneous distributions. For example, the median nerve can supply 3 or 4 digits, rather than three and a half (Fig. 12.182). Within an affected nerve or root all sensory modalities will be equally affected, with a boundary zone of partial loss in which appreciation of light touch is more disturbed than that of pain and temperature. In a peripheral neuropathy affecting sensory fibres, there will be a distal disturbance of sensory function which gradually merges into normality. A large-fibre neuropathy will tend to spare pain and temperature sensitivity. A small-fibre neuropathy, predominantly affecting pain and temperature, is rare. If pain fibres to the skin and joints are affected, consequences include painless skin ulceration, sometimes leading to amputation, and a severe derangement of joint function (Fig. 12.183a and b).

Spinal cord disorders

In a transverse cord lesion, for instance due to transverse myelitis, a sensory level is found approximating to the site of the spinal cord pathology. At this level there is often a narrow zone within which cutaneous stimulation, if sufficiently strong, can create a painful reaction (Fig. 12.184). In a unilateral cord lesion (Brown–Séquard syndrome) (Fig. 12.185) there is contralateral loss of pain and temperature to a level slightly below that of the lesion, along with ipsilateral weakness and depression of vibration and joint position sense. Causes include trauma and multiple sclerosis.

More localized spinal cord lesions occur. One confined to the region of the central canal will selectively disrupt crossing spinothalamic fibres but spare other sensory pathways. The result is a bilateral selective loss of pain and temperature over the affected segments (Fig. 12.186). Causes include syringomyelia and central cord tumours. Lesions confined to the dorsal columns interfere with vibration sense, proprioception, and two-point discrimination. If the cervical cord is affected, the patient sometimes experiences a curious electric shock sensation passing down the spine when the neck is flexed (Lhermitte's sign). At this level a lesion confined to the posterior columns will predominantly affect upper limb joint position sense.

External compression of the spinal cord is likely to spare those deeper fibres in the spinothalamic tract which come from segments immediately below the level of compression. Conversely a tumour spreading from the centre of the cord is likely to spare the superficial fibres emanating from sacral segments.

Brain stem and thalamic disorders

In the medulla, lateral lesions predominantly affect contralateral pain and temperature sensation, while medial lesions disrupt sensation served by the dorsal columns. Above this level pathological processes usually disturb all sensory modalities in the contralateral half of the body and cause ipsilateral facial sensory loss if the relevant part of the trigeminal nucleus is involved. Thalamic lesions affect all aspects of sensation in the opposite side of the body. In some cases spontaneous pains occur accompanied by intense burning sensations when certain cutaneous stimuli are applied (thalamic syndrome). The cause is almost always vascular (Fig. 12.187).

Cortical lesions

The cortex is concerned principally with the finer aspects of sensory appreciation. It allows definition of object size, shape, weight and texture. Loss of this facility is called astereognosis. The cortex allows both accurate definition of the site of contact and discrimination of single or multiple stimulation. It is closely concerned with the appreciation of joint position. Sensory suppression (see page 12.20) is a particular feature of cortical lesions. In non-dominant parietal lobe lesions, neglect of the contralateral limbs can be so profound that the patient denies their existence and tries to remove them as if belonging to another person.

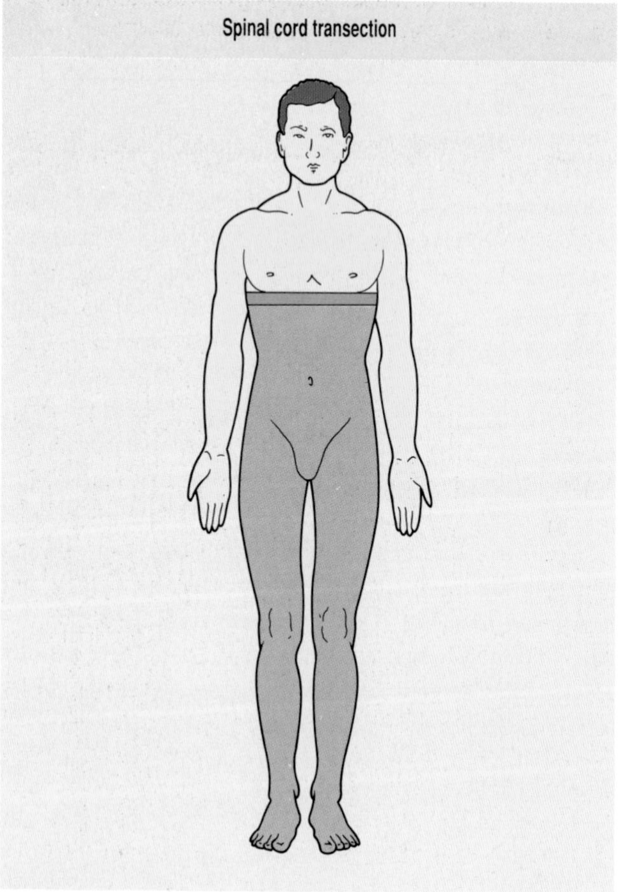

Fig. 12.184 Spinal cord transection at T5. There is complete loss of sensation below that level with a zone of altered sensation immediately above it.

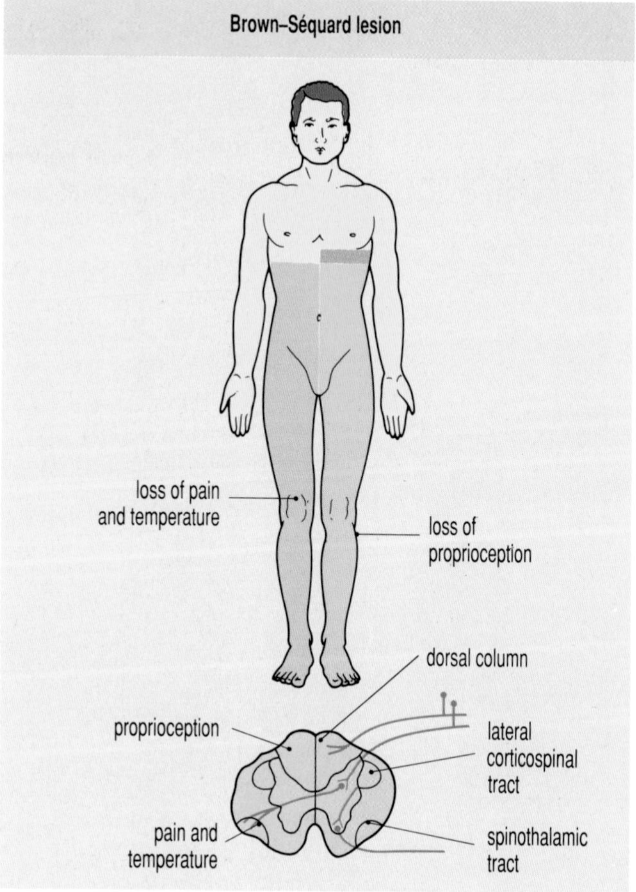

Fig. 12.185 Distribution of sensory and motor deficit in Brown–Séquard lesion.

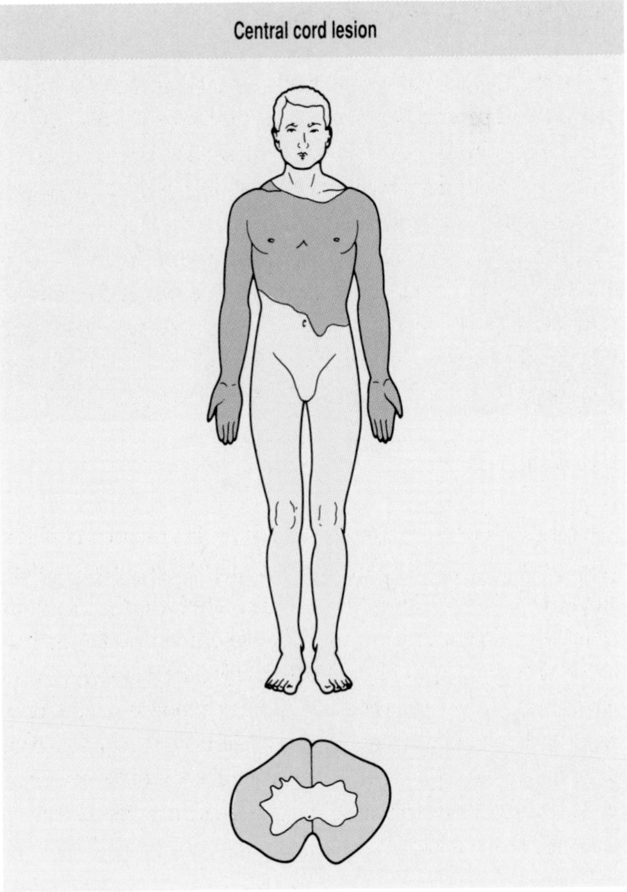

Fig. 12.186 'Cape' of selective pain and temperature loss due to a central cord lesion extending from about C3 to D10.

Non-organic sensory loss

The most common pattern of non-organic sensory loss is one in which cutaneous sensation to all modalities is affected, with little or no change in proprioception. Typically a single limb is involved, but sometimes the problem occupies one side or the lower half of the body (Fig. 12.188).

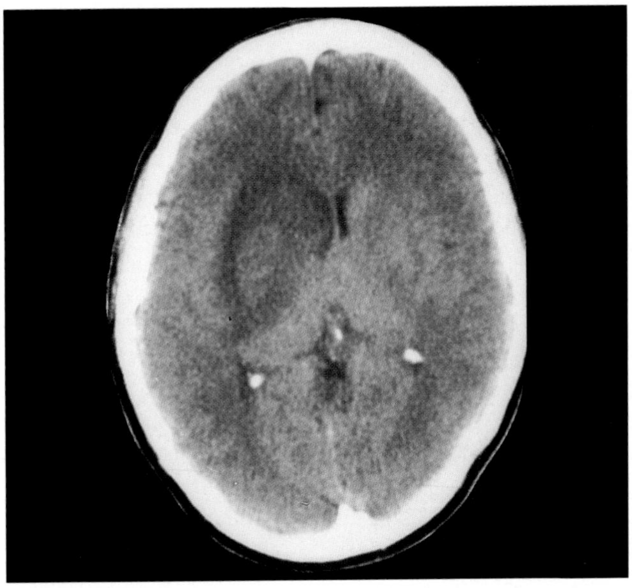

Fig. 12.187 CT scan showing a striatal infarct extending into the thalamus.

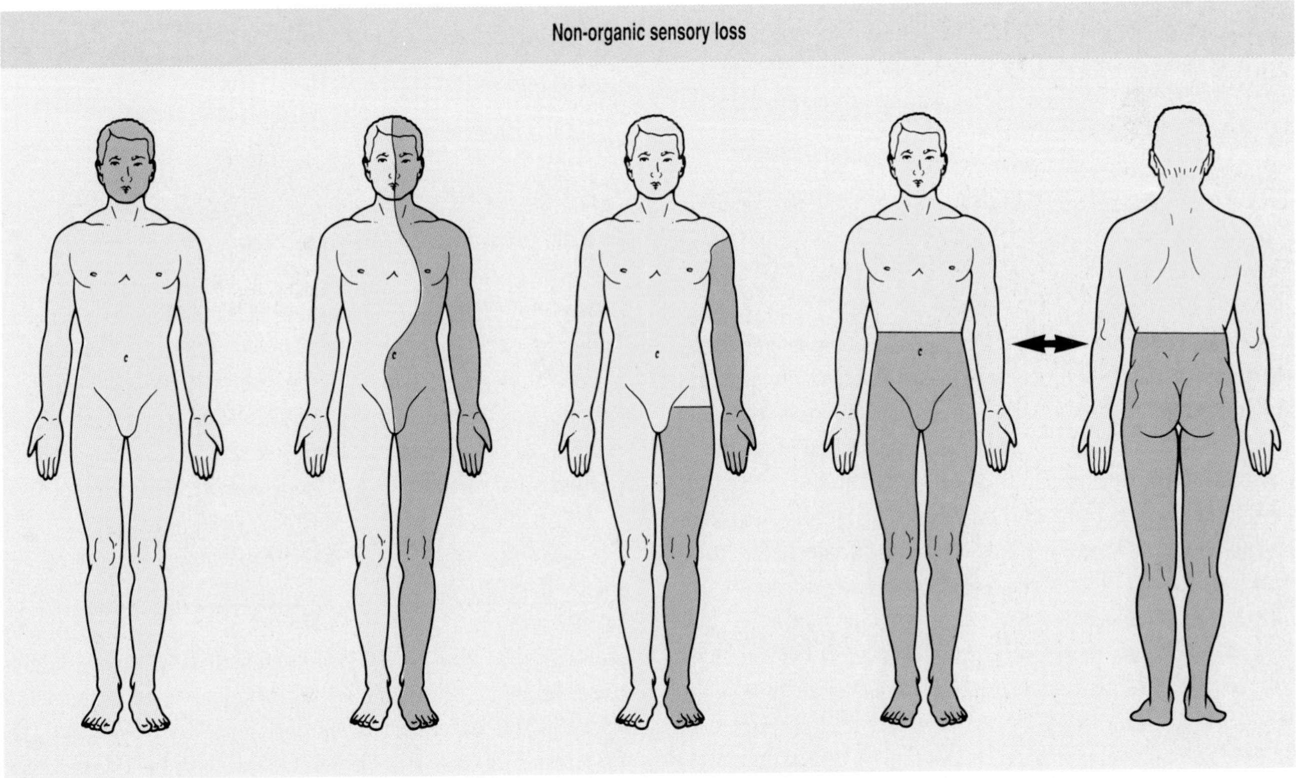

Fig. 12.188 Patterns of non-organic sensory loss.

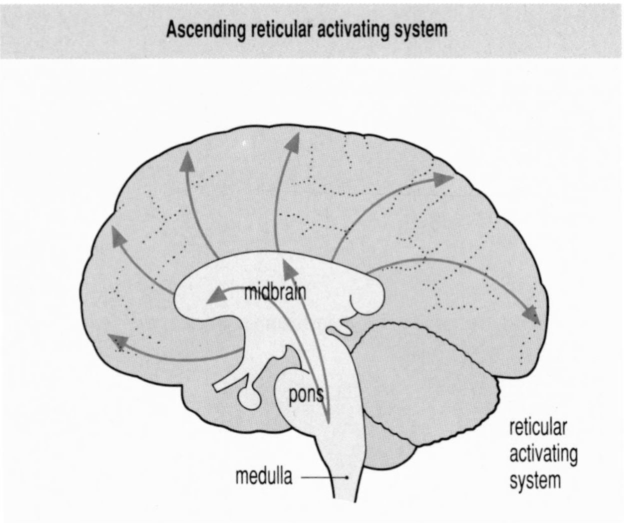

Fig. 12.189 The connections of the ascending reticular activating system.

Many patients with non-organic sensory loss perceive it as confined strictly to the limb. Consequently, sensation returns to normal at the shoulder, or above an approximately horizontal line at the level of the groin. Typically this transition is sudden, and the patient reacts adversely if a painful stimulus is being used. Rarely the patient will respond to stimulus in the intact limb by saying yes, and in the defective limb by saying no. Sometimes, when the patient turns into a prone position, the previously numb leg regains sensation on its extensor surface, having been transposed, so to speak, to the other side of the bed. Levels of non-organic loss can fluctuate, even within the course of a single examination. Hemisensory loss virtually never ceases at the midline, either straying beyond or falling short. Facial sensory loss, when not organically determined, has a tendency to be purely facial, following the hair line superiorly and the jaw line inferiorly.

THE UNCONSCIOUS PATIENT

SYMPTOMS

Lesions confined to one cerebral hemisphere seldom interfere with consciousness. Coma is the consequence either of extensive bilateral hemisphere disease, a unilateral hemisphere mass lesion, or more discrete pathology confined to certain parts of the brain stem. Critical in the development of coma, certainly in the second and third instances, is the integrity of the ascending reticular activating system (Fig. 12.189), which extends from the medulla to the thalamus. Disruption of this system above the pons is responsible for alteration of the conscious state.

Mass lesions in one cerebral hemisphere affect the conscious level by causing downward herniation of brain tissue through the tentorial notch, with secondary compression of the brain stem (Fig. 12.190). Two types of herniation are described, a central form, usually associated with slowly expanding, medially placed masses, and an uncal form, in which masses in the middle cranial fossa, particularly of the temporal lobe, cause displacement of the medial aspect of the uncus over the free edge of the tentorium. Pathological consequences of this herniation include ipsilateral third nerve compression, distortion of the contralateral cerebral peduncle, and paramedian brain stem haemorrhages.

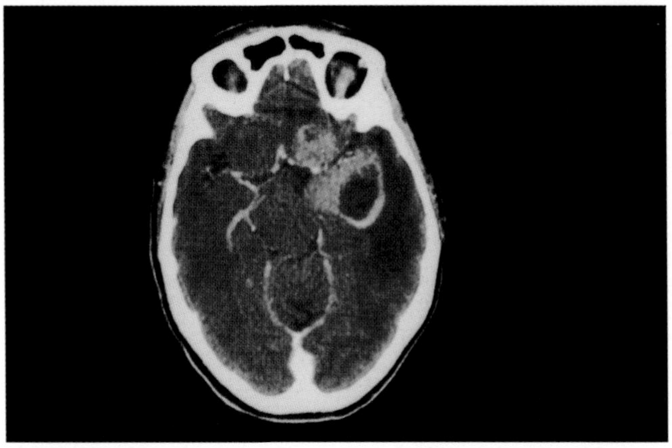

Fig. 12.190 CT scan showing herniation of a right temporal mass with distortion of the upper brain stem.

Some aspects of the clinical examination in the unconscious patient

1. Boggy scalp swelling
2. Alcoholic foeter
3. Spider naevi
4. Venepuncture marks
5. Hepatomegaly
6. Hypotension
7. Blood in the ear

Fig. 12.191 Aspects of the clinical examination in the unconscious patient.

EXAMINATION

Many aspects of the general examination can be performed in the unconscious patient (Fig. 12.191). Try to spend a few moments inspecting the patient before embarking on specific systems. The posture may be of value in diagnosis. Carefully examine the skin for signs of injury, petechial haemorrhages, or evidence of drug abuse.

Grading of coma	
1	Alert
2	Drowsy but reponds to verbal stimulation.
3	Unconscious – no response to verbal stimulation, but withdrawal response to pain.
4	Unconscious – decorticate responses to pain (flexion of upper limb and extension of lower limb).
5	Unconscious – decerebrate responses to pain (hyperextension of both upper and lower limbs).
6	Unconscious – no response to pain.

Fig. 12.192 Grading of coma.

	Patient's response	Score	08.00	10.00	12.00
Eye Opening	Spontaneous	4			
	To Speech	3			
	To Pain	2			
	None	1			
Best Verbal Response	Oriented	5			
	Confused	4			
	Inappropriate	3			
	Incomprehensible	2			
	None	1			
Best Motor Response	Obeying	6			
	Localizing	5			
	Withdrawing	4			
	Flexing	3			
	Extending	2			
	None	1			

Fig. 12.193 Glasgow coma scale.

Testing for neck stiffness

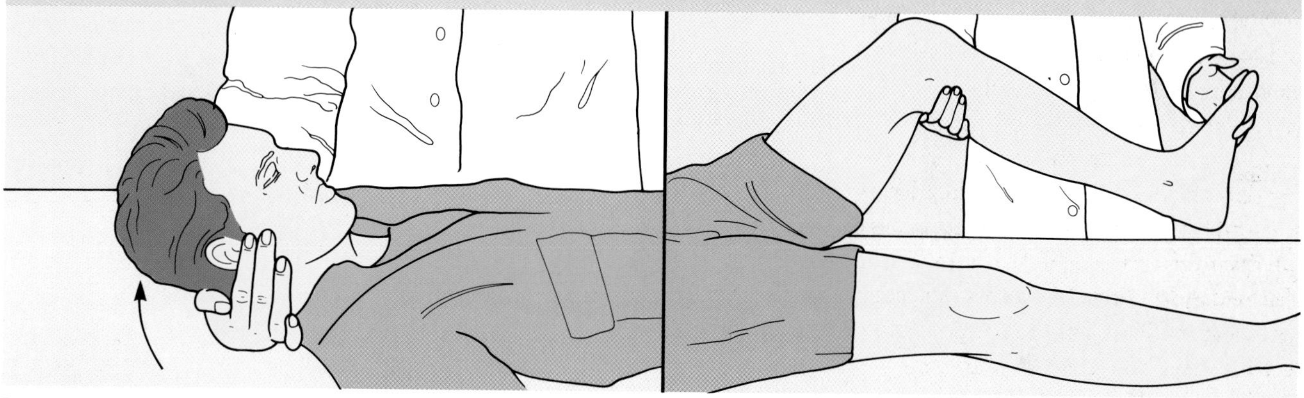

Fig. 12.194 Testing for neck stiffness (left), and eliciting Kernig's sign (right).

Skeletal system

Palpate the long bones for evidence of fracture. Note the presence of any localized scalp swelling indicating focal trauma, and inspect the external auditory meati for signs of bleeding, suggesting the possibility of a basal skull fracture.

Cardiovascular system

Perform a routine cardiovascular assessment, looking particularly for hypo- or hypertension, pulse abnormality, and abnormal heart sounds or murmurs.

Respiratory system

Assess respiratory rhythm and rate. Sometimes the patient's foetor, for example of alcohol, gives a clue to the diagnosis, but remember that in an individual who has been drinking the coma may have another cause (e.g. a head injury).

Gastrointestinal system

Palpate the abdomen. Is there hepatomegaly, suggesting primary liver disease, perhaps resulting in gastrointestinal haemorrhage from oesophageal varices? Look for other markers of liver disease, such as spider naevi.

Level of consciousness

Do not use terms such as stupor or coma to describe the patient's conscious state. Record the best level of response of which the patient is capable (Fig. 12.192). Having performed other aspects of the examination, you can then proceed to grade the conscious level using the Glasgow Coma Scale (Fig. 12.193).

Signs of meningeal irritation

Flex the neck to see whether there is any abnormal resistance to the movement, or a reaction on the part of the patient (Fig. 12.194).

Neck stiffness suggests meningeal irritation. Kernig's test is performed by flexing the leg at the hip with the knee flexed, then extending the leg at the knee. The patient may react as the leg is extended, or there may be an obvious reflex spasm in the hamstring muscles. With deepening levels of coma, these signs of meningeal irritation disappear.

The pupils

Examine the pupils for symmetry and size then test the direct light response using a bright pencil torch (Fig. 12.195). The presence of an optic tract lesion can sometimes be confirmed by finding a lack of response when light is shone into the eyes from the affected half field. A pathological process in the region of the pretectum will interrupt the pupillary light response. The pupils are mid-position in size and fixed to light. The ciliospinal reflex, elicited by pinching the skin at the side of the neck and dependent on sympathetic function, remains intact, leading to pupillary dilatation. Lesions of the oculomotor complex itself are likely to produce slightly irregular pupils fixed to all forms of stimulation. Disruption of the third nerve beyond the nucleus produces a characteristic eye position associated with a fixed dilated pupil.

In metabolic coma the pupils remain reactive and symmetric though often relatively small. Only in profound coma do the pupils become fixed. Certain drugs can influence pupil size or reactivity. Atropine will cause pupillary dilatation, as will over-dosage of amphetamines or tricyclic anti-depressants. Morphine derivatives, in excessive dosage, result in pinpoint pupils which retain their reactivity.

Ocular movements

First note any spontaneous eye movements. In many unconscious patients the eyes roam from side–to–side. The movements are usually conjugate but may occasionally become disconjugate. At other times the eyes should remain in the mid-position. Any deviation of one or both eyes implies a defect of oculomotor function unless there is a pre-existing strabismus.

Now assess eye movements. Having gently elevated the upper lids, firmly rotate the head laterally, then vertically (doll's head manoeuvre). If reflex eye movements are intact, the eyes move so as to leave them directed forwards. A more potent stimulus for reflex eye movement is achieved by caloric stimulation. Clear the external auditory meatus of any wax then inspect the tympanic membrane to ensure it is intact. Position the patient so that the head is elevated to about 30° above the horizontal, and using a soft rubber catheter instil ice-cold water into the external auditory meatus. A total volume of about 50ml suffices. Do not inject the water under pressure. If the brain stem reflexes are intact the eyes will tonically deviate to the side of the irrigated ear. It is usually not necessary to test reflex vertical movements – in order to do so, both ears have to be simultaneously irrigated with cold water (for down gaze) or warm water (for up gaze). Nystagmus is an unlikely finding in the comatose patient, but a variety of vertical movements can occur. Generally a rapid downward or upward conjugate movement followed by a gradual return to the mid-position (ocular bobbing and reverse bobbing respectively) is observed.

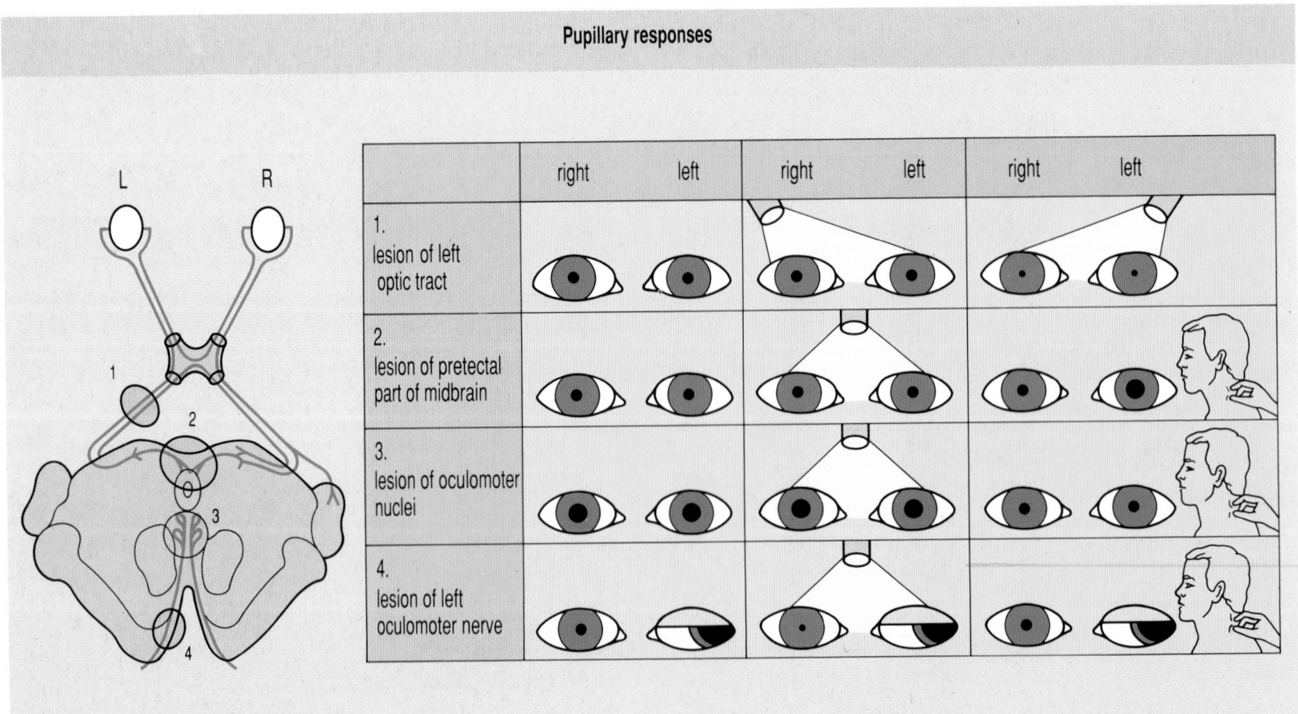

Fig. 12.195 Pupillary responses in the presence of lesions of the left optic tract, the pretectal part of the midbrain, the oculomotor nuclei, and the left oculomotor nerve. Ciliospinal responses are shown on the right.

Sustained horizontal ocular deviation indicates a frontal or brain stem lesion. In the former the eyes deviate away from the side of the accompanying hemiplegia. In a brain stem lesion below the decussation of the supranuclear pathway for horizontal gaze, the eyes deviate to the opposite side and hence to the side of an accompanying hemiparesis. Failure of upgaze occurs in the early stages of central transtentorial herniation.

Motor responses

Motor function in the limbs can be assessed partly by observing the patient's posture, and partly by assessing the response to a noxious stimulus, for instance pressure over the sternum, or, for assessing the limb response, squeezing the nail bed of a digit and the tendo Achilles. Always test bilaterally – an absent response from one side alone suggests the likelihood of an interruption of the pyramidal tract supplying that side of the body. An appropriate response is one which withdraws the limb from the stimulus. The two principal inappropriate responses are decorticate and decerebrate posturing (Fig. 12.196). In the former, the upper limbs flex and adduct, the lower limbs extend and plantar flex. This response typically follows an acute vascular event affecting the cerebral hemisphere or internal capsule. In decerebrate rigidity, the upper limbs are extended, adducted, and hyperpronated, with the lower limbs fully extended. This pattern appears with lesions in the region of the pons which separate lower brain stem structures from descending pathways, but it can also occur in some of the metabolic comas.

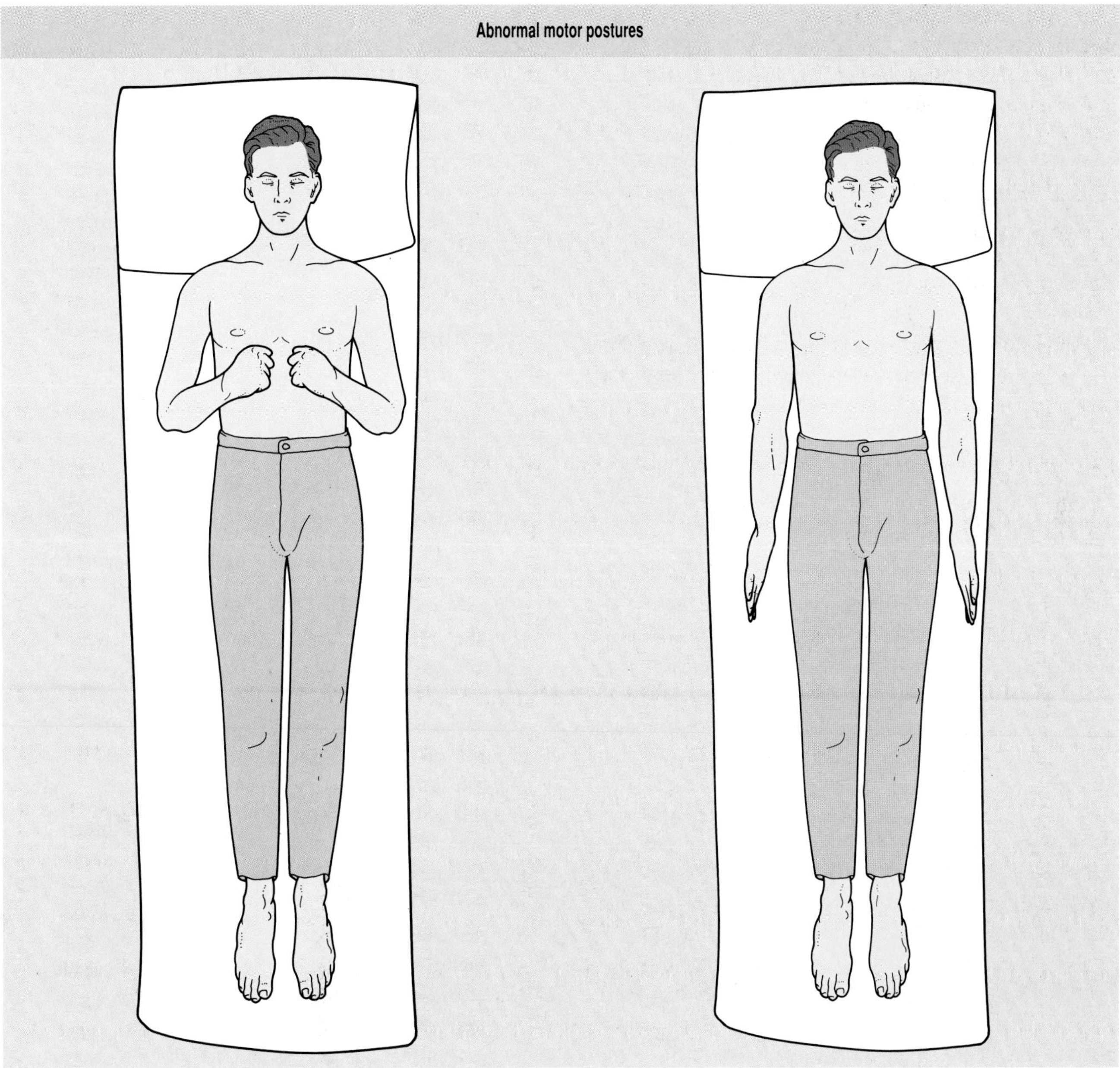

Fig. 12.196 Abnormal motor postures. Decorticate (left) and decerebrate (right).

Respiratory status

A number of abnormal respiratory patterns in the unconscious patient may allow localization of the lesion responsible for the coma (Fig. 12.197).

In Cheyne–Stokes respiration the respiratory rate waxes and wanes, with intervening periods of apnoea. The pattern is seen in metabolic coma, but also with bilateral deep hemisphere lesions. Central neurogenic hyperventilation consists of a persistently increased rate of relatively deep breathing. It is triggered by lesions lying between the lower midbrain and the lower pons. Apneustic breathing results in short periods of respiratory arrest on inspiration. Pontine infarction is the usual cause. Ataxic respiration is erratic in timing and depth and is triggered by disturbances of the respiratory centres of the medulla.

Respiratory patterns in the unconscious patient

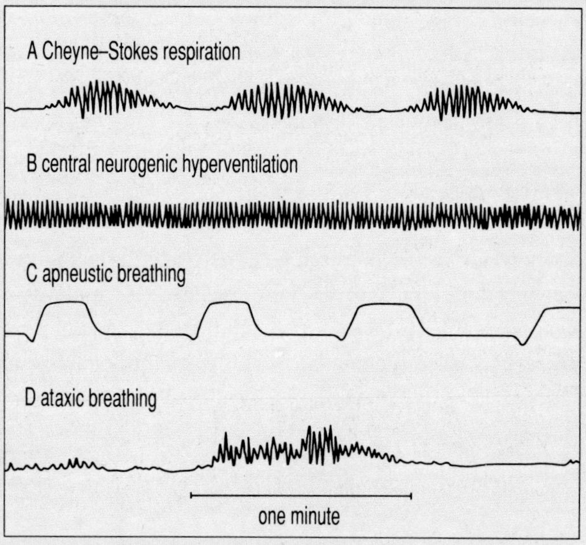

Fig. 12.197 Respiratory patterns and their anatomical correlates.

CLINICAL APPLICATION

There are significant differences between the neurological findings in patients whose coma has a metabolic basis and those in patients who have a structural lesion affecting the cerebral hemispheres or brain stem.

Metabolic coma

Patients in metabolic coma usually pass through phases of waning consciousness during which they become less alert, apathetic, and disorientated. The pupils remain reactive until the late stages of metabolic coma. The eyes remain central, but reflex movement, even that elicited by caloric stimulation, may eventually be lost. Apart from occasional cases showing conjugate downward deviation, the visual axes remain parallel and undeviated. The motor responses found in metabolic coma can mimic all of those seen in coma due to structural brain disease. Both generalized and focal motor seizures occur. Decorticate or decerebrate posturing are seen and some patients (e.g. those with hypoglycaemia) will display a hemiplegia which recovers when the metabolic abnormality is corrected. Myoclonic jerks occur in uraemia and in patients with hypercapnoea. Asterixis, or flapping tremor, is not seen in the unconscious patient but can be elicited in the drowsy stages of metabolic coma, particularly that associated with liver failure. If the hands are held outstretched, with the wrist and fingers extended, the fingers suddenly jerk downwards, then slowly return to their original position (Fig. 12.198). Almost any metabolic derangement, if sufficiently severe, can depress the conscious state. In addition to the features common to all of these types of coma, certain processes produce changes, which though not unique, are suggestive of the underlying mechanism. Focal motor deficit is particularly associated with hypoglycaemia but is also seen in patients with hepatic coma. In Wernicke's encephalopathy, the altered mental state is accompanied by ophthalmoplegia, nystagmus and ataxia. Papilloedema with intense retinal venous congestion is found in a small proportion of patients with respiratory failure. In drug-induced coma, though the doll's head and cold caloric responses are eventually lost, the pupils usually remain reactive until the very late stages.

Flapping tremor

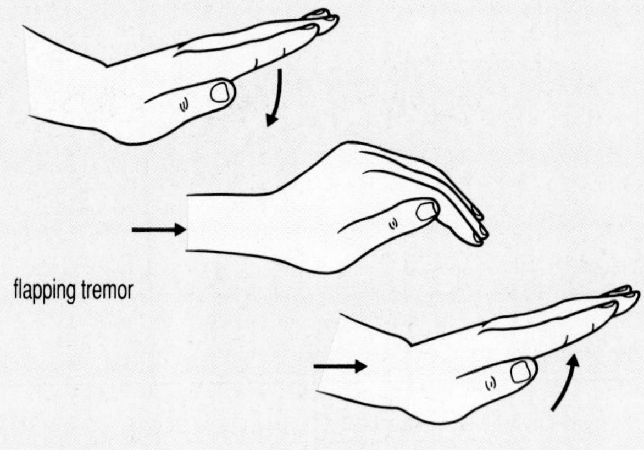

Fig. 12.198 Flapping tremor.

Structural causes of coma

When supratentorial lesions cause coma, the pattern of development of physical signs allows differentiation between central and uncal herniation. The pattern may alter according to the speed with which the size of a supratentorial mass increases.

With central herniation, as the conscious state alters, the first eye movement abnormality observed is impairment of reflex upward gaze. The pupils remain reactive. As a hemisphere lesion is present

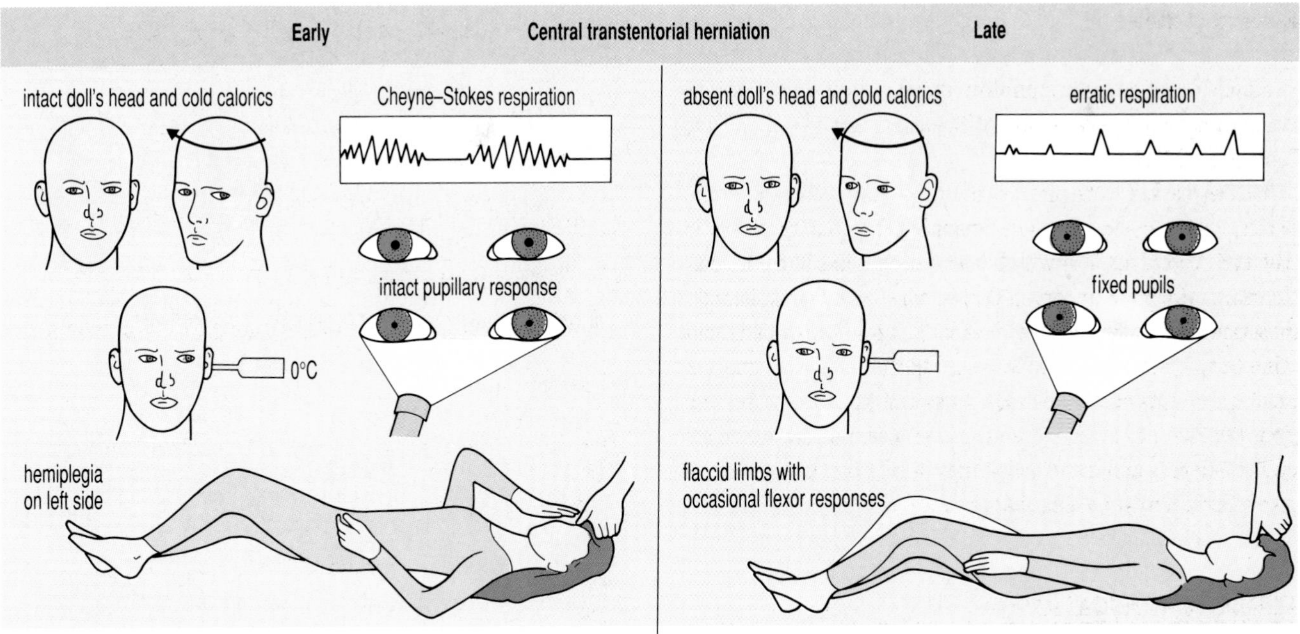

Fig. 12.199 Central transtentorial herniation.

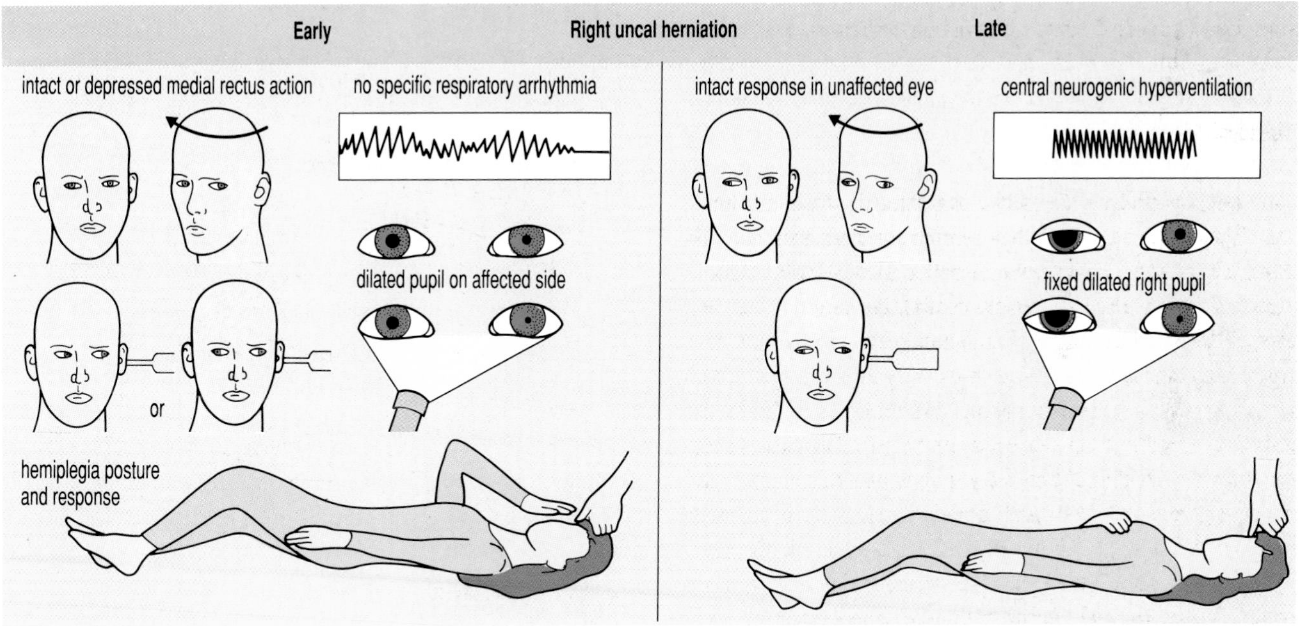

Fig. 12.200 Right uncal herniation.

there is likely to be a contralateral hemiplegia. The ipsilateral limbs may show a diffuse increase in tone, and the most likely respiratory arrhythmia is Cheyne–Stokes respiration (Fig. 12.199). Further signs appear as the transtentorial herniation proceeds. Horizontal eye movements become increasingly difficult to elicit, even using caloric stimulation. The pupils become fixed to light but remain mid-position in size. Decorticate posturing of the unaffected side becomes decerebrate and the most likely breathing pattern to emerge is central neurogenic hyperventilation.

Uncal herniation produces a different picture, at least initially. The pupil of the eye ipsilateral to the lesion becomes dilated, and this is followed by the development of an ophthalmoplegia. Initially the contralateral pupil remains reactive and the eye moves fully with reflex stimulation, but subsequently reflex movements are lost. The limbs ipsilateral to the lesion can develop a hemiplegic posture relatively early, due to compression of the contralateral cerebral peduncle against the tentorial edge (Fig. 12.200). Later bilateral decerebrate posturing appears. Central neurogenic hyperventilation is the most likely respiratory dysrhythmia.

The final stages of the two types of herniation are similar. Respiration becomes erratic and signs of cardiovascular instability emerge. Pupillary dilatation is a terminal event.

Supratentorial masses producing coma are usually vascular

rather than neoplastic. Causes include extradural, subdural, and primary intracerebral haemorrhage. The spectrum of pathological processes in the brain stem producing coma is considerably wider and includes infarction, tumour and haemorrhage.

BRAIN DEATH

The end point of many structural and metabolic insults to the brain is a state in which a deeply comatose patient maintains circulatory function providing that respiration is supported by artificial means.There is good evidence to suggest that if brain stem function can be shown to have ceased in such patients, there is no prospect for recovery (Fig. 12.201). Criteria of brain stem death have been devised to appraise this state, in order to identify those patients in whom further attempts at life-support are of no value (Fig. 12.202).

The first essential, when applying these criteria, is to ensure that the coma is not the consequence of a metabolic or drug-induced state which is potentially reversible. Usually retesting is performed after a period of at least 24 hours. This allows confirmation of the clinical diagnosis by another doctor and the positive exclusion of reversible factors. The responses to testing of brain stem function are likely to be depressed in the presence of hypothermia. The patient's body temperature must be above 35°C before testing is carried out. It must be clearly established that the patient's respiratory failure is not the consequence of neuromuscular blocking agents. Stimulation of a peripheral nerve can be carried out to confirm that neuromuscular conduction is intact. Finally a specific cause for the patient's coma must be identified. For most neurological disorders this will be evident from the patient's history or CT scanning. Identification of drug-induced or metabolic coma is likely to take longer.

Brain stem reflexes

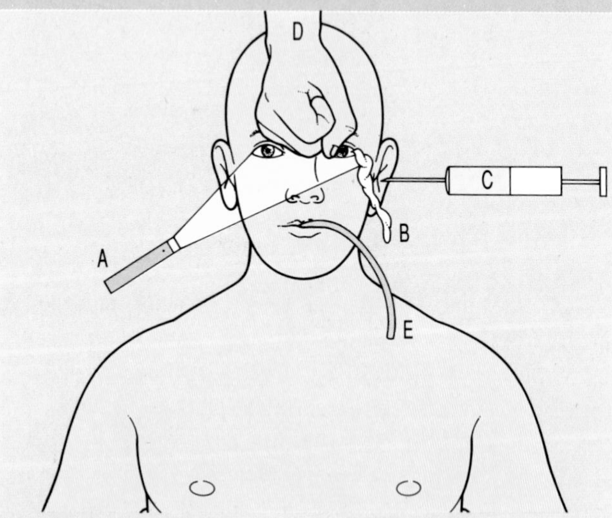

A pupillary light response.
B testing the corneal response.
C injection of ice-cold water to test the vestibulo-ocular reflex.
D stimulating the glabella with the knuckle.
E stimulating the trachea with a suction catheter.

Fig. 12.201 Testing brain stem reflexes.

Pitfalls

To avoid observer error, repeat testing is performed by another doctor after an interval exceeding 24 hours. There are certain spinal reflexes which can persist in the presence of brain stem death. These include the stretch reflexes, plantar responses or withdrawal, and flexion of the upper or lower limb triggered by neck flexion. The UK criteria for brain death no longer include the presence of an isoelectric EEG recording, though this criterion still receives support in other countries, for instanse the USA.

Criteria for brain death

1. Pupillary response

Use a bright torch (not an ophthalmoscope) to confirm that the pupils fail to respond.

2. Corneal response

Gently apply a wisp of cotton wool to the cornea. There should be no response. Note that repeated testing can readily traumatize the cornea.

3. Vestibulo-ocular reflex

Inspect the tympanic membrane to ensure that it is intact and not obscured by impacted wax. Insert a soft rubber catheter into the external auditory meatus and slowly inject approximately 50ml of ice-cold water. Repeat the test in the other ear. There should be no ocular deviation.

4. Motor response in cranial nerve distribution

This is most readily assessed by applying a painful stimulus to the glabella. The patient fails to respond.

5. Gag or tracheal response

Either stimulate the palate or pass a suction catheter into the trachea. The patient fails to show any response.

6. Respiratory reaction to hypercapnoea

First administer a combination of 95 per cent O_2 and 5 per cent CO_2 via the respirator until the pCO_2 has risen above 40mm Hg (6.0 kPa). Disconnect the respirator, but administer 100 per cent oxygen through a tracheal catheter at around 6 l/min. Observe if any respiratory response occurs when the pCO_2 exceeds 50mm Hg (6.7 kPa).

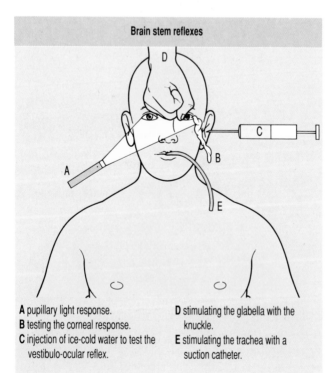

Fig. 12.202 Criteria for diagnosing brain death.

INDEX

D

E

F

G

T